The third edition of this highly successful postgraduate psychiatry text offers a comprehensive review of the characteristics, causes and treatment of the main psychiatric disorders. As with earlier editions it is subdivided into four parts: models and principles; origins, presentation and course of major clinical symptoms; psychiatry in the social, forensic and medical contexts; treatments both biological and psychological. It is also extensively referenced throughout and emphasises the relationship of research findings to clinical practice. The text has been extensively revised and updated in line with the most recent developments in psychiatric practice and thinking. In particular, more discussion is given to measurement issues, concepts of illness, brain imaging and neurophysiology. The highly distinguished team of contributors has also been enhanced through the introduction of one or two of the newer stars in the field. In this era of the multidisciplinary team approach to health care, psychiatrists now represent only a small proportion of postgraduate professionals dealing with the mentally ill. This new edition will without doubt be valued by all members of this team as well as general practitioners who seek an authoritative yet readable account of modern psychiatry.

D1332360

The Essentials of Postgraduate Psychiatry

The Essentials of
Postgraduate Psychiatry

Edited by

ROBIN MURRAY
PETER HILL
PETER McGUFFIN

Third edition

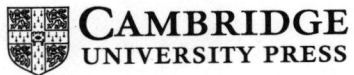
CAMBRIDGE
UNIVERSITY PRESS

PUBLISHED BY THE PRESS SYNDICATE OF THE UNIVERSITY OF CAMBRIDGE
The Pitt Building, Trumpington Street, Cambridge CB2 1RP, United Kingdom

CAMBRIDGE UNIVERSITY PRESS
The Edinburgh Building, Cambridge CB2 2RU, United Kingdom
40 West 20th Street, New York, NY 10011-4211, USA
10 Stamford Road, Oakleigh, Melbourne 3166, Australia

First published 1980
Second edition published by Grune & Stratton Ltd 1986
Third edition published by Cambridge University Press 1997

Printed in the United Kingdom at the University Press, Cambridge

Typeset in Postcript Times 10/13 pt

A catalogue record for this book is available from the British Library

Library of Congress Cataloguing in Publication data

The essentials of postgraduate psychiatry / edited by Robin Murray,
Peter Hill, Peter McGuffin. – 3rd ed.
    p. cm.
  Includes index.
  ISBN 0 521 44396 2 (hardcover). – ISBN 0 521 57801 9 (pbk.)
  1. Psychiatry.   I. Murray, Robin, MD, M Phil, MRCP, MRC Psych.
II. Hill, R. D. (Peter David)   III. McGuffin, P. (Peter)
RC454.E824   1997
616.89 – dc20   96–44256 CIP

ISBN 0 521 44396 2 hardback
ISBN 0 521 57801 9 paperback

Contents

6 Neurosis and personality disorder   145
Glyn Lewis and Simon Wessely

7 Eating disorders   192
Janet Treasure
A. ANOREXIA NERVOSA

B. BULIMIA NERVOSA

Contributors

Professor Louis Appleby, Senior Lecturer in Psychiatry, Department of Psychiatry, University Hospital of South Manchester, West Didsbury, Manchester M20 8LR, UK

Professor Paul Bebbington, Professor of Social & Community Psychiatry, Archway Site, Whittington Hospital, Highgate Hill, London N19 5NF, UK

Professor Alistair Burns, Professor of Old Age Psychiatry, The Department of Psychiatry, Withington Hospital, West Didsbury, Manchester M20 8LR, UK

Dr E. Jane Byrne, Senior Lecturer and Honorary Consultant Psychiatrist, The Department of Psychiatry, Withington Hospital, West Didsbury, Manchester M20 8LR, UK

Professor Anthony W. Clare, Medical Director, St Patrick's Hospital, James's St, Dublin 8, Ireland

Dr Ilana B. Crome, Consultant Psychiatrist – Senior Clinical Lecturer, North Staffordshire Combined Healthcare NHS Trust, Substance Abuse Unit, Ward 93, City General Hospital, Stoke-on-Trent ST4 6QG, UK

Dr Michael J. Crowe, Consultant Psychiatrist, Maudsley Hospital, Denmark Hill, London SE5 8AZ, UK

Dr Christopher Dare, Senior Lecturer and Head of Section of Psychotherapy, Department of Psychiatry, Institute of Psychiatry, De Crespigny Park, London SE5 8AF, UK

Professor Anthony S. David, Department of Psychological Medicine, Institute of Psychiatry, De Crespigny Park, Denmark Hill, London SE5 8AF, UK

Dr A. Davies, Senior Registrar in Psychiatry, Section of Perinatal Psychiatry, Institute of Psychiatry, De Crespigny Park, Denmark Hill, London SE5 8AF, UK

PROFESSOR ANNE E. FARMER, Advisor on Postgraduate Education, University of Wales College of Medicine, Division of Psychological Medicine, Heath Park, Cardiff CF4 4XN, UK

DR MICHAEL FARRELL, Consultant Psychiatrist, Addiction Research Unit, Institute of Psychiatry, De Crespigny Park, Denmark Hill, London SE5 8AF, UK

DR EMILY FINCH, Consultant Psychiatrist, Addiction Research Unit, Institute of Psychiatry, De Crespigny Park, Denmark Hill, London SE5 8AF, UK

PROFESSOR WILLIAM I. FRASER, Department of Psychological Medicine, University of Wales College of Medicine, Ely Hospital, Cowbridge Road West, Cardiff CF5 5XE, UK

PROFESSOR PETER HILL, Section of Child and Adolescent Psychiatry, St George's Hospital Medical School, Cranmer Terrace, London SW17 0RE, UK

PROFESSOR ROBERT W. KERWIN, Department of Psychological Medicine, Institute of Psychiatry, De Crespigny Park, Denmark Hill, London SE5 8AF, UK

PROFESSOR RAMESH KUMAR, Head, Section of Perinatal Psychiatry, Institute of Psychiatry, De Crespigny Park, Denmark Hill, London SE5 8AF, UK

PROFESSOR GLYN LEWIS, Professor of Community and Epidemiological Psychiatry, Division of Psychological Medicine, University of Wales College of Medicine, Heath Park, Cardiff CF4 4XN, UK

PROFESSOR SHON W. LEWIS, Academic Department of Psychiatry, Withington Hospital, Nells Lane, Didsbury, Manchester M20 8LE, UK

DR GEOFFREY G. LLOYD, Consultant Psychiatrist, Department of Psychiatry, Royal Free Hospital, Pond Street, London NW3 2QG, UK

PROFESSOR ROY J. MCCLELLAND, Professor of Mental Health, Department of Mental Health, Queen's University of Belfast, Whitla Medical Building, 97 Lisburn Road, Belfast BT9 7BL, UK

PROFESSOR PETER MCGUFFIN, Head of Division, Department of Psychological Medicine, University of Wales College of Medicine, Heath Park, Cardiff CF4 4XN, UK

DR R. J. MCIVOR, Senior Registrar in Psychiatry, Section of Perinatal Psychiatry, Institute of Psychiatry, De Crespigny Park, Denmark Hill, London SE5 8F, UK

PROFESSOR ANTHONY MANN, Professor of Epidemiological Psychiatry, Section of Epidemiology & General Practice, Institute of Psychiatry, De Crespigny Park, Denmark Hill, London SE5 8AF, UK

DR STIRLING MOOREY, Consultant Psychiatrist and Honorary Senior Lecturer, St Bartholomew's Hospital, West Smithfield, London EC1A 7BE, UK

PROFESSOR PAUL E. MULLEN, Professor & Director of Forensic Psychiatry Services, The Rosanna Forensic Psychiatry Centre, Private Bag No. 1, Rosanna, Victoria, Melbourne, Australia

PROFESSOR ROBIN M. MURRAY, Head, Department of Psychological Medicine, Institute of Psychiatry, De Crespigny Park, Denmark Hill, London SE5 8AF, UK

DR MICHAEL PHELAN, Clinical Lecturer & Assistant Director, PRiSM, Institute of Psychiatry, De Crespigny Park, Denmark Hill, London SE5 8AF, UK

DR LYN S. PILOWKSY, MRC Clinician and Senior Lecturer in Psychiatry, Department of Psychological Medicine, Institute of Psychiatry, De Crespigny Park, Denmark Hill, London SE5 8AF, UK

DR GERALDINE STRATHDEE, Head of Service Development, The Sainsbury Centre for Mental Health, 134–138 Borough High Street, London SE1 1LB, UK

PROFESSOR PAMELA J. TAYLOR, Professor of Special Hospital Psychiatry, Department of Forensic Psychiatry, Institute of Psychiatry, De Crespigny Park, Denmark Hill, London SE5 8AF, UK

PROFESSOR GRAHAM THORNICROFT, Senior Lecturer & Director PRiSM, Institute of Psychiatry, De Crespigny Park, Denmark Hill, London SE5 8AF, UK

DR JANET TREASURE, Department of Psychological Medicine, King's College Hospital, Denmark Hill, London SE5 9RS, UK

DR SCOTT WEICH, Senior Lecturer in Psychiatry, University Department of Psychiatry, Royal Free Hospital School of Medicine, Rowland Hill Street, London NW3 2PF, UK

PROFESSOR SIMON WESSELY, Department of Psychological Medicine, Institute of Psychiatry, De Crespigny Park, Denmark Hill, London SE5 8AF, UK

PROFESSOR GREG WILKINSON, Department of Psychiatry, 3rd Floor, Alexandra Wing, The Royal London Hospital, Whitechapel, London E1 1BB, UK

DR RUTH WILLIAMS, Senior Lecturer in Psychology, Institute of Psychiatry, De Crespigny Park, Denmark Hill, London SE5 8AF, UK

DR ALISTAIR B. WILSON, Consultant Psychiatrist, Greater Glasgow Community Mental Health Services, Riverside Resource Centre, 12 Sandy Road, Partick, Glasgow G11 6HC, UK

Foreword to the First Edition

This is the first general textbook of psychiatry to emerge from the Institute of Psychiatry and the Bethlem Royal and Maudsley Hospitals – known to the world at large as 'The Maudsley'. Until now an organization which every year produces a considerable crop of monographs, books on special subjects, reviews and original articles, has eschewed such a venture. Like all exciting enterprises, it carries a certain risk – the challenge of retaining the many flavours of Maudsley teaching while reducing the whole to more amenable proportions, and of persuading a number of highly individualistic soloists to take part in an ensemble.

Henry Maudsley himself was only 23 when appointed as Superintendent to the New Cheadle Royal Hospital. By the age of 32 he had published several articles and his 'Physiology and Pathology of Mind'. It is therefore most appropriate that the challenge of producing a book based on teaching at the Maudsley should have been taken up by a younger generation of psychiatrists. I knew many of them when they worked with me as a trainee psychiatrist, and have learnt much more from them than they ever did from me. Nor will it surprise the reader to learn that, during the period of the book's incubation, many of its contributors have been appointed to senior positions and have already distinguished themselves in a variety of different fields. The result of their labours is a very readable volume which provides up-to-date reviews of most of the important fields of psychiatry, with a plentiful supply of references for further reading.

The student who reads this book will find that it will illuminate many of his activities, be they clinical practice, teaching or research. He will become aware not only of important areas of knowledge, but also of areas of ignorance requiring further exploration. The latter aspect of a psychiatrist's education is often omitted, leaving a leaden lump of indigestible knowledge as an object for painful rumination. Yet it is the yeast which leavens the whole, and an essential ingredient for any serious student of psychiatry who values the Maudsley approach.

June 1979

J. L. T. Birley
Formerly Dean
Institute of Psychiatry
and of
Royal College of Psychiarists

Preface to the First Edition

In the past two decades the scientific foundations of psychiatry have been greatly strengthened by research into such areas as the epidemiology of mental disorder, the biological understanding of the psychoses and the rational application of pharmacological and psychological treatments. But psychiatric textbooks have seldom kept abreast of these advances and have, in particular, failed to meet the needs of the postgraduate student. This book is intended to provide the postgraduate with a portable general text that steers a middle way between unjustifiable dogmatism and obsolescent exhaustiveness, and integrates research findings into the general body of clinical knowledge. We believe that good clinical practice is grounded in and informed by the academic debate that surrounds it, and consequently have attempted not only to present the essential clincial information but also to show how it derives (or fails to derive) from rigorous scientific enquiry.

Multi-author books run the risk of inconsistency and repetition. However, since all but one of the contributors are, or have been, members of staff at the Maudsley Hospital, this volume presents a reasonably coherent point of view which emphasizes the critical approach for which that institution is renowned. This is not to say that readers should expect a narrowly uniform approach since many varieties of psychiatry are practised at the Maudsley.

From the outset we have tried to reflect the richness and variety of psychiatry as well as the need to anchor clincial practice in an objective framework. The chapters are divided into four parts, the first of which discusses different models of mental illness, and outlines the principles of phenomenology and measurement. The second part describes the origins, presentation and course of the major clinical syndromes, while the third examines psychiatry in its social, forensic and general medical contexts. The final part includes chapters on biological and psychological treatments. Throughout we have included liberal references in the expectation that readers will wish to have controversial statements supported and will feel sufficiently curious to read the originals for themselves.

In choosing to identify essentials of postgraduate psychiatry we assume a basic knowledge of such topics as routine clinical assessment, compulsory admission procedures and the ability to work within a team. We also presume multidisciplinary standards of clinical practice which we hope most psychiatrists would regard as reasonable, and levels of information which are amply sufficient for the candidate preparing for postgraduate qualifications in psychiatry.

Psychiarists now represent only a small proportion of the postgraduate professionals dealing with the mentally disordered since psychologists, social workers and nurses have all developed specialized skills indispensable to the multidisciplinary approach. But many feel that a lack of confidence in, or lack of knowledge of, the basis of clinical psychiatry hampers their response to the needs of the mentally ill. The editors believe that they will find this book valuable as will general physicians and general practitioners seeking an authoritative and yet readable account of modern psychiatry.

Maudsley Hospital
June 1979

Peter Hill
Robin Murray
Anthony Thorley

Preface to the Second Edition

We have been greatly encouraged by the response to this book, and the need for a second edition has provided us with the opportunity to introduce a number of significant improvements. In making these we have been particularly conscious of the fact that less than one-half of our readers are British, and have therefore further emphasized those aspects of practice which transcend national boundaries. In one review of the first edition a distinguished professor complained of the youth of the authors. If only that were true! Nevertheless, we have tried to maintain the freshness and enthusiasm of the first edition by introducing ten new contributors, and covering four new subjects (Adolescence, Atypical Psychosis, Self-Destructive Behaviour, and Disorders of Women).

June 1985   R. M.
Institute of Psychiatry

Preface to the Third Edition

Much has changed since the original publication of this book in 1979. Operational definitions of psychiatric conditions have become part of everyday clinical practice. The dramatic advances in neuroscience have had a major impact on psychiatry. Thus, our understanding of Alzheimer's disease has been transformed by molecular genetics, and novel techniques of functional brain imaging are providing new insights into the physiological basis of psychotic symptoms. Psychiatric epidemiology has successfully moved from being merely descriptive to employing analytical techniques to address questions of cause. Greatly improved drugs have been introduced for depression and now also for schizophrenia. Among psychological treatments, analytical psychotherapy has continued to lose ground to the behaviour therapies, and increasingly to cognitive therapy. The antipsychiatric movement has almost disappeared, but its legacy is the modern emphasis on community psychiatry, and on user involvement. This, our third edition reflects these trends. On the international scene, American psychiatry has largely abandoned its preoccupation with psychoanalysis, and the major continental academic centres have regained their confidence, while psychiatry in the former communist countries is fast recovering from its nightmare of isolation and abuse. These welcome changes have been accompanied by an almost universal swing towards the blend of the phenomenological tradition of classical European psychiatry and British empiricism epitomised in 'The Maudsley' approach to psychiatry. Paradoxically, this has meant that 'The Maudsley' itself has had to broaden its base to apply the new neuroscience techniques to psychiatry, and to greatly expand health service research; as a result it was recognised in a 1993 survey by the American magazine *Science Watch* as being the most widely cited psychiatric research centre in the world. We consider that 'The Maudsley' approach, as illustrated in this book, has much to offer as a counterweight to the commercial machines of the pharmaceutical industry and the American Psychiatric Association. We have a new publisher, and Peter McGuffin joins us as a new editor. Many of our original contributors from 'The Maudsley' have now, like two of the three editors, moved away to head their own departments. Their wider experience brings a new realism to the book while the younger contributors, who have rewritten many of the chapters, keep it right up to date. We hope that in this way, the book retains its original mixture of theory and yet immediate practicality, and conveys to the reader the enthusiasm of the contributors for their subject.

April 1997   Robin M. Murray
Peter Hill
Peter McGuffin

PART I

GENERAL PRINCIPLES

1

The mental state and states of mind

PAUL E. MULLEN

It is the duty, and should be the privilege of the medical examiner to spend several days in the examination of a lunatic before they pronounce a decided opinion

Theodric Beck (1823)

The injunction of Dr Beck may seem whimsical in these days of community psychiatry but clinical psychiatry without some curiosity and concern with the mental life of the patient would be an impoverished speciality. This is as true for those psychiatrists whose primary interest is in classification and diagnosis as for those who seek first and foremost to explore the meaningful connection and mental mechanisms of their patients' internal world. The information generated by such interest, if it is to be shared, requires to be expressed in an agreed language of sufficient clarity and precision. Putting names to things is an essential prerequisite to any meaningful discourse.

Abnormalities of mental state as symptoms

Abnormalities of mental state are frequently treated in psychiatry merely as symptoms that act as signposts pointing towards particular diagnostic conclusions. The theoretical structure underlining this approach is the familiar medical model.

Reservations can, however, be expressed about equating abnormalities of mental state with symptoms in a way analogous to symptoms in general medicine. In medicine itself the symptom can be seen as expressing the effect of the disease process. The pain down the left arm on exertion can reflect the physical changes accompanying cardiac ischaemia. The patient's complaint is a direct pointer to a physical lesion. The tone and quality of the patient's complaint may, in this situation, be affected by the character and culture of the individual, but still the symptom can be employed as a signpost to the disease. In psychiatry, even if one grants uncritically the claim that underlying disturbances of mental state are disorders of the brain, a straightforward expression of the disease by the symptom is less easily maintained. The so-called symptoms of psychiatric illness are virtually always disturbances of mental state. When patients give voice to their complaints, or more often try to express the disturbances in their experience of themselves and their world, there lies behind their statements the whole mental life of that particular individual. As Minkowski (1970) expressed it: 'behind confusion always lies the confused person, behind melancholy the depressed, behind the syndrome of influence the influenced'. Abnormalities of mental

3

state are not necessarily to be viewed as disordered fragments but, on the contrary, can be seen as reflecting the whole personality and mental functioning of that individual. This view suggests that the syndrome in psychiatry cannot so easily be equated with a simple association of symptoms, but becomes the expression of a profound modification in the whole mental life and personality of this individual.

The clear and precise definition of clinical symptoms has manifest utility and serves the medical model of psychiatric disorder admirably. There must, however, be some disquiet over the extent to which this detracts from the exploration and delineation of the patient's actual experiences. A hallucination can be defined as a perception without an object. Employing this definition, whether or not the particular patients has had a hallucinatory experience, can be determined by asking the right questions. Having established the presence of the hallucination, the psychiatrist may feel they have exhausted this area of enquiry but what has been defined is a symptom; what has not occurred is the elucidation of the patient's actual experience.

To take an example, hypochondriasis has been defined as painful or unpleasant worrying, specifically concentrated on the possibility of disease or malfunction that is beyond the subject's power to control and out of proportion to any actual illness or disorder that is present (Wing *et al*, 1974). Hypochondriasis so defined may present in very different ways in the context of very different states of mind: the severely depressed patient in a state of agitated despair who complains of the decay and decomposition within her; the dement who repeats interminably a cry for help and for a cure to some ill-defined malaise; the young man who travels from physician to physician with a bizarre account of physical disorder, which he says leaves him without feeling, without will, and unable to think of anything but his supposed malfunction; the woman who has moved from doctor to doctor for 30 years with a multiplicity of aches and pains and despite accumulating operations, vague diagnostic labels and innumerable courses of treatment, continues to complain bitterly of being plagued by ill health. The symptom hypochondriasis could be used for all. The context of the hypochondriasis in these particular cases could be further placed in the context of a syndrome such as Briquet's, or a psychiatric disorder depression, or even a clinicopathologic entity, Pick's disease. That further elaboration does not bring us much closer to understanding the state of mind that manifests in these four individuals through their worry and concern over the state of their physical health. If we have a real curiosity about the mental life of our patients and are not content to remain exclusively within the reductionism of the currently fashionable diagnostic labels, then the exploration of mental state must extend beyond symptom collection. Symptoms are constructs that do not exist in pure form but vary with the context, with the influence of other disturbances in mental state, with the situation in which they are experienced, with the cultural and personal background of the individual and even with the theoretical assumptions of the examiner who directs and constrains the patient's description.

Abnormal phenomena

In the following sections abnormal phenomena will be discussed. The emphasis will be in describing mental phenomena prior to their becoming part of the formulation of particular disorders but for convenience and coherence some common syndromes, such as mania, will be used to draw together the associated phenomena. Space allows only a restricted presentation; as neuropsychiatric disturbance such as memory, attention, and orientation are discussed elsewhere, they have been omitted. Similarly, conversion and dissociative states are not discussed

Perceptual disorders

Madmen are visionaries of the senses because they do not see things as they are and because they often see things that are not.

[Malebranche, 1674]

The sensory modalities are the special senses of sight, hearing, smell and taste, as well as the sensations of touch, pain, temperature, point discrimination, and position. Except in peculiar circumstances, we experience perceptions not sensations. Sensations are transformed into perceptions by their origin being experienced as arising from some external object. If I experience a smell without recognition or association it would be a simple sensation, but once it is referred to some external object, say a rose, it forms part of a perception. In perception we usually experience ourselves in relation to an object in the world. Objects are normally perceived as particular things. This is especially true of visual perceptions where, for example, if I look at a cube I tend to perceive it as a cube, though at most I can only immediately apprehend three of its sides and a possibility exists, until I have examined every aspect, that it is not truly a cube. Meanings tend, therefore, to be imminent in perception. Perceived objects stand bodily before us resisting and infused with a quality of reality. In that we believe what we see, we do so usually without any verification or consideration. Traditionally, theories of perceptions introduce into perception itself intellectual operations and a critical examination of the evidence of the senses to which we in fact resort only when direct observation founders in ambiguity. Clearly, however, when we deal with perception rather than sensation we are dealing not simply with the raw data itself, but with a process that usually involves a knowing what as well as a sensing of. In stating that he hears a voice, the patient is recognising the type and nature of what he hears.

Disturbance in sensory function

Disturbances in the sensory modalities themselves are largely the result of organic lesions and are dealt with in standard texts of neurology. Occasionally the absence of sensation (e.g. blindness or anaesthesia), the perversion of sensation (e.g. tingling paraesthesia), or the abnormal heightening of sensation (e.g. hyperacusis), may be complained of without any obvious explanation in physical pathology. This, for example, will be seen in certain conversion symptoms of a hysterical type. In some manic patients all sensation may appear heightened, as they may also be in the depressed, though for one it is the source of pleasure and delight, in the other an additional burden and imposition. A dulling of sensations with everything experienced as lacklustre and bleak may also accompany depression.

Disturbances in perception

Agnosias

The disturbed ability to organise sensory impressions so as to allow the recognition of objects (that is to perceive objects) is known as agnosia. Agnosias may obviously affect different sensory modalities and usually reflect cortical damage.

Micropsia and macropsia

The relative proportions of perceived objects may alter to render them enlarged (macropsia) or diminished (micropsia). Such changes may occur, for example, in severe fatigue, sleeplessness, toxic states, and temporal lobe epilepsy.

Synaesthesia

This is where perceptions in one modality, for example hearing, are simultaneously experienced as if they were also present in another modality, for example, the visual. This is encountered in some drug intoxications. The visual effects that occur concomitantly with music in states of cannabis intoxication are often highly prized by its habitués.

False perceptions

These are actual perceptual abnormalities and imply that the experience involved is of perceiving something, not just believing something.

(i) Hallucinations There is a long tradition of distinguishing between illusions and hallucinations (Van Den Berg, 1982), Esquirol (1833), held that:

> a person labours under an hallucination who has a thorough conviction of a sensation when no external object suited to excite this sensation has impressed his senses, whereas it is an illusion if the senses are deceived respecting the qualities, relations, and causes of impressions actually received and cause them to form false judgements respecting their internal and external sensations.

Hallucinations proper have the following characteristics:

1. They are actual false perceptions, not distortions of real perceptions.
2. They are experienced as being out there in the world and as inhabiting objective space.
3. They are experienced as having the qualities and force of the corresponding normal perceptions, being just as vivid, whole and immediate.
4. They are usually experienced alongside and simultaneously with normal perceptions (complex visions may be an exception).
5. They are as independent of our will as are any normal perceptions, in that they cannot be conjured up or dismissed.

The hallucination may show a greater independence from will and action than a normal perception for, though I can turn away from looking at the page before me or cease attending to the droning voice of a lecturer, my hallucinations will continue to force themselves to my attention. A hallucinated voice will usually penetrate the most efficient ear muffs, and one patient continued to be plagued by hallucinated voices even after he had destroyed his eardrums with needles, thus reducing the rest of the world to silence.

Hallucinations do not yield to argument, for the immediateness of the experience, like that of normal perception, permits of no doubt, but the experienced reality of hallucinations can vary. On more than one occasion I have had patients try to explain how the voices or visions differ from actual perceptions. It has been suggested that hallucinations owe as much to interpretation as perception, with the patient elaborating and constructing his or her experiences out of more basic hallucinatory events (Horowitz, 1978). Patients frequently find no difficulty in discriminating between their hallucinations and true perceptions. Hallucinations are usually confined to a single sensory modality and this or some other subtle difference from normal perception may make the patient aware of the false nature of the perceptions. The ease with which hallucinations are distinguished from real perceptions in some patients is illustrated by a telephonist who, despite being troubled by constant auditory hallucinations, continued to work efficiently, unerringly distinguishing them from the disembodied voices of callers. A particular patient may suffer simultaneously from hallucinations in several sensory modalities at the same time, but they will rarely be perceived as emanating from a single entity. Occasionally multi-modal or scenic hallucinations, are described, in which a complex visual and auditory hallucination is experienced, but if a patient reports a vision that also speaks, particularly if it answers back, the most likely explanations are malingering or hysteria.

Hallucinations can be subdivided by sensory modality:

(a) *Auditory hallucinations* may range from ill-defined sounds to highly organised perceptions where, for example, a voice recognisable to the patient as that of a relative or acquaintance will be heard talking at length. One of my patients was constantly plagued with the sound of the Beatles playing Strawberry Fields complete with full musical accompaniment, a phenomenon that despite his fondness for popular music palled after the first few weeks. True auditory hallucinations usually have a directional quality and the patient can describe from where they appear to be emanating. Certain modes of hearing voices were held by Kurt Schneider (1974) to be of special diagnostic importance in schizophrenia. The hearing of one's own thoughts read aloud, voices talking one with another, and voices that maintain a running commentary on the patient's thoughts and actions, were considered first rank symptoms. Occasionally tinnitus and other disturbances due to local disease of the ear may be confused with hallucinations.

(b) *Visual hallucinations* may also vary from ill-defined shapes and colours though clearly recognisable objects and persons to the complex visions that may, for example, accompany ecstatic states.

(c) *Olfactory and gustatory hallucinations* can occur separately or more commonly together. They are seen in some types of schizophrenic disorder, but may also be found in affective and epileptic disturbances. The persecuted patient may taste and smell the poisons placed in his food by his tormentors, the depressed may be assailed by the stench of his own decomposition, the over-sensitive may squirm in embarrassment at what he perceives as his overpowering odour (the distinction from illusion may often be difficult in these cases).

(d) *Tactile hallucinations* refer to cutaneous perceptions that vary from vague tingling or sensations of temperature change to perceptions experienced as being held, hit or caressed. In certain intoxications, typically cocaine, the patient may experience formication, where what is perceived seems like bugs crawling around, on, or under the skin.

(d) *Somatic hallucinations* may be difficult on occasions to distinguish from tactile hallucinations and, at the other extreme, merge into delusional beliefs about bodily change. One patient described having his semen drawn out of him by ghouls. Clearly connected with this bizarre delusional belief were tactile hallucinations involving the perceptions of being pricked with pins and tingling sensations around the base of his spine, but also somatic hallucinations involving the experience of his testicles and penis shrinking into his abdomen and his spine feeling as if 'hollow and cracking'. Somatic hallucinations may accompany epileptic activity. One such patient who described strange abdominal sensations that preceded his fits, perceived them as writhing movements and, in turn, interpreted that as snakes squirming around in his belly.

Disturbance of body image may occur in a variety of organic brain disorders, in some psychiatric disorders, and probably most commonly in normal individuals under the influence of sleep deprivation, exhaustion, or intoxication. The most common disturbances of body image are the perceptions of changes in size and shape of parts of the body (head and hands seem most common) or of the whole body. The reported alteration in body image in anorexia nervosa would appear a more subtle phenomenon.

(ii) Illusions. These are distortions of real perceptions in contrast to hallucinations, which arise without external stimulus. The perceptual stimulus, arises from an actual object and the illusion is formed by the perception's transformation. The other characteristics are identical with those listed for hallucination. Illusions do, however, usually exhibit a more transient existence than hallucinations and often vanish when attention is drawn to the misperception.

A common illusion occurs in the overwrought individual whose vision on a dark night distorts the branches blowing in the wind into a perception of an attacker moving towards him. A depressed patient out driving reported being frozen in horror at the sound of a child screaming in pain, only to realise later that she had misperceived the squeaking of the brakes of her own car. It is important in this example that the patient heard quite distinctly a scream of pain and did not misinterpret a squealing of brakes for the squealing of a hurt child. The patient with delirium tremens is often accosted by the transformation of the articles around him or her into terrifying illusions.

(iii) Functional hallucinations. These hallucinations, which may be confused with illusions, are rare phenomena where an hallucination occurs simultaneously and in association with a real perception. Thus hallucinatory voices may only be heard against the background of a running tap, and when the water is turned off this will abolish the hallucination. The noise of running water in this example is not transformed or distorted into

an hallucinatory voice, nor is it misinterpreted as such, for the functional hallucination is heard alongside and separable from the accompanying real perception. A man complained that when out driving he was assailed by insulting voices. These voices were only to be heard at traffic lights and were confined to periods when the amber signal was on. When the lights changed to red or green the voices ceased.

(iv) Pareidolia.   Another common and normal phenomenon, pareidolia are the perceptions conjured up by ill-defined sense impressions such as those that occur when staring into the dying embers of an open fire.

Phenomena related to false perceptions

(a) Misinterpretations

These are not false perceptions as are illusions, for they consist of a correct perception, the import of which is incorrectly deduced. Thus shiny metal may be mistaken by the weary prospector for gold, the perception of glitter being correct, its interpretation over-hopeful, Misinterpretations frequently arise in paranoid patients, where, for example, every creak and bang, though correctly perceived, may be misinterpreted as the approaching footsteps of the persecutor.

(b) Pseudohallucinations

Pseudohallucinations are a form of imagery as distinct from hallucinations and illusions, which are perceptual phenomena. An image is a product of thought and it is a reflection upon the world, unlike a perception where there is a sensing of something external in the real world. Though an image is a cognition it is experienced figuratively as if it were a perception. Pseudohallucinations are pathological images experienced as emanating from the mind, they are seen in the mind's eye, heard with the inner ear, not perceived by the actual eyes and ears. Pseudohallucinations inhabit subjective inner space, not the outside world of objects. They are the patient's own thoughts and there is a feeling of responsibility for them, though unlike the images of normal mental life, the morbid pseudohallucination is not under voluntary control. It confronts the patient as within their mind, it is not there at his or her behest, nor will it evaporate in answer to their wishes. Inner voices are the most commonly encountered examples, often being described as voices in the head or the voice of conscience.

A patient when first seen complained that she occasionally experienced a voice that said clearly 'work' or 'pull yourself together'. This she experienced as in her mind, in the subjective world of her imagining, and she attributed it to the voice of her conscience. It was thus a pseudohallucination. Some time later she described voices whispering to her at night from beneath the bed and behind the curtains and, though the voices were now indistinct and she could not be sure exactly what they said, she was sure they were not in her mind but were coming to her from particular locations in the outside world. In this case the patient would readily accept that the now hallucinated voices were due to something having gone wrong with her mind but nevertheless experienced them as true perceptions. In this particular case

9

the hallucinations became progressively more prominent and clearly enunciated and she was finally assailed by voices emanating from various points around her room laughing, talking about her, and instructing her on how she should behave.

Thoughts experienced as being read aloud are not pseudohallucinations if the thoughts are alienated from the individual and become an auditory perception confronting him or her as part of the external reality.

A problem is created by patients like the one just cited who say they know the voices or visions are in their mind, thus indicating that they have insight into the morbid nature of their experience. In such a case it is important to distinguish whether the phenomenon was experienced as a perception from objective space or really was an image within subjective space. Pseudohallucinations are sometimes characterised as pathological perceptions in which the sufferer is aware of their morbid nature and does not project them into the surrounding world. It seems unwise to this author to call hallucinations pseudohallucinations simply because the patient has insight into their morbid nature (Fish, 1967; Hare, 1973), for this is to make the classification of a perceptual disorder dependent on the patient's judgement at the moment of being interviewed and not on the nature of the experiences themselves.

(c) Eidetic images

Eidetic images are perfectly normal phenomena most frequently encountered in children. They are images of something once perceived, which can be conjured up with almost all the original details intact. Thus a page of a book previously read may be recalled as an image so vivid that the eidetic person can read out the text as from the original.

Perceptual disorders and pseudohallucinations occur in all forms of psychotic disturbance, in disturbed states of consciousness and with surprising frequency in normal individuals. (Slade & Bentall 1988; Posey & Losch 1983). During the phase that intervenes between the waking state and sleep many people experience illusions and hallucinations. The hallucinations on falling asleep are termed *hypnagogic*, and those on awakening *hypnopompic*. In the grief that follows a bereavement, hallucinations and pseudohallucinations of the lost one are a common and normal phenomenon. In situations of extreme stress, be it physical or emotional, where high levels of general arousal pertain, perceptual disturbances tend to become more frequent, albeit fleetingly. Sensory deprivation procedures have produced a wide variety of perceptual abnormalities including organised hallucinatory experiences. A variety of organic states are associated with perceptual disturbance and any major disruption of cerebral function can produce such phenomena, usually is association with the clouded consciousness of a confusional state. Meaningful auditory and visual hallucinations are particularly associated with temporal lobe dysfunction and it has been claimed that they may actually be produced by direct stimulation at or near the temporal lobe. Hallucinogenic drugs induce a wide range of perceptual disturbances, the form and content of which tend to be in constant flux, unlike the hallucinatory disturbances of schizophrenia, and they are predominantly visual in character.

Tactile and somatic hallucinations need careful attention. If the patient has a tactile hallucination, such as a strange tingling, he or she may say it is due to rays directed upon them or 'as if' there were some electrical current. The sufferer from disseminated sclerosis may similarly describe a true paraesthesia as if it were an electric current (Lhermitte's sign). Care must therefore always be exercised to distinguish odd ways of expressing true sensory disturbances from the elaborations, delusional or otherwise, of false perceptions. Further, it is wise not to forget that a bizarre interpretation, particularly of a somatic sensation in a schizophrenic, may mask the symptom of a physical disorder.

Feelings, emotions and affects

The terminology in this area is complicated, as several common usages often attach to each word. For example, feelings in everyday parlance can refer to sensations, beliefs, presentiments, considerations for others, and may even be employed as being synonymous with emotions. Despite the wide overlap in the various terms, some rough distinction and hierarchy is worth attempting.

Feelings can be taken to be basic experiences of pleasure and displeasure. Wundt (1903) suggested feelings vary according to their degree of pleasantness or unpleasantness, the extent to which they produce excitement and the degree of induced tension or conversely relaxation. A feeling need not be about anything, it is simply an account of an internal state.

Emotions can be thought of as involving a more complex state of mind than feelings, for they are usually intentional, being actively directed at something. If I am in love, it is love of someone and it is the charms of the beloved that I am aware of, not the dissociated experience of being in love. An emotional state such as sadness could, of course, become an object for consciousness, an abstraction on which it is possible to reflect, but as soon as it becomes again the emotion of sadness it is sadness about something. The distinction between feeling and emotion may be illustrated by anger. On arriving at work an individual discovers that the typing he had expected to be completed by his secretary is not on his desk and becomes angry – he is now experiencing the emotion of anger about being let down. A few moments later he discovers the typing placed on the filing cabinet: he can no longer be angry about being let down but the feelings accompany the emotion of anger – the sense of displeasure, palpitations and general perturbation – may continue for some time. This example also illustrates how a judgement, in this case of having been let down, is integral to an emotional experience and with judgement comes the possibility of choice (see Solomons, 1980). It also highlights the autonomic changes that accompany the more vehement of our emotions.

Emotions often involve what Frijda (1986) refers to as objectivity in that they are felt to occur to one, to come unbidden and to be independent of one's conscious choices. Emotions are experienced as happening to us and often as being irrational and uncontrollable reactions. Thus though emotions are usually intentional, in the sense of being a conscious orientation toward something, they may be experienced as unintentional, in the sense of being beyond or outside of conscious control. Emotions may involve not only feelings about something, but behaviour or, more exactly, a disposition to behave in a particular manner. Thus love would be associated with a tendency to approach or behave pleasantly towards the object of that affection, just as fear would lead to a tendency to recoil or flee from what was

11

feared. Fantasies are so intimately related to most strong emotions that they can be regarded as an integral element in the experience. Finally, what gives rise to emotions, how they are expressed and possibly even how they are experienced, are influenced by the social and cultural context that mold expectations (Harré, 1986; Mullen, 1991).

Romantic jealousy offers an example, (Mullen, 1990). It involves the experience of painful feelings associated with the fear related to loss and the anger towards the person believed to be guilty of infidelity. There is a cause in the sense of a state of affairs that has aroused suspicions and a judgement that the rights of the jealous have been infringed and disregarded. What constitutes fidelity and therefore infidelity is in part culturally determined. It has an object in that there is jealousy of someone and about something. Jealousy often brings with it vivid fantasies of the partner's supposed infidelities, sometimes described as visual images of such immediacy that it is like watching the actual event. There is a tendency to certain types of behaviour, including checking, cross-questioning, verbal, and even physical aggression. The 'acceptable scripts' determining jealous behaviours are culturally sanctioned.

Moods and affects designate more sustained and pervasive states of mind of which individual emotions may be a part. It is the prevailing tone within which the emotional life of the individual proceeds. Jaspers (1963) appears to argue that mood comes about with prolonged emotion but in practice it often appears as if the mood precedes and constrains the emerging emotional responses. Thus, within the affective state of depression, individuals may be predisposed to experience a variety of emotions – shame, fear, anger – just as they are rendered impervious to others, such as joy. Mood and affect are more global designations than emotion and represent a more complex conceptualisation of the person's psychic experience. Mood and affect define to a significant extent our orientation of the world. The horizons of our existence can be profoundly influenced by mood, for example depression brings with it a narrowing of possibility, a shrinkage of our sense of agency and effectiveness as well as a general dulling of experience.

Temperament is that aspect of the individual that may be taken to be a lifelong predisposition to particular kinds and types of emotional responses and affective states.

Thus a hierarchy moving from feelings through emotions, moods, and affective state to temperament involves increasing complexity in terms of state of mind and usually to an increasing duration of that state.

Pathology of feelings and emotions

The pathology of emotions may be considered, employing the model outlined, as involving alterations in:

1. The types and quality of events and intentions that call forth emotional responses.
   The alterations and pathologies involving the situations and intentions that call forth emotions are of considerable importance in psychiatry, but usually receive scant attention in terms of pathology of emotion. To use jealousy as an example once more, it is normally considered in terms of the abnormal ideas (delusions of infidelity) that call it forth. Clearly, however, there are types of jealousy where the degree of response, the types of

situations invoking it, and the intentions of the emotion can be grossly deviant within the accepted social and cultural norms, without any abnormal beliefs regarding the activities of the partner being involved. Intense doubts about the partner's fidelity may plague the individual, occupying a central part in his mental life, but except at moments of extreme distress insight into their excessive and morbid nature may be retained. The pathology of love could within this model be seen as occupying a wide range of disturbances including some of the sexual perversions (Boss, 1949).

2. The characteristics, tone and strength of feelings generated.

Traditionally the psychopathology of emotion has concentrated primarily on alterations in the tone and character of the feeling generated. This is in keeping with the view of emotions as occurrences that simply happen in or to us. The disturbances described in this area are:

(a) *Poverty of emotional responsiveness*, where there is a loss in the intensity of feelings evoked by events and the emotional life becomes flat and barren. This is seen in its most dramatic form in the chronic schizophrenic state and is part of the so-called negative symptomatology. The blunting of responsiveness should perhaps be distinguished from flattening though they often seem to be used interchangeably. *Blunting* strictly refers to a loss of sensitivity or indifference to the emotional import of an event as opposed to a poverty of response (Sims, 1988). Flattening, in contrast, is illustrated by those who are aware of the potential meaning of an event and the feelings it should evoke but lack the appropriate degree of response. One articulate young woman with schizophrenia described that when with others she would know she should be sharing their laughter, their interest, even their anger, but unlike them she could only perform emotions, not experience them.

(b) *Anhedonia* is a related phenomena where there is a loss of responsiveness specifically tied to the experience of pleasure, which can either be in physical experiences or the pleasures derived from social interaction.

(c) *Incongruity* is where the emotional responses of individuals to their experiences seems to outside observers to be inappropriate. Marked blunting or flattening can give the impression of incongruity though strictly the term should be restricted to situations where the emotion expressed is totally out of keeping with the situation.

(d) *Rigidity of emotional responses* is where the patient is still capable of demonstrating emotional responses but they tend to be limited and constricted in range and are relatively unresponsive to changes in context. Restricted affect is a term covering a similar range of phenomena. In poverty there is an absence of responses; in rigidity the response persists without altering to suit the changing situation.

(e) *Lability* is where sudden short-lived but often intense changes in feeling may occur in response to minor events. This is often encountered in manic states but may be seen in depression and can be a feature of a variety of brain disorders such as the post CVA syndromes.

(f) *Apathy* is where an indifference to the individual's situation is expressed. At first glance it may seem similar to the poverty of emotional responsiveness described, but it usually evokes a very different empathic response in the interviewer. In poverty, the interviewer senses a profound emptiness in the emotional responses; in apathy, it is a

13

sense of withdrawal and turning away from concern with the world rather than a loss of ability to respond. Apathy involves a giving up with a loss of the will and motivation to respond.

(g) *Ambivalence* is where contradictory emotions and intentions coexist at the same instant. In its common usage ambivalence refers to the relatively mundane experience of having a mixture of apparently contradictory emotions about someone or something that tend to alternate rapidly. The term has also been employed by Bleuler (1950) to refer to a far more fundamental split in the emotional life, where radically incompatible emotions and desires coexist at the same moment. Bleuler considered this more extreme form of ambivalence one of the fundamental symptoms of schizophrenia.

(h) *Alexithymia* is employed to describe a virtual inability to recognise or verbalise emotional experiences and a paucity of associated fantasies (Sifneos, 1972). The concept has been widely, if not wisely, applied.

3. The behavioural responses and coping mechanisms employed to deal with the emotions. The behaviour called forth by an emotion or affective state may be abnormal in its form and its degree. In explosive reactions there is a sudden discharge of strong emotion accompanied by ill-controlled and ill-considered behaviour. Such explosive reactions may occur in relatively normal individuals in situations of extreme emotional stress, or may be called forth by quite mundane emotional demands in those of poorly disciplined and self-indulgent temperaments. At the other extreme, strong emotion may induce an inappropriate inability to respond, the individual 'freezes' or is 'paralysed' by the emotion. In shy and self-conscious individuals the possibility of strongly desired social or sexual contact with another may induce not approaching or affectionate behaviour, but a total inability to act and even result in avoidance and flight. In some individuals the difficulty in accepting or coping with their emotions may lead to the exhibition of inappropriate behaviours: the man unable to express anger who becomes increasingly ingratiating and subservient as his internal rage mounts; the desiring man appalled by his own erotic needs who responds with coldness, anger and condemnation towards the person he desires. There can be few of us who are so blessed as always to exhibit the behaviour appropriate to our emotions and the vicissitudes that affect this area of function form a large part of the psychopathology of everyday life.

Pathology of Affect

(a) Depressive states

A search for a clear definition of symptoms rather than the description of phenomena dominates the discourse on depression. In part this reflects the clinical need to define a common and treatable disorder. The exploration of the experience of depression from which a phenomenology emerges may seem clinically irrelevant compared to a good diagnostic instrument on which sleep, mood, suicidal impulses and the like can be simply rated. After all don't we know what it is like to be depressed?

Kraepelin (1921) suggested that 'simple' depression could be understood as the various manifestations of an inhibition of mental life with slowed cognitions, physical activity and speech together with an associated impaired concentration and sense of enervation and exhaustion. This psychic inhibition can culminate in depressive stupor, where mental life drags to a virtual stop. Accompanying this slowing Kraepelin (1921) suggests that patients experience themselves as cut off from both their own thoughts and their own bodies; he writes 'thinking and acting go on without the cooperation of the patient; he appears to himself to be an automatic machine' (p. 75). Schneider (1959) emphasised a similar flattening of mental life, in which the world becomes valueless and the subject's own feelings are experienced as absent or alienated. Certainly in many depressives there is an oppressive sense of being slowed up mentally and physically so that every movement is a struggle and every thought seems to emerge only after prolonged effort. Equally, in a smaller proportion the depression is characterised by harried and agitated excitation in which the patient, tortured by ideas of guilt or hypochondriacal fears, is in a constant state of complaining restlessness (Leonhard, 1979).

One obvious aspect of depressives' experience is the hopelessness about themselves and their future. This involves not just a loss of optimism but a shift of horizon so that the depressive lives in an interminable present whose only prospect is the past. It is quite possible to regard the future as likely to be grim, or worse, without being depressed. In depression the hopelessness about the future is in large part a loss of any belief in a future. The past overwhelms the present, and it becomes a past that ceases to be a source of information and possibility for the future but a past that leads nowhere and can only be an obsessive and repeated lesson in failure and emptiness. To compound the problem is the sense of time slowing to a point where some patients experience themselves as frozen in time or outside of time. Jaspers (1963) writes of depressive patients feeling as if it is always the same moment, like a timeless void (p. 84). Curiously some depressives have a sense of time as something external and separated from themselves, which rushes past. Their day lasts an eternity but the world slips by in a flash.

A sense of permanence pervades severe depression. Depression is experienced as a reality that has no end and from which there is no escape; the past is transformed into a progression of memories infused with regret and responsibility, and the future is exhausted and empty (Minkowski, 1970). There is a block on becoming, a halt to the process of self-realisation, everything is final, everything is lost but equally there is often a sense of finally facing up to an immutable reality. Depression is real, all else was error and self-deception.

Associated with the experience of depression are what Kraepelin (1921) refers to as 'imperative ideas' focused on wickedness, worthlessness, persecution, degeneration and death. These themes impose themselves on the depressive and become not just concerns but overwhelming experiences. The mental content of the depressive may be dominated by ideas of inferiority with self-accusations, self-denigrations and fears of damaging others. The claims of guilt and sin can be tinged with grandiosity and hyperbole. Even mild to moderate depression is often associated with a sense of physical deterioration both in the fabric of the body and the fabric of the world. In it's most flamboyant manifestations this leads to hypochondriacal delusions and *ideas of annihilation* in which the whole world is either about to be destroyed or has already disintegrated leaving the patient surrounded by wraiths and phantoms.

One of the many paradoxes encountered in the depressed is the alternation between a suicidal despair, which disclaims any interest in survival, and an anxious hypochondria, which ruminates fearfully on potentially lethal conditions. These imperative ideas of the depressive often manifest both apparent depth and an overwhelming immediacy, but conversely, may have a peculiar ephemeracy. Thus one minute the agonised depressive grasps one's hand contorted with grief and guilt over past indiscretions and claiming a universal responsibility for the world's evils, and the next is complaining bitterly about the slights, lack of care and even active persecution by staff and fellow patients. No punishment too great but equally no service or kindness adequate to slake the depressives sense of entitlement.

One aspect of the phenomenlology of the depressed that is often missed or misinterpreted is the experience of persecution. Suspiciousness and persecutory ideas are to be found even in mild to moderate depression. This can become a dominant theme with complaints of being followed, talked about, deprived and disadvantaged, plotted against and even assailed by threatening voices. Sensitive ideas of reference and delusions of reference may be prominent, even obscuring the primary depressive disorder.

The prevailing mood in depression is often described as sad. In practice the gentle quietness of sadness is rarely encountered. Gloom, active distress, dull despondency and irritable complaint are more frequent. It is also worth remembering that some socially adept depressives present with a self-depreciatory irony that can disguise the underlying despair.

Central to depression are disturbances in biological processes, most particularly those concerning appetites and circadian rhythmicity. Sleep is disrupted. Attempts to link particular types to sleep disturbance, such as early morning waking, to particular types of depression are often misleading. In depression there is usually a combination of difficulty initiating sleep, an unstable and restless sleep and difficulty maintaining sleep with early waking. Early waking is usually more prominent in older subjects. Interest in food along with other pleasures is attenuated or lost and the libido shrinks to nothing.

(b) Manic states

There is a tendency to conceive of mania as the mirror image of depression, which though useful up to a point can miss many of the salient features. Jaspers (1963) characterised mania as 'primary, unmotivated and superabundant hilarity and euphoria; as a delight in life, a lively optimism' (p. 596). Though manics may evince these charming characteristics, for all except the mildest of cases a darker side alternates with, if not completely obscures, these elements of good cheer. Irritability manifests at the least frustration, intolerance lies imminent in the exaggerated and overbearing ambitions of the manic and the driven physical overactivity can all too easily explode into violence.

The manic is driven and buffeted by elevated and exaggerated emotions, desires and activities. There is an increased pace to existence but the price of this busyness is a dislocation in the inner unity that usually directs the coherent unfolding of our ideas, intentions and activities. The fragmentation and disruption in the manic's activities increase with the more severe forms of mania.

The mood in mania is heightened but with increased intensity comes an instability and lability. There can be sudden switches from jocularity to accusatory irritability, from exultation to despair. There may be an air of pompous superiority but unlike the similar demeanour found in some delusional disorders the manic's exaggerated self-confidence is usually a fragile and fugitive audacity.

States of *ecstasy* may occur in which the patient is transfigured by delight, often remaining relatively or even completely immobile. Such patients are difficult to distract from their delighted state, accounts of which can usually only be obtained retrospectively. They may be infused with a sense of joy and contentment, and may describe an 'oceanic feeling' in which they experience themselves as in some kind of mystical unity with humanity, life or even the universe. Religious connotations are, not surprisingly, attached to such experiences. One of my patients, a philosopher previously bereft of religious sympathies, was discomforted in a manic episode by such an ecstatic experience. He felt he had to in some way integrate this into his materialist world view. Like many who have ecstatic experiences, its intensity and 'realness' was too great to consign it to a symptom of illness. Manic patients on recovery may have a clear insight into the fact that they have been mentally ill but still cling onto the relevance of some of their experiences and revelations.

There is a sense in most manics of the tempo and profundity of their thought processes being enhanced. The speeding up is associated with difficulty sustaining attention and in more severe states the flight of ideas produces a dislocation and fragmentation sometimes termed secondary incoherence. The outward manifestation of pressured thinking is pressured speech and distractibility (see page 38).

There is a physical restless or *volitional excitement* in manics that can be impressive. One manic patient strode repeatedly around my room in a circuit that included clambering from chair to desk, across my desk and descending via the radiator. In severe mania, just as speech can disintegrate into disjointed words and phrases, so activities may descend to purposeless flapping. Even in mild mania many tasks are initiated but few completed.

Perception is heightened in mania. The world becomes a source of colourful and intense experiences but some patients describe a fragility and falseness to these perceptions. One young woman said it was like being on the set of some opulent stage show with everything multi-coloured and gleaming but that nothing seemed to have any real substance or robustness; she said 'it was as if I could reach out my finger and put it through walls, furniture even people'. Hallucinations, particularly visual and auditory, occur in more severe mania. Complex visions can accompany severe mania. One patient, on emerging from an ecstatic state, described being able to see a great distance and what she saw was a great copulation with people making love in some extended garden of carnal delights (less colourful visions are, however, more common).

A sense of physical well-being and enhanced strength is common in mania and may lead to a belief in invulnerability, which can precipitate dangerous activities. One patient drove for several miles down the wrong side of a busy freeway, happily bouncing his car against the sides of oncoming vehicles secure in the knowledge he was beyond injury or the law (in fact he turned out to be correct on both counts).

In even mild mania there is a tendency to grandiosity and an exaggerated sense of personal worth. It is important to relate the patient's claims and behaviour to what is usual for him. One of my patients who was employed as a lavatory attendant entertained the idea that he was a station porter, which for him was grandiose. Grandiose ideas and exaggerated expectations feed fleeting delusional notions and delusions of reference. They do have immense wealth from an inheritance that had previously slipped their mind; the latest pop song is adapted from a piece they strummed some years ago and the royalties will soon begin to flow; they are the repository of the economic wisdom that will solve their, and everyone elses, unemployment. In mania, delusions, like other mental contents, usually emerge rapidly but are not sustained. This being said, states of so called *delusional mania* occur where the dominant feature is a fixed and often extensively elaborated elusional system, usually of religious or grandiose content to which hallucinations and misinterpretations are often linked but in which excitement and elation are more muted. This state may have a remarkable tenacity and can create diagnostic difficulties. The elation and exaggerated sense of worth can produce fantastic claims and stories in which fantasy and fabrication combine to produce fluent confabulations. This can be difficult at first glance to distinguish from the fluent confabulations seen in association with some delusional disorders but the history of its emergence, the content and the evanescence of manic phenomena usually suffice to separate the phenomena.

In mania, heightened interest and engagement with the world go together with increased appetites of all kinds but most obviously in the sexual area. Increased and disinhibited sexual behaviour is common. Again it is essential to relate the emergent behaviour to what is normal for the patient. A vicar's wife showed, for her, the grossest of sexual disinhibition by tiptoeing around their suburban garden in the nude, albeit in the dead of night. A lack of prudence characterises the financial as well as the sexual activities of the manic. Inflated self-confidence, a sense of invulnerability, and heightened acquisitiveness can combine to produce flights of financial mismanagement that are ruinous not only to the patient but to anyone over whose money he can exert control.

Disturbed sleep is virtually universal and it is often the change in sleep pattern that is the harbinger of a manic episode. In severe mania the sleep pattern is totally disrupted with the patient having only brief naps or micro-sleeps.

States of mania exert a fascination and attraction not only for observers but retrospectively for some patients. Though some patients fear above all else the loss of control and the driven self-damaging behaviour of mania, others hark back nostalgically to the elation, self-confidence and activity of their previous mania. Not a few patients knowingly induce a manic episode in the mistaken belief that this time they will control it rather than letting it control them. Manic states can and do lay waste our patients' lives destroying their interpersonal, professional and economic existence.

(c) Anxiety states

Anxiety plays a fundamental role in mental disorders and we all partake of it from time to time. Nevertheless it is an experience peculiarly difficult to describe. It is relatively easy to speak of what makes us anxious, be it fear of failure, illness, crowds, snakes or whatever. The physical concomitants of anxiety such as palpitations, muscle tensions, tremulousness, hyperacusis are equally readily described. Attempts to capture the psychological state of being anxious often tend to produce only a list of similes such as worrying, dread, panic, terror and tension.

Anxiety occurs in response to the expectation of some approaching evil and in essence it is the experience of some feared future possibility brought forward to plague one in the present. Anxiety is a currently experienced distress at an apprehended future threat. In straightforward fear the arousal relates to an obvious and imminent possibility, such as the danger presented by the snake on the path or the rapidly approaching vehicle. In anxiety a more distant and ambiguous future calamity is brought forward to vex and distress. Severe forms of anxiety usually concern a more nebulous but nevertheless overwhelming threat that seems to impinge on one's very survival. The state of being anxious creates a sense of confusion and uncertainty that disrupts the individual's capacity either to escape the dread, or form, let alone realise, any effective intentions. Anxiety often focuses on a particular threat of personal or social annihilation, such as a heart attack or of exposure to overwhelming social embarrassment, but is not exhausted or coextensive with its chosen object. The fear is of the death consequent on the heart attack or the total social ostracism consequent on the exposure of the supposed or actual transgression. Pathological anxiety brings with it an inexhaustible vision of awfulness in the face of which we stand confused, incapable of action and crying out for help that will inevitably be inadequate.

Obsessive and compulsive phenomena

The essential feature of these phenomena was described by Lewis (1967) as 'the fruitless struggle against a disturbance that seems isolated from the rest of mental activity'. This places the emphasis on a conscious resistance to these 'homemade but disowned' impulses. A distinction is often drawn between *obsessions* as recurrent cognitions in the form of intrusive thoughts, impulses, ideas, or images and *compulsions* as repetitive seemingly purposeful stereotyped behaviours (APA, 1987; Rachman & Hodgson, 1980). In practice compulsions are behavioural responses to obsessions though not all obsessions lead to compulsions.

Central to the experience of an obsession is usually a fear or phobia. Typical fears are of death, contamination, acting violently and being blasphemous (Straus, 1948). The cognition, usually but not always a fear, is experienced in a very particular manner in that the sufferer recognises to some extent that it is irrational, or at the very least senselessly insistent. An act of will is usually made, to suppress or turn attention away from this preoccupying cognition. Occasionally the intrusive cognition will not appear to carry frightening connotations, as with an intrusive melody or an impulse to carry out some form of exercise of mental agility. Usually, however, on further elaboration these will either turn out to be performances aimed at warding off what is feared (compulsions) or displacement activities to blot out some feared cognition. One patient, referred because of increasing inability to function at work, reported an overwhelming preoccupation with mental arithmetic, which he felt impelled to carry out despite attempts to resist and return his attention to matters at hand. It was only later he acknowledged that he harboured the belief that only by the successful completion of increasingly complex arithmetical calculations could he prevent his wife's infidelity. The patent absurdity, if not of the fear of infidelity at least of the remedy, made him believe that if he revealed this notion he would be locked up as mad.

The fear not only keeps reverberating in the sufferer's consciousness but the world often becomes a source of constant reminders and provocations. Cut flowers conjure up images of death and decay, the sight of a wristwatch provokes a fear that it may have a luminous dial indicating the presence of the feared radiation, the knife is a potential weapon, the spanner is a potential weapon, the glass if broken could become a potential weapon, etc, etc. For the obsessional the sign or symbol of the feared is magically transformed into the presence of what is feared.

The compulsive element of the experience is usually secondary in that it develops to defend against the obsessing fear. Thus the hand-washing is a response to the preoccupying fear of contamination (which itself may be generated by a fear of bringing death or decay on oneself or others). As Lewis (1967, pp. 157–72) points out, the compulsions can themselves become obsessional, that is the patient has to struggle against them and may indeed develop defensive behaviours to ward them off. Thus one patient overwhelmed by compulsive hand-washing to fend off the feared contamination developed a complex set of hand movements and gyrations to defend against the impulse to keep washing.

The compulsions can become ritualised to create a magical counter charm to the intruding obsession. It is not enough for those obsessed by contamination to wash, they have to wash in a very particular and usually increasingly complex manner. Failure to complete the precise and stereotyped ritual, or more particularly the fear of an incorrect performance, leads to a compulsion to repeat the compulsion. The perfectionism so often found in the character of the obsessional combines with the magical thinking to produce a tangled web of obsessions, compulsions and rituals that enmesh the victim. In severe obsessional illness patients can become so isolated within the multilayered obsessions and compulsions that they are overwhelmed and their consciousness of the basic irrationality of their thoughts and actions, as well as their resistance to these phenomenon, may become so attenuated as to be at times invisible. Not surprisingly, some regard severe examples of these disorders as being close to, if not actually, psychotic (Insel & Akiskal, 1986).

Delusions

Socrates declared we do not call those mad who err in matters that lie outside the knowledge of ordinary people; madness is the name they give to errors in matters of common knowledge . . . we don't think a slight error implies madness but just as they call strong desire love, so they name a grand delusion madness.

Xenophon (1923).

Definition

Delusion involves abnormal beliefs that arise in the context of disturbed judgements and an altered experience of reality, such that it becomes a source of new and false meanings. In everyday language, the term delusion is simply used to designate a belief considered patently false. In psychopathology the implications of referring to someone as deluded goes far beyond merely indicating that they harbour false convictions, or have made false judgements on a particular topic. Delusion has long been regarded as one of the central characteristics of madness and involves more than false and arbitrary ideas developed without adequate proof.

Delusions usually have attributed to them the following characteristics:

1. They are held with absolute conviction and are experienced as self-evident reality, not as merely opinion or belief.
2. They are not amenable to reason nor modifiable by experience.
3. They are experienced as of great personal significance and usually preoccupy the person to the point of disrupting social and interpersonal functioning.
4. Their content is often regarded by others as fantastic or at the very least inherently unlikely.
5. They consist of convictions that are highly personal and idiosyncratic that are not likely to be shared even by those of similar social and cultural backgrounds.

These characteristics are not, however, sufficient to separate delusions from non-pathological beliefs and convictions. The addition of three further characteristics assists in making such distinctions:

6. They often emerge in a manner that suggests their pathological origins.
7. They often extend to contaminate a wide range of the patients' beliefs about themselves and their world.
8. They are usually self-referential in that they directly concern, and are primarily about, the deluded subject and their immediate relationship to the world.

These eight criteria need to be critically examined.

The absolute conviction in the truth of one's beliefs is not confined to the deluded subject. Further, the deluded patient may on occasions paradoxically combine an apparent total certainty with, at another level, an awareness of the delusional nature of his or her beliefs. The double-entry bookkeeping is illustrated by the patients who of their own volition come to psychiatrists to tell of their divine mission rather than to the relevant ecclesiastical body.

The imperviousness of a delusion to modification by reason or experience in no way distinguishes it from common error and opinion. Logical error is not the exclusive hallmark of delusion nor, sadly, is the failure to expose beliefs to the test of critical appraisal confined to the mad. The errors of most normal individuals are those common to their social group and take their origin from shared misconceptions. The errors of the deluded patient tend to be idiosyncratic in the extreme. Their origin is often to be sought in some as yet little understood disruption and change of mental function, which fundamentally alters the patient's knowledge of the world. The failure of deluded subjects to change their opinion when faced by contrary argument should perhaps occasion no surprise, for our own mistaken beliefs recede more before the changing structure of our environment, wrought by the slow passage of time, than they do before mere reason.

A subject's delusional system is usually a private and isolating series of beliefs about the world. It forms a central and overriding series of convictions that influences, if not dominates subjects' beliefs about themselves and their world. It is perhaps surprising that delusional systems that are nearly always pre-eminent in governing individuals' understanding of their experience are remarkably variable in the extent to which they direct actions. A study by Wessely and colleagues (1993) suggested a half of their deluded subjects had to some extent acted in a manner congruent with their morbid beliefs. Typical of the delusionally influenced behaviours were avoiding watching the TV, stopping going out socially and avoiding foods thought to be poisoned. The grandiose delusions in the sufferer with GPI or the extensive system of beliefs to be found in many chronic schizophrenics may, however, have little influence on the patient's behaviour. The delusions in affective psychoses more often call forth behaviour consistent with the beliefs. Manics, for example, may well act on their convictions, spending money they do not have, entering into impossibly ambitious projects and offering their unsolicited advice to all.

The content of delusions is often fantastic, but then inherently unlikely notions are not unknown even among psychiatrists. It is not the truth or falsity of the belief that defines a delusion in psychiatry, for delusions may on occasions partake of the truth. The potentially correct delusion is most commonly encountered in morbid jealousy. One patient had the infidelity of his wife conclusively revealed to him on Christmas Eve, when returning from work he noted that the lights on the festive tree in his front window were flashing on and off in synchrony with those of his neighbour's tree. The actual nature of the wife's relationship to this particular neighbour is not critical to the phenomenological analysis of this belief as a delusion, though it may, of course, be relevant to speculations about meaning. The way in which a belief emerges and the reasons for its acceptance are, therefore, part of the way we recognise delusions.

Delusions are not dependent on any defect in the patient's intelligence, nor of disruption in the faculties for reason and logical thought. An intelligent and articulate individual who becomes deluded will put these abilities to the service of the delusion and a luxuriant growth of bizarre ideas may result, which are argued and defended with all the subject's usual mental agility. An excellent example is provided by Schreber's (1955) memoirs.

Delusions can relate to the belief systems of normal individuals. False beliefs do not always indicate psychopathology. Idiosyncratic and unshared beliefs are not of necessity false, let alone morbid. Take an original concept in science. At the moment of its inception it could be confined to one individual and not shared by those of a similar social and cultural background. A concept in science would, however, be directed at a circumscribed area, would be understandable within the accepted and shared discourse of science and, though it might be of great personal significance to its instigator, that significance would be primarily in terms of what it explained about the world in general, not about the internal and intimate world of that individual. Such a belief might be termed delusional by the scientist's colleagues out of incredulity or even envy, but hopefully it would be unlikely to acquire the epithet delusional within a psychopathological framework. Religious belief, particularly sudden religious revelation, shares some of the characteristics of delusion, but again it would normally be distinguished by being recognisably part of an accepted area of religious experience and discourse. Totally private religious revelation, independent of any accepted theological context, could present considerable problems, separating from a morbid phenomenon.

In distinguishing between novel scientific ideas and religious beliefs, the dimension termed extension by Kendler and colleagues (1983) is of value. Extension describes the extent to which a delusional belief spreads to involve various area of the subject's life. A scientific idea, however fundamental, is unlikely to explain why the scientist's neighbours seem unfriendly, why a colleague wears a red tie, or why their food tastes bitter. A run of the mill persecutory delusion, on the other hand, can usually generate explanations for these and many other mundane events. Similarly, religious revelations, however fervently believed, usually limit their explanatory power to spiritual, ethical and moral issues whereas delusions are highly personalised and self-referential and often extend to reveal the meaning behind a wide range of apparently trivial occurrences.

Classification of delusion

A number of attempts have been made to classify delusions (see reviews by Arthur, 1964; Winters and Neale, 1983; Garety, 1985; Oltmanns and Maher, 1987). Perhaps the simplest division that has been suggested is dependent on the degree of conviction with which the beliefs are expressed (Wing *et al.*, 1974). Partial delusions are those where the individual is prepared to entertain the possibility of being mistaken, whereas delusions proper are held with a conviction that excludes the possibility of doubt. The problem with this division is that the way in which opinions and beliefs are expressed is largely a function of the interplay between educational and cultural background and the personality of the individual. Some of us express trivial and peripheral assumptions with force and conviction whereas others timidly advance their most heartfelt beliefs. Should delusion supervene this habitual method of presenting belief may mislead the observer as to the true level of conviction with which the ideas are adhered to. There is also considerable fluctuation in individual patients over time in how firmly they adhere to their delusional convictions.

Delusions have been divided into those judgements that arise in an understandable way from particular interactions or experiences and those that appear *de novo* like sudden intuitions or brain waves. Those delusions, where no connection can be comprehended between the emergence of the belief and any precursor, and which confront the observer as something absolute and irreducible, have been termed *Primary or autochthonous delusions.* Jaspers (1963), observed that in these primary delusions there occurs an experience radically alien to the healthy person that comes before thought, although it becomes clear only in thought. The primary delusion emerges in the context of a radical change or break in normal mental function and is indicative of a process at work. The primary delusion is thus assumed to be an eruption of an extra conscious process into the normal flow of intentional mental life. The primary delusion cannot be fully explained by an appeal to the meaningful connections that usually govern the stream of consciousness. On the contrary, it is an ultimately irreducible phenomenon not amenable to psychological understanding and only explicable finally in terms of the causal connections governing the presumed organic changes in the brain. Clearly this is an untestable hypothesis. It does not, of course, imply that the content of a primary delusion has no connection with the patient's past life or present situation; it merely claims that the emergence of the belief and part at least of its initial content will not be amendable to such an analysis. Once the primary delusion is established, the further elaboration of any delusional system will in principle be open to an analysis in terms of its meaningful connections.

An example of a primary delusion is a patient who, on asking a friend for a light for his cigarette, was passed a box of matches on which appeared the slogan 'the greatest match in the world'. This revealed to the patient in a moment of intensely experienced insight that he was the light of the world. This delusional brainwave made sense for the patient of many of his recent experiences and much of his prior life; he realised his failures had been trials, his rejections, persecutions, and his sexual inadequacy part of divine inspiration. A totally new perspective on the world overthrowing most of his previous concepts came with this revelation.

Secondary delusions or delusion-like ideas emerge understandably from other psychic events or the subject's interaction with the world (Jaspers, 1963). Their origin can be traced to affects, drives, fears, or some devastating personal experience. They are therefore amenable, at least theoretically, to analysis in terms of the meaningful connections of psychic life. A morbid alteration in a subject's mood may, for example, if it is towards elation, precede the emergence of delusions of grandeur or, conversely, a depressive swing may be followed by delusions of poverty or guilt. The hallucinated subject's perverted senses may be the starting point of a delusional development as may some real experience of injustice in a paranoid personality. A suspicious prickly individual with a propensity to self-reference was exposed to a series of personal disasters including loss of job, loss of money, and loss of his home following mortgage foreclosure. The events (partly self-induced) were explained by him initially as due to a generally ill-disposed world towards a man of his obvious but unrecognised talents. As he continued to ruminate on the events, a pattern became more and more obvious to him. Slowly over a period of many months a delusional system involving a complex plot by members of his family in league with the local constabulary and public health officials emerged. This delusional system became the focal point of his life, dominating from then onwards his thoughts and actions. The slow emergence of this secondary delusional system was in the context of immense personal stress, probably associated with an unrecognised depressive mood swing occurring in a person with a suspicious and over-sensitive personality structure.

There is obviously a problem in a classification that relies on as subjective a criterion as 'understandability'. Theoretically the division is attractive; in practice, it is often difficult and inconsistent of application (Koehler, 1979). The distinction also relies on the content of the phenomena rather than the form that goes against the aim of classifying by form rather than content. To try to some extent to circumvent this problem, Schneider (1959) divided delusions into two major forms, *delusional perception*, and *delusional notions*. Delusional perception, Schneider considered of particular significance in the diagnosis of schizophrenia. It was a two-stage phenomenon involving first, a true perception of a real object and secondly, the emergence of a delusional insight generated by the perception, this delusion having no easily comprehensible connection to the perception. This new knowledge does not derive from reflection upon the perception but is imminent in the perception the perceiving and the knowing are directly and immediately linked, the one is contained in the other.

These classifications of delusion pay little direct attention to the extent of the restructuring of the patient's knowledge of himself and his world that is involved. The type of knowledge involved is also only indirectly employed within these classifications. Delusion involves both the elements of beliefs or knowledge about something and the interpretation or, more precisely, the misinterpretation of occurrences or objects in the surroundings. It might be helpful to construct a hierarchical model according to the degree to which patients' views differ from normal convictions in terms of how firmly they are held, how idiosyncratic they are, and the extent to which they influence their views of themselves and their world. Delusion usually involves both belief and interpretation; the balance between these two elements varies and two hierarchies are possible, those predominantly involving morbid belief and those morbid interpretations.

Morbid interpretations

Self-consciousness is characterised by a heightened self-awareness. Individuals often believe that their own personal preoccupations with regard to appearance, actions, and even thought will be mirrored in the attention they receive from those around. Some minor facial blemish will not only be the centre of their attention, but that of all those they encounter. Their thoughts, particularly those involving sex and anger, will be embarrassingly obvious from their facial expression. Their actions will make them ridiculous in the eyes of all. Self-consciousness is the lot of most of us at some time or another. It is usually more marked in adolescence and when entering unfamiliar social situations. At the extreme it can produce extensive disruption of an individual's ability to function socially.

Sensitive self-reference is a propensity to interpret habitually the words and actions of others and incidental happenings of the world as being directly concerned with oneself. It is clearly related to self-consciousness and the two often occur together, though essentially the self-conscious individual is turned in on him or herself whereas the self-referring is painfully aware of his or her surroundings. In self-reference, not only is there heightened self-awareness, but a tendency to divine personal meanings in trivial and unrelated events. The world becomes centred on the individual, and the mundane words and actions of others are seen as being directed at the individual. Self-reference normally has a persecutory flavour, so the remarks and actions of others are invested with unpleasant and even sinister import. A couple laughing on the other side of a crowded room are laughing at the patient, the overheard snatch of conversation in a bus is about him or her, the shrug of the shoulders of the barman is a dismissive insult not a mere gesture, etc. In self-reference, individuals normally convinced at the time that the events they misinterpret were directed at them and them alone, but in retrospect will at least entertain the possibility of error. In self-reference the meaning attached to the action or event is not impossible nor even necessarily improbably, people could be laughing at them, passing remarks, intentionally obstructive, etc. It is the frequency of the self-reference and its extension into every area of social and personal interaction that leads to its recognition as morbid.

Delusional mood is characterised by an altered experience of the world where, in some intangible way, events take on an uncanny quality and tension. The events as well as the actions and words of others seem to hint at hidden meanings and are infused with a direct and personal significance. The precise nature of the meaning seems elusive and, though there is often a sense that a pattern of meaning is about to emerge, it remains just out of grasp. The individual in such a state often appears perplexed or frankly fearful. This state differs from self-reference in that it involves an attribution of meaning to a far wider area of the patient's experience of the world, everything is imbued with personal meaning. On the other hand, the precise meaning of the occurrences is far less clear than in self-reference. Thus, though a somewhat less clearly defined abnormal state of mind than self-reference, it is a more extensive and pervasive disturbance and is less easy to relate to normal experience. Delusions of reference may crystallise out of a delusional mood.

Delusions of reference have a similar structure to self-reference in that some event or aspect of the environment is taken to indicate a very personal and direct meaning for the patient. The interpretation placed upon the event in delusions of reference is more idiosyncratic and cannot so easily be seen as a possible, even if unlikely, interpretation. Thus a headline in a newspaper ostensibly about events in the Middle East Conflict was interpreted as a direct reference to the patient's homosexuality. The code numbers at the top of a banal communication from the tax inspector was interpreted as further evidence of a conspiracy. The colour of the tie worn by the doctor enables the patient to identify him as part of a sect dedicated to persecuting the patient. The television compere is understood as repeatedly making veiled references to the patient's sexual activity disguised as sports commentary. In delusions of reference the meaning derived from the event is incomprehensible to others in the patient's social group. The delusion of reference remains an interpretation, thus a meaning is attributed to an event, but it is not open to doubt, it is experienced as self-evidently true. The information contained in a delusion of reference, however bizarre, is essentially limited and restricted; it may form part of the patient's more extensive delusion system, but is only a part.

Beliefs about the world

Overvalued ideas have enormous personal significance out of all proportion to their overt content. They differ from the strongly held beliefs of the commonality in the degree of emotional investment and the focal part they play in the mental life of the individual. Clearly some types of convictions, particularly the religious and political, are often invested with great significance, but overvalued ideas normally concern more mundane and specifically personal matters. Despite their importance to the individual, they remain beliefs about the world not the articulation of self-evidence reality. The content, though often eccentric, is not entirely removed from what is regarded by their peers as conceivable. The overvalued idea often develops out of a conflict between a vulnerable personality and some elements in their environment (McKenna, 1984). Individuals, though strongly protesting the accuracy of their beliefs, will entertain the possibility of error, albeit only the dimmest and most distant possibility.

Simple delusions are true delusions, in that they are absolute convictions experienced as self-evident reality that are immutable in the face of contrary argument or experiences. They are highly personal and their content is often fantastic. They normally, however, concern a relatively limited aspect of the individual's beliefs about himself or his world. The depressive delusions of bizarre bodily afflictions, such as their blood drying up, their heart being absent, their bowels rotting away, are typical examples. The erotomanic delusions and circumscribed persecutory delusions, that attribute malevolent intent to specific individuals or groups and do not spread to affect the majority of the patient's relationships to others, are further examples. The impression given by patients with this type of morbid belief is that their beliefs about other aspects of the world are largely consonant with those of their fellows; except in the particular and often quite narrow area occupied by the delusions. This type of delusion may fluctuate in intensity and in the extent to which it preoccupies the patient. These fluctuations are often connected to factors that appear to be related to the genesis of the delusions. Thus as the mood fluctuates the delusions associated with an affective psychosis may wax and wane. In the persecutory delusions of some paranoid patients, interpersonal conflict may exacerbate the problem, and the removal of a source of stress may at least temporarily allow the beliefs to recede into the background.

Unsystematised delusions are characterised by a number of poorly organised and unintegrated delusional notions. The patient's account is often difficult to follow both because of the partial nature of the accounts provided and by the frequent shifts in focus. In some cases, despite the poorly articulated nature of the beliefs, they appear to have for the patient profound significance but in others there is a superficial and almost trivial quality to the fluctuating kaleidoscope of odd ideas and fragmented beliefs.

Systematised delusions involve a profound delusional restructuring of the patient's view of him or herself and surroundings. The delusional system contaminates wide areas of patients' beliefs about their world. There may appear a central core to the belief system, for example, personal divinity, a plot, some damage or injury sustained, but the delusional beliefs spread to contaminate wide areas of the patients' understanding of their position and relationships. The systematised delusions may grow gradually by accretion over months or years, or may emerge rapidly, transforming almost at a stroke the patient's mental life. Systematised delusions, perhaps because of their extended and extensive nature, change (if change they do) slowly over time rather than in obvious response to alterations in the patient or his or her environment. The systematised delusions offer no possibility or refutation; all new experience and information becomes incorporated within this morbid knowledge.

Systematised delusions may emerge on the basis of delusions of reference, either gradually or on occasion as an almost immediate and extensive restructuring of the patient's view of him or herself and his or her world. Systematised delusions are usually sustained and extended by misinterpretations, misperceptions, delusions of references and restructured, if not frankly delusional memories.

A final point is that at the centre of many delusional systems lies an altered world view from which the details of the system spread. In the persecutory view, the patients are acutely aware of the outside world and its impact upon them, where all occurrences are potentially threatening and destructive but above all, meaningful and personalised. In the depressive view, their own internal preoccupations with guilt, loss and disintegration come to colour the world in which they live and constantly confirm and reflect their internal reality.

Delusions and reality

The relationship of the patient's private delusional world to the shared reality varies (Scharfetter, 1980). In some cases the delusion comes to dominate the patient's mental life and he or she withdraws completely into a private world. In other cases, although the delusional reality is predominant, the patient continues to live to some extent within the shared social context. In some the delusional reality exists side by side with the shared reality without either seeming to affect, or contaminate, the other (Bleuler's double registration). Finally, delusional reality may be inextricably intermingled with the shared reality.

Delusions of specific content

Delusions are, on occasions, classified according to content. This is usually self-explanatory, e.g. delusions of grandeur, delusions of guilt, delusions of persecution, delusions of poverty, etc., but a few specific types require brief mention.

Nihilistic delusions involve a delusional belief that something is dead or non-existent. This may involve a belief that some organ or part of the body has gone or rotted away or that the individual is himself dead. The term nihilistic delusions is often employed loosely to cover all delusional ideas about bodily dysfunction and decay in depression. When nihilistic delusions form a prominent feature within the clinical picture, the term Cotard's syndrome is occasionally employed.

Erotomanic delusions are characterised by an exaggerated and irrational attachment, usually to someone who in reality has little or no relationship to the sufferer. They can be predominantly a conviction that the patient is loved by someone who has done nothing to encourage such a belief or be an intense and totally preoccupying infatuation that fixes on someone who had made clear their total lack of interest (Mullen & Pathé, 1994).

Delusions of possession in which the patient is convinced they are possessed by some spirit or force. These tend to be found among those whose cultural background provides some basis for beliefs in possession. That being so, it can be quite difficult to separate them from an overdramatic presentation of a culturally appropriate belief. Occasionally, in forensic practice, claims of being possessed are advanced to exculpate some offence. Among the possessors I have encountered are devils, holy spirits, dead relatives, warrior ancestors and the spirit of a dead rabbit (!). Beliefs in being possessed are distinct from the experience of being influenced by outside forces and the belief in being someone else. Thus one of my patients believed he was Elvis Presley and that an imposter was entombed at Gracelands whilst another believed she was on occasions possessed by the spirit of the departed rock star. In the state of possession a tension exists between oneself and the interloping possessor and even, as with holy spirits, when the possession is welcome it remains to some extent a separate and intruding presence.

Misidentification syndromes involve a conviction, often delusional, that the people encountered by the patient are not who and what they appear or claim to be (Coleman, 1993). This can involve denying the identity of familiar individuals or claiming that strangers or chance acquaintances are in fact relatives or significant figures from the patient's past life. The misidentification may involve a belief that familiar and often closely related individuals are not really who they appear, but merely have the same outward appearance, the inner psychological identify being different. This can lead to claims that the patient is being duped by doubles disguised as his relatives or, as in one patient of mine, that his family's bodies had been taken over by a race of aliens. Sometimes it is a physical identity rather than a psychological identity that is at issue and subtle differences discernable in the individual's appearance, seem to reveal them as imposters or chance or subtle similarities of appearance apparently vouchsafe identity. This phenomenon is not so uncommon in severe psychotic disturbance as the literature sometimes suggests. It is graced by the eponym of *Capgras syndrome* (Capgras & Reboul-Lachland, 1923; Christodoulou, 1977). Misidentifications can be quite bizarre when, for example, the patient seems utterly convinced that a young nurse is his dead mother, or ignoring minor issues of gender, that the man in the next bed is really his wife. More frequently, the delusional misidentification is based on some minor similarity of appearance or mannerism between the individual and who they are claimed to be by the patient. On occasion this type of misidentification is referred to as the *illusion of Fregoli*, but the term is misleading on several counts.

Delusions may come to be shared, usually with a family, and these shared delusions may be referred to as *folie à deux, folie à trois*, etc., psychosis of association, double or multiple insanity. Several variants have been described:

1. Simultaneous emergence of delusion in closely associated individuals, where the content is shared, probably as a result of shared environment, but the origin is independent.
2. Imposed delusions, where a dominant figure within a relationship or group imposes his or her delusional view on the others to such an extent that the delusional system seems eventually to be totally shared.
3. Communicated delusions, where two individuals living in close association, both of whom have a propensity to psychotic disturbance, come to influence and share each other's delusional world.

Delusional memory is a phenomenon where a delusional insight occurs not as an intuition about the world or as a change in knowledge of or about the world, but in the form of a memory. An example is provided by a patient who suddenly 'remembered' that a few weeks previously she had been attacked and raped by her brother and brother-in-law in the midst of a family gathering. The conviction that this had occurred emerged *de novo*, the lady could point to nothing that suggested such an event. On the contrary, she was constantly surprised that everything and everybody around her were so normal and apparently unaware of the terrible happening, even those she believed to have been involved. The belief continued without seeming to alter this lady's experience of her world or even her relationship to the central figures in the memory.

Dysmorphophobia is an intense and unshakeable conviction on the patient's part that an aspect of his or her appearance or body is misshapen and conspicuously ugly. This phenomenon is associated with an intense preoccupation with the supposed deformity on which the patient ruminates at length. The actual experience and perception of the individual's own body seems altered in that slight deviations from normal shape or size will be claimed by the patient to be gross and obviously different from normal. There is often associated despondency and this phenomenon can be secondary to depressive disorders. The narcissistic elements are usually obvious. This phenomenon can, in clinical practice, therefore partake in part at least in delusion, perceptual disturbance, obsessive ruminations, phobia, and mood disturbance.

Passivity phenomena (disturbances of ego boundary)

Passivity experiences are a group of phenomena disparate in many ways but having in common a disturbance in the experienced integrity of the self. They are sometimes referred to as disturbances of ego boundary because of this experience of the breaking down, or violation, in the unity of the self. The boundaries are breached between the patient's internal private world of thought and fantasy and the external world of objects and other people (including the internal thoughts, wishes, and intentions of others). These phenomena are occasionally classified as delusions (Spitzer & Endicot, 1978; Sims, 1988) presumably on the grounds that they constitute not an experience of, for example, influence or thought broadcasting, but a belief in being influenced or broadcasted. The distinction may on occasion be so subtle as to appear entirely academic but for most patients these are direct experiences not beliefs, though they may give rise to delusional explanations. One patient complained that a 'filthy word' was repeatedly inserted into her mind. This occurred several times a day and would occasion her considerable embarrassment. She had noted that these insertions tended to occur when she was near or in sight of a tower at a Salvation Army citadel. On the basis of this observation she had become increasingly convinced that she was being persecuted by the Salvation Army, who had a radio transmitter beaming the words into her brain. She experienced the thought insertion but she became convinced its origins lay in the transmitter in the tower. One is an experience, the other an explanatory belief. I have a pain in my belly. I am convinced it is an appendicitis. The experience of pain and explanatory beliefs are distinct phenomena.

These experiences are of two basic types in that they can be directed inwards or outwards. In the first there is an experience of influences or intrusion from the outside into the internal world. In the second group there is an experience of the thoughts, wishes or intentions of the individual diffusing or emanating out to influence, or become available to, others. These effects can involve the content of thoughts and fantasies, the intentions and actions, the emotions and desires of the patient.

The types of passivity experiences will now be discussed under the heading of thoughts, emotions, intentions, and actions.

Thoughts

Directed outwards

Thought diffusion and *thought broadcasting* involve a conviction on the patients' part that those around them know their innermost thoughts. It is not merely that they divine their secret thoughts from their words, actions, or facial expressions, but that the thoughts themselves are directly available and can be, in a real sense, read by others. There is a sense of having become transparent, making one's innermost thoughts open to direct observation. In florid form there can be the experience of one's own thoughts being shared and participated in by everyone around. This experience may lead to delusions of explanation. One of my patients described a complicated plot whereby a neighbour, who was a BBC journalist, would nightly broadcast her every secret thought to the nation; this explained why everybody knew about them and shared them.

Thought withdrawal occurs where patients experience their thoughts as removed or ablated by some outside influence. This experience has been claimed to underlie the abnormality of expressive behaviour known as *thought blocking* (Fish, 1967).

Directed inwards

Thought control involves the patients' experience of their innermost thoughts falling under external influence. *Thought insertion* occurs when alien thoughts are imposed upon them.

Intentions, Will and Actions
Directed outwards

The patient experiences him or herself as able to influence the apparently volitional acts of others. One patient explained to me he could make people move and speak as he wished and pointed out from the window of the office how he was willing the people outside to walk along the street. In another case a patient described how every move or action he initiated was simultaneously mirrored in those around him because his will controlled theirs but this disrupted his life because when, for example, he went shopping the shops were always full with others who because of his influence were on identical errands.

Directed inwards

The experience is of made impulses and made volitional acts. This can again involve the experience of the patient's intentions and will falling under outside control or of the imposition by an outside force of action upon him or her. An elderly and normally prim and proper lady periodically lifted her skirts and performed a brief dance. This she explained was nothing to do with her but was the result of the actions of a malevolent race of aliens she called 'fantasias' who were imposing the actions upon her. Here both the control of the acts and the acts themselves were alien. More commonly, what is experienced is simply a loss of control over will and action as a result of outside influence.

Emotions

Made feelings and emotions occur when patients experience their emotional lives as coming under outside influence, either in that they are made to feel a certain way or that alien emotions are imposed upon them. Patients more frequently report being robbed of feelings or of having their emotional responses blocked by alien influence.

Depersonalisation and derealisation

Depersonalisation and derealisation refer to experiences that, though most frequently encountered in those afflicted by depressive or anxiety disorders, can occur in normal individuals when they are overtired, stressed or intoxicated. The basic disturbance involves an alteration from the usual of both the experience of the self and of the world. It can manifest in such features as:

1. the surroundings take on a quality of strangeness;
2. a sense of unreality pervades not only the perceptions of the external world but one's own cognitions and conations;
3. the experience of the passage of time is altered by a slowing or slippage;
4. spatial relationships seem altered, which can produce distortions and may even be associated with micropsia or macropsia;
5. one's own body image may be altered, producing not only experienced unfamiliarity in one's physical being but a non-recognition of body parts;
6. emotions, feelings and affects lose their subjective impact,though the sufferer is not without emotion; on the contrary there is usually fear and agitation consequent in the changed experiences;
7. actions appear to be carried out automatically without personal involvement or intent as if as one patient put it, 'I was trapped inside a machine which I could only watch but not control'.

Depersonalisation is to be distinguished from passivity experiences in which there is an experience not of alienation from subjective experience but alien influences on such experiences. It is also to be distinguished from multiple personality, in which there is an alteration in subjectivities, as well as from an insight into actual changes in personality consequent on, for example, brain damage or the depredations of schizophrenia. Separation from dissociative experiences can be difficult and Fish (1967) seems to regard them as identical (p. 78) and DSM-IIIR (APA, 1987) sees depersonalisation as a specific form of dissociation. Taylor (1982) in an elegant paper on the topic, argues there is a doubling of the ego so that a subsidiary ego emerges, which observes the activities of the self.

In normal mental function there is only a tangential and passing awareness of the process of thinking or perceiving. We can by an effort of will reflect upon our experience and activities but it is neither usual nor sustainable. In depersonalisation there is an unbidden and unwanted self-awareness in that we become conscious of our mental activities. Perceptions are disrupted by sensations being separated from the meanings usually inherent in them and our cognitions and conations become objects of scrutiny not lived experiences. This pervasive self-reflection totally disrupts the normal flow of psychic life and imbues it with an alien character. We no longer reach out for the pen, we become conscious of the act of reaching out for the pen, we no longer see our reflection, we become conscious of seeing a reflection that we assume must be ours. In depersonalisation we remain conscious of our activities and they remain accessible to normal awareness, unlike dissociation where there is a separation or removal of selective mental events from consciousness. Depersonalisation and derealisation are a morbid exaggeration of self-awareness and self-reflection that disrupt the sense of being part of, and at one with, one's own cognitions, conations and actions.

Volition

The pathological disturbances of action and movement largely fall within the rubric of neurology, however, certain syndromes that include characteristic disturbances of motor behaviour require brief mention (see Lohr & Wisniewski, 1987) for a thorough review).

Tics

These are repetitive stereotyped movements involving voluntary musculature. Though usually capable of brief inhibition by an act of will and to some extent responsive to mood and situation, they are for the most part outside of the patient's control. Tics cover a spectrum from minor repetitive twitches involving the small muscles of the face to complex movements, which may involve several large muscle blocks. In *Gilles de la Tourett syndrome*, motor tics are combined with repeated vocalizations, often in the form of obscenities and profanity (coprolalia).

Catatonia

Catatonia, first delineated by Kahlbaum in 1874, is a syndrome that can be seen in both predominantly affective and schizophrenic disorders and may be mimicked by a number of organic disorders. It consists of disturbances in volitional movement and language. Several aspects of the syndrome seem to be polar opposites. There may be periods of incoordinate and violent over-activity (*catatonic excitement*); at the other extreme the patient may remain immobile for long periods, often appearing as if frozen to the spot. *Posturing* occurs where bizarre and uncomfortable poses may be held for long periods, as do reiterated *stereotyped movements*, where the same action is endlessly repeated. The normal fluidity of voluntary motor activity may be disrupted to produce an awkward and stilted quality, which is most obvious in the odd gaits encountered in this disturbance. *Automatic obedience* can be a feature with unhesitating compliance to any command or request without apparent conscious control, but so can the reverse, *negativism*, where there is a positive effort to resist and often do the opposite or some eccentrically unrelated performance rather than what is requested or required. *Ambivalence*, in the Bleulerian sense, may effect motor actions – the patient commences an act, then before completing it, reverses his or her movements and begins once more, only again to halt and reverse.

Echolalia and echopraxia occur where patients repeat or imitate the words or actions of those around them. In echolalia the repetition seems to occur in an automatic fashion without any apparent understanding. Echo phenomena are not confined to catatonic syndromes but occur in a range of pathological and even psychological conditions (Ford, 1989). Just as the fluidity of voluntary movement is disrupted, so the usual flow of speech is disrupted to produce hesitancy with a stuttering or explosive quality. *Verbigeration*, described by Kahlbaum (1973, orig. 1874) and speech composed of oft repeated, meaningless words and sentences, may also be present in catatonia. A characteristic disturbance of muscle tone, where there appears to be present a *waxy flexibility* (flexibilitas cerea), can accompany posturing and immobility in the catatonic syndrome. Pouting movements of the lips are also described to accompany catatonic states (*Schnauzkrampf*) as are facial grimacing and tics. Subtle catatonic disturbances are often either not recognised or dismissed as side-effects of antipsychotics.

Cataplexy

Cataplexy is a sudden partial, or complete, loss of tone in the voluntary musculature without disturbance of consciousness. It occurs in narcolepsy.

Stupor

Stupor describes a syndrome whose most prominent features are a gross reduction in voluntary movement (*akinesia*) and speech (*mutism*). There is a suspension of expressive and reactive movements. Incontinence may occur. In neurology, stupor is often used rather loosely to describe a state of reduced consciousness bordering on coma. In contradistinction, attempts have been made in psychiatry to define stupor as an absence of voluntary movement in presence of clear consciousness. This is helpful in as far as it distinguishes 'functional' from 'neurological' stupor, but the attribution of clear consciousness to functional stupor is clinically questionable (Berrios, 1981).

Kraeplein (1919) attempted to distinguish four types of stupor: depressive, manic, catatonic, and hysterical. In depressive illness, stupor usually follows a period of increasing motor retardation and withdrawal; the patient may still radiate a sense of melancholy by facial expression and by a passive turning away from proffered assistance. The refusal to eat and drink in depressive stupor may represent a total lack of interest, though one of my patients retrospectively described being convinced his insides had disappeared, so he felt anything that passed his lips would enter his abdominal cavity and kill him. In mania, stupor may supervene on the excited disturbances of delirious mania where extreme restlessness, hallucinosis and some clouding of consciousness give way to a state of mute immobility. In this state some signs of the previous gross overactivity may remain in brief outbursts of motor restlessness and in constant movements of the head and eyes. In schizophrenia, stupor may supervene on a catatonic picture. Retrospectively, schizophrenic patients can often provide quite detailed accounts of the happenings during the period of stupor and on occasion will give explanations of their immobility; for example, they were directed by God or under some external control. States of stupor can follow extreme stress and then can be conceptualised as dissociative states or as an extreme reaction, as if paralysed by fear. These latter may be encountered under battle conditions and following catastrophes.

Disturbance of language

Thought can never be directly observed. The attempt to study it must, therefore, rely on language in the form of speech, writing, or other symbolic creation. The entrenched tradition of speaking of thought disorder when actually confronted with disturbed language rests on the assumption that language directly mirrors thought.

Speech disorder is usually separated from language and thought disorder. It is confined to disturbance in the actual articulation, due to a disruption with the mechanics of speaking. Stuttering is a typical example and the lalling speech of cerebellar dysfunction would be another. A distinction between language as a system of symbol and sign formation, and thought as the content and import of those symbols and signs, is occasionally made. Thus, employing this division, thought disorder would include delusions and other disturbances of the content of thought. In this section we will be concerned with the disturbance of language.

The structure of language can be analysed in terms of semantics, which concerns itself with meaning, and of syntax, which are the rules governing the combination of words to form sentences. In most of the language disorders observed clinically by the psychiatrist, the disorder is in the area of meaning, the semantics, rather than the syntax, the latter being significantly disrupted only in the most florid forms of psychotic speech. Meaning lies not only in the words used, but also in the situational context of the utterances. Statements occur in particular spatiotemporal situations, which include speaker and hearer, the actions they are performing and the various external objects and events. Further, a shared knowledge of what has been said earlier and its relationship to current statements is assumed. Thus what Searle (1969) has termed 'speech acts' consist of language in its context that communicates to the receiver. This understanding of utterances in their context is referred to as pragmatics and it is argued that it is a derangement in this pragmatic function of language that characterises schizophrenic speech (Cutting, 1985).

In an ideal language, one word or sign would exist for one meaning. In practice there are many synonyms where a particular meaning is designated by several distinct words (e.g. hide, conceal, secrete) and frequent homonyms where single words signify more than one meaning (bank of river, Bank of England, trunk of elephant, trunk – a piece of luggage). Words may also be used literally or metaphorically (a man's head, the head of a company, a glaring light, a glaring error). In the language disorders encountered by psychiatrists there may be semantic disruption arising from a confusion of homonym, synonym and metaphor. A patient, for example, when asked if the pills were making him better, replied: 'Healed? I have no heels (glancing at the bottom of his slippers), I'm only brought to heel'. The word healed is employed as a synonym for getting better, then confused with its homonym, the heel of a shoe, and in this example the metaphorical use of heel is employed to produce a nice resolution that allows the patient to comment on his resentment at being compulsorily detained. Bleuler reports a patient who when asked if anything was weighing heavily on his mind replied: 'Yes, iron is heavy'. A patient in a group asked if he was down, immediately left saying: 'Yes, I need to lie down'. This taking of the literal rather than the metaphorical use of words was referred to by Goldstein (1944) as *concrete thinking*, though whether it is truly a preference for the concrete sense or just a tendency to associate to the commonest usage of a particular word is uncertain.

A word may be chosen in language disorder not because of its relationship to the meaning of the utterance, but because of an association of sound to a previous word or phrase. Thus, 'I feel like going out, stout, a drink would be nice, ice, I suppose I'll stay, lay down for a while', or 'everybody seems to revolve around me, involve and resolve around me' – this is termed a *clang association*.

Words may be invented in language disorders. These idiosyncratic words of no generally agreed significance are termed neologisms. They may consist of entirely new words, which even the patient may be hard pressed to explain, or be created by compressing or running together existing words. A patient referred to a 'mongery ridicule', and although he could spell the word, the only definition he offered was that it 'wasn't quite nice'. In this example the phonetic or sound structure is acceptable for a word in English. On occasion sounds entirely foreign to English phonetics will be emitted apparently as words. An example of a word created by condensing existing terms is 'amisachrist', which was used by a patient to describe a psychiatrist who misunderstood him (a mistaken psychiatrist). Jaspers (1963) suggested neologisms may arise from the patient's struggle to express unique and essentially incommunicable experiences.

Idiosyncratic similes and metaphors may be encountered. A schizophrenic patient of Bleuler (1950) announced her forthcoming pregnancy with 'I hear a stork clapping in my body'. A patient of mine replied to the enquiry about his religious views with 'I'm for the elected by a puff of smoke from the chimney', referring obliquely to the process that heralds the election of a new Pope in the Roman Catholic Church.

Words, phrases, and occasionally syllables seem to recur far more frequently in the language of the schizophrenic than in normals. This is in part connected to the phenomena of *stereotopy* and *perseveration*. In the perseveration of coarse organic brain disease identical words and phrases tend to be simply repeated. In those with schizophrenia it manifests as a repeated use of similar words and phrases in different contexts. An extreme example is provided by a patient who, when asked if he understood a question, replied. 'I see something like I might be wrong like, but there like the rules I don't like the rules turned upside-down and I don't know like and I was like as though the bed turned over'. A patient reported by Kraepelin (1919) would, when writing home to relatives, fill pages with similar words or phrases presented in varying orders interminably. A more restricted vocabulary is also said to be found in the language-disordered schizophrenic than in normals of a similar educational and intellectual background (Poverty of Language). The frequent repetition involves syllables and phrases as well as words, so the problem is more likely to stem from a tendency for the same speech elements to intrude repeatedly into the discourse rather than just a restricted repertoire of words.

The concept of redundancy has been borrowed from information theory and applied specifically to schizophrenic language disorder (Maher, 1972). Redundancy used in this technical sense refers to the likelihood that a particular word or letter will occur. The more predictable the word or letter is, the greater the redundancy, in that it conveys less information. Normal language has a high degree of redundancy in that many of the words and phrases are predictable to a high level of certainty from the context. In the schizophrenic the disruption of the context of the language and the reduced consistency and coherence within the expression of ideas leads to a decreased predictability of the words and thus to decreased redundancy. A *word salad*, for example, where there is a total breakdown in the contextual restraint, and words follow each other apparently at random, has no redundancy, for no given word can be predicted in advance from any preceding work or phrase; each word comes as a total surprise, free of the limitations of semantics or syntax. Experiments based on the redundancy concept have demonstrated that observers provided with transcripts of normal speech and schizophrenic speech, with every fifth word deleted, can correctly fill in the missing word significantly more often from the normal speech, confirming the decreased redundancy in the schizophrenic utterances. In related experiments it was suggested that speech-disordered schizophrenics are themselves less able to utilise contextual clues and redundancy in learning written passages. The specificity of these findings has been challenged, however (Rutter, 1979).

The meaning of language depends not only on the particular words but, as has been mentioned, the context of the utterance. In normal speech there is a tacit acceptance by speaker and hearer of all relevant conventions, beliefs, and presuppositions of the common speech community. In language disorder there may emerge, in conversation or writing, themes that are inappropriate to the context. Thus highly personal and idiosyncratic statements will be interposed with the more appropriate aspects of the discourse. This tends to produce in the listener a degree of confusion. The mixing in of snatches of conversation about unrelated matters into the ongoing discourse has been labelled *intermingling* (Harrow & Proson, 1979). This appears to reflect an impairment of the subject's ability to remain within the normal social constraints upon communication.

The disruption of context and the lack of sufficient connection between successive phrases is shown by a patient who wrote: 'I want to leave the trees are beautiful if only the food too long love'. In a single sentence the desire for discharge, the gardens, the food, and a greeting are all combined. There is a failure to keep separate ideas that are unconnected, and the patient's preoccupations are all jumbled together into a single statement. A patient replying to an enquiry as to how he felt, included the following: 'it doesn't really matter if you eat refined sugar as long as you can balance it by doing something else you or using your energy expending your energy in the best manner possible and I would really like to become a DJ you know I have a high sort of ambition this is why I would like a cigarette now. That's all'. The preoccupation with diet, physical fitness, job ambitions, and the desire for a cigarette become included in a response to a routine enquiry about health. This tendency was described as *over-inclusion* by Cameron (1944), because the patient is unable to prevent subsidiary and peripheral thoughts intruding and becoming included in the statement. A young librarian in the early stages of a psychotic episode was asked to reorganise the Divinity section of the library's filing system. This resulted in a total restructuring of the index with everything recatalogued under divinity. The young man had included all topics under Divinity, not from some insight into the ubiquitous nature of God, but from an inability to separate any category from the other, thus including all in one. Here over-inclusion was demonstrated in action, not speech.

Thought-blocking is evinced by a sudden stopping in mid-sentence, despite the subject's desire to continue speaking; after a pause the flow of speech may recommence, perhaps on some unrelated topic. There may be a perplexed silence and a complaint that his or her thoughts have been removed, stolen, blocked or have disappeared. This phenomenon can be quite dramatic in some schizophrenic patients and may be accompanied by considerable subjective distress. Blocking in the context of other signs of schizophrenic speech disorder is of diagnostic importance. When it occurs as an isolated event it is easily confused with the non-specific phenomenon of losing the train of one's thoughts, which occurs in normals, particularly when tired or under stress and as part of the speech retardation of depressive

37

states. The presence of schizophrenic language disorder should not be assumed on the basis of thought-blocking alone.

The clinical psychiatrist most frequently observes disturbance of language in the flight of ideas of the manic and the schizophrenic language disorder, often referred to as formal thought disorder. This being so, this section will continue by discussing these two specific language disturbances.

Flight of ideas

Flight of ideas is encountered in manic disturbances but is also mimicked by some organic brain syndromes, by one's more loquacious or intoxicated companions, and it can even appear in relatively pure form in some subjects, who on other criteria would be considered undoubtedly schizophrenic. There is an accelerated tempo of speech often referred to as *pressure of talk*. In addition to the increased rate of delivery, the language employed is characterised by a wealth of associations, many of which seem to be evoked by more or less accidental connections. The relationship between statements is disrupted by this chaos of association and the progress of speech ceases to be guided by the unfolding of a train of thought and comes under the influence of this plethora of new connections. The excited speech wanders off the point following the arbitrary connections, and the coherent progress of ideas tends to become obscured. The somewhat haphazard verbal associations become governed by sound, rhyme, associations to peripheral concepts, *double entendre*, etc. In classical flight of ideas, although the connections and associations are accidental or peripheral to the general sense of the statement, they are usually in themselves fairly obvious and unremarkable and would individually be acceptable in other situations. This is in stark contrast to schizophrenic language disorder, where the individual connections are often so opaque and personalised as to defy comprehension in any situation. Clang associations and puns are frequent. One manic patient I encountered attempted to speak exclusively in blank verse interspersed with long recitals from nineteenth-century poets.

In flight of ideas, a wide range of unusual connections drive on the rapid speech and the listener is often borne along by the flow and may even share in the amusement and pleasure the patient derives from the novel associations. The patient exhibiting flight of ideas often expresses a subjective sense of their thoughts racing and of new ideas forcing themselves on their attention.

Schizophrenic language disorder

Schizophrenic language disorder, or as it is sometimes termed *formal thought disorder* is characterised by disturbance in the area of semantics, though in advanced forms the syntax may also be disrupted. Bleuler (1950) considered the disturbance of association to be a fundamental symptom of schizophrenia that led to a disruption of the threads that guide thinking. Ideas fortuitously encountered are combined in a manner dependent on incidental circumstances rather than any train of thought. A patient, when asked where she lived, replied: 'I come from Somerset. Somerset is a lovely place, everyone stops up that way, you know, before they go back home for the weekend. I'm home on my weekends, but I was never really satisfied with myself nor my schoolwork'.

In those with schizophrenia whose language is disordered there are found *clang associations* and *condensations*. *Sterotopy*, evidenced by a tendency to return again and again to a single theme also occurs. The language disorder of schizophrenia can vary from a barely detectable disturbance to an almost total disorganisation of communication. Kurt Schneider (1950) considered that disjointed, fragmented, and inconsequential thought was commonly manifested in the speech of schizophrenics. However, he pointed out that milder degrees of such disturbance was not uncommon in normal people and this being so, however important these thought disorders might be for the theoretical definition of schizophrenia, they could not in practice hold much weight as diagnostic features. In ambiguous cases he held it was too difficult to pin down such phenomena as unmistakable schizophrenic symptoms, and in florid examples other more reliable diagnostic signs would be present.

Carl Schneider, in contrast, gave considerable attention to these phenomena in his *Psychiologie der Schizophrenen* (1930). He considered schizophrenic language to be characterised by: (1) an interweaving or bringing together of heterogeneous elements (*fusion*); (2) a mixing and muddling up of actual definite but heterogeneous elements (*substitution*); (3) a snapping-off of the chain of thought (*omission*); and (4) the disruption of the thought content with insertion of other thought contents in place of the true chain of thought (*derailment*). He described *transitory thinking* as characterised by derailments and omission in the train of thought by which both the semantics and syntax may be disrupted and *drivelling thinking* where there is a mixing and muddling of the thoughts (substitution), which obscures the meaning. In drivelling, the listener may obtain an initial impression that something meaningful is being said but soon realises that it is a flow of words and high-sounding phrases signifying little or nothing. A patient who talked at great length with slow, ponderous and heavily accentuated speech included the following in a monologue:

> In other words you said that you were coming, and I said to myself and I dismissed it from my thoughts. I suppose it wasn't exactly forgetting that she would be appearing but no to stress this all the time and he just wanted to come home and I was foolish over money and what have you, and you see now I could talk to him about that.

The language of schizophrenics may be weighed down with unnecessary detail and circumstantiality in much the same way, perhaps, as writers on the subject. Complex and intricate forms of expression may serve to obscure the train of thought and platitudes and proverbs may come to totally dominate their speech.

Andreasen (1979, 1986) suggested that all the many and various terms used to describe the communication difficulties of those with schizophrenia could be reduced to 20, she claimed, mutually exclusive terms. These are: poverty of speech production (laconic speech); poverty in the content of speech; pressure of speech; distractible speech; tangentiality; derailment (loosening of associations); incoherence (as in word salad); illogicality; clanging; neologisms; word approximations (where words are used unconventionally); circumstantiality; loss of goal (where the communication drifts apparently aimlessly); perseveration' echolalia; blocking; stilted speech (ponderous and overly formal); self-referential speech (where communications return repeatedly to the patient and their highly personal preoccupations);

phonemic paraphasis (mispronunciations because sound or syllables have slipped out of sequence); and semantic paraphrasis (substitution of inappropriate words – Malapropism). The most frequent abnormalities she noted in her patients were derailment, loss of goal and tangentiality, though these were also found in the communications of manic subjects. Poverty of speech was the abnormality found specifically in schizophrenic rather than manic utterances. There might, one would have thought, be problems in distinguishing a number of these categories, for example, word approximations from semantic paraphrasis.

An individual patient may be aware of the disruption of his or her thinking even though it is not obvious to the observer. Some patients become very concerned with words and the potential meanings hidden within these signs and symbols. The language disorder of one patient expressed itself in an extensive series of written productions about words, an extract of which is provided.

> RAYMOND = RAY-MOUND = hill of the ray = tower of the telepathic waves. Also it = RAY-MONDE, ray and world (French, Le Monde). The Germanic name which gives the modern Raymond was Regimund. Regin = strong, powerful; mund = protection. Thus my telepathy is a powerful protection. Mund = protection was often used with a word "beorg" = him to mean fortress. Regin is nearly the same word as the Anglo-Saxon Regn = rain. Thus one has Regn = rain and mund = fortress = fortress from which comes the rain, i.e. rain = telepathic waves.

This section has been concerned with language productions, but it is worth remembering that a number of reports have pointed out that in schizophrenia there occur abnormalities in the perception of speech and of short-term verbal memory. Such receptive defects could contribute to the language abnormalities.

A final point that needs emphasising is that a variety of brain lesions produce dysphasic speech, which may have superficial resemblances to formal thought disorder. For excellent accounts of the organic dysphasias see Lishman (1987) and Brain (1965).

Conclusion

Descriptive psychopathology attempts to orient the clinician towards the precise observation and description of his or her patient's state of mind. The descriptions can, in addition, form the basis for classification and for empirical studies. Careful observation and classification is the starting point for good clinical psychiatry and above all it provides the best protection for the patient from being wrongfully labelled as mentally ill and treated as such or, conversely, from being denied care when in fact needing it.

2

The disease concept in psychiatry

ANTHONY W. CLARE

Introduction

One of the more controversial aspects of contemporary psychiatric theory and practice concerns the very concept of mental disease. It appears to lack the objectivity, the hardness, the reliability and validity of physical disease, and permits a bewildering number of interpretations, some complementary, some contradictory. It seems inordinately sensitive to personal, social and political influence. It has been argued, most pugnaciously by Thomas Szasz, that the whole notion of mental disease is unsound given that disease, as it is widely understood, involves a disturbance of the function or structure of an organ or part of the body. The mind, insists Szasz (1960; 1974), is not an organ or part of the body and cannot therefore be diseased in the same sense as the body can. The great majority of disorders for which psychiatrists accept responsibility do not appear to manifest any reliable physical pathology, whatever the current confidence that many such disorders will soon be found to have underlying biological, including genetic, causes. Many of the defenders of the concept of mental illness (Wing, 1978a; Torrey, 1988; Blakemore, 1990), while challenging Szasz's criticisms, appear to accept his definition that disease implies some underlying organic abnormality. They argue instead that such abnormalities do occur in the case of mental diseases but have yet to be identified. Other critics, however, unimpressed by the evidence, established or putative, of any organic pathology, insist that mental disorders are ideological constructs (Boyle, 1990). A sociological perspective on psychopathology has developed with, as its main focus, the social effects of 'labelling' (Scheff, 1966; Erikson, 1964). In place of the mental disease concept, these critics argue that it would make better sense to speak of problems of living, faulty learning, maladaptions, communications disorders, social disturbances and identity crises.

At the heart of these criticisms of the disease model is the belief that it is narrow and reductionist. Maher, for example, while not eschewing the importance of biological factors, advocates behavioural disturbances that characterise many forms of psychiatric disorder (Maher, 1970). Other critics emphasise the need not merely to acknowledge the importance of behaviour in mental disorder but argue that the psychiatrist or psychologist has to discover its meaning by the process of understanding of the individual, his social and cultural context and the interaction between both (Jenner *et al.*, 1993; Littlewood & Lipsedge, 1982).

The lack of consensus concerning the concept of mental disease has led some to argue, like Lewis (1963), that medical criteria are safer, 'that is, criteria essentially concerned with the integrity of physiological and psychological functions'. However, this necessitates consideration of what precisely are the 'medical criteria' of mental disease.

The disease concept

The difficulty of defining disease is implicit in the very structure of the word itself (Dubos, 1968). So many different kinds of disturbance can make a person feel ill at east and provoke him or her to seek the advice of a physician that it is hardly surprising that the word sometimes appears to encompass most of the difficulties inherent in the human condition. Our current notions of disease, like so much of our science, medicine and philosophy, stem primarily from the Greeks who, as Bynum (1983) reminds us, elaborated on conceptual framework and vocabulary that permeated psychiatry until the last century and whose clinical attitudes are still of relevance today. In Homeric Greece the underlying assumption was that human beings are literally driven mad just as they are driven to acts of courage, cowardice, altruism and conceit. Hippocrates and his school, in contrast, regarded diseases as natural occurrences, amenable to materialistic explanations and responsive to the interventions of doctors combined with the body's own natural healing powers (Neuberger, 1943). For all its holistic quality, Hippocratic disease theory was frankly biological, as this excerpt from the treatise On the Sacred Disease makes clear:

> Men ought to know that from the brain, and from the brain only, arise our pleasures, joys, laughter and jests, as well as our sorrows, pains, griefs and tears. Through it, in particular, we think, see, hear and distinguish the ugly from the beautiful, the bad from the good, the pleasant from the unpleasant, in some cases using custom as a test, in others perceiving them their unity. It is the same thing which makes us mad or delirious, inspires us with dread and fear, whether by night or day, brings sleeplessness, inopportune mistakes, aimless anxieties, absentmindedness, and acts that are contrary to habit. These things that we suffer all come from the brain, when it is not healthy, but becomes abnormally hot, cold, moist or dry, or suffers from any other unnatural affection to which it was not accustomed.

Diseases were no longer the malignant creations of capricious gods or irrational forces but were regarded as natural phenomena developing in accordance with natural laws. The Hippocratic view of disease laid great emphasis on the need to base medicine on the natural sciences, on a profound knowledge of the biological phenomena of life in health and disease, on a recognition of the influence, beneficent and malign, of environmental factors, and on a realisation of the close interdependence of body and mind. Hippocratic writings represent the first known systematic attempt to explain the phenomena of disease in terms of natural laws (Dubos, 1968). They envisaged disease as a combination of signs and symptoms observed to occur together so frequently and so characteristically as to constitute a recognisable and typical clinical picture.

Such a *clinical-descriptive* or *syndromal* definition of disease was imaginatively implemented by Thomas Sydenham, the seventeenth-century English physician who, on the basis of precise and methodical recording of signs and symptoms, succeeded in differentiating a remarkable array of diseases including measles, scarlet fever, gout, smallpox and malaria. Sydenham, however, belonged to a contrasting tradition, sometimes termed Platonic, which envisaged diseases as specific and separate entities and he insisted that they could be reduced to 'certain and determinate kinds with the same exactness as we see it done by botanic writers in their treatises on plants' (Taylor, 1972). Diseases from this vantage point were conceived as having some form of autonomous existence with natural histories of their own, as beings invading the body from outside or as parasites growing within it. Such a reification of disease persists to this day despite the fact that it rests on a confusion of cause with its effect. In Taylor's words, 'the cause of a disease may be a concrete object entering the body of a human being, but the disease so caused is an attribute to the human being involved'. Shades of such confusion can be detected in a phrase such as 'the incidence of a particular disease' when what is actually meant is the incidence of *patients* with a particular disease.

Almost two centuries after Sydenham, Rudolf Vichow, the brilliant German pathologist, was to challenge this 'botanical' view of diseases and relocate the essence of disease *inside* the body. 'Diseases', he wrote:

> are neither self-subsistent, circumscribed, autonomous organisms, nor entities which have forced their way into the body, nor parasites rooted on it . . . they represent only the course of physiological phenomena under altered conditions.
> Virchow (1842).

Virchow identified social and environmental events amongst his 'altered conditions' and prescribed social reform as an antidote to disease but disease itself slowly became identified with cellular pathology and diseased organs became the focus for serious study. Pathological anatomy flourished although, as Weindling (1992) has pointed out, the biological approach to understanding disease during the latter part of the nineteenth century was accompanied by intensified measures to improve housing and environmental conditions on the basis of concepts such as 'natural immunity'. Nevertheless, the *disease-as-lesion* view came to dominate medical thinking over the past century and it is only within the past 30 years that its limitations have become apparent.

The notion of an abnormality or lesion is relatively uncomplicated as long as one is concerned with a departure from a recognised and standard pattern. The problem is that it is not always apparent where normal variation ends and abnormality begins. Conditions such as hypertension, diabetes, congenital abnormalities and anaemia are examples of disturbances that pose difficulties for the disease-as-lesion view. An even more serious shortcoming is that symptoms and signs, whose organic basis has yet to be established, strictly speaking cannot be acknowledged as diseases. There is no lesion. Thus migraine, Menière's disease, trigeminal neuralgia and obesity are among a host of conditions that require to be conceptualised in some other fashion. Indeed, in this regard it is worth noting that, as Kroenke & Mangelsdorrff (1989) have shown, the majority of patients attending hospital outpatient departments do not have any structural organic disease.

Yet the emphasis on disease-as-lesion has contributed to the tendency for some, doctors as well as patients, to view disorders that lack an established organic pathology as not real diseases at all but rather imaginary or 'all in the mind'. Patients who thus complain feel vulnerable to suggestions that they are not really ill. Commenting on the tendency of sufferers from chronic fatigue syndrome to identify the cause as viral, Wessely and his colleagues (1991) noted that such attribution 'conveys certain advantages, irrespective of its validity. It is simple, frequent and easily accepted'. In addition, it protects self-esteem by removing questions of guilt and blame. Such a simplistic view of disease contributes to the stigmatisation of psychiatric disorder in that many psychiatric sufferers are seen by others as not having real diseases. In turn, this leads to a situation whereby the very suggestion that a psychiatrist or psychologist be involved in the diagnosis or treatment of a condition leads some to conclude that the disease and the sufferer in question are not being regarded as genuine. Watts (1982) has argued that patients often 'have a crude dichotomy of aetiologies, believing they must either have genuine symptoms with an organic aetiology or that they have psychological symptoms that are simply "all in the mind"'. Doctors, too, as Wessely and his colleagues (1991), point out, often appear to regard suffering due to disorders that lack an established organic basis, such as myalgic encephalopathy (ME), as not suffering at all or, just as deleterious in the long term, 'react to such unhelpful views by totalling denying the possibility of psychological distress'. Ironically, one consequence of such views is that any improvement on the part of the patient that is not the result of some biological intervention is often interpreted by others, including doctors, as proof that the whole problem was 'psychological' after all and not therefore a 'real' disease!

The view that at the heart of every psychiatric disorder is a pathological abnormality waiting to be uncovered, be it a metabolic defect or a genetic abnormality, envisages abnormal mental symptoms and abnormal mental states not so much as diseases in their own right but more as epiphenomena of underlying physical disturbances. The view is stated with some pungency by Macalpine & Hunter (1974):

> The lesson of the history of psychiatry is that progress is inevitable and irrevocable from psychology to neurology, from mind to brain, never the other way around. Every medical advance adds to the list of diseases which may cause mental derangement. The abnormal mental state is not disease, nor its essence or determinant, but an epiphenomenon. That is why psychological theories and therapies which held out such promise at the turn of the century when so much less was known of localization of function of the brain, have added so little to the understanding and treatment of mental illness, despite all the time and effort devoted to them.

However, there have been those, such as Engel (1977) who have been harshly critical of such reductionism. Articulating arguments propounded by others (Comfort, 1972; Mahler, 1973; Illich, 1974), Engel suggests the replacement of the defective biomedical model by a 'biopsychosocial' model of disease, which would take into greater account environmental determinants, the patient's social context, and the complementary system devised by society to deal with the disruptive effects of illness, namely the physician's role and the health care system. Behind such views lies a conviction that the emphasis on the biological basis of disease results in a neglect of the wider psychosocial implications. The fact that environmental factors such as nutritional excess, insufficient exercise, emotional tension, smoking, and other deleterious habits can provoke vascular disease in persons with abnormal lipid and cholesterol metabolism is one that critics such as Engel emphasise to illustrate the extent to which the simple disease-as-lesion argument has been abandoned in general medicine itself.

These views had been anticipated by John Ryle, Britain's first professor of social medicine, who in a volume of essays entitled *Changing Disciplines* (Ryle, 1948), declared:

> We no longer believe that medical truths are only or chiefly to be discovered under the microscope, by means of the test-tube, or by clinical examination and increasingly elaborate pathological studies at the bedside. Psychological and sociological studies have an important part to play. Even so, it is not yet appreciated how intimately disease and social circumstances are inter-related. The whole natural history of disease in human communities, as well as in individuals, is ripe for a fuller and more exhaustive study.

A related view of disease as 'adaptation to stress' is associated with the name of Adolph Meyer, professor of psychiatry at Johns Hopkins early this century. Meyer based his concept on a 'psychobiology', which made no sharp division between psychological and physiological data but emphasised that many if not all diseases are the expression of both organic and psychic factors. Disease, from this perspective, is a 'reaction' of the whole organism to its environment. The individual being unique, his disease is unique. Such a formulation makes it difficult to construct a classification system wherein diseases can be classed in general. Nor is it easy to distinguish between those reactions of the organism that qualify as diseases and those that can be seen as natural and normal. What it does, however, do is re-emphasise the individual and personal aspects of disease and the role of environmental factors in its genesis and manifestations.

Disease can also be defined in terms of a *deviation from normal*, that is to say as a statistical concept. Such a formulation derives support from demonstrations such as that by Pickering and his colleagues (Oldham *et al.*, 1960) that essential hypertension is a graded characteristic depending, like height and intelligence, on polygenic inheritance and shading gradually into normality. Other physical disorders that can be conceptualised usefully in this way include cervical cancer, diabetes mellitus and sickle cell anaemia. However, as Kendell (1975) has pointed out, such a statistical definition of normality and abnormality fails to distinguish between those deviations that are harmful, such as high blood pressure, and those that are not and indeed that might actually be beneficial, such as superior intelligence. Scadding's (1967) attempt to meet this objection has merited much attention but it too leaves some major problems unresolved. Confronted by the shortcomings inherent in the various definitions of disease, Scadding (1967) proposes one of his own:

> A disease is the sum of abnormal phenomena displayed by a group of living organisms in association with a specified common characteristic or set of characteristics by which they differ from the norm for their species in such a way as to place them at a biological disadvantage.

Such a definition indicates the need to establish normal standards for relevant populations, no easy matter when psychological and behavioural standards are under scrutiny and implies a statistical basis to the concept of abnormality. Its reliance on the notion of biological disadvantage could be employed to justify restoring homosexuality to the status of mental disease, a status it held prior to 1974 when some 11 000 members of the American Psychiatric Association voted to declassify it. Where once homosexuality was regarded as psychopathological and requiring treatment, now it is seen as a minority sexual preference.

Lewis (1955), in an influential paper 'Health as a Social Concept', argued for the definition of mental disorder to be based on deviations from psychological norms. In physical disease, the diagnosis rests on establishing a deviation from agreed physical norms, such as those relating to cardiac size, respiratory flow, glomerular filtration rate, or whatever. Environmental and psychological factors, including social and cultural ones, play an often crucial role but the diagnosis of physical disease rests on a demonstration of a disturbance in an organ or a bodily system. In mental illnesses, Lewis argued, such a part-function disturbance occurs in one or more of the recognised psychological functions, functions such as perception, learning, remembering, feeling, thinking, motivation, impulse control, etc. Disturbances in perception or memory are the psychiatric equivalent of disturbances in, say, the liver or lymphatic system. Deviant, maladapted, non-conformist behaviour, on the other hand, is only pathological if it is accompanied by a manifest disturbance in one or more psychological part-functions. For mental disease to be inferred in Lewis's view

> disorder of function must be detectable at a discrete or differentiated level that is hardly conceivable when mental activity as a whole is taken as an irreducible datum. If non-conformity can be detected only in total behaviour, while all the particular psychological functions seem unimpaired, health will be presumed not illness.
> Lewis (1955).

Unfortunately, there are a number of areas, such as the personality disorders and the so-called sexual perversions, in which the presence or absence of a disturbance in psychological part-functions such as impulse control or learning may be suspected but cannot be established. One consequence is that highly disturbed individuals who appear to meet lay criteria of 'madness' by virtue of the strangeness or seeming motivelessness of their behaviour are deemed mentally well by psychiatrists adopting the Lewis definition of disease. Additionally, we know considerably less about psychological part-functions at the present time than we do about physiological part-functions so the comparison is not a particularly useful one. Lewis's insistence that social norms should not become a criterion of normality represents, in one critic's eyes, little more than an aspiration. 'In many areas if we are determined not to resort to social criteria, all we can do is defer judgement' (Kendell, 1975). In practice, of course, deferring judgement is precisely what many psychiatrists do. In those conditions, such as the major psychotic illnesses in which there are grounds for supposing the existence of some underlying somatic process and in which there is relatively clear-cut evidence of disturbed psychological functioning, most psychiatrists appear reasonably agreed as to the legitimacy of conceptualising such conditions as diseases. In other conditions, and most notably the personality disorders, in which evidence of disturbance in psychological part-function is conspicuously lacking and in which no underlying physiological disturbance can be reliably demonstrated, psychiatrists and psychologists adopt profoundly contradictory positions (Asubel, 1961; Szasz, 1972) while the more cautious among them refrain from committing themselves one way or the other.

In practice, the formulation of a named disease may be founded on little more than an isolated symptom or symptoms (e.g. tension headache, rheumatism, insomnia) in which case a *symptomatic* diagnosis can be made. It may rest on no more than a combination of clinical signs and symptoms observed to cluster together frequently and distinctively as a *syndrome* (e.g. migraine, phobic anxiety). It may depend on *morbid pathological* changes (e.g. an inflamed appendix, gallstones), *biochemical abnormalities* (e.g. porphyria, diabetes), specific *deficiencies* (e.g. pernicious anaemia, pellagra) or measurable *disorders of function* (e.g. respiratory emphysema). It may even be defined on the basis of some *chromosomal abnormality or change* (e.g. Down's syndrome, Turner's syndrome). Depending on the stage to which our understanding of disease has evolved, the formulation of a diagnosis can end in very different sorts of conclusions. One major purpose of diagnosis, however, is that it should permit reasonably accurate predictions to be made concerning aetiology, prognosis and response to treatment. Taken together, these aspects of the disease concept constitute some if not all of the elements of the so-called 'medical model'.

The medical model

The notion of the medical model is by no means unequivocal but is subject to much uncertainty and confusion. A number of definitions, some contradictory, some overlapping, are in current use. They have been admirably summarised by Macklin (1973). She identified four main versions. The first is a relatively neutral statement to the effect that according to the medical model, psychological ailments are held to be analogous to physical ones in so far as both sorts of ailments have ascertainable causes and the disease state is manifested in symptoms. No specification of the types of cause is provided (Sahakian, 1970). The second is similar but adds the important addendum that the medical model characteristically focuses on the causes of abnormal or maladaptive behaviour rather than the behaviours themselves and construes the 'real' disorder in terms of an underlying disease state of the organism (Ullman & Krasner, 1975). In this view the medical model involves not merely a conceptual characterisation of the nature of emotional disorder but also entails a certain sort of precedural process of diagnosis and treatment on the part of the clinician. The third version emphasises the view that the medical model in attempting to explain the origins of neurotic and psychotic behaviour, alcohol addiction, delinquency, marital difficulties, and school learning difficulties as 'sickness inside the person' make them 'discontinuous with normal behaviour'. The medical model, in other words, suggests that these conditions are among a number of discrete mental illnesses, each with a separate cause, prognosis, and potential treatment (Albee, 1969). Finally, there is the medical model as described by Szasz, which differs from the preceding three in that whereas Szasz attributes to the medical model the assumption of neurological and/or physicochemical causes, the first three definitions are neutral with respect to the types of causes presupposed by medical model theorists.

As Macklin (1973) has noted, with the exception of the first definition, which is the most neutral and general of all those cited, each characterisation of the medical model 'is propounded by a writer who is attempting to reject the model'. Thus the second definition is proposed by behaviourists who regard neurotic symptoms as simple learned habits. According to this *behavioural model*, eliminating the symptoms eliminated the neurosis. There is no underlying disease. There are symptoms. In this formulation, psychoses possibly, and neuroses and personality disorder certainly, are examples of abnormal behaviour that has been learned and is being maintained either because it leads to positive effects or avoids negative ones. The typical therapeutic response includes establishing the behaviour to be modified, the conditions under which it occurs, the factors responsible for the persistence of the behaviour, a set of appropriate treatment conditions and a schedule of retraining (Lazarus, 1968; Liberman & Raskin, 1972; Eysenck, 1975).

The third definition of the medical model proposed above primarily relates to social and institutional reform. Its criticisms of the medical model relate to its impact on the nature of the institutions developed for intervention and prevention and the kind of manpower used to deliver care. The so-called *social model* highlights the manner in which the individual functions in the social system. The mind–body dichotomy is regarded as spurious or irrelevant and the individual viewed as a unit, the condition, form and destiny of which are moulded primarily by environmental forces. Mental illnesses are seen as evolving processes, reactions to socially disruptive events such as bereavement, poverty, overcrowding, pollution and marital breakdown (Weiss & Bergen, 1968). Treatment consists of reorganising the patient's relation to the social system or of reorganising the social system itself.

As a generalisation, the social and behavioural models of psychiatric disturbance have grown up in contrast to the biological or medical model. The *psychoanalytical model*, on the other hand, has historical roots as deeply embedded in antiquity as those of the biological standpoint. In the view of one eminent psychiatric historian, 'modern dynamic psychotherapy derives from primitive medicine and an uninterrupted continuity can be demonstrated between exorcism and magnetism, magnetism and hypnotism, and hypnotism and the modern dynamic schools' (Ellenberger, 1970). According to this model, adult neuroses and vulnerabilities to stress are the consequence of early childhood deprivation, developmental fixations at certain crucial stages of maturation, distortions in early relationships and confused communications between parents and child. Therapy consists in clarifying the meaning of events, feelings, impulses and behaviours in the context of past and often forgotten or repressed events and experiences. A crucial aspect of this model is the doctor–patient relationship, the therapeutic alliance, which, it is argued, enables the patient to work through the disturbance and abandon familiar but destructive methods of coping with reality.

Other models have been described (Siegler & Osmond, 1974) including the *conspiratorial*, in which psychiatric illness exists only in the eye of the observer, the so-called patient being the victim of labelling, the *family interaction* model, wherein the entire family is deemed 'sick' and is brought for help by the 'index patient', who may well be the healthiest member, and the *moral* model, which portrays mental illness as identical with deviance and the mentally ill as responsible, autonomous, self-willed individuals to be held responsible for their antisocial activities. There is also the *psychedelic model*, popular in the sixties, in which mental illness is viewed as a metaphorical 'trip', the patient proceeding through a state of 'supersanity' and, if properly guided, emerging on the far side in a more enlightened and sensitive condition.

These are some of the models formulated to explain the phenomena subsumed under the term mental illness. Some of them are relatively discrete but the majority overlap one with the other. In practice a clinician may well borrow ideas and practices from many of them when handling particular problems or patients. But, given the dominance of the medical model, it is necessary to return to the discussion of what exactly it is. Hornstra (1962) has identified as its particular characteristics the following: a specific aetiology, a predictable course, manifestations describable in signs and symptoms and a predictable outcome modifiable by certain describable manoeuvres. Lazare's (1973) definition, which he derives from Slater & Roth (1969), is similar apart from the fact that it includes the proposition that 'there eventually will be found a specific cause related to the functional anatomy of the brain' for each abnormal mental condition. However, few proponents of the medical model believe that unicausation is an essential feature. There are, for example, very few doctors who would hold that cigarettes are the sole cause of cancer, excess lipids of arteriosclerosis and deficient insulin of diabetes. Multiple causation, including genetic, familial, somatic, psychological, social and cultural 'causes', has long been accepted in medicine though this has not prevented those, like Milton & Wahler (1969) from arguing that the locus of the disease process as postulated by the medical model is 'inside the person'.

A more serious criticism of the applicability of the medical model to psychiatry relates to the relative *unreliability* of psychiatric diagnoses. Diagnoses are of questionable value if useful predictions cannot be made from them. If the diagnoses themselves are subject to disagreement and discrepancy, the accuracy and hence the value of these predictions will be correspondingly reduced. Kendell (1975) summarises the issue when he declares 'the accuracy of the prognostic and therapeutic inferences derived from a diagnosis can never be higher than the accuracy with which, in any given situation, that diagnosis can itself be made'. Diagnostic unreliability can result from inconsistency on the part of the diagnostician (Ward *et al.*, 1962), differences in diagnostic significance attributed to elicited symptoms (Beck *et al.*, 1962; Katz *et al.*, 1969), inadequacies of the nomenclature (Cooper *et al.*, 1972), the influence of diagnostic 'set' and suggestion (Termelin, 1968; Rosenhan, 1973), lack of psychiatric experience on the part of the diagnostician (Schmidt & Fonda, 1956) and international variation in the way diagnostic categories are implemented (Pichot *et al.*, 1966; Rawnsley, 1967; Cooper *et al.*, 1972; Kendell *et al.*, 1974). Impressed by these diagnostic deficiencies, a variety of experts have suggested that the conventional descriptive diagnostic categories should be discarded altogether (Masserman & Carmichael, 1936; Colby, 1960; Menninger, 1963; Mannoni, 1973). However, others argue that with special efforts to control inter-observer variation, appropriate training, adequate acquaintance with an agreed rating scale or internationally accepted glossary of terms and the use of standardised psychiatric assessments, significant improvements in diagnostic reliability can be achieved (Wilson & Meyer, 1962; Wing *et al.*, 1967; Cooper *et al.*, 1972; WHO, 1973*b*).

When attempts have been made to improve reliability in this way, relatively high levels of diagnostic agreement between psychiatrists have been reported. Using an early version of the Present State Examination, Wing and his colleagues (Wing *et al.*, 1967) reported a concordance rate of 92% between two psychiatrists rating patients diagnosed as schizophrenic. Kendell (1973) found an average level of diagnostic agreement of 77% between Maudsley-trained psychiatrists asked to rate an unselected series of new in-patients with five minutes to spare for each interview and no additional information provided. Kreitman and his colleagues (1961) obtained a level of agreement of 75% for organic diagnoses and 81% for functional psychoses but only 28% for neurotic disorders, a finding that supports the general view that organic states produce higher concordance rates than functional states, and psychotic illnesses higher rates than neurotic illnesses and personality disorders.

However, even supposing it is accepted that a reasonable level of diagnostic reliability can be attained in psychiatry, how *valid* is the diagnostic process? The main *raison d'etre* of diagnostic categories is that they predict – be it course, outcome and/or treatment response. Indeed it is often advanced as an argument for the value of a diagnostic approach in psychiatry that differences in response to therapeutic agents such as ECT, tricyclic antidepressants, monoamine oxidase inhibitors, phenothiazines and lithium do occur to a demonstrable extent. In fact there is considerable overlap between treatments. The phenothiazines, for example, are used for their 'antipsychotic' effects in schizophrenia, their tranquillising effects in mania and to sedate in agitated depressions. Lithium has been advocated for use in aggressive states, alcoholism and affective psychoses. ECT, while recommended for seriously depressed patients, has advocates too for its use in catatonic schizophrenia and severe mania. At the present time, psychiatry clearly lacks treatments of such specificity as is possessed by substances such as cyanocobalamin or thyroxine in physical medicine. Perhaps the most appropriate analogy between psychiatric drugs and physical ones is with the steroids, a group of drugs exerting a wide variety of effects and used in a remarkable array of conditions. It is interesting to note, too, that many of the conditions in which the steroids are used, such as multiple sclerosis, ulcerative colitis, and the autoimmune disorders, are at a similar stage of development as diseases as most psychiatric disorders, namely the syndrome stage.

Most psychiatrists accept the validity of the distinction between schizophrenia and manic depression because the two conditions appear to have different courses and outcomes and different family histories. Yet, as Kendell (1989) admits, few psychiatric disorders have been adequately validated and 'it is still an open issue whether there are genuine boundaries between the clinical syndromes recognised in contemporary classifications or between these syndromes and normality'. Indeed considerable overlap between the two major psychoses continues to exist. While it has been possible to demonstrate a boundary between schizophrenia and other forms of mental disorder (Cloninger *et al.*, 1985), most attempts to demonstrate natural boundaries between different depressive syndromes or between affective disorder and schizophrenia have been unsuccessful. The more biologically minded look to the 'new genetics' to explain this variation while the phenomenologically minded such as Sass (1992) look to cultural factors as playing a crucial role in the genesis or the shaping of schizophrenic forms of psychopathology.

Another approach involves the application of *cluster analysis*, a generic term for a variety of statistical techniques designed to sort heterogeneous populations into groups or clusters of individuals similar to each other with regard to the ratings on which the analysis is based. While it has been possible to demonstrate a boundary between schizophrenia and other forms of mental disorder (Cloninger *et al.*, 1985), most attempts to demonstrate natural boundaries between different depressive syndromes or between affective disorder and schizophrenia have been unsuccessful. However, Everitt and his colleagues (1971) have been able to show that clusters representing the syndromes of mania, melancholia and schizophrenia were generated by two different clustering procedures from two different data sets, one American and one British.

Kendell (1989) has argued that only by being willing to investigate, either by prospective follow-up, therapeutic trial or family study, a cohort of subjects who have deliberately been selected to represent a population that is more comprehensive than any single diagnostic category are we likely to establish a sound validity for a psychiatric classification of conditions.

The sick role

One aspect of the medical model that has received much critical attention is the so-called '*sick role*'. It is a concept that is largely derived from the writings of the sociologist Talcott Parsons. Parsons (1951) described four features of the sick role that help distinguish it from orthodox deviancy. First, there is the exemption from normal social responsibilities. Such an exemption requires legitimization from a physician. People are sometimes reluctant to accept that they or others are sick. The physician may serve as a court-of-appeal. This is particularly true of psychiatric ill-health. Secondly, the sick person cannot be expected to get better by an act of decision or will but is in a condition that must be 'taken care of'. Of course the process of recovery may be spontaneous but while the illness lasts the patient cannot help it. His condition must be changed, not merely his attitude. It is not simply a question of 'pulling oneself together' or 'showing willpower'. Thirdly, implicit in the definition of the state of being ill is the view that illness is undesirable and unsought and the patient has an obligation to want to get well. Fourthly, there is the related obligation, proportional to the severity of the condition, to seek technically competent help, that is to say, in the most usual sense the help of a physician and to co-operate with the physician in the process of getting well.

The extent to which a mentally ill person is responsible for his actions is a question that crops up in a number of guises and most often in forensic settings. Only two models put forward an unequivocal answer – the 'moral' model asserting that the person is primarily responsible and an 'organic' model, often confused with the medical model, asserting that the person is not responsible at all. The most accurate answer probably varies depending on individual circumstances, psychological and social factors and the nature of the condition itself. What is clear, however, is that at the heart of the medical approach and the corresponding sick role is the belief that the psychiatrically ill person, in common with the physically ill one, is not fully responsible for being sick and, once sick, is unable without some form of professional advice and/or treatment to return to a state of health save in exceptional circumstances.

There are, however, a number of disconcerting aspects to the application of the sick role in psychiatry. In the rest of medicine, the sick role is for the most part voluntarily adopted by the patient. It is not, as it is in the case with a small but important minority of psychiatric patients, imposed. In the case of compulsorily detained psychiatric patients it is the doctor and not the patient who attributes a behavioural abnormality to mental illness. Scheff (1974; 1966), in his influential work on *labelling theory*, suggested that much of the disturbance manifested by many psychiatric disorders was a consequence of rather than a justification for psychiatric intervention. The disadvantages of psychiatric diagnoses or labels are reflected in the fears of stigmatisation and rejection expressed by discharged mental hospital patients (Link *et al.*, 1987) while Barham (1993) reminds us that for individuals with the diagnostic label of schizophrenia 'loss of confidence in the viability and value of their life projects, and the reconstruction of themselves as useless are as much as anything powerful determinants in the transformation of a potentially manageable disability into permanent social disablement and chronicity'. The political abuse of psychiatry has likewise given psychiatrists cause to be alert to the professional danger of being misused as agents of social control. Nor, as Cooper (1992) points out, is this a danger restricted to the former Eastern bloc countries. Western psychiatry, as Odegaard (1975) pointed out:

... tends towards conservatism in its attitude to the social order. Our tranquillising therapy does somehow 'help to maintain the capitalist system' while actually psychiatry should be a liberating force. The problem arises when one tries to decide what kind of liberation we, as psychiatrists, can recommend as good for mental health. Nevertheless, we should admit a responsibility not only for social *control*, but also for social *change*.

Summary

Psychiatrically ill individuals suffer from illnesses whose aetiology and pathogenesis at the biological, psychological, behavioural and social level remain obscure. In Kety's (1974) words, 'we have only unsubstantiated hypotheses of how to prevent them'. What is still required is research but research, to be fruitful, needs to be based on firm foundations. Psychiatry's nomenclature, its list of terms used to describe and record clinical observations, remains subjective and somewhat arbitrary. Its classifications are fragile. Nevertheless, there is a broad consensus within psychiatry, a consensus that has strengthened in recent years, to the effect that the advantages of the disease approach, the diagnostic process and the present, rudimentary classification system outweigh the disadvantages. Furthermore, the early results of attempts to improve the situation are encouraging.

3

Current approaches to classification

ANNE E. FARMER

Why classify?

In most of the rest of medicine the importance of diagnosis is rarely questioned. However, in psychiatry the diagnostic process is less clear-cut and its usefulness has sometimes been challenged. How psychiatric disorders are classified has been the subject of fierce debate, particularly in the middle of this century, and some have even argued for diagnosis to be abandoned in relation to psychiatry (Menninger, 1963). One of the main problems is that most diagnoses remain syndromal, i.e. for most disorders attempts to discover coherent links between clinical features and specific aetiological factors or biological tests related to pathogenesis have failed. Thus psychiatrists rely on clinical descriptions of signs and symptoms in making a diagnosis, a process of low epistemological ranking, and cannot rely on laboratory or radiological tests to confirm or refute their findings.

If diagnosis is at such a primitive stage why has so much effort been made to classify psychiatric disorder? Why not abandon diagnosis completely and agree with Menninger (1963) that all individuals must be considered on their own merits free from the 'pernicious restraints' imposed by disease categories? It has also been suggested that attributing a psychiatric diagnosis to a patient detracts from his or her dignity and is stigmatising; society reacts against him and the individual becomes permanently 'labelled' (Scheff, 1963). Indeed it has been shown that the presence of a psychiatric 'label' strongly influences general practitioner's decisions to refer depressed and anxious patients to psychiatrists (Farmer & Griffiths, 1992).

However, there are a number of major fallacies in the argument to abandon diagnosis (Kendell, 1975). If we fail to distinguish between different types of mental disorder or between mental illness and health we fail to separate the different needs of someone who has a psychotic disorder from another who has an anxiety state. In Menninger's time, treatment options for these disorders were more limited but in the past 30 years pharmacological and psychotherapeutic interventions have become increasingly sophisticated and the management of the two conditions would now be quite distinct. From the point of planning services it is also important to categorise individuals, since they are likely to share needs in common. For example, health planners setting up day-care facilities to provide for the needs of severely mentally ill patients will need to know whether they are providing such facilities for 20, 200 or 2000 individuals. Such issues cross cultures and national boundaries and the World Health Organization has sought to achieve international agreement regarding diagnosis. The International Classification of diseases, 10th edition '*Classification of Mental and Behavioural Disorders*' will be considered in detail later in this chapter. However, first the historical background to current developments in psychiatric classification will be considered.

Historical background

Current descriptions of mental disorders have their origins in French, German and British philosophical and conceptual thinking of the nineteenth century. Much of the terminology has changed its meaning over the intervening decades and this is probably most apparent with descriptions of disordered personality (Berrios, 1993). Much subsequent effort by researchers and clinicians over the past 150 years has been to try to group these syndromal descriptions into a meaningful nosology. The most recent attempt to do this has been the introduction of operational definitions of psychiatric disorder in the 1970s.

Around the turn of the nineteenth century, two main classes of psychotic illness were delineated by Kraepelin (1896a). Individual syndromes described by Hecker (hebephrenia – 1871), Kahlbaum (catatonia – 1874) and Kraepelin (dementia paranoides – 1913) were considered by the latter to be variants of the same disorder, which he termed dementia praecox. Kraepelin separated this disorder from '*folie circulaire*', the name given by French psychiatrists to a group of illnesses characterised by depressive and manic mood phases (Baillarger, 1853; Falret, 1854) and which he renamed 'manic depressive insanity'. Inherent in these early descriptions of the main categories of psychotic disorder was the considerable variation in clinical presentations that could occur. This phenotypic heterogeneity was implied by Bleuler (1911) when he introduced the term 'group of schizophrenias' for dementia praecox and persists to the present day in the numerous subtypes of affective disorder and schizophrenia in modern classifications (WHO, 1992a).

The term 'moral insanity' was introduced by Prichard (1835) to describe individuals who were neither insane nor intellectually impaired but who behaved socially in an abnormal way. Those whose behaviour caused problems for others, e.g. antisocial or asocial, were considered to have disordered or deviant personalities. The term 'psychopathic' was coined to describe such personality types (Koch, 1891). Where the socially abnormal behaviour caused distress to the individual the concept of 'neurotic reaction' or 'neurosis' slowly evolved.

Subsequent use of these terms, especially by the emerging psychoanalytical movement, changed their meaning and led to confusion about their definitions. For example, Kraepelin considered psychopathic personalities to be '*formes frustes*' of the psychoses or deviations from normal development due to genetic or organic aetiological factors. On the other hand, Koch described varieties of psychopathic personality that occurred as a result of a disease process, while in psychoanalysis these terms refer to deviation from the normal line of development that has occurred in childhood.

Jaspers (1963) attempted to clarify the distinction between neurotic and psychopathic behaviour and psychosis in terms of the 'understandability' of symptoms. He considered that psychopathic behaviour and neurotic symptoms were an extension of normal reactions and could therefore be 'understood' by an empathic observer. Psychotic behaviour or symptoms however could not be 'understood' in the same way. Despite these and subsequent attempts to clarify these concepts, confusion continued and their precise meanings failed to be defined. More recently these terms have been dropped from international classification (APA, 1994) although, in ICD-10 (WHO, 1992a) the terms psychosis and neurosis have been reintroduced but only to describe symptom profiles.

Another problem that bedevilled attempts to create a meaningful nosology for psychiatric disorder was the poor agreement between psychiatrists about diagnosis. As well as confusion about the precise definitions of the terms used (see above), classification was also considered less important during the 1930s and 1940s, probably due to the emerging influence of the psychoanalytic movement, especially in the United States. This was particularly noticeable for psychotic disorders. By the 1960s huge differences in first admission rates for schizophrenia and manic depressive illness were noted, both within the US and between the US and the UK. A series of studies, the US/UK diagnostic series (Shepherd, 1957; Bellak, 1958; Kramer, 1961) were undertaken to establish why this was the case. Research teams in the US and UK were trained to use a structured interview on all new admissions to establish psychopathology. The data obtained from the interviews was scored by computer, and a 'study' diagnosis was then compared with the admitting doctor's diagnosis in both sites. While the standardised diagnoses in the UK and the US showed good agreement for the rates of different psychotic disorders, the hospital diagnoses reflected the national differences shown earlier. These studies therefore indicated that the national differences in rates of schizophrenia and manic-depressive illness were due to the diagnostic practices and did not reflect true differences in incidence and prevalence of the disorders in the two sites. The studies also showed that training doctors to use a standardised interview could greatly improve the reliability between them (inter-rater reliability) (Cooper et al., 1972). A computerised diagnostic programme could also greatly assist the diagnostic process, by eliminating any personal diagnostic bias.

Subsequently, the degree to which diagnostic practice differed on a more global scale was investigated in the World Health Organization-sponsored International Pilot Study of Schizophrenia (WHO, 1973). As well as examining the incidence and prevalence of schizophrenia in nine countries, this study also compared local diagnostic practises. As in the US/UK diagnostic series a structured interview, the Present State Examination, was employed by the project team to elicit current psychopathology and cases were assigned to a single category according to the *International Classification of Diseases* 8th Edition (WHO, 1974), using a computerised diagnostic system CATEGO (Wing et al., 1974), A total of 1202 patients were interviewed in nine different countries, US, UK, USSR, Denmark, Formosa, Nigeria, Czechoslovakia, Columbia and India. Each patient received a clinical diagnosis from a local psychiatrist. Subsequently 360 additional items of information were gathered by the project team using the Present State Examination and were processed by the CATEGO program. The results of the study showed that for seven of the nine countries clinical diagnoses were consistent and largely in agreement with the project diagnosis. However, in two sites, Washington, US and Moscow, USSR, the local psychiatrist diagnosed schizophrenia more frequently than the project team, but for different reasons. Thus both the International Pilot Study of Schizophrenia and the US/UK diagnostic series examined the problems relating to clinical diagnoses that had been highlighted earlier. They confirmed that inter-rater reliability could be dramatically improved if a structured interviewing technique was used and if standardised diagnostic procedure such as a computerised scoring program was adopted.

Following these studies the great impetus in psychiatric classification was to improve the reliability, as reflected in agreement between raters. The next major advance therefore was with the introduction of operational definitions of psychiatric disorder. It was originally suggested by Carl Hempel (1961) that one way of overcoming the difficulties of psychiatric classification would be to adopt 'operational definitions' for the various categories of illness. The term operational definition was first introduced by a physicist, Bridgman, in 1927, who defined it as follows: 'An operational definition of a scientific term S is a stipulation to the effect that S is to apply to all and only those cases for which performance of test operation T yields the specific outcome O'. To translate this for application in psychiatry, operationally defining disease S goes as follows. Instead of stating that the typical features of a disease are features, A, B, C, D and E, etc., an unambiguous statement is presented in the operational definition defining precisely how much of A, B, C, D and E must be present (or about) to fulfil the definition, e.g. a disorder X may be diagnosed if the patient has one of the symptoms listed under A, two of the symptoms under B, one of the symptoms under C, etc. Thus proceeding operationally facilitates precise, reliable, unambiguous features of disorder to be defined.

The first operational definitions to be published were the St. Louis criteria (Feighner *et al.*, 1972). Interestingly the authors cited neither Bridgman nor Hempel but the formats used were recognisably suggested by Hempel. There followed a proliferation of other authors producing operational definitions for psychiatric illness, some for a broad range of disorders and some confined to schizophrenia (Carpenter *et al.*, 1976) or its subtypes (Tsuang & Winokur, 1974). The Research Diagnostic Criteria published in 1975 (Spitzer *et al.*, 1975) together with the St. Louis criteria influenced the development of the *Diagnostic and Statistical Manual*, 3rd Edition (DSM-III) of the American Psychiatric Association, published in 1980.

As will be noted from the above authors, the production of operational definitions of psychiatric disorder is largely a North American phenomenon. Having demonstrated excellent reliability and proved their worth in various research studies, operational definitions of psychiatric disorder became increasingly important and virtually mandatory for researchers wishing to publish their results in reputable journals. The American Psychiatric Association was the first national body to take on the enormous tasks of producing operational definitions for clinical as well as research use and make their use central to psychiatric diagnosis for all clinical practice within the US. The DSM-III criteria were produced by various committees whose brief was to focus on different aspects of the classification. In addition, field trials were held of draft versions of DSM-III around the United States to test their applicability. As well as producing clear operational definitions for all major psychiatric disorders, personality disorders were also operationally defined. In addition to these main categories the DSM-III criteria were multi-axial, Axis one being the main psychiatric syndromes; Axis two, personality disorders; Axis three, any concurrent physical health problems; Axis four, psychosocial stressors; and Axis five, the highest level of functioning in the year prior to evaluation. Using all five Axes allows a more holistic view of the patient and his or her main psychiatric problems to be put into the context of other aspects of their health and functioning. In practice, Axes four and five have been seldom used even in research and most clinicians focus only on Axes one and two. The revised version of DSM-III, DSM-IIIR was published in 1987. The impact of DSM-IIIR was less than its immediate predecessor and the differences between the two manuals are not great. In 1994, DSM-IV was published, which closely resembled its predecessors.

In 1993 the *International Classification of Diseases* 10th edition (ICD, 10) classification of mental and behavioural disorders was published, in a version that consisted of Diagnostic Criteria for Research. These operational definitions of all major psychiatric and personality disorders have been agreed internationally and also subjected to international field trials (WHO, 1993). These criteria are in addition to clinical descriptions and diagnostic guidelines (WHO, 1992*a*).

Advantages and disadvantages of operational definitions

Because of their unambiguous and precise format, operational definitions can be easily applied by clinicians. Agreement and communication between clinicians is facilitated and this has led to an improvement in inter-rater reliability for diagnosis. In addition, it has been relatively straightforward to incorporate each criterion into the format for a structured interview and to devise computerised scoring programs. Indeed, structured interviews can be written in such a way that they can be administered and scored with good reliability and validity by lay interviewers who have no psychiatric training (Robins *et al.*, 1988). This can provide a highly cost effective means of acquiring information about the incidence and prevalence of psychiatric illness in general population samples where the employment of clinicians would usually be considered far too costly. As mentioned above, the explicit nature of operational criteria can enhance agreement not only nationally but internationally (ICD-10). Lastly, most authors of operational definitions have tried to take an aetiologically atheoretical perspective. Thus operational definitions should be equally acceptable to behavioural, biological or psychodynamic schools of thought.

Balanced against these advantages are a number of disadvantages. Firstly, there are many different operational definitions, especially for schizophrenic and affective disorders, none of which have proven validity. As Brockington *et al* (1978) have pointed out, the 'previous state of inarticulate confusion in the diagnosis of schizophrenia has been replaced by a babble of precise but differing formulations of the same concept'. In the research setting it is possible to adopt a polydiagnostic approach and collect enough clinical information so that all operational definitions for the disorder in question can be fulfilled (Kendell, 1975). In order to facilitate the application of such a polydiagnostic approach for psychotic disorders, the OPCRIT computerised scoring system (McGuffin *et al.*, 1991) was devised.

Although operational definitions have been shown to be highly reliable (see Table 3.1)

Table 3.1. *Percentage agreement and kappas for five main operational criteria included in OPCRIT*

	Agreement (%)	Mean kappa
DSM-III	96	0.85
DSM-IIIR	90	0.74
Feighner	81	0.61
RDC	87	0.71
French	90	0.74

(P < 0.00001 all definitions)
Three raters, 54 case vignettes

there is a restriction in terms of the information that is used in the operational diagnostic process compared to the usual clinical situation. Previous psychiatric history, informant information, previous response to medication, as well as difficult-to-define commodities depending on 'clinical impression' are usually omitted from operational definitions. Thus, there is no room for clinical hunches or intuition on the part of the doctor. In addition, there is a tendency to focus on positive symptomatology rather than less easily rated negative items such as amotivation or anhedonia. Improved reliability has been largely brought about by the highly prescriptive 'top down' format of operational definitions, where a series of pre-set rules have to be fulfilled before the diagnostic category can be applied. Individuals who fail to fulfil one or more items fall outside the diagnosis and end up in 'not elsewhere specified' or 'atypical' categories. If the criteria are too narrow the majority of subjects end up in such a category, which can then be larger than the main diagnostic groups (Farmer *et al.*, 1992). Other problems with operational definitions include the absence of standardised severity ratings in some definitions, which therefore means that both mild self-limiting illness and severe life-threatening disorder are included within the same diagnostic category (e.g. DSM-III major depression). The absence of an explicit diagnostic hierarchy can also be problematic for the clinician as well as for some types of research such as genetic studies. While there may be strong arguments against the introduction of such hierarchies there is also a need for unequivocal guidance in some instances, which has so far been missing. The DSM-III, DSM-IIIR and DSM-IV criteria give only limited guidance for the rater to decide, in a case with an admixture of depressive and psychotic symptoms, whether the diagnosis is one of psychotic depression or schizophrenia. In practice this decision is left to the individual researcher or clinician's personal judgement and is therefore subject to the same potential types of prejudice and bias that the introduction of operational criteria was meant to overcome. Despite all these problems, however, these national developments within the United States have paved the way for the World Health Organization to produce the new *International Classification of Diseases* on the bedrock of experience gained in the use of operational definitions over the past two decades.

The development of an international classification of diseases

The first comprehensive nosology covering a whole range of disease and including a classification of mental illness was produced by the newly formed World Health Organization in 1948. A number of previous attempts to list causes of death as well as to classify disease and injury had been unsuccessful in obtaining international use and this revision, entitled the 6th, although recommended for use by all the member states of the WHO, also failed to gain universal acceptance. Following a large enquiry into the state of classification undertaken on behalf of the WHO by Stengal (Stengal, 1959) a new edition was finally published in 1965, which was entitled the 8th Edition of the International Classification. (The 7th Edition, published in 1955, had the same mental disorders section as the 6th revision.) As well as introducing a glossary of definitions for the first time the section for all psychiatric disturbances was made self-sufficient, in Section 5. For the first time all major contributors to the psychiatric literature with the exception of France, were officially committed to using the same classification. The 9th revision was published in 1975 and came into use in 1978. Only minor changes were made from the 8th Edition. This classification continued to be the main system in use in the United Kingdom until April 1994. However, in view of all the rapid advances made in psychiatric nosology, with the introduction of operational definitions this classification became increasingly outdated and many psychiatrists within the UK became more familiar with the North American 'DSM' series of classifications, both in their clinical as well as their research practises. The publication of ICD-10 was therefore eagerly awaited.

The International Classification of Diseases 10th Edition: Classification of Mental and Behavioural Disorders

As discussed above, the World Health Organization has a responsibility for producing regular revisions of the *International Classification of Diseases* for use internationally. As well as providing international communications about statistics of morbidity and mortality, the ICD classification also acts as a reference for national and other psychiatric classifications. Additional uses include scientific research, clinical work and service development and psychiatric education. Thus ICD-10's classification on mental and behavioural disorders had to be acceptable to a wide range of users in different cultures, practical to facilitate understanding, easy to use and translate into different languages and versatile, so that it is possible to apply it to different work settings and/or by a variety of different professionals. With this in mind, Chapter 5 (F) on mental and behavioural disorders consists of a family of documents. The first of these, 'the blue book' (WHO, 1992*a*) consists of the clinical descriptions and diagnostic guidelines for service use as well as the discussion on the concepts upon which the classification is based. The second part, 'the green book' is the operational criteria version entitled the *Diagnostic Criteria for Research*. Unlike the US national classifications, clinical guidelines are kept quite separate from the more narrowly prescriptive operational criteria. The third document is a shorter, more simple version of the clinical descriptions, which will be used in the primary care. Lastly, a multi-axial system is being produced. Unlike previous international classifications, extensive consultation was undertaken with several hundred expert psychiatrists from many countries regarding the classification between 1984 and 1990. A draft version of the 'clinical diagnostic guidelines' was circulated widely and field trials were undertaken in 110 clinical centres in 37 countries, in which 700 clinicians took part.

Wherever possible in Chapter 5 (F) ICD-10 is a descriptive classification, like its predecessors ICD-9 and DSM-III and DSM-IIIR. However, aetiology does form some part of the organisation of the classification in some areas, particularly regarding organic brain syndromes and substance-related disorders.

ICD-10 has an alphanumeric coding scheme based on codes with a single letter followed by two numbers, e.g. A00–Z99. Further detail is provided by decimal numeric sub-divisions at the four-character level. Mental and behavioural disorders are included in Chapter 5 F00 to F99. This allows up to 100 sub-divisions within mental illness, although a proportion of numbers are left unused for the time being so that the introduction of changes to the classification can be undertaken without the need to redesign the entire system. The way Chapter 5 is sub-divided is shown in Table 3.2.

The classification uses the term 'disorder' to avoid difficulties in the use of terms such as 'disease' and 'illness'. Disorder is defined as the existence of a clinically recognised set of symptoms or behaviour, associated in most cases with distress and with interference with personal function. Terms such as psychogenic and psychosomatic have been omitted from the classification. Other terms such as 'impairment', 'disability', 'handicap' are used according to the WHO (1980) definitions. The main innovations in ICD-10 will now be discussed.

ICD-9 employed a neurotic/psychotic conceptual dichotomy, which is largely avoided in ICD-10, although the terms 'neurotic' and 'psychotic' are still retained as descriptive terms, e.g. 'Neurotic, stress related and somatoform disorders' (F40–F48); 'Acute and transient psychotic disorders' (F23). In using the term 'psychotic' in the latter, no assumption is being made regarding putative psychodynamic mechanisms, it merely indicates presence of delusions, hallucinations and some abnormalities of behaviour. Disorders in ICD-10 are arranged in groups according to major common themes or descriptive likenesses. For example, cyclothymia (F34.0) is in the affective disorder block F30–F39 rather than in F60–F69, disorders of adult personality and behaviour and schizotypal disorder previously regarded as a personality disorder are included in F26–F29 (schizophrenic illnesses).

All disorders associated with psycho-active substance misuse are grouped together in F10–F19, regardless of severity (Table 3.3). Indeed substance misuse is organised primarily according to substance (F10–F19) and type of disorder is shown after the decimal point, e.g. acute intoxication .0, harmful use .1, dependent syndrome .2 etc.

F20–F29 is entitled 'schizophrenia, schizotypal and delusional disorders'. New categories have been added such as 'undifferentiated schizophrenia', 'post schizophrenic depression' as well as including 'schizotypal disorder'. Schizoaffective disorder is also found in this section (F25), as is an expanded section on acute short, duration psychoses, since these are commonly seen in developing countries.

Table 3.2. *Chapter V (F) ICD-10: List of Categories*

F0	Organic including symptomatic mental disorders
F1	Mental and behavioural disorders due to psychoactive substance use
F2	Schizophrenia, schizotypal states and delusional disorders
F3	Mood (affective) disorders
F4	Neurotic, stress-related and somatoform disorders
F5	Behavioural syndromes and mental disorders associated with physiological dysfunction and hormonal change
F6	Abnormalities of adult personality and behaviour
F7	Mental retardation
F8	Developmental disorders
F9	Behavioural and emotional disorders with onset usually occurring in childhood or adolescence

Table 3.3. *ICD-10 Mental and behavioural disorders due to psychoactive substance use*

F10	Alcohol	Acute intoxication
F11	Opioids	
F12	Cannabinoids	Harmful use
F13	Sedatives or hypnotics	Dependence syndrome
F14	Cocaine	
F15	Other stimulants (including caffeine)	Withdrawal state ± delirium
F16	Hallucinogens	
F17	Tobacco	Psychotic disorder
F18	Volatile solvents	
F19	Multiple, Other, Unidentified } Substances	Amnesic syndrome, Residual or late psychotic disorder

Mood disorders are categorised in F30–F39. The nomenclature 'bipolar' has been adopted instead of 'manic depressive' used in ICD-9. There is now much research evidence to suggest that a bipolar–unipolar dichotomy is a more appropriate way to classify mood disorders (Farmer & McGuffin, 1989). Bipolar disorder is characterised by the presence of an episode of mania within the lifetime course of the illness, while unipolar disorder consists of single or recurrent episodes of depression. In ICD-10, mania is sub-divided to severity into hypomania and mania with or without psychotic symptoms. Similarly, depression is divided into three severity states: mild, moderate and severe. In addition, it is possible to categorise a depressive episode as with or without somatic symptoms, or with or without psychotic symptoms. Classifying a common condition such as depression according to severity as well as according to symptom profile is clinically very relevant. Persistent mood disorders such as cyclothymia and dysthymia are also included in this section, as is recurrent brief depressive disorder (Table 3.4).

F40–F49 includes anxiety disorders such as phobic disorders, panic and generalised anxiety, obsessive-compulsive disorder as well as reaction to stress, adjustment and dissociative disorders. The increasing evidence for somatoform disorders and chronic

Table 3.4. *ICD-10 Mood (Affective) Disorders F30–F39*

Category	Severity rating (mild/moderate/severe)	Symptom type*
Manic episode	✓	P
Bipolar disorder	✓	S + P
Depressive episode	✓	S + P
Recurrent depressive disorder	✓	S + P
Persistent mood disorders (cyclothymia/dysthymia)		
Other and unspecified mood disorders		

*S, = somatic symptoms; P, = psychotic symptoms

fatigue syndrome (as neuraesthenia) has ensured that these disorders also have their own categories in ICD-10.

Behaviours, syndromes and mental disorders associated with physiological dysfunction and hormonal change, such as eating disorders, non-organic sleep disorders and sexual dysfunction, are categorised in F50–F59. The greater detail included in ICD-10 compared to its predecessor is on account of the increasing importance of such disorders in liaison psychiatry.

F60–F69 includes disorders of personality as well as of adult behaviour such as pathological gambling, fire-setting and stealing. While F90–F99 covers only those disorders that are specific to childhood and adolescence (behavioural and emotional disorders with onset usually occurring in childhood and adolescence), dysfunction that can occur in persons of almost any age should be applied to children and adolescents when required, for example, disorders of eating (F50), sleeping (F51) and gender identify (F64).

As described above, the rules of taxonomy require that each patient be restricted to the membership of a single diagnostic category. While in theory this is highly desirable in practice, clinicians frequently encounter patients who they consider cannot be adequately described without using two or more categories. Thus the authors of ICD-10 recommend that clinicians should follow the general rule of recording as many diagnoses as are necessary to cover the clinical picture. However, if more than one diagnosis is recorded it is best to give one precedence over the others by specifying it as the main diagnosis and to label others as subsidiary or additional diagnoses. It is also recommended that precedence should be given to that diagnosis most relevant to the purpose of which the diagnoses are being collected. In clinical work this is often the disorder that gave rise to the consultation or contact with health services. On other occasions it may well be the main 'lifetime' diagnosis. However, if there is any doubt, a useful rule is to record the diagnoses in the numerical order in which they appear in the classification, which has an in-built hierarchy (F0, organic disorders, through to F9, behavioural and emotional disorders occurring in childhood).

ICD-10 is the main classification for all national purposes in the UK from April 1994. The Royal College of Psychiatrists has recognised the need to train all clinicians in the new classification in advance of this date and have run training workshops for divisional representatives so that they in turn can train other consultants and junior staff within their divisions.

ICD-10 and structured interviews

For the first time in its history, the World Health Organization have also supported the development of structured diagnostic interviews at the same time as producing a new international classification. Three structured diagnostic interviews have been produced to accompany ICD-10 and DSM-IV. These are the Composite International Diagnostic Interview (CIDI) (Robins *et al.*, 1988), the Schedules for the Clinical Assessment of Neuropsychiatry (SCAN) (Wing *et al.*, 1990) and the International Personality Disorder Examination (IPDE) (Loranger *et al.*, 1991). As well as covering major diagnoses according to ICD-10 and DSM-IV, all three interviews have been developed for use in a variety of cultures, countries and settings. Each has been translated into all major languages and back-translated into English. Special training in the use of each interview is required. All have computerised scoring programs and their acceptability and reliability has been internationally tested.

The CIDI has been specifically designed for epidemiological use and includes additional modules for the specific examination of individuals who misuse substances (the CIDI Substance Abuse Module). CIDI has a highly structured format, which enables it to be used by lay interviewers who do not have any clinical background.

Both the CIDI and the SCAN are discussed in greater detail in Chapter 8. Here it is sufficient to say that the SCAN interview consists of three main parts. Part 1 covers questions for non-psychotic disorders, part 2 psychotic disorders and part 3 observations of speech affect, etc. Clinical expertise is required for its use and SCAN is based on the PSE-CATEGO series of examinations and computerised scoring programmes.

The IPDE assesses the phenomena and life experiences that are relevant to the diagnoses of personality disorder in DSM-IV and ICD-10. The examination is arranged under six headings, consisting of work, interpersonal relationships, affects, reality testing, impulse control and behaviour at interview. An item-by-item scoring manual defines each criterion and the examination is scored according to a three-point scale. Informant information can also be used. The concurrent production of a new classification plus three structured interviews has been a highly innovative move by the World Health Organization.

Other matters of coding and mental health information systems

The NHS reforms and the development of community-based multi-disciplinary care for the mentally disordered and mentally distressed require much more than the routine collection of diagnostic information only. More comprehensive information systems are required to enable the measurements of needs and outcomes, to audit clinical practice and to address issues of service quality in the purchaser/ provider contracting process and the development of NHS Trust Hospitals. Indeed the need to develop information systems capable of recording and analysing health and social functioning of mentally ill people has been recognised in the 'Health of the Nation' document produced by the Department of Health. A review of the current approaches has recently been undertaken on behalf of the research unit of the Royal College of Psychiatrists (Shanks, 1992). Computerisation within the NHS enables a wide range of clinical data to be systematically collected and analysed. As well as diagnosis, issues such as mobility, incontinence and employment status can also be recorded. As well as ICD-10 and structured clinical interviews such as SCAN (see above) there are two other coding systems currently available. These are the Read Codes and Functional Analysis of Care Environment (FACE).

The Read Codes have provided a glossary of terms used by the medical profession and relate mainly to primary health care teams. To date, the Read system has not included terminology in classification in psychiatry, but this work is currently being undertaken. However, the Read system offers little over and above the comprehensive ICD-10 classification.

The Face Recording and Measurement system, however, is much more ambitious. This complex computerised system allows two types of information to be collected: 'presentations', which are clinical signs and symptoms and 'activity', which records information regarding interventions. In addition, the FACE system should facilitate the production of realistic service specifications, the measurement and management of resource use and outcome, the assessment of clinical needs, care planning and enable medical and clinical audit to be carried out. Both systems require the gathering and entering of considerable amounts of computerised data and the motivation of mental health professionals in undertaking such a process will be the main factor in utilising each system to its maximum potential.

4

Measurement in psychiatry

SCOTT WEICH, MICHAEL PHELAN
and ANTHONY MANN

A. PSYCHIATRIC AND SOCIAL INSTRUMENTS

Principles underlying measurement in psychiatry

Standardised instruments are now commonly used in psychiatric research and practice, where they serve four principal functions, namely: (1) identification of psychiatric 'cases'; (2) improvement of the accuracy of assessment and diagnosis; (3) assessment of the severity of psychiatric symptoms (or social disabilities); and (4) the evaluation of change that may be in response to specific interventions.

In contrast to other branches of medicine where phenomena are often quantifiable by physical observation (e.g. pulse rate, blood pressure), psychiatry usually depends on the assessment of subjective thoughts, feelings and perceptions. Psychiatry also differs in employing systems of classification based entirely on descriptive phenomenology, whereas in other branches of medicine specific aetiologies can often be invoked. Since there are no absolute criteria against which psychiatric diagnoses can be validated, scientific progress in psychiatry has been based on, firstly, establishing a consensus among clinicians about the signs and symptoms that constitute specific psychiatric disorders, and, secondly, operationalising clinical practice. To a considerable extent, current systems for classifying psychiatric disorders and standardised rating scales for identifying and quantifying the severity of these conditions have been developed simultaneously.

Choice of instruments

The choice of an instrument will be determined by the purpose for which it is intended. For example, a screening or case finding instrument may be a poor indicator of severity or response to treatment. The condition under investigation, and the setting in which the study will take place, are equally important, since instruments are usually developed for particular applications and settings, and misleading findings may arise if these conditions are breached. Having decided on the purpose for which the instrument is to be used, a further choice must be made between (i) self-report; (ii) interview-based; and (iii) observational assessments. While certain psychotic conditions, particularly mania, may not be suitable for assessment by self-report owing to a loss of insight, it is debatable whether such measures are always inferior to those based on interviews, as is sometimes assumed. If conducted by a clinician, an interview-based measure has the advantage of allowing the subjects' responses to be challenged and probed, in a manner consistent with clinical evaluation (Spitzer *et al.*, 1992). Self-report measures, including highly standardised instruments delivered by a lay interviewer, are characteristically cheaper and quicker to administer, and are free from observer bias (see below). Since there are strengths and weaknesses of all three methods, the decision will depend on the nature of the information to be gathered, the sample size, and the time available for data gathering. If an interview-based measure is to be used, a further choice must be made between an instrument suitable for use by lay interviewers and one that requires specialist clinical skills. Examples of all three types of instrument can be found later in this chapter.

Psychiatric instruments are further characterised by the type of rating scale employed. Interview- and observer-based measures in psychiatry nearly always use *Likert scales* to quantify attributes which, like attitudes or the severity of specific symptoms, can be treated as continuous variables (Thompson, 1989; Kline, 1993). These scales usually appear as statements followed by 5- or 7-point rating scales indicating the extent of agreement or disagreement, or symptoms followed by a scale indicating severity. Although self-report instruments most often use Likert scales, an alternative approach is the *visual analogue scale* (McCormack *et al.*, 1988). This method comprises verbal cues separated by a 10 cm straight line, on which the respondent is required to indicate, for example, where they believe they lie on the dimension of mood between very happy and very sad. Though easy to administer and score, visual analogue scales are used much less frequently than Likert scales. One reason for this may be difficulty in demonstrating acceptable levels of agreement with established measures of psychopathology.

Information bias

All of the instruments used in psychiatry depend on human judgement, whether that of the subject, an independent observer, or both. As such, all are unavoidably prone to information bias. Information bias refers to any systematic (non-random) error of measurement, of which there are two types: subject bias and observer bias. Bias can never be eliminated completely, but it can be minimised; the point is to consider its likely effect on the measurement in question (Hennekens & Buring, 1987).

There are specific forms of information bias that reflect human psychology and are common to all instruments (Kline, 1993). A subject's response to any questions is influenced by both the content of the question and the way in which it is asked. Self-report measures are especially prone to the tendency for some subjects to answer all questions in the same way. Six different phenomena have been identified: always saying 'yes' (*acquiescence*), always saying 'no' or giving unusual answers (*deviance*), always giving the answers that put the subject in the best light (*social desirability*), always giving *extreme responses*, or never giving extreme responses (*bias towards the middle*), and giving the same responses to all the questions, in keeping with responses to the first few questions (*response set*). Most of these can be countered by careful phrasing of questions, and balancing items so that agreement sometimes requires a negative response. The lie scale incorporated in the Eysenck Personality Inventory (Eysenck & Eysenck, 1964) can be used to assess the extent of social desirability bias. The *halo effect* describes a type of observer bias, namely the tendency to rate individual items in accordance with a global judgement about the subject. Thus, having ascertained that a subject has one biological symptom of depression, a rater may be more likely to rate other similar symptoms as present. This error is most likely to affect instruments that rely heavily on clinical judgement, but can be countered by interspersing items from different subscales, and by training and supervision.

Psychometric properties of individual instruments

The psychometric properties of psychiatric instruments can be considered under the headings of reliability and validity. Since there are no 'gold standards' by which to assess the validity of instruments, great store has been set by developing instruments that are reliable. It is important to remember that while important, reliability is really of secondary importance: it is necessary but not sufficient for establishing the validity of an instrument.

(i) Reliability

This refers to the repeatability of measurement, and has little to do with 'accuracy' (Morley & Snaith, 1992). A reliable instrument is one that produces the same results on repeated administration. There are three formal criteria by which the reliability of instruments are traditionally assessed: *inter-rater*, *test–retest*, and *split-half reliability*. Inter-rater reliability refers to the level of agreement between two raters, and is assessed either by comparing independent ratings made simultaneously during a single interview, or at consecutive interviews with a single subject. Test–retest reliability measures the agreement between scores for the same subject made over a period of time. Since psychiatric symptoms are likely to fluctuate, this type of reliability is most important for instruments that claim to measure relatively stable traits. Split-half reliability is a measure of the internal consistency of an instrument, which involves dividing an instrument into two equivalent halves and comparing a subject's scores on each half. Strong positive correlation between half scores suggests that all the items are indeed measuring the same construct. Since there are a large number of possible split halves, a further statistic may be calculated, *Cronbach's alpha coefficient*, which is equal to the average correlation between all possible combinations of items into two half-tests (Carmines & Zeller, 1979).

Though often treated as such, reliability is not a fixed attribute of an instrument, but varies between individuals, populations and settings. For example, the reliability of a measure may differ according to the age, gender and ethnicity of subjects, the setting in which it is administered, or the identity and experience of raters. This variability was first explored by Cronbach *et al.* (1972), and led to *Generalisability theory*. These authors have argued that reliability and validity are dependent on the particular use for which an instrument is intended, and recommend re-validation for every new application (Rust & Golombok,

1989). According to this approach, test construction and application are integrated. The innovative aspect of generalisability theory is the quantification of the contribution of different sources of error to the variability in test results, using analysis of variance. As a result of its theoretical and practical complexity, this work has had a minimal impact on research methods in psychiatry.

(ii) Validity

This is best defined as the extent to which an instrument measures what it claims to measure. There are five main types of validity: *face*, *content*, *criterion*, *construct* and *predictive validity*, though clearly all of these will not be relevant for all instruments. It is important to be clear about the intended use of an instrument, since an instrument may be valid for some purposes but not for others.

Face validity is unquantifiable, and refers only to the general appearance of the instrument. For example, a measure of depression that included items about both cognitive and biological symptoms could be said to have face validity. *Content validity* is also largely subjective, and refers to whether an instrument appears to be a balanced and comprehensive measure of the phenomenon of interest. Since there is often disagreement about the cardinal features of psychiatric disorders, *item bias* refers to the extent to which an instrument includes, say, more questions about the biological than the cognitive symptoms of depression. *Criterion validity* is a measure of agreement between an instrument and an external criterion. For example, a measure of the availability of social support could be said to have criterion validity if subjects' responses were highly correlated with an independent account of the frequency of contact with friends and relatives. Since there are few recognised 'objective' criteria against which to validate psychiatric instruments, new instruments tend to be compared with existing measures of the same construct. If there is evidence of agreement, the new instrument is said to have *concurrent validity*. A second type of criterion validity is *predictive validity*, or the extent to which scores on an instrument are predictive of some future event. For example, a valid measure of IQ might be expected to predict future educational achievement. *Construct validity* means that results obtained from an instrument are consistent with theoretical assumptions underlying its design. This is perhaps the most important but least accessible form of validity.

Instruments in common use in psychiatry

The remainder of this chapter is devoted to a discussion of some of the instruments commonly used in psychiatric research and clinical practice. Lengthier discussions are available elsewhere (Ferguson & Tyrer, 1989a; Thompson, 1989). Instruments designed for assessment of children, the elderly, drug and alcohol misusers, and those that measure cognitive or intellectual ability are beyond the scope of this chapter.

Case finding

The aims of epidemiological investigation include estimating the frequency and distribution of disorder in populations, and searching for potential aetiological risk factors. Any such enquiry requires a definition of 'caseness', and instruments capable of accurately identifying 'cases' (Williams *et al.*, 1980). Since most populations contain subjects with symptoms ranging from the transient and minor to the severe and chronic, any definition of 'caseness' amounts to the imposition of a threshold value on a continuous distribution (Robins, 1985; Rose & Barker, 1986).

Prior to the 1979s, surveys estimated prevalence of disorder using ratings by experienced clinicians or proxy measures such as hospital admissions. Cultural and historical variation in the sorts of patients seen by psychiatrists, and criteria used for diagnosis, meant that such findings were difficult to interpret. The debate on 'caseness' during the 1970s and 1980s (Wing *et al.*, 1981) coincided with revisions of diagnostic classification and the development of standardised instruments. The problem of defining caseness was resolved by placing the greatest possible emphasis on reliability. Thus one definition of a 'case' of psychiatric disorder is that the patient's symptoms fulfil the operational criteria of DSM-IV (American Psychiatric Association, 1994) or ICD-10 (World Health Organization, 1992*a*).

The impracticality of clinician-administered diagnostic schedules for large-scale surveys has led to the development of self-report questionnaires and standardised instruments for use by lay interviewers (Lewis & Williams, 1989).

The most widely used case finding instrument in the UK is the *General Health Questionnaire* (GHQ) (Goldberg, 1972), a self-administered questionnaire 'aimed at detecting psychiatric disorders in community and non-psychiatric clinical settings' (Goldberg & Williams, 1988). The GHQ was developed on the assumption that there are undifferentiated subjective experiences of psychiatric disorder that distinguish all such subjects from those who are well. The questionnaire was originally intended for use in primary care settings, and enquires about recent changes in functioning. The resulting score amounts to a quantitative assessment of the likelihood that an individual would be identified as a psychiatric case by a psychiatrist.

The GHQ has been used in over 50 validation studies, in about 40 languages. It performs equally well in these diverse settings, with only minimal modification. In addition to the original 60-item versions, 30-, 28-, 20-, and 12-item versions have been produced following principal components analysis, with minimal effect on psychometric properties (Goldberg & Williams, 1988). All except the GHQ-28 exclude original items endorsed by physically ill subjects. Though it has proven difficult to assess test-retest reliability in an instrument that responds to transient change, Cronbach's alpha coefficient is reported between +0.82 and +0.93. Criterion validity has been demonstrated by comparing the GHQ with interview measures of psychiatric morbidity, most commonly the Clinical Interview Schedule (Goldberg *et al.*, 1970). In 22 studies, the median correlation between scores on these measures was + 0.70, and the sensitivity and specificity of case finding for all versions of the GHQ were between 70% and 90%.

The GHQ is highly acceptable to the general population, as evidenced by its frequent use in large-scale surveys in clinical and non-clinical settings (Mann, 1977; Tarnopolsky *et al.*,

1980; Blaxter, 1990; Taylor, 1992*b*). The GHQ has been used most commonly to estimate the prevalence (Williams *et al.*, 1988), presentation (Bridges & Goldberg, 1985; Craig *et al.*, 1993), detection (Marks *et al.*, 1979) and outcome of psychiatric disorder among primary care attenders (Johnstone & Goldberg, 1976; Mann *et al.*, 1981*a*). Its extensive use has tended to conceal its principal limitations, namely high rates of 'false negatives' among those with chronic psychiatric disorder (Goodchild & Duncan-Jones, 1985) and 'false positives' among the physically ill (Finlay-Jones & Murphy, 1979; Benjamin *et al.*, 1982).

An alternative case-finding instrument is the *Self-Reporting Questionnaire (SRQ)* (Harding *et al.*, 1980), a 24-item questionnaire developed by the World Health Organization for use in general medical settings in developing countries. Comparison with the GHQ suggested similar effectiveness in case detection (Mari & Williams, 1985), and yes/no response categories make it particularly suitable in settings where literacy may be poor.

Assessment of global psychopathology

Standardised interview schedules that enquire about a broad range of possible symptoms can be divided into those that provide a quantitative *description* of their nature and severity, and those that generate *diagnoses* according to leading systems of classification.

Descriptive instruments

(i)   The *Clinical Interview Schedule (CIS)* (Goldberg *et al.*, 1970) was the first standardised interview designed specifically to assess common mental disorders in community settings, among subjects who may not see themselves as psychiatrically disturbed. The original schedule, intended for use by experienced clinicians, resembled a formal psychiatric examination. In addition to enquiring about past medical history, past psychiatric history and family history, the interviewer asked standardised questions about ten non-psychotic symptoms, and made separate ratings of the presence and severity of 12 possible 'manifest abnormalities' observed at interview. Finally, the interviewer judged whether the subject was a psychiatric case, and decided on an appropriate diagnosis. High reliability was obtained among trained raters.

   The CIS has been revised for use by lay interviewers (Lewis *et al.*, 1992), by removing all but the systematic and highly standardised enquiry into non-psychotic symptoms. Elimination of the 'manifest abnormality' section means that it is largely free from observer bias and is less dependent on training. While extending its applicability in non-psychiatric settings, Lewis & Williams (1989) found that these changes did not alter the validity of the CIS. The CIS-R has recently been used in the UK national survey of psychiatric morbidity (Department of Health, 1993*b*). A computerised version of this instrument has been shown to possess psychometric properties similar to the original (Lewis, 1994).

(ii) *The Brief Psychiatric Rating Scale (BPRS)* (Overall & Gorham, 1962; Overall, 1974) was designed as an efficient and clinically valid means of assessing efficacy in psychopharmacological research, and has been used most widely among patients with psychotic disorders. The BPRS consists of 18 separate symptom constructs, each of which is rated on a seven-point scale of severity. Though in theory it can be used to evaluate specific treatment effects (Snaith, 1993), Manchanda *et al.* (1989) have highlighted serious shortcomings. Reliability is high among clinically experienced raters within centres, but the lack of cues for rating severity leads to variation between centres. The most serious drawbacks are the overlap between items and their lack of correspondence with current psychopathological concepts, making ratings particularly susceptible to the halo effect.

Diagnostic instruments

(i) *The Present State Examination (PSE)* was first published in 1967 (Wing *et al.*, 1967), and has now reached its tenth edition. The prime aim of the PSE system is to 'describe clinical phenomena clearly, precisely and reliably', and it was not originally developed as a diagnostic instrument (Wing, 1983). However, a computer programme, CATEGO, was developed in 1971 to produce standardised diagnostic groupings. The PSE is designed to be used by psychiatrists after a specified period of training, although trained interviewers without clinical experience have also used the instrument successfully. Interviewers are trained to discover whether each of a comprehensive list of symptoms is present, and if so with what degree of severity. For most symptoms, questions are suggested, but interviewers are free to clarify with their own supplementary questions when necessary. For the ninth edition of the PSE an index of definition (ID) was constructed based on the number, type and severity of symptoms elicited. The index specifies eight levels of definition of disorder, and the threshold for 'caseness' is set between levels 4 and 5 (Wing *et al.*, 1978). The PSE is designed to examine subjects with psychiatric rather than personality disorders. Nevertheless the PSE has enabled great strides to be made in comparing psychiatric diagnoses throughout the world, and has been used in a wide range of psychiatric research.

PSE 10 has been incorporated into the *Schedule for Clinical Assessment in Neuro-psychiatry (SCAN)*, which has been developed along with the Composite International Diagnostic Interview (CIDI) (see below) by the Task Force on Psychiatric Assessment Instruments (Wing *et al.*, 1990). SCAN was developed with the aim of producing a comprehensive procedure for clinical examination, which could also generate ICD-10, DSM-IIIR and more recently DSM-IV categories. A major addition to PSE 10 is the inclusion of sections on eating disorders, somatoform disorders and alcohol and substance abuse, which were absent from PSE 9. As well as PSE 10, SCAN contains a 59-item group check-list, which consists of groups of symptoms rather than individual symptoms, and a clinical information schedule. Information for these are obtained from case records, clinicians and other informants. SCAN also gives the option of supplementing information on present state by rating a secondary period, which can be a previous representative episode of illness, or a lifetime ever rating. Data is processed using the CATEGO-5 programme.

(ii) *The Composite International Diagnostic Interview (CIDI)* is a highly standardised instrument designed for use in epidemiological studies in cross-cultural settings where interviews by clinicians would be unfeasible (Robins & Sartorius, 1993). The CIDI combines the first 40 items and certain psychotic symptoms from the PSE with the *Diagnostic Interview Schedule (DIS)* (Robins *et al.*, 1981), a standardised instrument designed for use by lay interviewers in the Epidemiologic Catchment Area study (Robins *et al.*, 1984). In combination with a computer programme, data gathered by lay interviewers using the CIDI is sufficient to make reliable ICD-10 and DSM-IIIR diagnoses (Wittchen *et al.*, 1991). Both the DIS and CIDI ask first about lifetime prevalence of symptoms, before enquiring about timing of onset and duration to arrive at lifetime, one-year, six- and three-month prevalence rates. The main advantages of CIDI are its standardisation, extensive field testing in diverse settings and languages, and exceptionally high reliability (Wittchen *et al.*, 1991). Despite concern about disagreement between clinicians' assessments and results of the DIS during the ECA Study (Anthony *et al.*, 1985; Folstein *et al.*, 1985), there is substantial evidence that both the DIS and CIDI are valid for use in epidemiological studies (Helzer *et al.*, 1985; Robins, 1985). Although the CIDI depends on subjects' self-assessment and not the judgement of the interviewer, high degrees of reliability were obtained for classification of psychiatric syndromes and quantification of the severity of psychiatric disorder when PSE items incorporated in CIDI were compared with the PSE (Farmer *et al.*, 1987). The main drawbacks of the CIDI are the time needed for training – five days (Essau & Wittchen, 1993) – and the duration of interview. The schedule comprises nearly 300 items, and takes over two hours in a third of interviews (Wittchen *et al.*, 1991).

(iii) In contrast to the work of Lee Robins and colleagues (above), Robert Spitzer and his colleagues have remained committed to the view that '. . . the most valid diagnostic assessment still requires the skills of a clinician' (Spitzer *et al.*, 1992). The *Schedule for Affective Disorders and Schizophrenia (SADS)* (Endicott & Spitzer, 1978; Hasin & Skodol, 1989), a semi-structured interview for use by experienced clinicians, was the most widely used diagnostic instrument in psychiatric research in the USA prior to the advent of DSM-III. This interview was designed for use with psychiatric patients, and provides a comprehensive assessment of the symptoms of disorders defined by the Research Diagnostic Criteria (RDC) (Spitzer *et al.*, 1978a). The full SADS interview enquires separately about the time of maximum symptom severity during the current episode, the severity of symptoms in the past week, and lifetime experience of symptoms. Each symptom is rated on a seven-point scale, according to explicit criteria. The interview takes between one and three hours to administer, in addition to time spent interviewing informants and consulting case records. When the assessment has been completed the rater makes a diagnosis on the basis of RDC criteria. Additional versions of the SADS are available, of which the two most frequently used are the SADS-L (lifetime version) and the SADS-C (change version). The SADS-L assesses both current and lifetime psychopathology, but enquires about the former in less detail than the full SADS and was designed for use among non-patient or community samples. The SADS-C comprises those items from the full SADS concerned with symptoms in the past week, and is suitable for repeated administration with the same subject.

(iv) To keep pace with changes in diagnostic practice following the introduction of DSM-III

(American Psychiatric Association, 1980) and DSM-IIIR (American Psychiatric Association, 1987), Spitzer and his colleagues developed the *Structured Interview for DSM-IIIR* (SCID) (Spitzer *et al.*, 1992). In doing so they sought not only to produce a DSM-IIIR compatible version of the SADS, but to develop an instrument that required less training and was more user-friendly (Hasin & Skodol, 1989). Unlike the SADS, which enquires about all possible symptoms and requires the interviewer to arrive at a diagnosis after the interview, the SCID incorporates diagnostic algorithms within the interview. Questions are grouped by diagnosis, and if any criterion essential to a diagnosis is not met the interviewer is instructed to skip the remaining questions about that diagnosis. Since the SCID was designed for use by experienced clinicians, interviewers are trained to challenge subjects and ask supplementary questions, as necessary. Like the SADS, interviewers are encouraged to gather information from as many sources as possible. To facilitate its use in research settings, the SCID is organised into modules, each of which corresponds to a major DSM-IIIR diagnostic class. Versions of the SCID include SCID-II, which assesses personality disorders, and is preceded by a self-report questionnaire, SCID-P (patient), for use among those identified as psychiatric patients and SCID-NP (non-patient), for use where subjects are not necessarily seeking help for psychiatric disorders, as in community surveys. A large multi-site reliability study found kappa values in excess of 0.6 for all major current and lifetime diagnoses among psychiatric patients, but lower levels of reliability among non-patients (Williams *et al.*, 1992).

(v) *The OPCRIT system* (McGuffin *et al.*, 1991) is a diagnostic tool that can be completed from written material alone, without the necessity of an interview with the subject. Standardised ratings for psychotic disorders are obtained using a 90-item checklist, and diagnoses are generated by a computerised scoring programme. The system allows multiple operational criteria to be applied to large numbers of subjects, and for the relationship between different operational definitions to be examined.

Assessment of the severity of specific conditions

The instruments described in this section are designed for the assessment of individual psychiatric disorders. These instruments are constructed on the assumption that a score representing the number and severity of the symptoms elicited will fluctuate with the intensity of the condition. The development of effective interventions for specific conditions has created demand for instruments that are sensitive to small changes, and that can be used repeatedly in the same individuals. To maximise sensitivity to change, preference is often given to items concerning symptoms that are not only common in the conditions under study, but are likely to vary in the short-term. Instruments that were designed to assess severity or change of specific disorders (such as Hamilton Rating Scale (HRSD), see below) are not in themselves diagnostic, and should only be used once the specific diagnosis has been made. It cannot be assumed that a high score on either the HRSD or the Beck Depression Inventory (BDI) is diagnostic of depression. Misleading findings may arise where subjects with different symptoms achieve similar global scores (Cooper & Fairburn, 1986). Although not a diagnostic instrument, many researchers have treated it as such, using a threshold score to determine the presence or absence of depression.

Depression

More instruments have been developed for the assessment of depression than for any other psychiatric disorders; a recent review identified over 30 in the English language alone (Snaith, 1993). The diversity of existing instruments partly reflects continuing disagreement concerning the core constructs of depression (Snaith, 1987). Since different scales assess different aspects of depression, the choice of instrument will directly affect both the study outcome and the extent to which findings may be compared with those of other studies (Bowling, 1991; Snaith, 1993). Thompson (1989) summarised the statistical methods used to evaluate the internal consistency of rating scales for depression: factor analysis, item-total correlation, and latent trait analysis.

(i) The Hamilton Rating Scale for Depression (HRSD) is an observer scale consisting of 17 (or, less commonly, 21) items scored on a combination of five- and three-point scales. One of the first measures designed to assess depressive illness (Hamilton, 1960, 1967), it has since become widely accepted as the 'gold standard' measure, particularly in drug trials. Designed for use by experienced clinicians, training in the use of this instrument is necessary. Information from sources other than interview with the subject may be used to arrive at ratings. There are no standardised questions, but a detailed glossary is provided. The instrument assesses cognitive and behavioural aspects of depression but places particular emphasis on somatic symptoms.

Considerable attention has been given to the strengths and weaknesses of the HRSD (Hedlund & Viewig, 1979; Maier & Philipp, 1985; Thompson, 1989; Bech, 1992). Inter-rater reliability has been found consistently to exceed 0.85. Despite findings to the contrary (Bech, 1981; Maier et al., 1988a,b), the balance of evidence suggests that the scale is a valid measure of the severity of depression (Hedlund & Viewig, 1979; Thompson, 1989). HRSD scores correlate highly with psychiatrists' global ratings of severity of depression (Bech et al., 1975; Feinberg et al., 1981), and most factor analyses have identified a dominant general severity factor on which all items load positively (Hamilton, 1967; Mowbray, 1972). Critics of this instrument have highlighted its relative insensitivity to change (Montgomery & Asberg, 1979), heterogeneity, poor transferability (Bech et al., 1981; Bech, 1992) and high somatic content (Snaith, 1993). The time taken to complete the assessment, and its reference to the 'past few days', make it unsuitable for frequent use on the same subject.

(ii) The Beck Depression Inventory (BDI) consists of 21 categories of symptoms and attitudes with four or five statements of severity for each; the patient selects the statement that most closely matches his or her current experience (Beck et al., 1961). In addition to sadness, anhedonia and suicidal ideation, ten items concern the negative cognitions that the author believes characterise depression, such as sense of failure, expectation of punishment and self-dislike, and seven items address the somatic manifestations of depression. Though originally intended to be administered by an interviewer, the BDI is most often used as a self-report measure. Like the HRSD, the BDI should only be used to assess severity once a diagnosis of depression has been made. No training in its use is necessary, and it is suitable for frequent use on the same subject. In common with other self-report measures, the BDI has been criticised as inferior to observer scales in assessing severity of depression (Kearns *et al.*, 1982) and prone to subject bias (Langevin & Stancer, 1979). A comprehensive review by Beck *et al.* (1988a) found evidence of satisfactory psychometric properties.

(iii) The Montgomery-Asberg Depression Rating Scale (MADRS) was specifically designed to assess change in severity of depression (Montgomery & Asberg, 1979). The MADRS contains no somatic or psychomotor items. Although it is an observer scale, the MADRS consists of only ten items. Its brevity, high inter-rater reliability, and sensitivity to change (Kearns *et al.*, 1982) account for the widespread use of the MADRS in treatment studies (Thompson, 1989).

(iv) The Hospital Anxiety and Depression Scale (HAD) (Zigmond & Snaith, 1982) was originally intended for use in general medical settings, where scores on other instruments may be contaminated by symptoms of physical illness. The HAD comprises two seven-item self-report scales. Items on the depression scale are largely restricted to the assessment of anhedonia, though anxiety items enquire about autonomic symptoms. While it is recognised that anxiety and depression frequently coexist, especially in community settings (Eaton & Ritter, 1988), opinion differs over whether these are separate 'disorders' (Stavrakaki & Vargo, 1986; Lewis, 1991). Despite the authors' protests (Snaith & Owens, 1990), studies among medical out-patients (Lewis & Wessely, 1990) and general practice attenders (Wilkinson & Barczak, 1988) combined subscale scores into a global measure of 'mood disorder' and found that the HAD was as good as the General Health Questionnaire at case identification. The authors caution against using the HAD in this way, and are supported by findings among medically ill subjects. Zigmond & Snaith (1982) found that both subscales were highly correlated with independent global ratings, and poorly correlated with each other. In a study of 575 patients with early-stage cancer, Moorey *et al.* (1991) identified two distinct factors that corresponded to the anxiety and depression subscales. The HAD should be used with care in applications other than that for which it was designed.

Mania

In contrast to depression, there are few rating scales for mania. Since characteristic symptoms such as grandiosity and lack of insight preclude accurate self-report, valid ratings of mania can only be made by observers. The best known measure is the *Manic State Scale (MS)* (Beigel *et al.*, 1971), designed for use by nurses. This instrument consists of 26 items, each of which is rated on separate five-point scales for frequency and intensity. Though time consuming to score, satisfactory inter-rate, reliability and construct validity have been demonstrated (Bech, 1981). Blackburn *et al.* (1977) produced a modified version of this instrument (the *Modified Manic Scale (MMS)* for use by psychiatrists. This scale provides a detailed assessment of psychopathology, and comprises 28 items, six of which are completed after consultation with nursing staff. All items are rated on a six-point scale of severity. Brief instruments are the *Bech–Rafaelson Scale for Mania* (Bech *et al.*, 1979) the *Mania Rating Scale* (Young *et al.*, 1978), for use by psychiatrists, and the *Manchester Rating Scale for Mania* (Brierley *et al.*, 1988), for use by nurses. All three are easy to use and have adequate psychometric properties.

Anxiety

The main application for anxiety-rating scales has been in the evaluation of potential anxiolytic drugs (e.g. Cross-National Collaborative Panic Study, 1992). Such instruments are rarely used in clinical practice, mainly because of the inability of anxiety-rating scales to discriminate between anxiety and depression. The measurement of anxiety is complicated by difficulties in distinguishing between trait and state anxiety, and in combining intensity and duration in a single index of severity. Although specialised instruments have been developed to assess phobias and panic disorder, the validity of differentiating these from other anxiety disorders has been questioned (Sheehan & Sheehan, 1982).

(i) The most commonly used measure of state anxiety is the *Hamilton Anxiety Scale (HAS)* (Hamilton, 1959). This observer scale comprises 14 items, seven of which assess somatic or autonomic symptoms. Like the HRSD, this instrument was designed for use by experienced clinicians, and takes at least half an hour to complete. Consistently high reliability has been found between trained raters. Apart from Hamilton's identification of two orthogonal factors, a general factor and a bipolar factor of psychological versus somatic symptoms, relatively little data exists concerning the validity of the HAS. Studies suggest that this instrument is unsuitable for assessing anxiety among depressed subjects, where it is unable to distinguish between those with and without coexisting DSM-IIIR anxiety syndromes, or between anxiolytic and antidepressant drug effects (Gjerris *et al.*, 1983; Maier *et al.*, 1988c). These findings underline Hamilton's original disclaimer that the HAS was only to be used in subjects with a diagnosis of 'neurotic anxiety state'.

(ii) The *Clinical Anxiety Scale (CAS)* (Snaith *et al.*, 1982) was designed by identifying HAS items that were most strongly correlated with a combined clinical and self-report judgement of the severity of anxiety among 51 psychiatric patients with an ICD-9 diagnosis of anxiety neurosis. Ten items were chosen after excluding those that might be influenced by depression or drug side-effects, though a six-item version appears equally valid. Though based on the HAS, more explicit guidance is given on the administration and scoring of the CAS, the content of which concerns psychic tension rather than somatic symptoms. The authors reported that the CAS was superior to the HAS as both an indicator of the severity of anxiety and as a measure of change. Like the HAS, this instrument is only valid among those with a diagnosis of an anxiety disorder.

(iii) Self-report measures of anxiety have not been widely used. The *Spielberger State–Trait Anxiety Inventory* (Spielberger, 1983) is the best known of these, and comprises separate state and trait schedules. Scores on the trait scale correlate satisfactorily with other measures of trait anxiety, and are more stable on re-testing than those on the state scale (as expected). Little psychometric data exist on the validity of the state scale, which has not been compared with other anxiety-rating scales. Strong correlations have been found between scores on both scales and BDI scores, an association that is strongest for trait anxiety. Although the *Beck Anxiety Inventory (BAI)* (Beck *et al.*, 1988*b*) was designed specifically to discriminate between anxious and depressed subjects; a high prevalence of panic disorder in samples chosen for the development and evaluation of this instrument may explain why 16 out of 21 items concern somatic manifestations of anxiety (Fydrich *et al.*, 1992).

Obsessive-compulsive disorder

The *Leyton Obsessional Inventory* (Cooper, 1970) was originally designed for a study of obsessional traits and symptoms among housewives. This measure requires subjects to sort 69 questions on individual cards into 'yes' and 'no' replies, and can be administered by lay interviewers. Although Murray *et al.* (1979) found that it distinguished between obsessional patients and normal controls, it has proven rather too cumbersome for widespread use. A briefer instrument is the *Maudsley Obsessional Questionnaire* (Hodgson & Rachman, 1977), which consists of 30 yes/no items framed to prevent an obsessional acquiescent response set. More recently, researchers have eschewed these composite state/trait instruments in favour of separate brief measures of rituals, obsessional thoughts, compulsions and avoidant behaviour (Marks *et al.*, 1980, 1988).

Eating disorders

As both anorexia and bulimia have become more widely recognised, so numerous instruments have appeared claiming to identify these syndromes and their underlying psychopathological features. This field has recently been succinctly reviewed by Szmukler (1985, 1989) and Halmi (1985).

The *Eating Attitudes Test (EAT)* (Garner & Garfinkel, 1979; Garner *et al.*, 1982) is a self-report instrument consisting of 26 items covering both cognition and behaviour. Principal components analyses in clinical and community settings suggest that EAT score is dominated by a 'dieting' component, making it difficult to interpret except among those who are thin or pathologically preoccupied with their weight (Wells *et al.*, 1985). Although validated as a measure of the severity of anorexia nervosa, the EAT has also been used inappropriately for case identification in community surveys. Used in this way, the EAT has a positive predictive value of around 10%, since the prevalence of this disorder is less than 1% (Williams *et al.*, 1982). In common with all self-report measures, the EAT is further limited by the tendency of anorexic subjects to deny their illness.

Personality disorder

The measurement of personality disorder has, until recently, been neglected by psychiatric researchers (Tyrer *et al.*, 1991). Inventories to define personality were devised by psychologists to measure individual differences in a series of dimensional scores, postulated to represent traits or facets of personality. Thus, every individual could be located in a multidimensional matrix, and abnormality inferred from the extent of the deviance of an individual's responses from population means. A widely used example of these inventories is the *Minnesota Multiphasic Personality Inventory (MMPI)* (Burgos, 1972), which is most widely used in the United States. Five hundred and fifty statements are grouped into nine scales, some of which have apparent clinical labels such as depression, hysteria and paranoia, whereas others appear to represent personality factors such as 'ego strength'.

The MMPI is, perhaps, cumbersome and time-consuming, but extensive normative data is available. The *Eysenck Personality Inventory (EPI)* (Eysenck & Eysenck, 1964), is the personality questionnaire most widely used in Britain. Its 48 questions measure two major orthogonal factors: extraversion/introversion (E) and neuroticism (N). The test also incorporates a lie scale that enables the tester to assess the extent to which the subject has 'faked good'. There is a vast amount of research data published based upon this inventory. Eysenck and others have attempted to put these personality dimensions on a biological footing by bringing evidence from genetic and psychophysiological sources to be associated with scores. Twin studies demonstrate that both E and N are moderately heritable.

At least at first sight, the dimensional view of personality does not fit easily with the categorical model of abnormal personality used in clinical psychiatric practice. Clinical research in personality disorder has been further handicapped by the vague and inconsistent diagnostic criteria found in earlier versions of International Classification of Diseases (ICD). Now, DSM-IIIR, DSM-IV and ICD-10 have each attempted to improve the situation by specifying operational definitions of the common features of abnormal personality and a threshold of possession of criteria for a diagnosis to be allowed. Standardised interviews based on these operational definitions, such as the *Personality Assessment Schedule (PAS)* (Tyrer & Alexander, 1979; Tyrer *et al.*, 1988), have allowed systematic research into the prevalence rate of personality disorders, their impact upon outcome for other clinical disorders, and the validity of the various sub-categories of personality disorder (Pilgrim & Mann, 1990; Tyrer *et al.*, 1991).

Both self-report and interviewer administered instruments now exist for the assessment of personality disorder, and derive information from the patient, from an informant or both (Ferguson & Tyrer, 1989*b*). Many instruments have recently been published, so that full data on their psychometric properties must be awaited. Until then, clinicians should choose between the various instruments according to the practicalities – the time taken, the availability of informants, etc. However, it is worth considering some of the principles underlying an assessment instrument and against which the published instruments should be judged.

(a) Who is providing the data?

In clinical psychiatric practice, it is usual to interview the informant for data on personality, because patients' abnormal mental states may distort self-concept (Hirschfield *et al.*, 1983). Most personality measures are designed for use with the patient rather than an informant, and a recent study using a semi-structured interview found no evidence that anxiety or depression affected the description of premorbid personality (Loranger *et al.*, 1991). Nevertheless, agreement between patient and informant rating is often poor (Zimmerman *et al.*, 1986). One reason is that informants may provide more information, allowing more frequent diagnosis of personality disorder (Stangl *et al.*, 1985). On the other hand, informants could be biased and may not be available. Acceptable inter-informant agreement of the *Standardised Assessment of Personality (SAP)* (Mann *et al.*, 1981b) has been reported for anankastic and self-conscious personalities (Pilgrim *et al.*, 1993).

(b) What is being measured?

ICD-10 and DSM-IV define thresholds of criteria that need to be present for a personality disorder to be diagnosed. In addition, both require some evidence of social impairment and personal distress. Although these two aspects are not clearly defined, the purpose of including them is to separate a concept of personality disorder from an intermediate state where abnormal traits may be present. The majority of the instruments in current use aim to classify, according to ICD-10, DSM-IIIR/IV or both. The results of their measurement will only be as good as the taxonomy itself. There remains much research to do to be sure that the two major systems meet criteria for a good taxonomy, i.e. the categories are mutually exclusive yet exhaustive of all possibilities. Data derived from a range of patients in general practice, medical and psychiatric settings will be needed to test the accuracy of the current categories.

(c) How reliable is the instrument?

Personality assessment must be capable of generating good inter-rater reliability amongst its users. Well-designed questionnaires with clear definitions and directions, combined with preliminary training, will help reliability. Good inter-rater reliability figures are shown for existing instruments. However, inter-rater reliability may be artificially enhanced where this is defined as the agreement between two or more ratings of the same interview recorded on audio or video tape, or by having two co-raters present in the interview room. A better approach would be to have the second interviewer assess the patient immediately after the first, although independently. This in turn could introduce errors of its own, from informant boredom, which might lead to fewer affirmative responses to probe questions in order to speed up the interview (Loranger *et al.*, 1991).

(d) What is the evidence for validity?

Personality disorder, by definition, should be stable and should be apparent to observers in a range of settings. Evidence of good reliability and stability over time (test–retest reliability) and between information derived from more than one informant (inter-rater reliability) would help confirm validity. However, criterion validity must also be demonstrated – from concurrent validity with other forms of personality assessment or predictive validity that a personality category is associated with specific biological, behavioural or illness variables.

Instruments of social psychiatry

Social psychiatry is concerned with relationships between mental health and the social environment. Instruments used in this type of enquiry are best considered under the three broad headings suggested by Brugha (1989): (1) measures of an individual's social functioning; (2) measures of social resources; and (3) measures of environmental adversity.

Assessment of social functioning

The instruments so far described in this chapter have been concerned with measuring the symptoms of mental disorders. The emphasis on symptoms is understandable, since patients usually complain about symptoms, diagnosis is dependent on symptoms, and treatment is usually aimed at reducing symptoms. Nevertheless, social disabilities associated with a disorder may well be more distressing for a patient than specific symptoms. Social impairments are often longer lasting and harder to treat, and social functioning may be a better predictor of service utilisation and cost of care than either diagnosis or symptomatology (McCrone & Phelan, 1995). Such areas must therefore be considered when evaluating specific interventions. There is a bewildering range of instruments to choose from and only a representative sample can be discussed here.

Before examining individual instruments it is important to consider the inherent difficulties concerning their validity. Ensuring the content validity of a measure of 'social functioning' requires that a large number of areas be included, though this must be matched against the need to keep the schedule to a practical length. Most instruments measure functioning that is below normal, and are based on a consensus of what constitutes a normal level of functioning. Many instruments do not allow for the specific cultural and situational factors that determine what is normal for an individual. For instance, in some societies it may be seen as entirely normal for a man to be unable to cook his meals. Concurrent validity is therefore difficult to establish in the absence of a 'gold standard' measurement of social functioning. The construct validity of social functioning depends on interactions between the many diverse factors that contribute to the concept, e.g. personality, intelligence, physical abilities, social environment, social support, expectations of others and rewards. With these limitations in mind we can now examine some of the approaches taken to measure social functioning.

(i) Global functioning

The *Global Assessment of Functioning Scale (GAF)* was introduced as axis V of DSM-IIIR to provide a measure of 'a person's psychological, social, and occupational functioning' (American Psychiatric Association, 1987). The GAF is a modified version of the *Global Assessment Scale (GAS)* (Endicott et al., 1976), which has been widely used in both research and clinical settings, and has established reliability (Dworkin et al., 1990). The GAF is a 0–90 scale. With the aid of nine anchor points describing different levels of symptoms and functioning, the rater decides on a single number to summarise a person's overall condition.

The simplicity of the GAF makes it attractive to both clinicians and researchers. The major limitation is that it combines both symptoms and functioning in a single rating. Clearly this will, at times, be inappropriate. A person may well have severe symptoms but still be functioning at a high level, or else be severely disabled with quite minor symptoms. In view of this problem it has been suggested that symptoms and functioning should be rated separately (Goldman *et al.*, 1992).

(ii) Social attainments and roles

A crude measure of a person's social functioning can be summarised by examining major social attainments and fulfilment of social roles. The *Psychiatric Epidemiology Research Interview* (Dohrenwend *et al.*, 1981) covers occupational, marital and parental attainment. Although such attainments may suggest a degree of social functioning in the past they do not necessarily reflect current performance. The lack of attainment may also be influenced by external factors, such as a high unemployment rate, rather than individual disability (Wykes, 1992).

A more precise measure of current functioning is obtained by examining a person's recent performance in specific social roles. An example of this approach is the *MRC Social Role Performance Schedule (SRP)*. In this instrument the threshold of what is deemed to be abnormal was set to try and be appropriate across cultural boundaries, and 87% of the general population had no serious problem in any of the roles incorporated into the instrument (Hurry & Sturt, 1981). However, some roles will always be inappropriate for certain populations. For instance, prisoners or institutionalised patients will not have the opportunity to fulfil domestic, sexual or financial roles.

(iii) Social behaviour

These instruments, which focus on specific behaviours, rather than the attainment of social roles, have the advantage of being more sensitive to change and are particularly appropriate for people with severe disabilities. The *Social Behaviour Scale (SBS)* (Wykes & Sturt, 1986) measures a range of behaviours, mainly on five-point scales. It has established psychometric properties, having been used in numerous studies of patients in different settings and cultures. *REHAB* (Baker & Hall, 1988) was designed specifically for people who are 'living in, or attending, a residential or day care institutional setting'. Again, psychometric properties have been established and normative data for over 800 patients are available. The *Life Skills Profile (LSP)* (Rosen *et al.*, 1989) is a carefully developed instrument, and though designed for people with schizophrenia, it can be used for people with any serious psychiatric disorder.

Resources in the social environment

The 'social environment' comprises the social context in which an individual exists, and is partly determined by immutable characteristics of the individual, such as age, ethnicity and parental social class. More mutable factors, such as occupation or housing, are sometimes considered as 'social resources', though relative impoverishment (however defined) in any of these domains can be construed as 'social adversity'.

Social support, defined broadly as 'those aspects of relationships thought to confer a beneficial effect on physical and psychological health' (Brugha, 1988), has attracted considerable attention recently. Research has been impeded by the difficulties of conceptualising and measuring social support (Bebbington, 1991). Although the social support literature is characterised by conceptual diversity, there is general agreement that social support comprises both practical and emotional forms of 'positive' support, and the absence of 'negative' or undermining interactions with others (Payne & Graham Jones, 1987; Brugha, 1988). There is now consistent evidence of an association between the perceived adequacy of social support and non-psychotic psychiatric disorder (Brown & Harris, 1978; Henderson et al., 1981, Brown et al., 1986; Brugha et al., 1987), though the nature of this relationship has not been fully elucidated (Alloway & Bebbington, 1987). Interpretation of such findings is also beset by difficulty in differentiating between dissatisfaction with social support, personality and depressed affect (Brugha, 1988). A lack of social support may reflect a negative response set, an inability to make friends or even the occurrence of a life event involving the loss of someone close.

Establishing adequate psychometric properties for any measure of social support is especially difficult, since there is no 'gold standard' for comparison. Standard criteria for evaluating reliability have also been questioned: for example, ratings that are too stable over time may reflect the respondent's personality rather than any quality of the relationship in question (Waring, 1985). Since concurrent validity is less conclusive than in other areas of psychiatric measurement, one approach is to demonstrate criterion validity be assessing correlations between responses given by subjects and independent information provided by those identified as sources of support, and between social support and more objective indices, such as frequency of contact and physical proximity (Stansfeld & Marmot, 1992). Most measures of social support assess both the quantity and quality of social interactions, though some place particular emphasis on enumerating subjects' social network, while others are more concerned with intimate dyadic relationships. A further distinction is between instruments employing lengthy semi-structured interviews, and structured self-report questionnaires suitable for large-scale epidemiological enquiry. Examples of the former are the *Self-Evaluation and Social Support Schedule (SESS)* (Brown et al., 1986) and the *Interview Schedule for Social Interaction (ISSI)* (Henderson et al., 1981), while a recent example of the latter is the *Close Persons Questionnaire (CPQ)* (Stansfeld & Marmot, 1992). All three instruments have satisfactory test–retest reliability, internal consistency and criterion validity, though both the SESS and the ISSI are time-consuming to administer. The ISSI comprises 52 questions about availability and satisfaction with support in six domains, most notably attachment and social integration. The SESS emphasises very close relationships, and like its companion measure, the LEDS (Brown & Harris, 1978) (see below), employs ratings made by an independent panel. The SESS attempts to assess the social behaviour of subjects and significant others independent of subjective perceptions, and to differentiate between 'available' and 'actual' support. The CPQ, a self-report instrument developed for a longitudinal cohort study of 10 000 British civil servants, quantifies subjects' social networks and enquires about practical and emotional support from up to four close persons.

Environmental adversity

Perhaps the most widely known and accepted research finding in social psychiatry is the association between the experience of recent threatening life events and the onset of psychiatric disorder, particularly depression (Paykel & Cooper, 1992). Ever since the advent of the first standardised rating scale (Holmes & Rahe, 1967), the familiar debate between self-report and investigator-based methods has raged more fiercely than in any other area of psychiatric measurement. Paykel (1983) and Katschnig (1986) argue against self-report measures of life events on theoretical and empirical grounds,emphasising the importance and difficulty of quantifying the 'stress' associated with any particular event.

The most widely and successfully used measure for assessing life events is the *Life Events and Difficulties Schedule (LEDS)* (Brown & Harris, 1978), a detailed semi-structured interview. Trained interviewers elicit information about the timing of 38 specific events in relation to both the onset of disorder and the context in which they occur. The severity of threat posed by events is rated by a panel who are 'blindfolded' to the subject's mental state, on the basis of a vignette presented by the interviewer. The severity of threat is rated according to both the nature of the life event itself and the social context of the subject. The panel also provides ratings of whether events are judged to be dependent or independent on the subject's actions, and whether the principal focus of the threat is the subject or someone else. The use of explicit rules ensures high inter-rater reliability (Tennant *et al.*, 1979). Katschnig (1986) compared the LEDS with the earliest and best-known checklist of life events, the *Schedule for Recent Events (SRE)* (Holmes & Rahe, 1967), among depressed patients and found satisfactory correlation between numbers of life events identified by each instrument in the sample as a whole, but very poor agreement for individual patients or specific events. Katschnig concluded that the self-report checklists were wholly inadequate for the further elucidation of the mechanisms by which specific psychosocial stressors precipitate psychiatric disorder in vulnerable individuals. While accepting the superiority of semi-structured interviews, Brugha *et al.* (1985) developed a brief 12-item inventory-based interview, the *List of Threatening Experiences (LTE)*, which is suitable for use in epidemiological surveys. The LTE accounted for 83% of all life events, and 77% of events rated by the LEDS as having severe or moderate long-term threat in a community survey. In a study comparing newly referred psychiatric out-patients with matched controls recruited from general practice, Brugha & Conroy (1985) found that events in the preceding six months identified by the LTE were more strongly associated with depression than those identified using a longer and more exhaustive checklist. The LTE is particularly suitable 'where adversity is not the sole major issue of interest' (Brugha, 1989), and has recently been used by the OPCS in the UK national survey of psychiatric morbidity (Department of Health, 1993).

Other measures relevant to psychiatry

Quality of life

Improving the quality of life of patients is a universal aim of all health professionals, and quality of life is recognised as an important outcome measure for all types of health care

(Fitzpatrick *et al.*, 1992). However, quality of life is an abstract concept, which is hard to define. The major components are the absence of symptoms, adequate social performance, and the ability to engage in satisfying activities. Two examples of quality of life measures suitable for people with mental disorders are the *Quality of Life Interview* (Lehman, 1982) and the *Lancashire Quality of Life Schedule* (Oliver, 1991).

Needs assessment

People with serious mental illness frequently have a complex mix of medical and social needs. In the UK, recent government policy has placed great emphasis on the assessment of individual need, prior to the planning and delivery of care (House of Commons, 1990). Regular clinical assessments of patients' needs are essential for the appropriate targeting of care. Measurement of met and unmet need is a powerful outcome measure for any mental health service evaluation. The *MRC Needs for Care Assessment (NCA)* was designed to identify potentially remediable areas in which a patient's level of functioning is at or below a minimum specified level (Brewin *et al.*, 1987). If problems are identified for which no potential remedy exists, the NCA indicates that there is 'no meetable need'. The NCA was designed to measure the needs of those with long-term mental illness living in the community.

The *Camberwell Assessment of Need (CAN)* is a more recently developed instrument that is briefer than the NCA, and is suitable for use by untrained raters. This instrument covers 22 social and clinical needs. Levels of met and unmet need are recorded, along with measures of the amount of help received from informal carers and health professionals. Each item is rated independently by the subject and his or her key worker. Separate research and clinical versions are available.

Patient satisfaction

If patients are satisfied with their care they are more likely to comply with treatment, resulting in better outcome (Kalman, 1983). Patient satisfaction is therefore an important aim for any psychiatric service. Most research in the area has been conducted with non-standardised instruments without established psychometric properties, and the results are not generalisable. An example of a satisfaction instrument that does have established psychometric properties is the *Verona Service Satisfaction Schedule* (VSSS). This instrument was designed in Italy (an English translation of the schedule is now available), and it is primarily for the assessment of community-based psychiatric services (Ruggeri & Dall'Agnola, 1993).

Conclusions

The development of rating scales, standardised interviews and self-report question-naires has been a significant contributing factor in the scientific advance of psychiatry over the past 20 years. Use of these instruments means that work in different centres is much more comparable than before, and findings can now be replicated. There is, however, a tendency towards the uncritical acceptance of results obtained using psychiatric instruments, particularly once psychometric data has been published. It must be remembered that the reliability and validity of an instrument are not fixed characteristics, but are both user and population-dependent. There is a need to re-evaluate continuously the performance of instruments, particularly if used in new settings. This has traditionally proven to be rather unattractive, with researchers choosing instead to develop yet more instruments to measure the same constructs (Snaith, 1993).

Existing psychiatric instruments represent nothing more than an attempt to operationalise clinical practice, by replacing subjective judgement with explicit rules. As such, the assessment of psychiatric instruments has always attached the greatest importance on achieving high reliability, while validity has proven much more elusive. Given that psychiatric taxonomy remains essentially descriptive, the relationship between psychiatric instruments and diagnostic categories should in theory be dialectic. Knowledge about the nature of psychiatric disorders has developed by a continuous process of refinement in the light of new findings using specific instruments, and vice versa.

Having established reliable, and as far as is possible, valid measures of psychiatric symptoms, the next task for psychiatric measurement is the development of instruments to assess 'quality of life'. Current developments in this sphere are being driven partly by the realisation that the outcome of psychiatric disorder entails much more than symptomatic recovery, and partly by the need to evaluate the cost-effectiveness of competing interventions. There is now a more pressing need to develop and refine measures for assessing objective and subjective social circumstances, social functioning and satisfaction with care.

Measurement in psychiatry

SHON W. LEWIS

B. BRAIN STRUCTURE AND FUNCTION

Introduction

Modern, non-invasive brain imaging techniques allow in vivo measurement of the structure and functioning of the human brain. Structural imaging has revolutionised diagnostic neurology, but has yet to make a major impact in the day-to-day practice of clinical psychiatry, although a large body of research has accrued. Unlike neurology, where the brain pathology is often gross and qualitative, with focal radiological lesions, controlled studies in psychiatry have shown that the pathology, where present, tends to be quantitative and relatively minor. The two broad modalities of brain imaging, structural and functional, can be thought of as assessments of form and content respectively. This chapter will review the principles and applications of current imaging techniques in psychiatry.

X-ray imaging

Structural brain imaging began with the plain skull X-ray. X-rays (and gamma rays) represent the extreme of the short-wavelength end of the electromagnetic spectrum, with the highest frequency and highest energy photons. X-ray production is by means of an X-ray tube. Initial beam intensity is a product of the number of photons in the beam and the energy of those photons. The X-rays produced interact with biological materials in two main ways. Photons are either absorbed, or scattered. *Absorption* involves the X-ray photon displacing an electron from an atom, which is thus converted to a positive ion. The degree of absorption is related to the atomic number of the tissue and is expressed as an attenuation coefficient.

A good imaging system will produce images that are sharp, and also have good resolution. *Resolution* is a measure of the ability of the system to produce clearly separate images of small objects that are close together. Effective, safe imaging is a trade-off between the desire to obtain as good as image as possible and the need to keep radiation dosage to the patient to a minimum. X-ray imaging systems whether traditional or CT produce their image from those X-ray photons that are transmitted through the target issues. The denser the tissue, the more X-rays are absorbed and the fewer transmitted. With plain X-ray imaging, the transmitted photons hit a silver bromide film, causing it to darken. High density tissue, such as bone, will leave the film white because few X-rays are transmitted.

The traditional cranial X-ray investigation in psychiatry was the plain lateral skull X-ray, which usually gave little information. Abnormal areas of calcification could be seen and skilled radiologists could deduce raised intracranial pressure. There is little indication in clinical psychiatry today for routine skull X-rays. The potentially risky procedure of *pneumoencephalography* involved introducing some air into the cerebrospinal fluid via a lumbar puncture, then tilting the patient so as to use the air pocket to outline the boundaries of the ventricular system. This has been superseded by computed tomography.

Computed tomography

Computed X-ray tomography (CT) was developed in the early 1970s, earning Hounsfield, its inventor, a Nobel prize. Its development depended more upon the arrival of appropriately fast computers rather than any special radiological advance.

In cranial CT, a narrow beam of X-rays is produced in bursts as the X-ray tube is moved around the subject's head in a transverse plane. Opposite, a sensitive radiation detector measures the amount of radiation emerging at many different projections. In this way, multiple projections (about a million) of the object are obtained, allowing its internal structure to be reconstructed. This reconstruction takes the form of a grey-scale (white to black) image of the distribution of attenuation coefficients within the object.

The X-ray beam is 'collimated' (focused) through an aperture first at the tube source and again at the detector, in order to reduce the blurring effects of scatter. To make the image, information from the many projections is entered into a stepwise, iterative image building process known as 'back projection': an initial estimate of the image is adjusted repeatedly with new information from each successive projection. The final image of a two-dimensional slice is made up of a matrix of small square elements, typically 256 x 256 in number. Each square, or *'pixel'*, has its own attenuation coefficient, derived from a succession of many X-ray projections that have undergone a mathematical (Fourier) analysis. Each pixel actually has a third dimension of depth, the thickness of the slice, and this cuboid volume is called a *voxel*. Pixels are displayed on a grey scale according to attenuation coefficient, with high attenuation (e.g. bone) appearing white. Attenuation coefficients are corrected to that of water being zero, the result being called the 'CT number' or Hounsfield unit (Table 4.1).

The digital data from the CT scan can be stored on magnetic tape or disk and is converted into analogue form for display. Final image quality depends on a variety of factors. Spatial resolution of about 0.5 mm is possible with most current CT scanners. Increasing the matrix size to 512 x 512 will increase resolution but requires a greater X-ray exposure. Under some circumstances, an intravenous contrast agent can be given to enhance resolution of particular vascular structures. A constraint on resolution for all computerised imaging techniques is the 'partial volume' artefact. This arises where a pixel (or voxel) straddles the

Table 4.1. *CT numbers for cranial tissue*

Bone calcification	+1000
Muscle	+50
Chronic subdural	+25
Grey matter	+18
White matter	+15
Cerebral oedema	+10
CSF	+8
Fat	−100
Air	−1000

interface between two structures of different densities. The final pixel CT number represents a mean of these two structures, appearing as a grey intermediate between two extremes. This gives rise to a visible 'fuzziness' of the structure interface on the final image. The partial volume effect compromises measurement, particularly of structures that are small or that have convoluted boundaries not perpendicular to the CT slice. Movement of the patient will also impair image quality and is made less likely by having brief scanning times.

Magnetic resonance imaging

Magnetic resonance imaging (MRI) is the second main medium in use for imaging brain structure. Compared to X-ray CT it has several advantages (Table 4.2) and the resulting brain image shows much more useful detail, for instance in differentiating clearly white from grey matter, which CT is poorly able to do.

Although the final steps of image reconstruction, into a matrix of pixels on a grey scale, are similar to CT, the principles of MRI are different and are based on nuclear magnetic resonance (NMR). NMR as a technique for analysing chemical compositions of substances, rather than an imaging technique, was discovered in the 1940s, earning its early investigators, Bloch and Purcell, a Nobel prize.

Where CT involves transmission (of X-rays), MRI involves a more complicated mixture of transmission and emission (of radiowaves). The basic property of atoms that is being imaged in MRI is the 'paramagnetic' property of some nuclei, such as sodium-23 or phosphorous-31, or hydrogen. These are nuclei that contain unpaired protons that are spinning, and thus exert a magnetic field. In most nuclei, paired protons will be spinning in opposite directions and thus cancel out any net magnetic field. Hydrogen, however, contains just one proton in its nucleus. In practice, by far the most abundant such atom in biological tissue is hydrogen and the resulting image essentially is a map of the distribution and concentration of the protons of hydrogen atoms, in the form of water (two H atoms per molecule) and organic compounds.

Like tiny bar magnets, hydrogen nuclei will line up with their axes of spin more or less parallel when exposed to a sufficiently strong magnetic field, and this is the first step in MRI. Next, a second property of these spinning protons is exploited. Whilst spinning, the protons

Table 4.2. *Advantages of cranial CT and MRI compared*

CT	MRI
Widely available; cheaper	No ionising radiation
Better for imaging calcification; safe in presence of ferrous metals	Good tissue contrast
	High resolution
More comfortable procedure	Multiplanar imaging

Table 4.3. *Physical tissue factors determining image in CT and MRI*

CT	MRI
1 Number of atoms per unit volume of tissue	1 Number of protons (H nuclei) per unit volume of tissue
2 Atomic number of atoms	2 Spin-lattice (T1) relaxation time
	3 Spin-spin (T2) relaxation time
	4 Movement of protons

will 'wobble' slightly around the axis of spin, usually likened to the wobbling of a spinning top or gyroscope as it starts to slow down. The technical term for this is 'precession'. If pulses of energy are now applied at radio-frequencies similar to the precession frequencies, these will 'resonate' with the precessing protons, which will absorb the energy of these pulses and tilt, by up to 180°, within the field. When the pulse switches off, the protons will 'relax' back to their original orientations to the field, releasing the stored energy again, which induces small currents in nearby detector coils. These currents make up the signal from which the image is constructed. The intensity of the signal depends firstly on the density of protons in the tissue examined and secondly on the time taken for the protons to 'relax' back to their original positions (Table 4.3). This relaxation time has itself two parameters, which are influenced by the surrounding chemical environment: so-called T1 and T2. T1 relaxation ('spin-lattice') represents the rate at which the disturbed protons realign with the field and is a measure of the overall loss of energy. Different tissues show different T1 relaxation times: relatively long for cerebrospinal fluid, for example, and short for white matter, whose hydrogen nuclei realign more quickly. T2 ('spin-spin') relaxation time refers to the part of the signal decay caused by the individual precessions of the realigning protons becoming less exactly in phase with one another as they were when in their 'tilted' state. This is a measure of the exchange of energy between adjacent protons. Again, different tissues have different T2 times. Every magnetic resonance image contains both T1 and T2 information, but by preselecting particular timing and length sequences of the radio-frequency pulses, the final image can be weighted so that it represents mainly T1, or mainly T2 relaxation information, or mainly proton density information. 'Inversion recovery' sequences are strongly T1 dependent and give good anatomical images: 'short T1 inversion recovery' (STIR) is a variant that incorporates T2 information. 'Spin echo' sequences are mostly T2 weighted. The choice depends largely on what one is interested in viewing in the final image. In a T1 weighted image, CSF will look dark (low signal), grey matter grey, and white matter light. In a T2 weighted image, CSF will look light (high signal), as will grey matter, and white matter look dark.

One of the requirements of an MRI scanner is a very high field strength, typically between 0.2 and 1.5 tesla: some 10 000 times the strength of the earth's magnetic field. This usually requires an electromagnet made of an alloy cooled by liquid helium to very low, superconducting temperatures. The high field strengths pose no known biological hazards so long as magnetic materials (pacemakers, aneurysm clips, etc.) are kept well away: such objects are subjected to forces in excess of 20 G near a 1.0 tesla magnet.

Quantitative measurement of brain structure

The main objective of CT and MRI is to produce valid anatomical images for clinical interpretation. However, in neuropsychiatric research the variables of interest are usually not focal lesions nor gross deviations from normality, but quantitative measures of area or volume. In early CT research, these measures were made using crude methods such as using tracing paper or mechanical cartographic instruments ('planimetry') on the CT film itself to calculate areas of particular structures. With the area of the lateral ventricles, this was by convention expressed as a percentage of the measured area of the entire brain on the same transverse slice, in order to correct for differences in head sizes: the ventricular brain ratio (VBR). Subsequently, a variety of interactive software packages run on computer workstations has become available, which allow highly reliable measurement from the original digital data. MRI makes quantitative measurements more flexible by enabling clear separation of white from grey matter and making possible image reconstruction in many planes. Given a full set of contiguous slices, interactive programmes can calculate volumes of particular compartments, such as CSF or cerebral cortical grey matter.

Functional imaging: brain activity and emission tomography

Radioactive isotopes tend to change their nuclear composition to a lower energy, undergoing radioactive decay. This process involves emission of particles or rays. Gamma rays are one form of electromagnetic radiation, like light or X-rays, with sufficient energy to knock electrons from atoms (ionisation). They are the basis of nuclear functional imaging techniques. Gamma-ray detection systems have as their basic component a crystal of fluorescent sodium iodide, which emits scintillations of light when struck by gamma radiation. In front of this, a high-density (such as lead) tube acts to focus the gamma-ray beam from the subject. Behind the crystal is a photomultiplier to boost the weak scintillations into measurable pulses of electric current. Finally a 'pulse height analyser' filters out pulses of the wrong energy levels that are likely to represent scattered rays that have lost some of their energy.

To be useful in clinical imaging, radioactive isotopes must have several properties. One is a radioactive half-life that is neither too short to allow practical delivery and measurement, nor so long as to continue emitting extensively once the examination is over. The radioactive half-life ($T_{\frac{1}{2}}$ is defined as the time taken for half the initial radioactive mass to decay on its exponential decay curve. In clinical practice, the effective decay time is also influenced by a biological half-life arising from natural washout of the radioisotope from the living tissue. Another desirable property is the ability of the radioisotope to be chemically tagged onto another molecule to make a 'radiopharmaceutical' designed to travel into the target tissue (brain), or bind to the target receptor.

Increase in activity in a particular brain region means increased work, demanding increased oxidative metabolism (glycolysis) and increased local arterial blood flow. This notion that, like muscular activity, central nervous activity results in a proportionally increased metabolism and blood flow is generally attributed to Ray & Sherrington (1890). Their idea was overlooked for much if this century, and until recently, the notion of an active, locally responsive cerebral blood supply was rejected. Mechanisms that mediate the local vasodilatation are unclear, but may involve nitrous oxide released postsynaptically following increased synaptic activity.

Like a plain lateral skull X-ray, an unelaborated static gamma detector system passively viewing a patient will produce a two-dimensional image in which tissues are superimposed with no clue as to depth, and furthermore where there is no correction for gamma-ray attenuation with distance. The solution is analogous to X-ray CT, with a focused detector taking a circumferential set of many one-dimensional projections, which are then reconstructed mathematically by filtered back projection into a two-dimensional slice made up of pixels. Iterative techniques can also correct for depth-dependent attenuation. The two main systems to use this method are, firstly, single photon emission tomography (SPET or SPECT) and, secondly, positron emission tomography (PET). The difference between the two systems lies essentially with the type of radioisotope used: single photon emitters or positron emitters.

Single photon emission tomography

The most common SPET instrument in use today in clinical nuclear medicine is the rotating gamma camera. For regional cerebral blood flow (rCBF) imaging, however, it is not ideal and has limited sensitivity and resolution: head-dedicated, multi-detector scanners are better. Radiopharmaceuticals for use with SPET need to combine a good gamma emitter, with a suitable half-life of a few hours at most, such as iodine-123 or technetium-99, with a molecule that allows transfer across the blood–brain barrier. ^{99}Tc-labelled hexamethyl-propyleneamine oxime (HMPAO: Amersham) crosses the blood–brain barrier proportionately to rCBF, enters the brain cells and becomes 'trapped' because of a change in ionisation at intracellular pH. A static 'snapshot' image of brain rCBF in the first minute or two following intravenous injection is thus produced. 'Dynamic' SPET giving sequences of rCBF images over time can be produced using xenon-133 gas which the subject inhales, although the images obtained are of poor quality.

Radiolabelled receptor ligands can be used with SPET (and different ones with PET) to image particular receptor sites, such as dopamine D2 receptors (iodobenzamide with SPET; raclopride or methylspiperone with PET), 5-HT$_2$ receptors (ketanserin) or GABA receptors

S.W. LEWIS

(iodomazenil; flumazenil). Usually given intravenously, these bind to specific receptors and the gamma radiation produced can be used to estimate the site, number and density of available receptor sites. This technique can be used in psychopharmacological experiments to look for abnormal numbers of receptors in untreated psychiatric disorders, or investigate the mode of action of psychotropic drugs.

Positron emission tomography

The principles of PET are similar to those of SPET. However, PET uses positron-emitting radioisotopes such as fluorine-18, oxygen-15, or carbon-11. These decay by emitting a positron, which almost immediately collides with an electron to give a pair of gamma rays emitted in diametrically opposite directions. Pairs of detectors mounted opposite one another around the head are programmed to pick up this simultaneous arrival of two gamma rays from one point and a relatively high resolution image (in the order of 5 mm) can be built up. Oxygen-15 is used to measure rCBF and fluorine-18 labelled deoxyglucose can be used to give similar maps of regional cerebral metabolism. The practical drawbacks with PET are that the radionuclides have half-lives of only a few minutes and they need an on-site cyclotron for their production. However, PET is more versatile and informative than SPET. With PET (and to a lesser extent SPET) rCBF imaging, a powerful strategy is to compare rCBF patterns at rest with those while the subject is engaged in a specific cognitive tasks. Subtracting the first from the second will give a map of those brain areas activated during the task.

Other functional imaging techniques

New magnetic resonance techniques are being developed, which in time will become the definitive functional, as well as structural, brain imaging modalities. *Magnetic resonance spectroscopy* can detect small shifts in the signal from protons or other paramagnetic nuclei such as phosphorus, when they are in particular chemical environments. Spectra are produced with different peaks corresponding to different molecules at different concentrations: with phosphorus, for example, this can be used to assess ATP turnover or membrane phospholipids. *Functional MRI* (fMRI) can also measure rCBF by using the principles of MRI to detect the small paramagnetic changes that occur when oxyhaemoglobin becomes deoxygenated in active cortex, the blood oxygen level dependent (BOLD) technique, which promises rCBF measures in the future without the need for radioisotopes. fMRI needs very fast scan times to be useful and these are made possible using new techniques such as echoplanar imaging.

EEG mapping techniques, such as brain electrical activity mapping (BEAM) can give three-dimensional maps of surface electical activity across the scalp. Magnetoencephalography is a similar technique. The main strengths in these techniques is their potential for detecting very rapid changes in real time. Problems include artefacts and low spatial resolution.

Clinical applications: dementias

The clearest clinical application for structural brain imaging in psychiatry is in the diagnosis and assessment of dementias and focal organic brain syndromes. Either CT or MRI examination is mandatory in the clinical assessment of presenile dementia and many would argue that senile dementias presenting between the ages of 65 and 75 also deserve routine structural brain imaging. The purpose is firstly to rule out treatable although rare causes of dementia such as slow growing tumours, chronic subdural haemorrhage and normal pressure hydrocephalus. In Alzheimer's disease (AD), findings on CT are of progressive enlargement of lateral and third ventricles and cortical sulci, which is earliest and most marked in medial temporal lobe regions (Pearlson, 1994). The appearances of cerebral atrophy are supportive of a diagnosis of dementia in the presence of clinical features and alongside other investigations such as neuropsychological evaluation and EEG. However, normal ageing is accompanied by reduction of brain volume by 5–10% by the age of 80, with enlargement of lateral and third ventricles and cortical cerebral sulci. Thus, the presence of cerebral atrophy on CT or MRI alone in diagnosing the presence of dementia is not a definitive diagnostic sign. A significant proportion of false positive (apparent cerebral atrophy in normal subjects) and false negative (appearances within the normal range in definite dementia) are found. Follow-up rescanning, looking for progressive change, makes for a more accurate diagnostic test (Burns & Pearlson, 1994). Furthermore, high resolution MRI with quantitative measures of hippocampal atrophy appears to be a promising and sensitive marker for AD, successfully distinguishing cases from elderly controls or depressives in about 90% of instances.

On MRI, small areas of high signal subcortically, known as white matter hyperintensities, appear in about a third of healthy elderly subjects (Boone et al., 1992). Multi-infarct dementia similarly shows the appearance of generalised cortical atrophy, along with radiological evidence of deep lacunar infarcts in about 70% of cases (Cummings & Benson, 1992). There is a large overlap with Alzheimer's disease appearances. In Huntington's disease, there is progressive atrophy of the caudate nuclei. Basal ganglia volumes have been noted to be decreased in presymptomatic individuals who are gene marker positive (Pearlson, 1994), although this is insufficiently sensitive to be of practical value. In HIV disease, structural imaging can be used firstly to exclude intracranial opportunistic infections such as cytomegalavirus, and lymphomas, and also to disclose the cerebral atrophy and periventricular white matter changes seen in the AIDS–dementia complex.

Functional imaging can also be valuable in the assessment of dementia, although it is not widely used. The evidence is that in Alzheimer's disease bilateral temporo-parietal blood flow deficits pre-date gross structural changes; SPET is the most appropriate investigation for this. Magnetic resonance imaging is useful in particular neurological disorders that may have psychiatric consequences: it is the method of choice to show the plaques of demyelinating disorders such as multiple sclerosis. Recent research (Wallis et al., 1993) suggests that MR of the hippocampus may become a more useful diagnostic tool in complex partial epilepsy of temporal lobe origin than is conventional EEG. Hippocampal atrophy in comparison to the unaffected side can usually be demonstrated with careful measurement. Ictal blood flow changes in the temporal lobe can be shown in epilepsy with SPET.

The psychoses

In schizophrenia, minor enlargement of lateral and third ventricles and cortical sulci have been shown on CT in comparison with matched healthy controls, although these are too small and non-specific to be of any diagnostic use in individual cases. This also goes for the reduction in medial temporal lobe structures, including hippocampus and amygdala, which can be seen on quantitative MRI. In 5% of cases there will be static, neurodevelopmental lesions, which will be of little significance to the management of the illness (Lewis, 1990). There is a good case in an illness as severe as schizophrenia for performing routine CT or MRI in all first episode cases. This is mandatory if there is a history of neurological symptoms (such as seizures) or focal signs on examination. Severe affective disorders can also show minor degrees of ventricular enlargement. Structural imaging is indicated in refractory or atypical cases to exclude occult neurological disease.

Functional imaging has little clinical role as yet in the diagnosis and management of the psychoses. In a research context, PET studies have shown correlations with patterns of symptoms. In particular, negative symptoms in schizophrenia and psychomotor retardation in depression seem to share a similar cerebral functional deficit, with decreased activity in left dorsolateral prefrontal cortex (Liddle et al., 1992).

Future developments

Magnetic resonance applications will become increasingly important in psychiatry. High resolution structural imaging will become central to the early diagnosis and staging of primary dementias and may become a more important tool in helping determine prognosis in schizophrenia. Advances in image analysis will allow routine co-registration of structural and functional MR images. This will lead to refinements in understanding the action of new pharmacological and psychological treatments in schizophrenia and other psychoses, with the prospect of designing optimum treatment packages tailored to the symptom patterns seen in individual patients.

PART II

CLINICAL DISORDERS

5

Child and adolescent psychiatry

PETER HILL

Introduction

Child and adolescent psychiatry (child psychiatry for short) is the general application of psychiatry to an age group, taken here as being those under the age of 18. It is concerned with children who suffer from emotional symptoms, whose psychosocial development is distorted, whose personal relationships are impaired or whose extreme behaviour gives rise to distress to their family or other caregiving adults. Such children are colloquially considered as psychologically disturbed when their condition is not easily understood or managed. The lay observer seeks single causes or simple explanations and when these fail, assumes a psychological fault within the child, a mental flaw akin to an illness. In contrast, the psychiatrist recognises a complex, multifactorial causality that commonly yields symptoms (a term generally used to include signs) that often differ from normality by degree rather than type. Symptoms or behaviours pathognomonic of psychiatric disorder in childhood are unusual: more commonly it is their frequency, severity, persistence or occurrence at an inappropriate age that indicate pathology.

Childhood is not a homogeneous epoch and children change with age. Many psychiatric conditions in childhood are distortions of psychosocial development. The child's disorder must therefore be appraised in a developmental context. An influential conceptual approach emphasising this and thereby forging links between the study of development and psychiatric disorder is termed developmental psychopathology. This concerns itself with explanations as to why variations between children arise in emotional, behavioural and cognitive development, examines the continuities and discontinuities between normality and abnormality, and considers interactions between genetic and environmental influences. Disorders are understood to be the outcome of complex interactions between aetiological factors rather than resulting from single disease processes.

Psychosocial development necessarily takes place within an interpersonal setting within which the quality of attitudes and relationships is crucial. The family is the principal crucible for this process in childhood and peer group influences are added to this as the child matures. The origin of the child's symptoms may lie within the family or its response to them may maintain the problem. In addition, parents are in a position of power over their children and are thus central to processes such as engaging mental health services or implementing treatments on their behalf. Not surprisingly, child and adolescent psychiatrists are as concerned with families and family dysfunction as they are with individual children.

However, the child is not passive. Genetic endowment shapes emotions and behaviours and these affect the child's family members (Scarr, 1992). Their responses also elicit and moderate further responses on the child's part. The child influences his environment which also influences him (the male pronoun is used in this chapter since boys are more likely to exhibit disorder). There is an intimate and mutual interaction between the child and his caregivers, which must be included in formulation, treatment and the assessment of prognosis. This interaction is ongoing and makes a simple statement about causation difficult (Blanz et al., 1991). It is necessary to consider Predisposing, Precipitating and Perpetuating factors and, with respect to the latter, to take a systemic view and examine reciprocal effects between child, family and a wider environment. These are often self-sustaining yet can have a perverse effect upon the child who exhibits maladaptive behaviour or experiences distress.

It has often been said, aphoristically, that at the heart of an emotional or behavioural problem of a child there is a child trying to solve a problem. In adapting to a stressor, the child may respond in a way that is intended to relieve stress but actually exacerbates it or causes major distress to others. The analogy is with inflammation. While not always an adequate explanation for psychiatric disorder in the young, the aphorism makes the point that a number of emotional and behavioural disorders arise out of environmental adversities to which the child must actively adapt. Such adversities may be continuing, such as persistent marital discord between the parents, or they may be discrete and termed life events. Most commonly, several adversities of both types can be seen to operate when a child is a clinical case. Usually they do more than add up; they interact so that each multiplies the effect of another. Children who are exposed to adversity yet do not become clinical cases may have experienced less adversity or may possess or experience protective factors such as high intelligence or a warm emotional relationship with a parent. Alternatively they may show a positive adjustment to stress, which can subsequently prove to be a steeling experience, prompting the development of new skills or knowledge that can confer resilience. But some children are vulnerable and develop adjustments to adversities that are associated with substantial personal distress, are self-defeating or are problematic for their caregivers. If sufficiently persistent these may be included among the range of psychiatric disorders.

Classification

There have been four major approaches to the definition of psychiatric disorder in childhood.

1. The recent European tradition has been to identify its presence when emotional or behavioural deviation from the norm is associated with significant suffering or with impaired personal functioning or impaired development. That is to say that the child is handicapped by his symptoms or their effect (the impairment criterion).

2. The North American clinical approach has been to identify disorder when there are

enough clinical features of sufficient duration and severity to qualify as a particular identified disorder within the DSM classificatory system. This approach has also been implicitly adopted in ICD-10 though the introduction to Chapter V of this book invokes the necessity for an impairment criterion too. In parallel, DSM now includes an impairment criterion for most categories in its fourth revision. Both systems are, of course, categorical. In other words, disorders (not children) are recognised by possessing certain characteristics in common. Assigning a child's condition to a diagnostic category enables predictions about aetiology, course, and treatment to be made.

3. An older tradition identifies normal developmental trajectories, relationships and mental mechanisms in terms of psychoanalytic metaphor and recognises disorder when these are considered faulty.

4. Within the research arena, dimensional approaches have had some influence, especially that arising from the application of multivariate statistics to scores on the Child Behaviour Checklist (see Achenbach & Edelbrock, 1978) within populations of children. For many clinicians such approaches differ little from the categorical approach at an early level of analysis since they tend to identify major groups of internalising and externalising behaviours that correspond to emotional and conduct disorders respectively. At further levels of analysis, groupings tend to depend upon the statistic selected and some rare conditions are omitted. There is also the possibility that extremes of dimensions are actually different from lesser deviations, as in severe mental retardation (Plomin et al., 1991).

Within ICD-10 there is both a section devoted to behavioural and emotional disorders with onset usually occurring in childhood and adolescence and a section of disorders of psychological development which also are evident in childhood. Children can also suffer conditions described in other sections. The structure of ICD-10 is not entirely consistent and its introduction points out the inconsistency of listing anorexia nervosa and gender identity disorders within the 'adult' section even though they usually have an onset in childhood or adolescence.

In general, disorders tend to be more precisely defined and differentiated with increasing age throughout childhood and adolescence. The range of conditions in late teenagers is much more like the range encountered in an adult population but the disorders of pre-school children are quite different. In between there is a transition that is exemplified by considering the pattern of disorders in adolescence. In the early teens, the range of conditions and problems is generally similar to that in middle childhood so that, for instance, hyperkinetic disorder, separation anxiety disorder or faecal soiling would readily be found within a group of clinic attenders but manic depressive disorder, substance abuse, eating disorders or schizophrenia would be rare. By the age of 17, these latter conditions would have become much more frequently encountered and the former have themselves become rare. In parallel with this, there is a shift from a male predominance among affected young teenagers to an excess of girls in middle and late teens, a phenomenon mainly do to the increase with age of depressive and anxiety disorders (Cohen et al., 1993).

There is a serious problem with comorbidity in child and adolescent psychiatry: many children display a clinical picture that fulfils the diagnostic criteria of more than one condition (Caron & Rutter, 1991). In part this is understandable since the causation and maintenance of psychiatric disorders in the young is complex and interactive; a number of adversities and vulnerabilities are general rather than specific in their effects. But there are also insufficient hierarchical rules in the main classificatory systems to indicate how one condition can trump or subsume another pattern of clinical features.

For the last two decades it has been customary for academic departments of child and adolescent psychiatry to organise linear classificatory systems such as ICD-9 into a multi-axial classificatory system to ensure full description of the child's condition. That practice became mainstream for psychiatry with the advent of DSM-III but ICD-10 is still principally a linear, monaxial system though there is a multiaxial version for child and adolescent psychiatric disorders in press. It contains axes for

- clinical psychiatric syndromes
- specific developmental disorder
- intellectual level
- physical disorders
- level of adaptive functioning
- psychosocial factors

Epidemiology

The above considerations make generalisations about the frequencies of psychiatric disorders in childhood and adolescence difficult. Furthermore, the use of an impairment criterion means that a condition will be less frequently diagnosed and ICD-10 will therefore identify conditions less frequently in a given population than did DSM-III, even though the conditions described in each classifactory system are qualitatively very similar. There are difficulties in knowing how best to combine information from several sources. Lastly, the type of interview used will alter detection threshold: structured schedules that score responses and sum these will differ in sensitivity from those that require the interviewer to evaluate responses and make a judgement (Breslau, 1987). With this in mind, there may still be value in considering the epidemiology of child and adolescent psychiatric disorder as a whole.

The overall rate of psychiatric disorder varies according to criteria, locality and age range. Several large epidemiological studies have been carried out, particularly in the UK, US, Canada, Puerto Rico, New Zealand and Sweden, which demonstrate both common ground and variation. There are some salient findings (see Costello, 1989; Brandenburg et al., 1990; Rutter, 1989a,b).

An overall rate of 7% for severe emotional and behaviour problems in preschool children was provided by the Waltham Forest study of three-year-olds (Richman et al., 1975). A further 15% had less severe, though appreciable, psychological problems of similar type. For the group of affected children, taken as a whole, there were associations with poor quality of parental marriage, maternal depression and delayed language development. Chronicity was remarkable. Two-thirds of the affected children continued to show emotional and behaviour problems five years later (Stevenson *et al.*, 1985), a finding echoed by the 54% persistence rate over three years in the Martha's Vineyard study (Garrison & Earls, 1985).

In middle childhood, the classical studies on the Isle of Wight (Rutter *et al.*, 1970) and in South London (Rutter *et al.*, 1975) used a two-stage design: questionnaire detection followed by interview (the child and parents in the Isle of Wight (IOW) study and teachers in the London one). A rate of 6.8% for psychiatric disorder among ten year-olds on the semi-rural island was doubled, when questionnaire data were compared, in a urban part of inner London. In each case an impairment criterion was employed. DSM-criteria yield much higher figures for psychological morbidity. Offord *et al.* (1987) using DSM-III criteria in a study of 4–11-year-olds in Ontario employed a two-stage study including cut-off criteria derived from interviews with a subsample of children. They found 19.5% of boys and 13.5% of girls to be cases of conduct, emotional, somatisation or attention deficit disorder. Cohen *et al.* (1993) suggested that most recent studies indicate an approximate prevalence rate of 20% for DSM-III diagnoses among school-age children. Most of these are strikingly persistent over time. The point that DSM-III will yield higher prevalence rates than a system using an impairment criterion needs to be borne in mind; DSM rates seem very high to a European-trained psychiatrist.

Studies of psychiatric disorder in adolescence are bedevilled by at least two problems. One is the fact that adolescence is not a homogeneous epoch, as pointed out above. The other is the ambiguous standing of information derived from the adolescents themselves, rather than their parents or teachers. For instance, if parent and teacher information is relied upon, Rutter *et al.* (1976) found an overall rate of 8% but this rose to 21% when data from the adolescents were included. This latter figure, although thought to be unrealistically high at the time, is supported by the Ontario study, which yielded rates for psychiatric disorder (DSM-III criteria) among 12–16-year-olds of 19% of boys and 22% of girls (Offord *et al.*, 1987). These figures are generally in line with an overall rate of 22% with DSM-III disorder among 15-year-olds interviewed in the Dunedin study (McGee *et al.*, 1990). Slightly more conservative figures have been suggested by reviewers who place emphasis upon impairment criteria and Hill (1989), for example, suggested that studies carried out before DSM-III yielded some consensus around a prevalence rate of 15%.

Within the overall figures, the prevalence rates for individual disorders are masked but a host of studies have yielded figures for these, conveniently listed by Wieselberg (1993). Some of these are cited within specific sections of this chapter.

It is possible to make some general remarks about risk factors for child psychiatric disorder. By and large they derive from large sample studies of middle childhood, within which the two groupings of emotional/internalising and conduct/externalising disorders numerically swamp all other diagnoses. For instance, in the IOW study (Rutter *et al.*, 1970), these two conditions accounted for 2.5% and 4% of all children respectively and thus 96% of all disordered children in that survey. At that time, British child psychiatry was dominated by a child guidance system that was closely linked with education and predominantly addressed the needs of 7–14-year-olds. Contemporary clinical practice addresses a wider age range and the problems of pre-school children and teenagers are given as much weight as those of middle childhood. Finer discrimination within the major diagnostic groupings is now reflected in more diagnostic categories in classificatory systems. There are also age differences with respect to size of effect. Family adversities are less powerful aetiological factors in adolescence (Blanz *et al.*, 1991). Nevertheless, there is some virtue in listing overall risk factors:

- In the individual child
  - boys are more prone to disorder than girls up until the mid teens
  - the rate of disorder increases progressively with lowering of overall intelligence
  - chronic physical illness (double the risk on the IOW)
  - brain damage (increased the risk fivefold on the IOW)
  - difficult temperament
  - general and specific genetic factors
- In the family
  - discordant, openly hostile or argumentative family relationships
  - child abuse or neglect
  - criminality in another family member
  - psychiatric disorder in a parent, particularly the mother
  - divorce, bereavement, repeated separations from parents or other family disruption
- In wider society
  - social disadvantage (but not social class in all psychiatric disorder is considered together)
  - inner urban living

Many of these, listed as variables in studies, are simplifications of complex processes within which various aetiological and maintaining mechanisms operate (see Rutter, 1989). Clinical practice is involved with detail at this level; family therapy, for instance, is concerned with the fine grain of relationship dynamics and behaviour patterns that cannot be reflected in epidemiology. Research, too, is as interested in, say, the genetic origins of individual disorders and the micro-environment of the families of conduct-disordered boys, as it is in overall statements about risk, adversity, vulnerability or resilience.

Further identification of risk, or indeed protective, factors includes the effects of one condition on the likelihood of another. Some such conditions can be conceptualised as disorders: for instance, hyperkinetic disorder increases the risk of subsequent conduct disorder (see below) or specific reading disorder in middle childhood, which is associated with elevated rates of conduct disorder in some (but not all) studies. Others are attributes of the child: difficult temperament or, more complicatedly, poor peer relationships, both risk factors for disorder or poor prognosis.

The power of the social psychiatric model that draws upon developmental psychopathology is its ability to accommodate such an interplay of aetiological factors. Cox (1993) provides an elegant exposition of current knowledge, emphasising the power of environmental adversity in producing child psychiatric disorder. Accordingly it has been tempting to apply the concept of adjustment disorder to a large number of psychiatrically disordered children because the concept of reaction to adversity has such wide application. Yet, as Hill (1994*a*) pointed out, the central tenets of adjustment disorder are illogical and the term persists only by habit. It is not a concept that is developed in this chapter.

Development and disorder

Childhood and adolescence are developmental epochs characterised by rapid change. The relative prevalence and clinical picture of childhood psychiatric disorders vary according to age. Furthermore, development itself can be distorted and produce extreme variations that may be regarded as disorder. Knowledge of psychological development is necessary. Thus it is important, for instance, to have a grasp of attachment theory in order to understand the problems of pre-school children, particularly those associated with anxiety, for whom the attachment relationship is an important source of reassurance and dysphoria management generally. Indeed, the dual function of parents as attachment, anxiety-relieving figures on one hand and socialising agents on the other is what makes it so difficult for some children and some parents to learn how to cope with unwelcome rules and alarming situations. Many of the problems of young children – sleeping difficulties, feeding problems, temper tantrums and disobedience – can be traced to a tension between whether a parent is primarily a source of emotional security or a disciplinarian. The child cannot understand how someone who at other times provides comfort can also insist upon a disciplinary requirement that produces discomfort. Attachment is also a prerequisite for adequate social functioning among peers so that insecure or abortive attachments are associated with peer rejection, a further risk factor for psychiatric disorder.

The fundamental issues of attachment and temperament are not addressed here but are described in child development textbooks, in the earlier edition of this book (Hill, 1986), or in review papers (Prior, 1992; Rutter, 1995). Some of the vicissitudes of attachment are classified as disorders. Thus *separation anxiety disorder* refers to a markedly severe version of normal separation fears with excessive clinging and preoccupations about abandonment, the possibility of a disaster affecting a parent or irrational fears of kidnappers. *Reactive attachment disorder* is indicated by a combination of anxious avoidant attachment with hypervigilance and poor ability to maintain peer group interactions; it is seen as a consequence of parental maltreatment. *Disinhibited attachment disorder* is the pattern of diffuse and unselective attachment behaviour, indiscriminate friendliness and attention-seeking found in children who have been unable to form selective attachments during infancy.

These are severe distortions of development. It is important not to confuse common or minor developmental difficulties with psychiatric disorder. Indeed, the confusion of disorder with development itself was typical of several decades of thinking about adolescence. It is now well known that although minor psychological symptoms are common in adolescence (as they are in early adult life), most adolescents do not have a psychiatric disorder and disorder in adolescence is to be taken as seriously as at any other epoch (see Hill, 1989). Yet development can regress as well as progress and a regression in development (such as the appearance of separation anxiety in a young teenager) can be an important symptom of distress or dysfunction.

The professional preoccupation with development can create difficulty. Because children and adolescents are by definition immature and are still seen as having developmental potential, some diagnoses such as personality disorder are made with reluctance. Yet a number of children seen clinically have manifest disturbances of personality and it becomes difficult to characterise their condition. A few diagnostic categories such as Asperger's syndrome are available but otherwise the use of terms that concentrate upon one feature of the condition (describing abnormal attachment, conduct or hyperkinesis) predominates. On occasion there is no adequate term in general use by child psychiatrists; for instance to describe disproportionate social immaturity or self-centred callousness.

Nevertheless, the child and adolescent psychiatrist always has to consider developmental needs and status. They influence assessment, so that interviewing parents is always necessary and interviews with the child must attend to communicative and cognitive maturity level. They govern the selection of treatment intervention, so that children are usually managed on an out-patient basis in the care of their parents rather than being admitted to hospital. They influence prognosis when maladaptive behaviours and attributions in a young child become ingrained in a general response style or world view (as in abuse victims).

Child abuse and neglect

The concept of child abuse has expanded from the original 'battered baby' image to a notion of severe parenting failure which includes (1) physical abuse; (2) emotional abuse; (3) sexual abuse; and (4) neglect. Definitions of these can be attempted but with two caveats: that most of those that have been coined define abuse in terms of perpetrator behaviour, and that any definition is relative to local and contemporary cultural standards of child care. Indeed, a recent form of words, frequently used in discussion, is that the child has been treated in an unacceptable way by an adult in a given culture at a given time. This describes the concept but does not define the limits of acceptability. Such limits are hard to delineate because exactly what parents have to do in order to rear children adequately is not known in detail. We do know the general principles of adequate child-rearing and we recognise that parents do not have to be perfect, but 'good enough' in Winnicott's phrase (see Adcock & White, 1985). Yet different children make different demands upon parents for protection and support in development so an interactive approach is inevitable. For such reasons, studies and practice have concentrated upon extreme instances. Nevertheless the problem is not rare: Skuse & Bentovim (1994) have suggested that 4% of UK children will be notified to child protection agencies at some time in their childhood. Meadow (1989a) has stated that four UK children die each week as a result of child abuse.

One clinical problem is that many children who have experienced abuse have suffered several forms. Nearly all physical abuse by parents is also emotional abuse because the abusing parent negates the trust placed in him or her by the child. The subcategorisation of abuse makes it possible to handle it bureaucratically (for child protection registers) but such a typology does not necessarily predict prognosis or treatment; the whole picture must be taken into account and multiple forms of maltreatment and neglect are common. Child abuse is not a diagnosis. A situation in which a child is abused will evoke medical interest at several levels: the child, the effect of non-abusing parents, and the perpetrator. All may need treatment; the child may also require medical appraisal to provide evidence as to whether there has been abuse for legal purposes. The phenomenon of abuse involves knowledge that the abusive act has been perpetrated and that the child has been harmed, the two components of the concept of 'significant harm'; a term coined in the English Children Act 1989. Psychiatrists from different specialties therefore have various interests and responsibilities in all this but all also need to have a knowledge of working with child protection procedures alongside social services departments, the police, probation service and the courts. There will be local arrangements for this. Within England and Wales the legal framework is the Children Act and various advisory documents such as *Working Together under the Children Act* (Department of Health, 1991*d*) support this.

Physical abuse

The definition usually adopted of 'non-accidental injury (NAI) which results from acts or omissions on the part of parents or guardians and which violates community standards of adequate child care' rests upon judgements based upon norms which will vary locally and historically. Physical injury resulting in tissue damage is often held to be the threshold of unacceptability but this would not necessarily include intentional poisoning or suffocation. Annual incidence rates in various countries vary according to local criteria and there are obvious difficulties in the reliable estimation of population rates of a phenomenon which is already hard to detect. Some agreement exists that a minimum of about 0.5% of children under three years of age will suffer *serious* injury as a result of physical abuse each year (see Parke & Collmer, 1975) but the rate for abuse of adolescents is thought to be higher than among small children (Garbarino, 1989). The survey by the US National Center on Child Abuse and Neglect (1988) suggested an annual rate of 2.5%, though this included a majority of cases of neglect. It was lower than the figure of 4% obtained in a cross-cultural study between Sweden and the US (Somander & Rammer, 1991) but this included some mild cases in which there was a risk rather than actual injury.

Abuse does not necessarily associate with generally inadequate child care. An outburst of helpless rage against a persistently crying baby may coexist with otherwise reasonable child care. Nevertheless, habitual violence towards a child is often a feature of chronic polymorphous child abuse (physical, emotional, and sexual) and neglect. Parents who physically abuse their children are more likely to be socially disadvantaged, lack social support systems, have experienced an excess of recent adverse life events, have high stress levels, and use an authoritarian parenting style coupled with a lack of involvement with their children. In Skuse & Bentovim's (1994) terms there is a picture of 'worried parents, with little enjoyment of parenting, little satisfaction with and expressed affection for their child, isolation from the wider community and a lack of encouragement for the development of autonomy . . . in their child . . . yet (they) also expect high standards of achievement'. Detection of physical abuse will rest in the first instance upon an adequate degree of suspicion. The characteristics of suspicious injuries are primarily a concern of paediatricians and general practitioners and are not detailed here.

A remarkable variant of physical abuse is the systematic poisoning of children by a parent, apparently thereby to obtain psychological gain, for instance by being admitted to hospital with their child and becoming involved with professional carers. Known as 'Munchausen syndrome by proxy' (see Meadow, 1989), it has a different mode of presentation (bleeding, neurological signs, rashes, glycosuria, etc.) and is associated with rather different family dynamics to the more familiar forms of physical abuse. It may also present as enforced invalidism. A notorious instance is the partial suffocation of a baby by the mother or nurse who then claims the child suffered an apnoeic episode (Southall *et al.*, 1987) though sometimes the suffocation proves fatal and presents as cot death. The vast majority of cot deaths are not caused by such suffocation.

The immediate results of physical abuse include a 10% mortality rate among instances of serious battering (Baldwin & Oliver, 1975), but it is the longer-term consequences which are more frequently the concern of psychiatrists, usually because of psychological consequences of the experience of abuse and concomitant neglect. Note, however, that shaking a baby can cause cerebral cortical microhaemorrhages, which in turn produce cognitive or language delays.

In the medium term, abused children will display psychological symptoms, the extent of which has been well reviewed by Aber *et al.* (1989). They will typically be unhappy, wary, untrusting, angry and indifferent to others' distress in peer-group relationships, and either excessively inhibited or grossly aggressive and provocative when dealing with adults. Lacking in self-esteem, some will, when older, exhibit poor academic achievement. A few may act in a pseudo-mature way, even being solicitous towards their abusing parents – presumably to guard against any failure to meet parental expectations, which could trigger a violent outburst. A number of affected children will fulfil the criteria for reactive attachment disorder. Physical abuse suffered in early childhood has a powerful link with later aggressive behaviour (Dodge *et al.* 1990). Many of the reported sequelae of physical abuse are actually a consequence of the inevitable emotional abuse that follows the betrayal of the child's trust in the parent coupled with the fact that physical and separate emotional abuse commonly co-occur in any case.

Intervention that goes beyond measures to secure child protection by using the relevant legislation in concert with social services departments, is usually to try to reduce the chance of repetition by training parents in parenting. However, the success rates of such interventions in the US (see Cohn & Daro, 1987) or the UK (Smith & Rachman, 1984; Nicol *et al.*, 1988) has not been impressive and re-abuse or drop-out from treatment are not at all uncommon. Psychotherapeutic work with the victims is unevaluated and some psychotherapists specifically exclude physical abuse victims from treatment on the basis that they are too damaged by their childhood experiences. Primary prevention studies have usually targeted high-risk groups and in a fairly comprehensive review MacMillan *et al.* (1994*a,b,*) considered that home visitation programmes held some promise of moderate effectiveness.

Emotional abuse

All forms of abuse by parental figures include emotional harming. The concept of emotional abuse isolated from the other forms of abuse and neglect is poorly defined. Some aspects of emotional cruelty can be displayed when ordinary parents are exasperated and once again it is of degree or persistence, coupled with demonstrable damage of the child that defines abuse. Glaser (1993) has provided a helpful overview that includes a categorisation of inappropriate parental behaviour and the following subcategories are a simplification of her scheme:

Persistent negative attitudes
- overt rejection or blame, attributing inherent badness to the child
- unremitting verbal abuse
- sadistic terrorising by threats of severe violence
- excessive non-physical punishments such as prolonged isolation, refusing to speak to the child, or exposure to feared stimuli
- belittlement, denigration or mocking and taunting

Use of guilt and fear as the predominant disciplinary practices
- threats of abandonment used as disciplinary tool
- making continued care conditional upon the child's behaviour or gratitude
- induction of guilt or terror to promote compliance

Ignorance or exploitation of the child's immature developmental status
- inappropriate expectations or imposed responsibilities
- incorrect accusations or motivations such as persecution or wilfulness
- use of mystification or intentional bewilderment

Distorted recognition of the child's individuality
- using the child to obtain vicarious satisfaction for the parent or to fulfil other parental needs other than ordinary parental pride and satisfaction
- involvement of the child in delusional or coercively applied ideological systems

Clearly such practices exploit the natural dependence, loyalty and credulity of children and are not confined to parents. Many are mediated verbally. This means they can be observed directly as compared to physical or sexual abuse, which are detected retrospectively by observation of wounds, behaviour or as a result of disclosure. The essential feature is the patients' active abuse of their child's emotions, which goes beyond the neglect of a child's emotional needs for adequate development.

The signs of emotional damage to the child are not specific to abuse. They include abnormal attachment behaviour patterns, persistent free-floating guilt or anxiety, poor self-esteem, incorrigible stealing from home, covert attacks on parents' possessions, placement of urine or faeces as if to exert revenge, compulsive eating of sweet foods, social withdrawal and underachievement (often colloquially described as 'depression') or angry misbehaviour, apparently in self-confirmation of a 'bad' role identity. Such children are nearly always shunned by their peers (see Mueller & Silverman, 1989).

A child may be relatively protected from emotional abuse by having a warm relationship with another non-abusive parent or grandparent and the ability to perceive an abusing parent as nevertheless benevolent (Farber & Egeland, 1987).

Interventions in emotional abuse need not follow the pathway prescribed for intrafamilial physical or sexual abuse: investigation and confirm, protect the child, treat. Rather, a trial of treatment of the parent–child relationship (which will include advice and training to the abusing parent) should be initiated to test response. Protection procedures need only be instigated should this fail.

Sexual abuse

This is a composite term for the sexual exploitation of a child by a sexually mature individual. It includes abuse by adults or older children in a position of trust, especially those with parental responsibilities, as well as so-called strangers who are in fact quite often known to the child, such as babysitters or teachers. The term incest is narrowly defined in law and refers to vaginal intercourse with a first degree female blood relative. Child sex abuse (CSA) is a broader concept and includes both homosexual and heterosexual encounters involving any of a range of activities that sexually arouse the abuser: exposing, peeping, fondling, masturbating, oral–genital contact and penetrative sex. These can occur in affectionate as well as coercive or violent settings, within and outside of the family.

Given such a broad concept, prevalence figures inevitably vary. Further uncertainty is produced by the variety of enquiry methods used by surveys and different approaches to sampling. More sophisticated studies (e.g. Anderson *et al.*, 1993) provide different rates for different types of abuse. Smith & Bentovim (1994), reviewing existing knowledge, suggested that 15–30% of women will have been subjected to unwanted sexual contact during childhood and probably twice that number to a sexual experience not involving contact. Of the contact group, some 5% (i.e. roughly 1–1.5% of all women) have experienced penetrative sex. Community samples show a female to male ratio among victims of about 2.5:1, a smaller gender difference than applies in clinical samples. Girls are more likely to have been abused within their families, boys by strangers. The mild association between CSA and socio-economic disadvantage reported in some clinical samples disappears for girls (though possibly not for boys) in community samples. Although exhibitionism and fondling are the commonest forms of CSA, nearly half of boy victims are masturbated or buggered by a perpetrator. First abuse is most usual between the ages of 8 and 12. Many children are subject to several types of sexual abuse and there may be coexisting physical abuse in 15–25%. Men are the usual perpetrators and in clinical studies fathers the commonest subgroup. Stepfathers, although numerically fewer, are proportionally over-represented.

Intrafamilial abuse is the more likely form to come to clinical attention and probably the more severe variant since it involves a breach of trust and family relationship dysfunction, which may exert an additional aetiological influence on psychopathology. It also tends to involve repeated abuse whereas stranger abuse in not uncommonly a single episode. Within clinical samples, which are thus more likely to include girls and protracted abuse, the clinical effects on the individual child include:

- heightened sexual activities: public masturbation, seductive behaviour towards adults, sexual abuse of younger children or, less commonly, inhibition of normal age-appropriate sexual activity.
- a sense of guilt about, and responsibility for, the abuse
- a sense of powerlessness, social isolation and poor self-esteem
- anger towards either the abuser or the non-abusing parent (who should have protected them)

- intrusive memories and thoughts about the abuse with anxiety, insomnia, hypervigilance concerning the perpetrator, and avoidance of situations that are reminiscent of the abuse, sometimes to the extent of post-traumatic stress disorder
- a range of somatic symptoms (aches and pains) and possibly elevated rates of eating disorders
- an increased rate of self-harm (overdoses, self-cutting, running away)
- a decline in school achievement
- (mainly boys) increased aggressive antisocial behaviour, especially bullying, perhaps to overcome feelings of vulnerability

Probably CSA increases the rate of most psychiatric symptomatology in children as a non-specific risk factor; most, but not all, abused children are symptomatic (Monck *et al.*, 1995). Psychopathology is more likely to ensue if CSA is

- repeated
- coercive
- penetrative
- perpetrated by a parent
- met with maternal hostility when disclosed to her
- preceded by stressful experiences

In subsequent adult life, depressive and anxiety disorders, marital and sexual problems and low self-esteem have a higher than expected rate (Mullen *et al.*, 1988; Bifulco *et al.*, 1991).

The management of CSA is often inextricably linked with child protection issues. It can come to light in three main ways: spontaneous disclosure by the child, the presence of a physical complication such as unexplained pregnancy or a sexually transmitted disease, or as a result of questioning by a professional who suspects the possibility. The child's account of the abuse is central since physical findings are only detected in a minority (no more than 40% in the view of the Royal College of Physicians, (1991), though many would think this is a high estimated rate and a more widely accepted figure is 20%). Disclosure to anyone but an experienced investigator should be met by a few questions to confirm the likelihood of abuse, followed by a request for assistance from a senior colleague before activating local child protection procedures if appropriate. Investigative interviews to detect CSA are a skilled process and experienced interviewers are more effective and more reliable (Lanktree *et al.*, 1991; Wiseman *et al.*, 1992) The use of anatomically correct dolls is controversial and their role takes second place to an approach that is supportive to the child, structured and balances facilitatory and non-directive techniques (Vizard, 1991; Jones, 1992). It is usual practice to videotape the interview.

Helping a child to overcome CSA, once child protection issues have been resolved, will include assisting emotional processing by helping the child to recollect her experiences within a supportive individual or group context while teaching coping strategies such as relaxation, cognitive reframing, and covert self-reassurance. The issue of responsibility is dealt with by repeated explanations. Hypersexualisation needs control by establishing norms and providing age-appropriate sexual knowledge; it may need to be dealt with as a disciplinary issue by carers or teachers.

Rehabilitation within the family is occasionally successful and requires intensive family work, which necessarily includes open discussion of family issues. Most known CSA victims require alternative family care in the homes of relatives, foster families or children's homes so that the effects of family breakdown dictate additional therapeutic work with the affected child.

Neglect

This is plainly a matter of degree. The child's parents fail to act to ensure his or her nutrition, health, safety and adequate development. Emotional unavailability, by intent or as a result of parental depression, may be included here or, according to some authorities, under the heading of emotional abuse. Parental shortcomings are usually multiple and persistent. Neglect is usually inferred from pathological consequences: failure to thrive in infancy, retardation of language development, or impaired development of selective interpersonal affectional bonds. Rarely, children are kept in appalling conditions of multiple privation and emerge with severely compromised development (see Skuse, 1988).

Most, but not all, non-organic failure to thrive in infancy arises from deviant parent–child interactions that compromise adequate feeding, though most such children will not be abused in other ways (Skuse *et al.*, 1992). Growth failure may be permanent and result in psychosocial short stature ('deprivation dwarfism'), in which bodily proportions are immature but weight is normal for height. Stunting of growth is commonly accompanied by ravenous feeding and searching for food, even at night. Sleep is disturbed independently of this with an abnormally small amount of slow-wave sleep and frequent wakings. Cognitive capacities are generally poor and intelligence is typically in the mild mental retardation range with concomitant language delay. Mood is lowered and apathy a common problem. Relationships with others are shallow, unselective and unfulfilling, with importunate approaches to others, social disinhibition and true attention-seeking behaviour. This is the consequence of impaired attachment development and may fulfil the criteria for disinhibited attachment disorder.

Procedural issues

Developed societies have procedures for ensuring the prompt protection of an abused or neglected child; in England and Wales this is the emergency protection order, which allows the child to be removed to a place of safety, usually by the police or social services, or kept in hospital following presentation there. Further action is taken by local social services working together with medical and police services and eventually a multidisciplinary case conference is called to determine further action and to consider placing the child's name on a child protection register. A care plan that goes beyond assuring the child's safety and attempts to remedy the home situation or find alternative parenting for the child can be planned between the various agencies. Some longer-term legal framework is usual to maintain protection and ensure the best interests of the child are met; in the UK by a Care Order, made by a court of law.

Anxiety disorders

The classification of anxiety disorders in children and teenagers uses a number of categories. Phobias, predominantly those of single objects or defined situations, are well recognised as *phobic anxiety disorder of childhood* or simple phobia disorder (DSM-IV). By current convention, fear of strangers or social encounters is separately recognised as *social anxiety disorder* or social phobia (DSM-IV). Separation anxiety, a normal phenomenon during attachment formation in early childhood, is *separation anxiety disorder* if overwhelming. Children can receive a diagnosis of *generalised anxiety disorder* according to the same criteria as adults. Panic attacks in the setting of other childhood anxiety disorder are, of course, well-recognised. Although, for practical purposes, classical *panic disorder* occurs infrequently in prepubertal children (Klein *et al.*, 1992), in adolescence the prevalence of panic disorder is about 1% (Ollendick *et al.*, 1994). There are also particular patterns of anxiety-related pathology: school refusal, elective mutism and post-traumatic stress disorder, which are classified separately. Obsessive-compulsive disorder is classified separately because of the developing view that it is not an anxiety disorder.

The difficulty is that there is insufficient evidence to justify anything more than tentative category boundaries. Anxiety is distributed throughout the general population in varying degrees of severity and it is not certain that severe anxiety can validly be regarded as a separate anxiety disorder. Klein (1994) suggests that four conditions be met before diagnosing any anxiety disorder:

- the child continues to be abnormally anxious or apprehensive in the absence of anxiogenic stimuli;
- the child's ability to participate in age-appropriate social and academic activities is compromised;
- there is an inflexibility of affective response so that a variety of situations that are not intrinsically anxiogenic for other children provoke a high level of anxiety or apprehension;
- there is a desychronisation from normal development, e.g. separation anxiety in an adolescent.

These are akin to the familiar impairment/suffering criterion referred to earlier. Such an approach suggests that anxiety disorder cannot be diagnosed by questionnaire alone and anxiety questionnaires for children have not achieved satisfactory validity (Perrin & Last, 1992).

Furthermore, there is extensive comorbidity among the various categories of anxiety disorder in childhood. In various epidemiological studies using DSM-III, a substantial minority (roughly 20–40%) of children with anxiety disorders received more than one anxiety disorder diagnosis (Kashani & Orvaschel, 1988; McGee *et al.*, 1990). There is also an appreciable (30–80%) comorbidity rate with depressive disorder though anxiety usually precedes depression chronologically (Bird *et al.*, 1988; Kovacs *et al.*, 1989). A subgroup of children with hyperkinetic disorder also have pathological levels of anxiety (Pliszka, 1989).

Clearly there is work to be done in teasing out the subcategories within pathological anxiety. The problem may be inflated by increased comorbidity, which will affect any clinical sample. Anxious children are a minority among clinic populations yet in two-stage epidemiological studies of the general population they form one of the commonest diagnoses. Benjamin *et al.* (1990) have reported a rate of 5.4% for all anxiety disorders among 7–11 year olds and Kashani & Orvaschel (1988) a rate of 8.7% among 14–16 year olds. In epidemiological studies there is no consensus as to which subcategory is the commonest, though in those studies including parental accounts, simple phobias usually appear as the commonest and avoidant disorder/social phobia the least common. Yet simple phobias are rare in clinical practice, which is more concerned with separation and generalised anxiety disorders. Clearly there is considerable selection of clinic cases from the general population.

The clinical presentation of anxiety varies with age. In preschool children, tearfulness and clinging are the predominant signs and anxious preoccupations may appear in the content of play. In middle childhood, tears and clinging can still be seen but irritability or even aggressive behaviour are not infrequent. Regression and manipulative behaviour in order to control environmental stimuli or coerce parents, are typical. Apprehensive questioning and demands for reassurance are common. Anxious adolescents resemble adults in the presentation but may, like younger children, lack an adequate vocabulary to express their subjective emotional state in words. Thus, throughout childhood, the signs of high psychophysiological arousal can be the presenting features: hyperventilation and its consequences, abdominal pain, vomiting, headache, urinary frequency, bedwetting and sleep disturbance. These foment hypochondriacal fretting, which may also be the presenting feature. Panic attacks are increasingly common with age and affect nearly half of all adolescents (Ollendick *et al.*, 1994).

The aetiology of childhood anxiety disorders is obscure. Levels of anxiety within the normal range seem to be under some genetic control (Stevenson *et al.*, 1992) but the inheritance of anxiety disorders in childhood has been little studied.One study (Last *et al.*, 1991) suggested higher rates of anxiety disorders among the families of anxious children compared to the families of hyperactive children. Kagan's work on inhibited temperament (shyness, caution and timidity; Kagan *et al.*, 1988) identified a group of inhibited children who were assessed some years later and found to have high rates of anxiety disorders (Hirschfield *et al.*, 1992). This suggests a link with temperamental traits but how specific this is is debatable. For instance, temperamental inhibition is also found to be disproportionably prevalent among the children of adults with affective disorders (Rosenbaum *et al.*, 1988).

On first principles it would seem reasonable to consider both causes of high anxiety and causes of insufficient anxiety management but this has not been done systematically. Anxiety management in the young child is a function of the attachment dynamic (mother's proximity provides relief) so it is unsurprising that there is a close relationship between pathological anxiety and unresolved or insecure attachment as revealed by age-inappropriate separation anxiety. However the evidence is equivocal as to whether some aspect of mother's behaviour can cause childhood anxiety. Although it is usually assumed that overprotective maternal handling could provoke anxiety in the child or impair its waning with age, it might also be a response to it, or both the child's anxiety and the mother's overprotection might be expressions of a familial trait.

Certain experiences can produce enduring anxiety and studies of children with post-traumatic stress disorder provide an instance of this. Yet many children with pathological anxiety do not seem to have a history of adverse experiences so that it seems unlikely that this is universally necessary. One is left with a suspicion that multifactorial causation with an interplay of elements and various aetiological pathways to a final common state is a likely model.

Timidity and anxious concerns are relatively more common among children than adults. The traditional assumption is that emotional disorders of childhood have a good prognosis. Accordingly, some suggest that anxiety disorders in children do not deserve clinical attention. Such a position ignores the suffering of the young person. Also there are good grounds for thinking that pathological anxiety is a problem that deserves early intervention from a prognostic viewpoint. About half of the group of adults with anxiety disorders had an onset of their anxiety disorder in childhood (see Klein, 1994).

Selecting a treatment for an anxiety disorder rests mainly on clinical experience. Individual psychotherapy has a long history of application and the general principles are well-recognised (e.g. Lewis, 1986) although the scientific evidence for its effectiveness is slight. Behavioural treatments are the approach of choice for specific fears and have been described in detail (Morris & Kratochwill, 1983). A number of clinics use family therapy but there is a lack of evidence for its efficacy in anxiety conditions. Medication has been little studied and although different clinicians use benzodiazepines, selective serotonin re-uptake inhibitors (SSRIs) and buspirone, there is again no hard evidence that these approaches are especially effective. An initial vogue for tricyclics has waned and initial positive results have not been replicated (Berney et al., 1981; Klein et al., 1992b).

Instances of pathological anxiety associated with specific behavioural syndromes are considered separately below.

School refusal

The term school refusal, loosely synonymous with school phobia, refers to an inability to attend school because of anxiety. A child may not be at school for various reasons. Ordinary physical illness provides sanction for absence but may mislead the unwary. An anxious child may focus upon the psychophysiological concomitants of anxiety (palpitations, nausea and vomiting, tension headache, etc), which present as a physical complaint. If so, an anxiogenic origin is indicated by a peak on schoolday mornings and an absence at weekends or during the holidays.

Truancy, wilful and unjustifiable absence from school on the child's initiative, may be distinguished by the fact that the parents do not know where their child is when he should be in school. The distinction between school refusal and school truancy is real. Hersov (1960a, b) was able to demonstrate important differences between school refusers and truants seen at a psychiatric clinic. Truancy was associated with antisocial behaviour, poor academic attainments, and a family background marred by disharmony and disciplinary inconsistency. Conversely, school refusal was typically manifested by children who were dependent, inhibited, and timid. Their academic attainments were appropriate or even superior, their school behaviour exemplary. Unlike the truants they came from families characterised by parental overprotection and with a history of neurotic disorders.

Parental concern about a child who remains at home when he or she should be at school usually indicates school refusal. The exception is the wilfully disobedient adolescent, well beyond parental control, who does as he pleases in all aspects of like. Some such spoilt youngsters are fearful of school, but not all.

Most children at some time or other become anxious about attending school but parental pressure ensures that they do attend. The clinical picture of school refusal is based on those whose school attendance has broken down and these are uncommon in clinics. The sex incidence is equal and the commonest age at presentation is 11 years (Smith, 1970).

In addition to a refusal to go to or remain at school in the face of parental pressure, entreaty, or threat, the child may display overt panic at the time to leave for school. Alternatively he may later run home from school in panic. In young children an acute onset is characteristic in contrast to the more insidious development often seen in adolescents. Precipitating events often include changes of teacher or school, illness or bereavement in the family, a move of house, or the departure of a close friend.

Such behaviour may be a realistic response to bullying or a symptom of various psychiatric disorders and reflect differing mechanisms; it is not a diagnosis. Particularly amongst younger children, the problem is less that of a phobia of school, more a fear of separation from an attachment figure. This is a frequent underlying pathology, though certainly not universal (Hersov, 1985). Parents who have never achieved satisfactory separation from their families or origin, or who had unfortunate school experiences themselves, find corresponding difficulties promoting their children's separation and school attendance in the face of protest by the child. There may, of course, be an underlying genetic predisposition affecting both parent and child.

Children with pathological separation anxiety frequently express fears of harm befalling a parent. There may have been overt parental threats of suicide or departure expressed directly to the child or overheard in a quarrel between the parents. When separation anxiety is mooted as fundamental it should be demonstrated in other separation situations and be relieved by the presence of attachment figures. To complicate matters, separation fears may be activated by a depressive disorder. Specific fears should be enquired about; these encompass realistic apprehension in the face of bullying or exclusion as well as frankly phobic disorders. These include anxiety about reading aloud in class or surviving assembly without fainting.

Older children usually present a more chronic picture. Some have longstanding difficulties adapting to situations that place new demands upon their competence. They demand excessive reassurance (and earn parental irritation) before exposing themselves to untried situations. Others have chronically low self-esteem, which may predispose to depressive disorder. The increasing demands of school life, both educational and social, are met by maladaptive responses characterised by withdrawal into the family, though this is often at the expense of worsening parent–child relationships with acrimonious recrimination, stubbornness and wilful protestation by the child replacing earlier compliance.

The management of school refusal involves recognition (thus avoiding multiple, unnecessary physical investigations or prolonged convalescence where somatic symptoms exist) and correction of inappropriate class or school, unnecessary games etc. The principle is to return the child to school as quickly as possible and treat underlying conditions once this is achieved. Severe depressive disorder is an obvious exception to this rule. For acute cases (usually under age 11) most authorities agree on an enforced return to school on an early, decided date with firm, consistent action from both parents and educational welfare officers/educational social workers supported by the psychiatric team acting in liaison with the school (Kennedy, 1965). The analogy is with a flooding procedure in adult anxiety disorders.

Where there is a longer history or an older child, the initial assessment leads to a programme of graded return to the school negotiated with the child once the principle of inevitable return is accepted. This is more akin to a desensitisation or graded exposure paradigm. There will be brief trips to the vicinity of the school, the completion of schoolwork at home, collecting books from school, going to a classroom for selected activities and so on progressively according to a hierarchy of threatening situations. There is no coercion of the child. The aim is ultimately to hand over to the parents all responsibility for maintaining the child's attendance. Thus, at the same time as the child is working through the steps of a graded return, the parents receive guidance in their handling of the re-entry to school, particularly an encouragement of firmness in the face of attempts by the child to remain at home.

Medication is generally unhelpful. In spite of earlier claims, tricyclic antidepressants are only effective when school refusal arises out of a depressive disorder (Berney et al., 1981). In the most severe cases admission to a psychiatric in-patient until will allow intensive treatment of underlying disorders, and ensures continued education. This may need to be followed by boarding school placement if adverse family factors are not correctable. A home tutor should be regarded as the last resort.

More than two-thirds successfully return to school (Baker & Wills, 1979). Good prognosis is related not only to younger age (adolescents seem to have more serious individual and family pathology), but also to the stability of the home. Berg (1982) has reviewed long-term studies of how school refusers fare in adult life. Approximately one-third of adolescent school refusers may be expected to continue to suffer from neurotic symptoms and social impairment in young adult life, though only about 5% of the most severe cases will develop agoraphobia (see e.g. the paper by Boreham, 1983).

Elective mutism

A persistent refusal to talk outside the home or other than among a small group of close associates is a rare condition generally considered to be anxiety-based. Speech is adequate for communication, though Kolvin & Fundudis (1981) were able to demonstrate an excess of developmental articulation defects and speech delay within their sample. They also noted negativistic stubbornness in half of the children and sensitive or submissive qualities in the remainder: substantial personality variations that were likely to associate with poor peer relationships, sphincter problems, separation difficulties, and a range of behavioural disorders. The mean IQ of the group was low (85). There was a high rate of psychiatric disturbance in their families, particularly abnormalities of personality. Follow-up studies revealed a poor prognosis in about one-half of all cases.

Hayden (1980) identified four sub-groups. *Symbiotic* mutism referred to clinging, shy but manipulative children. *Speech phobic* mutes were a rare group of children with obsessive compulsive rituals surrounding their own speech. Reactive mutes were withdrawn, miserable, and speechless following a traumatic experience such as rape. *Passive-aggressive* mutism was characterised by the use of silence as a defiant manoeuvre. Clinical experience suggests it may be most typical of adolescent elective mutes.

Hayden remarked on the common associated findings of tenser stiff bodily movements, other associated fears and nervous habits, and timidity outside the home coupled with a stubborn and demanding manner within it. The passive-aggressive group was an exception to the latter, being generally antisocial. High rates of pathology, including a past history of child abuse, were discovered within the families of these electively mute children. Sexual abuse is particularly common (MacGregor *et al.*, 1994).

The treatment of elective mutism tends to be empirical and involves a behavioural approach whereby fear-inducing people or situations are faded in gradually, whilst the child is praised or otherwise rewarded for reading or talking. Alternatively, operant methods may be used to shape up speech production in a constant situation (see Kratochwill, 1981, for an overview of treatment). Any abnormality of family relationships will require simultaneous treatment.

Post-traumatic stress disorder (PTSD)

Children can develop a reaction to catastrophic or terrifying events that is essentially the same as PTSD in adults. Repetitive, intrusive memories (flashbacks) of the traumatic experience are coupled with hypervigilance, hyperarousal and avoidance of stimuli reminiscent of the original trauma. The current definitions emphasise the presence of emotional numbing yet this is hard to demonstrate in children (Frederick, 1985). Yule (1994), on the basis of his clinical experience, has described additional features: separation difficulties, irritability, problems with concentration and learning new material, survivor guilt, sleep disturbances, a sense of a foreshortened life, and other anxiety and depressive symptoms. Affected children experience a pressure to talk about the experience but simultaneously find it difficult to do so. Themes related to their traumatic experience emerge in repetitive play or drawings. Their schoolwork is adversely affected.

The type of experience most likely to produce PTSD is one that is sudden, unpredictable and dangerous. It is particularly likely to occur in war and children exposed to political violence show a high rate of PTSD (Richman, 1993). Most studies, however, have been of disasters affecting a number of people and two points need to be made. Firstly, PTSD is only one consequence of such traumata. Other children show less differentiated anxiety or depressive reactions, sometimes referred to as adjustment disorders. The intensity of PTSD seems to bear a close relationship to the horror of the experience and within a group of children there may therefore be a shading off into other patterns of response; the boundaries of the condition are vague. Secondly, experiences affecting individual children can produce PTSD, notably sexual abuse (Goodwin, 1988) or witnessing the murder of a parent (Black & Kaplan, 1988).

The prognosis of PTSD is poor in the short term so that children show little improvement over several months but generally improve subsequently though the pattern of symptoms changes with a relative decrease in flashbacks and an increase in anxiety and depression. Treatment approaches include exposure to the trauma through recollection assisted by a therapist. Some children who are particularly troubled by memory flashbacks in bed at night benefit from masking by listening to music or a tape-recorded story. Medication is not much used. Adolescents who have shared a traumatic experience can benefit from group discussion (Galante & Foa, 1986) and this can be conducted very soon after an incident as a debriefing (Yule & Udwin, 1991).

Dissociative and somatoform disorders

Dissociative reactions in children are most likely to be abnormalities of gait, sense organs or apparent seizures. Commonly the child has experienced illness affecting the organ system in question and the diagnosis of dissociative disorder by total exclusion of organic illness is incorrect. Taylor's (1979) formulation of an enactment by the child of his or her idea of sickness in order to resolve a predicament is helpful. In this respect, direct questioning about abuse is wise. The treatment of chronic dissociative disorder is based on dealing with the predicament and providing sympathetic, gradual rehabilitation without the child feeling that loss of face is inevitable. To that end, debates about how much is psychological, how much physical, how much unconscious, etc. are unhelpful.

Somatic complaints are common in anxiety, but whether one can always turn the proposal around and infer anxiety or a stress response when physical symptoms cannot be found to have physical pathology is doubtful. Recurrent central colicky abdominal pain, for instance, rarely has a demonstrable physical basis that could be revealed by physical investigation but only a proportion of cases can be clearly shown to be anxiety-based. The psychiatrist's contribution is sometimes to handle the anxiety of the paediatrician and counsel fewer rather than more investigations. An association with stress needs demonstration by diary keeping. Some affected children clearly use complaints of pain to communicate mental distress to their parents but it would be unwise to assume this usually to be the case. It is easy to overlook the child's suffering if all that is done is to reassure the parents that the condition is not physically serious.

Depression

Over the last two decades there has been a movement towards the increasing recognition of depression as a disorder that can affect the young, predominantly those over the age of 11. Debate about the pathoplastic effects of developmental stage continues but a common convention is to assume that the basic criteria for diagnosis are essentially the same for adults, adolescents and children; this is the case in both ICD-10 and DSM-IV.

Distinguishing depressive disorder from situational misery caused by adversity is not straightforward. Nor is it always easy to differentiate it from temperamental attributes such as ingrained pessimism and low aspirations. Current categorisation approaches using descriptive diagnostic criteria do not necessarily help.

Further complications arise because of the common association of depressed mood or depressive disorder with other psychiatric conditions, notably anxiety disorders and conduct disorder. Many studies of depression in the young use adult-derived RDC or DSM criteria, which appear to recruit a mixed bag of patients including the situationally miserable, the oppressed and those with other conditions as well as a depressed mood. For instance, Kovacs et al., (1989) found that 41% of depressed youngsters also had an anxiety disorder according to DSM criteria. Conversely, Last et al. (1987) found rates for depressive disorder varying between 25% to 56% in groups of young people with various anxiety disorders. About 20% of adolescents with depressive disorder also fulfil criteria for conduct disorder (see e.g. Kashani et al., 1987) and a similar proportion of juvenile delinquents will also be depressed (Alessi et al., 1984). The fact that DSM has not, until DSM-IV, included an impairment criterion means that it has probably identified a larger and less severely affected group than would otherwise be the case. There is thus a suspicion that DSM depression is a symptom complex rather than a unitary condition of depressive disorder. Nevertheless, most of recent research has used DSM criteria so some suspension of scepticism is practical in order for rough principles to be established. Therefore the term depression is taken here to be equivalent to major depressive disorder and it is acknowledged that it is an umbrella concept.

Cases of depression identified by structured interview and those identified by scores of self-report questionnaires are not the same. Using questionnaires, between 8 and 18% of the general young adolescent population are considered depressed at any one time, whereas interview methods identify 3–5% (Reynolds, 1994). Most studies do not include a dysfunction or impairment criterion, an exception being that of Kashani et al. (1987), who found a general population prevalence rate for major depressive disorders of 4.7%. The ratio of affected girls to boys is about two to one, though the ratio alters with age and the maximum gender difference occurs in the mid-teens (Cohen et al., 1993).

Moderate depression and depressive symptomatology are therefore quite widespread among the young and common in clinical practice (see Kolvin et al., 1991). They are associated with a range of psychiatric disorders, particularly anxiety disorders, conduct disorder, substance abuse and are common among the victims of parental abuse (Downey et al., 1994) or sexual assault (Frank et al., 1988). Yet depressive mental states in adolescents are under-recognised by conventional services. Indeed, in Cooper & Goodyer's (1993) school-based study none of the identified cases were known to services.

Although identified by adult-derived criteria, the high rate of comorbidity and age-related variations in the clinical picture mean that adolescent depression appears to differ in a number of ways from depression in adult life. However, there are grounds for thinking that there are similarities too. DSM depression is very much more common among the adolescent offspring of parents with affective disorder than those without (e.g. Warner et al., 1992). Depressed children and adolescents have higher than expected rates of depression in adult life (Harrington et al., 1990), unless the childhood depression is combined with conduct disorder. This may explain why though such continuity is greater for girls and women (Kandel & Davies, 1986). If the most severe cases of depression in the young are taken, then similarities with adult depression are stronger. For instance, Hill (1994) was able to show that, contrary to received wisdom, sleep abnormalities in severe adolescent depression correspond to those in depressed adults.

Table 5.1. *Differences from adult depression*

More common than in adults	Less common than in adults
social withdrawal	delusions
irritability	suicide
running away from home	altered libido
separation anxiety	sleep disturbance
pain in head, chest or abdomen	weight loss
decline in school work	

There are important ways in which immaturity colours the form of depression and it is important to employ a developmental perspective. This is reflected not just in the clinical features but in assessment procedures: the need to include parents' accounts in appraisal, the relevance of school, and recognition of age-appropriate ways of handling distress such as regression, especially in terms of attachment behaviour (e.g. following parents around).

Compared with the picture in adults, depression in older children and adolescents is more likely to show certain features (Table 5.1) and less likely to show others. Bipolar disorder is rare before puberty and, perhaps because of this, can be misdiagnosed, especially in manic presentation (Carlson, 1990). For instance, Isaac (1992) found eight out of 12 adolescents who were considered to have treatment-resistant externalising disorders actually fulfilled criteria for bipolar disorder. Typically it has an abrupt onset and may present with such severity that schizophrenia is diagnosed. Cyclothymic mood swings of lesser severity are present in perhaps one-quarter of the adolescent children of parents with bipolar disorder (Klein *et al.*, 1985).

The aetiology of depression in children and adolescents almost certainly depends upon contributions from both genetic and environmental adversities. Parental, especially maternal, psychopathology is quite common and most likely to be depressive disorder (Goodyer *et al.*, 1993). The lifetime prevalence of depression in the relatives of depressed children is raised and in Harrington *et al.*'s (1993) study it was doubled. Yet about half of the parents of depressed adolescents do not have current or past psychopathology (Goodyer *et al.*, 1993) and it is accepted that environmental factors alone can precipitate depression. These may be acute life events or chronic adversities. There are interactions in that acute events are more likely to occur in the setting of chronic problems (Wilde *et al.*, 1992) and the presence of a depressed parent can increase the likelihood of adverse life events. The type of adverse life event does not seem usually to be crucial, though bereavement and peer rejection seem especially potent (Patterson & Stoolmiller, 1991). There is a little evidence that physical maltreatment as a chronic problem is likely to produce depression in about 20% of victims (Famularo *et al.*, 1992).

The detection of depression in clinical practice necessitates an individual interview with the adolescent. This must include a mental state examination and appraisal of suicidal intent. Many adolescents are secretive, even ashamed of their state of mind. They will not readily admit to despair in front of a parent for fear of alarming them or out of a wish to preserve face. Good practice involves the clinician 'reaching out' to make contact with concealed feelings and ideas. Some words used by teenagers such as 'bored' and 'fed up' need exploration as a monosyllabic adolescent will not bother to explain anhedonia at length. Sometimes a self-report questionnaire allows the adolescent to admit to depressive symptoms more readily than does an interview. The Childrens Depression Inventory (CDI) and the Reynolds Adolescent Depression Scale (RADS) are the most widely used in clinical practice (see Kazdin, 1990). Accounts from the parents and school are crucial but not sufficient in themselves. Social withdrawal is an important sign (Cooper & Goodyer, 1993) as is loss of interest in previously enjoyed pursuits. Situational mood fluctuation should not disqualify the diagnosis.

When treating depression, most clinicians use antidepressants but the evidence that they are more effective than non-specific measures is lacking and there are several studies of treatment using tricyclic antidepressants with negative results (Puig-Antich et al., 1987; Geller et al., 1992; Hazell et al., 1995), partly because of high placebo response rates. There is a suspicion that tighter diagnostic criteria and larger doses of antidepressants would enable an effect to emerge. Because of the risk of fatal overdose, many clinicians use lofepramine or an SSRI but with one exception (a rather sparsely described study by Simeon et al., 1990) reports of the latter have been open trials or case reports of unusual children. There is insufficient experience with moclobemide but occasional reports of favourable response to older MAOIs (e.g. Ryan, 1990). Lithium is used in adolescents in a way comparable to adult psychiatry but has been little studied. There is evidence that it can treat adolescent depression resistant to tricyclics (Ryan et al., 1988) and reduce the risk of relapse in teenage bipolar disorder (Strober et al., 1990). Ambrosini et al. (1993) provide a review of pharmacological interventions.

There has been a surge of interest in psychological interventions. Interpersonal or psychodynamic psychotherapeutic approaches have rarely been specifically evaluated though have their advocates (e.g. Mufson et al., 1993). Cognitive-behavioural and similar approaches (such as rational emotive therapy) have been subject to comparative evaluation from which it is possible to draw the conclusion that they are moderately effective but not always more so than rather non-specific approaches such as relaxation training (Reynolds, 1994). Harrington (1992), in a useful review of treatments, considers that the case for psychological treatments has only so far been made for milder forms of depression.

ECT is rarely used for adolescent depression, nearly always as a last resort for relentlessly suicidal patients with very severe depressive illness who have not responded to other methods of treatment. Report of its use in such instances indicate it can be very effective (Bertagnoli & Borchart, 1990).

There are no grounds for thinking that depression in adolescence has a benign course. Typically, its natural history is to persist for months (Strober et al., 1993) or, in an appreciable minority, several years (Kovacs, 1985). Among girls (but not boys) who kill themselves, it is the commonest diagnosis to be made on psychiatric post-mortem (Shaffer & Piacentini, 1994) and the commonest single diagnosis to be made in adolescents who take overdoses (Sadowski & Kelley, 1993). The prognosis for a particular episode of depression is quite good; three-quarters will recover within a year (Kovacs et al., 1984a). However, the chance of relapse is high and in the study by Kovacs and her colleagues (1984b), 70% had a further episode within the next five years. The risk of depression in adult life is increased compared both with other childhood psychiatric disorders and the general population (see above).

Overdoses

It is unusual for children to take overdoses before puberty. Between two-thirds and three-quarters of teenagers who take overdoses are girls. Analgesics or psychotropic agents are the preferred agents (Sellar *et al.*, 1990). The previously increasing rate of overdoses among UK teenagers may have reached a plateau (Alderson, 1985). Most instances are precipitated by interpersonal crises but these often occur against a background of family conflict or indifference, which may be seen as more dysfunctional by the teenager than her parents (McKenry *et al.*, 1982). As a group, teenagers who take overdoses have experienced a higher number of adverse life events than depressed or normal controls (De Wilde *et al.*, 1992) and more likely to have experienced sexual or physical abuse.

Depressive episodes, conduct disorder and substance abuse are all common among overdosing teenagers but the figures provided by various studies vary widely. Probably depression is the commonest psychiatric pathology with a reported prevalence of between one- and three-quarters of all cases (see above). As with adults, it is unwise to assume that suicide is the prime motive for an overdose since clinical experience suggests a range of reasons (see Hill, 1989). Nevertheless, some who take an overdose intend to die (Brent, 1987) and to rely on the cliché that the action is a 'cry for help' is unwise (Hawton *et al.*, 1982). For many, however, it is a demonstration or communication of the intensity of their feelings. Appraisal of suicidal intent is therefore mandatory and admission to hospital is conventional not merely to treat physical complications but in order for such evaluation to be carried out by interviewing teenager and parents before further decisions are made about treatment and when the teenager should return home.

Treatment generally takes the form of joint meetings between parents and the teenager to promote appreciation of the young person's distress and improve family communication. Some teenagers will benefit from specific treatment of depression or cognitive interventions to improve social problem solving. The exercise is hampered by a low compliance rate and many adolescents or their families fail to return for out-patient treatment.

The specific prognosis for further overdoses may be a little better in teenagers than adults, so that Hawton (1982) suggests a repeat of 10% over the following year. The risk of repetition rises with a history of previous attempts, substance abuse, living away from home, presence of psychiatric disorder, poor peer relationships, male sex and early parental loss. In a long-term follow up, Otto (1972) found an eventual suicide rate of 4%, the risk being substantially higher in boys and those who have psychiatric disorder at first contact and are in their late teens.

Suicide

It is exceptional for prepubertal children to kill themselves though they make threats to do so. Rates of suicide in the UK and the US increase in linear fashion from the age of 13 to 24 and in recent years there has been a increasing rate in the 15–19-year-old males in both countries, accounting for 13–14% of all deaths in this age group (see e.g. Department of Health, 1994). This increase has been linked to substance and alcohol abuse by Brent *et al.*

(1987) and Shaffer & Piacentini (1994), which may also partly explain why suicide is commoner among boys.

Most UK adolescent suicides are the result of hanging, overdoses or jumping from a height. They are most likely to be committed while awaiting punishment for a misdemeanour or, less commonly, after reading or hearing about a suicide, after a humiliation, or when a relationship is threatening to break up. A number have no precipitant, occurring in the setting of a depressive disorder. There is accumulating evidence that suicide can be precipitated by the suicide of prominent individuals or dramatised suicide on television (e.g Wasserman, 1984; Gould & Shaffer, 1986).

Psychiatric autopsy studies use interviews with relatives in order to reconstruct the dead teenager's mental state. Earlier series were small but Shaffer & Piacentini (1994) report a large study in New York, which identifies psychiatric disorder in two-thirds of adolescent suicides and psychiatric symptomatology short of diagnostic criteria in the remainder. Important findings include:

- About half had previous contact with a mental health professional.
- Roughly one-third of each sex met criteria for anxiety disorders.
- Major depressive disorder affected approximately one-third of girls and one-sixth of boys.
- Nearly half of the boys had either or both conduct disorder and drug or alcohol abuse.
- Two-thirds of older (age 17–19) male teenagers had a significant alcohol abuse problem.

There were, in this study, three common patterns:

1. An irritable, impulsive, volatile group, over-sensitive to criticism.
2. A perfectionistic group, anxious about forthcoming events, who found it difficult to adapt to new circumstances.
3. A depressed group, mainly girls.

The above findings enable predisposed individuals to be characterised. They will have the personality traits described or be clinically depressed. Suicide is most likely after a stressful event has provoked powerful emotion and when judgement is impaired by alcohol or drugs. It will be even more probable if the suicide of a glamorous figure has recently been portrayed or reported on television and the means for killing oneself are readily available.

Obsessive-compulsive disorder (OCD)

True obsessive-compulsive symptoms should be distinguished from the magical rituals common in middle childhood: not walking on cracks, counting objects, etc. These are not accompanied by any anxiety or a sense of compulsion and are not regarded by the child as senseless. On the other hand, true obsessional symptoms and compulsive rituals can be observed from the age of about ten onwards, occasionally earlier. Resistance is not easy to elicit in many cases, particularly in contamination rituals, which may be energetically justified by an articulate teenager. As with adults, secretiveness about obsessions means that clinical enquiry needs to be specific and persistent.

Epidemiological data are therefore understandably sparse and most studies are of a clinical series. Flament *et al.* (1988), using DSM-III criteria for OCD in a well-conducted study of 5 000 American high school students, found a prevalence rate of 0.35%, whereas Esser *et al.* (1990), Thomsen (1993) and Zohar *et al.* (1992), using broad criteria and no impairment criterion, found prevalence rates for obsessive symptoms of about 4%, among which repetition of thoughts was the commonest symptom. This suggests a continuum of severity so that a moderate amount of obsessional mental activity is not that uncommon but full-blown OCD remains relatively uncommon. There is no difference between sexes and no relation between age and type of preoccupation (Thomsen, 1991).

In clinical series, contamination concerns and rituals are the commonest preoccupation, followed by fears of harming others (or rituals to ward off disaster), death and sex. Primary obsessional slowness is rare. What evidence there is for cross-cultural variation suggests it is minimal (see Thomsen, 1994*a*).

Most studies show a predominance of cases from higher social classes and an as yet unresolved question arises as to whether this can be explained entirely by referral bias. Thomsen's (1994*b*) catchment area study suggests it may not. Apart from this, there is an absence of positive systematic findings of family or cultural influence on obsessional preoccupations. Most, but not all, studies that have examined obsessionality in relatives have found an elevated rate of obsessional traits and in some studies rates for full OCD in first degree relatives are as high as 24% (Swedo *et al.*, 1989). Remarkably, the type of obsession in a parent bears no relation to the type in the affected child.

The relationship of OCD to other psychiatric conditions is not clear-cut. In anorexia nervosa, obsessional traits and an obsessive approach to food are well-recognised but it is also true that true obsessions with their content unrelated to food are commoner than expected (Rothenberg, 1986) and both bulimia and anorexia nervosa are commoner than predicted in adolescents with OCD (Flament *et al.*, 1990). Similarly, true obsessions are disproportionately common in both Tourette's patients and their relatives (Robertson, 1994), while tics are correspondingly commoner than predicted in children with OCD who are followed up (Leonard *et al.*, 1992). Indeed the distinction between a tic and an obsession can sometimes be hard to make.

The term 'obsession' is sometimes used to describe repetitive activities or rigid preoccupations in autism and Asperger's syndrome but these are not obsessive-compulsive in form. However, true OCD may well be over-represented in pervasive developmental disorders. Szatmari *et al.* (1989*a*) found rates of 10% and 8% in high-functioning autism and Asperger's syndrome respectively. Conversely, children and adolescents with OCD not uncommonly have social empathic difficulties and peculiar interests in childhood (Thomsen & Mikkelsen, 1993). Such findings have led to speculation about the links between anankastic personality disorder, OCD and pervasive developmental disorders.

The fundamental mechanisms underlying OCD are unclear. Studies of EEG and soft neurological signs in adolescents do not demonstrate specific abnormalities compared to other psychiatric controls. Rapoport (1991), synthesising information from neuropsychological studies, suggests that there is a dysfunction of pathways linking basal ganglia, thalamus and frontal lobes. She speculates, usefully, that these pathways are linked to forms of self-protective behaviour such as grooming and checking so that some compulsive rituals can be seen as an excess of partial forms of these.

Treatment of OCD in children and adolescents is often complicated by the fact that young patients are ambivalent about it, claiming that if left to their own devices they can master the problem. Furthermore, other family members are often drawn into rituals and find it easier to comply rather than face a tantrum. Obtaining an agreement to treat is not always easy. Most cases will be handled as an out-patient in the first instance and the two approaches known to be effective are clomipramine (Flament et al's, 1985), and a behavioural package combining exposure to anxiety-provoking stimuli and response prevention (Bolton et al., 1983). Some parents find the latter difficult to implement and see it as inhumane. In such cases, treatment in an in-patient unit may be more acceptable to them.

Indeed, admission to an in-patient unit is not uncommonly followed by a dramatic remission, which can be protracted and not relapse until the child returns home. Overall response rates are probably more encouraging than published series, which tend to be drawn from in-patient units though in most series there is a group of patients who do poorly. This is reflected in follow-up studies of affected children, which suggest a picture similar to that found in studies of adults. Three broad groupings appear: those who continue to have unremitting and handicapping OCD, those whose symptoms abate but incompletely leaving subclinical or episodic firms, and those who become symptom-free. In the studies of Rapoport's group (e.g. by Flament et al., 1990) there were roughly equal numbers in each group.

Conduct disorder

A child displaying antisocial, aggressive or defiant behaviour that violates social expectations for a child of that age, presents as an enduring pattern of behaviour, and is associated with impaired social functioning in other areas is regarded as having a *conduct disorder*. Antisocial behaviour can be insufficiently severe or not be associated with a general impairment of social functioning: the mere presence of bad behaviour is not sufficient grounds for a diagnosis of conduct disorder. Nor is delinquency (a synonym for law-breaking behaviour) the same thing. An adolescent with a conduct disorder will probably break the law frequently but some antisocial behaviours (lying, bullying) are not necessarily illegal. Most juvenile delinquents are infrequent offenders and do not have conduct disorders though recidivist offenders are likely to.

There is a range of antisocial behaviours including disobedience, defiance, excessive fighting, bullying or other aggressive behaviour; lying, firesetting, stealing, vandalism, truancy, running away from home, cruelty to animals, and malicious teasing or provocation. Commonly, children with conduct disorder are also angry, irritable, rude, anti-authoritarian, have a low frustration tolerance and show rages or severe tantrums. They tend to blame others for their own problems, are mistrustful and may misinterpret ordinary social overtures from others as hostile.

Severe and persistent antisocial behaviour can be associated with other psychiatric symptomatology. When emotional symptoms are particularly prominent, *depressive conduct disorder*, and *other mixed disorder of conduct and emotion* are the relevant diagnostic categories. If marked disturbance of activity and attention coexists with persistent antisocial behaviour, the diagnosis is *hyperkinetic conduct disorder*. Emotional symptoms are common in conduct disorder (Rutter *et al.*, 1970) and even when they are sufficiently severe to warrant a mixed diagnosis, the associated features of the condition resemble conduct disorder more than an emotional or neurotic disorder. It may be that hyperkinetic conduct disorder is a common development of hyperkinetic disorder, arising from a coincidence of aetiological factors, in other words a comorbidity of two conditions rather than a separate condition in its own right. It may also reflect an assumption that hyperkinetic disorder is a common vulnerability for the later development of conduct disorder (Loeber, 1990).

Conduct disorder as a primary diagnosis can be subdivided into various categories, which are probably points on a continuum of severity:

• oppositional defiant disorder (ODD)
   characteristically found in young children who are hostile, provocative, defiant, angry, resentful, irascible and disobedient but whose behaviour does not violate the rights of others. The mildest or earliest form of conduct disorder.
• conduct disorder confined to the family context
   antisocial and aggressive behaviour that goes beyond oppositional, defiant behaviour and violates the rights of others but is only evident within the family. Stealing from parents, cutting up the clothes of family members or destruction of furniture are common patterns.
• socialised conduct disorders
   persistent antisocial behaviour that includes both oppositional behaviour and violation of the rights of others outside the home but is associated with good integration into a peer group and sustained friendships with children of a similar age.
• unsocialised conduct disorder
   antisocial behaviour extending beyond the family, often carried out on a solitary basis, associated with a pervasive abnormality of relationships with other children. This commonly includes unpopularity and rejection by them with a consequent lack of sustained, confiding peer relationships

If the above subcategories are pooled,then a rate of about 5% of children will be regarded as having a conduct disorder. In most instances this will be present from an early age though DSM-IV distinguishes between child-onset and adolescent-onset, the former being more severe. Boys outnumber girls by about four to one, a closer ratio than was the case two decades ago.

The aetiology of conduct disorder, taken as a unitary entity, is complex (see Earls, 1994). There is no single cause of conduct disorder and it is usually assumed that there is an interaction between elements in the child and factors in the family, school and peer group. Yet is has been remarkably difficult to demonstrate robust vulnerabilities in affected children. Hyperkinetic disorder is a clear risk factor but most cases of conduct disorder are not hyperactive. Various studies have identified adverse temperament, neuropsychological deficits and autonomic reactivity as risk factors but with little replication of findings. There is a pool of rather imprecise evidence about the genetic contribution to persistent criminality or aggressive behaviours but no firm findings about conduct disorder itself. This may hinge upon the age of the probands, since there is some evidence that the impact of genetic effects increases with age when compared to environmental affects (see Simonoff *et al.*, 1994). Some common associates of conduct disorder (reading difficulties, negative attributions as to other children's motives, poor interpersonal problem-solving) may be consequences rather than causes.

There is, however, massive confirmation of the aetiological importance of family factors for most cases, particularly those of early onset (Blanz *et al.*, 1991). The parents of most children with conduct disorders show erratic, punitive, inconsistent disciplinary practices with poor supervision and a tendency to use threats or multiple instruction, which are not followed through, in a setting of negative, nagging verbal interactions. Children in such circumstances can learn to escalate negative behaviours to escape parental criticism that elicit further negative actions from parents until the efforts of both parties are reinforced by relief that follows as one party gives in and angry exchanges cease. This is the coercive family process identified by Patterson (1982). The parents of children with conduct disorder are also more likely to be less positive or emotionally warm to their children, be depressed (Williams *et al.*, 1990), socially isolated (Wahler & Dumas, 1985), alcoholic or criminal (Frick *et al.*, 1989) and to quarrel between themselves. Discordant relationships at any level of the family are associated with conduct disorder. Divorce rates are high among families containing children with conduct disorders but it is the discord promoting the divorce, rather than the divorce process itself and the presence of aggressive conflict within the discord, that are relevant (Jouriles *et al.*, 1989). Almost certainly it is the way in which poverty or overcrowding induce stress, and a high rate of daily hassles with disrupted parenting as a consequence, that underlies the association between social disadvantage and conduct disorder (Webster-Stratton, 1990).

It is evident that, once antisocial behaviour is established, its maintenance will be enhanced by the negative responses not only of parents but of peers and teachers (Campbell & Ewing, 1990; Ladd, 1990). The child becomes surrounded by negative responses that undermine his self-esteem and thus reduce the chance of him becoming less suspicious, exhibiting generosity, learning new social or academic skills, or acquiring self-restraint.

The treatment of conduct disorder has historically been viewed pessimistically. However, in the last decade or so a consensus has emerged that it is now possible to reduce antisocial behaviour substantially, certainly in the home setting, if a combination of methods are used. Parent training in using a behavioural approach equips parents with handling skills for defiant, aggressive behaviour on the part of their child. This can be enhanced by attending to parental demoralisation, social isolation and marital dissatisfaction. Current enthusiasm is for the use of a group setting in which parents discuss videotape vignettes of handling difficult child behaviour with a therapist. This procedure avoids blame and concentrates on which factors maintain problematic behaviour rather than what originally caused it (Webster-Stratton & Herbert, 1993, have provided an excellent overview). It is enhanced by a parallel programme for the child and most experience has been gained with teaching the child a cognitive-based strategy for social problem-solving, self-control and developing empathy. Kazdin *et al.* (1987) have developed a successful programme for young adolescents and Webster-Stratton (1991) has a programme for 4–8-year olds. Such a multi-modal approach is in use in a few US and UK centres but has not been sufficiently widely adopted to be regarded as mainstream. The results are undeniably positive but not all families obtain large reductions in their children's antisocial behaviour. Clinical experience suggest that anti-authoritarian attitudes and a lack of proactive organisational skills on the part of a number of parents remain major problems. Nevertheless, energetic attempts are being made to apply similar techniques to children and their families in an attempt at prevention or escalation (Tremblay *et al.*, 1991; Greenberg & Kusche, 1993).

In the longer term, the conventional wisdom is that rather less than half of all conduct disordered children will continue to be seriously antisocial adults though this is something of an oversimplification. Aggression persists as a behavioural trait and is comparable to IQ in its stability over time (Olweus, 1979). Zocolillo *et al.* (1992) were able to demonstrate that children with conduct disorders had deficits in a number of areas of social functioning in adulthood. Substance abuse, at least in men, seems to be a particular problem, though retrospective enquiry implies that conduct-disordered girls are prone to depression in adult life (Robins & Price, 1991). About 10% of children with conduct disorder will die from violent means before middle age (Rydelius, 1988).

Hyperkinetic disorder

The terminology of clinical problems associated with inattentive restlessness in childhood continues to evolve. It may help to note that the phenomenon of pervasive hyperactivity, in other words inattentive restlessness in several types of situation associated with a quality of impulsivity, is quite common and affects about one in four primary school-age children (McArdle *et al.*, 1995) but a psychiatric disorder in which hyperactivity is predominant to handicapping degree is less prevalent. With respect to disorder, attention deficit disorder (ADD), which is an abbreviation of the old DSM-III term, has gained widespread currency but the newer DSM-IIIR/IV term attention deficit hyperactivity disorder (ADHD) is more of a mouthful. The ICD-10 umbrella term hyperkinetic disorder would seem apposite but is the umbrella term for a pair of principal conditions, one of which (disturbance of activity and attention) refers to pure hyperactivity but with a limp title. All point specifically to the crucial importance of attention problems. The text of ICD-10 implies that 'hyperkinetic disorder' and 'disturbance of activity and attention' are equivalent terms and so the briefer term is used here. ICD-10 requires both inattention and restlessness to be present but ADHD can be diagnosed if only one of these is evident and thus identifies a larger group of children.

One of the more important advances in this area has been the application of a pervasiveness criterion. In other words, the cardinal features of restlessness and impaired attention must be present in more than one situation, e.g. at home and in the classroom. There are three necessary criteria for the diagnosis of hyperkinetic disorder.

- onset in the first five years of life;
- pervasive restlessness, particularly in structured situations requiring self-restraining;
- inability to sustain attention long enough to complete assigned age-appropriate tasks.

Additionally, children with a hyperkinetic disorder are frequently impulsive, distractible, noisy, talkative, reckless, and socially disinhibited. Their activity is not just excessive – it is ill-organised and poorly regulated. In the view of some authorities (Barkley, 1990) the difficulties affected children have in curbing their tendencies to be distracted and in controlling impulsivity are central and the unofficial term behavioural inhibition disorder has been invoked accordingly.

In judging whether a child has a hyperkinetic disorder, some threshold is required, since the problems are at the extreme end of a continuum that blends into the range of normal variation. If the diagnosis is made on the basis of evident activity and difficulties with sustained attention, then a surprising number of children are identified. For instance, in North America several questionnaire-based studies using ADD(H) or ADHD criteria have indicated point prevalence rates in the 10–20% range. Szatmari *et al.* (1989*b*) found 9% of primary school boys were above threshold for ADD(H) using rating scales previously calibrated to reflect clinical caseness. In one county in the USA, some 6% of elementary school pupils were receiving treatment for attention deficit disorder (Safer & Kruger, 1988) and there appears to be a trend towards the more frequent diagnosis of the problem in other countries (Rey & Hutchins, 1993). The manual for DSM-IV suggests a prevalence of 3–5%. Yet in the UK, using ICD-9 criteria, the diagnosis is restricted to a smaller number: 1.7% of primary school boys in Taylor *et al*'s (1991) study. Taylor (1994) has suggested that an ICD-10 criterion will yield a prevalence figure of 0.5% for all children (boys outnumbering girls 4:1) though this is likely to be lower than the rate for the broader concept of ADHD. Given differing diagnostic habits, the ordinary clinician will find the criteria of pervasiveness and impairment useful in differentiating pathological from normal. In other words, does the inattentive restlessness manifest itself across situations and does it impair the child's normal developmental progress or ability to engage in ordinary childhood activities?

Comorbidity is a significant problem when hyperkinesis is studied. A number of hyperactive toddlers become conduct-disordered children and this is a commonly recognised sequence in routine clinical practice. It seems more likely to occur in families with interpersonal discord and who experience social adversities. By school age both conditions can be recognised and ICD-10 recognises this by the taxon *hyperkinetic conduct disorder*. Most children with hyperkinetic disorder are of normal intelligence though the average IQ is lowered and there is a general statistical association between hyperkinetic disorder and a variety of neurodevelopmental delays including specific reading disorder (less impressively so with ADHD). This is the basis for the discredited concept of minimal brain dysfunction, abandoned because of poor coherence of the full clinical picture though partly resuscitated by Gillberg *et al.* (1983) as DAMP: disorders of attention, motor and perception. Children with severe hyperkinesis are quite likely also to have poor motor planning of 'soft' motor signs, delays in speech development, and specific reading difficulties.

The cause of hyperkinesis is poorly understood, despite the fact that the condition is the most intensively investigated of all childhood psychiatric disorders with over a thousand scientific publications extant. Difficulties in sample definition account for substantial differences between studies and in general associations are more commonly found when severe (ICD-10 rather than DSM-IV) cases are studied. Comorbidity, particularly with conduct disorder, confuses the picture.

The vast majority of cases do not have obvious brain damage. Various biological markers have been reported but proved hard to replicate. Most workers consider a genetic aetiology likely and there is confirmation of an effect from twin studies (e.g. those of Goodman & Stevenson, 1989) but a significant non-genetic effect is present. It is not possible to tie this down to any specific environmental factor. Diet, allergy or toxins are significant in only a tiny minority of affected children and the findings of high rates of parental psychopathology are mainly found in older studies in which hyperkinesis with conduct disorder (a common association) was not differentiated from pure hyperkinesis. The direction of effect may, of course, be from difficult child to fraught parent and may be more relevant to the persistence of hyperkinesis than its initial cause.

If fundamental mechanisms rather than causes are studied, the picture is little clearer (see Taylor, 1994). Neurotransmitter studies yield contradictory results though noradrenaline and dopamine have been much studied. Brain imaging shows no pathognomonic structural changes but functional imaging shows reduced blood flow and glucose take-up in frontal areas. EEG and evoked potential studies suggest normal resting autonomic activity but inefficient alerting responses and under-reactivity to novel stimuli. Perinatal abnormalities are a little more common than expected in cases of severe hyperkinesis but only apply to a minority of cases (Chandola *et al.*, 1992). Maternal smoking in pregnancy and low birth weight show a significant but weak association with subsequent hyperkinesis.

Psychological studies have been equally obscured by sample definition problems. Attention deficits have been most elusive to pin down and the hypothesised deficit appears to be related to higher-order difficulties in self-monitoring and self-control rather than any simple perceptual or information-processing problem (Douglas, 1988). Impatience, rather than impulsiveness, seemed a more accurate concept in Sonuga-Bark *et al.*'s (1992) neuropsychological study; the hyperkinetic children investigated had an aversion to delay so that they opted for a shorter wait and a smaller reward rather than a larger reward obtainable by waiting longer. In experimental situations hyperkinetic children almost always react more quickly, less accurately and without taking the whole stimulus array into account.

With all this in mind it is not surprising that hyperkinetic children do badly at school in both academic and behavioural terms, even when no specific developmental disorder of academic skills is also present. Referral may be prompted by disruptive behaviour in class or poor academic performance.

Pre-school children are characteristically lively and often do not moderate this according to the situation. This leads some parents to regard them as 'hyper' and may provoke medical consultation. Assessment needs therefore to seek specific instances across situations. Hyperkinetic children of any age may suppress their overactivity in a brief clinic assessment and the tyro will take this as evidence against the condition. A period of observation of at least 40 minutes, during which tasks requiring attention are set, is a minimum. Reports from school are mandatory. The parents can be asked to complete the Conners' questionnaire (Conners, 1973), which contains a hyperactivity factor, and responses loading on this can be scored. Although cut-off scores on this have been used in research studies they are based on parental rather than professional judgement and there is an appreciable false positive rate. A better use of the instrument is to provide a baseline for evaluating treatment interventions.

Treatment must be multi-modal. The attitudes and handling methods of parents and teachers will need careful appraisal and, usually, modification not just to make the child more quiet and tractable but in order to limit damage to the child's self-esteem. Hyperkinetic children live their lives to a soundtrack of persistent criticism and negative injunctions and can rapidly lose a sense of self-worth. Educational deficits will need correction. Poor skills in making and keeping friends may respond to social skills training (but usually do not). Specific methods to promote attention, self-monitoring and impulse restraint include behaviour modification techniques implemented by parents and teachers as well as, in a few children, cognitive methods such as covert self-instruction. The difficulty with the latter is that it is possible to teach children the technique but hard to get them to use it *in vivo*. This exemplifies the problem of hyperkinesis: it is not so much a skills deficit but an inability to deploy, in ordinary situation, the skills that are possessed.

Medication is the most powerful treatment but is never enough alone. A variety of agents promote attentiveness and on-task behaviour for short periods after their administration but do not produce lasting change. Methylphenidate is the least likely to provoke unwanted effects and is given in divided doses with a starting daily dose of 0.3 mg/kg. Insomnia is the main problem so that doses are given in the morning, which means that teachers see the benefit more than do parents. Anorexia is also a common problem growth though retardation, dysphoria, exacerbation of tic disorders and abdominal pains are occasional problems. Similar agents include dexamphetamine, pemoline, even caffeine. Their nomenclature as stimulants causes raised eyebrows among parents but their ability to calm overactivity and promote attentive behaviour extends to normal children too (Rapoport *et al.*, 1980). Dependency is not a problem among hyperactive children. Other drugs known to be effective include imipramine (which is weaker but does not cause insomnia), clonidine, moclobemide and low-dose (less than 3mg/day) haloperidol. Medication for hyperactivity has been very thoroughly researched. It produces undoubted short-term gains but whether it should be continued for long periods to minimise the risk of secondary problems cannot be decided on present evidence (Jacobvitz *et al.*, 1990).

The type of diet that aims to eliminate a string of foodstuffs thought to contain colourants or preservatives ('cutting out the E numbers') is of no therapeutic benefit. A drastic form of exclusion diet that reduces intake to three basic foods and then includes other foods one-by-one, discarding those that exacerbate hyperkinesis, has been shown to be effective in some children (Carter *et al*, 1993) but is not very powerful, extremely arduous and impractical for many families. It requires a dietician to supervise it.

A number of behaviour modification techniques have been employed but the gains in real-life situations have been small and less impressive than medication. The two main components are parent training and cognitive self-control and these complement each other but do not seem to interact (Horn *et al.*, 1991). It is likely that behavioural approaches affect rather different behaviours than does medication. In a classroom study by Wolraich *et al.* (1978), methylphenidate moderated restlessness and focused attention whereas behaviour modification improved academic performance and social behaviour.

It is important to attend energetically to other comorbid conditions and academic difficulties since these can affect prognosis. Although family and individual psychotherapy are ineffective in altering restless inattentiveness, they may be needed as supplementary interventions to promote healthy individual and family functioning.

The natural history of the condition is for overactivity to decline in the early teenage years but for impulsiveness and inattentiveness to persist. By adolescence, the impact of these handicaps will often have been overwhelming so that poor self-esteem, educational failure, desertion by friends and delinquent behaviour or conduct disorder are all likely consequences. The chances of this happening increase if the initial clinical picture was severe, if antisocial behaviour is evident, and there is family discord, parental psychiatric disorder or paternal delinquency (see Taylor *et al.*, 1991). Treatment using stimulants, whatever its short-term benefits, does not prevent this (Barkley *et al.*, 1990), presumably because it is necessary to attend to parenting practices, social relationships and low self-esteem as well. These are possible mediators for social and education failure and need therapeutic attention in their own right.

By adulthood, the prognosis has improved for many, though some will continue to show signs of immaturity in personal functioning, often with persisting impulsivity and explosive reactions to frustration (Weiss & Hechtman, 1986). A much smaller number can reasonably be regarded as still consistently showing signs of hyperkinetic disorder equivalent to those evident in childhood though it is not clear that they can be helped by stimulant medication (Shaffer, 1994*a*).

Enuresis

In this section, as in everyday clinical practice, enuresis (which is more correctly defined as involuntary urination and may thus be termed nocturnal or diurnal) means bedwetting and is usually considered only to be a problem when it affects children over the age of five. It affects roughly 10% of UK children at the age of five years, 5% at age 10 and 1% at age 18.

The normal development of diurnal bladder control is thought to result from social training: intensive, early, and with use of warm praise for appropriate voiding. How this relates to nocturnal continence is frankly mysterious. Nevertheless, it is assumed that the following social factors, which are commonly associated with nocturnal enuresis, operate by diluting or interfering with some aspect of continence training or learning:

• Large family
• Social disadvantage
• Institutional upbringing

These react with constitutional factors and the following are over-represented within an enuretic population (see Shaffer, 1994*b* for specific references):

• Male sex
• Genetic component:
    (a) 70% of enuretics have a first degree relative who wet(s) the bed,
    (b) greater concordance in MZ than DZ twins,
• Immature circadian rhythm of urine osmolality,
• Immature configuration of the vesical base plate,
• Psychiatric disorder

In a small number of enuretic children, the incontinence relates to substantial intellectual retardation, spinal dysraphism, concurrent urinary tract infection, neuroleptic administration, or encopresis. No association has been shown with any particular abnormality or stage of sleep, though it is unusual to wet the bed during REM sleep. Like normals, children with enuresis show a lightening of sleep as their bladder fills but they do not seem to make the final move from light sleep to waking (Watanabe & Azuma, 1989).

No psychiatric disorder is found in the majority of enuretic children, though a small correlation exists between psychopathology and enuresis, particularly among girls and children who wet during the day. Whereas enuretic children are about twice as likely to be psychiatrically disturbed than the general child population, no specific psychopathological picture emerges (Shaffer, 1973).

Conventionally, enuresis is classified into primary (never dry and predominantly 'developmental') and secondary (onset after a dry period in response to stress or psychological disorder). However, longitudinal studies (e.g. Fergusson et al., 1986) show that many enuretics, subsequently termed primary, achieve periods of dryness lasting several months in early childhood, which is subsequently forgotten by their parents. Moreover, there is very little evidence to show that children with primary enuresis are less likely to manifest psychiatric disorder than their secondary counterparts, though children who go on to develop secondary enuresis have more psychiatric symptoms in the first place (McGee et al., 1984). The distinction is not very useful.

Enuresis may follow, cause, or have common origin with psychiatric disorder. All three mechanisms have face validity. Most clinicians are familiar with the global improvement in self-esteem, irritability and compliance of the mildly disturbed child whose bedwetting is successfully treated symptomatically. Yet more serious psychiatric disorder will not resolve (Moffat et al., 1987). Similarly, the familiar picture of a recently bereaved child who begins to wet the bed (van Eerdewegh et al., 1982) supports a notion of emotional stress operating causally in some instances. The similarity between those psychosocial and individual factors that predispose to both enuresis and psychiatric disorder in general suggest a common aetiology to both.

Successful management of the enuretic child and his family necessitates scrupulous attention to detail (see Hall et al., 1994). Initial assessment includes a history and examination, with particular attention to the possibility of a spinal dysraphism, as well as sending urine for microscopy, bacteriology, protein, and glucose screening. Individual interviews with parents and child should include consideration of sleeping arrangements and parental attitudes towards the child and possible treatment approaches. Explanation and reassurance are always needed. A star chart should be employed to achieve a baseline record and is often sufficient treatment in its own right.

Tricyclic antidepressants, oxybutinin and desmopressin (a synthetic anti-diuretic hormone analogue) all produce dryness within a few days in a majority of cases but a relapse on discontinuation is very common, thus restricting their use to 'first aid' measures – holidays, or pending arrangement of bedrooms to enable to use of an alarm. Imipramine, the most widely used antidepressant, is dangerous in overdose and desmopressin is therefore preferred. It may have a lower relapse rate than imipramine (Miller & Klauber, 1990). The 'bell and pad' enuresis alarm is the most effective treatment, 80–90% achieving dryness, failures usually ascribed to faulty technique. Modern alarms use a moisture sensor worn in a perineal pad (or wedged between two layers of underpants) and a buzzer worn on a pyjama jacket. The alarm method takes several weeks to work. Rather more than one-third of patients subsequently relapse during the following months or years but can be successfully re-treated. It has been shown that 'over-learning' by giving the newly continent child a fluid load at bedtime while continuing the alarm will reduce the likelihood of relapse (Young & Morgan, 1972), as will treating most but not all nights. The efficacy of the actual alarm is best understood in terms of avoidance learning or a punishment paradigm, rather than a classical conditioning paradigm, as the end result of treatment is usually a continent child who sleeps through the night rather than one who wakes to micturate. To be effective the alarm must wake the child and it seems that this is a mildly aversive experience, avoided by the development of continence.

The practical aspects of alarm treatment require meticulous attention to ensure that the child is woken adequately, does not interfere with the apparatus, and does not suffer false alarms. Careful demonstration and child–parent co-operation are vital. Any associated psychiatric disturbance or bacteruria requires attention in its own right.

Elaboration of the alarm technique into the package known as 'dry bed' training (Azrin *et al.*, 1974) involves fluid loading, frequent waking with requests to delay urination, praise for dry sheets, and an over-correction element of linen changing should the child wake and the alarm sound. Parental involvement is intense, yet it is still unclear whether the package is an advance over the conventional regime. It is quicker but no more effective overall.

Faecal soiling

Nearly all children achieve faecal continence by the age of four years. The subsequent prevalence rate for soiling in childhood is about 1%, boys predominating over girls. Involuntary soiling may result from:

1. Unsuccessful training

   slack techniques
   elements within the child (low intelligence, autism)
   precarious continence lost in the face of stress

2. Faecal escape on account of

   diarrhoea secondary to organic bowel disease
   urgency, especially associated with fear

3. Retention of faeces within the rectum, the consequence of

   obstruction (partial Hirschprung's disease or asynchronous anal sphincter operation)
   painful anal fissure
   lifelong constipation (Coekin & Gairdner, 1960)
   psychological inhibition of voluntary defaecation

   Retention is by far the most common mechanism encountered in soiling children seen in psychiatric clinics. Difficulties derive from the interaction of a vulnerable constitutional diathesis with coercive or anxiety-provoking toilet training, particularly at the hands of a tense parent or one preoccupied with cleanliness (Anthony, 1957).

There appears to be a spectrum within this group. At one end are children who view the pot or lavatory with apprehension at not being able to defaecate to parental order and are unable to let go, particularly when letting go has in the past resulted in soiling and consequent parental wrath. Once away from the anxiety-creating situation, the child relaxes and defaecates either involuntarily in his pants or secretively in a private receptacle such as a cupboard or secluded corner: 'respite defaecation'.

Moving along the spectrum of retention locates habitual retention, which distends the rectum so that voluntary defaecation becomes difficult because the loaded rectum inhibits anal relaxation. Furthermore, the over-stretched rectal wall habituates and fails to inform conscious awareness of its condition; the call to stool is muted. Faeces are eliminated passively in response to mechanical pressure from new colonic contents arriving in the rectum, or in response to spontaneous involuntary rectal contractions, especially following exercise. Once again the child may find he has soiled himself and hide the offending faeces out of shame. Long-standing retention leads to the formation of scybalic rocks with massive colonic distension, an inability to defaecate and fermentation of rectal contents leading to offensive liquid seepage through the anus.

The term encopresis has given rise to much disagreement as to its meaning and is probably best avoided. Some authors reserve it for the rare problem caused by a child who intentionally defaecates in sensitive places in order to wreak revenge on others, usually parents or foster parents. A normal consistency, normally formed stool has clearly been placed for effect; a rather different situation from the involuntary soiler who tries ashamedly to hide a bundle of soiled underpants under his bed or in a cupboard.

Recent studies have drawn attention to abnormal anal sphincter functioning in a number of children with chronic constipation and soiling (Loening-Baucke & Cruikshank, 1986; Wald et al., 1986). It is argued that such children have difficulty expelling faeces as their external anal sphincter contracts instead of relaxing though the problem of differentiating cause and effect is clear. Some centres now carry out anorectal manometry on chronically constipated soilers (Clayden & Agnarsson, 1991).

No single group of psychological characteristics reliably defines the soiling child or his family, though many observers comment on the frequency of discord and rejection within family relationships and the predominance of covert aggression and denial within the child. Although sexual abuse has been highlighted as a possible cause (Boon, 1991), it is only occasionally encountered. With such a chronic disorder, the debate as to whether family pathology is cause or consequence is less relevant than identifying those family issues that maintain the problem.

Management of retention-based soiling hinges on three components:

1. Informing the child and parents of the pathophysiology of the condition and endeavouring to reduce anxiety, minimise negative attitudes and reduce concerns about cleanliness in child or parents to manageable limits. Clayden & Agnarsson (1991) provide an informative booklet.

2. Emptying the rectum with oral laxatives or microenemata.

3. Education of appropriate defaecating habits according to a simple operant programme wherein appropriate use of the toilet is systematically rewarded. Continuing the laxative speeds the acquisition of skills by increasing the number of opportunities to learn. Involvement of the parents allows faulty parent–child patterns of interaction to be corrected.

Enuresis, a commonly associated condition, often clears with successful management of the soiling. Difficulty with managing hostility may require individual or family psycho-therapy as additional elements in a flexible yet rational approach to treatment, generally successful on an out-patient basis, but very occasionally requiring an in-patient setting.

Tic disorders and Tourette's syndrome

A tic is a quick, sudden, purposeless co-ordinated movement, which mimics a fragment of normal behaviour, tends to recur at the same place in the body and can be imitated by the affected person. Typically, it is greatly diminished or absent during sleep and is most prominent when the child is either underaroused and passive or highly aroused by anxiety or excitement. Older children will describe how a local irritant sensation or a mental discomfort occurs spontaneously, accompanied by the knowledge that performing a tic will reduce the discomfort (Leckman *et al.*, 1993). A tic may be suppressed voluntarily at the expense of mounting tension.

Simple tics (*transient tic disorder*) are quite common in middle childhood, occurring in about 5% of children with boys outnumbering girls by 2 to 1. The mean age of onset is seven years, with the head and neck most commonly affected (blinks, grimaces, throat clearing) and a wholly benign prognosis usual. In a more persistent variant (*chronic tic disorder*) tics appear and disappear, replacing each other over the months and waxing and waning in severity. This can continue for years.

Multiple tics coupled with the appearance of vocal tics (grunts, yelps, squeals, barks or verbal utterances) form *Gilles de la Tourette's syndrome*. This has been found to have a prevalence among older children and teenagers of about 3–5/10 000 and a more marked male predominance (about 9:1) than is the case for transient tic disorder (see e.g. Caine *et al.*, 1988). Children with Tourette's syndrome may develop more complex vocal tics including coprolalia, echolalia and palilalia (foul utterances, repetition of a question posed by another person, and repeated repetition of the final syllable of one's own utterance) but these only affect a minority. More common are complex repetitive behaviours (complex tics) such as squatting, pirouetting, eye-poking or slapping one's body. Typically, tics, whether simple or complex, occur in bouts that may be of remarkable intensity with large numbers of tics being executed within a few minutes. Some cases display compulsive activities such as repetitive touching, sniffing objects, compulsive counting or 'balancing' (e.g. doing the same action with one hand after is has been carried out with the other). These behaviours and ideations are sometimes indistinguishable from obsessive-compulsive phenomena. A number of young people with Tourette's syndrome also have restless inattentive behaviour and fulfil

135

criteria for hyperkinetic disorder and there is a greater than expected association with pervasive developmental disorders (Comings, 1990).

The aetiology of tic disorders is only partially unravelled. There is a powerful genetic component (see Robertson, 1994) as revealed by family and twin studies. Studies of family pedigrees also emphasise the close connection with obsessive-compulsive disorder. The underlying neurophysiology has been investigated by neurotransmitter assay and by functional imaging, but without a consensus interpretation emerging. There seems to be an imbalance of dopamine and noradrenaline functioning centring upon the basal ganglia but a variety of disparate findings defy simple interpretation (Leckman & Cohen, 1994 and Robertson, 1994, have provided overviews).

Identifying a tic is rarely a problem but differentiation from a simple habit, the involuntary movements of Sydenham's chorea, certain focal seizures and Wilson's disease occasionally cause difficulty. The process of full diagnostic appraisal of a severe tic disorder is quite often complicated by denial or dissimulation so the full picture may take time to establish.

Treatment of transient tic disorder is essentially explanation and reassurance since the prognosis is nearly always benign. A follow-up appointment is wise since apparent transient tics occasionally progress to a more severe variant, and the vocal tics of Tourette's syndrome often appear a year or two after simple motor tics have established themselves. Chronic tic disorder has a less favourable short-term prognosis and children may benefit from learning relaxation and having a structured day to keep them busy. A few will need haloperidol if their tics provoke teasing or restrict their pursuit of an ordinary life. The purpose of pharmacotherapy is not to abolish tics but to facilitate normal development.

Tourette's syndrome virtually always requires medication; haloperidol, pimozide and probably sulpiride are the first-line drugs (Shapiro et al., 1989). Clonidine can help some children who cannot tolerate neuroleptics and may be especially useful for those with hyperkinetic symptoms, since stimulants exacerbate tics in some cases (Leckman et al., 1991). Medication is likely to be required for years and the problems of tardive dyskinesia and gynaecomastia can supervene. The dose should be reviewed frequently as changing environmental circumstances and the natural tendency of tic disorders to wax and wane in severity alter the balance between dose and benefit. An earlier enthusiasm for behavioural methods such as massed practice has waned and these are no longer widely used.

Severe tic disorders tend to improve with passage through adolescence. About one-third of Tourette's syndrome cases remit by adult life and a similar proportion are much improved. The remaining third will continue to show multiple tics during adult life but coprolalia may disappear (Robertson, 1989; Bruun & Budman, 1992).

Specific learning disabilities

Some children have difficulty learning to read in spite of having an adequate IQ and intact sense organs. Their specific reading disorder is developmental in origin but they form a heterogeneous group (Hooper & Willis, 1989). It is possible to make a few generalisations: they are relatively likely to be boys, to have a history of delayed speech development, to have auditory processing and auditory memory impairments, to find discrimination between right and left difficult (note there is no excess compared with normal controls of 'crossed laterality', which refers to a lack of consistency in dominance between hands, eyes and feet), to have minor motor planning and coordination problems and a family history of poor reading. The basic deficit is probably one of phonological analysis and there is a strong hereditary element (DeFries *et al.*, 1987; Pennington *et al.*, 1991).

How far such reading difficulties differ from the low end of a normal distribution of reading ability is unresolved. Some studies find a 'hump' on the tail of the distribution curve (Stevenson, 1988), other do not (Shaywitz *et al.*, 1992). Stanovich (1994) has argued that the definition of the problem in terms of a discrepancy between reading ability and IQ means this issue has never been adequately addressed and there is no evidence for a qualitatively different disorder. Certainly the term dyslexia is to be used with caution in that it implies just this as well as hinting at a unitary condition; a concept that is unsustainable. Some children with specific reading disorder have abnormal brains: disturbed cortical architecture (Galaburda *et al.*, 1985) or an atypical asymmetry of the planum temporale (Larsen *et al.*, 1990) but this has not been shown to be consistently present. There is some impact of social circumstances, since the rate is higher in inner urban settings (Berger *et al.*, 1975). There are moderately strong associations with conduct disorder and hyperkinetic disorder (see Maughan & Yule, 1994, for a discussion).

The reading difficulties are remarkably persistent and the treatment is the provision of skilled, intensive reading tuition. There is some evidence that the effect of this is enhanced by the GABA analogue pracetam (Wilsher & Taylor, 1994) but it is not used in normal clinical practice. Spelling difficulties commonly emerge later. Specific spelling disorder suffers by virtue of not being associated with reading difficulties and the spelling tends to be more phonetically accurate. *Specific disorder of arithmetical skills* is quite likely to be linked with visuo-spatial difficulties; otherwise relatively little is known about these conditions.

Childhood autism and other pervasive developmental disorders

The pervasive developmental disorders are characterised by impaired and abnormal reciprocal interpersonal interactions which go beyond abnormalities that can be explained by developmental delay. There is always some abnormality in communication, using the term broadly, and a constant impoverishment of interests and activities. The term pervasive refers to the fact that these disabilities are pervasive across situations, not that there is a pervasive impairment of development in all modalities.

Childhood autism is the best known pervasive developmental disorder but its clinical picture varies with age and intelligence. Classical descriptions focus on middle childhood and near-normal intelligence, yet autism is a life-long handicap and is commonly associated with limited intelligence: roughly 70% of people with autism have an IQ below 70 though a few have normal or even superior intelligence. Awkwardly, the commonest form of autistic social behaviour is found in association with low intelligence, in which setting the determination to preserve environmental sameness, a criterion for the diagnosis of childhood autism, is often absent. Thus if there are autistic social and communicative

Table 5.2. *Behavioural abnormalities in childhood autism*

(A) Impairments of social interaction
  – Aloof and indifferent to other people
  – Poor gaze contact
  – Inability to maintain reciprocal social interactions (conversation, co-operative play)
  – Absent or very weak emotional attachments to parents
  – No persisting friendships
  – Lack of empathy, poor perception of others' emotions and motivations
  – Indifference to social conventions
  – No sharing of interests with others
  – Poor social imitation
(B) Impairments in communication
  – Absent speech in about half
  – Abnormal speech in remainder: – delayed acquisition
                                    – immediate echolalia
                                    – repetition of learned phrases without grammatic
                                      transformation (e.g. pronoun reversal)
                                    – immature syntax, often telegrammatic
                                    – neologisms
                                    – concrete, pedantic content
                                    – poor pragmatics (appreciation of social context)
                                    – unusual delivery of intonation
  Abnormal response to sounds
  – Poor comprehension of speech and gesture
  – No imaginative play in which invisible qualities and motives are attributed to toys
  – Poor use of symbolic toys
(C) Restrictive, repetitive and stereotyped patterns of behaviour
  – Rigid 'play': lining up toys
  – Watching regular actions, e.g. washing machines
  – Resistance to imposed change with preservation of sameness of timetable or environment
    (routines, furniture arrangement etc.)
  – Attachments to particular, non-cuddly, objects or collections of useless objects
  – Tantrums when frustrated by denial of above
(D) Additional abnormalities, not constantly present and not required for the diagnosis
  – Toe-walking
  – Flapping hands, spinning objects
  – Self-injurious or self-stimulating behaviours (head-banging, body rocking, etc.)
  – Unpredictable fears, hostile attacks or outbursts of laughter
  – Circumscribed, unshared, sterile fascinations (railway timetables, lists, etc.)
  – Isolated skills (jigsaws, calendrical calculation, etc.)

impairment but not detectable constraint of interests and activities beyond that predicted by intelligence, the picture is termed *atypical autism* whereas childhood autism is, by ICD-10 criteria, dependent upon the presence of all of four criteria:

1. Onset before the age of 3 years.
2. Qualitative impairments of reciprocal interaction.
3. Qualitative impairments in communication.
4. Restricted, repetitive and stereotyped patterns of behaviour, interests and activities.

These are expanded upon, descriptively, in Table 5.2. Usually there is no period of normal development before the condition becomes manifest to professionals but an onset over a period of weeks is evident in a minority and tends to be associated with subsequent lower levels of functioning (Burack & Volkmar, 1992). An onset between ages two and three may be classified as atypical autism or as *disintegrative disorder*, the latter label describing autistic social behaviour and a severe regression in language and play, which may develop at any age between two and middle childhood and is usually accompanied by a severe decline in intelligence. In practice its clinical presentation shades into autism and an underlying aetiology is unlikely to be discovered through physical investigations. To what extent it merits a separate label is unclear. The differential diagnosis of autism is from global developmental delay (which often co-exists), higher order specific language impairments of developmental origin, which not infrequently have impaired attachment behaviour and symbolic play, and Rett's syndrome, which affects girls only and has an onset in the second year of life. The latter is characterised by a loss of language and play with the appearance of hand-wringing mannerisms, vacant gaze, hyperventilation and slowing of head growth. Affected girls are severely mentally handicapped and eventually develop various motility problems affecting trunk and legs. Epilepsy quite frequently supervenes.

Classical ('nuclear' or 'Kanner') autism is rare with prevalence rates around 2–5/10 000, depending upon the criteria used. Earlier reports that children from middle-class families are commoner than expected in samples largely reflect referral bias but whether such a class bias still holds for community samples is unresolved. Recent whole population studies have not shown any social class bias (e.g. those by Steffenburg & Gillberg, 1986). Males are affected approximately three times more commonly than females.

The precise aetiology of autism is debatable but there is no doubt that it is a neurobiological condition. Evidence for a powerful genetic influence exists from family and twin studies (see Bailey *et al.*, 1995) and there is a little evidence that a locus on chromosome 15 may be implicated, at least in some cases (Baker *et al.*, 1994; Bundey *et al.*, 1994). Although autistic children are more likely to have suffered perinatal complications this is now thought to be a reflection of an abnormal foetus, since children experiencing these are also likely to display minor congenital physical abnormalities implying foetal maldevelop-ment (Rutter *et al.*, 1993).

Earlier assumptions that fragile-X was a cause of a significant number of cases of autism seem unlikely to be true. The abnormal social behaviour associated with fragile-X is typified by anxious gaze aversion and social apprehension and can be distinguished from autism (Turk, 1992). The fragile-X anomaly can only be found in about 2% of cases of tightly defined autism (Bailey *et al.*, 1993). Whether autism can profitably be regarded as a behavioural syndrome with a number of underlying causes, demonstrable on investigation, is controversial. Gillberg (1992) has claimed that 37% of his sample had a definable physical condition that could be causal; other authorities (e.g. Rutter *et al.*, 1994) point to a rate of about 10%, which is in line with my clinical experience. The difference probably hinges upon the inclusion or exclusion of atypical autism and the level of enthusiasm for full investigation. Associations with underlying conditions are weak and generally found in studies of children in which the diagnostic criteria for autism are broad and in which the children are of low intelligence. They are probably strongest for tuberous sclerosis, phenylketonuria, rubella embryopathy, and herpes encephalitis though a full list of 18 conditions is suggested by Gillberg (1992).

Within this group with no evident underlying neuropathology, neurophysiological, neuroimaging and neurochemical studies have yielded mixed results and no consistent, replicated picture has emerged (see Lord & Rutter, 1994 for a brief review). Rather more productive have been the parallel programmes of investigation that have tried to characterise the fundamental psychological deficits. Hobson (1993) has demonstrated the poor ability of autistic individuals to recognise emotions in other people and interpret gesture, facial expression and vocal inflexion. Following Leslie (1987), a number of investigators, notably Baron-Cohen (e.g. Baron-Cohen et al., 1993) have investigated autistic children's 'theory of mind', i.e. their ability to assume that other people have independent private motivations, memories and ideas. Generally, autistic young people have handicaps of varying degree in this area and their disinterest in other people and lack of interest in communication become understandable. The theory of mind account cannot, however, explain all abnormalities in autism (Happé, 1994).

After a period of nosological uncertainty a consensus has developed that Asperger's syndrome is a term that can be used to describe the social abnormalities seen in autism when these are present in a person who has near-normal speech development (Cox, 1991). In fact, the social use of language (pragmatics) and the ability to use metaphor are constrained so that affected individuals show poor ability to converse reciprocally, use a mechanical and monotonous tone of voice, lack empathy and think concretely. Commonly they have circumscribed, sterile interest patterns such as railway timetables or compiling long lists of computing. It is possibly ten times as common as childhood autism (Gillberg, 1992) and may be predisposed to by structural abnormalities of the cerebellum and corpus callosum (Berthier, 1994).

The management of autism is essentially the management of a devastating handicap: there is no cure. Social and communicative development should be fostered actively and secondary problem behaviours such as tantrums, self-injurious behaviour or unacceptable sexual behaviours will need prompt attention along behavioural lines. The parents and siblings need continuing support, not least in advice as how to evaluate the trends in ineffective 'miracle' therapies (holding therapy, facilitated communication, diets, fenfluramine, etc), which plague the field. By and large, education is the most powerful influence for improvement in autistic children. Special education is inevitable and may require placement in a school for autistic children which includes a curriculum emphasising language development and social skills within a structured, timetabled environment.

Autistic children grow into autistic adults. They will generally improve a little socially as they move through adolescence but the core handicaps never disappear. About one-third develop epileptic tonic-clonic seizures in adolescence but these are not uncommonly infrequent and may not require anticonvulsants. Good indicators of improvement in social adjustment are an IQ over 50 and the development of useful communicative language by the age of five. In adult life, autistic individuals need a range of provisions. Some will live in special residential communities, others at home with parents, often attending a local training centre. Only a small minority, possibly less than 10%, will have the skills to work and sustain an independent life.

General principles of treatment in child and adolescent psychiatry

The selection of treatment intervention will, of course, be influenced by the type of disorder, but comorbidity and available skills in any particular clinic will also need consideration. Furthermore, for some conditions, the choice between several treatments cannot be based on hard evidence for efficacy and a recourse to clinical experience or general principles is inevitable, as in the rest of medicine. There are thus some general points about treatment that should be made.

When child and adolescent psychiatry is located within the broader concept of a child and adolescent mental health service, it can sensibly be understood as a multi-disciplinary activity dealing with the most complex cases or as an intervention carried out by psychiatrists working alone, especially when providing consultation to other agencies. Thus in the currently advocated UK model it is located in the upper levels of a tiered system that includes four tiers including primary care interventions, mental health professionals working solo, out-patient teams, and in-patient units or highly specialised clinics (Department of Health, 1995; Hill, 1994; Williams & Richardson, 1995). This model seeks to unite primary care work, community (child guidance) clinics, clinical psychology services and hospital-based psychiatric services. It allows a coordination of efforts at prevention and limits the duplication of local child mental health services. It is parallelled by a move towards evidence-based interventions based on local health needs (Wallace *et al.*, 1996).

Given the impact of family relationships upon childhood psychopathology, the fact that referral to child mental health services is often at the parents' initiative, and the social power parents have over their children, it is not surprising that child psychiatry treatments nearly always involve parents. This may be at various levels: providing information or straightforward advice to parents, supporting their efforts, or changing their attitudes and behaviours, especially when they have maltreated their child. Such direct work with parents is common but goes largely undescribed though the work of trained health visitors with the parents of preschool children has been shown to be moderately effective in the short term (Nicol *et al.*, 1993).

The central concept of family therapy is that the child's symptoms or problematic behaviour are a manifestation of family relationship dysfunction. The whole family, or at any rate the entire household, thus become the focus for treatment. This does not necessarily mean that the family dysfunction initiated the problem but that it seems important in maintaining it. The actual treatment methods and philosophy used – Milan systemic, strategic, structural, behavioural, etc – may then be selected according to therapist skill rather than the characteristics of the case. Overall, there is some indication that family therapy is effective (Jenkins, 1990) but the evidence tends to come from meta-analytic appraisals of small studies or the application of a specific technique to a group of children defined by their disorder. The enthusiasm for family therapy as an approach that can be applied to virtually all disturbed children has evolved into a more discriminating approach though precise indications and contraindications remain elusive. It is still enormously

141

popular with professionals but not always with parents since it can give the impression that family relationships cause the clinical problem and parents feel blamed accordingly.

Children may be seen individually for discussion of their problem and situation. When this is based on the realities of the child's situation it is counselling, an approach quite widely used but essentially unevaluated. Studies that have attempted to do so (e.g. those of Adams, 1961) have quite often reported positive findings. Individual psychodynamic psychotherapy with children, in earlier years the principal psychiatric intervention, can be informed by various philosophies and metaphors of mental functioning. All place prime significance on the inner mental world of the child, linking this to emotions, attitudes and behaviours that are seen as problematic or unhealthy. Earlier professional preoccupations with psychological defences against anxiety caused by fantasies have evolved into a concern with perceptions of family relationships. Rather than verbal disclosure, the thematic content of play is the preferred mode of communication with pre-pubertal children and is the main source of information about the young child's preoccupations. It is assumed that he is unaware of some of these and the therapist endeavours to make interpretations that demonstrate how unconscious themes and forgotten memories influence current feelings and behaviours. In protracted treatments of more than a dozen sessions or so, the nature of the relationship with the therapist is usually considered crucial material for reflection and explanation because it mirrors both earlier and current family relationships.

Individual approaches to children also include cognitive treatments, though these are largely at an experimental stage. Although social problem-solving techniques have been taught to primary school-age children as a preventive measure, cognitive methods to treat disorders are generally applied to older children such as adolescents with depression, low self-esteem, general anxiety or who have problems with self-control.

Group approaches to children fall into two major categories. Social skills groups tend to be concerned with social repertoire and major abnormalities of social interaction. Talking groups are quite widely used for a range of disorders in adolescence and there is evidence for their efficacy with mild to moderately severe disorders (Kolvin et al., 1981). Sexual abuse victims are frequently treated by a composite approach that includes a talking group. There is no good evidence that talking groups are effective with young children.

Behavioural approaches are quite widely applied as part of a treatment package as opposed to a whole treatment in their own right (Hill, 1990). There is an extensive literature on both assessment and treatment and there are important distinctions from adult psychiatric practice. Parents are commonly recruited as co-therapists, for instance in the dispensation of praise, sticky stars or beads as tokens, or tangible reinforcers, and close inspection of operant programmes often reveals that the covert purpose of a programme is first to change parental behaviour in order, secondarily, to change the child. Compared with adult practice there is more use of operant approaches, to build, diminish or replace behaviours. Positive contingencies are generally preferred but the use of time out (from positive social reinforcement) and the enuresis alarm are instances of aversive consequences, widely employed. Flooding is less used because the powerless state of children raises ethical issues and the poverty of their coping responses can leave them traumatised. Graded exposure or full desensitisation, commonly in vivo, are treatments of first choice for a number of phobias. The overall efficacy of behavioural approaches is hard to demonstrate but since most behavioural interventions are individually tailored according to an applied science model, it is an intervention that evaluates its own efficacy. The steps are:

1. definition of problematic response;

2. collection of baseline data to quantify it;

3. hypothesis as to its relationship to environmental variables or skills deficits;

4. manipulation of environmental variables or skill building;

5. reassess problem quantitatively;

6. form new hypothesis if no improvement.

Medication has historically been little used by psychiatrists though general practitioners have been less tentative (Adams, 1991). Clomipramine in obsessive-compulsive disorder, stimulants and tricyclics in hyperkinetic disorder, haloperidol and pimozide in Tourette's syndrome, and mainstream treatments for adolescent depressive disorder or schizophrenia are all well-recognised and documented. Sedation of small children with anti-histamines and the use of imipramine for enuresis are two approaches quite widely practiced in primary care but eschewed by psychiatrists except for brief respite. There is growing interest in the area of childhood psychopharmacology (see e.g. Gadow, 1992) but relatively little soundly established indications for medication as first line treatment apart from the above situations.

Treatment approaches that aim to alter the child's living context have always been part of the psychiatric repertoire. Recommendations about special educational needs, alternative family placement or the provision of social services and forensic resources are part of the work. The provision of formal mental health consultation to other professionals without assumption of direct professional responsibility is increasingly in demand though its evaluation is problematic. In a rather similar vein, the provision of reports to courts and other agencies is part of indirect promotion of child mental health or the amelioration of psychiatric disorder through guiding environmental manipulation.

Coda

There has been a growing realisation that neither childhood nor adulthood are homogeneous epochs when the continuity of psychopathology between them is considered. Some conditions are remarkably persistent: autism is a case in point. Others become less prevalent with age and are relatively common in early childhood but have disappeared by adolescence: feeding and sleep onset difficulties in pre-school children for instance. Hyperkinetic disorder is most evident in middle childhood, usually burns out in late adolescence (Mannuzza et al., 1993) but can persist into adult life. It is quite commonly associated with the development of conduct disorder or delinquency, presumably because of demoralisation and disillusionment, particularly because of academic failure and deteriorating peer relationships. The co-existence of discordant family relationships seems a more relevant determinant of adult prognosis than the hyperactivity per se (Weiss & Hechtman,

1986). A typical age of prominence is also shown by Tourette's syndrome, which commonly presents in early adolescence and continues into the late teens, at which point there is some chance of recovery though many cases of Tourette's syndrome and of early adolescent schizophrenia will persist throughout the teens and throughout adult life as chronic conditions. Then there are disorders that appear in late childhood or adolescence and may clear up temporarily only to recur in adult life: obsessive-compulsive disorder, some cases of schizophrenia, bipolar disorder and depression are instances (Zeitlin, 1986). Certainly for schizophrenia and bipolar disorder, an early onset is a poor prognostic marker.

More intriguing is the manner in which some childhood disorders predict different adult disorder. Conduct disorder, for instance, is not only a forerunner of dissocial personality disorder in adulthood in nearly half of all cases but is also a predictor of adult alcohol or substance abuse in men and depression in women (see above and von Knorring *et al.*, 1987). A neurotic disorder in childhood (ICD-8), sufficiently severe to require admission to hospital, was found by Thomsen (1990) to predict a higher rate than expected of hospital admission in adult life with a diagnosis of personality disorder, but not neurosis, in adult life. This may be an artefact of admission policies as Zeitlin (1986) found that a diagnosis of an emotional disorder in out-patient children was followed in adult life by depression or neurotic disorder in three-quarters of cases. It is increasingly accepted that childhood symptoms offer a better indicator of adult mental state than do childhood diagnoses.

One reason for continuity is the persistence of adversity, particularly adverse family relationships, which are notoriously persistent. Pathways linking child and adolescent psychopathology can be conceptualised in various ways (Rutter, 1989)

- continuing social adversity;
- shaping one's own environment which then acts back, continuing to influence development;
- persisting lack of positive coping strategies;
- retention of perverse internal working models of relationships;
- development or continuation of low self-esteem or learned helplessness;

Active treatment or prophylaxis have made the natural history of untreated childhood psychiatric disorder somewhat less important. It is no longer a simple matter to make statements about the adult mental health implications of childhood psychiatric disorder. Furthermore, a general appreciation that children and teenagers deserve treatment in their own right, not just because of the consequences for their later life, is overdue.

6

Neurosis and personality disorder

GLYN LEWIS and SIMON WESSELY

General aspects of neurosis

Introduction

The clearest definition of neurosis is simply the antithesis of psychosis, hence neurotic disorders are those psychiatric conditions in which there is no overall loss in the perception of external reality. Even this has inconsistencies, since by convention eating disorders and substance misuse are excluded from neurotic conditions, whilst some subjects with either obsessive-compulsive disorder or hypochondriasis may have only the most tenuous grip on external reality in some areas of their life, yet are still considered with the rubric of neurosis. An impairment of insight is a feature of all psychiatric disorder and even of the psychopathology of everyday life. The impairment of insight in neurosis is less marked, and less disruptive on overall functioning in neurosis than psychosis. Another definition of neurosis is aetiological – there is a frequent implication that psychosocial factors are more important in the aetiology of neurotic disorders and that they are more understandable in terms of the patient's predicament. There is some evidence for a continuum between neurotic and psychotic depression (Kendell, 1968) and perhaps it is inadvisable to attempt too rigid a distinction between the concepts.

In practice, neurosis as an overall term has tended to be superseded by the use of separate diagnoses, which are discussed below, or in community and primary care studies by the concept of 'common mental disorders', which are mostly various admixtures of depression and anxiety. No definition of neurosis can compete in rigour with the standardised criteria for the individual disorders.

The authors of DSM-III (American Psychiatric Association, 1980) have abandoned the term neurosis altogether, largely because of the failure to integrate the different concepts of neurosis held by the psychodynamic and phenomenological schools. This view has been maintained in DSM-IV (APA, 1994). However, for many the loss of the resonant term neurosis is too high a price and like many terms in psychiatry we suspect that it will outlive its obituarists. ICD-10 represents an uneasy compromise – neurosis is retained, but depressive neurosis disappears within mood disorders. In this chapter we will continue to list arbitrarily certain disorders that are traditionally grouped under the term neurosis, but for which we acknowledge that the links may primarily be historical.

If one chooses to retain the category of neurosis, many would regard the majority of cases of depression as falling within the rubric of neurosis. However, following the current division of disorders within ICD-10 and DSM-IV, depression is discussed in Chapter 11 on the affective disorders. We therefore concentrate to a large extent on disorders where anxiety forms an important component of the symptomatology.

History

Neurosis is derived from the Greek word for nerve, which reminds us that neurosis began with a radically different meaning from that now used. It was introduced by Edinburgh physician William Cullen in two books published in 1769 and 1777. It covered a wide range of conditions, associated with disorder of the nervous system. As used by Cullen, and later Pinel, it included a wide range of disorders, such as epilepsy, tetanus and paralysis. During the nineteenth century these and other disorders for which gross pathological changes could be discerned were removed.

Although neurosis then covered a range of emotional disorders not dissimilar to current usage, its suggested aetiologies were very different. Following a series of major advances in the natural sciences, such as the discovery of the electrical nature of the nervous impulse, and the spinal reflex, neurosis was assumed to be a somatic disturbance of the nervous system. Several other closely related conditions, such as neurasthenia, neurospasm and spinal irritation were also recognised at the time. The suggested aetiologies differed, with the favoured mechanisms first involving the peripheral nervous system (the reflex hypothesis) and later the central nervous system (as in failures of cerebral blood flow or energy supply). However, the flourishing of the natural sciences, especially neurophysiology and neuropathology, mean that none of these hypotheses could be sustained.

The name of Sigmund Freud will always be associated with the fundamental change in the understanding of neurosis that occurred at the end of the nineteenth century. The revolution took two forms. First, the origins of neurosis shifted from physical to psychogenic – hence the term psychoneurosis. Second, the classification of neurosis was altered, and recognisably modern conditions such as phobia, anxiety and obsessive compulsive disorder began to emerge from over-stretched categories such as neurasthenia. In Freud's key paper (Freud, 1895) he described anxiety disorder and panic attacks, and argued they should be separated from neurasthenia. In the light of subsequent events, it is worth noting that he did not suggest separating anxiety and panic. Of course, Freud was by no means solely responsible for this change. Charcot and later Janet and Bernheim were as influential.

The reasons for these changes are complex, and should not been seen as an inevitable progress from ignorance to enlightenment, as occasionally portrayed by psychoanalytically influenced historians. Numerous social, professional and economic factors played their part in the transfer of the care of the nervous patient from the physician to the psychiatrist (Oppenheim, 1991; Shorter, 1992).

Classification of neurosis

Psychiatric classification has largely been developed from hospital-based practice. The resulting categorical classification systems have many limitations, and in particular do not correspond with psychiatric disorder as found in the community. In consequence, often fierce arguments have developed about the classification of neurosis.

Only a small proportion of psychiatric disorders seen in primary care or community settings are seen in specialist hospital practice. Goldberg & Huxley (1992) estimate that only about 7% of all those with psychiatric disorder are seen by psychiatrists in the UK. Though there is an overlap in the severity of conditions seen in primary and secondary care, it has been observed that the disorders seen in hospital settings are more discrete than those seen in primary care. It is not clear whether this clinical observation is true, nor whether the reason for the difference, if it exists, is the result of referral bias on the part of the primary care physician. Various terms have been used to describe the less differentiated syndromes – undifferentiated neurotic syndrome, minor psychiatric morbidity (although often it is not minor at all), or even just psychiatric 'caseness'.

Most primary care physicians do not use the complex standardised criteria that have recently become fashionable within psychiatric services. It is questionable whether such definitions will ever become widely used in primary care. Critics would argue that diagnostic schema have become far too long and over complex and not related to the primary task of diagnosis, namely helping doctors improve treatment for patients. As we shall see below, there is now evidence that antidepressants provide effective treatment for both depressive and anxiety disorders. If the main therapeutic option for anxiety and depression involves the same therapeutic agent it is difficult to argue that the 54 pages of the ICD-10 chapter on neurotic disorders and the 17 sub-classifications of depression found therein will be of much use to most primary care physicians or indeed most psychiatrists.

Relationship between anxiety and depression

The distinction between anxiety and depression is fundamental to attempts to classify minor psychiatric disorders in general practice and the community. There is still much controversy about the relationship between the two emotional states (Stavrakaki & Vargo, 1986; Tyrer, 1989) and the evidence is confused, confusing and often contradictory.

The 'Newcastle' group of Roth and colleagues are associated with the idea that anxiety and depression are separate disorders (see the paper by Roth et al., 1972) on the basis of principal components analysis of clinical ratings. Other pieces of evidence have also been proposed to support the distinction, including the observation that loss events precede depression, danger events precede anxiety, whilst loss and danger events led to mixed states (Finlay-Jones & Brown, 1981). Both family history and twin studies (Noyes et al., 1983; Torgersen 1985) provide some evidence for the dichotomy and a different prognosis has also been claimed, being better for depression than panic disorder (Coryell et al., 1983).

The opposing view, of a continuum of disturbance rather than two discrete entities, is associated with names of Aubrey Lewis and Edward Mapother, and was given experimental support by the work of Robert Kendell, who failed to identify a point of rarity between the two subgroups, as well as finding change in diagnosis over time (Kendell, 1975). Kendell suggested that data presented by the Newcastle group may have been influenced by studying the atypical group of patients who are admitted.

Other studies have demonstrated an overlap of symptoms that seems at odds with Roth's view. A number of studies have shown high rates of depression in those with agoraphobia and other anxiety disorders. For example, in a Swiss population study, Angst & Dobler-Mikola (1985) showed that approximately one-third of subjects with either major depression or anxiety disorders had both disorders. Patients with anxiety neurosis have a high rate of depressive symptoms, and vice versa (see the paper by Breier *et al.*, 1985).

Dimensions or categories

One of the long running debates within medical classification concerns the distinction between categories and continua. It has been persuasively argued (Rose & Barker, 1978) that a dimensional approach is a more useful description of disease, particularly in population-based studies. However, doctors often find categories useful in clinical work because decisions, for example, about treatment are all-or-none. The purpose of classification is to provide a useful description of the natural world. From the point of view of an epidemiologist studying disorder in the community a dimensional approach is the most valuable.

Few would argue that there is no overlap of symptoms but psychiatrists still disagree about the extent to which anxiety and depression co-vary or on the rather metaphysical question of whether they are two separate 'disorders' or 'entities'. The model adopted by Goldberg & Huxley (1992) amongst others is of two dimensions, one representing anxiety, the other depression, which are allowed to be correlated with each other. In other words both anxiety and depression are conceived as dimensions, but people with depressive symptoms can also be more likely to have anxiety symptoms. This simplifies the question into the magnitude of the correlation between the two dimensions.

Leff (1978) has demonstrated that psychiatrists perceive anxiety and depression as less closely correlated than their patients and so there are grounds to suppose that there may be a potential bias to perceive anxiety and depression as more distinct, as least amongst some doctors. This hypothesis is supported by the observation that self-report measures of anxiety and depression, which should reduce observer bias, are more closely related than those requiring clinical judgement (Lewis, 1991). In general, factor analytic studies of self-report questionnaires show poor separation between the symptoms of anxiety and depression (Williams *et al.*, 1968; Mendels *et al*, 1972). In contrast Roth and colleagues (Roth *et al.*, 1972; Mountjoy & Roth, 1982) have repeatedly found separate anxiety and depression factors using observer rating scales or clinical interviews. Goldberg *et al.* (1987) found two separate anxiety and depression factors but they were highly correlated ($r = 0.74$).

There are two main explanations for these contradictory findings. Firstly, as suggested above, some psychiatrists may regard anxiety and depression as separate conditions with separate treatments, and this view may bias an assessment. Secondly, it can be argued that a clinician can distinguish between anxiety and depression whereas the subject completing a self-report scale cannot, or uses the terms less precisely. Lewis (1991) has provided some evidence that these discrepant results occur because of observer bias in measurement scales requiring clinical judgements on the part of the observer.

There is also some evidence that questions the traditional view that anxiety and depression have different pharmacological treatments, Johnstone *et al.* (1980) in a group of neurotic patients did not find that the symptoms of anxiety and depression predicted differential response to a tricyclic antidepressant or a benzodiazepine. Similarly Tyrer *et al.* (1988) reported that tricyclic antidepressants (and placebo) were better than a benzodiazepine in the treatment of neurotic disorders irrespective of diagnosis (panic, generalised anxiety disorder and dysthymia). The Cross-National Collaborative Panic Study (1992) also found equal efficacy of the benzodiazepine alprazolam and the tricyclic imipramine in the treatment of panic disorder and Wilkinson *et al.* (1991) in a meta-analysis concluded that antidepressants were as effective as anti-anxiety medication in panic disorder. The distinction between anxiety and depression is therefore difficult to make on the grounds that they respond to different classes of pharmacological agents.

Cognitive theories of anxiety are also very similar to cognitive theories of depression (Beck *et al.*, 1985). According to the theory, if a person predicts that some adverse event will definitely happen, the result is a depressed mood; if an adverse event might happen the result is anxiety. Such a view would predict a considerable overlap between the symptoms of anxiety and depression. One might also expect considerable week-to-week variation in the symptoms depending upon the degree of belief attached to the patients' cognitions.

A reasonable conclusion would be that there is an overlap between anxiety and depression, and those who experience one tend to experience the other. There is, however, a subjectively different experience between depression and anxiety and in some individuals one or other dominates at any given time. As Tyrer (1989) has argued, categorical classifications of neurotic disorders only work if a rigid hierarchy of diagnostic precedence is imposed. Both Tyrer (1989) and Andrews (1991) have argued for a separate diagnostic category of General Neurotic Syndrome to deal with the overlap discussed above. This idea has not found general acceptance, though many are sympathetic with their approach. As these authors recognise, a categorical classification sits uneasily with the empirical data in the area of neurosis.

Comorbidity

We have argued above for regarding neurotic symptomatology as continua, especially within community studies. The opposing view, that has tended to dominate the diagnostic manuals, is to provide a categorical system of classification. Since the development of operationalised criteria for diagnostic categories, it has become increasingly apparent that many individuals meet the criteria for more than one disorder. This phenomenon is referred to as comorbidity.

The diagnostic manuals have increasingly abandoned the hierarchical diagnostic systems that were either explicit or implicit in psychiatric practice. For example, DSM-III did not allow generalised anxiety disorder (GAD) to be diagnosed in the presence of major depression, whereas DSM-IIIR, DSM-IV and ICD-10 now allow this. There has therefore been increasing work calculating the overlap between various neurotic disorders.

One of the main findings is that neurotic disorders occur more often together than one could explain by chance. In the US National Comorbidity Survey (Kessler *et al.*, 1994), 59%

Table 6.1. *Prevalence (%) of subjects with neurotic symptoms defined by the CIS-R in the OPCS National Survey of Psychiatric Morbidity (Meltzer et al. 1995)*

Symptom	Men	Women
Fatigue	21	33
Sleep problems	21	28
Irritability	19	25
Worry	17	23
Depression	8	11
Depressive ideas	7	11
Anxiety	8	11
Obesessions	7	12
Concentration and forgetfulness	6	10
Somatic symptoms	5	10
Compulsions	5	8
Phobias	3	7
Worry about physical health	4	5
Panic	2	3
Sample size	4859	4933

of those with at least one psychiatric disorder met the criteria for three or more disorders. Of those with GAD, 38% also had major depression and 27% had agoraphobia (Wittchen *et al.*, 1994).

From the point of view of those who tend to 'lump' diagnoses rather than 'split' them, the growth in research in comorbidity is a reflection of the limitation of viewing psychiatric diagnoses as categories. It also reveals a tendency towards reification of diagnostic categories once a committee has come up with the operationalised criteria. If a single dimension of neurotic symptomatology accounts for most variation in the community (Lewis, 1992), then one would expect that subjects with more symptoms would have a more severe disorder and therefore be more disabled, receive more attention from the health service and receive more diagnoses. This is one of the results emerging from studies of comorbidity but can be explained more parsimoniously by a much simpler unidimensional model.

Descriptive epidemiology

In community surveys, the majority of the population have at least one neurotic symptom at any one time. For example, in the British Health and Lifestyle survey (Cox *et al.*, 1987), 70% of the population reported at least one of the symptoms on the General Health Questionnaire (GHQ; Goldberg, 1972). In that sense, the abnormal individuals are those without neurotic symptoms. Table 6.1 gives the prevalence of the 14 symptoms estimated using the revised Clinical Interview Schedule (CIS-R; Lewis *et al.*, 1992) from the results of the OPCS National Survey of Psychiatric Morbidity conducted in Great Britain (Meltzer *et al.*, 1995). Fatigue is the most common symptom, and is present in about 25% of the population (see also Lewis & Wessely, 1992). Irritability and worry are also commoner than

Table 6.2. *Prevalence (%) of neurotic disorders from three population surveys, and from primary care*

Disorder	ECA, 1 month prevalence[a] (US, 5 sites)	OPCS National Survey of Psychiatric Morbidity[b] (UK), 1 week prevalence	US National Comorbidity Survey[c], 12 month prevalence	WHO Psychological Morbidity in Primary Care[d], 12 month prevalence
Depression	2.4	1.7	10.3	10.5
Phobias–total	6.7	1.8		
Agoraphobia	7.6[e]		2.8	1.5
Social phobia	3.2[e]		7.9	
Specific phobia	15.1[e]		8.8	
Panic disorder	0.5	0.8	2.3	1.1
Obsessive-compulsive disorder	1.3	1.3		
Generalised anxiety disorder	1.3	2.9	3.1	7.9
Mixed anxiety–depression		7.1		
Diagnostic criteria	DSM-III	ICD-10	DMS-III-R	ICD-10

Notes: [a] Robins & Regier, 1991; [b] Meltzer *et al.*, 1995; [c] Kessler *et al.*, 1994; [d] Ormel *et al.*, 1994; [e] lifetime prevalence.

depression and anxiety. In Goldberg *et al.*'s (1976) primary care study 82% of the subjects complained of either anxiety or worry.

In the OPCS National Survey of Psychiatric Morbidity (Meltzer *et al.*, 1995), 17% of the population had a neurotic psychiatric disorder in the week before interview. The threshold in this study indicates a degree of symptomatology that would generate concern amongst a primary care physician. Of those studies in the multinational WHO study of common mental disorders in primary care 21% fulfilled one or more ICD-10 diagnosis, mostly neurotic conditions (Ormel *et al.*, 1994). Table 6.2 gives the prevalence of the main neurotic disorders from three population-based studies and the WHO study of primary care. There are quite marked differences in prevalence between the surveys. These result from using different diagnostic criteria, different assessments for psychiatric disorder and geographical and temporal variation.

It has been estimated that, in the UK, over 90% of people with a neurotic disorder will consult a primary care physician in the course of a year. This is because about two-thirds of people consult their GP every year and neurotic disorder increases the likelihood of consultation (Goldberg & Huxley,1992).

Published incidence rates vary, depending upon methodology, case definitions and length of follow up. The better studies suggest annual incidence rates of 1% (Stirling County, Canada; Murphy *et al.*, 1988), 2% (Lundby, Sweden; Hagnell *et al.*, 1994), 3% (Otago, New Zealand; Romans *et al.*, 1993) and 4% (ECA, USA; Eaton *et al.*, 1989).

Gender

Neurotic disorders of whatever type are commoner in women, with only two exceptions, social phobias and obsessive-compulsive disorder. Women are more likely to consult doctors for health problems including mental health problems. Kessler *et al.* (1981) have argued that this is mostly due to women being more likely to label themselves as having a psychological problem.

There are a number of possible explanations for the increased prevalence of neurosis in women. Many of the studies are cross-sectional and so the excess prevalence may result from either a higher incidence in women or a longer duration of illness, though longitudinal studies have usually confirmed a higher incidence in women. The difference between the sexes may result because women are more likely to divulge details of their emotional life or be more aware of them. One other possibility is some underlying inherited abnormality, for example, related to endocrine differences. Alternatively, differences between the sexes may result from differences in vulnerability related to environmental factors in development. For example, sexual abuse is commoner in female than male children.

One of the most likely explanations for the gender difference concerns the different social roles occupied by men and women. Women are more likely to be in low status jobs and are also more likely to have too many roles. For example, most women continue to provide child-care and homekeeping while out at work. Studies on relatively homogenous groups of men and women, for example civil servants of the same grade, find that there is no gender difference in psychiatric disorder (Jenkins, 1985; Wilhelm & Parker, 1989). These studies argue for the importance of current social role and circumstances in determining the differential rates in women and men.

Socio-economic status

Neurotic disorders are commoner in those with lower socio-economic status. In the UK National Psychiatric Morbidity Survey (Meltzer *et al.*, 1995), overall rates of neurotic disorder were 18.2% in social class 5 and 10.0% in social class 1 (Registrar General's classification). Indices of lower disposable income and wealth, such as housing tenure, were also associated with neurotic disorder (local authority renters 23.8% versus home owners 13.6%).

Public health aspects

Major depression is associated with profound morbidity and social impairment, equal to or in excess of that seen in many chronic physical illnesses (Wells *et al.*, 1989). Panic disorder, phobic disorders, generalised anxiety and neurasthenia are also associated with occupational and social disability (Davidson *et al.*, 1993; Ormel *et al.*, 1993, 1994) – often, especially in the case of neurasthenia and phobic disorders, severe. Recent community studies in the United States have studied neurotic disorders that do not meet the full criteria for DSM-III disorders and hence are rarely seen in secondary settings. The results show that depressive and other neurotic symptoms below the criteria for major depression lead to more disability, in aggregate, than major depression itself (Broadhead *et al.*, 1990; Johnson *et al.*, 1992); although major depression is more disabling for the individual affected there are more individuals with the less severe disorders. This public health point has repeatedly been made with a variety of other disorders (Rose, 1992). Even individual symptoms such as fatigue are very common and have a public health impact (Kroenke *et al.*, 1988; Lewis & Wessely, 1992).

Neurotic disorder also increases the likelihood of consulting a primary care physician, and is associated with sickness absence and increased labour turnover. There is considerable impact on industry of neurotic disorder as well as direct costs on the health service (Croft-Jeffreys & Wilkinson, 1989; Smith *et al.*, 1995). Neurotic disorders are less disabling to the individual than psychotic disorders. However, because they are more common, in aggregate they lead to as much disability and have important economic consequences.

Geographical variation in the rates of disease can help provide clues to aetiology and are also useful in planning services. There have been many reports that neurotic psychiatric disorders are commoner in urban areas, at least in Western societies (Blazer *et al.*, 1985; Lewis & Booth, 1994). The reasons for this are not understood, though Brown and his colleagues found that stressful life events were commoner in South London than North Uist in the Outer Hebrides, Scotland (Brown *et al.*, 1977). There is also evidence for regional variation in the rates of neurotic disorder within the UK (Lewis & Booth, 1992).

In the long-term, preventive strategies for neurotic disorder will need to be based upon sound epidemiological findings concerning the environmental cause of the conditions. At the moment a public health approach towards preventing these conditions is premature but an important priority for research must be to understand more about the aetiology of these conditions and translate the findings into practical preventive strategies.

Psychological and physiological aspects of neurosis

Phenomenology of anxiety

Like the other symptoms of neurosis, anxiety is a normal emotional experience, and no clear-cut distinction can be made between those with 'normal' anxiety and those in whom anxiety is a significant and disabling symptom. Anxiety can be distinguished from worry. Worry is the phenomenon of unpleasant, recurrent thinking about a problem or concern. There is therefore a clear mental or cognitive element to worry. In contrast, anxiety refers to the somatic and emotional aspects of anxiety that can exist independently of any conscious awareness of worrying thinking. Though worry is usually found in people who are also anxious, Wing *et al.* (1974) argue that worry is also a non-specific symptom present along with other symptoms, especially depression. Anxiety is characterised by the following features:

Somatic symptoms There are a number of prominent somatic symptoms of anxiety that result from autonomic arousal, muscular tension and hyperventilation. Autonomic arousal can lead to palpitations, muscular tremor, perspiration and abdominal discomfort ('butterflies in the stomach').

Patients with anxiety complain about feeling out of breath and many hyperventilate. Hyperventilation provides a possible explanation for many of the symptoms of anxiety and panic-overbreathing leads to hypocapnia (a low pCO_2). The resulting alkalosis in turn leads to cerebral vasoconstriction, nervous hyperirritability, paraesthesia, chest pain, headache, dizziness and faintness. However, not all hyperventilators report anxiety (see below).

Subjective muscular tension is also a prominent feature of anxiety. Starting with the early studies of Sainsbury & Gibson (1954) there have been claims that many of the local symptoms of anxiety are related to muscle activity and tension, but the results have not always been replicated. Two of the more interesting studies have related chest wall muscle activity to chest pain in subjects with panic attacks (Lynch *et al.*, 1991), and increased muscle tension in the paravertebral muscles of patients with back pain when emotionally arousing subjects were discussed (Flor *et al.*, 1985).

Cognitive symptoms The cognitive element of anxiety is difficult to determine and often patients are not able to give an account of any thoughts when anxious. When patients do describe the thoughts accompanying anxiety it is usually concerned with predicting some fairly catastrophic event. For example, fear of public ridicule in social phobia, or of collapse, death or loss of control in a panic attack.

Emotional symptoms There has been a long-running controversy about the labelling of emotions and whether there is an 'emotion' that can be identified independently of the somatic and cognitive symptoms of anxiety (see below). In clinical settings patients complain of feeling anxious in addition to the symptoms given above.

Psychological theories of anxiety

The James-Lange (James, 1890) theory, articulated towards the end of the nineteenth century, turned the common-sense view of emotion on its head. Rather than the internal state of anxiety leading to the behavioural and physical symptoms, they argued that the behavioural and physical symptoms were interpreted by the person and labelled by the individual as anxiety. However, Cannon (1927) suggested that the autonomic nervous system was too slow and stereotyped to explain the wide variety of emotional experience and the rapidity of the development of anxiety.

The first psychological theory of phobia was that of Watson, in which he induced a conditioned fear of a tame white rate in 'Little Albert' (Watson & Rayner, 1920). More recently, Mowrer (1960) and other two-stage learning theorists have developed a psychological model based upon animal learning theory that is a synthesis of the behaviourism of B.F. Skinner and the reflexology of Pavlov. Phobias result from the experience of traumatic events associated with the consequent unpleasant stimuli and fear (classical conditioning). This state is maintained by subsequent avoidance of these stimuli, which act as a negative reinforced (operant conditioning).

Two-stage theorists argue that stimuli associated with certain events (reward, punishment, absence of expected reward or frustration, etc.) lead to internal states that in humans are called emotions. There are a number of problems for this extrapolation to human life. For example, the implications are that hunger (a stimulus associated with food) is an emotion. Furthermore, the number of possible emotions are relatively small, in contrast, to the subjective experiences of human life. The clinical range of phobic fear is also limited to a fairly restricted and non-random set of stimuli. Little Albert was conditioned to show fear to a white rat, but subsequent efforts to induce a little girl to develop a conditioned response to a toy duck were a failure (English, 1929). These and other observations led to theory of 'preparedness' – that humans are 'prepared' to develop fear responses to only a limited range of stimuli (Seligman, 1970).

Human beings are rational, thinking beings, not passive, reflexive organisms responding in an unthinking way to the events and situations in which they find themselves. The application of animal learning theory to human problems is therefore bound to be limited. Cognitive psychology (Anderson, 1980) has now become accepted as the main approach towards understanding human perception, motivation and behaviour.

Schacter & Singer's (1962) famous experiment found that the injection of epinephrine affected the intensity of emotion rather than the label that was applied to it, which depended upon the context. They concluded that there was an important cognitive element in the labelling of emotion by subjects, similar in some ways to the point James was making at the end of the nineteenth century.

Beck's (1976) introduction of cognitive psychology into thinking about psychiatric disorder is of great importance. His theory suggests that the emotions of depression, anxiety and anger result from the individuals' interpretation of the outside world and depression in particular results from negative thoughts about the self, world and future – the cognitive triad (see Chapter 25). Though there is still controversy about the primacy of thought over affect, cognitive psychology now appears to be the most promising approach towards understanding the psychological mechanisms of neurosis.

Neurochemistry of neurosis

The effectiveness of benzodiazepines in the treatment of anxiety have focused attention on the role of GABA (gamma-aminobutyric acid), since benzodiazepines are known to increase the affinity of GABA for its binding sites. Flumazenil, a benzodiazepine antagonist, increases anxiety (Nutt et al., 1990). Both serotoninergic and noradrenergic systems have also been implicated in the aetiology of pathological anxiety. Evidence for a role for serotonin in anxiety comes largely from empirical treatment studies. Drugs found to have anxiolytic properties include serotonin reuptake inhibitors, buspirone (a 5-HT$_{1A}$ agonist), M-CPP (a 5-HT$_2$ agonist), and ritanserin (a 5-HT$_2$ antagonist). Interestingly, the role of serotonin has also been inferred from the other clinical observation that drugs that block serotonin re-uptake also produce acute anxiety, known as the 'jitteriness' syndrome (Pohl et al., 1988). As Nutt (1990) has pointed out, these observations, like those of all provocation tests, cannot imply causality, since it remains unclear whether it was the agent itself that

155

directly provoked symptoms, or whether it was the subject's cognitive response to the procedure that generated anxiety.

The noradrenergic system has been implicated by studies reporting that yohimbine, a blocker of presynaptic inhibitory α_2-adrenoreceptors, causes anxiety, whilst clonidine, an α_2-adrenoreceptor agonist, reduces it. Subjects with yohimbine-induced panic attacks show large increases in noradrenergic activity and a blunted growth hormone response to clonidine, suggestive of noradrenergic dysfunction involving subsensitivity at the αa_2 adrenergic receptor (Charney et al., 1992). The model is thus that an overactive noradrenergic system causes the subject to produce an excessive emotional response (anxiety and/or panic) to a stimulus that would normally be innocuous (Nutt, 1990).

How do these neurochemical findings relate to the structure and function of the brain? In a series of animal studies, Jeffrey Gray (1982) has highlighted the role of the septohippocampal region, whose function he suggests is to receive information and to match this 'actual' information with what was 'expected'. His animal model of anxiety is based upon the idea of a psychological mechanism for behavioural inhibition elicited by fearful and frustrating situations (see Gray, 1982). The physiological substrate for this is the septo-hippocampal system and the associated monoamine pathways.

Aetiology – environmental factors

Most studies of the aetiology of neurosis have concentrated on studying depression. We will briefly discuss these and point out any findings that are relevant to anxiety disorders when they are available.

Childhood experience

Parental loss and separation   The seminal studies of Brown & Harris (1978) suggested that loss of mother before 11 increased the risk of adult depression. Subsequent studies have produced contradictory findings (Parker 1992). Tennant et al. (1981a) have argued that parental–child separations were not associated with depression, but to seeking help for depression. Separation or loss of a parent rarely occurs in isolation and any association with neurotic disorder may be confounded by other variables. For example, childhood parental loss is often followed by socio-economic disadvantage and inconsistent or inadequate parenting by alternative caregivers. Other events, aside from actual parental loss, including both parental indifference (Brown & Harris, 1993) and lack of care (MacKinnon et al., 1993) are also both associated with adult depression, whilst a history of parental conflict was associated with all neurotic diagnoses in the Zurich longitudinal study (Angst & Vollrath, 1991). Parker's work from Australia has also linked type of parenting during childhood to later depression, but also, albeit to a lesser extent, anxiety (Parker, 1979). Adverse early experiences are associated with adult anxiety disorders in London (Brown & Harris, 1993), Florence (Farravelli et al., 1985) and South Carolina (Tweed et al., 1989). In all the studies the strongest associations were found in panic disorder, and the weakest for generalised anxiety disorders.

Other early experiences   There has recently been considerable interest in the possibility that child sexual abuse increases the risk of neurotic disorder in adulthood. Community-based studies find that adults with a variety of neurotic diagnoses report increased rates of early traumatic sexual encounters (Angst & Vollrath, 1991; Brown & Harris, 1993). Disentangling the links between abuse and adult disorder is not easy, since child sexual abuse does not happen randomly, and is associated with other adversity, including poverty, parental discord, inadequate parenting, and physical abuse. However, child sexual abuse was independently associated with adult psychiatric disorder in a community survey from New Zealand (Mullen *et al.*, 1993*a*).

Although childhood experiences are important in the aetiology of adult neurosis, there is no simple relationship between childhood and adult neurotic disorder. Most emotionally disordered children do not become neurotic adults, and most neurotic disorders develop in adult life (Rutter, 1972). However, there is a striking continuity between depression as a child and depression as an adult (Harrington *et al.*, 1990).

Adolescent experiences   In general, the literature on the social aetiology of neurosis concentrates on childhood predictors of adult disorder, and adult experiences. Mental health in childhood is also frequently addressed (see Chapter 5), but the change from childhood to adulthood has received less attention. Specific issues such as unemployment (Banks & Jackson, 1982) and acute life events have been addressed (Goodyer *et al.*, 1987). A recent community based study showed that 17% of girls living at home showed evidence of psychiatric disorder – independent risk factors were maternal distress and the quality of the parental marriage (Monck *et al.*, 1994).

Adult experiences

Life events   The relationship between life events and neurotic disorder has been extensively reviewed elsewhere (see Bebbington, Chapter 18). This body of work has provided some of the most convincing evidence for establishing psychosocial environmental stresses as important causes of depression. In particular, George Brown's work has been influential in arguing that the social context of life events and the meaning attached to them by the individual is also an important determinant of the likelihood of developing depression. Brown & Harris, and many others, concluded that events involving loss and humiliation are more often the proximate triggers for depressive episodes (Brown *et al.*, 1995), but those involving danger (by which they mean the anticipation of imminent future loss or deprivation) are more likely to precede anxiety (see Finlay-Jones, 1989). The latest findings from the Bedford College group suggest that anxiety occurring in the absence of depression is linked to childhood, but not adult, adversity (Brown *et al.*, 1993).

One of the limitations of the life event approach is that it seems to have a limited relevance to public health. Life events, such as bereavement, are an inevitable part of the human condition. Though other life events such as redundancy could in principle be influenced by economic policy it is more likely that the context of the life event is more amenable to policy changes than the occurrence of life events themselves. Future research should include the role of the context of life events, for example, poor housing, financial problems or

157

inadequate child care, in the hope of drawing conclusions that could potentially influence government policy.

Social support and social networks   One consistent finding is an association between poor social support and neurotic disorder. Brown & Harris (1978) found that women who lacked an intimate or confiding relationship had an increased risk of depression (in the presence of a life event) and Scott Henderson and colleagues (1980) in Australia went on to find a more general association between neurotic disorder and lack of satisfaction with the social network. In the ECA all anxiety disorders were commoner among the separated or divorced (Regier *et al.*, 1990), whilst in New Zealand females who were widowed, separated or divorced were more likely to have neurotic disorder than those currently married (Romans *et al.*, 1993).

There are two areas of controversy in this area. The first is the rather technical point of whether social support interacts with life events in increasing the risk of depression, in other words whether there is a stronger association between life events and depression in the presence of poor social support. This issue depends upon the nature of the statistical model that is being used by the researchers (Alloway & Bebbington, 1987). Of more importance, however, is the question of whether the association between poor social support is causal or results from either a personality attribute or measurement bias resulting from depression. Henderson has argued for the latter while Brown maintains the former position.

Unemployment   Unemployment is associated with higher rates of all forms of psychiatric disorder (Bebbington *et al.*, 1981*b*). Warr (1987) has conducted some elegant studies showing that men made unemployed are at increased risk of developing neurotic disorder and their mental health improves when they return to work. The situation for women is more complicated because of the expectation of work within the home.

Physical illness

Physical and psychiatric illness are associated more than by chance alone. In general there is a three-fold increase in psychological disorder in patients with medical illness (see Lloyd, Chapter 21). The relationship between physical and psychological illness is complex. Psychological disorder may result from illness or chronic disability. Sometimes physical and psychological illness may have a common aetiology, for example, diseases of the central nervous system are more likely to have a coexistent psychiatric disorder. There may also be a Berksonian or referral bias that leads to the association seen in health care settings. However, the commonest reason for the association between physical and psychological illness is somatisation. Illness behaviour has its effect on symptoms reporting (see Stansfield *et al.*, 1933).

Aetiology – personality

It is widely assumed that personality characteristics are an important risk factor for developing neurotic disorder. Eysenck's (1952*a*) neuroticism scale is claimed to be such a dimension, those scoring high on neuroticism having an increased risk of developing neurotic illness. However, there is a considerable overlap between the questions asked by neuroticism scales and the actual symptoms of neurotic disorder. A number of studies (Coppen & Metcalfe, 1965; Kendell & DiScipio, 1970; Hirschfield, 1983) have found that neuroticism scale scores are closely correlated with measurements of neurotic disorder and change with recovery from depression. Katz & McGuffin (1987) found that neurotic illness was a better predictor of depression at follow-up than neuroticism scale scores. Duncan-Jones *et al.* (1990) have also argued, with evidence from statistical models, that the neuroticism scale is effectively measuring the same thing as the average level of neurotic psychiatric disorder measured by the General Health Questionnaire.

For these reasons it is difficult to be confident that associations between neuroticism and increased incidence of neurotic disorder are a reflection of the neuroticism scales' ability to measure an underlying personality construct. It is likely that the neuroticism scale is merely measuring sub-threshold degrees of psychiatric morbidity. Therefore, an association between neuroticism and psychiatric disorder will result from the fact that both scales are measuring the same construct.

An alternative approach would be to use the theories of personality developed by social learning theorists. For example, Warr's (1987) work on unemployment has demonstrated that 'commitment to work' is related to poor mental health during unemployment and good mental health in employment. Warr and colleagues could demonstrate some predictive value for the scale, both when adolescents became unemployed and in predicting worsening of mental health in middle-aged men as unemployment continues. Work commitment was assessed by a short and simple scale incorporating a handful of attitudinal questions such as 'If you had won a million pounds would you still want to work?' This series of studies provides a model for studying personal attributes and their relationship with mental illness and shows an interaction between personality and the impact of a life event. They also illustrate the link between an individual's attitudes and societal norms, in this instance, the social and economic importance of the 'work ethic' (Weber, 1930).

Other personality constructs have been suggested to underlie the vulnerability to depression in some individuals. These include attributional styles that focus on fixed, internal attributions for adverse events (Abramson *et al.*, 1978), coping styles (emotional rather than reality, focused; Lazarus & Folkman, 1984) and self-esteem (Brown *et al.*, 1986). At present there is little consensus about the important personality variables that presumably increase vulnerability to depression.

Gavin Andrews (Andrews, 1991) has developed an overall theory of neurosis that suggests that adversity is the trigger for the onset of disorder, but there are also underlying vulnerabilities, in particular trait anxiety levels and the pattern of coping style.

Aetiology – genetics

There has long been interest in the relative contribution made by genetic and environmental factors in the neuroses. It would, however, be reasonable to say that the answers are far from clear, despite some recent advances. The difficulties in defining neurotic disorder are particularly relevant in genetic studies where lifetime prevalence is of interest.

Criticisms of the validity of lifetime prevalence estimates obtained from cross-sectional data, such as those articulated by Gordon Parker (Parker, 1987), should thus be remembered when considering genetic investigations. In addition, until recently most studies were of hospital ascertained cases and were thus biased towards the more severe end of the spectrum.

There is some agreement that neurotic depression has a low familial loading. The genetics of depression are considered in greater detail in Chapter 11. The evidence is more confusing for anxiety disorders. Most studies have found familial contributions to panic disorder. For example, Crowe *et al.* (1983) found a substantial increase in the risk of definite and probable panic disorder in the relatives of 41 patients with panic disorder (but no increase in generalised anxiety disorder). Other studies have concurred with his. However, the population-based twin register study of Andrews and colleagues (1990), using sophisticated methodology including researchers blind to both the zygosity and diagnosis of the co-twin, found no differences in MZ/DZ concordance for panic disorder with or without agoraphobia. Perhaps this reflected the differences in severity between clinical and population-ascertained subjects already alluded to. However, in a second population-based study of 2163 women selected from a twin register performed by Kendler and colleagues in Virginia the estimate of the heritability of panic disorder was of the order of 40% (Kendler *et al.*, 1993*a*).

Matters do not become any simpler when the question of comorbidity is addressed. Because most of the neurotic and affective disorders have high rates of comorbidity, establishing genetic vulnerability to individual disorders becomes difficult. Thus family members of unselected subjects with panic disorder have increased rates of not only panic disorder, but also depression, phobic disorders and alcohol abuse (Leckman *et al.*, 1983). Improvements in methodology and sample selection have led to some discrimination; relatives of probands with panic disorder are at increased risk of panic disorder and social phobia, but probably not other psychiatric disorders (Goldstein *et al.*, 1994). Panic disorders are not increased in the first degree relatives of probands with generalised anxiety disorder (GAD), and vice versa – GAD is not increased among the relatives of those with panic (Crowe *et al.*, 1983; Kendler *et al.*, 1993*a*).

The genetic component to GAD is unclear. Family history studies of subjects with GAD recruited by newspaper advertisement found that GAD is increased amongst first degree relatives of cases of GAD (Noyes *et al.*, 1987). Kendler *et al.* (1992), using the Virginia Twin Register, demonstrated a significant genetic liability to GAD in women. However, a large population survey in Norway reported a far less substantial genetic contribution to GAD (Tambs & Moum, 1993). These conflicting results may imply either confusion about the definition of GAD, or heterogeneity, or both. However, at present it appears that the genetic basis to GAD, whatever that may be, does not overlap with that for panic and phobic disorders. Kendler now argues that GAD and major depression have the same underlying genetic liability.

Turning to the phobias, the studies of Kendler and his group in Virginia using their large twin registry have shown familial aggregation of all the phobias, which they demonstrated are due to genetic liability, rather than shared environment. However, environmental influences are far from discounted, with childhood phobia-specific events being associated with the common, simple phobias, but non-specific environmental stressors linking with the less common, but more clinically relevant, agoraphobia and, to a lesser extent, social phobias (Kendler et al., 1993b). Environmental factors also are pinpointed by another Australian twin study that studied the twin pairs on five occasions (MacKinnon et al., 1990). Genetic factors again influence the liability to develop symptoms, but the intensity of symptoms varied according to current social circumstances.

The genetics of social phobia are particularly unclear, since many early studies chose to group all the phobias together. However, a recent family study found a marked increase in social phobia in the relatives of probands (Fyer et al., 1993).

Taken as a whole one can see some similarities emerging between the genetics and social psychiatry literature. Looking particularly at the work of Kendler and colleagues, and that of Brown and colleagues, a pattern can be discerned in which non-specific early adversity (which can involve parental indifference, parental separation, sexual or physical abuse) increases the risk of the more serious of the anxiety disorders, such as panic disorder and agoraphobia. The general experience of early social adversity has less to play in the aetiology of the mild phobic and simple phobic disorders. Genetic factors contribute to the liability to all the phobic disorders, but the evidence for a single major locus is unconvincing, and multifactorial inheritance seems the most likely model.

Prognosis of neurosis

The prognosis of neurotic symptoms in the community is relatively good but there are still a significant proportion of people with chronic neurotic disorders. Tennant et al. (1981b), found that over half of all cases of mental disorder identified in a community survey had remitted a month later, of which most were related to adverse life events. Tennant et al. commented that such syndromes may be conceived as normal distress responses. Mixed neurotic conditions, as seen in general practice, also have a reasonable prognosis. Looking at 'minor affective disorders' Catalan et al. (1984) found that two-thirds recovered from the acute episode within one month, irrespective of treatment. Mann et al. (1981) found that 24% improved after 1 year, 52% had a fluctuating and 25% a chronic course. Chronicity was associated with severity of illness, being older, presence of physical illness and receiving psychotropic medication – diagnosis had little influence in this or another study. (Huxley et al., 1979). However, Murphy et al. (1986) in a 17-year follow-up did not find any influence of age or severity; 56% of community cases had experienced one or more further episodes, and 25% had never been free of symptoms.

The more severe phobic, panic and obsessive compulsive disorders seen in specialist settings tend to run chronic courses. On average, patients have had symptoms for about 10 years at the time they present to some specialist services (Marks, 1987). Untreated the social phobias rarely recover (Davidson et al., 1993).

It is well known that depressive disorders are associated with a substantial mortality from suicide and accidents (see Chapter 11 McGuffin). However, neurotic disorders in general, and anxiety disorders in particular, are also associated with increased mortality. A recent long-term follow-up of all those admitted to Swedish psychiatric hospitals with a diagnosis of an anxiety disorder confirmed a five-fold increase in mortality due to suicide, with other increases in deaths from alcohol and smoking-related diseases (Allgulander, 1994). The

Stirling County studies found that mortality was increased in neurotic disorder, with Standardised Mortality ratio of 150. Neurotic disorders are associated with physical illness and the total increase in mortality cannot be solely explained by suicide, accidental death or smoking-related diseases (Murphy *et al.*, 1987; Sims, 1987).

Management

The management of the neurotic disorders will be discussed in the next part of the chapter under the rubric of each neurotic disorder. We will confine ourselves to general comments at this stage.

Pharmacological treatment of neurosis

Benzodiazepines are undoubtedly effective in the short-term treatment of anxiety. Their actions are mediated by specific benzodiazepine receptors in the central nervous system, which are an integral part of the GABA-A receptor, and thereby increase the functional consequences of GABA activity. They reduce sleep latency (the time from awakeness to full sleep), and are effective hypnotics. Their use is now very limited as there is considerable evidence of tolerance to the effects of bnezodiazepines and that a proportion (about 10–15%) of people will become dependent and show clinically significant withdrawal symptoms, even after as little as four weeks of treatment (Lader, 1989). The side-effects of benzodiazepines include impairment of psychomotor, cognitive and memory functions, which can also be a problem when the effects of hypnotics last over to the following morning.

At present the UK consensus views benzodiazepines with displeasure, and, other than for the very briefest period, sees them as having little or no role in the management of neurotic disorders (see Tyrer & Ashton, 1989, for two opposing views). As a result tricyclic antidepressants are increasingly being used to treat anxiety and phobic disorders and there is now evidence that they are of equivalent efficacy in the longer term (see Chapter 8).

β-blockers reduce the physical symptoms of anxiety by blockade of peripheral β-adrenergic receptors. They have a limited role but are helpful in performance anxiety, for example in musicians (James & Savage, 1984). Buspirone has complex actions, inhibiting serotonin function whilst increasing noradrenaline function. It is claimed to have an anxiolytic effect without the sedation accompanying benzodiazepines. It is relatively slow acting and has troublesome side-effects, which reduce its value.

Psychological treatment

There are a vast number of psychological treatments. They can be divided into three broad groups. First, behaviour therapies based upon exposure. Second, those treatments with manuals or guides that provide recommended techniques, for example cognitive therapy, and finally those based upon psychodynamic theories and without the explicit structure and directiveness of the 'manualised' therapies. Some recommendations can now be made that certain treatments work better for certain categories of neurotic disorder though much work is needed in order to inform such clinical decisions (see Chapter 25).

Dynamic psychotherapy is commonly used in treating those with neurotic disorders. Controversy over the effectiveness of this approach is well aired but in many parts of the world dynamic psychotherapy is often the most available form of treatment. There has recently been a rapid increase in the number of counsellors in British primary care, many of whom will be using a dynamic approach (Sibbald *et al.*, 1993). In the UK, NHS specialist psychotherapists who use a psychodynamic approach generally see the more disabled individuals who would often come under the rubric of personality disorder.

Social treatment

The general principles of social management apply to neurotic disorders. Assessment should include an evaluation of housing, relationships with the patient's immediate family, day-time occupation and use of leisure time. Financial circumstances and debts are also important stressors. Social interventions are varied and could include recommending attendance at a day-centre or a self-help group for single parents, arranging day care for children, or encouraging participation in an evening class. Involving the partner or spouse in therapy might be appropriate, either to counsel and support them or to consider marital therapy. Referral to social work colleagues may be necessary in more complex cases or where child protection issues are important. Voluntary and self-help groups are especially valuable in providing support and debt counsellors and citizen's advice bureaux can provide guidance.

Physical versus psychological treatments

There have been a number of studies comparing physical and psychological treatments. It is difficult to make any general statements about their comparative efficacy and if there are clear messages these are referred to elsewhere in the text. The psychological therapies tend to be more expensive in the short term, but these extra costs could be justified by a better response to treatment in the longer term (e.g. Evans *et al.*, 1992). The simultaneous use of psychological and physical treatments is still a source of controversy. Most clinicians tend to adopt a pragmatic approach and be prepared to use both modalities simultaneously. However, some practitioners of psychological treatments hold strong views about the potential for interference with psychological treatment when patients are simultaneously given pharmacotherapy, particularly benzodiazepines. Most trials do not support any adverse effects of combining, for example, antidepressants and cognitive therapy when treating depression. We would recommend that combined treatments in anxiety are probably as, if not more, efficacious than either psychological or pharmacological treatments used singly.

The neurotic disorders

Generalised anxiety disorder

In ICD-10, generalised anxiety disorder (GAD) is a disorder characterised by anxiety, most days, for at least several weeks at a time and usually for several months. Patients should not meet criteria for phobic anxiety, panic or obsessive-compulsive disorders. It can therefore be loosely summarised as what is 'left over anxiety when phobias and panic has been removed' (Tyrer & Hallstrom, 1993). The rather vague definition may explain the wide variations in reported prevalence. Of all the anxiety disorders, GAD shows the most overlap with depression.

Differential diagnosis

Physical illness The prominent physical symptoms of anxiety can sometimes be confused with other physical disorders. Thyrotoxicosis, hypoglycaemia and the rare phaeo-chromocytoma can present with complaints of anxiety. Complaints of breathlessness could also perhaps be confused with asthma and pulmonary embolus. It is more difficult to distinguish physical conditions from anxiety without clear situational precipitants.

Substance abuse Withdrawal from a number of drugs, such as alcohol, opiates and benzodiazepines, is accompanied by prominent anxiety. Anxious patients may also use alcohol to overcome their symptoms. However, Bernadt & Murray (1986) showed that as many patients admitted to the Maudsley Hospital with minor depression or anxiety had decreased their drinking before admission as had increased it. Longitudinal studies such as those conducted by George Vaillant (1986) in the United States found that neurotic disorder is more often the consequence of alcohol dependence than its cause.

Depression The difficulties in distinguishing depression and anxiety are partly a matter of nosology. As the earlier sections have shown, the overlap between the two conditions is considerable.

Management

Psychological treatments are frequently used, such as relaxation, biofeedback and cognitive therapy, frequently combined in anxiety management packages. At present cognitive therapy seems to offer some advantages in skilled hands (Butler *et al.*, 1991), particularly when longer term outcomes are measured (Durham *et al.*, 1994 see Chapter 25).

The current UK practice is generally to avoid prescribing benzodiazepine drugs for more than two weeks because of the risk of dependence. Tricyclic antidepressants are as effective in the longer term (after about four weeks or so). One compromise might be to prescribe both benzodiazepines and tricyclics at first and withdraw the benzodiazepine after two weeks.

Phobias

A phobia is an irrational fear or anxiety associated with avoidance of the feared situation or object. A phobia should have three characteristics: (1) anxiety should be out of proportion to the real threat of the situation; (2) the anxiety cannot be reasoned away and is beyond voluntary control and (3) the desire to avoid anxiety also leads to behavioural avoidance of the feared situation.

Phobias were the commonest specific neurotic disorder in the ECA study. The age-standardised one month prevalence was 3.8% for males and 8.4% for females (Regier *et al.*, 1990), although this is elevated by the high rates of simple phobia, which have not been replicated elsewhere and may be artefactual.

The commonest phobia encountered in specialist clinical practice is agoraphobia, representing 60% of phobics referred to the Maudsley Hospital (Marks, 1987). There is a female excess for most phobic conditions, with the exception of social phobia, with a sex ratio of unity. Specific phobias are commoner in the community but these are often not particularly disabling.

Classification of phobias

The most controversial area of classification concerns the relationship with panic disorder (see below). We will follow ICD-10 and European practice in regarding agoraphobia with panic attacks under the heading of phobia. There is reasonable agreement over the following three groups of phobias:

1. Agoraphobia
   A characteristic group of fears, including fear of public places, crowds, enclosed spaces and public transport. Typically agoraphobics are worse when alone, exposed to bright light, away from home, and in situations lacking an easy exit.

2. Social phobia
   The fear of situations in which other people may see the person, or form an opinion of them. Typical fears include being afraid of eating and drinking in front of people and speaking in public or social gatherings. The patient is often anxious or shaking, blushing, vomiting or otherwise looking ridiculous.

3. Specific (isolated) or simple phobias
   Simple phobias are commonly found for such stimuli as spiders, heights, dogs, snakes, thunder and lighting. Whereas social phobia has a mean age of onset of 19 years, and agoraphobia 24 years, animal phobias have a mean age of onset of four (Marks & Gelder, 1966). Specific phobias of animals or insects are common in children by age four, but, with the exception of snake phobias, most subside (Holmes, 1936).

In addition to these three categories, two other categories of phobia are sometimes also described. First, blood phobia, a particular form of specific phobia in which blood and injury are the stimulus. It is argued that this should be a separate category from specific phobias because in most phobic patients the heart rate increases in the phobic situation. However, blood phobics develop vagal inhibition after the sight of blood, which leads to loss of consciousness. Unlike other phobics, blood phobics actually faint (rather than fear fainting). It has a strong genetic component (Torgerson, 1979). The second category is illness phobia, in which patients show intense fears of specific illnesses such as cancer, heart disease or sexually transmitted disease. These are better thought of as specific forms of hypochondriasis as there is no avoidance component.

Management

The most effective element of psychological treatment for most phobias appears to be graduated, *in vivo* exposure to the feared stimulus (Marks, 1987; Clum *et al.*, 1993). It is no longer necessary to commence with exposure in imagination, nor routinely to use symptom reduction strategies such as relaxation. Longer exposure is more effective than shorter exposures. Some critics of behaviour therapy argue that it increases coping behaviours but does not influence panic attacks. However, behaviour therapy appears to decrease the frequency of all the symptoms of phobias, including panics (Marks *et al.*, 1993). Other critics suggest that behaviour therapy is limited in situations where avoidance is not a principal feature. It is of course true that 'pure' behaviour treatment cannot treat anxiety without some behavioural precipitant (or response as in obsessive compulsive disorder). In practice most therapists would use a cognitive-behavioural approach. The long-term results of behaviour therapy are very good and most patients who improve seem to maintain improvement for many years after treatment has ended (Munby & Johnston, 1980).

Most of the research on pharmacological approaches to phobias have involved patients diagnosed with panic disorder. For example, 75% of the subjects in the Cross-National Collaborative Panic Study (1992) also showed some avoidance. In that study imipramine and the benzodiazepine alprazolam were of equal efficacy over eight weeks of treatment. However, Marks *et al.* (1993), studying patients with agoraphobia with panic, concluded that exposure was more effective than alprazolam in the longer term, particularly after withdrawal of the medication. In view of the problems with dependence it seems advisable to avoid benzodiazepines, though a tricyclic such as imipramine may be of value.

Management of social phobia   When first introduced, monoamine oxidase inhibitors (MAOIs) such as phenelzine enjoyed immense popularity in the treatment of neurotic disorders. The Newcastle group, for example, argued strenuously for a specific effect of MAOIs on what they chose to call 'phobic anxiety disorder', in which depersonalisation also played a prominent role. However, dissatisfaction with this classification, specific criticisms of the clinical trial evidence, and fears concerning the risks of MAOIs, meant that these drugs fell out of favour by the 1980s.

Recently there has been a reappraisal of the role of MAOIs in anxiety disorders. The Columbia group in New York, led by Michael Liebowitz, have suggested that MAOIs are more efficacious then tricyclics in atypical depression. However, the overlap between this concept and that of social phobia led the Columbia group to argue that MAOIs are particularly useful in social phobia (Liebowitz *et al.*, 1985).

Some cognitive techniques such as self-instructional training and rational emotive therapy have been shown to be as effective as behaviour therapy in the social phobias (see Emmelkamp *et al.*, 1985). In general these require more in the way of therapist time and training that the simpler behavioural approaches already reviewed (see Chapter 25). Cognitive theorists also suggest that excessive fears of negative evaluation by others are at the core of social phobia and that it often coexists with depression.

Panic

Panic disorder is a category that was introduced in the USA but has been slow to gain acceptance as a useful addition to psychiatric nosology in other parts of the world. ICD-10 now includes panic disorder and it is defined in ICD-10 as 'recurrent attacks of severe anxiety (panic) which are not restricted to any particular situation or set of circumstances and which are therefore unpredictable'. There is usually an accompanying cognitive component, usually a fear of dying, losing control or going mad. The attacks are intensely unpleasant, usually last a few minutes and the patient attempts to terminate the attacks as quickly as possible.

In the ECA the one month prevalence was 0.3% (males) and 0.7% (females) (Regier *et al.*, 1990). In the UK OPCS Survey, there was a one-week prevalence of 0.9% in women and 0.7% in men (Meltzer *et al.*, 1995). There are a larger number of individuals in the community who experience panic attacks but do not meet the research criteria of panic disorder. 3% of women and 2% of men reported at least one panic attack in the last week in the UK National Survey of Psychiatric Morbidity (Meltzer *et al.*, 1995).

Differential diagnosis

Panic attacks can be confused with epilepsy, particularly partial complex seizures. This confusion is more likely if there are no situational precipitants for the panic attack.

Classification of panic and situational anxiety

The principal transatlantic difference in the psychiatric nosology of neurosis is the importance given to panic disorder in North America. DSM-IV states that 'Agoraphobia is not a codable disorder' as it is subsumed largely under the heading of panic disorder, though the diagnosis of agoraphobia without panic can still be made. ICD-10 regards panic attacks that occur in an established phobic situation as an expression of the phobia, which is given diagnostic preference. In ICD-10 panic disorder is reserved for individuals without phobic symptoms. Fortunately for international collaboration, the categories are comparable; 'F40.01 Agoraphobia with panic disorder' in ICD-10 should include the same individuals as '300.21 panic disorder with agoraphobia' in DSM-IV.

There are a number of sources of controversy surrounding the classification and presumed mechanisms underlying panic attacks and panic disorder.

Primacy of panic The view underlying the DSM approach to panic is the suggestion that agoraphobia is a conditioned response to a sudden onset of spontaneous panic attacks. There are a number of arguments that have been used against this position. First, panic disorder is less common that agoraphobia (Regier *et al.*, 1990), which does not support the concept of the primacy of panic. Second, panic should precede the onset of avoidance behaviour but it is common to see patients who do not give such a history. Lelliott *et al.* (1989) reported that the onset of panic was preceded by phobic avoidance or affective symptoms in 70% of cases whilst Eaton and Keyl (1990) found that 79% of new cases of agoraphobia had no history of panic. Panic attacks are also seen in a variety of psychiatric disorders including GAD, major depression, agoraphobia, social phobia, specific phobia and obsessive compulsive disorder (Barlow *et al.*, 1985). Perhaps the salience of panic attacks may increase the likelihood of patients' recall above other less vivid events. Panic attacks in agoraphobic subjects may also be associated with seeking treatment, rather than the onset of disorder and give the clinical impression that they preceded the avoidance.

Spontaneous panic attacks The DSM view of panic rests upon the distinction between spontaneous and situational panic. However, there appear to be few phenomenological distinctions between them (Margraf *et al.*, 1987). Cognitive theories of panic have become influential within recent years and these suggest that so-called spontaneous panic attacks may be set off by misinterpretation of bodily symptoms.

The cognitive view of panic suggests that the process begins when a person becomes aware of either a non-pathological somatic symptom, such as a missed heart beat or post-exertional chest discomfort, or perhaps an abnormal sensation of pathophysiological origin, such as those produced by hyperventilation. If this is erroneously interpreted, and especially if attributed to a sinister cause ('catastrophising'), anxiety and panic is the result (see Clark, 1986). It is supported by experimental evidence showing that artificially increasing the heart rate, or giving false feedback concerning the heart rate, can trigger panic in predisposed individuals. At the very least these ideas are a persuasive challenge to the idea that all non-situational panic attacks are 'spontaneous'.

Neurochemical precipitation of panic attacks One of the main stimuli of biological research in the aetiology of panic disorder has been a series of observations that a number of agents can provoke panic attacks in predisposed subjects.

a) Lactate

The classic studies of Da Costa, Thomas Lewis and Paul Wood led to the observation that patients with anxiety disorders (formerly neurocirculatory asthenia or effort syndromes) have poor exercise tolerance and produce excessive lactic acid in response to exercise. This led to the study of Pitts & McClure (1967), who found that 13 out of 14 patients with anxiety disorders, but only 2 out of 10 controls, developed anxiety symptoms after the direct infusion of sodium lactate, a finding that has been consistently replicated using the more modern criteria of panic (Liebowitz *et al.*, 1984). A recent paper showed that lactate administered during sleep provokes greater fluctuations in cardiac and respiratory activity in panic-prone subjects than normal controls (Koenigsberg et al.,

1994). The finding cannot therefore be attributed to anticipatory anxiety.

Lactate precipitation of panic disorder is specific (i.e. lactate infusion does not precipitate other disorders) and is blocked by agents such as imipramine and MAOIs, but not B-blockade. The mechanism by which lactate precipitates panic is controversial – possible explanations include metabolic alkalosis, cerebral vasoconstriction, and increased sensitivity of the medullary chemoreceptors to carbon dioxide. However, there are also some phenomenological differences between lactate-induced panic and clinical panic attacks (Nutt, 1990).

b) Hyperventilation

Overbreathing leads to hypocapnia (a low pCO_2) and thus to some of the symptoms associated with anxiety and panic. Training habitual hyperventilators to breath appropriately has therapeutic benefits (Salkovskis et al., 1986); the basis of the well known 'paper bag' treatment of acute anxiety so beloved of casualty officers. However, not all hyperventilators are anxious (see Bass & Gardner, 1989) and hyperventilation per se does not always provoke panic (Papp et al., 1993). Treatments aimed at controlling breathing also improve panic attacks in those who do not hyperventilate (Hibbert & Chan, 1989). Ambulatory monitoring of transcutaneous pCO_2 shows that although some panic attacks are indeed associated with lowered pCO_2, others are not (Hibbert & Pilsbury, 1989). Hibbert and Pilsbury argue that hyperventilation is the consequence, and not the cause, of panic.

The role of carbon dioxide is further complicated because although reducing pCO_2 can trigger panic, so does increased pCO_2. Inhaling CO_2 acts like lactate to produce respiratory stimulation and provoke panic, perhaps related to an altered central 'suffocation' alarm monitor (Klein, 1993; Gorman et al., 1994). Thus although hypocapnia and hypercapnia have different effects on, for example, the cerebral circulation, they both cause anxiety-related symptoms. These findings seem more consistent with the cognitive theory of panic resulting from a misinterpretation of bodily symptoms, whatever the physiological significance of them.

c) Other pharmacological precipitants

A number of other pharmacological agents have been reported as provoking panic susceptible subjects. These include caffeine, cholecystokinin, yohimbine (an α_2-adrenoreceptor antagonist), clonidine (an α_2-adrenoreceptor agonist), fenfluramine (a 5-HT agonist) and flumazenil (a benzodiazepine antagonist) (Nutt et al., 1990; Nutt and Lawson, 1992). It is presumed that whereas hyperventilation and lactate produce panic via a peripheral mechanism, flumazenil and the serotonergic and noradrenergic agents act centrally.

In a recent review Klein has elegantly integrated reports of both respiratory and psychological dysfunction to propose that panic results from the combination of an unstable respiratory system (centrally, and presumably genetically, mediated) linked with cognitive distortions of the meaning of the resulting symptoms (Klein, 1993).

Pharmacotherapy of panic The division of anxiety disorders into generalised anxiety disorder and panic began with Donald Klein's (1964) finding that imipramine was effective in treating panic attacks, but not generalised anxiety disorder, whilst benzodiazepines did the reverse. He suggested that that this differential response to treatment implied a biological distinction between panic and generalised anxiety disorder. However, the differences in treatment response between panic and anxiety are not as clear-cut as they first appeared.

The large Cross-National Collaborative Panic Study (1992) found that imipramine and alprazolam were equally efficacious in treating panic and Wilkinson *et al.* (1991) concluded, on the basis of a meta-analysis, that there was little difference between the effects of panic of anti-anxiety and anti-depressive medication. Tyrer *et al.* (1988) also found that dothiepin, a tricyclic antidepressant, was better than diazepam at treating both panic and generalised anxiety disorder in the longer term. Other have claimed that imipramine is effective for phobic and anticipatory anxiety, but not panic (Mavissakalian & Perel, 1985).

Another area of controversy surrounds the possibility that tricyclic antidepressants work because of the mood-elevating properties in patients with comorbid depression. Zitrin and other workers from Donald Klein's group have shown that imipramine is effective in the treatment of panic disorder even in the absence of depression (Zitrin *et al.*, 1983). For example, in one study (Zitrin *et al.*, 1980) there was no correlation between response to drug and initial levels of depression. Marks *et al.* (1983) challenged these findings – they failed to find any effect for imipramine, which they attribute to the low levels of baseline depression in their study. There are also reports that the selective serotonin re-uptake inhibitors (Black *et al.*, 1993) also have anxiolytic properties.

Conclusion   At present the concept of panic disorder does not seem to add very much to our understanding of the classification and treatment of anxiety. The concept has stimulated a great deal of research but it is difficult to draw any very confident conclusions. Those with a phobia and panic are probably still best dealt with by treating the phobia. Patients with panic, in the absence of avoidance, can be thought of as having particularly severe anxiety. The absence of any clear-cut evidence that panic disorder has a specific treatment, as originally suggested by Klein, also makes the concept less valuable. However, panic attacks are an important aspect of the presentation of a patient and probably help in thinking about management and it is potentially useful to distinguish this group from other anxiety disorders.

Management

One of the complications in reviewing this literature is that the DSM-IV approach towards diagnosing panic means that the majority of the subjects in the North American trials have agoraphobia or other phobias with panic. Following ICD-10, we are using panic disorder to refer to patients without a phobia. It is therefore difficult to disentangle this group from the broader group of panic patients studied in the US trials. However, in view of the problems with dependence on benzodiazepines, it is probably advisable to prescribe imipramine or another tricyclic agent as a pharmacological treatment (Clum *et al.*, 1993).

Cognitive therapy for panic disorder involves identifying and challenging patients' misinterpretations of bodily sensations. It is too early to comment on the long-term efficacy of cognitive therapy for panic disorder, but preliminary evidence is promising, and suggests that although both relaxation therapy and imipramine are superior to placebo in treating panic, the effects of cognitive therapy are more long lasting and gains more likely to be maintained beyond the end of active treatment (Margraf *et al.*, 1993; Clark *et al.*, 1994). Further details are contained in Chapter 25.

Obsessive compulsive disorder

An obsession is a repetitive thought that is unpleasantly distressing and which the patient resists thinking. It is recognised as coming from within the person but is also seen as irrational and unwanted. The content of obsessive thoughts are usually seen as repugnant and senseless, for example, aggressive thoughts in a person who takes pride in lack of aggression or blasphemous thoughts in a religious person.

Compulsions are repetitive and stereotypic acts carried out in order to relieve or prevent some perceived unwanted outcome that would cause anxiety. For example, compulsions involving checking doors, windows, and ovens are probably most common in the community. Cleaning compulsions are common in clinical practice. Compulsions are not pleasurable, are usually seen as senseless and are resisted by the sufferer. In practice there is a continuum from the classic patient described above to those who hold their beliefs are valid and do not resist them to any notable extent (Kozak & Foa, 1994). The term rituals tends to be used to describe more complex acts of a compulsive nature.

Carrying out obsessive rituals usually results in sufferers taking a considerable time to complete everyday tasks. Slowness is usually secondary to recognised avoidance strategies or rituals, but if unaccompanied by rituals has been labelled 'primary obsessive slowness' (Rachman, 1974) and is remarkably treatment resistant.

The ICD-10 category of obsessive-compulsive disorder (OCD) requires obsessional symptoms or compulsions to be present on most days for at least two successive weeks. Most clinical cases have a mixture of obsessions and compulsions. It is relatively uncommon for compulsive rituals to be present in the absence of obsessional thoughts.

Until recently OCD was considered a relatively unusual disorder with a prevalence of around 0.1%. However, the ECA reported a one month prevalence of 1.1% (males) and 1.5% (females) (Regier *et al.*, 1990). The most likely explanation for this finding is that obsessional symptoms are very common, though the severe and disabling disorders seen by psychiatrists are much less so. OCD shares with social phobia the distinction of being the only neurotic disorder with nearly equal sex ratio. About a quarter of cases of OCD have premorbid obsessional traits.

Differential diagnosis

Depression Depressive symptoms and obsessive compulsive symptoms commonly co-exist. Kendell & DiScipio (1970) found that 30% of inpatients with major depression had obsessional symptoms that worsened during episodes of depression, but not to the same degree as in primary OCD. Conversely, 30% of patients with typical obsessive compulsive disorder satisfy criteria for major depression (Coryell, 1981) and the depressive and obsessional symptoms tend to worsen or improve in parallel. It is probably better to provide a patient with two diagnoses, if that is appropriate, rather than ignore one element of their clinical picture.

Schizophrenia   The bizarre nature of some of the rituals and beliefs held by sufferers from OCD can lead to confusion with psychotic illness including schizophrenia. A psychotic diagnosis will be favoured when there is a lack of resistance and lack of insight – most sufferers with OCD recognise their beliefs as senseless.

Neurological abnormalities and OCD

There have been many reports that OCD is accompanied by increased rates of soft neurological signs, including speech and gait abnormalities, clumsiness and delays in specific actions, such as in initiating limb movements, switching from one motor programme to another and carrying out two motor acts simultaneously (Hollander *et al.*, 1990; Hymas *et al.*, 1991). There is also an increased rate of OCD in several organic conditions, including post-encephalitic Parkinson's syndromes, Huntingdon's Chorea, Sydenham's Chorea and Gilles de la Tourette Syndrome. A recent follow-up study of children diagnosed with OCD found an increased rate of Gilles de la Tourette syndrome (Leonard *et al.*, 1992).

Physiological and neurochemical abnormalities

The evidence for serotonin dysfunction in OCD rests on the observations that serotonergic agents have some effect in OCD, whilst serotonin agonists such as meta-chlorophenyl-piperazine (M-CPP) sometimes, but not always, worsens it (Charney *et al.*, 1988; Hollander *et al.*, 1992). New scanning techniques have shown that previous theories of a primary serotonergic dysregulation, based on the efficacy of serotonergic reuptake inhibitors, are simplistic (Hollander *et al.*, 1992). Attention has thus shifted to the role of neuropeptides. CSF levels of corticotrophin releasing hormone (CRH), vasopressin and somatostatin are increased in OCD, and reduced after treatment with clomipramine (Altemus *et al.*, 1994).

The similarities between some features of OCD and those of movement disorders have led to several investigations of the basal ganglial structures. One CT study showed caudate atrophy, but this has not been confirmed by the more sensitive MRI techniques (see Insel, 1992). A PET study of cerebral metabolic function compared the effects of both behavioural (response prevention) and pharmacological (fluoxetine) treatment. Subjects who responded to either of the treatments were found to have altered glucose metabolism in the right caudate nucleus, which normalised after treatment (Baxter *et al.*, 1992). Recent PET studies have used patients as their own controls by studying cerebral blood flow whilst provoking the onset of obsessive compulsive behaviours. An increase in cerebral blood flow in the right caudate nucleus, together with the left anterior cingulate cortex and the bilateral orbitofrontal cortex was reported in one study (Rauch *et al.*, 1994), while another found increases in the right striatum and orbitofrontal cortex (McGuire *et al.*, 1994). Overall, the functional imaging data points to an association between striatal and orbito-frontal activity and obsessive-compulsive symptoms.

Genetics

Early studies reporting substantial genetic contribution have not always been replicated. The more recent family history studies show increased rates of other neurotic disorders in the first degree relatives of probands, but are inconclusive as regards OCD itself. In a well conducted twin study Clifford *et al.*, (1984) demonstrated a clear genetic contribution to obsessional traits and symptoms, but McKeon & Murray (1987) found no evidence of increased risk of OCD in the relatives of patients attending for treatment, nor of a genetic contribution to obsessional traits, but did find an increased risk of other psychiatric disorders. Black *et al.* (1992) also found evidence of clustering of other psychiatric disorders, but not for OCD. Lenane *et al.* (1990), whose probands were children with OCD, did find familial aggregation of OCD itself. One possible explanation is that children have a particularly severe form of OCD, with a poor prognosis, and thus the different results reflect heterogeneity.

Management

Behaviour therapy is an effective treatment for compulsions. Rituals are treated by exposing the patient to the environmental cues that trigger the ritual, but preventing carrying out of ritual. About 60–70% of patients will improve with exposure and response prevention treatments. This improvement is usually maintained at two-year follow up, and there is no evidence of symptom substitution (Balkom *et al.*, 1994).

The most studied pharmacological agent is clomipramine, a potent tricyclic that acts as a serotonin presynaptic re-uptake inhibitor. The arguments about its efficacy are reminiscent of those surrounding the drug treatment of phobias. There is no doubt that clomipramine, and also other serotinergic agents such as fluoxetine and fluvoxamine, reduces the symptoms of OCD, but is this simply because of its effect on mood disorder? Marks & O'Sullivan (1989) concluded that clomipramine does reduce the symptoms of OCD, especially, but not entirely, in those with concurrent mood disorder. Drug treatment is associated with significant side-effects, whilst exposure treatment seems to offer better protection against relapse. The combination of behaviour therapy and antidepressants has not been well studied, but there is some suggestion of increased efficacy for combined treatment (Balkom *et al.*, 1994).

Most studies of psychosurgery were carried out before behaviour therapy and drug therapy became a routine part of treatment. If there is a place for psychosurgery, usually bimedial leucotomy or stereotactic limbic leucotomy, it is as a last resort.

Post-traumatic stress disorder

Post-traumatic stress disorder (PTSD) is diagnosed when certain psychological symptoms develop after exposure to a traumatic event. Essential for the diagnosis is some form of re-experiencing of the original trauma in the form of thoughts, dreams or reliving the original experience ('flashbacks'). In addition there may be numbing of emotional feelings, associated with attempts to avoid reminders of the experience, both external and internal. Finally, symptoms of depression, anxiety and irritability are common. The term is new,

173

introduced into DSM-III in 1980 in recognition of the psychological distress experienced by veterans of the Vietnam war, but the condition must be as old as warfare itself. Its origins lie not only in soldiers' reactions to combat (e.g. shell shock) but also transport accidents (e.g. railway spine) and, more recently, has been extended to the traumatic reactions to events such as being taken hostage or rape.

Community surveys in the United States give point prevalences in the range 0.5 and 2.0%. In the St Louis branch of the ECA study the lifetime prevalence of PTSD was about 1% (Helzer et al., 1987) – whilst the lifetime prevalence in South Carolina was 1.3% (Davidson et al., 1991). This prevalence rises in high risk groups – for example, 30% of Australian bush fighters, 60% of children exposed to a sniper attack, and the majority of children surviving the Armenia earthquake (Pynoos et al., 1993).

Aetiology

Most of the ICD-10 and DSM-IV eschews using aetiology in the criteria for psychiatric conditions and PTSD is distinctive in requiring a cause for the diagnosis to be made. The ICD-10 definition states that the stressor is an event 'of an exceptionally threatening or catastrophic nature which would be likely to cause pervasive distress in almost anyone'. This definition is included to distance PTSD from other psychiatric conditions by implying that it is a 'normal' reaction and also that the traumatic incident itself is a necessary and sufficient cause for the disorder. However, PTSD does not develop in everyone exposed to trauma, no matter how severe.

The role of the traumatic incident is called into question by the studies of McFarlane (1998a,b) of psychiatric morbidity in a group of firefighters who had intense exposure to an Australian bush fire. Against his expectations, he found that neither the intensity of exposure, the perceived threat nor the losses actually sustained during the disaster, were associated with the development of PTSD. Instead, characteristics such as personality and both past and family history of psychiatric disorder were significantly associated with the development of PTSD. Feinstein & Dolan (1991) in another prospective study also found no association between the severity of the stressor and the development of post traumatic stress disorder. However, others have claimed such a link (Breslau & Davis, 1987), and it is also true that victims who are amnesic for the period of trauma do not develop PTSD (Mayou et al., 1993).

Epidemiological studies find that the development of PTSD is associated with a history of childhood behavioural problems, parental divorce, poverty, physical abuse and current unemployment (Helzer et al., 1987; Davidson et al., 1991). A large twin study of Vietnam veterans has also provided convincing evidence of the role of genetic liability (True et al., 1993). Intriguingly, a recent case series describes patients who have all the features of PTSD, but without any exposure to trauma (Scott & Stradling, 1994).

Recent research has also moved away from the previous preoccupation with the results of high profile disasters, to study instead more mundane and individual traumas such as road accidents. Malt (1988) conducted a Norwegian cohort study of 107 victims of individual accidents. Twenty-two per cent developed psychiatric illness during a two-year period, but only one was diagnosed as PTSD, the rest being largely accounted for by depressive disorders. In general he felt that the effects of trauma were similar to the effects of other physical illnesses, such as myocardial infarction or burn injury. Mayou *et al.* (1993) reported a higher prevalence of PTSD in a follow up study of consecutive road accident victims in Oxford. Ten per cent fulfilled the criteria, but other psychiatric symptoms were more common, in particular phobic anxiety about driving or being a passenger. Looking at train drivers who had experienced a person jump under their cab, Farmer *et al.* (1992) noted 16% to have PTSD, but all also fulfilled criteria for depressive illness.

PTSD is thus found in combination with a range of other psychiatric disorders, comorbidity in the current jargon. Those with PTSD also have higher rates of a number of other diagnoses, particularly alcohol abuse, anxiety, depression and OCD (Helzer *et al.*, 1987). In consequence 'almost any statement about the relationship of PTSD to other psychiatric disorders can be supported' (Davidson & Foa, 1991). One reason is that, almost alone in psychiatric nosology, PTSD is an aetiological classification that sits uncomfortably with the majority of psychiatric diagnoses, which are descriptive.

Thus it is still questionable, and indeed doubtful, whether a single post-trauma syndrome exists across all cultures, and in response to all traumas. The boundaries between PTSD and other more familiar psychiatric syndromes that become manifest after adversity are blurred.

Neurobiology

Investigations into the neurobiology of PTSD began by observing that combat veterans showed a pattern of a dysregulated sympathetic nervous system, with both higher and more labile heart rates, blood pressure and so on, particularly in response to traumatic imagery, all of which are assumed to indicate chronic psychophysiological arousal in response to uncontrollable trauma (see Orr *et al.*, 1993). Two studies have also found some evidence of an altered hypothalamic–pituitary–adrenal feedback mechanism, with low urinary cortisol and enhanced cortisol suppression to dexamethasone, which should be contrasted with the characteristic findings in major depression (Yehuda *et al.*, 1991). If substantiated, this suggests that tests of biological response may differentiate PTSD from other neurotic syndromes. However, similar abnormalities have been claimed in other conditions, such as seasonal affective disorder and chronic fatigue syndrome (Demitrack *et al.*, 1991). There is little doubt that psychic trauma can produce neurochemical and perhaps neuroanatomical changes, but, just as in other neurotic disorders, claims for specific neurobiological aetiologies can be taken too far – one author notes that officers seem less liable to develop PTSD than other ranks, and attributes this to the greater neuronal network of the former (Kolb, 1987)!

Management

At present there is a paucity of properly conducted treatment trials. A variety of physical and psychological therapies are used as some have found that denial and/or avoidance is associated with the syndrome. Cognitive and behavioural approaches are frequently employed and appear to be the most successful, particularly in reducing the intrusive symptoms of PTSD (Solomon *et al.*, 1992).

PTSD and the law

There is a considerable amount of work relating to litigation and compensation in cases of PTSD. Trimble (1981) has shown how views on post-traumatic syndromes swing from psychogenic to somatic, always influenced by the role of compensation. Whichever school is in the ascendancy (post-traumatic stress disorder being the current one), is more a reflection of social pressures than objective evidence. The recognition of PTSD in psychiatric classification was in response to social pressure, and has led to a series of well-publicised legal claims in this country and the United States. Few can doubt that much of the interest in the condition has been stimulated by litigation. It is also clear that litigation can itself become a factor shaping illness experience and prognosis. However, the occasional view that PTSD is manufactured to obtain compensation, and that symptoms will resolve after litigation, is likely to be as inaccurate as similar claims regarding other aspects of so called 'compensation neurosis'.

Neurosis and physical complaints

Somatoform disorders

The classification of somatoform disorders is also a confusing area. It can be approached in three ways:

1. Somatic symptoms of psychological origin

Somatic symptoms such as fatigue, chest pain and headache are extremely common in the community (Kroenke & Price, 1993; see Table 6.1). Most are not associated with clear-cut physical causes, and are hence frequently known as functional somatic symptoms. Some are associated with psychiatric diagnoses such as anxiety or depression. Others will attract such syndromal labels as irritable bowel syndrome or chronic fatigue syndrome, particularly in specialist practice (see Chapter 21).

When the somatic symptoms are particularly severe and numerous, some subjects will fulfil criteria for somatisation disorder, also known as Briquet's syndrome or Briquet's hysteria. This diagnosis, first proposed by researchers in St Louis, is given to those who experience multiple physical symptoms affecting multiple organ systems, arising before the age of 30, and not explained by organic disease (Guze, 1975). The St Louis group have also provided evidence linking somatisation disorder in women with antisocial personality disorder in men (Cloninger et al., 1975). Somatisation disorder itself is commonest in, but not restricted to, women (Golding et al., 1991).

Somatisation disorder is relatively rare in the community, with a prevalence of around 0.1% but is far from rare in general medical clinics. Between 8–12% of general medical out-patients fulfil criteria for somatoform disorders, chiefly somatisation disorder itself (van Hemert et al., 1993). Clinical and management aspects are discussed by Lloyd (Chapter 21).

If somatisation disorder according to the classic criteria is relatively unusual in the population, patients with unexplained somatic symptoms are extremely common, and in recognition of this cases with many of the same characteristics of the full somatisation disorder, but who have fewer symptoms, have been labelled as 'abridged somatisation disorder' (Escobar *et al.*, 1987). In many respects, and in particular the tendency for excessive use of the medical, as opposed to mental health, services, the two syndromes are alike. As has been argued throughout this chapter, somatisation disorder, like the rest of the neuroses, represents a spectrum of severity (Katon *et al.*, 1991).

The current classification of the somatoform disorders is unsatisfactory. We concur with the suggestion of the Oxford group that the best approach is multi-dimensional. They have suggested the following classification (see Sharpe *et al.*, 1995).

1. Symptoms (number and type)

2. Psychiatric diagnoses (depression, anxiety, panic etc)

3. Cognitions (fear or conviction of disease)

4. Behavioural and functional impairment

5. Pathophysiological disturbance (hyperventilation, inactivity, etc).

2. Somatisation as a process

Goldberg & Bridges (1988) have suggested an influential definition of somatisation, seeing it as a process by which patients gain access to medical care. They define somatisation as occurring when a patient with a psychiatric disorder consults with physical symptoms, which are attributed to a physical cause. Finally, treatment of the psychiatric disorder would be expected to reduce or eliminate the physical symptoms.

Defined in this manner, somatisation is a very common process by which patients present with psychological disorders to their doctors. Twenty per cent of new attenders in general practice are somatisers, in contrast to the 5% who present with solely psychological symptoms (Goldberg & Bridges, 1988; see Chapter 19). Contrary to popular prejudice, somatisation is not associated with class, gender, intelligence or ethnicity. Instead, comparing somatic with non-somatic presentations, a Manchester study found that somatisers were less depressed, had less social dysfunction, but had more unsympathetic attitudes to mental disorder. In common with other investigators, they reported that somatisers were more likely to have received previous medical care both as an adult and as a child (Bridges *et al.*, 1991; Craig *et al.*, 1993).

Why do patients somatise? This should be addressed as two linked issues. The first is why do people develop medically unexplained symptoms, the second is why they then present these to doctors? Both psychological and physiological mechanisms exist to explain at least some of the factors underlying the production of somatic symptoms (see Sharpe & Bass, 1992). Some are straightforward – hyperventilation producing physical symptoms has already been discussed. Inactivity leads to muscle fatigue, whilst over-exertion causes delayed fatigue and myalgia. Psychological traits such as excessive attention to bodily sensations, patterns of symptom monitoring and a tendency to negative, disease-linked interpretations of symptoms have all been described, and all are exacerbated by affective disturbance. The excessive attention paid to internal sensations may also have a physiological, as well as a psychological bias. Impairment in the ability to filter out irrelevant stimuli,and hence an abnormal perception of internal sensations has been suggested on the basis of neurophysiological and evoked potential studies (Horvath *et al.*, 1980; Gordon *et al.*, 1986), although such studies need replication.

Having become aware of these symptoms, many factors then lead to the choice to present to the doctor using a physical, rather than a psychological, idiom. These include the stigma of mental illness, the failure to link emotional distress and physical symptoms, understandable concern about the possible cause of physical symptoms, and the belief (frequently correct) that doctors prefer to deal with physical, rather than psychological problems, early experience of illness, either in the patient or the family, is also implicated. Finally, Goldberg & Bridges argue that somatisation provides a mechanism by which those unsympathetic to the idea of mental distress can occupy the sick role, without loss of self-esteem. They also consider it as a means of blame avoidance.

Somatisation as a process is not a diagnosis, but a useful way of understanding attributions, illness behaviour and referral patterns. Somatisation is not a discrete category, but overlaps with the somatoform, affective and anxiety disorders.

3. Somatisation and health service use

Patients with persistent somatisation have considerable public health importance. They have long hospital careers – in one case register study being associated with a median number of 22 admissions (Fink, 1992*a*), and consume vast quantities of medical and surgical resources for little or no benefit (Fink, 1992*b*). The same, if less extreme, tendencies to use medical in preference to mental health services, and to have high rates of disability and occupational impairment, have been noted in those who fulfil criteria for either abridged somatisation disorder, or simply functional somatic symptoms (Escobar *et al.*, 1987; Katon *et al.*, 1990).

The phenomenon of somatisation has important implications for primary care. The majority of people with neurotic disorder attending a primary care clinic do not complain of psychological but of physical symptoms. This phenomenon may be different from the persistent 'doctor shoppers' who repeatedly complain of presumed psychogenic physical symptoms. It is probably more readily understood in terms of the relative importance to the patient of the physical and psychological symptoms and the widely held view that medical intervention will not help psychological symptoms. It is likely that those patients who present physical symptoms in the presence of neurotic disorder receive inappropriate treatment for their physical symptoms and have a better prognosis if they are recognised (Goldberg & Huxley, 1992).

Hysteria

Hysteria is another of those stubborn terms that, despite its many deficiencies, remains in clinical usage, and, in Aubrey Lewis's words, 'outlives its obituarists' (Lewis, 1975). However, even if it still exists, it is no easier to define. Freud used the term conversion (although not invented by him – see Reynolds, 1869), to refer to the process by which psychological distress is held to be repressed or 'converted' into a physical symptom, usually of neurological origin, such as fits or paresis. However, the rediscovery of the work of Pierre Janet, and the dramatic increase in interest in the so-called 'dissociative disorders' in the United States led to the introduction of the composite term dissociative (conversion) disorders into ICD-10, partly to avoid the problems of the term hysteria (see below), and partly to reflect the change in American psychotherapeutic practice. This links two processes; dissociation is an alteration or narrowing of consciousness associated with a lack of awareness of events and selective amnesia, whilst conversion refers to a limitation of motor or sensory function by the so-called processes of repression and conversion.

The most commonly encountered clinical syndromes include amnesia, fugue, paralysis, convulsions and sensory losses (Marsden, 1986). The diagnosis is difficult and most cases probably present to neurologists. In ICD-10 the diagnosis of a dissociative or conversion disorder is made when there is no physical cause for the symptom and there is evidence for a psychological causation, such as a relationship with a stressful event. This diagnosis of hysterical or dissociative disorders thus depends first upon a diagnosis of exclusion, and second of finding a particular psychological association that is assumed to be aetiological. It is not surprising that, even without considering the considerable difficulties of conveying the diagnosis to the patient or relatives, clinicians find it difficult to be confident about the diagnosis.

Multiple personality disorder is usually included as a dissociative condition and now appears in ICD-10 and DSM-IV. It is characterised by the presence of two or more personalities in a single person, usually referred to by separate names. In the United Kingdom it is usually seen as an iatrogenic condition when a suggestible patient with dissociative traits meets a therapist interested in the condition. Transitions from one personality to another often occur during sessions with therapists.

The concept of hysteria

In recent years the concept of hysteria has come under renewed pressure for several reasons:

1. Hysteria as a misdiagnosis of known organic disease Slater mounted one of the strongest attacks on the status of hysteria. His study was a 7-year follow up study of 85 patients diagnosed as hysteria at the National Hospital for Nervous Diseases, in London (Slater, 1965). He found that 30 had definite organic disease, such as multiple sclerosis, glioma and so on, of which eight were dead. Thirty-four now had obvious psychiatric disease, such as depression or schizophrenia, of which four had committed suicide. Only 22 out of 85 still had hysteria. Slater concluded 'if in our patients we find the signs of hysteria and no more, then these are signs that we have not yet looked deeply enough'. This provides the empirical basis for the aphorism taught medical students 'when the GP diagnoses hysteria, send for the undertaker'.

This study has, however, been somewhat misinterpreted. First, the setting was a tertiary referral centre for neurology, and the patients had been referred there, often by other neurologists, for a neurological opinion. One would therefore expect a high rate of organic disorder in the sample. Second, the presence of organic disease is not incompatible with hysteria – for example, epilepsy increases the risk of non-epileptic seizures, and hysterical symptoms are common after brain injury (Eames, 1992). Third, even in this sample, hysteria remained the only diagnosis in a substantial minority. Thus one should beware of over-interpreting this admittedly seminal study, and not follow the example of Slater's colleagues Ida MacAlpine and Richard Hunter (1966) who suggested, with Slater's research very much in mind, that the march of psychiatry is always from the psychological to the organic, from 'psychology to neurology, from mind to brain and never the other way round', describing a irreversible tide in which diseases once thought to be of psychological origin are admitted to the Pantheon of real diseases and their previous adherents mocked. Instead, it is salutary to recall the equal and opposite flow as floating kidneys, visceral proptosis and autointoxicating colons are revealed to originate in social and psychological disturbances. Slater's study is a cautionary tale about making the diagnosis of hysteria rather than arguing that hysteria does not exist.

Hysteria has, in the past, been said to be associated with certain clinical features, chiefly *belle indifference* and secondary gain. However, *belle indifference* is rarely present. Far from being indifferent, psychophysiological studies have shown that levels of general anxiety are high (Lader & Sartorius, 1968). It is also difficult to separate secondary gain from the general advantages of the sick role.

2. Pejorative diagnosis A series of authors, particularly those writing from a cultural or historical perspective, have outlined how hysteria is frequently used to describe patients who are difficult, complaining, awkward or female (see Chodoff, 1982; Micale, 1990).

3. The unconscious One important reason for the loss of the word hysteria from the current diagnostic manuals is its association with the Freudian concept of hysteria. Freudian criteria for hysteria rested upon an underlying unconscious mechanism; the repression of unwanted unconscious desires and the conversion into a loss of function, corresponding to the subject's idea of physiological dysfunction. This idea, though lacking conventional empirical support, is still a useful one in clinical psychiatry. In many ways it lives on in the present writings about somatisation – the idea that some physical symptoms have a psychogenic origin. However, the idea that somatic symptoms, whether in hysteria or somatisation, act as a 'defence' against the experience (as opposed to the willingness to admit to) psychological symptoms is untrue – epidemiological studies have demonstrated beyond doubt the linear nature of the relationship between somatic and psychological symptoms – the more one experiences the former, the more one experiences the latter. (Simon & VonKorff, 1991; Wessely et al., 1996).

4. The disappearance of hysteria Another argument used against the concept of hysteria is that, like schizophrenia, it seems to be disappearing. The florid seizures and bizarre contractures and paralyses of yesteryear are no longer seen, or at least only in rural, unsophisticated communities (Critchley & Cantor, 1984). However, this frequently reported observation should not be taken at face value (see Micale, 1993) – it is the socially created diagnosis of hysteria that changes over time. As already mentioned, hysteria continues to be diagnosed in 1% of admissions to the National Hospital for Neurology (Marsden, 1986). Pseudoseizures remain the stock-in-trade of the average neurologist. Shorter (1992) has argued that although the more bizarre sensory and motor expressions of hysteria have changed, perhaps because modern neurological investigations are adept at quickly establishing the non-organic nature of such florid hysterical phenomena, the symptoms of hysteria are now the more indefinable complaints of fatigue, exhaustion, poor memory and so on. This argument emphasises how modern hysteria overlaps with the general expressions of somatisation and somatic distress, as presumably anticipated by the St Louis group, who synthesised the old concept of hysteria into the modern concept of somatisation.

Modern views

The current concepts of hysteria now give a greater importance to factors outside the individual, such as the role of the family, and wider cultural and social matters,including the increasing medicalisation of distress, and the continuing stigmatisation of psychological disorder. Robert Kendell has emphasised how hysteria may develop as a distortion of the normal doctor–patient relationship. Kendell (1983) pointed out the 'manipulative behaviour of the hysterical patient is a strategy for achieving power in a role which does normally provide it'. The writings of Mechanic and Pilowsky have also been influential in developing the concept of illness behaviour, and hence abnormal illness behaviour, in understanding the use of the sick role in hysteria (see Pilowsky, 1978; Mechanic, 1986).

In conclusion, hysteria is a concept that doctors cannot do without. Hysteria will not disappear, but will continue to reflect changes in the ideas of acceptable illness held by doctors and patients alike (Mechanic, 1986; Stewart, 1990; Shorter, 1992). Anyone who uses it, however, must be aware that they will be contributing to a rich, and continuing, legacy for present and future historians of medicine.

Hypochondriasis

Hypochondriasis is a fear of physical illness. This is normal – a person experiencing chest pain may reasonably fear the possibility of heart disease. Hence the second part of the definition of hypochondriasis, that such fears must persist despite appropriate medical reassurance. The diagnosis is thus the only one in the psychiatric dictionary that involves the action of a doctor before the diagnosis can be made.

Hypochondriasis has a complex phenomenology. It can be an overvalued idea, a delusion, an auditory hallucination, or an anxious or depressive preoccupation. Kenyon's view that hypochondriasis is álmost invariably secondary to another psychiatric disorder, such as depression or anxiety, has been influential (Kenyon, 1964). There is no doubt that hypochondriasis is most often a symptom of another psychiatric disorder, and in particular anxiety (Barsky et al., 1992).

Clinicians in general hospital practice will also be familiar with patients who present with a single unshakable belief of physical illness (such as being infested by a parasite). These are regarded as a form of delusional disorder (Munro, 1980a). Other hypochondriacal beliefs arise in the course of delusional depression or schizophrenia. Treatment of these, and other

181

secondary causes of hypochondriasis, should, as usual, be directed towards the underlying disorder.

However, in recent years a place has been found for the diagnosis of primary hypochondriasis. Barsky (1979) has been influential in drawing attention to the common phenomenon of amplification of normal somatic symptoms, and its relationship to hypochondriasis (see Barsky, 1979). This is, as we never tire of saying, a dimensional response, but at the end of the spectrum are a small group of patients, uncommon in psychiatric but not medical practice, who fulfil the criteria for hypochondriasis in the absence of any other psychiatric disorder (Noyes et al., 1993).

Specific treatments for hypochondriasis itself have been developed. These rely on the general principles of dealing with all somatoform disorders, but in addition include a cognitive behavioural component that sees hypochondriasis as a health-related anxiety, associated with numerous cognitive distortions about the meaning of symptoms and disease. Treatment is directed at challenging automatic thoughts and dysfunctional assumptions about physical illness, and by reducing reassurance-seeking and abnormal illness behaviour (Warwick & Salkovskis, 1990). Of course, hypochondriasis depends upon doctors not just for its diagnosis, but also for its perpetuation, and will continue to be an unwelcome consequence of the current medical culture that views high technology investigations as anxiolytic, and not anxiogenic, in the management of patients with medically unexplained symptoms.

Like adults with somatisation disorder, those with hypochondriasis have increased rates of childhood trauma (sexual abuse, violence, parental disharmony), linked with increased rates of early childhood illness (Barsky et al., 1994). The links between early experience and either somatisation or hypochondriasis are unclear. However, it is likely that future studies will need to differentiate between those risk factors associated with neurotic disorder in general (such as childhood trauma, parental discord), and factors such as childhood exposure to illness and parental illness behaviour that may predict the subsequent style of presentation of neurotic symptomatology and illness behaviour.

Neurasthenia

Neurasthenia is another term with a long history. Originally referring to nervous weakness, it was at one time the generic term for almost all the neuroses. As outlined in the earlier part of this chapter, it gradually lost its meaning and disappeared from psychiatric practice, at least in Western society. Recently there has been a revival of interest in the condition, stimulated by the reawakening of interest in fatigue syndromes (see Wessely, 1990). Neurasthenia has reappeared in ICD-10, and now refers to an illness characterised by profound physical and mental fatigue and fatigability, but in which evidence for anxiety or depression is not prominent.

Subjects fulfilling various criteria for neurasthenia or neurasthenic syndromes are common. In the Swedish longitudinal study of the Island of Lundby the lifetime prevalence of fatigue syndrome (defined again as excessive fatigue in the absence of clear cut features of anxiety or depression) was 33% for women and 21% for men (Hagnell et al., 1993). Merikangas & Angst (1994) reported figures for ICD-10 neurasthenia of 6% for men and

10% for women in the Zurich Longitudinal survey. In the recent multinational WHO study of mental disorder in primary care the prevalence of ICD-10 neurasthenia was 5.5% (Ormel et al., 1994). Neurasthenia is also associated with substantial disability that equals that reported for depression (Ormel et al., 1994; Wessely, 1995).

Neurasthenia is thus common, but many of those cases will equally fulfil criteria for psychological disorders, especially depression and anxiety. Easy fatigability, poor concentration, irritability and the sense of increased mental effort appear in many of the criteria for both neurasthenia and common neurotic disorders. In both the community and in specialist practice there is no doubting the close relationship between, on the one hand, neurasthenia or chronic fatigue syndrome, and, on the other, psychiatric disorders (Wessely et al., 1996). The WHO study of mental disorder in primary care reported 71% comorbidity between neurasthenia and psychiatric disorder (Ormel et al., 1994), exactly the same as reported in a primary care study of chronic fatigue and chronic fatigue syndrome (Wess, 1995).

In hospital studies about one-third of those presenting with a label of chronic fatigue syndrome or its local variants do not fulfil criteria for standard psychiatric disorders, such as depression or anxiety, and thus are pure cases of neurasthenia. The distinction between neurasthenia and chronic fatigue syndrome is more a matter of illness attribution than symptoms – whereas the former is usually seen as a psychological disorder, the latter is frequently associated with a firm belief in a physical aetiology (Wessely, 1994).

Personality disorder

There is more controversy over personality disorder than almost any other area of psychiatric practice. It is a confusing area and one that attracts very little research attention. It is an important clinical area about which we know very little.

What is personality?

The difficulty of defining personality and its use as a lay term has added unnecessarily to the arguments over the nature of personality. Personality can be defined in different ways. A very general definition might be: any psychological attribute (excluding intelligence) of a person that varies between individuals. In the recent controversies over the nature of personality, no one doubts that people differ from one another in their psychological attributes. However, personality is also used in a much more specific way: personal attributes, as above (e.g. honesty), that are seen across different situations (e.g. at home and at work), which are related to other attributes (e.g. conscientiousness) and endure over someone's whole lifetime. Within experimental psychology, this more specific view of personality is associated with those who conceptualise personality as 'traits' (e.g. Eysenck, 1952a; Cattell, 1957) but a similar view of personality underlies psychodynamic personality theories (e.g. Storr, 1979) and the categorical classification of personality disorders used in psychiatry.

Criticisms of trait theory have come from those experimental psychologists who emphasise the national, cognitive determinants of social behaviour, which includes both social learning theorists (Mischel, 1968; Bandura, 1977a) and cognitive psychologists (Anderson, 1980). Mischel (1968) in particular has argued that this more specific trait view of personality needs empirical support. One cannot begin to study personality if it is defined in a way that implies an unproven theory of personality.

Another point should be made. Personality traits can only be a description, they cannot explain or cause behaviour though the concept is sometimes used as though it can. Gilbert Ryle (1949) has lucidly argued against this sort of 'explanatory' statement as creating a 'ghost in the machine'. Furthermore, personality traits are usually defined using behavioural measures so it is tautologous to say that a trait caused the behaviour that was used to define the trait in the first place. Wootton (1959) has made a similar point about the use of the term psychopathic or antisocial personality disorder to explain criminal behaviour, when the criminal behaviour has been used as grounds for the diagnosis.

Lay personality theories

It is a truism to say that ordinary people have their own concept of personality. Allport (1937) found over 11 000 trait terms in English (e.g. outgoing, shy, nervous, intelligent etc.), and in ordinary social interaction we often ask 'What sort of person is this?' a question that is often answered with a trait term. Allport's list, rooted in lay psychology, formed the basis of Cattell's (1957) and other trait theorists' ways of measuring personality. Subjects were asked to rate themselves or others on a variety of trait terms and the results were subjected to factor analysis. Cattell, Eysenck and others interpreted such findings as revealing the underlying dimensions of personality but one can also interpret the results as reflecting the theory of personality used by ordinary people.

This interpretation is supported by the key experiment of Passini and Norman (1966). In the late 1950s and 1960s one group had shown that factor analysis of trait ratings from a variety of different studies all produced a similar 5 factor result (Norman, 1963). But Passini and Norman (1966) found an almost identical 5 factor solution when raters who had only seen people for less than 15 minutes and had not spoken to each other were asked to rate the subjects as they imagined they would be. This '5 factor personality structure' therefore appeared to reflect the way ordinary people characterise each other, rather than representing the underlying structure of personality. Tyrer and Alexander (1979), though, argue that the similarity of the factor structure in those with and without personality disorders supports the idea that PD is an extreme variant of normal, but it could merely reflect the 'personality theories' used by the informants and interviewers.

Situations

One of the central issues in the personality literature has been the assertion that behaviour is influenced by the situation as well as by personal factors. Trait rating scales already imply cross-situational consistency and to examine whether people really do behave similarly in different situations needs direct behavioural measurement.

A number of such studies have been done and Mischel (1968) amongst others has pointed out that the correlation coefficients in these studies (with the exception of intelligence) are usually very modest, less than 0.3, and account for less than 10% of the variance. For instance, Hartshorne and May's (1928) study of schoolchildren found that the average correlations between cheating on four different tests was only 0.26, though the correlation between cheating on the same test on different occasions was 0.66. Mischel and Peake (1982) conducted two delay of reinforcement studies on the same group of children that only differed in a single respect, in one group the experimenter remained in the room. The correlation coefficient between the two was only 0.22.

Mischel's conclusions have been challenged (e.g. Epstein, 1979) but the data against substantial cross-situational consistency seems overwhelming. Broad behavioural consistencies must exist (a correlation coefficient of 0.3 is significant if the sample is large enough) but are too small to be of any use in predicting the behaviour of individual people.

When a thinking and reasoning person enters a situation it would be unlikely, indeed maladaptive, for broad personality traits to have a strong influence on behaviour. Perhaps cross-situational consistency should be regarded as a sign of an 'abnormal personality'? Indeed, Tyrer et al. (1979) have suggested that cross-situational consistency is more apparent in those classified as personality disordered.

The medical concept of personality disorder therefore rests on the rather shaky foundations of traditional trait-based personality theory.

Personality disorder: history and terminology

Pinel made the first reference to the concept that has become known as personality disorder. In 1801 his manie sans deliré referred to a group of patients who displayed the usual signs of 'insanity' but did not experience hallucinations or impairment of consciousness. Prichard's 1835 idea of 'moral insanity' was somewhat more narrowly defined as a 'morbid perversion of the feelings, affections and active powers, without any illusion or erroneous conviction' but probably still included the majority of the currently classified functional disorders and almost certainly included the neuroses. In the second half of the nineteenth century Lombroso was the first who explicitly linked personality with an inherited predisposition to criminality. Kraepelin introduced the more modern terminology of psychopathic personality though moral insanity continued to be used in Britain until the 1920s (Lewis, 1974).

Kretschmer introduced the notion that psychopathic personalities could be minor forms of major mental illnesses, for example, paranoid and schizoid. He also described 'sensitive' personalities who experienced ideas of reference under stress. Henderson (1939) also attempted to classify within the psychopathic personality group, proposing the aggressive, inadequate and creative subtypes. K. Schneider (1950) provided a more finely grained classification based upon the predominant clinical feature, including hyperthymic, depressive, explosive and asthenic. However, it is important to realise that Schneider did not distinguish between neurosis and personality disorder.

The current classification and concept of personality disorder thus has a confused parentage. Several ideas, including Kretschmer's (1918) concept of minor forms of illness and Schneider's classification based upon the predominant clinical features, have provided subtypes to the current ICD and DSM classification. Likewise the relationship between

Table 6.3. *Categories of personality disorder common to ICD-10 and DSM-IV*

Paranoid	Sensitive to what are seen as humiliations and rebuffs. Misconstruing neutral or friendly actions as hostile. Tenacious sense of personal rights. Excessive self-reference and self-importance
Schizoid	Emotional coldness and detachment. Withdrawal from close relationships and an autistic preference for fantasy. Eccentricity
Dissocial	Disregard for social obligations. Lack of feeling for others. Behaviour not readily modifiable by experience, including punishment. (Synonyms: antisocial, sociopathic)
Borderline	Tendency to act impulsively. Outbursts of anger and violence including self-harm. Emotional instability. Self-image unclear or disturbed. (Synonyms: emotionally unstable, borderline type)
Histrionic	Self-dramatisation, theatrically and exaggerated expression of emotions. Persistently manipulative. Suggestibility. (Synonym: hysterical)
Dependent	Weak inadequate response to the demands of daily life. Encouraging others to assume responsibility for major life areas. Undue compliance with the wishes of others. (Synonyms: asthenic, inadequate)
Avoidant	Persistent feelings of tension, apprehensiveness. Preoccupation with being criticized or rejected in social situations. Belief one is socially inept, inferior to other people
Anankastic	Indecisiveness, doubt and excessive caution. Perfectionism and excessive attention to detail. Rigidity and stubbornness. (Synonyms: compulsive, obsessional)

personality disorder and neurosis has often been unclear. It should also be pointed out that European psychiatrists tend to use psychopathy to refer to all personality disorders while in the British tradition, psychopathy tends to have a more restricted use for those with antisocial personalities, particularly when the person has committed criminal offences.

Classification

The ICD-10 and DSM-IV have different classifications of personality disorder. The changes between ICD-9 and ICD-10 have not been based upon advances in knowledge but rather on the results of discussion by a committee. Those categories that are included in both ICD-10 and DSM-IV are in Table 6.3. In addition, DSM-IV has the schizotypal, narcissistic, and passive-aggressive categories. Of particular note is borderline personality disorder, characterised by impulsivity, rapidly swinging moods, unstable relationships and repeated incidents of self-harm (Tarnopolsky & Berelowitz, 1987). ICD-10 has introduced the idea of 'trait accentuations' as a minor form of personality disorder.

Some have suggested that individual subtypes of personality disorder have an increased susceptibility to mental illness, for example, for those with anankastic personality disorder are more likely to develop an obsessional-compulsive disorder. However, this is not true of hysterical personality and hysterical conversion symptoms. The DSM-IV concept of schizotypal personality disorder is thought of as a minor form of psychotic illness along the lines of Kretschmer.

The subtypes described in ICD and DSM seem to be little used clinically. The exceptions are possibly the borderline and antisocial categories. DSM have suggested that the different categories of personality disorder are grouped into three clusters. Cluster A, the 'odd' or 'eccentric' group, includes paranoid and schizoid. Cluster B, 'dramatic' or 'erratic', includes histrionic, antisocial and borderline. Cluster C, 'anxious', includes avoidant, dependent and anankastic.

Current clinical use of personality disorder

Most contemporary psychiatrists use personality disorder in their clinical work and in 1986 7% of those occupying psychiatric beds in the UK had been given such a diagnosis (Smith *et al.*, 1995). The diagnosis of personality disorder can be made when the current clinical picture has been present since adolescence. The most reliable information will be obtained from an informant who has known the patient since adolescence and many psychiatrists would be reluctant to make the diagnosis without such evidence. Another important criterion for diagnosing personality disorder is that there should be evidence of significant subjective distress and/or social disability resulting from the clinical features justifying the diagnosis. The notion that lack of response to traditional treatment indicates a personality disorder is not justifiable in the absence of evidence for abnormalities since adolescence.

Epidemiology

Problems with classification and concerns about the concept of personality disorder have limited the number of epidemiological studies. de Girolamo & Reich (1993) have reviewed the prevalence studies. The more recent studies suggest a prevalence as high as 10% in the community (e.g. Casey & Tyrer, 1986; Reich *et al.*, 1989) though studies based upon clinical diagnoses seem to provide much lower estimates, of less than 3% (Dilling *et al.*, 1989).

Lee Robins' (1966) classic study illustrates that antisocial behaviour as a child is a powerful predictor of antisocial behaviour as an adult. Antisocial behaviour as a child increases the risk of marriage breakdown, however, marriage to a stable partner appears to protect against further criminality. This provides evidence for the increasingly popular view that the continuities observed between childhood and adult disorders are often dependent upon a chain of events in which the childhood psychopathology can have an adverse influence on subsequent life events.

Personality disorder and psychiatric disorder

The relationship between personality disorder and other psychiatric disorders is a source of some controversy. There are probably four options:

1. Personality disorder and other psychiatric disorders cannot occur simultaneously. This is probably supported by few psychiatrists though the diagnostic process sometimes implies that the two options are mutually exclusive.

2. All people with a psychiatric disorder also have a personality disorder. This is probably true in the sense that those people who develop a functional psychiatric disorder have some underlying vulnerability, which probably includes some personal characteristics. However, the severity of the underlying personality disturbance in many if not most of

those who develop a psychiatric disorder is rarely of a severity to justify the diagnosis of personality disorder as currently conceived.

3. Some people with personality disorder develop psychiatric disorder but psychiatric disorder and personality disorder can occur separately. This approach is now the commonest view of the relationship between personality disorder and other psychiatric disorders. This is formalised in DSM-IV that includes personality disorders in Axis II, making it easier to diagnose both a personality disorder and psychiatric disorder. It is important to note that it is especially important to confirm the diagnosis of personality disorder using informants if a coexistent psychiatric disorder is suspected.

4. Personality disorder is a chronic neurotic disorder. The symptoms of personality disorder are often, though not always, the same as those of neurotic disorders. This position holds that personality disorders are chronic neuroses starting in adolescence, and are therefore more severe than the chronic neuroses that start later in life.

Amongst all the controversy there is, surprisingly, one area of relative agreement: that personality disorder is not a mental illness (Lewis, 1974). Though Henderson (1939) and Cleckley (1976) disagree, more recently PD has increasingly been distinguished from illness. This has led at times to an unhelpful dichotomy between those with mental illnesses who deserve sympathy and care and those with personality disorders who are rejected and held responsible for their condition and behaviour (Lewis & Appleby, 1988). It would be unfortunate if the category of personality disorder were used to justify therapeutic nihilism or to prevent more research into the possibility of developing effective treatments.

Clinical management

The traditional view is that there is little one can do to alter the course of the underlying personality disorder, though the subjective distress and social disability tends to improve slightly with age. The management of this group therefore is primarily one of containment and treating any additional psychiatric disorders that are present. Management of personality disorders is particularly challenging and as a group they have a substantial suicide rate.

Deciding upon the presence or absence of another psychiatric disorder can be difficult, particularly distinguishing episodes of depression from temporary crises provoked by a life event. Particular attention must be paid to extracting information from reliable informants about any recent change of mental state or behaviour.

Despite the importance of personality-disordered patients and the clinical problems they pose, there has been very little research into effective treatments using randomised controlled trials (Dolan & Coid, 1993).

Pharmacological treatment

The conventional wisdom is to eschew pharmacological treatments in personality disorder. There are few randomised controlled trials conducted with this group of patients and any improvement could, in any case, be attributed to the coexistence of other psychiatric disorders. Most clinicians therefore use pharmacological treatments on an 'experimental' basis with each patient, often on a symptomatic basis and particularly if other psychiatric disorders are present. For example, if there are symptoms of depression a trial of antidepressants may be indicated. In patients with long histories one may find a long series of unsuccessful trials of various pharmaceutical agents. Benzodiazepines should be used sparingly if at all because the long-term nature of the problems probably raise the possibility of dependence.

Low dose neuroleptic treatment has been advocated, particularly for antisocial and borderline patients, without any convincing evidence from randomised studies. Similarly antidepressants have been advocated, particularly for borderline patients. Soloff *et al.* (1986) in one of the rare randomised studies found haloperidol was slightly better than amitryptilline and placebo in a sample of borderline patients. There have been claims that selective serotonin reuptake inhibitors are of particular help in those with personality disorder but at present there is no convincing empirical evidence to support their use over the less costly tricyclic antidepressants.

Psychological treatments

Both dynamic psychotherapy and schema-focused cognitive therapy (Beck & Freeman, 1990) claim to treat the underlying personality disturbance but convincing empirical evidence for their effectiveness is still poor. Behavioural and cognitive-behavioural treatments are worth trying on a symptomatic basis if the patient's cooperation can be enlisted.

In-patient treatment

In-patient treatment at a general psychiatric unit is rarely indicated for those with personality disorder except for brief admissions over a crisis. There has, however, been considerable interest in long admissions (1–2 years) to therapeutic communities as a treatment for personality disorders. This approach was developed in the UK and proponents argue that the underlying personality is being treated using this method (Jones, 1953*b*) though there are no convincing studies at present suggesting this approach is effective (Dolan & Coid, 1993). Outside these specialist settings the aims of in-patient admission should be for a brief respite to attempt to reduce suicide risk over a short period. If a patient is asking for admission, it is usually better to see him or her frequently as an out-patient, as admission can sometimes be quite stressful and undermining.

The Henderson Hospital in the UK is a therapeutic community that requires the patient to want to be admitted to the unit and engage in a challenging but supportive community (Norton, 1992). One of the key elements of the approach is a democratisation of the relationships between staff and patients along with a culture that examines all incidents, interactions and relationships within the setting. Though it is usually stated that patients have to want to be part of the community, some units in prisons also accept compulsory patients (e.g. the Dr Henri van der Hoeven Clinic in the Netherlands).

189

Social management

The general principles of rehabilitative psychiatry apply to those given the diagnosis of personality disorder. Attention to suitable housing, the family environment and ensuring occupational activity during the day are all of potential value.

Problems with the concept of personality disorder

Relationship between personality and neurosis

Many of the symptoms experienced by those who are given the diagnosis of personality disorder are similar or identical to those characteristic of neurotic disorders. Even when neurotic symptoms are not the overwhelming clinical feature, they are usually present on direct questioning (e.g. Lazare & Klerman, 1968; Slavney & McHugh, 1974; Gunn & Robertson, 1976; Thompson & Goldberg, 1987). This had led to the suggestion that personality disorders are best conceived as a chronic neurosis.

Eysenck and similar personality trait theorists make the distinction between state and trait. Social learning theory does not need to make this distinction. All behaviour, whether exhibited over a great length of time or only covering a short period, would have the same basis in beliefs and attitudes and their interaction with the environment (Mischel, 1968; Beck, 1976). Some personality inventories, particularly the scales measuring 'neuroticism' appear to correlate markedly with measures of mental illness, and change with recovery from depression (Coppen & Metcalfe, 1965; Kendell & DiScipio, 1968; Hirschfeld et al., 1983). The distinction between trait and state may be an attractive simplification but there is still no way of distinguishing a neurotic trait from a neurotic state, nor a personality disorder from a chronic neurosis. Shepherd et al. (1968) in their international study of diagnostic habits noted that personality disorder in one culture was neurosis in another.

Replacing this concept of personality disorder with the simpler and more comprehensible idea of chronic neurosis would fit the available evidence, but some features of personality disorder are not neurotic symptoms. For instance, the concept of antisocial PD, at least in DSM-IV, includes committing crimes. But many critics have pointed out the legal and philosophical difficulties of psychiatric explanations of crime (e.g. Wootton, 1959). There are therefore definite advantages if psychiatrists abandon the impulse to explain all deviant behaviour.

Personality disorder as a pejorative label

The most serious of the reservations expressed with the personality disorder concept is that it is a derogatory moral judgement (Gunn & Robertson, 1976). Lewis & Appleby (1988) have argued that this results from the exclusion of personality disorder from the category of mental illness. Whatever mental illness means (Lewis, 1953; Farrell, 1979), it implies amongst other things a lack of control over behaviour and a lack of responsibility for action. The inference that an action is not under control has been linked with sympathy and willingness to help (Weiner, 1980). In the context of a psychological abnormality, mental illness can be seen as a label conferring reduced responsibility for behaviour, legitimising medical care and encouraging sympathy. Lewis & Appleby's (1988) study provided some evidence for this based on questionnaire responses to case vignettes given the diagnosis of personality disorder. Compared with control vignettes, cases with PD were seen as manipulative, attention seeking, less sympathetic, not deserving health service resources, and not being mentally ill. Someone who has a personality disorder is seen neither as normal, nor as mentally ill. Classifying these individuals as suffering from chronic neuroses would rely less on precarious theories of personality, would not be attempting to explain all deviant behaviour and hopefully would eliminate a pejorative term from the psychiatric taxonomy.

Reliability

Trait ratings require global judgements based on ambiguous data. This vagueness must contribute towards the unreliability of personality assessment, and the trait ratings themselves can be very unreliable even in research settings (Gunn & Robertson, 1976). There is now a striking contrast between the mental illness section of DSM-IV or ICD-10 with its exactly specified operational criteria and the section on personality disorder, with its rather vague trait descriptions. Antisocial PD continues to be the most reliable of all the categories (Mellsop *et al.*, 1982) possibly because the criteria include behavioural items (mostly about infringements of the law) as well as trait terms. It is ironic that the most reliable of all the PD categories has also attracted the most controversy about its validity (Wootton, 1959; Frances, 1980).

Standardised assessments of personality have been developed however, and these can produce a more reliable assessment (Standard Assessment of Personality, Mann *et al.*, 1981; Personality Assessment Schedule, Tyrer & Alexander, 1979; Personality disorder Examination, Loranger *et al.*, 1987). They are discussed in Chapter 4).

Validity

Pre-existing beliefs or schemata can influence perception, memory and social inferences (Anderson, 1980) and in general the bias acts in order to confirm such beliefs (Nisbett & Ross, 1980). Trait ratings are particularly susceptible, and such a confirmatory bias challenges the validity of trait ratings in assessing personality and in part explains why trait theories of personality continue to make intuitive sense. As Mischel (1968) has asserted, trait rating scales lead to information about what is in the mind of the rater, as well as, or even instead of, the behaviour of the rated.

These biases may also influence clinical assessment. For instance, suicidal thoughts in someone with a PD could be seen as manipulative or histrionic, and therefore attract less sympathy and importance than the same complaints in someone regarded as 'ill'. Walton and Presly (1973) drew attention to the tendency for men to be given a diagnosis of antisocial personality while the women were given the hysterical personality label.

7

Eating disorders

JANET TREASURE

A. ANOREXIA NERVOSA

Introduction

The eating disorders, anorexia nervosa and bulimia nervosa, have become serious public health concerns. Anorexia nervosa is now the third most common chronic illness in teenage girls (Lucas *et al.*, 1991). Bulimia nervosa appears to be displacing depression as the symptomatic expression of psychic distress in young women. The lifetime prevalence in Westernised women is 4% and rising. Profound effects on physical as well as psychological health are common to both disorders. Although there is a tendency to group anorexia and bulimia nervosa together under the title 'eating disorders' there are important differences in terms of antecedent factors, course and management.

Classification

The criteria for anorexia nervosa in DSM-IV and ICD-10 are shown in Table 7.1. Much of the psychopathology in current definitions is culture-bound. One feature that has already failed to stand the test of time is body image distortion (Hsu & Sobkiewicz, 1991). This entered classification systems in DSM-III (APA, 1980) and was ardently pursued by researchers in the 1980s, but like the treasure at the end of the rainbow was never found. It is replaced in DSM-IV criteria by 'overconcern with body size and shape'. Describing oneself as fat when one is painfully thin may be one facet of the more central phenomenon of denying the severity of illness or disability

The morbid fear of fatness, which is present in current diagnostic systems also, may not be fundamental to the illness (Russell & Treasure, 1989; Schmidt & Treasure, 1993a; Theander, 1994; Russell, 1995). It is the current explanation for the failure to eat. In the past, fasting has been understood as an act of piety/to compensate for sins and ward off evil. In this context young women with anorexia nervosa were possibly seen as saints. St Catherine of Sienna would be one example (Bell, 1985; Rampling, 1985). Later cases of probable anorexia

Table 7.1. *Criteria for classification of anorexia nervosa*

DSM-IV (307.1)	ICD 10–F50
Refusal to maintain body weight over a minimal norm/leading to body weight 15% below expected or failure to gain weight during growth	Significant weight loss (BMI < 17.5 kg/m^2) or failure of weight gain or growth Weight loss self-induced by avoiding fattening foods and one or more of the following (a) vomiting (b) purging (c) excessive exercise (d) appetite suppressants (e) diuretics
Intense fear of gaining weight or becoming fat	A dread of fatness as an intrusive overvalued idea and the patient imposes a low weight threshold on herself
Disturbance in the way in which one's body weight, size or shape is experienced e.g. 'feeling fat' (denial of seriousness of underweight or undue influence of body weight and shape on self evaluation)	
Absence of three consecutive menstrual cycles	Widespread endocrine disorder (a) amenorrhoea (b) raised growth hormone (c) raised cortisol (d) reduced T$_3$
Binge/purging type: binge eating or vomiting/misuse laxatives diuretics	

nervosa aroused interest as freaks of nature. These women appeared to defy science by surviving with little or no food, for example the case of Martha Taylor described by John Reynolds (1669). Currently in Hong Kong, vague abdominal distress is the usual rationalisation for not eating (Lee *et al.*, 1989). This resembles the presentation in nineteenth-century France where women with anorexia nervosa at that time hinted that food was injurious to them. Marce described this symptom as a form of dyspepsia. Given that much of the psychopathology is subject to pathoplasticity, what are the core features? Russell (1995) recently defined them as 'self imposed reduced nutrition in the context of psychosocial stress'. Szmuckler & Patton (1995) have also proposed a definition of anorexia nervosa free from cultural colouring 'subjects who became emaciated through restricting their dietary intake for whatever reason. This restriction is deliberate and the resulting state is positively valued by the subject'.

What sort of condition is anorexia nervosa? Richard Morton (1946) described the illness in his treatise on the consumptions, noting that 'nervous cares' were frequent antecedent factors. Marcé (1860) termed anorexia nervosa a hypochondriacal delirium, whereas Lasègue (1873) classified it as a form of hysteria. The Anglo-Saxon name is derived from Sir William Gull (1874). He initially called the syndrome 'apepsia hysterica' but four years later he replaced 'apepsia' with 'anorexia' as he observed that food, if taken, was digested indicating that the stomach was not at fault. He later argued that because men could be afflicted and the deficit was central rather than peripheral that nervosa was a better term than hysterica. Gull toyed with this problem for several years. He initially stated that anorexia nervosa was due to a 'morbid mental state' and later that it was a 'perversion of the ego'.

The controversy continues. The vogue to argue for anorexia nervosa as an atypical variant of affective disorder (Cantwell *et al.*, 1977) has now passed as the evidence accrued was unconvincing. A few (but not all) studies have found a higher incidence of depression in relatives. However, the converse, that is a greater risk of anorexia nervosa in families of depressed probands, has never been found (Strober *et al.*, 1990).

A more recent proposal is that it is a form of obsessive-compulsive disorder (OCD) (Rothenberg, 1986; Fahy, 1991). There is some support for this in terms of family history and antecedent factors: (a) obsessive compulsive disorder is significantly higher in the first degree relatives of anorexia nervosa patients than with controls (Halmi *et al.*, 1991); (b) obsessional traits are common antecedents (Rastam & Gillberg, 1992) and (c) women with obsessive compulsive disorder commonly have a history of anorexia nervosa (Kasovits *et al.*, 1986; Fahy *et al.*, 1993). However it is uncertain whether this represents core anorexia nervosa or whether patients with OCD have been recruited to swell the ranks. The psychopathology of OCD may have undergone pathoplastic change. In the West we now fear food. It makes you fat (with all the connotations of laziness, greed and powerlessness that this evokes); it also gives you heart attacks, cancer, hyperactivity and germs such as BSE, listeria, salmonella. It is one small step from the cultural fear to the terror in OCD.

Yet another model is that anorexia nervosa is a form of addiction, a dependence on starvation (Szmukler & Tantam, 1984). In South America, anorexia nervosa has been classified as a psychosis because of the delusional conviction with which sufferers' beliefs are held.

Historical case presentations

Vivid clinical descriptions of anorexia nervosa date from the mid-seventeenth century. Richard Morton described two patients whose illness appeared to be due to voluntary food restriction. One was a 18-year-old girl who:

'fell into a total suppression of her Monthly Courses from a multitude of Cares and passions . . . From which time her appetite began to abate . . . she was wont by her studying and continuing pouring upon Books to expose herself both day and night . . . she was like a Skeleton only clad with skin.'

This girl died. However, the second patient, a 16-year-old schoolboy, who:

'fell gradually into a total want of appetite, occasioned by studying too hard and the Passions of the Mind . . .'

was cured by advice to:

'abandon his studies, to go into the country air, and to use riding and a milk diet.'

A young French psychiatrist, Louis-Victor Marcé, wrote in 1860 of

> 'young girls who at the period of puberty become subject to inappetancy carried to the utmost limits . . . these patients arrive at the delirious conviction that they cannot or ought not to eat . . . All attempts made to constrain them to adopt a sufficient regimen are opposed with infinite strategies and unconquerable resistance.'

Sir William Gull (a physician at Guy's Hospital) and Charles Lasegue (a French psychiatrist) between 1868 and 1888 brought the illness to the attention of the medical community with articles and case presentations. Lasègue's (1873) account is particularly vivid and well observed:

> '. . . gradually she reduces her food further and further, and furnishes pretexts for so doing . . . the abstinence tends to increase the aptitude for movement.'

He describes the lack of insight into the dangerousness of the weight loss and gives a typical repost when confronted:

> 'I do not suffer and therefore must be well.'

Epidemiology

Most of the estimates on the incidence of anorexia nervosa are based on data from psychiatric case registers and are hence limited to cases referred for psychiatric care. Approximately 70% of cases of anorexia nervosa presenting to primary care are referred on to specialist care (Hoek, 1993). Not all are referred to psychiatrists; some are referred to paediatricians and general physicians. Databases held in primary care also do not detect all cases. On the other hand, community screening surveys are never large enough to detect more than one or two cases. It has been found repeatedly that cases of anorexia nervosa are missed if preliminary screening questionnaires are used. (It is uncertain whether this is unconscious denial or deliberate cunning!). The incidence of anorexia nervosa derived from these various methods is shown in Table 7.2. The most detailed survey was that of Lucas *et al.*, 1991), who screened all the medical records from the Mayo clinic using additional probes such as amenorrhoea, vomiting, weight loss, etc. Over half the cases of anorexia nervosa they detected had not been diagnosed as such.

It is uncertain whether there has been an increased incidence rate of anorexia nervosa. Psychiatric case registers have shown an increase but this may reflect increased recognition and a change in referral practices. The meticulous study from the Mayo clinic in the period 1930–1990 does not suggest there have been major time trends in incidence. Williams & King (1987) argue that the increased incidence of anorexia nervosa is a medical myth resulting from the relative increase in young women and an increased readmission rate to hospital. The latter may arise because the course of the illness may have changed over time becoming more chronic, leading to an increased prevalence rate.

Studies that have estimated the prevalence of anorexia nervosa are shown in Table 7.3. They are subject to the same inaccuracies as were described for incidence. The exception is a study from Sweden. All children born in 1970 from Gotenberg were screened aged 15, using a

Table 7.2. *Incidence of anorexia nervosa per 100 000 population*

Study	$n \times 10^6$	Period	Source	Incidence
Szmuckler *et al.* (1986)		1978–82	Case register	4.06
Lucas *et al.* (1991)		1935–84	Medical records	8.2
Hoek (1991)	0.15	1985–86	General practitioners	6.3

Table 7.3. *Prevalence of anorexia nervosa in young people*

Study	$n \times 10^3$	Age	Method	Prevalence
Gillberg *et al.* (1994)	2	15–17	School nurse	1.08 female
				0.09 male
Lucas *et al.* (1991)		15–19	Medical records	0.48
Hoek *et al.* (1991)		15–29	General practice	0.16

two-stage procedure, growth charts and school-nurse records followed by an interview (Rastam *et al.*, 1989). The survey was repeated when they were aged 18 (Gillberg *et al.*, 1994). The research team stated that they were certain that they missed no cases.

Aetiology

Research or speculation into aetiology has often failed to differentiate between anorexia nervosa and bulimia nervosa (see Brumberg, 1988; DiNicola, 1990) despite there being enormous differences in epidemiology and clinical features that need to be explained. It is highly probable that sociocultural factors account for these differences and are of more relevance to bulimia nervosa than anorexia nervosa.

A. Sociocultural factors

Feminist issues

The female preponderance has to be explained. (This is even more marked for bulimia nervosa than anorexia nervosa.) Conflict associated with female roles in society may be relevant (sexual experience: Bruch, 1978; powerlessness and inequality: Palazzoli, 1974; Orbach, 1978).

Dieting

In contrast to bulimia nervosa (see below) there is, as yet, no direct evidence that dieting increases the risk of anorexia nervosa. The relevant epidemiological studies have not been done because the lower frequency of anorexia nervosa makes such a project a formidable task.

The indirect evidence to support dieting as a risk factor is:

(a) Clinically, dieting often precedes onset.
(b) Groups with high levels of dieting behaviour have a greater incidence of anorexia nervosa.

Evidence against dieting as an important risk factor is:

(a) Marked changes in the incidence of anorexia nervosa have not occurred despite great cultural changes in dieting behaviour.
(b) No models of self-starvation after food restriction exists.

Dieting may act as a risk factor in the context of a more specific genetic or biological vulnerability, and it is probably an important maintaining factor.

B. Family factors

Minuchin developed a model of 'psychosomatic families'. Anorexia nervosa was the prime example. His idea was that these families show characteristic patterns of interaction that include enmeshment, overprotectiveness, rigidity and lack of conflict resolution. As aetiological theory it has found to be lacking. Family factors do affect the course of the illness (Szmuckler et al., 1985; Van Furth, 1991). For example, the level of expressed emotion predicts outcome. However, overall expressed emotion is low in the relatives of patients with anorexia nervosa, i.e. critical comments are few and hostility is low.

C. Psychological factors

Depression and recent severe life events, such as death of first degree relatives, were among the commonest identifiable antecedents in the Swedish community case-control study described above (Rastam & Gillbert, 1992). Over three-quarters of a clinical sample have had serious life stress in the year before presentation (Schmidt et al., 1993a,b).

Slade (1982) has suggested that stress triggers the development of an eating disorder if underlying vulnerability factors such as perfection, maturity fears and general dissatisfaction are also present. Indeed obsessionality, perfectionism and asceticism are common in anorexia nervosa. Over half of the children who developed anorexia nervosa had premorbid obsessional traits (Rastam & Gillbert, 1992). High levels of asceticism and perfectionism persist despite recovery (Lovell, 1994). There is less evidence that some of the features noted by Bruch (1978), such as interceptive awareness, ineffectiveness and maturity fears are relevant. A variety of psychodynamic models have been developed. However, in a recent review, Dare & Crowther (1995) suggested that these may be of value in understanding the patient rather than being of aetiological importance.

D. Heredity and biological hypotheses

Several strands of evidence point to a specific genetic risk for anorexia nervosa:

(a) female relatives of probands with anorexia nervosa have a tenfold greater risk of developing an eating disorder than the general population (Strober *et al.*, 1990); overall the incidence rate in relatives is 7%;

(b) twin studies in anorexia nervosa have found higher levels of concordance in identical compared to non-identical, same-sex twin pairs (Treasure & Holland, 1988).

The mechanism for such a genetic vulnerability is a matter of speculation. One possibility is that it is an abnormality in body weight control that may only be revealed by weight loss or psychosocial stress. Supporting this is the clinical finding that weight loss from whatever cause, as part of a grief reaction, due to glandular fever or even political action (two sisters who were IRA hunger strikers developed anorexia nervosa that continued when their political action was over), may trigger anorexia nervosa. In identical twin pairs discordant for anorexia nervosa the affected twin had higher levels of life events prior to onset. On the other hand, the genetic risk might be for certain temperamental features, for example obsessionality. Perfectionism and body dissatisfaction were vulnerability factors found in the twin study (Treasure & Holland, 1993). We can, however, safely rule out the possibility of it being a variant phenotype expression of a non-specific neurosis gene (depression, anxiety, alcoholism).

In animals, certain strains can develop analogues of anorexia nervosa. 'Thin sow syndrome' affects young pigs (Owen, 1990). Rats can develop progressive weight loss in the context of time-limited feeding and a running wheel (Epling & Pierce, 1984). A different animal model is that seen in social colonies such as the mole rat. In these there is one dominant female who is big and fertile with small sister infertile rats who live in the colony to help feed the young (Demaret, 1991).

Russell, 1970, suggested that anorexia nervosa may be caused by abnormal hypothalamic function. Indeed, there have been many case reports of brain lesions in this area presenting like anorexia nervosa. Increased serotonin activity in the hypothalamus could account for the anorexia, obsessionality and psychosexual inhibition characteristic of anorexia nervosa (Treasure & Campbell, 1994).

Clinical features

The median age of onset is 17 years but cases as young as eight and as old as 60 have been described. Less than 10% of cases are male. Case registers have not confirmed the common belief that anorexia nervosa is confined to the upper social classes. However, there is an association with high educational achievement.

All too often the onset is insidious. Family members may ignore the weight loss or even praise it. The eating behaviours follow trends in dietary fashion, with fat replacing carbohydrate as the enemy of dieting people. Family and patient may protest that she is eating large amounts. Indeed her plate may be piled high with large quantities of vegetables, salads or other low calorie foods.

A useful diagnostic feature is the contrast between the degree of emaciation and the level of overactivity and protestations that there is nothing wrong. Parents may describe a change in their daughter's temperament. Their 'good girl' has become difficult, emotional, irritable and excessively conscientious. Loss of menstruation is a good marker of nutritional insufficiency, although in a few cases it occurs before there is any weight loss. The equivalent feature in men is loss of erections on waking. It can be more difficult to make the diagnosis in prepubertal children when there is a failure to grow rather than weight loss.

Physical assessment

The facial features appear gaunt, with the rest of the body hidden in layers of bulky clothes. The hands, feet and nose are pinched, blue and cold. The skin is dry and downy, lanugo hair may be present on the cheeks, nape of the neck and forearms and legs. The head hair may become thinned and dry so that it breaks off and sticks out. The pulse rate is slow and blood pressure low (90/60 mmHg). A proximal myopathy may be present in severe cases. Test for this by asking the patient to get up from a squat without using her hands as leverage.

Comorbidity

Depressive and obsessional symptoms are common and in part can be explained by weight loss, as they are a feature of involuntary starvation. Many of the so-called biological features of depression are also present in anorexia nervosa. It is unusual, though, for patients with anorexia nervosa to express suicidal thoughts or to see their behaviour as leading towards death. The strength of the resistance to weight gain is also a good distinguishing feature between depression with weight loss and anorexia nervosa with depression. In older (over 30) women the two features may be more tightly intermingled with pronounced depressive features and severe weight loss with a reluctance to gain weight. In these cases the onset usually follows severe life events. The obsessional behaviours in anorexia nervosa are usually focused around food, eating and exercise. In approximately 10% the obsessional behaviour is more generalised and includes cleaning, checking and counting.

Avoidant, anankastic and emotionally unstable personality features are present in approximately half of those referred for psychiatric treatment (Gartner et al., 1989; Wonderlich et al., 1990). However, most of these appear to be state-related as they vanish after recovery. The purging subtype of anorexia nervosa is frequently associated with a borderline personality and other impulsive behaviours such as stealing, alcohol abuse and self-harm.

Some personality traits are more persistent. These include poor self-esteem with little self-confidence regarding academic abilities or personal attractiveness. Perfectionist traits are usual; flawed work may be destroyed and repeated, or personal belongings strictly ordered.

Measurement

A structured interview, the Eating Disorder Examination, which assesses the relevant psychopathology and has similarities to the Present State Examination has been developed (Cooper & Fairburn, 1987). Several self-report questionnaires are also in common use. The eating attitudes test (EAT) is a self-report questionnaire that has been validated in clinical samples but has poor sensitivity and specificity when used in the community (Garner & Garfinkel, 1979). The Eating Disorder Inventory is also a self-report questionnaire, produced later by the same group (Garner *et al.*, 1983), which incorporates factors from the EAT and in addition personality dimensions.

Somatic effects

Anorexia nervosa affects all systems of the body. A detailed exposition can be obtained from recent reviews or books (Bhanji & Mattingly, 1988; Sharpe & Freeman, 1993; Treasure & Szmuckler, 1995). In this chapter we outline major abnormalities of relevance for differential diagnosis or management.

Endocrine system

Two hypotheses account for the abnormal endocrine features in anorexia nervosa: (1) a hypothalamic abnormality; (2) a secondary effect of starvation. Most of the evidence supports (2); although the exception is that in a minority of cases amenorrhoea presents before weight loss. The pattern of hormonal abnormality is shown in Table 7.4.

Reproductive system

Regression to a prepubertal status occurs, the uterus and ovaries shrink and multiple small follicles appear in the ovaries. Many patients are concerned about their long-term fertility and this can be a motivating factor. Full recovery restores reproductive potential. However, partial recovery is associated with an increased miscarriage rate, low birth weight, increased perinatal morbidity and feeding and parenting problems in childhood.

Gastrointestinal systems

Gastric emptying is delayed but improves with refeeding (Szmukler *et al.*, 1990) and may act to maintain the illness. Gastrointestinal problems such as ulcers and irritable bowel may persist after recovery.

Central nervous system

Brain scans show that the ventricular spaces are increased and neuropsychological deficits are present.

Skeleton

Bone substance is lost with increased duration of illness. Pathological fractures develop. Poor nutrition rather than oestrogen deficiency is probably the primary abnormality. Stunting occurs if the onset is early (Gillberg *et al.*, 1994; Russell, 1985).

Table 7.4. *Changes in hormonal status in anorexia nervosa*

Increased	Decreased
Cortisol	LH
GH	FSH
CCK	Oestrogen
	T_3
	TSH
	Noradrenaline

Cardiovascular system

The QT interval increases, which may lead to the development of arrhythmias (Cook *et al.*, 1994).

Haematology

Anaemia and white cell counts of less than 4000 are common. Platelet suppression is rare but is a sign of dangerous weight loss. The ESR is low and usefully excludes inflammatory bowel disease.

Comorbidity with a physical illness such as diabetes, thyroid disorder or Crohns can lead to management difficulties and an increase in complications.

Assessment

The diagnosis of anorexia nervosa rarely poses difficulties except in atypical cases such as children, males and older females where the psychopathology may be somewhat different. A crucial step at the first assessment interview is to develop a therapeutic alliance. Denial and ambivalence are characteristic features of anorexia nervosa. Developing a good relationship is perhaps more difficult that in any other field of psychiatry. More often than not the patient is unforthcoming and angry at being coerced into seeing a doctor by concerned relatives and friends. It is important to establish an individual relationship with the sufferer.

Motivational interviewing as exemplified by Miller & Rollnick (1991) is a useful intervention. Detail how eating difficulties have caused problems or concerns for their health (physical and psychological), career or social life. A straight enquiry about the history of their anorexia nervosa may be met by the sulky reply 'I haven't got anorexia nervosa'. The following are a list of questions that are helpful in starting the interview.

1. Problem recognition
   What difficulties have you had in relation to your eating?
   What makes you think your eating is a problem?

In what ways has this been a problem for others?

How has your eating problem stopped you doing what you want to do?

2. Concerns

Who is most concerned about your eating problem?

What is it about your eating that other people might see as reasons for concern?

What do you feel about your eating and weight? In what way does it concern you?

What do you think will happen if you don't make a change?

3. Intention of change

The fact that you are here indicates that at least part of you thinks it's time to do something.

What are the reasons you see for making a change?

If you were 100% successful in overcoming your problem and things worked out how you would like, how would your life change?

What are the advantages/disadvantages of making a change?

4. Optimism

What makes you think if you decide to change you could?

What do you think would work for you if you decided to change?

Once the patient's concerns have been established, a weight and diet history will need to be obtained to establish whether there is any degree of stability and control. Both the rate of change of weight as well as the absolute level are markers of dangerousness. Patients with the restricting form of illness usually maintain a regular meal pattern whereas those who are in the prodrome of the bulimic form will have prolonged periods of abstinence. Avoid any comments that could be interpreted as critical or hostile, as the patient is acutely sensitive to these.

The rest of the assessment can be a routine psychiatric examination. A physical examination including weight and height and some investigation is essential. Table 7.5 details the weight thresholds to fulfil WHO ICD-10 criteria for anorexia nervosa and those that indicate that weight loss is severe. Table 7.6 details the investigations that are valuable in managing anorexia nervosa.

Offer management plans, in the form of choice if at all possible, even if this means including 'second best' options. If too rigid a proposal of treatment is offered it is likely that patients will rebel and not fully comply. If they are unable or unwilling to follow treatment recommendations they think they have failed, or they will reject all that has been said as inapplicable to them. A range of alternative approaches may lead to a more active collaboration.

Motivating the patient involves many of the techniques of standard psychotherapeutic practice: expression of empathy, provision of advice, encouraging the setting of goals and the promotion of self-efficacy and hope. It is necessary to tread a fine balance between coercion and collusion. Too much confrontation or coercion leads to a build-up of resistance. Avoid being pressed into the position of insisting on change. Insistence could engender rebound opposition even if this is not openly expressed. On the other hand, to watch passively as the patient continues to lose weight or binge could be considered negligent. The answer is to work with the patient so that the resolution to change comes from her.

Table 7.5. *A chart of weight thresholds for use in anorexia nervosa*

	5' 0"	5' 2"	5' 4"	5' 6"	5' 8"
Normal range BMI (20–25) kg/m²	45–56 kg	48–60 kg	51–64 kg	54–68 kg	58–72 kg
Weight threshold for anorexia nervosa BMI 17.5 kg/m²	39 kg	42 kg	45 kg	51 kg	
Medical danger BMI < 13.5 kg/m²	30 kg	33 kg	34 kg	37 kg	39 kg

Table 7.6. *Investigations in anorexia nervosa*

1. Physical examination
   –Skin for petechial rash/lanugo hair/Raynaud's/chilblains/callus on hand/self-mutilation
   –Mouth and teeth for caps/loss of enamel/abrasions
   –Lying and standing blood pressure for dehydration and circulatory failure
   –Abdomen for constipation
   –Ability to rise from a squat for proximal myopathy

2. Blood count
   –Anaemia (Hb 9–12 g/l) (usually normocytic normochromic)
   –White cell count in the range 2000–4000
   –Platelet deficiency (rare)
   –ESR normal

3. Blood chemistry (urea and electrolytes are usually sufficient unless there are other indications)
   –Urea usually low in restricting anorexia nervosa but can be increased with vomiting and laxative abuse
   –Potassium <3.5 mM/L (vomiting or laxative abuse)
   –Bicarbonate <30 mM/l (vomiting: <18 mM/l (laxative abuse)
   –Aspartate transaminase, alkaline phosphatase, gamma glutamyl transaminase may all be increased
   –Cholesterol >6.5 mM/l
   –Amylase (salivary isoenzyme) increased (bulimia, vomiting)
   –Phosphate levels decreased
   –Carotene increased
   –Protein usually normal

4. Blood hormones (these are of no use diagnostically and do not need to be performed routinely)
   –See Table 7.4
   –Basal TSH normal (delay response to TRH)
   –Basal ACTH normal (decrease response CRH)
   –Basal insulin reduced (increased sensitivity to insulin)

One of the first steps in engaging the patient in treatment is to gain some understanding of the reasons underlying her ambivalence. Often several of these maintaining factors act in concert. Examples are outlined in Table 7.7.

Motivating the patient to change may take a long time. It may be helpful to involve the supporting network if no progress is made on an individual basis.

Table 7.7. *Reasons for ambivalence*

(a) Social (e.g. fashionably slim, attributes of power and success)
(b) Familial (e.g. vulnerable, powerful, revenge)
(c) Physiological – tolerance (e.g. stomach emptying, ketones)
(d) Behavioural – conditioning (e.g. fat aversion)
(e) Psychological – (e.g. control over food as a coping strategy, concentration on food avoids a focus on difficult issues)

Treatment

There have been major changes in the way anorexia nervosa has been managed over the last few decades but these changes have rarely followed scientific progress. This is in contrast to progress made in the development and evaluation of psychological treatments for bulimia nervosa (Fairburn *et al.*, 1991). Part of the difficulty is that the condition has an average duration of five years and treatment has to be prolonged. Also medical emergencies may interfere with any planned course of treatment.

In the past, treatment recommendations from all sources were remarkably similar and centred upon removing the patient from her family and home surroundings:

> 'The hypochondriacal delirium, then, cannot be advantageously encountered so long as the subjects remain in the midst of their own family and their habitual circle: the obstinate resistance that they offer, the sufferings of the stomach, which they enumerate with incessant lamentation, produce too vivid an emotion to admit of the physician acting with full liberty and obtaining the necessary moral ascendancy. It is therefore indispensable to change the habitation and the surrounding circumstances and to entrust the patients to the care of strangers' (Marcé, 1860).
> 'Recovery at home is rarely possible, but with removal to suitable surroundings, close supervision, and insistence on adequate food intake many of these cases may be restored to physical and mental health' (Ryle, 1936).

These authors indicate that recovery after such treatment was good. This is no longer the case. The relapse rate after discharge is high; up to a third fail to show any improvement at follow-up (Garfinkel & Garner, 1982).

Case registers from psychiatric and general medical clinics have shown admission rates for eating disorders for the United Kingdom, Denmark, Switzerland, the Netherlands and Czechoslovakia of approximately 5 per 100 000 inhabitants per year (e.g. Szmukler *et al.*, 1986; Nielson, 1990; Willi *et al.*, 1990; Hoek, 1991; Krch, 1991). If an adequate out-patient service is available the admission rate can be decreased to 1 per 100 000 total population per year.

Weight gain remains a critical component of treatment. In-patient care in a specialised unit leads to reliable weight gain but this is by no means the only way. Rather than forcibly separating the patient from the family, the family has been used as an ally in treatment (Russell *et al.*, 1987; Perednia *et al.*, 1989), particularly in the early stages of illness. Day patient treatment offers an interesting alternative and has been developed in Toronto and Edinburgh (Piran & Kaplan, 1990).

In 1983, Morgan and colleagues provocatively questioned the place of in-patient treatment:

> 'whilst admission to hospital might make the situation safe for a while, especially when weight is very low and there is a suicidal risk, it can also involve considerable disruption in the patient's management: it may represent a counterproductive retreat from confrontation with certain life difficulties and signify confirmation of the sick role in the eyes of relatives who then dissociate themselves from active participation in therapy. It is not always a major therapeutic step forward to admit a patient to a hospital ward, and our findings suggest that criteria for hospital admission in anorexia nervosa should always be scrutinised carefully.'

In the United Kingdom and the United States of America, consensus treatment recommendations have been made (Royal College of Psychiatrists, 1992; American Psychiatric Association, 1993). In these reports a graded approach to treatment has been advocated (see Table 7.8 and Royal College of Psychiatrists Report, 1992a).

It has been difficult to evaluate treatments in anorexia nervosa, as treatment requires time and emergencies may confound the planned interventions. Therefore the recent study at St George's Hospital is to be commended (Crisp et al., 1991). The design was ambitious: to compare out-patient with in-patient treatment. Patients were randomly allocated to one of four programmes: (I) admission to hospital; (II) combined individual and family therapy as an out-patient; (III) group therapy; or (IV) a control condition which consisted of one out-patient assessment. The methodological difficulties encountered and surmounted in this work have been discussed in an earlier paper (Gowers et al., 1988). The constraints of the design led to a need to be selective about which patients could be involved in the study. For example, the patients had to have a duration of illness of less than ten years, to live near the hospital and not have had prior treatment within the department. These conditions led to low recruitment (21/68, i.e. 31% in 1986; Gowers et al., 1988). This means that the results cannot, perhaps, be generalised to all patients.

The remarkable finding from this study was that in terms of global measurements of improvement on the Morgan & Russell scales there were no differences between groups. On individual subscales there were a few differences: for example, the nutritional outcome in the subset who had complied with their allocation to in-patient treatment was better than the 'no treatment' group. No other differences between the group allocated to in-patient treatment and the group given 'no treatment' were found. This replicates the findings from Bristol (Morgan et al., 1983) in which it was found that an early out-patient intervention was effective.

A major difficulty in interpreting the results from Crisp et al. (1991) was the poor adherence to treatment. Only 18/30 allocated to in-patient treatment accepted this option and all but six of those allocated to 'no treatment' sought treatment elsewhere (six in-patient treatment; five out-patient hospital treatment; three received regular support from general practitioners). Also a large number of those allocated to out-patient treatment 'dropped out' before their treatment was completed.

The results of this study are somewhat surprising given the huge differences in resources allocated to each treatment condition. A cynical interpretation would be that specialist treatment is unnecessary. The authors argue that all subjects were given a specialist's

Table 7.8. *A stepped care approach to anorexia nervosa*

Phase of illness	Treatment	Care provider
Excessive dieting	Education (nutritional, weight, clinical), weight monitoring	General practitioner, community psychiatric nurse, school counsellor, specialised voluntary organisations
Clinical anorexia nervosa	Specific psychotherapy (educational, behavioural, cognitive, problem solving)	General or child psychiatrist, clincial psychologist
Anorexia nervosa > 1 year duration	Specific out-patient psychotherapy (family or cognitive analytical)	Specialised eating disorder unit
Anorexia nervosa with life-threatening complications or treatment resistant to out-patient care	In-patient or day patient treatment	Specialised eating disorder unit

assessment and reformulation, which of itself may have a therapeutic impact. Also, because of the vagaries in compliance, all groups received treatment. Specialist treatment does appear to confer some benefits, as the mortality in patients referred to a specialised centre was significantly decreased when compared to an area with no specialist services (Crisp *et al.*, 1992).

Individual therapy

Hall & Crisp (1987) compared two brief (12 sessions) out-patient interventions with a sample of 30 patients. The psychotherapy condition delivered an unspecified blend of psychodynamic and family therapy: the dietary advice programme involved nutritional counselling. Modest gains occurred in both groups: the dietary group gained more weight and the psychotherapy group made greater strides with social and sexual adjustment. The majority had continuing therapy. Another small study compared behavioural, cognitive beavioural and standard out-patient treatment (Channon *et al.*, 1989). There were no differences between the groups and again the majority required continuing treatment after the six month intervention. Most of these have involved young patients with a short duration of illness, the group with the best prognosis.

The standard model of CBT (Cognitive Behavioural Therapy) needs modification for use with patients with anorexia nervosa. Forging a collaborative relationship with patients is difficult and the therapy may need to be prolonged. One pilot study has used cognitive analytical therapy, a model of treatment that combines cognitive techniques with some exploration of the past to identify how maladaptive schema (problem procedures) have developed. Fifteen patients were randomised to either cognitive analytical therapy or educational management. At one year there were no differences between the groups apart from self-evaluation of recovery, which was higher in the group given cognitive analytical treatment (Treasure *et al.*, 1995).

Family therapy

In the 1970s there were enthusiastic reports of the efficacy of family therapy in the treatment of anorexia nervosa. A randomised control trial, which compared family therapy with individual treatment, indicated that family therapy was more effective at preventing relapse following in-patient treatment in the subgroup whose illness had begun before the age of 18 and was of short duration (Russell *et al.*, 1987). Individual therapy was more effective than family therapy in older patients. These research findings thus support clinical pragmatism, in that it is helpful to involve the family of a young adolescent who lives at home. It remains unclear what specific components of family therapy are of value. A recent pilot study found that parental counselling combined with individual treatment was as effective and more acceptable than the more formal therapy approach (Le Grange *et al.*, 1992). A review by Hodes *et al.* (1991) details various forms of family therapy used in the management of anorexia nervosa.

It often comes as a surprise to many parents that they need to set firm limits over eating. Both parents are encouraged to work together as a team on this problem. If one parent takes sole responsibility for the illness a collusive relationship can develop. At times it may be necessary to refer one or both parents for counselling or support as caring for their daughter can be exhausting.

As in individual therapy, education is an important component of treatment. The family should be informed about the medical, psychological and social ramifications of anorexia nervosa. It is helpful to dispel the mistaken beliefs about aetiology, for example that it is caused by stubbornness and naughtiness on the part of the sufferer or that the behaviour of the family is causal. Such mistaken attitudes merely perpetuate guilt, recrimination and criticism and make treatment difficult. The parents are helped to find ways in which they can encourage their daughter to eat; this may entail direct supervision with firm limit setting. Parents are encouraged to take control over their daughter's health and welfare; this requires them to negotiate a consistent plan of management. Once this first phase is finished, with weight loss less of a critical issue, the next phase, which often centres about interpersonal issues within the family, begins. Finally, control over eating is handed back to the child and parents and child adjust to independence and separation.

Indications for admission

The proportion of patients treated as in-patients has gradually decreased over the last decade as more patients are treated as out-patients and as the proportion of patients with bulimia nervosa increases. In the majority of cases the main reason for admission is for refeeding and weight restoration. Another reason is for a diagnostic assessment. Medical or psychiatric co-morbidity such as diabetes, self-harm, depression, obsessional symptoms or severe purging behaviour may make an admission necessary. Finally, in-patient treatment is necessary if out-patient treatment has failed.

Table 7.9. *Clinical and psychiatric grounds for admission*

A. *Medical indications*
1. Body mass index below $13.5 \, \text{kg/m}^2$ (or a rapid rate of fall > 20% decrease in six months)
2. Syncope
3. Proximal myopathy
4. Hypoglycaemia
5. Electrolyte imbalance, e.g. $K^+ < 2.5$
6. Petechial rash and platelet suppression.

B. *Psychiatric indications*
1. Risk of suicide
2. Intolerable famly situation
3. Extreme social isolation
4. Failure of out-patient treatment

Emergency admissions

Immediate treatment is required if the patient's physical or mental state is dangerous or if there are contraindications to out-patient treatment. An outline of some of the physical complications that signal the need for urgent treatment and other clinical factors are given in Table 7.9.

A common approach in specialised in-patients units is for the nurses to take control of eating away from the patient at first. Food portions are gradually increased to obtain a steady rate of weight gain, with snacks and drinks between meals. The daily calorie content of meals starts at about 1000 calories and gradually increases to 3000 calories. Often the amount of choice offered to the patient is limited so that patients will not be able to maintain their restrictions on the amount of fat, protein and fibre needed to achieve the appropriate amount of calories.

Medical problems that can arise with refeeding

1. Acute gastric dilatation
2. Low phosphate
3. Refeeding oedema

Acute gastric dilation is a rare but a potentially lethal complication. It is the practice of many units to gradually build up the quantities of food prescribed to avoid this complication. It presents with vomiting, abdominal pain and distension. On examination, a succussion splash can be heard, other bowel sounds are absent. Risk factors include hypokalemia and a rapid increase in food intake. If recognised early it responds to nasogastric aspiration and intravenous feeding. It can, however, be complicated by stomach rupture, which has a high mortality.

Hypophosphataemia may become apparent upon refeeding when the increased metabolic demands for phosphate outstrip reserves. It has been called the nutritional recovery syndrome. It may be symptomless or delirium, status epilepticus, cardiac abnormalities and suppression of the haematological system and respiratory failure can occur. Risk factors include severity of emaciation, intravenous feeding and alcoholism.

Weight gain of 1 kg per day can mark the beginning of refeeding oedema. This is most common if purging and diuretics have been used. Measures such as avoidance of extra salt with meals and elevation of the limbs are usually sufficient and diuretics rarely, if ever, should be used.

If possible, intravenous fluid or salt replacement should be avoided. Alarmingly low potassium levels of 2.5 mMol per litre are frequently seen but gradual oral replacement is safest. If the parenteral route is used then regular monitoring of sodium, potassium, calcium, magnesium and phosphate levels are needed. The ECG may also need to be monitored as prolongation of the QT interval is common and increases the risk of a serious arrhythmia developing.

Difficulties in management

Occasionally a patient will lose insight into the dangerousness of her condition. The reasons for implementing involuntary treatment using the Mental Health Act are to (1) safeguard life and (2) improve mental state.

Physical treatment

Trials of various forms of psychoactive drugs have been undertaken: amitryptiline, chlorpromazine, sulpiride and pimozide have failed to show any beneficial effects. Cyroheptidine, an antiserotoninergic drug, was found to be marginally superior (Vigersky & Loriaux, 1977; Goldberg et al., 1979; Halmi et al., 1986).

Drugs may have some role in alleviating symptoms of anxiety and depression. The depressive symptoms that accompany anorexia nervosa unusually may not improve or may even worsen during weight gain. In such cases treatment with a tricyclic antidepressant may be helpful. An atypical subgroup who may benefit from antidepressants are middle-aged women who, in the course of a major depressive illness, lose a great deal of weight not simply from a depressive want of appetitive but because they develop typical anorexic attitudes of food avoidance and over-concern with weight. Merely administering an antidepressant often fails to remedy their depression and their weight loss. On the other hand, combining the antidepressant with a weight gain programme is most likely to restore such patients to their former health. Chlorpromazine has been used in small doses to reduce anxiety and guilt.

Overall, for restricting anorexia nervosa, the benefits of drug treatment are small and need to be balanced by the finding that a significant proportion of the mortality found in anorexia nervosa is a result of an overdose of antidepressant medication (Patton, 1988). It must be noted, however, that in modern clinical practice compliance with medication is usually poor, perhaps because this represents sacrificing control. Alternatively, the patient may discover from her own research that weight gain is a side-effect of such medications.

Outcome

Russell (1977) stated that anorexia nervosa is an illness that must run its course and has cycles of recovery and relapse and that a reliable expectation of outcome can only be

Table 7.10. *Prognostic factors for anorexia nervosa*

A. *Illness Related:*
1. Long duration resistant to treatment
2. Lower minimum weight
3. Age of onset (lower gives better outcome)

B. *Premorbid Adjustment:*
4. Personality difficulties
5. Poor relationship with family
6. Social difficulties

made after four years has elapsed. Even when the outcome is favourable, the illness usually lasts two to three years. Factors that affect the prognosis are shown in Table 7.10.

The course of anorexia nervosa is variable and can range from a mild transient episode to a severe, chronic and relapsing condition (Theander, 1970, 1985; Steinhausen *et al.*, 1991). Approximately 50% recover completely although the problem may last for three years or more. Twenty percent have residual minor problems. Up to a third of cases of anorexia nervosa follow a chronic course despite appropriate attempts at treatment. Such cases may require support over many years and may need interventions to ameliorate the psychological, social and physical consequences of their disorder.

Patients who require in-patient treatment have a poor prognosis and relapse is common. A recent five-year follow-up of 112 patients after their first admission to hospital with anorexia nervosa in New Zealand found that 43% were readmitted (McKenzie & Joyce, 1992). The cumulative length of stay in hospital was only exceeded by patients with schizophrenia and organic disorders. In recent years there has been an increase of readmission rates (Williams & King, 1987; Nielson, 1990) with anorexia nervosa, which suggests that the course of the illness has worsened.

The mortality rate for anorexia nervosa is approximately 0.5–1% per year of observation (Herzog *et al.*, 1992) with a standardised mortality rate six times of the normal population. The mortality rate was 15 times higher if weight had fallen below 35 kg (Patton, 1988). Suicide has been the commonest cause of death, followed by infection, gastrointestinal complications and emaciation.

B. BULIMIA NERVOSA

Introduction

It is rare for a new illness to be defined. Bulimia nervosa is one such case and yet it has not remained an esoteric, small-print subject but has spread rapidly amongst young women of the world.

Classification

Bulimia first entered classification systems in DSM-III (APA, 1980). The criteria were tightened, and the name changed to bulimia nervosa in DSM-IIIR (APA, 1987). The criteria have been further defined in DSM-IV and are very similar to those of ICD-10 (WHO, 1992a). (Table 7.11). Although initially bulimia nervosa was seen as a late manifestation of anorexia nervosa it is now recognised to also develop in the context of personality and psychological difficulties.

Bulimia nervosa is perhaps the best example of how pathoplastic factors have affected the form of psychiatric illness. In nineteenth-century Vienna, Freud discovered that sex was a source of much neurosis. Food has now replaced sex as the neurotic focus of much of our culture. Russell (1985) wrote about this phenomenon: 'The increased population of patients with eating disorders probably represents a population of vulnerable individuals who in earlier times would have developed different forms of neurotic illness – possibly hysteria or anxiety states'.

History

Bulimia nervosa was defined in 1979 by Gerald Russell although similar case reports had appeared earlier (Wulff, 1932; Binswanger, 1959). Russell defined bulimia nervosa as an ominous variant of anorexia nervosa. Gradually the clinical picture has changed so that the majority of cases of bulimia nervosa have not had a previous episode of anorexia nervosa. It took Russell six years to collect his 30 cases, yet today the condition is very common, indicating that the prevalence has increased rapidly over the last three decades. A recent proposal is to define an additional syndrome, commonly found in obesity, binge-eating disorder (Spitzer et al., 1993).

Epidemiology

The short history of bulimia nervosa means that there are little data on its incidence. Bulimia nervosa was only recognised in the World Health Organization International

211

Table 7.11. *Criteria for the classification of bulimia nervosa*

DSM-IV Bulimia Nervosa 307.51	ICD-10 Bulimia Nervosa (F50.1)	DSM-IV Binge Eating Disorder
Recurrent episodes of binge eating: (1) large, amount of food in 2 hours, (2) loss of control	Episodes of overeating	Recurrent episodes of binge eating: (1) large, (2) no control Binge eating associated with at least 3 of the following (a) rapid eating (b) uncomfortably full (c) eat without hunger (d) shameful, solitary eating (e) disgust, guilt, depression after overeating
Regular use of methods of weight control (a) vomiting (b) laxatives (c) diuretics (d) fasting/strict diet (e) vigorous exercise	Methods to counteract weight gain (a) vomiting (b) laxatives (c) fasting (d) appetite suppressants (e) metabolic stimulants (f) diuretics	Marked distress after binge eating
Minimum average of 2 binges a week in 3 months		Binge eating on average at least 2 days a week for 6 months
Self-evaluation is unduly influenced by body weight or shape	Morbid fear of fatness with a sharply defined weight threshold	
The disturbance does not occur exclusively during episodes of anorexia nervosa	Often a history of anorexia nervosa	Disturbance not exclusively present with anorexia nervosa or bulimia nervosa

Purging type: regularly use vomiting, laxatives, diuretics after binge eating
Non-purging type: no vomiting or laxative abuse

Table 7.12. *Incidence of bulimia nervosa per 100 000 population*

Study	$n \times 10^6$	Period	Source	Incidence
Hoek	0.15	1985–6	General practitioners	9.9

Table 7.13. *Prevalence of bulimia nervosa in young females*

Study	$n \times 10^3$	Age	Method	Prevalence
Rastam *et al.* (1989)	2	15	School nurse	0.14
Whitehouse *et al.* (1992)	0.5	–	Screen GP attendees	1.5
Bushnell *et al.* (1990)	1.5	18–44	Two-stage screen	1.0
Hoek (1991)		15–29	General practice	0.17

Classification of Diseases in 1992 and so has not had a separate code on case registers or hospital data in the United Kingdom. In the USA, the diagnostic systems have evolved from bulimia to bulimia nervosa over the last decade and thus the cases defined by epidemiological studies have also been in transition. Table 7.12 shows the incidence figures from registers within primary care. In Holland, the incidence in 1989 had increased to 11/100 000. Over half of the cases detected by these general practitioners were referred on for specialist psychiatric care. An excellent study on a community sample of twins found that the risk of bulimia nervosa has increased in cohorts of young women born after 1950 (Kendler *et al.*, 1991).

Several studies have investigated the prevalence of bulimia nervosa. Many of these have involved a two-stage screening approach that appears to be more successful than is the case for anorexia nervosa. The shame and disgust that many patients feel about their symptoms makes them less likely to confide in their general practitioners. It is not easy to make a spot diagnosis of bulimia nervosa as can be done with anorexia nervosa. The prevalence figures for bulimia nervosa from a variety of populations are shown in Table 7.13.

Very little work on the sociodemographics of bulimia nervosa has appeared. This is because many of the studies have been on selected populations. Males are rarely affected (4%) (Hoek, 1993). It appears to be a problem of urban rather than rural communities (Hoek, 1991). Bulimia nervosa is now common in Eastern Europe and in Japan. Certain ethnic minorities within the United Kingdom (Arab: Nasser, 1988 and Asian: Mumford & Whitehouse, 1988; Mumford *et al.*, 1991) appear to have rates of bulimia nervosa higher than the native population.

Aetiology

Any aetiological model of bulimia nervosa must explain:

(a) the rapid increase in incidence in cohorts born after 1950;
(b) the female preponderance;

(c) the clinical features;
   (i) inevitable weight loss preceding onset;
   (ii) higher premorbid BMI.

A sociocultural model of aetiology could account for these features.

A. Sociocultural factors

Dieting

Dieting is a major risk factor for bulimia nervosa. Several lines of evidence support this claim:

(a) The most powerful was the finding from a prospective study of London schoolgirls (Patton et al., 1990). Dieting increased the risk of developing eightfold bulimia nervosa.
(b) The fashion for thinness has developed in the last half of the twentieth century (Silverstein et al, 1986; Garner et al., 1980). This has fostered a booming dieting industry (Weightwatchers began in 1963 in the USA, 1967 in the UK; Slimmer's magazine launched in 1969). Such is the success of the slimming industry that it is now the norm to be 'on a diet'. This parallels the time course of bulimia nervosa.
(c) Bulimia nervosa is higher in populations where the prevalence of dieting is increased such as dancers (Hamilton et al., 1985).
(d) Binge eating is commonly seen in the context of dietary restraint (Herman & Mack, 1975), starvation and famine (Keys et al., 1950). It is a physiologically understandable mechanism in the control of nutritional homeostasis (Blundell & Hill, 1993).

However, although dieting is an important risk factor, other factors must account for individual susceptibility. One hypothesis put forward is that subjects with eating disorders may be more sensitive to media messages (Beumont et al., 1995) but this only begs the question, why?

B. Psychological Factors

Ruth Striegel-Moore (1993) has explored the question of 'why women' and 'why young women'. Two aspects of the contemporary sex-role stereotype may be important in increasing women's vulnerability to develop a bulimia nervosa: (1) women are expected to be, and are, more interpersonally orientated and are therefore more vulnerable to the opinions and behaviours of others and (2) beauty is a central component of femininity. These two factors interact and increase the value of cultural stereotypes of beauty. Again this is common to all women, so what are the factors that increase individual vulnerability?

In some, the family or school culture places undue emphasis on slimness, with mothers who diet or specialist ballet or drama schools. Others are insecure about their identity because of inadequate parenting or traumatic life events such as sexual abuse. The majority of patients with bulimia nervosa have experienced adverse events in childhood: parental separation, abuse or neglect (Schmidt et al., 1993a) and have suffered life events prior to onset (Schmidt et al., 1993b). Adverse developmental factors and poor parenting may lead to a poor sense of identity and low self-worth. Media role models may be used for self-definition. However, media images are carefully crafted fantasy and are full of inconsistencies or unrealistic expectations and almost prescribe bulimic behaviour. Super-women can somehow obtain bliss by eating large quantities of calorie laden ice-cream and yet remain thin.

Bingeing leads to positive immediate consequences, the hedonic effect of food and relief or distraction from distress, both emotional (stress, low self-image) and physiological (hunger). Negative consequences are delayed and are hence less effective in controlling behaviour. Five models have been developed to explain the psychology of binge eating: the addictions model, the conditioning model, the affect-regulation model, the escape model and the dieting model. None of them can explain all cases and so a catch-all biopsychosocial model has evolved (Polivy & Herman, 1985).

C. Heredity and biological factors

Differences in the concordance rates between identical and non-identical twins in bulimia nervosa have been found (Kendler *et al.*, 1991) and a genetic model can be sustained. However, the genetic risk of bulimia nervosa is less strong than that for anorexia nervosa and the results can be explained by environmental factors (Treasure & Holland, 1995).

It is possible that any genetic tendency towards bulimia nervosa is part of a non-specific liability to depression, alcoholism or impulsivity. Women with bulimia nervosa have a significantly (three- to fourfold) higher prevalence of affective disorder among their first degree relatives. An excess of alcoholism and substance abuse has also been found. Obesity is also increased in the families of bulimia nervosa (Treasure & Holland, 1995).

Clinical features

The median age of onset of bulimia nervosa is 18, slightly later than that of anorexia nervosa, female sufferers predominate, and all social classes are affected. Patients are usually of a normal body weight. Approximately a third have a history of anorexia nervosa and another third a history of obesity.

Preoccupation with weight and shape is the driving force behind the abnormal eating behaviours. Such is the strength of this overvalued idea that it can profoundly effect the quality of life. A history of weight loss preceding onset is typical and there is usually an attempt to follow a strict diet with protracted periods of fasting. The content of binges varies from an array of 'forbidden' palatable foods to foodstuffs that would be normally treated with disgust: leftovers, or food from the dustbin. The usual precipitants for binges are transgressions of self-imposed dietary rules or feelings of depression, anxiety, loneliness and boredom.

Binges are followed by some form of reparation. In the majority of cases this is self-induced vomiting, or abuse of laxatives and diuretics. Others fast for several days or have punitive exercise routines.

Medical assessment

At first glance the patient with bulimia nervosa may appear unremarkable. However, you may spot the characteristic dental signs, the teeth may appear small and smooth with the upper front teeth worn into an arch shape; alternatively the teeth may be deceptive even if they have been crowned. The side of the mouth may be cracked. The face may appear rounded due to swelling of the parotid gland. This is due to hypertrophy. Scars over the knuckles of the hand (Russell's sign) suggest that fingers have been used to induce vomiting. The hand may go into tetanic spasm when a tourniquet is applied to collect blood. There may be evidence of fluid and electrolyte imbalance with faintness or periorbital or ankle oedema.

Physical consequences of bulimia nervosa

Teeth

Vomiting leads to a progression of dental damage, starting with loss of enamel, smoothing surfaces and eroding cusps, leading to yellowing as dentine becomes exposed and eventually causing pulp necrosis and abscesses (Bishop et al., 1994).

Gastrointestinal System

Traumatic damage to the oesophagus and throat frequently occurs. Rarely, acute gastric distension occurs. Laxatives may produce melanosis coli, severe constipation and rectal prolapse. Gallstones also appear to be more common. Pancreatitis has been reported after binges but the most common cause for raised amylase levels is parotid hypertrophy.

Salt and Water Balance

Most of the purging techniques lead to loss of potassium both from the gut and via the kidneys. Potassium can fall to as low as 2.0 mM although this severity of depletion usually only occurs in the context of poor nutrition and anorexia nervosa. Bicarbonate levels rise because of loss of hydrogen ions from the stomach and kidney. Sodium levels fall with severe dehydration, in some cases as low as 120 mM. Although the level of these abnormalities is alarming it is important to remember that the deficit has arisen gradually and so rapid correction is rarely necessary and may be dangerous. Dehydration may be so severe that it leads to acute renal failure. Kidney stones appear to be common.

Cardiovascular System

Low blood pressure arises as a result of dehydration. Arrhythmias can occur.

Reproductive System

Abnormalities in the reproductive system are common and probably correlate with the degree of weight loss and so mirror those seen in anorexia nervosa. Approximately 60% have amenorrhoea or anovulatory cycles.

Measurement

The interviews and schedules in use for anorexia nervosa can also be used for bulimia nervosa. The Bulimia Investigatory Test, Edinburgh (BITE, Henderson & Freeman, 1987) is a self-report questionnaire that is widely used.

Differential diagnosis

As discussed in the historical section, binge eating can accompany a variety of medical conditions. A tendency to gluttony has been described in frontal lobe dementia (Erb *et al.*, 1987). Prader Willi syndrome is also associated with gross episodes of overeating, as is the Kleine–Levine syndrome.

Comorbidity

Additional psychiatric features are common. Depressive and anxiety symptoms predominate (Laessle *et al.*, 1987; Bushnell *et al.*, 1994) and drug and alcohol abuse (Russell, 1979) are common in patients with bulimia nervosa and may lead to treatment difficulties. These patients often have disorders of impulse control: self mutilation (10%), suicide attempts (30%), promiscuity (10%), shoplifting (20%). Alcohol abuse occurs in 10–15% and conversely up to a third of female alcoholics have a history of an eating disorder (Lacey & Moureli, 1986; Peveler & Fairburn, 1990). Patients often fulfil the criteria for 'borderline personality disorder', however, binge eating is one of the criteria for borderline personality disorder, so the argument is circular. Recent surveys using structured interviews have found that approximately 20% have abnormal personalities within the dramatic cluster; 13% of them so-called 'borderline personality disorder' (Yates *et al.*, 1989; Sunday *et al.*, 1993).

Assessment

Treatment should only take place after a comprehensive evaluation. Eating pathology and the methods of weight control used need to be fully assessed. A physical examination and a screen for electrolyte abnormalities is required if potentially damaging weight control measures are employed. The combination of vomiting and laxative abuse can lead to an unusual combination of low potassium and acidosis. The presence of any comorbidity should be established. Social difficulties and current life stresses should be sought as they may play a role in maintaining the illness. The formulation will often encompass trauma during childhood and persisting difficulties and stresses.

Patients with bulimia nervosa are initially less ambivalent about treatment than those with anorexia nervosa. However, when they later realise that treatment may entail a sacrifice of their control over weight and eating, the situation may reverse, leading to poor compliance. The initial assessment should focus on the patient's reasons for 'giving up bulimia', as when treatment is commenced these reasons can be used to encourage her to persevere.

Overview of treatment

There is little evidence of spontaneous remission of clinically relevant bulimia nervosa (Treasure *et al.*, 1994). Most authorities agree that out-patient treatments are most appropriate for sufferers of bulimia nervosa. Psychological treatment is the treatment of choice.

Psychoeducation is one of the cornerstones of treatment. Less severe cases may respond to this alone. Nutritional education was found to produce a better outcome than stress management (Fichter *et al.*, 1992). Olmsted and colleagues from Toronto (Davis *et al.*, 1990; Olmsted *et al.*, 1991) found that six sessions of psychoeducational seminars produced an abstinence rate of 20–30% (equivalent to the recovery seen by fluoxetine). Two self-treatment books for bulimia nervosa that provide information and use cognitive behavioural principles have been developed (Cooper, 1993; Schmidt & Treasure, 1993*b*). Twenty per cent of patients randomised to receive a self-treatment manual succeeded in controlling their symptoms (Treasure *et al.*, 1994) whereas the majority of patients in the waiting-list condition remain unchanged. A self-treatment manual can usefully supplement therapy and decrease the number of treatment sessions necessary.

Cognitive behavioural therapy was introduced for the treatment of bulimia nervosa by Fairburn (1981). It is now regarded as the 'gold standard' in view of its good performance when given either individually or in groups (Fairburn, 1985; Freeman *et al.*, 1988; Garner *et al.*, 1987 for an overview) but it is costly in therapist's time and training. The amount of therapy time has varied. At the top of the range is the 60 hours or more package from the group in Minnesota, spread over several evenings a week (Mitchell *et al.*, 1990). Standard cognitive behavioural treatment has been delivered in 16–20 sessions with twice weekly meetings initially.

Agras (1993) has reviewed the effectiveness of cognitive behavioural treatment (CBT). The overall level of abstinence found in the treatment studies completed to date is 40%. The dropout rate is 16%. Agras concludes that CBT is far from the ideal treatment for bulimia nervosa. However, alternative, 'manualized psychotherapies' had a dropout rate of 17% and an abstinence rate of 24%. But these results must not be dismissed prematurely, as Fairburn and his group (1993) found that the abstinence rates achieved by interpersonal therapy continued to accumulate in the year following treatment. At one year the abstinence rates following interpersonal therapy are equivalent to those of CBT and are superior to those of behavioural therapy, in which the results drop off after treatment has finished. Agras concluded that a sequential or combination model of the different types of therapies may be most appropriate.

Group approaches in general have been found to be less effective than individual therapy. A variety of formats have been used (educational/behavioural/psychodynamic: Lacey, 1983;

Table 7.14. *A tiered approach to treatment for bulimia nervosa*

	Cumulative % responders
Self-treatment, manual or self-help group	20
Individual therapy (CBT or IPT)	50
Combined therapy (Drug and BT/CAT/IPT)	75
Day-patient or in-patient treatment	80

cognitive behavioural: Freeman *et al.*, 1988; psychoeducational: Olmsted *et al.*, 1991). Although group treatment appears to offer a cost-effective way of administering treatment, the organisational problems involved in forming a cohesive group suitable for each member's needs can be formidable (Freeman *et al.*, 1991).

At the moment, our knowledge about which treatment suits which patient is incomplete. Tobin (1994) has suggested that a rigid focus on behavioural goals is ineffective in patients with personality difficulties. On the other hand, to practice in a psychodynamic manner and neglect the symptomatic behaviours may either convey the idea that the therapist lacks expertise or interest. Tobin suggests that the two approaches should be merged. Early intervention may prevent the symptom pattern becoming established. A stepped care approach to treatment in which additional elements are added as patients fail to respond or only show partial improvement is a rational development that can satisfy the service requirements (Garner *et al.*, 1986; Fairburn *et al.*, 1991).

An outline of the approach that developed at the Maudsley Hospital is shown in Table 7.14. It is important to develop an effective therapeutic relationship in which the patient is an active collaborator in her own treatment with responsibility for her actions. There is sometimes a tendency to try to please the therapist and to deny that symptoms are still present or to rebel and refuse to do homework, etc. The therapist should anticipate these two responses and explore their origin and meaning with the patient.

Patients who fail to respond to education alone will need a more complex therapeutic approach. Motivation difficulties and self-defeating attitudes or patterns of thinking may block change. It is beyond the scope of this chapter to do more than outline some of the basic components of cognitive behavioural treatment. The plan of treatment is outlined in Table 7.15. A basic outline of CBT is shown in Table 7.16 and examples of some of the common cognitive distortions seen in bulimia nervosa are shown in Table 7.17. Readers who are interested in further details should read the publications by Tiller *et al.*, 1993; and Freeman, 1995.

Medication

The combination of both pharmacotherapy and psychotherapy may improve the long-term outcome (Agras *et al.*, 1992, 1993). The choice is between a 5HT re-uptake inhibitor such as fluvoxamine or fluoxetine (Fluoxetine, Bulimia Nervosa Collaborative Study Group, 1992) or a tricyclic antidepressant such as imipramine. This decision may be

Table 7.15. *Schedule for cognitive behavioural treatment for bulimia nervosa (CBT)*

Stage 1	Assessment, education and motivation (1–6)
Stage 2	Cognitive and behavioural techniques (6–12)
Stage 3	Schema work (12–18)
Stage 4	Relapse prevention (18–20)

(Numbers in parenthesis indicate sessions.)

Table 7.16. *Content of cognitive behavioural treatment for bulimia nervosa*

Time limit	15–20 sessions over 3–4 months
Structure	(1) Agenda
	(2) Homework
Content	(1) Problem orientated
	(2) Scientific method
	(3) Not historical
Therapeutic relationship	(1) Collaboration
	(2) Open therapeutic process
	(3) Socratic questioning
	(4) Active and directive
Model	(1) Maladaptive learning

based on patient tolerance of side-effects. For example, fluoxetine may be of advantage in the overweight patient as it appears less likely to cause weight gain. Fluoxetine should probably be prescribed at a dosage of 60 mg/day while tricyclics should be prescribed at standard antidepressant dosages (e.g. 200–300 mg/day desipramine). The optimum duration of treatment is unknown but six months is generally regarded as appropriate (Walsh et al., 1991).

In view of the tendency for patients with bulimia nervosa to act impulsively, the potential risk of self-harm by overdosage needs to be borne in mind. Medication should not be prescribed for those patients who are unlikely to comply with follow-up or monitoring of side-effects or for those with a history of repeated overdoses. However, if medication is indicated for the treatment of depression, admission should be considered.

Patients who have severe symptoms and comorbidity may require brief periods of hospitalisation at time of crisis or for treatment of associated conditions, e.g. depression or alcohol abuse. Such admissions may serve as a break in the pathological eating pattern, but improvements are unlikely to generalise to the outside environment without additional treatment. Patients with severe electrolyte disturbance of physical illness may benefit from day-patient care prior to out-patient CBT to enable them to control their vomiting and to regularise their electrolyte imbalance.

Relapses should be expected and patients encouraged to view each one as a learning

Table 7.17. *Abnormal cognitions in bulimia nervosa*

Selective abstraction	The only way I can succeed is to control my weight
Dichotomous reasoning	If I eat any chocolate then I have failed and may as well eat three bars
Overgeneralisation	I was unhappy before I went on a diet. If I stop dieting I will be unhappy again
Magnification	If I eat a bar of chocolate I would be a glutton
Superstitious thinking	If I weigh 8 st I will be happy. My day is ruined if I weigh 8 st 1 lb
Personalisation	What will people think if they see me eating this?

experience. The relapse prevention model proposed for other addictive problems (Marlett & Gordon, 1985; Wanigaratne *et al.*, 1990, pp. 564–7) can be usefully applied in the context of eating disorders.

Outcome

In the clinical population the illness runs a relapsing and remitting course with a recovery rate of 40–70% after 2–5 years' illness (Fichter *et al.*, 1992). At ten year follow-up the figures are similar with just over half having fully recovered, approximately 10% continuing to suffer the full syndrome and the remaining 40% continuing to experience some symptoms (Collings & King, 1994). Cases of multi-impulsive bulimia have a poorer prognosis (Fichter *et al.*, 1994). Conflicting reports of the course of cases of bulimia nervosa within the community have been recorded; little improvement was found in one study (King, 1991), whereas approximately 40% improvement was found in other studies (Yager *et al.*, 1987; Patton et al., 1990).

The mortality from bulimia nervosa is probably lower than for anorexia nervosa but it is nine times that of a control population (Patton, 1988). Approximately 15% of cases of bulimia nervosa have significant medical complications (Hall *et al.*, 1989).

Prognostic factors

No clearcut prognostic indicators have emerged in investigations of the course of bulimia nervosa.
The following factors are associated with a poorer outcome.

1. Psychiatric comorbidity
2. Mixed anorexia and bulimia nervosa
3. Severe symptoms
4. Low social support

8

Drugs use and drug dependence

MICHAEL FARRELL and EMILY FINCH

Introduction

Drug dependence problems continue to grow and to make significant demands on a range of health and social services. The size and nature of the problem has changed dramatically in the UK and internationally since the last edition of this book. With the growth of the problem has come a growth of responses and a modest growth in knowledge. The criminal justice system, the public health sector and social services all have a role in their understanding and perspectives on the drug problem, although this chapter will concentrate on the aspects of the field impinging on the general and specialist addiction psychiatrist. The terminology on the subject continues to be refined, with a particular emphasis on the use of terms that aim to be objectively descriptive and do not contain a value judgement on the described behaviour.

Dependence and problems

The original description of clinical dependence concerned alcohol (Edwards & Gross, 1976) and has been applied to nicotine, benzodiazepines and other sedatives, opioids, stimulants and a wide class of psychoactive drugs. At the core of the concept is a strong desire or sense of compulsion to take the drug as manifested by drug-seeking behaviour that is difficult to control and is persisted with despite the adverse consequences resulting from this behaviour. Tolerance and withdrawal as consequences of drug exposure are not sufficient in themselves for a positive diagnosis of dependence. The distinction between physical and psychological dependence is difficult to make, can be conceptually confusing and has been abandoned in ICD-10, where the emphasis is placed on the characteristics of drug-seeking behaviour. Operational and diagnostic guidelines for the diagnosis of dependence have been outlined in ICD-10 and in DSM-IVR. The definition of drug dependence used in the 16th WHO Expert Committee report also incorporated the emphasis now placed on primary drug seeking (Edwards et al., 1981).

'A cluster of physiological, behavioural and cognitive phenomena of variable intensity, in which the use of a psychoactive drug (or drugs) takes on a high priority. The necessary descriptive characteristics are preoccupation with a desire to obtain and take the drug and persistent drug seeking behaviour. Determinants and the problematic consequences of drug taking may be biological, psychological or social and usually interact'.

The relationship between dependence and harmful or problematic use is complex yet there is an increasingly clear distinction between them. The World Health Organization Expert Committee on Drug Dependence at its 28th meeting in 1992 chose to use the term harmful use in preference to drug abuse. Harmful use is defined as a pattern of psychoactive drug use that causes damage to health either mental or physical. Such harmful use may impact on the user's family, community or society in general. ICD-10 specifically includes a diagnosis of drug-related harm. DMS-IV and ICD-10 adopt a multiaxial approach, making a distinction between consumption, dependence symptoms and adverse consequences.

Drummond (1990) has argued that dependence rather than consumption produces problems. Gossop *et al.* (1994) have described a relationship between severity of opiate and cocaine dependence, route of administration and risk-taking behaviour. Future work will use standardised measurement instruments to clarify the relationship between consumption, problems and dependence across a range of substances.

The measurement of dependence and withdrawal

In the UK the Severity of Opiate Dependence Questionnaire (SODQ) provides an operational measure of dependence in opiate users (Sutherland *et al.*, 1987). However, this instrument relies on a considerable number of withdrawal-related items and is specific to opiates. The Severity of Dependence scale (Gossop *et al.*, 1994) covers all types of drugs and in particular provides a useful measure of cocaine and amphetamine dependence. It contains five items covering a drug users' feelings of impaired control and preoccupation with their drug taking.

The measurement of withdrawal is best established for alcohol and opiates. The Short Opiate Withdrawal Scale (Gossop *et al.*, 1986) provides a brief scale that can be used clinically to monitor progress in the management of opiate withdrawal.

Harm reduction

Harm minimisation or harm reduction as a concept is not new (ACMD, 1984). In some countries harm reduction strategies are viewed as tacitly condoning drug use and of failing to emphasise adequately the need to reduce drug use. Harm reduction strategies define what practical interventions can be mobilised to reduce adverse health consequences of drug users' risk taking behaviour (Farrell & Strang, 1992) and prevent young drug users from acquiring life-threatening illness during a phase of drug use that may be transient. This involves a hierarchical approach, which firstly discourages people from taking drugs (Department of Health, 1991*a*). If they do take drugs, then it is suggested they avoid injecting; if they do inject it is suggested they use sterile injecting equipment and that they avoid sharing it with other drug users. If they do share then it is suggested that they clean the equipment.

Part of the HIV-prevention strategy has involved providing widespread advice and information on injecting risks and ensuring adequate access to sterile injecting equipment (Farrell & Strang, 1992). A network of needle and syringe exchange schemes has been developed across the UK. This has been extended to community pharmacies, as suppliers of sterile injecting equipment to drug users (Glanz *et al.*, 1989). There is now a body of international evidence that indicates that injecting drug users have significantly modified their behaviour in response to the risks posed by HIV (Stimson, 1995).

History

Like herbs and spices, drugs such as cannabis, nicotine, opiates and cocaine have been an international trading commodity for centuries. In the UK prior to the turn of the century there were no regulations controlling the supply and consumption of opiate and other dependence-inducing drugs (Berridge & Edwards, 1987). During the First World War the Defence of the Realm Act was invoked to restrict the supply of cocaine, as it was feared that this drug was impairing the war effort. The 'roaring twenties' in the US witnessed a substantial cocaine epidemic (Musto, 1987). In the UK in the 1920s the Rolleston Committee (1926), reported on the treatment of morphine and heroin addiction and stated that opiate addiction was a disease that was amenable to treatment. This medical perspective was significantly different to the approach taken in the US at the same time. There, the key control measures were criminal sanctions and control of supply, so many opiate addicts were incarcerated. (Musto, 1987).

The problem in the UK remained minimal up until the mid-1960s. Concerns began to arise about the prescribing practice of a small number of private practitioners (Strang & Gossop, 1994). The Brain Committee (1965) recommended the introduction of Drug Dependence Units (DDUs) and an addicts' notification index. The right to prescribe heroin and cocaine was restricted to specialist doctors but other opiate prescribing for the treatment of dependence by general practitioners was permitted. Approximately 3000 patients were taken on by these specialist DDUs and much of the treatment practices in the 1970s centred upon these DDUs (Mitcheson, 1994). In the late 1970s early 1980s a new heroin epidemic swept through the UK. The Advisory Council on the Misuse of Drugs (1982) recommended the establishment of community-based teams to work closely with generic and specialist services. A central funding initiative spearheaded the establishment of community-based teams in the mid-1980s (McGregor *et al.*, 1991). The advent of HIV and the risk of transmission of HIV through injecting drug use added extra impetus to the expansion of community drug services so that by the early 1990s there was over 300 community-based drug treatment and advice centres throughout the UK. During the late 1980s and early 1990s specific emphasis was put on the containment of the spread of HIV and the reduction of drug-related harm (ACMD, 1988, 1989, 1993). By the mid 1990s as the containment of HIV appeared to have been moderately successful (ACMD, 1993), concerns appeared to be shifting to law and order rather than health-related issues.

Epidemiology

The problem of drug misuse presents a specific challenge to epidemiology because of the illicit nature of the behaviour involved. Both direct and indirect information is now gathered in an attempt to develop a picture of the pattern of drug misuse in communities. In the US, Germany and Holland, national household surveys include questions on drug use. Such national data collections provide information on population trends in drug use over time and are particularly useful in providing a picture of patterns of cannabis, hallucinogen, stimulant and opiate use. The high school surveys in the United States have provided a picture of falling levels of illicit use among young people, yet other indicator data suggest that the size of the chronic heavy drug using population continues to grow. Because of the low prevalence of chronic heavy problematic drug use, population studies have difficulty assessing the size of this group. Other sources that have been helpful in estimating its size includes treatment service reporting systems such as the Home Office Addicts Notification Index (1994) and the Regional Drug Misuse Database (1994) in the UK, and the Drug Abuse Warning Network in the USA. Criminal justice data such as police arrest data, police and customs seizure date, are indicators of trends in drug using activity.

In an effort to take account of local variation, considerable effort has been made to provide a picture of the pattern of drug misuse within local communities (Hartnoll *et al.*, 1985). Methods used include:

(a) Multi-enumeration methods, which attempt to collate a range of data derived from hospitals, police, etc. From this local prevalence and incidence of various types of drug taking are estimated. This is used to develop indicator trends, which provide indirect estimates of the problem. There are several limitations, including problems of integrating conflicting information about trends from different indicators. The multi-enumeration method has been used in a number of places in the UK.
(b) Information-based field work using privileged access interviewing by interviewers who have access to the study population through their own lifestyle and behaviour. This has provided details on patterns and trends in drug use but lacks generalisability.
(c) Capture/recapture methods (Frischer *et al.*, 1992) have been used for estimating the size of animal populations in the wild and this method has been applied to the study of 'difficult to access' populations such as drug users. It is possible to develop denominators for the injector population and estimate the number of problem drug users in given populations.

Few national surveys have been conducted in the UK but recently the Wellcome Sexual Health and Lifestyle Survey (Johnson *et al.*, 1994) included questions on drugs, as did the British Crime Survey (1994) (Mott & Mirlees Black, 1995). The Health Education Authority have also conducted two large-scale school surveys (1992*a,b*).

While such surveys have limitations, there is a consistent finding that one-third of young adults have tried illegal drugs. According to the Health Education Authority survey (1992*b*), 25% of 16–19-year-olds have tried cannabis, 6% have tried LSD and 3% have tried ecstasy; 5% have tried amphetamines, 3% have sniffed solvents and less than 1% have tried heroin, cocaine or crack. The 1990s has seen substantial growth in the levels of cocaine use, and amphetamines have remained a substantial problem. The growth of the dance drug scene has resulted in increased levels of LSD and MDMA use. Ten years ago 1–2% of school children reported having ever tried LSD but it is now estimated that 5–6% have tried LSD or MDMA.

Available data suggest that less than 1% of the UK population have injected drugs and it is estimated that there are at least 150 000 injecting drug users in the UK (Johnson *et al.*, 1994). Over 20 000 treatment notifications were recorded to the Home Office in 1993 (Home Office, 1994).

Studies in older populations show a broadly similar picture to that in young adults, with high levels of ever having used cannabis but significantly smaller proportions involved in regular use; overall there is probably less than 1% prevalence of dependent illicit drug use (excluding cannabis). Problematic drug use may be concentrated in inner city localities and in severely economically deprived housing setting (Home Office, 1994).

The containment of HIV among the injecting drug user population in the 1980s and 1990s in the UK is a story of considerable success, by contrast to many of its European neighbours who have estimated average HIV seroprevalence among injecting drug users, ranging from 15% to 30%. The estimated HIV seroprevalence figure among injecting drug users for England excluding London was 1% and the figure for London was 6–10% (ACMD, 1993).

Studies of the prison population indicate that in most European prisons approximately one-third have a history of drug-dependence. In the UK, 11% of the male sentenced prison population and 25% of the sentenced female population have used drugs. (Maden *et al.*, 1991). It is estimated that this problem may be even larger among the remand population. This concentration of dependent and injecting drug users is associated with high levels of risk-taking injecting behaviour and presents a specific challenge for HIV prevention strategies (Farrell & Strang, 1992)

Overall the lack of good epidemiological data has been a serious obstacle to the analysis of trends and assessment of the success or failure of policies related to drug misuse. Epidemiological information at a national and a local level is needed to estimate the size of the population in need of prevention and treatment strategies. From survey data in the US it was estimated that 0.7% of the population were clearly in need of treatment (Gerstein & Harwood, 1990).

Aetiology

Drug misuse is a heterogenous behaviour. To identify aetiological processes there is a need to define clearly the field. This may include factors predisposing to the initial drug experimentation, factors influencing levels of consumption, factors influencing shifts in routes of ingestion, factors influencing development of dependence or factors influencing the development of harm related to drug consumption.

There is a need to clarify when drug use shifts from being a dimension or indicator of broader deviance into the arena of clinical concern, Jessor (1976) has reported high correlation between drug use, delinquency and precocious adult behaviour. Longitudinal study of these dimensions of behaviour as adolescents mature into adults indicates a high correlation between these different dimensions of behaviour. There is a reduction in deviance scores on all dimensions as adult relationships and working patterns are adopted.

There are over 40 distinct aetiological theories or models of drug misuse (Lettieri *et al.*, 1985). These include two major conceptual frameworks for attempting to understand the initiation and continuation of adolescent drug use. One is the model of underlying psychological disturbance, which holds the view that the individual consumes drugs to cope with intra- or interpersonal difficulties (Khantzian, 1985). The alternative model looks at the interaction between the individual and the environment and focuses on the functional role of drug-taking behaviour. This focuses on variables such as drug availability, environmental pressures to consume drugs, and sociocultural influences such as peer pressure. (Smart, 1980; Backman *et al.*, 1984). One of the most attractive models has been that of Jessor *et al.* (1991) whose problem behaviour theory sees drug use as a dimension of social deviance or social nonconformity, and argues that the behaviour has functional value within its social setting.

Animal studies have been important in understanding drug misuse, particularly in defining the individual properties of drugs and their abuse liabilities. Classical and operant models for explaining the reinforcing nature of drugs are now generally accepted (Wikler, 1965; Bandura, 1977*b*). Drug consumption is learnt behaviour. Most of the drugs that are misused can be readily self-administered by animals and studies generally report that 80% of experimental animals learn to self-administer intravenous cocaine or heroin (Deneau *et al.*, 1969; Yokel, 1987). The important implication of this type of study is that it suggests that pre-existing conditions such as psychopathology, etc. are not necessary for a drug to exert its control on behaviour and that continued exposure to the drug is adequate to motivate drug-taking behaviour.

Research on the biology of reinforcement, craving and tolerance or neuroadaptation continues to grow. A detailed neural mechanism underlying reward systems has been postulated for the psychostimulants and the depressants (Wise, 1987). This model outlines the neural mechanisms that govern reward and emphasises that drug dependence is an extreme form of motivational and appetitive behaviour. Animal studies now locate reward pathways within the mesolimbic system (Bozarth, 1991). The complex psychopharmacology of brain receptor mechanisms is adding rich scientific dimensions to the understanding of mechanisms of dependence (Edwards & Lader, 1992). The description of the range of opiate receptors, endogenous opioid agents and cannabinoid receptors has been a significant scientific advance but to date has had limited clinical or service application.

Natural history of drug use

There are differing opinions on whether to refer to the longitudinal pattern of drug use as a career or a natural history. The career description is preferred within a sociological approach that implies multiple routes and multiple options and is felt to be less deterministic, whereas the natural history model implies a pre-set course (Strang *et al.*, 1989). The actual difference between these two approaches may be more cosmetic than actual but, given the heterogenous nature of the behaviour, the description of pathways of behaviour and their longitudinal study have provided important insights into patterns of drug use (Kandel *et al.*, 1986; Newcomb & Bentler, 1988). The staging or sequencing of patterns of use may be divided into experimental, recreational and continual or compulsive. However, even at an early stage it is possible for an individual drug-taking episode to represent a high risk to the individual, as is the case with solvent-related mortality during experimental use.

Experimental drug use may now be a form of normal adolescent risk-taking behaviour (Hammersly *et al.*, 1990). The drug is taken occasionally in order to learn about its effects. The nature of the initial experience and peer group influences are likely to determine whether somebody moves from experimental to more regular use. The consumption of one drug increases the likelihood of consuming other drugs, so that those who consume tobacco are more likely to take cannabis and those who use cannabis are more likely to consume other illicit drugs (Kandel *et al.*, 1986) but this relationship is neither causative or predictable.

Regular, occasional or controlled drug use may mean that a drug is being used, for instance, every weekend and is not associated with any significant degree of dependence. Habitual use may or may not be associated with dependence. Daily use of alcohol in small quantities, while habitual and reinforcing, is not often associated with dependence. Daily use of tobacco is more likely to be associated with nicotine dependence with only a small number of people reporting controlled regular use of nicotine. Heroin and cocaine are similar to nicotine in their reinforcing properties and regular use is more likely to be associated with dependence. Dependence implies that there is a degree of neuroadaptation, which in the absence of drug consumption will result in receptor readaptation, which gives rise to a physical withdrawal in the case of opiates but not so with stimulants. Dependent drug use will be driven by the primary reward effect of drug consumption as well as by the desire to avoid or reduce adverse effects such as drug withdrawal.

The longitudinal study of patterns of drug use and its impact on other aspects of the life trajectory are difficult to conduct and sometimes hard to interpret. Despite this a number of key longitudinal studies from early adolescence into early adulthood (Newcomb & Bentler, 1988; Jessor *et al.*, 1991) suggest that the level of drug use is a predictor of future drug use and that initiation before 15 is associated with more developmental disruption. Jessor's work indicates that indices of a conformity such as church going and not smoking tobacco are highly correlated with not using drugs. The longitudinal study of the Jessor cohort indicates that growth into adult responsibilities or jobs, marriages, and children is a convergence towards social conformity, which is associated with less drug use and less problem drug use. This is postulated as the maturing out hypothesis by Winick (1962).

At the more problematic end of the spectrum, a 20-year follow-up of 100 heroin addicts in New York, found that 23% were dead, 35% were stable and abstinent and 25% have continued using opiates (Vaillant, 1973). In a recently completed twenty-two year follow-up study of London heroin addicts, 56% were off opiates, 21% were using and 10% were dead (Oppenheimer *et al.*, 1994; Stimson & Oppenheimer, 1982). Most long-term follow-up studies do seem to agree on a large excess death rate in heroin addicts over time – the Oppenheimer study reported that 34% of the original cohort of 128 addicts were dead at 22-year follow-up. The excess death rate was highest at the beginning of the study, and varied over time. The largest group of deaths in this study were caused by drug overdoses.

Other studies have looked at the complex influences on cessation of drug use and have studied untreated populations. The classic study of Robins (1993) studied the pattern of drug use among American soldiers prior to enlistment, in Vietnam, and on return home after the war. Despite high levels of opiate dependence in vietnam the majority stopped all opiate use on return. Robins has argued that her study demonstrates that the dangers of heroin are overstated but others have argued that the unique setting of this study makes it difficult to extrapolate conclusions into more day-to-day settings. Other studies, which have looked at the patterns of cessation of drug use without treatment (Biernacki, 1986; Brunswick *et al.*, 1990) indicate that stopping is associated with a complex set of changes in lifestyle. The large population-based studies of quitting smoking report that the majority of the population stop without assistance, those who try numerous times alone and fail then seek assistance. Those who then seek assistance are likely to double their chance of quitting but are also twice as likely to fail to stop as their counterparts who have stopped without assistance. Another long-term study of entrenched opiate addicts comments that eventual cessation of use is unlikely to occur if addicts are still using in their late thirties (Hser *et al.*, 1993). All studies agree on the very high mortality from drug use among long-term ongoing street heroin addicts.

Medical complications of drug misuse

Drug use, in particular injecting drug use, is associated with serious medical complications (Farrell, 1992). Such complications may present to Accident and Emergency Departments and general practitioners. The complications of drug misuse can be usefully divided into two groups – the acute and chronic complications of drug consumption, and the complications specifically related to the route of administrations such as injecting.

Drug complications

Overdoses may be accidental or deliberate. Opiate overdose is a medical emergency resulting in respiratory depression and requiring immediate resuscitation (Jaffe & Martin, 1990). Naloxone, a short-acting opiate antagonist, will in adequate doses reverse opiate-induced respiratory depression and precipitate opiate withdrawal. Any unconscious drug-user may be given naloxone to establish whether or not opiates are the cause of the unconsciousness. Barbiturate overdoses, which are more rarely seen, are associated also with respiratory depression and in this case the user will require artificial ventilation until the effects of the drugs have worn off. Cocaine overdose is characterised by epileptic seizures, cardiac arrhythmias, hyperpyrexia and, occasionally, sudden death (Cregler & Mark, 1986). Management of cocaine overdoses will require the monitoring of vital functions. Cocaine smugglers who conceal the drug in their body (so called body packers) die of acute cocaine toxicity when one of the concealed packets ruptures.

Withdrawal seizures are associated with alcohol, benzodiazepine and barbiturate use. Appropriate management of withdrawal usually prevents them, but if convulsions do occur they can constitute a life-threatening medical emergency requiring medication to control the seizures.

Hazards of injecting

Injecting drug use poses specific problems related to the levels of hygiene of injecting practice and also to the hazards of parenteral forms of drug administration (Farrell & Strang, 1992).

The transmission of viral and other contaminants through the use of communal injecting equipment continues to be one of the critical risk factors for the transmission of HIV, hepatitis B and C and others (Brettle *et al.*, 1990; Strang & Farrell, 1990). In the UK, specific targets have been set in the Government white paper *Health of the Nation* (Department of Health, 1991*a*) to reduce the levels of sharing of injecting equipment from 20% of injectors reporting sharing in the past month in 1990, to 5% by 1997.

Injecting also gives rise to site complications such as local cellulitis or abscesses. Infections that do not remain localised may result in systemic infections such as endocarditis, septicaemia, brain abscesses and osteomyelitis. Septicaemia needs appropriate antibiotic management. Infective endocarditis, classically affecting the tricuspid valve, can naturally occur in either heart chamber without an underlying valve abnormality. Endocarditis needs to be considered in any injecting drug-user with an unexplained pyrexia. Early identification of two-dimensional echocardiography and treatment targeted at the causative organism will result in a good recovery rate, though if injecting continues a high recurrence rate with a high mortality results (Robins & Michelson, 1988).

Long-term injectors experience problems finding a vein and may inject in deep veins, giving rise to thrombosis and pulmonary embolism. Secondary to long-term deep vein problems, a drug user may begin to suffer from varicose veins, varicose eczema and eventually varicose ulcers. These will all be complicated by continued injecting. Acute vascular events have been described recently following the injection of temazepam, either from extravasation of injected materials into the tissues or from accidental injection into an artery. This may result in compartment syndromes, which may require surgical intervention or occasionally the amputation of a limb (Barr, 1988).

Tuberculosis has become a problem among substance misusers and the homeless population and a major public health problem in many US and European populations of drug users. The screening and identification of TB is likely to become a significant task in the drug services of the late 1990s (ACMD, 1993).

Substance misuse and mental health issues

Mental health problems may cause or follow drug misuse. The nature of the relationship requires elucidation. Substance misuse problems are relatively common among general psychiatric populations and psychiatric problems are also common among people with substance-related problems. In both populations substance misuse is likely to aggravate functional impairment.

1. Psychiatric disorders secondary to drug use

Psychotic disorders

Up to 80% of regular cocaine users experience euphoria, impaired judgement, grandiosity, impulsiveness, increased sexual interest, compulsively repeated actions and marked psychomotor agitation. This state may be clinically indistinguishable from hypomania or mania but subsides within about thirty minutes (Strang *et al.*, 1993). With continued use of cocaine, the subject may experience hallucinations, both visual and auditory. Classically, but not diagnostically, tactile hallucinations, such as feeling insects under skin (formication), are felt. The user may also become paranoid, leading to panic and aggressive behaviour. Prolonged or high-dose use of cocaine may produce a full-blown toxic psychosis with persecutory delusions and hallucinations. In this state the user may lose insight and be violent. This mental state usually remits within 24 hours.

Amphetamines may produce similar toxic reactions, the psychosis may last longer than a cocaine-related psychosis but will usually resolve in a few days (Connell, 1958).

Management of stimulant psychoses may simply require reassurance. If the patient is agitated, oral diazepam (10–20 mg) may be useful. More severe cases of psychotic disturbances may need intramuscular haloperidol (10 mg). Diagnoses of stimulant-induced psychotic states can usually only be made retrospectively when results of a urine test confirm the use of drugs.

In the United States, acute psychological and physical illnesses resulting from cocaine use form 20% of all admissions to emergency treatment rooms (Cregler & Mark, 1986). Inner city acute psychiatric services in the UK are seeing more cocaine related acute psychotic reactions.

Psychiatric symptoms associated with cannabis use

Anxiety and panic attacks are common adverse reactions to cannabis consumption. Symptoms may include restlessness, depersonalisation, derealisation and paranoia. These usually respond to reassurance alone (Thomas, 1993).

High doses of cannabis can result in an acute toxic confusional state. The phenomenology of this reaction is indistinguishable from other toxic confusional states and is transient and self-limiting. There is substantial variation in the prevalence figures for acute psychotic reactions to cannabis. Variation in the strength and type of cannabis consumed may account for some of this.

Some acute psychotic reactions may occur in clear consciousness and be clinically indistinguishable from a schizophrenia-like psychosis. It is difficult to determine, however, whether such illnesses represent relapse in previously psychotic patients who are users, are precipitated in subjects who are vulnerable, or are psychiatric problems that are essentially toxic reactions to the ingestion of cannabis.

Cannabis may also contribute to a transient mood disturbance. This is usually depression and is mild and transient. There is no substantiated evidence that cannabis can produce more serious or prolonged mood disturbances.

There is some doubt as to whether cannabis can produce a long-term psychotic illness or indeed has any causal relationship to schizophrenia. Andreason studied 45 570 Swedish conscripts and followed them up over 15 years (Andreason *et al.*, 1987). They found an association between cannabis use and schizophrenia. Other studies have found that cannabis appears to enhance or magnify positive symptoms of schizophrenia in those with pre-existing disease. However, the case for a causal link between cannabis and schizophrenia is certainly not proven.

The term 'amotivational syndrome' has been used to describe a group of heavy cannabis users thought to show personality changes. Subsequent studies have not supported the existence of this syndrome but note that heavy cannabis consumers can be listless and apathetic.

2. Psychiatric comorbidity

There is a substantial literature on the types and prevalence of psychiatric disorders found in drug users. The psychiatric disorder found in the drug user may be related in various ways to their addictive behaviour (Meyer, 1986). Firstly psychiatric disorders may be a risk factor for addictive disorders. For example, antisocial personality disorder may predispose to developing dependence. There is also some evidence that some drug users with psychiatric symptoms may be using drugs to treat those symptoms – the 'self medication hypotheses' (Khantzian, 1985). Khantzian found that opiates were used by those with psychotic symptoms in order to control impulses and disorganised thinking and that cocaine was used by those who were depressed to control their dysphoric mood. Secondly, psychopathology may modify the drug user's course or career. Clients with antisocial personality disorder may do worse once they have become involved in substance misuse. A recent study in Australia, however, showed that in methadone maintenance, clients with symptoms of antisocial personality disorder complied with treatment just as well as control clients (Darke *et al.*, 1994). Depressive symptoms or syndromes may also modify the course and pattern of drug use, possibly by worsening prognosis. Lastly, substance abuse and other psychopathology may coexist in the same person coincidently. The risk of suicide or completed suicide after episodes of parasuicide are increased with a history of substance misuse.

Prevalence of psychiatric disorders

There have been many studies attempting to define the prevalence of psychiatric disorders in an opiate-dependent population. In 1985, Khantzian and Treece found that 93% of drug users had a DSM-III disorder, primarily depression and personality disorders. Prevalence estimates for current depression alone in opiate addicts have varied from 56% to 17% (Khantzian & Treece, 1985; Mirin *et al.*, 1988). Prevalence estimates of anti-social personality disorder have varied from 60.8% to 18% (Rounsaville *et al.*, 1982; Woody *et al.*, 1983; Darke *et al.*, 1994). If rates of any personality disorder are used, up to 91% of polydrug users have been found to have a mean of four DSM-IIIR axis 2 disorders (De Jong *et al.*, 1993). Prevalence estimates for anxiety and panic disorders also vary widely. A study of cocaine users found similarly high levels of psychopathology using the SADS-L: 55.7% had a current psychiatric diagnosis other than substance abuse and 73.5% a lifetime psychiatric diagnosis (Rounsaville *et al.*, 1991).

These estimates are of doubtful validity, because of the many methodological problems involved in obtaining appropriate samples to study and in diagnosing psychiatric illness in drug users. Firstly, studies use different diagnostic criteria. The studies described above attempt to diagnose psychiatric syndromes, mainly using RDC (research diagnostic criteria) and DSM-IIIR criteria and other studies have looked at psychiatric symptoms using instruments such as the GHQ (General Health Questionnaire, Goldberg & Williams, 1988) and the Beck Depression Inventory (Ross & Glaser, 1989; Darke *et al.*, 1992). Studies also include drug users in different stages of their addiction careers and there is some evidence that drug users' levels of depression (as measured by the Beck Depression Inventory) drop on starting methadone (Strain *et al.*, 1991; Finch *et al.*, 1995). This means that a treatment sample would be expected to have a much lower prevalence of depression. There are genuine difficulties with the symptoms of psychiatric disorder and their relation to drug use. The DSM definition of antisocial personality disorder includes criminal behaviour, which is almost invariably associated with any severe drug dependence. Drug use is often associated with sleep disorders and these are one of the DSM-IIIR criteria for depression. Symptoms of anxiety and panic may be due to drug withdrawal or intoxication and not a true psychiatric disorder.

The general psychiatric patient who uses drugs

Chronically ill psychiatric patients who use drugs are a difficult group to treat. There is evidence that some schizophrenic patients use drugs, especially cannabis, and this may influence the outcome of their illness (Mueser *et al.*, 1990; Turner & Tsuang, 1990; Mathers *et al.*, 1991). Cannabis may provide subjective relief from some of the negative symptoms of schizophrenia and stimulants may have a short-term effect on depressive symptoms. Opiate, cannabis or cocaine or alcohol abuse associated with coexisting major psychiatric illness may significantly impair social and personal function and increase rates of acute psychiatric hospitalisation.

Comorbidity and HIV risk behaviour

Over the last five years drug users have substantially modified their HIV risk behaviour. However, moderate levels of risk-taking behaviour persist and there is some evidence that comorbid psychiatric diagnoses may be associated with higher levels of risk-taking behaviour. Brooner and colleagues (1990) found that antisocial personality disorder was associated with HIV risk behaviour and similarly, Metzger found that high score on the BDI were associated with risk behaviour (Metzger *et al.*, 1991).

HIV-related illness

HIV-positive drug users and those who progress to AIDS may develop depressive illnesses and acute psychotic reactions. AIDS-related dementia requires substantial work to support an affected substance misusing patient. Issues of differential diagnosis will arise where heavy alcohol or heavy benzodiazepine use is implicated, since these may compromise cognitive functioning.

Treatment of drug users with comorbid psychiatric disorders

The drug-using patient with a psychiatric diagnosis may have a worse prognosis when treated for drug abuse problems though antisocial personality disorder may be an exception (see above). Studies looking at the treatment of depressive symptoms in drug users with antidepressants have failed to find conclusive evidence that they are useful (Kleber *et al.*, 1983). Antidepressants have, however, been found to help in depressive symptoms associated with cocaine withdrawal but may be less useful in decreasing cocaine use in patients on methadone (Gawin *et al.*, 1987; Arndt *et al.*, 1992; Kosten *et al.*, 1992).

Methadone itself may reduce depressive symptoms, although this may of course be associated with increased stability of lifestyle and reduction of psychosocial stresses. Woody *et al.* (1983) showed that psychotherapy was beneficial in drug users with evidence of depression.

Mental health professionals involvement in drug services

There are striking variations in the professional mix of staff delivering drug services across Europe. Medical, social and criminal justice models are applied with varying emphasis. A focus on behaviour change means that professionals whose skills are directed to that end should have an important role to play.

Over the last ten years there has been some question as to the role of the psychiatrist in the treatment of addictive disorders, as many treatments are essentially psychological and the medical care for HIV and HIV prevention has become the role of GPs and general physicians. Problem drug use spans a wide range of problems from the physical to the psychological; from the social to basic pharmacology. The psychiatrist as a behaviourally and scientifically trained clinician has a potentially major role in integrating the diverse range of issues that require addressing. Psychiatrists are also needed to assess and determine management strategies for addicts who are at a high risk from psychiatric problems and as drug use becomes more prevalent in the UK we will see more acute psychiatric disorders associated with drug use. The psychiatrist is needed to examine risk for continued HIV risk behaviour if it is found to be associated with psychiatric disorders. In the context of the specialist service, the psychiatrist in the UK is frequently the leader of a multi-disciplinary team and is responsible for service planning and organisation and with improving active liaison with GPs, general psychiatrists, general physicians and public health professionals.

Treatment

General treatment

This section will initially provide an overview of assessment and counselling strategies and will then look at aspects of treatment for specific drugs.

Advice and treatment for drug-related problems is generally conducted in a multidisciplinary setting. The task of assessment, goal setting and developing strategies in alliance with the patient to achieve these goals is the backbone of approaches to the treatment of addiction problems.

The purpose of treatment for drug users is to confer maximum health gain by addressing the health-related and social problems and by assisting in the reduction or elimination of drug use. Opportunities will be available to improve the physical, psychological and social well-being of the drug user before achieving a drug-free state. An intermediate goal, such as the cessation of injecting and sharing by encouraging a move from injectable to oral drug use, will confer significant health improvement, even though dependence on the drug may continue. A particular type of treatment may promote progression from one intermediate goal to another. Treatment interventions may confer substantial health gain without resolving the problem and the comparative value of a variety of interventions in achieving such gain needs ongoing evaluation (Gerstein & Harwood, 1990; Department of Health, 1996).

Assessment of the drug user

Drug users may present to services for various reasons in a variety of settings with differing needs. They may be asking for specific help with their drug problems, or they may present with a physical problem and their needs as a drug user have then to be taken into account. Whatever the setting, it is important that the drug user is appropriately assessed and their needs defined (Farrell *et al.*, 1996). The range of patients under consideration includes the dependent drug user, the injecting drug user, the intoxicated user, the experimental drug user, or the recently abstinent drug user.

The assessor should ascertain the type of drug/s used, the quantity, the frequency and the route/s. He should assess the evidence of tolerance, dependence, or withdrawal and ask specifically about alcohol and benzodiazepine use. The history must also contain some information about the patient's knowledge of HIV, whether needles have been shared and if so, with whom. For instance, many clients will share needles with a sexual partner only and not consider that this constitutes sharing behaviour. Sources of sterile needles and syringes and knowledge of cleaning methods should be clarified. Injecting site and physical problems as a result of injecting should be specified. The assessor should establish whether sexual activity is safe or unsafe, whether the patient is engaging in prostitution and, for a woman, whether she is pregnant. Past medical and past psychiatric history may be important and in many cases a forensic history may be relevant, for instance a patient may typically present for treatment when he or she has a court case pending. A full drug and personal history should be used to help the patient audit the impact of drugs on their life to date. It is important to attempt to gather information from other independent sources, for instance family, friends and other professionals involved, to corroborate the patient's self-report.

Physical examination is an essential part of the assessment of the drug user. This should include examination for vein puncture marks in the arms, groin, legs or ankles. There may be evidence of previous abscess scars and pigmentation over areas of habitual injection. The pupils may be markedly constricted or dilated. The patient's behaviour may also suggest drug use, he or she may be unaccountably drowsy, elated or restless or obviously suffering from intoxication or withdrawal symptoms. Examining for evidence of physical morbidity is also important; a consultation may be a chance to check for concurrent hepatitis B or C and offer HIV counselling and testing.

Laboratory analysis

A full drug-screen urine sample taken at the first consultation can be a good source of information when there is suspected drug-induced psychosis or when prescribing of substitute medication is being considered. Analysis usually involves thin-layer chromatography and either gas chromatography or EMIT (Enzyme Multiplied Immunoassay Technique) techniques. Positive results may be difficult to interpret without detailed knowledge, for instance there may be a positive response to cannabis for many days or weeks after one substantial intake, whereas cocaine may only give a positive result for 24 hours after use. Heroin is detected by the presence of morphine in the urine, but other opiates may also give morphine-positive results. Other laboratory techniques for the detection of drug use are available. There has been interest recently in hair analysis, which although still in the research stage does seem to provide good information about drug use over the longer term (Strang *et al.*, 1989).

Therapeutic assessment

Drop-out rates are high in drug treatment, so the initial interview is important. The manner in which the initial interview is conducted may have a profound influence on the options that the drug taker considers and on the course he or she subsequently follows. The initial interview should be treated as if it were the only interview (and indeed, it may be).

Miller (1983) first described the style of interviewing that attempts to capitalise on early opportunities. This technique, called motivational interviewing, requires the therapist to influence the personal decisions being taken by the client. The therapist has a covert goal – to generate a critical dissonance in the drinker or drug taker so that they become willing to consider alternatives to their continued alcohol or drug use. Miller describes this as a complete therapeutic process but the approach can be included within a total package of treatment. Prochaska & DiClemente (1983) have constructed three categories of change: the precontemplator, who may have thought at some stage about modifying his or her behaviour; the contemplator, who is ruminating on change but has yet to act; and the person in the action phase who is actively changing. The contemplation and action phase are driven by resolution formation, which can be actively shaped during the assessment and treatment phase.

Relapse prevention

Relapse prevention is a cognitive behavioural approach specifically designed to enhance the individual's capacity to maintain his or her chosen changed behaviour (Marlett & Gordon, 1985). The drug user is taught to identify particularly high risk situations and break down the process of relapse into various stages. He or she is then taught to develop specific coping skills both for preventing further episodes of drug use and also for reducing the catastrophic nature of relapses when they do occur. It is argued that over-investment in absolute abstinence may itself contribute to the catastrophic nature of relapse when it occurs. Specific treatment approaches include the teaching of skills and awareness by re-enacting past relapse situations, role playing and then *in vivo* visits to high risk situations themselves, initially accompanied and then subsequently alone. Episodes of drug use are viewed not as evidence of failure but as opportunities for learning about personal vulnerabilities for which existing skills must be enhanced.

Behaviour therapy

Behavioural approaches have been used in the alcohol field and there have been some attempts to apply the same principles to drug users. Individual signals or cues for drug use are identified and followed by systematic exposure of drug users to these cues (while the user is abstinent) while assisting the drug user in avoiding a response (drug use) (Childress *et al.*, 1986). The cues may be a variety of things. They may be internal feelings, such as anxiety or depression, or they may be external events, such as the sight of the drug or apparatus or meeting a group of other drug users. The work is initially carried out in a laboratory with the presentation of a stimulus without the response allowed until there is an eroding of the strength of the cue–response relationship. The work then moves from the laboratory to the world outside and the responses become real ones. There is evidence of powerful conditioned responses in heroin users and the relationship can be broken in a laboratory setting. However, there is some doubt as to whether this can be generalised to a clinical setting and be a clinically useful way of working with drug users (Dawe *et al.*, 1993).

Family work

The recruitment of families into the treatment process may be difficult though, if accomplished, family therapy is useful in helping a family deal with a member using drugs (Stanton & Todd, 1982). Using a systems-based approach, work with the family starts by agreeing its treatment aims. A contract of treatment is then drawn up, which includes basic rules on who will attend. Emphasis is placed on regular drug-free attendance. The therapist will aim to help the family to change rather than directing the family. This is done by reframing feelings such as self-blame as concern and helping to change the balance of power in the family. A family group will also allow the ventilation of feelings and reduce feelings of isolation and help a family understand how they may inadvertently facilitate drug use. Relapse may occur during family therapy although the crisis can be used as a learning experience for the whole family and they may be able to examine interactions that may have precipitated the relapse.

Family support is also available through family support organisation such as Families Anonymous and ADFAM.

Psychotherapy

Most individual work with drug users concentrates on achieving a drug-free state. As described above, this tends to use behavioural approaches such as relapse prevention and other techniques that are very focused. However, in some cases drug users may require more specific psychotherapy, such as cognitive therapy for depression or behaviour therapy for a specific anxiety state. Woody *et al.* (1983) has argued that the drug dependent population with associated psychiatric morbidity may benefit from adjunctive non-specific psychotherapy. Dynamic or insight-orientated psychotherapy is usually only useful when the addict is drug-free, has a stable lifestyle and is aiming for further consolidation of his or her drug-free state. This may be a useful way for drug users to deal with early trauma in their lives. Aspects of dynamic therapies are frequently incorporated into approaches to group therapy with drug users (Falkowski, 1991) and into broader approaches within residential therapeutic communities.

Narcotics Anonymous and Twelve Steps programmes

The growth of the self-help movement such as AA (Alcoholics Anonymous) and NA (Narcotics Anonymous) has been remarkable in the past two decades (Wells, 1987). The approach of NA has all developed from the original Alcoholics Anonymous groups. The Twelve Steps refer to the stages of growth through which the individual must progress in order to maintain sobriety. The philosophy of AA or NA is that there is no cure for addiction. The emphasis on chronicity tends to cause confusion but it may more usefully be seen as part of a practical strategy for ensuring continued vigilance rather than a statement with scientific origins. Narcotics Anonymous was started in San Francisco in 1953 and has slowly grown to become a large international movement with substantial growth in Europe during the 1980s. There are now a number of offshoots of NA including Cocaine Anonymous (CA) and Methadone Anonymous for those users of methadone treatment programmes who wish to refrain from other illicit of licit drug use.

Initially people are encouraged to attend NA meetings regularly. These begin as open meetings and they provide a setting for mutual support and self-help. Participants give their life story and the group then gives comments and suggestions and adds many of their own experiences. Several cities in the UK now have a wide network of meetings that take place on a daily basis, so it is possible for an addict in recovery to attend at least one meeting a day.

Residential rehabilitation programmes

There is now an international network of therapeutic communities, the majority run by the non-statutory or voluntary sector agencies (Rosenthal, 1991). They generally use self-help approaches within a drug free environment and the residents play a major role in the day-to-day running of the house. Progress is usually structured, with goals that the residents attempt to attain during their stay. The therapeutic sessions are often confrontational and feedback is provided on behaviour, often by other residents. The first therapeutic communities for drug users were set up in the late 1960s, based on successful projects in the

238

USA. The most famous of these is Phoenix House (De Leon *et al.*, 1973) and they are usually termed 'Concept Houses'. The resident stays 9–18 months in the main house or in an after-care hostel and treatment consists of progression through a structured hierarchical programme in which privileges and responsibilities increase as the resident becomes more senior. Despite the encouragement to stay 9–18 months, only a minority of residents actually stay this length of time.

A number of therapeutic communities in the UK are run on Christian lines and there is usually a gentler and more supportive environment, aligned for gradual recovery. Some of these houses regard Christian faith as an essential component to recovery and others do not. This gentle programme approach may be suitable to the most vulnerable drug users.

A network of Twelve Step residential programmes have been established internationally (Cook, 1988). These work to a much shorter time scale: about 2–3 months with an option of follow-up care.

A small number of half-way houses have been established in the community, in which there is an explicit attempt to involve the drug users in the community during rehabilitation. The recovering addict makes close links with the community and often contributes to good works and support.

Treatment evaluation

A substantial literature now exists on the evaluation of drug treatment (Gerstein & Harwood, 1990). The rigorous evaluation of interventions requires a good baseline knowledge of the natural history and the spontaneous patterns of cessation of drug use; to demonstrate efficacy there is a need to demonstrate that treatment interventions promote levels of behaviour change greater than those occurring spontaneously. The multi-modal nature of treatment and the process of client selection limits the comparability of treatment approaches. Reasonable evidence for effectiveness exists for methadone maintenance, residential therapeutic communities, out-patient treatment and Minnesota-method treatment. Much of the evidence for discussion is drawn from two longitudinal American studies: the DARP (Drug Abuse Reporting System) – a 12-year follow-up of a 1970s treatment cohort, and the TOPS (Treatment Outcome Prospective Study) – a five-year follow-up of a large national treatment sample. A large-scale prospective treatment outcome study (NTORS) looking at the outcome of over 1100 patients is presently underway in the UK (Gossop *et al.*, 1996). Other randomised and controlled trials have been conducted on methadone maintenance. The most extensive evidence supports the benefits of methadone maintenance yet there is a suggestive level of evidence in support of therapeutic communities and out-patient treatment. It is also clear that a particular treatment modality may vary substantially in how well it actually works in practice (Ball & Ross, 1991) and factors influencing this type of treatment variation need to be taken into consideration when planning services.

Specific drugs and related treatments

Opiates

Opiates (Jaffe & Martin, 1990) may be derived from the opium poppy or made synthetically. The extract from the poppy is opium, and is a milky juice oozing from the poppy seed pods. Once it has dried it is scraped off and left to dry further, during which time it darkens and hardens. It is then processed, first to yield opium paste and later boiled with acetic anhydride to produce diamorphone. The heroin is then further refined by adding caffeine or strychnine. This product is then used by drug users as illicit heroin.

The action of opiates ranges across a spectrum from pure agonist to pure antagonist activity. The analgesic property of opiates is the key action and is primarily effected at the mu, kappa and delta receptor sites (Jaffe & Martin, 1990). The dominant receptor site appears to be the mu site, which produces analgesia, drowsiness, respiratory depression, pupillary constriction, bowel motility, feelings of well-being (euphoria) and, during initial exposure, nausea and vomiting.

Heroin, a short-acting opiate agonist, is the drug used most commonly by illicit drug-users presenting to services in the UK. Drug-users will also use many other different opiates, usually in the context of poly-drug use. Other opiates such as dihydrocodeine and the partial opiate agonist buprenorphine have been commonly used. Methadone is a long-acting opiate agonist used as an opiate substitute during the treatment of drug users, is also used illegally and supplies are almost certainly obtained by diversion from treatment sources.

Heroin can be injected, smoked or 'chased' (vapour inhaled from heroin sublimated by a direct heat source on silver foil) but many other pharmaceutical opiates are either swallowed in tablet form or crushed and injected. Over the past decade the dominant route of initiation into heroin use appears to have shifted from injecting to smoking (Griffiths *et al.*, 1994). The main effect of heroin and other opiates is euphoria, especially when injected intravenously. Users report a brief and intense rush within a few seconds after taking the drug. Over the next few hours they report feelings of well-being and relaxation. With repeated use a tolerance develops to many of the effects of heroin, especially to the euphoric effects. Tolerance to constipation and miosis may be less.

The physical withdrawal syndrome is similar across all opiates but the time course and intensity is influenced by the opiate used. With heroin the withdrawal syndrome starts after six to eight hours and reaches a peak between 36 and 48 hours. The methadone withdrawal syndrome is much longer, starting up to about 36 hours after the last dose, reaching a lower peak and finishing after one to two weeks. The symptoms tend to be abdominal cramps, nausea, diarrhoea, piloerction (gooseflesh – hence 'cold turkey'), sweating, sleeplessness, irritability, rhinorrhoea, excessive lacrimation and uncontrollable yawning. In the long-term addict a subtle protracted disturbance of mood and sleep may persist for several months after acute withdrawal symptoms have disappeared.

Prescribing for opiate users

Prescribing long-acting mu opioid agonists such as oral methadone should be considered in one of four contexts (Department of Health, 1991*a*).

Table 8.1. *Commonly abused opiates and their methadone equivalents*

Drug	Dose	Methadone equivalent
Street heroin	$\frac{1}{4}$ g	20 mg (only an estimate as street purity varies substantially)
Pharmaceutical heroin	10 mg tablet or ampoule	10 mg
	30 mg ampoule	50 mg
Methadone	(1 mg in 1 ml) 10 ml	10 mg
	(2 mg in 5 ml) 10 ml	4 mg
	(10 mg in 1 ml) 10 ml	100 mg
	(formulations may vary)	
Morphine	10 mg ampoule	10 mg
Morphine sulphate (MST)	10 mg tablet	3.25 mg
Dipipanone (Diconal)	10 mg tablet	4 mg
Dihydrocodeine (DF118)	30 mg	3 mg
Dextromoramide (Palfium)	5 mg tablet	5–10 mg
	10 mg tablet	10–20 mg
Pethidine	50 mg tablet	5 mg
	50 mg ampoule	5 mg
Buprenorphine (Temgesic)	200 microgram tablet	5 mg
	300 microgram ampoule	8 mg
Pentazocine (Fortral)	50 mg capsule	4 mg
	25 mg tablet	2 mg
Codeine linctus 100 ml	300 mg codeine phosphate	10 mg
Codeine phosphate	15 mg tablet	1 mg
	30 mg tablet	2 mg
	60 mg tablet	3 mg
Gee's linctus 100 ml	16 mg anhydrous morphine	10 mg
J. Collis Brown 100 ml	10 mg extract of opium	10 mg

Source: Department of Health (1991*a*) *Drug Misuse and Dependence. Guidelines on Clinical Management*. London. HMSO.

1. Rapid detoxification over the course of one or two weeks. Such detoxification approaches in the in-patient setting (Gossop *et al.*, 1989) may achieve up to an 80% completion rate. Subsequent support and rehabilitation facilities will influence the number who remain drug-free.
2. Gradual out-patient withdrawal over several weeks or months. This is the commonly employed approach in an out-patient drug treatment service. Completion rates for detoxification with this modality are in the range of 15–20% (Dawe *et al.*, 1991).
3. Maintenance, in which the goal is stabilisation of opiate intake on prescribed oral methadone so as to promote and encourage a stable lifestyle away from the illicit drug scene. The bulk of the evidence of the benefits of methadone maintenance derive from controlled trials and outcome studies of structured oral methadone maintenance programmes (Ward *et al.*, 1992).

Methadone is usually prescribed in a form of methadone linctus, 1 mg in 1 ml, and the dose is taken once daily. In prescribed doses it does not give an opiate 'high'. Table 8.1 gives approximate conversion factors for other types of opiates but these are very rough conversion guides and if there is any doubt, a low dose of methadone should be given initially, which should be increased until signs of withdrawal are abolished. In the UK doses vary, from about 40–100 mg daily. Recent research has suggested that higher doses (60–120 mg) of methadone are associated with better outcome in treatment (Capelhorn *et al.*, 1993). A range of programme factors such as clinical leadership, programme organisation and staff skill significantly influence the overall efficacy of methadone treatment programmes (Ball & Ross, 1991). Maintenance may be short-term or indefinite and varies across treatment programmes.

Globally there is virtually no injectable prescribing for the treatment of drug dependence except in the UK, where a significant minority of long-term opiate addicts in treatment are prescribed injectable methadone or heroin. There are also two pilot projects in Holland and Switzerland. There has been one study comparing injectable heroin to oral methadone (Hartnoll *et al.*, 1983). This study found little difference between the two approaches. There is no evidence that injectable methadone offers added benefit over oral methadone and it is certainly associated with the complications of injecting (Strang *et al.*, 1994). However, in very few cases it may be impossible to achieve stabilisation without using injectable methadone, but its prescription is best undertaken by specialists with experience in the field. There has been some interest in the use of opiates other than as substitutes for opiate users. A wider range of substitute prescribing options exists, ranging from short-acting agents such as heroin (diamorphine hydrochloride) to buprenorphine (Farrell *et al.*, 1994), through to the long-acting methadone analogue LAAM (levo alpha acetyl methadol). There is considerable current interest in developing a varied range of drugs for substitute prescribing.

In the UK, any doctor can prescribe methadone for the treatment of addiction. In order to prescribe heroin, dipipanone, cocaine and some other drugs for the purpose of treatment of addiction a special licence has to be obtained from the Home Office. In the community, most methadone is prescribed to be picked up daily from a local pharmacist. These prescriptions are written on a pink FP10 if from a hospital or a blue FP10 from a GP and allow for instalment prescribing, which enables the pharmacist to dispense daily from a single prescription.

There is also interest in non-opiate alternatives to treat withdrawal in opiate users (Farrell, 1994). The α adrenergic agonist clonidine and newer drugs such as lofexidine seem to be effective in suppressing the autonomic features of the opiate withdrawal syndrome, although postural hypotension may result. Clonidine, therefore, should be used mainly on an in-patient basis for withdrawal. Doses typically start at between 0.2 and 0.4 mg daily and increase incrementally up to a maximum of 2 mg daily, depending on the development of postural hypotension.

Specific opiate antagonists exist and they can be used in several ways. Naltrexone can be taken by mouth and has a duration of action of 48–72 hours (Gonzalez & Brogden, 1988). Naltrexone opiate receptor blockade will block any positive subjective effect from opiate use. Total blockade lasts 36–48 hours and gradually wears off. Naltrexone simply blocks the positive effect and has a few adverse side-effects. Studies have used naltrexone to compress the opiate withdrawal period with the addition of clonidine to ameliorate some of the autonomic withdrawal effects. This has usually been done on an in-patient basis and has not been systematically evaluated. Finally, naloxone a shorter-acting antagonist can be used to treat opiate overdoses.

Stimulants

Amphetamine is still the most widely consumed stimulant drug in the UK and results in a larger number of arrests than heroin in the UK. After cannabis it is the most commonly used illicit drug. It is taken orally, snorted or injected intravenously and is usually taken either as illegally manufactured amphetamine sulphate or pharmaceutical dexamphetamine. 'Ice', a smokable methyl-amphetamine, is very occasionally seen in the UK. The recent dance drug scene in the UK finds amphetamines being used to sustain stamina for all-night dancing and makes it likely that its commonest style of use is intermittently at weekends.

The US experienced a major cocaine epidemic in the 1980s but in the UK cocaine was snorted or injected by a more limited range of drug users. In the mid-1980s there was an increase of cocaine smoking in the form of freebase cocaine (cocaine heated with bicarbonate and known as crack) (Gossop *et al.*, 1994). Subsequently there has been an increase in the use of crack-cocaine in the UK. Cocaine smoking now seems to be the main route of initiation and is associated with an increased severity of dependence and increased problems compared with intranasal use (Gossop *et al.*, 1995).

Cocaine taken intravenously results in euphoria, followed by a period of alertness and increased energy. If the cocaine is snorted the effect takes 20/30 minutes to start. Freebase cocaine, which is usually taken by inhalation of the vaporised drug, results in a fast euphoria, similar to intravenous injection.

The pattern of cocaine use varies substantially from occasional use to compulsive binges, lasting three to four days at a time. Stimulant use may be accompanied by use of a depressant drug such as an opiate or benzodiazepine to regulate the degree of activation resulting from the stimulant drug. During those binges cocaine may be taken as often as every ten to 20 minutes. Frequent cocaine injecting is associated with high levels of risk-taking behaviour.

Dependence on cocaine is seen, but may not necessarily be associated with daily use. Abstinence is followed by a 'crash period', which is a complex mixture of withdrawal symptoms and post-binge hangover. During the crash the user is characteristically sleepy, tired, anxious and agitated. This phase is followed by a purer withdrawal state with significant depressive symptoms, with low energy and social withdrawal. This may be accompanied by marked cravings for cocaine, at their most intense at the end of the first drug-free week.

The management of stimulant users

Cocaine and amphetamine detoxification is associated with considerable sleep disturbance, mood lability and sometimes suicidal ideation in the first two weeks of withdrawal. Both amphetamine and cocaine users can withdraw safely as out-patients by stopping using the drug and receiving appropriate psychological support. However, cocaine withdrawal can be very uncomfortable and psychologically difficult to tolerate and there has been substantial interest in the development of drugs that will treat the effects of the immediate post drug 'crash' phase. Tricyclic antidepressants have been evaluated, but after an initial enthusiasm now appear to have a limited role. Other drugs include bromocriptine and lithium, although the results of these have been even more doubtful (Strang *et al.*, 1993*a*). The key interventions remain that of psychological support and strategies to enhance motivation and develop alternative coping strategies.

There has been some interest recently in prescribing substitute amphetamines, such as dexamphetamine, for injecting amphetamine users. This has not been systematically evaluated but some clinicians report clinical benefit from this approach.

Hypnotics and tranquillizers

During the 1980s there was a rise in the problematic use of benzodiazepines (Strang *et al.*, 1993*c*). They are mainly seen in the context of poly-drug use and very high doses (above 200 mg diazepam equivalent) may be used. The most commonly used types of benzodiazepines are diazepam and temazepam but it is suggested that the shorter-acting drugs (e.g. lorazepam) may have more potential for abuse.

Benzodiazepines may be taken orally or injected. The commonest injected benzodiazepine in the UK is temazepam (Strang *et al.*, 1994). Temazepam use is commonly episodic, with binges followed by periods of abstinence. The problems of benzodiazepine abuse are intoxication, dependence, withdrawal and high rates of risk-taking behaviour related to injection technique (Klee *et al.*, 1990; Darke *et al.*, 1994*a*). Up to one-quarter of people presenting to community drug services report benzodiazepine abuse. A proportion of those will be benzodiazepine dependent and will require detoxification, for which purpose it is preferable to shift from short-acting benzodiazepines such as temazepam and flunitrazepam to longer-acting drugs such as diazepam.

LSD, ecstasy (MDMA) and other hallucinogens

LSD made a colourful contribution to psychiatry and counterculture in the 1960s and then appeared to fade away. During the late 1980s and early 1990s many countries witnessed a revival of hallucinogenic drug use including LSD, MDMA, MDEA, MDA, etc. among young people in the club dance culture.

An LSD trip begins about half an hour after taking a dose, peaks from two to six hours and fades out after about twelve. The effects of the drug may be determined by the expectations of the user and the situation in which the drug is used (Jaffe, 1990). Users often report visual and auditory illusions associated with alterations of experience of time and space. Self-awareness is heightened and feelings of dissociation from the body are commonly reported. Occasionally unpleasant reactions may result, especially if the user is unstable, anxious or depressed. Physical withdrawal phenomena do not occur after cessation of intake of LSD and although tolerance does develop, sensitivity to the drug returns rapidly. Flashbacks are an unusual but troublesome complication and may result in substantial functional impairment. These are usually some aspects of the original trip, although often milder and of a shorter duration. It is not clear if this is related to some central serotonergic mechanism or simply occurs because of a vulnerability to anxiety disorder. Cognitive-behavioural treatment strategies are useful for symptomatic management.

Ecstasy or MDMA is classed as an hallucinogenic amphetamine (Steel *et al.*, 1994) and is one of a large family of phenylethylamines (Schulgin & Schulgin, 1991). It is associated with feeling of heightened awareness, euphoria, well-being and occasionally hallucinations. Similar to LSD, MDMA appears to be weakly reinforcing. Initial experiences, while varied, seem to be associated with empathogenic effects and repeated use without substantial drug-free periods is associated with predominantly stimulatory effects. There are anecdotal reports of acute and chronic psychotic reactions and flashbacks associated with its use (Creighton *et al.*, 1991; McGuire & Fahy, 1991). There have been a number of high profile reports of sudden death associated with its use (Henry, 1992).

There are many other hallucinogens available, notably mescaline, peyote and psilocybin. Some of these have been used for traditional tribal religious and ceremonial purposes, which seem a vast distance from the heaving body mass of the rave scene of the 1990s.

Cannabis

Cannabis is by far the most widely used illicit drug in the UK, accounting for more than three-quarters of arrests for possession of drugs by the police. It is most commonly smoked as dried leaf alone, or as is the case with resin, mixed with tobacco. There are many psychoactive components in cannabis but the most active is delta tetrahydrocannabinol – often abbreviated to THC. In different cultures cannabis is also eaten mixed with foodstuffs, drunk or, very rarely, injected. It is a weakly reinforcing drug but some users report patterns of use consistent with dependence. There is a vast literature on the adverse health effects of cannabis (Hollister, 1986).

Most users experience mild euphoria, impaired co-ordination and altered perception of the passage of time. These effects depend greatly on the circumstances of use and the subject's initial psychological state. Occasionally short-term adverse reactions occur as anxiety states, panic attacks and paranoid ideas. Psychotic reactions do occur, although these are commonly of short duration and respond to symptomatic relief. There is some dispute over whether cannabis causes a more chronic psychosis but there is as yet no firm evidence for this. Most subjects experience no ill effects from taking cannabis but it is worth remembering that cannabis interferes substantially with motor performance and may result in impaired driving abilities over a relatively long period of 24–48 hours after use of the drug. Cannabis is eliminated slowly because it is fat soluble and so urine tests can remain positive for several weeks.

Volatile substance abuse

There are a vast array of volatile substance that may be inhaled. Adhesive is poured into small plastic gags, such as an empty crisp packet, and the vapour is inhaled. Typewriter correcting fluid and other liquids may also be inhaled, usually after being poured onto fabric. Gases in pressurised aerosol cans and in butane gas cigarette lighter fillers may also be inhaled. Volatile substance abuse may be initiated at a younger age than tobacco or any other substance use. It gives rise to pleasurable sensations such as feelings of well-being and euphoria. Heavier use results in changes in perception, such as hallucinations and tinnitus. The neuropsychiatric consequences of long-term use remain uncertain; cortical and cerebellar changes appear to reverse on cessation of use and some of the change may also be related to alcohol and other drug use (Chadwick *et al.*, 1989). Acute high doses may lead to unconsciousness and risk of death. There has been a continued high death rate from volatile substance abuse in the UK throughout the last 15 years, resulting from acute toxic effects such as cardiac dysrhythmias or from accidental deaths related to intoxication. There have been various attempts to reduce the abuse of volatile substances, including the 1985 supply of Intoxicating Substances Act, which makes it an offence to sell substances to people under 18, if there are grounds for believing they are likely to be inhaled. The main thrust of prevention has been in education, warning not only children, but also parents and teachers of the effects and dangers of volatile substance abuse.

Organising a treatment and advice service

Because of the varied nature and range of drug problems and populations involved in drug use there is a need for a diverse range of generic and specialist services with an overall emphasis on a flexible patient-orientated and family-orientated service that matches the problem to an appropriate response. The first-line response should be primary care and community-bases responses involved in a wide range of social agencies including social services, probation services, housing, etc. General medical and general psychiatric services will respond to the acute medical and psychiatric problems and will require the backup of specialised services, which should be involved in shared care with both primary care and general medical services. There is a need for links between the criminal justice system and the treatment system in order to divert drug users from custodial settings into appropriate treatment and rehabilitation channels (ACMD, 1994). The range and size of a service response will depend on the nature and scale of the problem and will exist in the context of a coherent national policy on the prevention and treatment of drug misuse.

9

Alcohol problems

ILANA B. CROME

Diagnosis and classification

Over two hundred years ago physicians recognised that alcoholism was within their remit – in America, Benjamin Rush (1785); in Britain, Thomas Trotter (1804); and in Sweden, Magnus Huss (1849). The term alcoholism was coined by Magnus Huss as he defined it as 'those disease manifestations which without any direct connection with organic changes of the nervous system take on a chronic form in persons who, over long periods, have partaken of large quantities of brandy' (Institute of Medicine, 1990). Despite the fact that this term is widely used by professionals and the public, there is little agreement as to its precise meaning.

Perhaps this has arisen because of the vast array of clinical presentations of alcohol abuse. Acute and chronic intoxication may be associated with psychological symptoms such as anxiety, parasuicide, suicide, paranoid ideas and insomnia. Gastritis, gout, accidents and trauma, and impotence are among the physical difficulties encountered. Absenteeism, child abuse and neglect, decreased productivity, public drunkenness and aggression, assault and homicide are related social problems. Regular heavy drinking is associated with homelessness, unemployment, delirium tremens, dementia, misuse of other drugs, cirrhosis, hepatic carcinoma, pancreatitis, cancer of the gastrointestinal tract, cardiomyopathy, neuropathy, myopathy and infertility, amongst others.

In *The 'Disease Concept of Alcoholism'*, Jellinek (1952, 1960) proposed that alcoholism was a phasic condition, and he described five patterns of alcoholism: alpha; beta; gamma or loss of control; delta or inability to abstain; and epsilon or episodic use. He considered only 'gamma' and 'delta' to be 'diseases'. He realised too that there was a wide range of differing patterns and problems associated with drinking. The key features of such a disease model (Pattison *et al.*, 1977) are that alcoholism is a unitary phenomenon where alcoholics differ from the rest of the population, where alcoholism is an irreversible condition with a progressive downward path manifest by loss of control, craving, compulsion to drink and inability to stop drinking. Critics commented on the methodological shortcomings of Jellinek's formulation, and experiments that took account of cognitive and environmental factors showed that loss of control need not necessarily be associated with alcoholism (Mello

Table 9.1. *Comparison between ICD-10 and DSM-IV*

	ICD-10 Dependence	DSM-IV Dependence
Compulsion to use	+	–
Impaired capacity to control use	+	+
Withdrawal state or relief	+	+
Tolerance	+	+
Neglect of pleasures, behaviours, interests	+	+
Persistent use despite evidence of harmful consequences	+	+
Great deal of time spent in activities related to obtaining, using or recovering from the substance	–	+

	Harmful use	*Abuse*
Evidence of psychological or physical harm caused by substance use	+	
Failure to fulfil major role obligations		+
Legal problems		+
Recurrent social or interpersonal problems		+
Use in physically hazardous situations		+

& Mendelson, 1971). Nevertheless, Jellinek's formulation rooted 'alcoholism' firmly in the clinical and research world.

The term alcoholism incorporates chronicity and harm attributed to alcohol. Thus the terms alcohol abuse, problem drinker, harmful drinking, pathological drinker, excessive drinker and alcoholic are unsatisfactory because it is not clear as to whether they denote dependence or the consequences of intoxication, regular heavy drinking or dependence.

A new era began in 1976 when Edwards and Gross (1976) described the 'alcohol dependence syndrome'. This biopsychosocial perspective defined the syndrome as having the following characteristics: a narrowing of the drinking repertoire; salience of drinking over all other activities; increased tolerance to alcohol; repeated withdrawal symptoms; repeated relief drinking or avoidance of withdrawal symptoms by further drinking; subjective awareness of a compulsion to drink; and reinstatement after abstinence. They stressed that these components could vary in degree and they suggested a separation of alcohol dependence from alcohol-related disabilities, i.e. the physical, social and psychological problems that may or may not occur in conjunction with dependence (Edwards *et al.*, 1977).

This delineation of a syndrome has contributed to a revision of terminology in the World Health Organization (1987) ICD-10 (International Classification of Diseases) as well as in the *Diagnostic and Statistical Manual* of the American Psychiatric Association, DSM-IV (American Psychiatric Association, 1987, 1994). ICD-10 has adopted the terms alcohol dependence syndrome and harmful use, while DSM-IV uses dependence and abuse. Table 9.1 illustrates the similarities and differences.

The evolution of the dependence syndrome concept has been useful in that it provides a basic set of criteria for diagnosis, and thus improved communication between professionals. It has some predictive power in that follow-up studies have indicated that generally severely dependent patients are very unlikely to return to normal drinking (Drummond, 1990).

On reflection, it becomes clearer that at different times the different scholars, quoted above, have appreciated that there is a diversity of alcohol problems, although superficially the idea of heterogeneity appeared to be subsumed under the general term and category 'alcoholism'. This heterogeneity manifests itself in the type of problem, the pattern of drinking, the presentation of problems associated with intoxication, withdrawal and dependence, the course of problems, the constellation of problems and the interaction, the causes, and the response to treatment. This distinction and definition of alcohol dependence and related disabilities marks an acceptance of the complexity of the field, and permits a more sophisticated understanding for developing better treatment options.

Alcohol-related disabilities

Psychological consequences

Alcohol may precipitate psychological symptoms as a result of intoxication, withdrawal and dependence (Helzer et al., 1985; Helzer & Pryzbek, 1988; Edwards, 1989; Glass & Marshall, 1991). Any relationship of psychological difficulties to alcohol use must be set in the context of a general psychiatric history. Recognition that there is an association dates back to Trotter and Rush.

In a study carried out at the Maudsley Hospital (Glass & Jackson, 1988) 10% of psychiatric patients were found to have an alcohol problem. Forty per cent of these patients had a dual diagnosis, i.e. additional psychiatric illness. The relationship between two disorders may simply be coincidental, or alcohol may exacerbate a psychiatric disorder, or patients may drink as a consequence of developing a psychiatric problem. Isolating and identifying associations is a complex matter, since many additional factors need to be considered, e.g. personality, drug use and period of assessment, that is during the withdrawal phase.

Alcoholics often present with symptoms of depression, e.g. dysphoria, agitation, apathy, suicidal ideation, loss of libido, early morning waking, loss of appetite, weight loss. Clinical experience dictates that treatment for coexisting affective disorder be withheld until the patient has been abstinent for 4–6 weeks. The relationship between suicide and alcohol is well established. The same risk factors may be involved in their aetiology. Adelstein & White (1976), in a cohort study of over 2000 hospital patients with a diagnosis of alcoholism, found significantly raised suicide in men, SMR (standardised mortality ratio) = 329, and women SMR = 230. Fifteen per cent of alcoholics may eventually commit suicide (Hawton, 1987). Alcohol may also increase the likelihood of a successful suicide as alcohol use is common immediately prior to or during suicide attempts. Particular risk factors for alcohol abusers include adverse life events, previous deliberate self-harm, depressed mood and serious physical complications.

Neurosis and personality disorder

Although note of the relationship between neurotic and personality disorder is often made, data on prevalence and natural history is limited. Anxiety and phobic symptoms may be causal factors as patients may attempt to control their symptoms by drinking but the alcohol consumption may then in turn exacerbate the anxiety or phobia. It is important to attempt diagnosis on the basis of multiple information sources and temporal sequencing of symptoms. This has implications for treatment since phobias, for example, may be amenable to behavioural modification (Stockwell & Bolderston, 1987).

Schizophrenia, alcoholic hallucinosis and pathological jealousy

The relationship between schizophrenia and alcohol problems is more tenuous than had been once supposed. Bernadt & Murray (1986) analysed drinking patterns in 317 psychiatric admissions and demonstrated that, on average, schizophrenics drank less than other psychiatric patients. Natural history studies suggest that very few cases of alcoholic hallucinosis develop into schizophrenia. Alcoholic hallucinosis is a condition in which a chronic drinker complains of auditory hallucinations of a persecutory nature. This may follow abstinence, reduction of consumption or even occurs during the course of drinking. There is an absence of thought disorder, a complex delusional system, a family history of schizophrenia, delirium, and physical symptoms of withdrawal. Differentiation from schizophrenia and an acute confusional state arising from drug or alcohol abuse can be made on the basis of history and urinary drug screen (Glass, 1989a;b). Twin and adoption studies serve to demonstrate that there is a separate predisposition to alcoholism and schizophrenia (Kendler, 1985). Pathological jealousy is an unpleasant and destructive syndrome that can develop on the backdrop of heavy drinking, but also as part of depression or schizophrenia.

Physical consequences

The physical complications of alcohol use are manifold. These relate to the pharmacological effects of alcohol, withdrawal, toxicity and deficiency syndromes as a result of chronic abuse.

Central nervous system

At blood alcohol concentrations (BAC) of 25 mg% euphoria is apparent, lack of co-ordination occurs at levels of 50–100 mg%, unsteadiness at 100–200 mg% and stupor at 200–400 mg%. Novice drinkers, females and children will exhibit such signs at much lower levels than a hardened drinker. *Intoxication* can lead to death from coma and respiratory depression at about 400 mg%. Intoxication may precipitate or be exacerbated by head injury, infection or hypoglycaemia. Alcoholic coma is a fatal condition in 55% of cases. Toxicology analysis is thus mandatory in such cases, and the expertise of physicians is essential.

Withdrawal syndromes may be mild or severe. Mild withdrawal presents about six hours after the last drink, and consists of nausea, vomiting, diarrhoea, insomnia, sweating, tremor, mood disturbance, anxiety and agitation. This state may continue for two to three days, and then abate slowly up to a week. Transient hallucinations, illusions or hyperacusis may occur. It may be compounded by delirium tremens, an acute confusional state, which usually presents with disorientation in time and place, predominantly visual but also auditory hallucinations, secondary paranoid delusions, extreme fear, sweats, shakes, hypertension and tachycardia. Convulsions may occur as part of this syndrome, i.e. 'rum' fits, but also secondary to intoxication or trauma, or as a toxic effect of alcohol. Delirium tremens has a mortality of about 5%. Severity is generally related to a previous history of delirium tremens, to heavy alcohol consumption, and to the presence of physical illness. The condition begins two to three days, and peaks at about a week, after abstinence (Chick, 1989). The CIWA (Clinical Institute Withdrawal Assessment for Alcohol) (Naranjo & Sellers, 1991) and the SSA (Selective Severity Assessment) (Gross *et al.*, 1971) have been developed to assess and monitor the severity of withdrawal.

Nutritional deficiency syndromes must be considered in alcohol abusers (Lishman, 1990). The most important is the Wernicke–Korsakoff Syndrome, which is consequent on thiamine deficiency. The common pathology is neuronal loss in the mamilliary bodies, vermis, anterior cerebellar lobules, aqueduct and fourth ventricle. Wernicke's encephalophy presents as opthalmoplegia, ataxia and confusional state. It is thus crucial to disentangle the contribution of symptoms of a withdrawal state from the possibility of Wernicke's as the two may co-occur. Korsakoff's psychosis presents as lack of insight, apathy, antegrade and retrograde amnesia with confabulation. It may or may not improve with vitamin replacement.

The initial presentation may be of peripheral neuropathy and cardiovascular disorder, e.g. hypotension or high output cardiac failure (e.g. beriberi) in combination with oral inflammation, and this is the result of thiamine deficiency. Peripheral neuropathy may be caused by toxicity and vitamin deficiency and may be mild peripheral or a severe incapacitating sensori-motor neuropathy. Lower limbs are affected more than upper, but foot and wrist drop, distal muscle weakness, and wasting may be noted. Alcohol abuse may be associated with other forms of neuropathy, e.g. vascular, trauma, viral and carcinoma. Pellagra (niacin and protein deficiency) and scurvy (vitamin C deficiency) are less common. Treatment usually consists of multivitamin preparations intramuscularly or intravenously early on, and then orally.

Alcohol *toxicity*, probably causing neuronal loss, results in cerebral dementia. Initially this may only come to light following psychological testing or the observation of dilated ventricles and cortical atrophy on MRI or CT scans. Reversibility can occur with abstinence. Alcoholic cerebellar degeneration presents as gross ataxia and the pathology is that of cell loss. It may respond to thiamine in the early stages. Central pontine myelinolysis, a rare condition, results from demyelination, presents with pseudo-bulbar palsy, and may be fatal. Marchiafava–Bignami syndrome results from demyelination of the corpus callosum.

Liver disease and gastrointestinal disorder

Alcoholic liver disease is a very common cause of morbidity and mortality in the developed world (Saunders, 1981; Peters, 1996). Fatty liver is generally asymptomatic and is

251

detected by abnormal liver function tests. It may, however, present with right abdominal pain, nausea and vomiting, which resolve on abstinence. Alcoholic hepatitis and cirrhosis result from chronic alcohol abuse. Alcoholic hepatitis produces liver cell necrosis and inflammation. This presents with jaundice, pyrexia, right abdominal pain, ascites and encephalopathy. Cirrhosis involves a permanent loss of liver cells, which are replaced by fibrosis. It may be asymptomatic (as may hepatitis) or present with gastrointestinal symptoms, ascites, encephalopathy and oesophageal varices, which may cause haemorrhage. Obviously abstinence and good nutrition are mandatory. Treatment of ascites is by diuretics and sodium restriction; of encephalopathy by protein restriction and lactulose; and variceal haemorrhage by transfusion, vasoactive drugs, oesophageal tamponade and sclerosis of the varices. Propylthiouracil has been shown to improve prognosis in chronic alcoholic liver disease.

Acute and chronic pancreatitis and gastritis and peptic ulcer are other gastrointestinal consequences of alcohol abuse. Chronic pancreatitis, which develops after long-term heavy alcohol abuse, may in addition result in diabetes and malabsorption syndrome.

Cancer

That there is an association between alcohol and cancer has been suspected for some time (Doll & Peto, 1981; MacSween, 1982). Heavy drinkers are more likely to be heavy smokers, and the increased risk from each substance problem appears to be potentiated by the combination. Steadily accumulating evidence indicates that alcohol consumption may be linked to cancers of the oral cavity, pharynx, oesophagus, liver, rectum, colon and breast (Garro & Lieber, 1990). The risk of developing cancer of the oesophagus if 50 times greater in heavy drinkers and heavy smokers than those who abstain. In one-third of patients who die with alcoholic cirrhosis, death results from liver cancer. Some, but not all, studies show an association between heavy alcohol consumption and cancer of colon and rectum, with N-nitrosamines in beer being a possible carcinogenic agent.

Cardiovascular and respiratory disease

The circulatory and respiratory systems are affected by alcohol. There has been much debate regarding the protective effect of low level alcohol consumption, e.g. two units per day, on cardiovascular disease. However Marmot & Brunner (1991), who reviewed the studies, state: 'the balance of harm and benefit does not weigh in favour of making recommendation to the public to increase consumption in order to prevent coronary heart disease'. Alcohol is an established risk factor for hypertension, and 30% of 'essential' hypertension may be related to alcohol abuse. There is a dose–response relationship. Furthermore, risk of stroke is increased in heavy drinkers and there is also a marked excess of chronic bronchitis and emphysema in this group. Alcoholic cardiomyopathy occurs in beer drinkers, and prognosis is poor, as 80% who continue to drink are dead in three years.

Haematological, musculoskeletal, endocrine and metabolic disorders

Alcohol is toxic to bone marrow, with resultant macrocytosis and thrombocytopenia. Gout, osteoporosis and avascular necrosis are recognised associations with alcohol abuse, as are acute and chronic myopathies. Alcohol produces a range of metabolic disorders: lactic acidosis, ketoacidosis, hypoglycaemia, hyperlipidaemia and disturbances in electrolyte and acid–base balance. Pseudo-Cushing's syndrome caused by alcohol is characterised by hypertension, obesity and bloated facies. Gonadal atrophy, as a result of direct toxicity to gonads and suppression of the hypothalamic–pituitary axis, causes impotence and diminished fertility.

Epidemiology

The information gathered is by no means conclusive because of different definitions, methods of data collection and problems in the reliability of reporting in the samples used (Mann & Smart, 1990). Epidemiological studies have shown that an intake of 4–6 units a day (up to 50 g) for 10 years may increase the risk of cirrhosis six times relative to consumption of 2–5 units (20 g) (Lelback 1975; Pequignot *et al.*, 1978). An increased risk to women above a daily intake of 2.5 units (20 g) has been demonstrated (Saunders & Williams, 1983). Marmot (1981) demonstrated an increased mortality for men consuming more than 30 units of alcohol a week. Similarly, relationships between overall alcohol consumption and alcohol-related problems have been demonstrated in the UK (Kendell, 1984), Sweden (Romelsjo & Agren, 1985) and the USA.

Britain

On this basis, it is estimated that 1.4 million people in the UK are drinking at levels regarded as harmful to health, i.e. more than 50 units per week for men, more than 35 units for women. An estimated seven million are drinking more than the recommended sensible limits by a public health education strategy, i.e. 28 units per week for men, 21 units for women. Men and women in the younger age groups have high consumption, those in the oldest have the lowest. There are regional variations with consumption in men, highest in North and North West England (Crawford, 1986).

Although it is difficult to estimate the total excess mortality due to alcohol misuse in the UK, several studies have shown this to be between 5000–40 000 per annum (McDonnell & Maynard, 1985; Royal College of Physicians, 1987; Anderson, 1988; Royal College of General Practitioners, 1986). In 1989, 185 000–224 000 life years (a measure of the effect of alcohol on life expectancy lost) were estimated to be lost due to alcohol use (Godfrey & Maynard, 1992; McDonnell & Maynard, 1985). Deaths from liver cirrhosis, a broadly accurate indicator of health problems related to alcohol, have doubled since 1968 (OPCS, 1991). Eight hundred people were killed in drink-driving accidents in 1990, and 92 820 people were convicted or cautioned for drunkenness offences in 1989.

Alcohol is estimated to have cost British industry £2122 million in 1990. The number of days lost through drink-related absenteeism is twice that of industrial action: 8–14 million days each year. Alcohol misuse costs British society, at a conservative estimate, £2.46 billion per annum. This estimate includes costs to industry, costs to the health service amounting to £149 million, and financing research and national alcohol bodies, which costs a parlous £1.24 million.

The 'Health of the Nation' strategy (Department of Health, 1992) and the 'Tomlinson Report' (Tomlinson, 1992) into London's health service, medical education and research both highlight substance problems as a target for action. The Tomlinson report noted that 30% of acute general hospital beds in London are filled with patients with alcohol problems. This is similar to an average of 23% in American studies (McIntosh, 1982), though a figure of up to 55% has been quoted. 'Health of the Nation' aims to reduce the proportion of men drinking more than 21 units of alcohol per week from 28% in 1990 to 18% by 2005, and the proportion of women drinking more than 14 units of alcohol per week from 11% to 7% by 2005.

These targets have focused on alcohol consumption, which has doubled from 4.4 litres of 100% alcohol per head in 1960 to 9.0 litres of 100% alcohol per head in 1991. Beer is the most common drink (54%), followed by spirits (22%), wine (20%) and cider (3.5%). There has been an increase in the popularity of wines and spirits (The Brewers' Society, 1992). In real terms this is a 123% increase in alcohol consumption overall between 1960 and 1987. More is spent on alcoholic drinks than on clothing and food in the UK. Drinking and driving offences have increased from 18 000 in 1968 to 93 000 in 1990. Screening with breathalysers has increased, though those with a positive test reached a peak in 1974, and had declined to half by 1990. Drunkenness offenders peaked in the late 1970s, and decreased until the late 1980s. Although the UK appears to have a low level of consumption compared to most European countries, the statistics quoted above indicate there is no cause for complacency.

Europe

According to the *Brewer's Society Statistical Handbook* (1993), most countries in the European Community have increased consumption of alcohol in the last 20 years (Powell, 1987) but France, Spain and Italy have decreased overall consumption. Furthermore, there is a changing pattern of alcohol consumption: per capita consumption of beer and spirits has grown in all countries, but wine consumption decreased in France and Italy, the two main wine-producing countries. It is important to recognise that the above data do not include home-produced alcohol, duty-free purchases, or non-recorded beverages e.g. cider in France. Since the strength of drinks are assumed to be the average, existing consumption data need to be standardised.

Even within Western Europe there are considerable differences in consumption of alcoholic beverages that may result from cultural factors (Pyorala, 1990; Hupkens *et al.*, 1993). Denmark, West Germany, the Netherlands, the UK, Ireland and Belgium are 'beer' countries, but between 1961 and 1988 per capita increase in wine increased more than beer and spirits in these countries. France, Italy, Greece, Spain and Portugal – 'wine' countries – showed a decrease in wine consumption, beer consumption increased, and spirits remained the same.In the European Community on average 10.8% males and 22.3% females were abstinent (UK 13.7% and 23.5% respectively). Males drank in five or six situations per week and females in three. The context of drinking differs in that Southern Europeans drink wine mainly at meals. Northern Europeans drink wine less often with meals than Southern Europeans, but they drink wine more at meals than outside meals. For instance, the Dutch, British and Irish mostly drink beer outside meals. In southern countries, where beer is a new beverage, younger people drink beer more often than older people. In northern countries, too, more younger people drink beer than older people. People of higher educational level consumed the new beverage type, while people of lower education level consumed traditional beverage type in greater numbers and more frequently than those of higher educational level.

United States

In the United States the apparent (based on tax records) consumption of alcohol, which had been rising during the 1960s and 1970s, has been decreasing in recent years. The largest decline has been in the consumption of spirits, which has fallen to its lowest level since 1958. Beer consumption has been dropping slightly, but wine consumption has remained fairly steady. The drop in spirits consumption may be as a combined result of ageing of the population, a decrease in the acceptability of heavy drinking, increasing concern about health and availability of lower alcohol beverages.

Authorities differ considerably in their estimates of the total costs of alcohol problems in terms of treatment, morbidity, mortality and lost productivity in the United States, ranging from $85 billion in 1988 to $136 billion in 1990. In 1987, 105 000 alcohol-related deaths occurred in the USA. A 1984 national US survey found 7% of all adults experienced moderate levels of alcohol dependence symptoms and 10% reported moderate levels of adverse social or personal consequences from drinking (Cahalan, 1992).

As mentioned earlier, estimates of costs to the country vary from 86 billion dollars in 1988, to 116 billion dollars in 1983 and 130 billion dollars in 1990. Ten billion dollars is spent on treatment for alcoholics, and alcohol-related crime and violence costs 2 billion dollars. One hundred thousand deaths per year are due to alcohol-related causes. These statistics are likely to be underestimates. Helzer (1987) cites Warhelt and Auth who reviewed twelve US surveys conducted between 1946 and 1982. These surveys indicated that 20–25% of men, and about 40% of women abstain from alcohol, that 12–33% of men and 2–5% of women drink heavily, and that 10% or more of men and 2–3% of women have experienced alcohol-related problems. The rates varied widely because of different methodology, definitions and samples.

In what is perhaps the largest comprehensive epidemiologic survey ever done in the field, the Epidemiologic Catchment Area (ECA) survey, 10 000 respondents were interviewed to estimate lifetime and current prevalence of mental disorders. The rates for current prevalence were similar to Warheit and Auth. Eighty four per cent of those who met DSM-III lifetime criteria for alcoholism reported no alcohol problems in the last year. Thus, rates of remission were found to be high, although estimates of lifetime prevalence were also remarkably high (up to nearly 30%) in men. In other American settings, e.g. general hospital in-patient population, the prevalence of alcohol problems is an average of 23%. The

255

emergency room attracts alcohol problems ranging from 10–32% of samples taken in casualty. People with alcohol problems are highly likely to have problems with tobacco use and quite likely to have problems with drug use.

Course and natural history

Death rates for treated and untreated alcoholics are higher than the general population and range from an annual rate of 1.7 to 3.7%. Deaths amongst alcoholics are due to cardiovascular disease, cirrhosis, neoplasms, accidents and suicide.

It is difficult to establish a consensus regarding a 'typical' course of the alcoholism. This is partly due to the paucity of studies of untreated groups and in the long-term (10 or more years). Taylor (1994) reviewed 13 treatment samples, which demonstrated remission rates of 21–80% over follow-up periods of 8–20 years. Especially in the longer term, improvements in drinking behaviour appeared to be related to improvements in psycho-social functioning. Most clinic samples demonstrate a degree of improvement, but six months of a year of abstinence does not necessarily equate to longer term abstinence. Fillmore & Midanik (1984) reported 17% abstinence over 14 years. Calculations indicate that relapse occurs at the rate of 25%–35% per annum.

Taylor et al. (1985) followed up male alcoholics for 10 years. While 25% were described as being in a 'troubled drinking' category, and 12% were abstinent, the majority moved between these two states and occasionally into social drinking. Only 4% remained abstinent over the period of the study.

Vaillant (1983) prospectively followed men from age 20 to 50 years old. One hundred and sixteen men developed symptoms of alcohol abuse. Onset of alcoholism was at about 31 years of age, though well before that time men had begun to move from a pattern of social drinking. In their early forties, men either died or began to abstain. Of the 116, 48 had achieved 1 year of abstinence, and 22 had returned to normal drinking. Eleven of the men who had achieved a year of abstinence relapsed to chronic abuse. Eighty-two per cent of those who became abstinent were gamma or loss of control alcoholics, compared to only 12% of those who returned to social drinking. Indeed, those who eventually became drinkers had low drinking problem severity scores. Those who achieved abstinence for a year had a wide range of problem severity scores including at the severe end of the spectrum. In this study, Alcoholics Anonymous, religious involvement or some substitute for alcohol that bolstered self-esteem appeared to be responsible for recovery in some people. Thus treatment was interpreted as being only one factor in the wider social context in which drinkers deteriorate or improve.

Polich et al. (1981) reported treatment of drinking problems over four years. Outcome was related to the orientation of the treatment agency towards abstinence or harm minimisation. The abstinence-oriented agencies achieved more total abstinence (29% compared to 22%) but less 'normal' drinking (14% compared to 46% and more 'problem' drinking (57% compared to 32%). Not surprisingly, social resources, coping skills and premorbid stability predict better outcome. Length of abstinence is predictive of lower relapse rate.

Schuckit (1989) suggests that establishing a diagnosis of 'primary alcoholism' makes it possible to predict the course of the disorder to some degree. Primary alcoholism is diagnosed when serious alcohol-related problems occur without evidence of psychiatric disorder or other substance misuse. In these patients major alcohol-related life problems are experienced in their mid-twenties to early thirties, with half of patients diagnosed as alcoholic fulfilling these criteria by the age of 31. Presentation for treatment, however, is usually in their early forties. Schuckit's view is that the drinking pattern fluctuates over time, in that the alcoholic will alternate between periods of abstinence, moderate drinking and severe misuse. Few remain consistently intoxicated and in any given month 50% of alcoholics will be abstinent, with a median of four months' abstinence over a one to two year period. In his experience 10–30% of alcoholics abstain or significantly decrease consumption without formal exposure to treatment.

Thus, recent research views the course of the disorder as a process that is in 'flux', i.e. that is transient and recurrent rather than one that is necessarily progressive.

What drives drinking behaviour?

There is no one single cause of alcohol problems, and many approaches have provided insights into the genesis of the difficulties that arise. People say they drink for a wide range of reasons, often multiple; for example, to prevent boredom, to relax, to socialise, to give confidence, and to relieve withdrawal symptoms are but a few. The challenge is to uncover what chain of events produces the individual problem drinker.

Various models have been proposed. These may be described as moral, disease, symptomatic, learning, social and biopsychosocial.

(a) The moral model blames the drinker for the problem, which is regarded as a sin due to weakness. The drinker is responsible for the consequences of his or her actions, and thus variants of this model are the 'legal' and 'spiritual' model. The former relates to the ability to control behaviour, the latter to the need for some powerful alliance to aid the alcoholic overcome temptation.

(b) The disease model espoused by Jellinek post-dated that of Rush, Trotter and Huss, and even Kraeplein and Alcoholics Anonymous. It shifted attitudes from the strictly pejorative view of the alcoholic. This had important political and social consequences in that alcoholics were no longer punished and denied access to help.

(c) The symptomatic model suggests that alcoholism is the result or symptom of some underlying psychological problem, personality difficulty or anxiety. This is now regarded as relatively simplistic, although interrelations between mental disorder and alcohol problems do exist.

(d) The learning model supposes that normal and abnormal behaviour are subject to the same learning processes. Thus, rather than identifying and isolating behaviour as different or deviant, this offers a way forward for changing behaviour by analysing, measuring, monitoring, and setting goals and so to change drinking behaviour. This implies a continuum of alcohol problems with a continuum of goals, including social drinking (Heather & Robertson, 1985). Recent cognitive behavioural formulations have taken account of processes such as expectancies, emotional state, experience, special situations, coping strategies, perceptions of feelings of control, and pharmacological factors.

(e) The social model seeks explanation in the environment of the individual rather than internal characteristics. Thus the culture, the values, the regulatory controls on alcohol, the workplace, the community, and the family in which the drinker is placed, may strengthen or diminish the resolve to drink.

(f) The biopsychosocial model attempts to integrate knowledge about psychological and biological vulnerabilities in a broader cultural, social and historical context. This model emphasises the dynamic interaction of the multiple components.

Significant studies that have underpinned some aspects of these models will be reviewed briefly.

Genetics

A variety of research methodologies have been adopted to examine the relative contribution of genetic and environmental factors (Ball & Murray, 1994).

Family studies

Cotton's view of family studies (1979) demonstrated that parental alcoholism was six times more likely in alcoholics, although 47–82% of alcoholics did *not* come from families with parental alcoholism. Guze *et al.* (1986) showed that the rate of alcoholism was almost twice as high in relatives of alcoholic probands (15.3%) than controls (8.7%). Dawson *et al.* (1992) reported that the odds of alcohol dependence was increased by 167% in individuals if both first and second degree relatives were affected, by 86% in those with a first degree relative affected, and by 45% in those with second or third degree relatives affected..

Twin studies

Difference in rates of alcoholism between monozygotic and dizygotic twins have been used as a measure of heritability. This is because monozygotic twins have the same genetic make-up whereas dizygotic twins share only 50% of their genes. Thus, any differences that occur in rates of a disorder between monozygotic and dizygotic twins are presumed to be genetic. This of course assumes the impact of environmental factors to be similar for each twin in a pair.

Since 1960, five studies in Sweden, the UK and USA have reported on concordance rates for mono- and dizygotic twins. Kaij (1960) found concordance rates for drinking behaviour in monozygotic and dizygotic twins were 53.5% and 28.3% respectively, while for chronic alcoholism rates were 71.4% and 32.3% respectively. The ratio of rates for monozygotic to dizygotic twins was 1.9 for drinking behaviour and 2.2 for chronic alcoholism. Hrubec & Omenn (1981) demonstrated a ratio of 2.2 for a diagnosis of alcoholism, while Gurling *et al.* (1981) using WHO diagnostic criteria of alcohol dependency was the only study to find a ratio of 0.8 (21% concordance in monozygotic twins and 25% concordance in dizygotic twins). The latter study demonstrated higher rates in males than females as one might expect. In males, the concordance rates for monozygotic twins was 33%, and that of dizygotic twins was 30%. For females, the rates were 8% and 13% respectively (Gurling & Murray, 1984).

Pickens *et al.* (1991) used a diagnosis of alcohol abuse and/or dependence, and found in males the concordance rate was 76% monozygotic twins and 61% for dizygotic twins. In females, rates were 36% and 25% respectively. If, however, a strict diagnosis of alcohol dependence is used, the rates for males are 59% for monozygotic twins and 36% for dizygotic twins (ratio 1.6) while for females the ratio is 5.0, since the rate for monozygotic twins is 25% but that for dizygotic twins is 5%. Estimates of heritability for alcohol dependence were 0.59 and 0.42 for males and females respectively. When Kendler *et al.* (1992) took a narrow definition of alcoholism, the ratio of monozygotic (26.3%) to dizygotic (11.9%) concordance rates were 2.2. It fell to 1.5 when a broad definition was used (46.9% concordance rate in monozygotic twins and 31.5% in dizygotic twins). The studies varied in the criteria used for determination of zygosity: appearance, direct questioning, serological status, and as mentioned earlier, diagnostic criteria. Nevertheless the overall results indicate a modest genetic susceptibility to alcoholism.

Normal drinking has also been examined in twins. Partanen *et al.*'s study (1966) in male twins showed that amount consumed and frequency of alcohol use was genetically determined, in contrast to lack of control and social problems, which were subject to environmental factors. Clifford *et al.* (1984) examined consumption in 494 twin pairs. Approximately one-third of the variance in alcohol consumption appeared to be genetic in origin. Concordance rates were greater in twins living together than in those living apart, pointing to how different environmental conditions affect consumption. Thus, there are problems surrounding the interpretation of twin studies such as the differential shared environment of monozygotic versus dizygotic twins or the effect of living with a heavy drinking twin.

Half-siblings and adoption studies

Schuckit (1987) found that 20% of half-siblings of alcoholic in-patients were also alcoholic. Two-thirds of the alcoholic half-siblings had an alcoholic biological parent compared with 20% in the non-alcoholic half-siblings. The time spent in an alcoholic environment for both sets of half-siblings was similar. Although Roe's study (Roe & Burks, 1945) showed no difference in drinking behaviour between adopted children of alcohol abusers and controls, it has been disregarded because of imprecise diagnostic criteria and small sample size. Goodwin *et al.* (1973) compared 67 male adoptees separated from their parents (one of whom was alcoholic) at 6 weeks with a control group. There was more than a three-fold increase in the likelihood of developing alcoholism in the adopted group (18%) compared to the control group (5%). Cadoret & Gath (1978) found increased alcoholism in adoptees with a first or second degree relative, as did Bohman (1978), who confirmed the threefold increase in alcohol abuse in adopted-away sons of alcoholic parents.

On the basis of Bohman's sample (Bohman *et al.*, 1981), Cloninger *et al.* (1981) claimed to have identified two types of alcoholism: milieu limited (Type 1) and male limited (Type 2).

The milieu limited type was characterised by age of onset over 25 years of age and no criminality or treatment for alcohol problems in the biological parents. This contrasted to the male limited type where school age of onset was under 25 years old and where alcohol abuse, criminality and treatment were extensive in the biological father. Loss of control (or psychological dependence), guilt and fear about dependence, harm avoidance and reward dependence were described in Type 1; inability to abstain, aggressive behaviour, and novelty-seeking personality traits were frequent in Type 2.

Despite misgivings about reliability of diagnostic criteria and interpretation of results, the increased rate of alcoholism in adoptees with an alcoholic biological parent is regarded as the most robust finding in support of a genetic contribution to the development of alcoholism.

Molecular genetics

The unpleasant flushing reaction in some Oriental people after alcohol is thought to be responsible for the low prevalence of alcoholism in this population (Yoishida et al., 1984). This is explained by the fact that ALDH2 (aldehyde dehydrogenase), the enzyme responsible for the majority of aldehyde oxidation, exists in two forms, one of which is inactive, ALDH2-2. This inactive form exists in varying frequencies in different populations. As a result of its low activity, acetaldehyde levels increase in the blood after alcohol consumption. Drinking leads to the accumulation of acetaldehyde, which results in to a disulfiram-like reaction, i.e. flushing, nausea, palpitations. Shibuya & Yoshida (1988) genotyped individuals with a diagnosis of alcohol-related liver disease and compared them to controls. The allele frequency for the low activity enzyme was higher (0.35) in the control group than the experimental group (0.07). The presence of this mutation in Japanese, Chinese and Koreans confers a protective role because of the aversive reaction to alcohol consumption, and divides these populations into those at risk of becoming alcoholic and those not at risk.

The dopamine neurotransmitter system is now a focus of interest (Tabakoff et al., 1988). Blum et al. (1990) claimed there was susceptibility to alcoholism attributable to variation in the dopamine D2 neurotransmitter receptor gene (DRD2). In alcoholics compared with controls an increased allele frequency of the A1 allele of the DRD2 gene was found. Six studies have now been done, and four have been significantly positive for association or linkage between the A1 allele and alcoholism. (Noble et al., 1991; Noble, 1991, 1993) has reviewed the work on A1 and B1 alleles of the dopamine receptor genes. His conclusion is that the dopamine receptor gene is the most important single gene determinant of susceptibility to substance abuse. Others are sceptical (Cook & Gurling, 1994).

Family history positive studies

Begleiter's group (1984) has investigated P3 (or P300s) event-related potentials in alcoholics and their sons. These potentials are presumed to reflect information processing in the brain. Offspring of alcoholics display P3 abnormalities, i.e. reduced response, in some studies but not all (Pollock et al., 1983; Polich et al., 1988). Similarly, Schuckit (Schuckit & Gold, 1988; Schuckit et al., 1991) have examined body sway after alcohol challenge in drinking men with a family history of alcoholism, and found this group to be less responsive than controls. The family history positive group were less sensitive and felt less intoxicated. A meta-analysis has confirmed a decreased intensity of reaction to alcohol as a characteristic more often seen in family history positive than family history negative subjects (Pollock, 1992).

Responsivity of serotonin systems to alcohol has also been studied. Family history positive young men differ significantly from family history negative young men. Family history positive men appear to have a higher uptake of serotonin, thus reducing availability of this neurotransmitter (Rausch et al., 1991). Lower levels of serotonin appear to be related to higher levels of alcohol intake (Naranjo & Sellers, 1985).

A similar strategy has been effected with neuropsychological testing. Children of alcoholics differ in their cognitive profile with regard to abstract reasoning and logical performance in some studies (Drejer et al., 1985; Knop et al., 1988; Tarter et al., 1989). Not all researchers are in agreement (Workman-Daniels & Hesselbrock, 1987). Schuckit et al. (1987) demonstrated equality of performance in these two groups on tests of verbal and total intelligence scores, memory, cognitive styles and school achievement. Whipple & Noble (1991) reported an atypical personality profile, i.e. more compulsive and fearful, in sons of alcoholics. Thus, this body of research indicates that a lower intensity of response to alcohol may place an individual at risk of developing alcohol-related problems in an environment where alcohol is freely available (Schuckit, 1994).

Environmental risk factors

Environmental factors that play a part in the aetiology of drinking behaviour may be divided into those factors that influence the availability of alcohol and those that render the individual vulnerable to the use and abuse of alcohol. The evidence regarding those social, economic and physical factors that affect availability, e.g. real price of alcohol, advertising, number of outlets, minimum drinking age and opening times, is discussed in the section on policy. Other environmental risk factors are discussed here. These include employment, culture, family interaction, peer group pressure, social class, and stress.

Peer affiliation

Adolescents with alcohol and drug-using friends are more likely to use the same substances themselves than those who associate with non-consumers (Hawkins et al., 1992). This relationship is not as simple as it might seem, in that sometimes alcohol and substance use appear to precede group membership and peer pressure, whereas in other settings, the opposite is the case (Mosbach & Leventhal, 1988). Thus there may be self-selection into high risk groups by vulnerable individuals who may be identified by high levels of sensation and risk-taking. Thus the motivation and reasons for joining a particular group may have clinical and treatment implications.

Family interaction

Positive parental attitudes to alcohol and drug use have a major influence in shaping use in children. It is thus self-evident that where one or both parents abuse alcohol, families manifest higher levels of conflict, disruption, economic difficulties, breakdown and impaired mother–child attachment (Holmes & Robins, 1987; Velleman & Orford, 1993; Zeitlin, 1994; Gorman, 1994). Close family involvement and support, on the other hand, are protective against initiation and later alcohol use (Brook *et al.*, 1986). Inconsistent discipline and disharmony as well as impoverished bonding increases risk of misuse and other psychological and behavioural dysfunction. The role of 'families' in 'causing' alcohol and drug problems has developed from a simple 'modelling' or 'initiation' model to one that suggests targeting of interventions at amelioration of communication styles and family cohesion, as well as education to alter parental attitudes to alcohol.

Employment

Employment can affect drinking in a variety of ways. Research demonstrated that particular occupations predispose to the use of alcohol. These are where alcohol is freely and cheaply available, where social pressure facilitates drinking, where people are separated from normal social relationships, where there is little supervision of drinking and colleagues collude in ignoring alcohol-related problems. Thus the alcohol industry, the armed forces, the entertainment industry, the medical profession, journalism and business are prime examples (Plant, 1979; Murray, 1980).

Where occupation is used as an indicator of socio-economic status, lower social class is related to greater alcohol abuse (Breeze, 1985). Alcohol-related problems, too, are more frequent in the socially deprived (Blane *et al.*, 1990). There is an element of self-selection into these occupations in that those with a degree of vulnerability might opt for a certain occupation because of the opportunities it affords. Since employment may also protect against alcohol abuse, the effects are not clear-cut.

Culture

Cultural factors operate from a young age. In a study on young Americans, 49% of white youths were initiated to alcohol by the 5th grade, compared to 40% of black youths, and 17% of Asian Americans. In Vaillant's study (1983) in the USA, the Irish subjects demonstrated high rates of alcoholism, they drank in pubs, and familial alcoholism did not influence the later development of dependence. In other ethnic groups, drunkenness was considered unacceptable, drinking was more frequent in the family setting, and alcohol dependence occurred more frequently if they had alcoholic relatives.

According to Bales (1946) the level of stress, norms governing substance use, and a substitute means of coping with stress were the three elements that determined how groups differed with regard to alcohol use. Linsky *et al.* (1987) tested this hypothesis by examining alcohol use in the USA. They demonstrated an inverse relationship between level of cultural approval of drinking (restrictions on use, religious attitudes to drink) and level of consumption and cirrhosis rate. Interestingly, the more permissive the norm, the lower the rate of arrests, probably because laws governing use are less prohibitive.

Psychological theories, personality and psychiatric syndromes

To examine the impact of a variety of factors in precipitating and maintaining drinking, Vaillant and colleagues (1983) and Beardslee *et al.* (1986) investigated background data, e.g. family history, ethnicity, family dynamics and psychological problems. Seventy-one men met DSM-III criteria for alcohol dependence and 32 for sociopathy. This study found that antisocial behaviour in youths (i.e. truancy, school behavioural problems) predicated alcoholism, which had an early onset. An unhappy childhood predicted poor mental health, but not alcoholism, and, furthermore, depression followed alcohol abuse, not vice versa. Hence, the previously held conclusion that alcohol abuse was symptomatic of personality problems, an unhappy upbringing or psychological problems was not warranted.

It is recognised that the alcoholic population is heterogenous in terms of personality structure, and that certain pathological personality types, e.g. antisocial personality and borderline personality, have prognostic value (Cloninger, 1987). Furthermore, proper assessment of individual personality traits may be advantageous in relation to assignment of appropriate treatment, e.g. those who are disorganised may prefer structure and may therefore find Alcoholics Anonymous acceptable. Those who are better suited to unstructured therapies are likely to be well-organised, and those who find confrontational approaches useful, are likely to have high self-esteem. The interaction of psychiatric illness and drinking behaviour is discussed in the section on alcohol-related problems. Coexistence of certain problems such as neurotic disorders, depression, schizophrenia, drug dependence and antisocial personality may affect outcome for alcohol problems (Rounsaville *et al.*, 1987; Kadden *et al.*, 1990).

Conditioning models, e.g. classical conditioning, tension-reduction or operant conditioning, provide additional approaches (Drummond *et al.*, 1990; Winokur & Coryell, 1991). Classical conditioning theory suggests that exposure to cues previously associated with heavy drinking or withdrawal symptoms produces a conditioned response, in this case withdrawal symptoms or craving. Tension-reduction theory explains alcohol consumption in terms of diminishing the stress associated with fear, anxiety, frustration or conflict. Operant conditioning takes account of antecedent events and consequences in explaining drinking behaviour. In this model, positive reinforcement might be associated with the euphoria or relaxation which results from drinking. The negative reinforcing effect of alcohol is associated with relief of boredom, withdrawal symptoms or anxiety and anger. Cognitive factors serve an important mediating function in alcohol consumption. The expectation or belief that a drink contains alcohol produces effects similar to alcohol even where there is none.

The pharmacological effect of alcohol interacts with the person's psychological state. Increased tolerance, decreased tolerance, the development of withdrawal symptoms that are relieved by drink, and brain damage will alter the manner in which alcohol is metabolised. Blood alcohol levels in the heavy drinker reach levels that would severely incapacitate, or even prove fatal, to the novice drinker. A history of chronic alcohol abuse may affect the capacity to make decisions about abstinence as a goal. Withdrawal symptoms and craving may override choices and steer people into a vicious spiral of increasing alcohol intake.

In summary, multiple dynamic factors govern alcohol use and abuse. The dose of alcohol, taken at a particular time of day, with a given frequency, in the company of a particular group at a particular place and occasion, which has a particular meaning with a given expectation of the effect of the drink, will contribute to drinking behaviour of an individual. The age, role, gender, social group and peer pressure, the family, marital, community and occupational environment as well as overall cultural values and controls on alcohol will inform drinking behaviour (Cochrane & Bal, 1990; Catalano *et al.*, 1992). The individual's genetic make-up, personality, sense of control and efficacy, degree of dependence, the presence of brain damage or psychiatric problems, reaction to internal and external cues or stimuli, financial state and the values of a treatment programme will all affect attempts to change drinking.

Treatment: assessment

History taking

A thorough substance use and misuse history should always be elicited in the context of a full psychiatric history (Glass, 1994). A detailed assessment has come to be seen as increasingly important for several reasons. First, there is considerable evidence that generalists spend little time doing so. Secondly, assessment is the first stop on the treatment map, i.e. the process of systematic information gathering and interaction between individuals may in itself be therapeutic (Edwards, 1987). This has particular relevance to the focus on brief intervention as the substantive therapy for alcohol problems. It is vital, also, for decisions regarding choice of appropriate treatment options. A high index of suspicion is a prerequisite, as is the recognition that this is often a difficult area for both doctors and patients. Finally, it should be borne in mind that persons with alcohol problems do not necessarily give inaccurate information regarding their drinking behaviour.

It is mandatory for each practitioner to draw up a mental checklist of those questions pertinent to alcohol problems. A personal history that incorporates information about the person's birth, developmental milestones, scholastic achievement, educational and occupational opportunities, family social and marital history will set the scene for relationships between lifestyle and social problems and alcohol use to be explored. Likewise, a family history must indicate to what extent a history of psychiatric or substance problems were a feature in grandparents, parents, siblings, children and often close relatives. Cautious probing is often necessary to uncover a hidden problem. A special note should be made of the intelligence and cognitive state of the individual as this too has consequences for treatment; blood alcohol level at the time of interview is a factor to take into account. It is useful to get a picture of level of alcohol consumption in units in the past 24 hours, past month and over the past 6 months. A unit is equivalent to 1 glass of table wine, or $\frac{1}{2}$ a pint of beer, or 1 measure of spirits, or 1 measure of sherry. As discussed earlier, a consensus emerged that a 'safe limit' for women is 14 units a week, and for men 21 units per week. The 'new' safe limit is 21 units per week for women, and 28 units per week for men. At levels above, damage may ensue.

Information about the person's drinking career, history and pattern of use, the age at which the person first tasted alcohol, moved onto weekend drinking first irregularly and then regularly, drank every evening, then every lunchtime, and finally, when regular morning drinking became established. The age at which withdrawal symptoms started is an important milestone. Whether other dependence features are present and when they began should be noted, along with episodes of delirium tremens. It is customary to take a history of the pattern of other drug use and complications, e.g. nicotine, cannabis, benzodiazepines, stimulants or opiates.

If there have been abstinent periods, the extent and possible reasons should be noted. A detailed history of treatment options approached, rejected, or valued should be gathered. This includes those agencies specifically directed at the alcohol problem and those tangential to it, e.g. general hospital in-patient unit for treatment of gastritis or social services involvement because of child neglect. A past, recent or present history of alcohol-related disabilities whether physical, social, or psychological must be elicited. The personality profile of the individual may also contribute to the assessment, and appropriate treatment possibilities. This may be linked to the life situation as measured by social network, abstinent friends, employment, financial status, housing and other interests.

Information on the relationship of the person's forensic background (e.g. violence, drinking and driving, being drunk and disorderly) to alcohol consumption must be sought. Similarly, the impact of drinking behaviour on occupational development, family life and sexual behaviour, including HIV risk, is an integral part of characterising the client.

This kind of practical schedule should provide the practitioner with a picture of the person's problem in quantitative and qualitative terms to set a baseline for communication to the person and to other practitioners. Information about use of alcohol, as well as the signs and symptoms and consequences of alcohol use, permits effective management.

Questionnaires and instruments

Screening may be achieved by the Alcohol Clinical Index (ACI) (Skinner et al., 1986), the CAGE questionnaire (Ewing, 1984) or AUDIT (Saunders & Aasland, 1987). Many scales to measure severity of alcohol dependence have been developed: the SADQ (Severity of Alcohol Dependence Scale) (Stockwell et al., 1979), SADD, i.e. Short Alcohol Dependence Data (Davidson et al., 1989) and ASI, i.e. Addiction Severity Index (McLellan et al., 1980). Scores on the SADQ correlate with indices of withdrawal symptom severity as assessed by a physician in patients attending a detoxification unit. The MAST (Michigan Alcoholism Screening Test), the ASI (Addiction Severity Index) and AUI (Alcohol Use Inventory) elicit information about the consequences of alcohol use.

Quantity/frequency questionnaires probe the frequency of drinking over, for example, a week, month or year and the amount of different types of drink each day. This allows calculation of the average weekly drink. Drinking diaries provide more accurate information than quantity frequency measures.

Computerised assessments appear to elicit more reliable information, especially at high levels of consumption, and frees time for an assessor. Deciding upon the correct mix of face-to-face interviewing, and self-report questionnaires, computerisation of questions and scoring is probably useful, especially if clients are disabled or speak a foreign language (Bernadt et al., 1982; Skinner et al., 1986).

Biological indicators

Routine laboratory tests should include haemoglobin, mean corpuscular volume, erythrocyte sedimentation rate, white cell count, gamma glutamyl transferase (GGT) aspartate aminotransaminase, alkaline phosphatase, uric acid, blood lipids, blood alcohol concentration, albumin, bilirubin and proteins. Raised GGT has proved to be one of the most sensitive tests for early liver disorder. The exact mechanism underlying the rise is not known, but it is assumed to be related to enzyme induction. GGT has been reported to be raised in 60–80% of clinic sample populations. GGT can also be affected by factors other than alcohol use, e.g. other drugs, diabetes, pancreatic, cardiac and renal disorders. An excess of false-positive readings may therefore be observed in clinic populations. Kristenson *et al.* (1983) have demonstrated that raised GGT identified only 30% of alcoholics in a health screening investigation. Abnormalities began to return to normal within 2 days of abstinence.

Enlarged red blood cells without anaemia produce a raised MCV (mean corpuscular volume), and this is raised in 50–60% of clinic populations. If two or more markers are used, sensitivity rises to about 80%. The value of more specialised tests, e.g. urinary dolichols (substances involved in the formation of certain protein carbohydrate compounds), carbohydrate-deficient transferrin (CDT), the blood metabolite of AST, 2, 3-butanediol, acetaldehyde and acetaldehyde adducts (AAs) as potential markers of alcohol consumption, remain inconclusive.

Biochemical tests are useful in a general hospital setting, but a combination of screening tests to include self-report questionnaires, a full history and clinical examination as well as biochemical tests is probably the best.

Management: pharmacological treatment

Medication is used for alcohol problems for three reasons:

1. to treat withdrawal, i.e. detoxification;
2. in the longer-term, during rehabilitation for relapse prevention;
3. treatment of additional psychiatric illness, or to alleviate the effects of alcohol.

Mild withdrawal can be managed with support, reassurance and counselling (Moskowitz *et al.*, 1983). Those patients who experience greater mood disturbance, profuse sweating, obvious tremors and who have a history of withdrawal seizures or delirium tremens, merit medication as well as treatment of concurrent physical illness.

Benzodiazepines are the mainstay of treatment due to their cross-tolerance with alcohol, relatively low dependence potential and toxicity if prescribed in short courses, as well as their anticonvulsant and anxiolytic properties. Longer-acting drugs, e.g. diazepam and chlor-diazepoxide, are the preferred option. Lorazepam and oxazepam can be used in patients with impaired liver function. For chlordiazepoxide the following regime is appropriate: 40 mg q.d.s. for two days; 30 mg q.d.s. for two days; 20 mg q.d.s. for two days; 5 mg q.d.s. for two days.

An alternative is chlormethiazole, which can be administered as three capsules (192 mg chlormethiazole per capsule) t.d.s. or q.d.s. reducing over no more than nine days because of abuse potential. Because of the latter, it has become a less attractive option, although intravenous use and higher doses are appropriate in severe withdrawal. Carbamezepine (Tegretol, 100 mg) starting at 200 mg per day, is suggested as an alternative as it has no abuse liability. It should be increased to 400 mg per day by day 3, and gradually decreased by day 8.

Vitamins orally, intramuscularly or even intravenously as thiamine hydrochloride are appropriate in patients with Wernicke–Korsakoff syndrome. Vitamins are often given to any severely dependent alcoholics.

Prophylactic treatment is recommended for patients with a history of withdrawal fits and delirium tremens. Benzodiazepines in doses higher than are usually administered may be appropriate. Some clinicians suggest phenytoin in divided doses over a week. If patients are in the acute phase of delirium tremens or having convulsions, intravenous chlormethiazole or diazepam respectively should be given. In these cases, medication should be given by slow infusion to avoid respiratory depression.

Drugs are used to prevent relapse. Alcohol sensitising drugs disulfiram and calcium carbamide inhibit aldehyde dehydrogenase, the enzyme that converts acetaldehyde to acetic acid. In the presence of alcohol, the accumulation of acetaldehyde results in nausea, vasodilation, flushing, hypotension, tachycardia, coughing and shortness of breath. For disulfiram the starting dose is 500 mg daily for one to two weeks, and a maintenance dose of 250 mg daily. The reaction can occur up to a week after cessation. It is most appropriate for people who have decided to abstain, but find an extra prop useful. Only experienced clinicians should prescribe this treatment, and as part of a total treatment package.

Since psychological symptoms are a feature of intoxication and withdrawal from alcohol, it is important if possible to delay any definite diagnosis of additional psychiatric illness till the patient has abstained from alcohol for 4–6 weeks. Tricyclic antidepressants are effective in depressive illness. Monitoring plasma levels is suggested to capitalise an optimal dose and avoidance of toxicity.

Anxiolytic agents may be administered to patients who experience anxiety disorders separately from any problems related to alcohol. However, it is vital to prescribe short courses where symptoms are closely monitored, and in combination with psychological treatments. Longer acting benzodiazepines are preferred because of lower abuse liability, though day-time drowsiness and cumulative toxicity is a problem.

According to several studies, lithium blocks the 'high' precipitated by alcohol and early indications are that serotonin uptake inhibitors (fluoxetine, fluvoxamine) may reduce alcohol consumption. Likewise, follow-up studies on bromocriptine and apomorphine (dopamine antagonist) and homotaurine (GABA receptor antagonist) may provide some alternative strategies in reducing desire to drink or craving.

Naloxone, and naltrexone, opiate antagonists, which are administered for detoxification and relapse prevention in opiate addicts, have recently been passed by the Food and Drug Administration for treatment of alcoholism.

Antipsychotic agents must be carefully selected, as hepatic and neurological side-effects may make them inappropriate in patients with alcohol problems. Low doses should be prescribed.

Management: psychological treatments

The process by which change occurs in people with addictive problems is complex. Prochaska & DiClemente (1985) have described at least four stages:

i   Pre-contemplation stage, where the problem user does not intend to change in the near future.
ii Contemplation stage, where costs and benefits are being reappraised.
iii Action stage, where a decision to change has been taken and positive steps in that direction made.
iv Maintenance stage, where a high state of vigilance prevails in order to prevent relapse.

Behavioural therapy

The components of the behavioural analysis to be undertaken for problem drinking include:

i   The frequency, intensity and pattern.
ii The 'triggers' or antecedents.
iii The factors that maintain or reinforce drinking behaviour.
iv The 'reinforcement hierarchy', i.e. the whole range of environmental factors that reinforce behaviour.
v   Points for intervention to environmental factors.

The range of treatments is broad, and they are discussed in greater detail in other parts of this volume. However, a brief review of these are (Hodgson, 1993):

Social skills training

The drinker is taught specific behavioural skills, often assertiveness training in groups in an effort to form and maintain interpersonal relationships.

Self-control training

Reduction or avoidance of alcohol intake is achieved by functional analysis and the development of specific strategies such as goal-setting, self-monitoring, learning of coping skills.

Motivational counselling

This intervention focuses on not confronting the individual but instead negotiating behavioural change in the context of the patient's state of readiness for it (Anderson, 1996; Miller & Rollnick, 1991).

Marital therapy

Involves couples, in groups, or simply together. The objective is to improve communication and problem-solving and so improve positive communication.

Community reinforcement approach

Aims at altering the environment so that abstinence becomes more rewarding than drinking (Azrin, 1976). Counselling may be directed towards employment, problem-solving, improving relationships and increasing leisure activities.

Stress management

Trains individuals in relaxation techniques, systematic desensitisation and cognitive strategies.

Aversion therapies

Based on induction of conditioned avoidance of alcohol by pairing images of alcohol with unpleasant experiences, for example, covert sensitisation, i.e. imaged adverse consequences.

Contingency management

Organise contingencies, e.g. punishment of drinking or rewarding behaviour unassociated with drinking through contracts.

Cognitive therapy

Recognises that thoughts or beliefs may precipitate drinking and their modification may alter drinking patterns. Relapse prevention strategies that stress cognitive processes, e.g. self-efficacy and expectancies, are one type of therapy.

Psychodynamic interventions

General psychotherapeutic principles are often a component of multimodal approaches, and appropriate psychotherapy may be advised or offered to particular individuals or groups.

Group psychotherapy

This is probably the most commonly used treatment, since it is offered as part of residential programmes, Alcoholics Anonymous, and out-patient programmes, again in the framework of a general service provision. The value is seen to be the sharing of experiences and identification of behaviour. This meeting is facilitated by staff, with a session daily or 2–3 times a week, and an optimum 8–10 members. Treatment programmes often utilise the general principles of group dynamics for other elements of the programme, e.g. physical, recreational and educational activities.

Alcoholics Anonymous

Self-help groups, primarily Alcoholics Anonymous (AA), A1-Anon and Alateen have worldwide acceptance. In 1987 membership was estimated as 1.5 million in 73 000 groups. Belonging to AA demands participation in a programme of recovery, called 'working the twelve steps'. The twelve steps are guides to the process of change needed to achieve and maintain abstinence. Members participate in meetings where experiences are shared and support provided. Finding a sponsor (a more experienced member who engages in 'twelfth-stepping') who provides help at times of crisis, is encouraged. A1-Anon and Alateen provide similar support for spouses and children of alcoholics. The use of AA techniques are incorporated to greater or lesser degree in most treatment programmes in the UK and USA. Thus AA can aid recovery, be part of formal treatment, or sustain recovery achieved by formal treatment. AA is considered by many lay persons and professionals to be the most successful treatment for persons with alcohol problems despite the lack of research to support this view (Bradley, 1988; Emrick, 1989; Ogborne, 1989). Research has indicated that not all who are introduced to AA affiliate, and not all who affiliate benefit. Indeed, it has been estimated that only 20% of those referred to AA ever attend meetings regularly. Given its impact, it is unfortunate that AA have not been the subject of more empirical research until recently (Ogborne & Glaser, 1981; McCrady & Miller, 1993).

Eclectic therapy

Family therapy comprises a wide range of differing conceptual models and settings. Psychodynamic behavioural or systems approaches for families have been used in in-patient treatment, out-patient and day patient, but as described earlier, studies of effectiveness are not forthcoming. This is partly because of difficulties in defining what constitutes objectives, treatment and the family constellations and the stage at which intervention is sought. What research has been done seems to point to the benefit of family involvement in treatment retention and consumption reduction of the problem drinker.

Cost-effectiveness

In 1991 Holder et al. reviewed randomised clinical trials and were able to show evidence of:

(i)   Great effectiveness resulting from studies on social and marital relationships, especially where family stability, cohesion and social support are present.
(ii) Effectiveness of self-control and stress-management training. Cue exposure techniques might improve results.
(iii) Promising results for covert sensitisation, behaviour contracting, non-behavioural

marital therapy, cognitive therapy and hypnosis. Further research is warranted.
(iv) Some approaches that are commonly used, but for which there is either insufficient or no evidence of effectiveness. Residential treatments and Alcoholics Anonymous are examples of the former. Aversion therapy, educational techniques, and psychodynamic therapy are examples of the latter.

This has important consequences for cost-effectiveness since there are a number of low-cost techniques that are effective, e.g. those that emphasise coping skills and relationships. Other high-cost interventions, e.g. residential treatments, were not effective. However, this should not lead to a total exclusion of treatment strategies that offer help and hope to the seriously dependent patient with complications. The issue now remains, who is likely to benefit from such intervention or, in the parlance, who is best matched?

Treatment outcome research

In the complex area of outcome research, 250 new studies have been carried out since 1980. Sixty of these studies have used controlled designs. Vaillant's seminal study quoted earlier demonstrated that outcome in 100 treated patients followed up for eight years was no different from the untreated group. This triggered interest in what the optimum duration and intensity of treatment might be (Saunders, 1989).

Research on duration and intensity

The central issue that defined the 1980s in terms of treatment research was work on duration and intensity of treatment. In the UK, Edwards and colleagues (1977) stimulated curiosity about the value of brief or minimal intervention when they studied 100 married men who were assigned to one brief advice and counselling session with their wives or the Maudsley Hospital's usual treatment package, i.e. regular out-patient follow-up, in-patient admission if necessary, and referral to Alcoholics Anonymous. Analysis after one year did not yield differences between the two groups.

In Sweden, Kristenson et al. (1983) studied 585 healthy middle-aged men who on general health screening were identified as heavy drinkers (i.e. more than 40 g alcohol per day) or moderate drinkers (i.e. 20–40 g alcohol per day). Seventy-six per cent of those heavy or moderate drinkers had a raised GGT on two occasions; this group was then randomised into a treatment or control group. The control group were informed by letter that they had impaired liver function, advised to cut down, and asked to attend for tests in two years. The intervention group were advised to cut down but also had a detailed examination and interview, were offered regular follow-up appointments when GGT was repeated, and once GGT decreased, follow-up was reduced. After four years the GGT had declined significantly in both groups. However, alcohol-related problems and mortality, hospitalisation and absenteeism had decreased only in the intervention group.

In Edinburgh, Chick et al. (1985, 1988, 1989) studied the effectiveness of brief intervention in 165 heavy drinkers in a general hospital setting. Patients were randomly assigned to a

271

control group, where no intervention was made al all, and an intervention group, where the patient was counselled by a nurse and given a booklet about ways of reducing consumption. At 12-month follow up both groups had reduced consumption significantly. For the treatment group, though, there was a 41% decrease in alcohol-related problems compared to 14% in the control group. Fifty-two per cent of the treatment group had definitely improved compared to 34% of the control group. Thus extended treatment reduced harm.

In 1988, Wallace *et al.* reported 999 patients recruited from 47 general practices. The treatment group were counselled and followed up by their general practitioners, whereas the control group received no unsolicited advice. At one year a significant reduction of drinking and GGT has occurred in treated men. Twenty per cent of excessive drinkers had reduced consumption overall, so that if general practitioners simply counselled their patients, 150 000 men and 67 500 women in the UK would decrease their drinking.

In New Zealand, Elvy *et al.* (1988) assigned drinkers in surgical and orthopaedic wards to two groups. The treatment group were counselled while the control group received no help. At one year the counselled group reduced alcohol intake and related problems. Chapman & Huygens (1988) assigned patients to in-patient programme or out-patient programme or a single interview. At 18 months there was no difference. In the US, Longabough *et al.* (1983) showed no significant differences in drinking or related problems at two years in patients assigned to day patient or in-patient treatments. Miller & Hester (1986) reviewed controlled out-patient versus in-patient treatment studies and concluded that in-patient care was not more successful. When they reviewed out-patient trials, more intensive treatment was no more advantageous.

Outcome research using non-pharmacological agents

Much research effort has focused on 'behavioural self-control'. Results are conflicting. In a controlled study, Brown (1980) showed significant reduction in drinking in a group of drunk drivers given help of this kind as compared to education only. Foy *et al.* (1984) found the opposite in a group of in-patient alcoholics given training in controlled drinking. Sanchez-Craig *et al.* (1984) assigned out-patient problem drinkers to abstinence or alcohol reduction but no differences were forthcoming. There is some evidence supporting behavioural marital therapy as an additional component to treatment, but the differential effect of variety of treatments on the alcoholic couple and family has not been evaluated.

Only one of the three controlled studies of relapse prevention has shown a small effect on treatment outcome (Annis *et al.*, 1988). Studies of treatment programmes which, on the whole, comprise a combination of techniques, have been uncontrolled (Cook, 1988*a,b*). As mentioned above, when Miller & Hester (1986) reviewed all controlled studies, they reported the effectiveness of aversion therapy, stress management, marital and family therapy and community reinforcement. Outcome research on insight-oriented psychotherapy, education interventions and Alcoholics Anonymous has either not been carried out or has not yielded clear evidence of benefit (Smart & Mann, 1993).

Outcome research using pharmacological agents

Studies of disulfiram and calcium carbamide (Fuller *et al.*, 1986; Peachey & Annis, 1985) show some evidence that in a highly compliant group, an improved outcome results. Zimelidine, a serotonin uptake inhibitor, was shown to reduce alcohol intake in animal and human studies but it was withdrawn because of neuropathy and influenza-like symptoms. Fluoxetine, also a serotonin uptake inhibitor, might affect initiation of drinking behaviour, so therapeutic trials on fluoxetine are underway in heavy drinkers.

Most studies have demonstrated that lithium is not effective in either depressed or non-depressed alcoholics (Dorus, 1988; Peck *et al.*, 1981; Pond *et al.*, 1981). Compliance, however, is more likely to be associated with abstinence. Furthermore, despite the fact that it seems feasible to treat additional psychiatric illness with psychotropics, this is unproven (Rounsaville *et al.*, 1987).

Special groups

Women

The stereotyped picture of the irresponsible impetuous female drinker is beginning to change (Plant, 1990; Royal College of General Practitioners, 1992). Research indicates that for women with alcohol problems the origins and patterns of drinking behaviour are heterogenous (Blume, 1986). In the Epidemiological Catchment Area (ECA) survey, the 'prevalence of alcohol abuse and/or dependence' during the year prior to interview was 11.9% for men and 2.2% for women. National prevalence rates for alcohol dependence and problems indicate that differences in alcohol consumption exist between men and women, a 2:1 ratio in general population studies and a ratio of 3:1 or 4:1 in treated populations, e.g. psychiatric hospitals. Women drink less frequently, in smaller quantities and different types of drinks.

Women are more likely to become intoxicated compared to men. Women have been shown to have increased bio-availability of alcohol compared to men and this may explain their vulnerability to complications (Frezza *et al.*, 1990). For example, women are more likely to develop brain damage as a result of their drinking (Acker, 1986; Jacobson, 1986; Hewett *et al.*, 1991). This is associated with shorter drinking histories, lower peak alcohol consumption, poorer performance on psychometric testing and more evidence of brain damage on scanning. Alcoholic liver disease also progresses more rapidly in women with a lower mean alcohol consumption compared to men (Saunders, 1981). Moderate alcohol intake has been associated with breast cancer (Willett *et al.*, 1987). Women more commonly present with an additional psychiatric illness (Thom, 1986, 1987); depression, anxiety and eating disorders predominate (Beary *et al.*, 1986; Pelever & Fairburn, 1990).

The fetal alcohol syndrome (FAS) is characterised by growth retardation, mental handicap and abnormal features of the head and face (Jones & Smith, 1973). The cardiac and neurological abnormalities, finger print and palmar crease abnormalities, genito-urinary problems and behavioural problems are termed fetal alcohol effect, or alcohol-related birth defect. Recent epidemiological data suggests worldwide prevalence of FAS of 1–3 per 1 000 live births. There is no clear safe limit as yet, and also no guarantee that social drinking is without risk of damage, since the mechanisms of damage are ill understood at present. Since it is probably the major preventable cause of learning difficulties, identification and treatment is vital (Streissguth, 1990).

Virtually all biological research, e.g. genetic, electrophysiological and hormonal studies, has focused on men. This imbalance needs to be redressed (Glass-Crome, 1994). The view that women have a poorer prognosis has not been rooted in substantial studies. Much research that has been replicated or reviewed points to women doing no worse, or better than men. Women are at a disadvantage in terms of pre- and post-treatment characteristics, e.g. accessibility, stable social support and increased prejudice about their drinking problem (Dahlgren & Willander, 1989). Some recent studies show greater improvement and involvement in programmes matched to women's needs (Copeland & Hall, 1992). Thus services must be geared to recognise, identify and treat female drinkers who present in a variety of settings (Jarvis, 1992; Sanchez-Craig et al., 1991).

Elderly

Alcohol problems may mimic many of the common presentations to a geriatric unit (Atkinson, 1991). These include falls, non-compliance with medication, malnutrition, generalised weakness, burns, hypothermia, confusional states and neglect. The more obvious presentations (e.g. liver disease or psychotic illness) may still be attributed to general decline and intellectual deterioration.

Prevalence data are difficult to come by and is usually based on 'safe limits' surveys and questionnaires not specific to the elderly. These are often irrelevant in that the rate at which alcohol is metabolised decreases with age as may the types of alcohol-related problems, e.g. the elderly are rarely employed and may be widowed. A UK study puts those at risk at 13% in a community survey (Bridgewater et al., 1987; Bristow & Clare, 1992).

The research that has been done defines two types: early onset – chronic drinkers who have aged – and late onset – those who begin to drink in late life. The latter often relates to the problems besetting the elderly: psychiatric and physical illness, financial insecurity, bereavement, retirement and isolation. The former group are more likely to have severe complications and personality problems.

The young

Among British secondary school children (age 11 years or more), 60–90% drink alcohol regularly and 10% drink heavily; about 35 000 children under the age of 16 consume alcohol in excess of the sensible limit recommended for adult men and women. Age of induction is at about 11 years, which is of concern as the earlier a substance is used, the greater the risk of progression to more dangerous patterns of use and behaviour and social problems (Swadi, 1988; Swadi & Zeitlin, 1988). Robins et al. (1986) delineated alcohol problems in parents, school failure and early smoking as special risk factors.

Occupational groups at risk

That occupational environment affects drinking has been demonstrated. For example, publicans in the UK have a mortality rate 15 times the average. Reasons are self-evident: easy availability, social pressures, separation from family and social restraints. Men in the drinks industry have the highest consumption per person employed, i.e. 38 units weekly in comparison to the national average of 20 units weekly. Other high-risk groups are men at sea, hoteliers, financiers, armed forces, journalists and medical practitioners.

Brooke *et al.* (1993) have analysed case records of 144 doctors who attended the Maudsley Hospital over 20 years. Personality problems, i.e. poor adult adjustment and limited coping strategies, anxiety or depression were the most common routes into substance misuse. A history of neurotic disorder was associated with early onset of substance misuse. Consultant grade doctors had later onset of substance problems and fewer career difficulties. The need is primarily for confidential expertise (Lloyd, 1990).

Public health, policy and prevention

It has almost become a cliché to talk of prevention of alcohol problems in terms of 'everyone's business'. A comprehensive prevention policy comprises a range of overlapping components. These include controls on price, availability, the use, and marketing of alcohol, as well as educational and mass-media information campaigns. Evidence for their effectiveness has been gained from a number of countries. The findings suggest that no single measure or approach is sufficient to produce change, that some policies, e.g. taxes, may need to be internationally agreed. The host of professionals whose concerted effort is required to underpin such a movement make it not only the domain of health care providers and purchasers, but also government administrators, educationalists, research analysts, workplace management, community workers and others (Babor *et al.*, 1986; Royal College of General Practitioners, 1986; Royal College of Psychiatrists, 1986; Royal College of Physicians, 1987; Moskovitz, 1989; Moser, 1991).

The 'Health for All' targets of the European member states of WHO (1992*c*) state that 'By the year 2000 the health-damaging consumption of dependence producing substances such as alcohol, tobacco and psychoactive drugs should have been significantly reduced in all Member States' and 'alcohol consumption should be reduced by 25%'.

The British 'Health of the Nation' document (Department of Health, 1992) focused on the opportunities for reducing excessive consumption, and stated that:

1. 'Health will be one of the factors which the Chancellor of the Exchequer will take into account in deciding the appropriate level of alcohol duties in any one year.'
2. 'The commitment within the framework of the family health service to the promotion of the sensible drinking message will be strengthened.'
3. 'An agreed format for the display of customer information on alcohol units at point of sale will be considered jointly with the alcohol trade association.'

4. 'There will be a new initiative to monitor the penetration of the sensible drinking message.'
5. 'Employers will continue to be encouraged to introduce workplace alcohol policies and to evaluate their impact.'
6. 'The expansion and improvement of voluntary sector service provision will be supported.'

The recognition that the relationship between per capita consumption and alcohol misuse and harm, which implied that most problems are rooted in the general population of drinkers rather than only in the severely dependent alcoholic, stimulated a new review of the ways and means by which reduction in consumption could be achieved (Kendell, 1979; Kendell *et al.*, 1983).

Price controls are one way. For, if all things are equal, an increase in the price of alcohol precipitates a decrease in consumption and harm. Furthermore, it is likely to be the heavier drinkers who are affected to a greater extent than moderate drinkers. On the other hand, it is estimated that harmonisation of taxes in the European community might lead to an increase of 30% in alcohol consumption in the UK.

Availability may be limited in a number of ways. Age limits for legal purchase of alcohol usually parallel voting age. The objective of an age limit is to limit damage resulting directly from alcohol and increase age of first use, thus diminishing the risk of later use. In North America increasing the minimum age has led to reduction of road traffic accidents in young drivers. Time of sale is another method of control. The increase in licensing hours in England and Wales in 1988 did not appear to affect alcohol consumption. However, in Sweden and Norway, Saturday closing produced decreases in public disorder, whereas Sunday opening in Australia increased traffic accidents. If retail outlets are limited, or sales curtailed dramatically, consumption and related problems decrease. A powerful example is the anti-alcohol campaign in the USSR between 1985 and 1987. Furthermore, if sales to intoxicated persons are barred, alcohol-related traffic accidents drop. Enforcement of controls can reduce alcohol-related problems, e.g. drunk driving and work-place campaigns can reduce accidents.

Research on the effect of advertising is equivocal and views as to how to curtail alcohol advertising conflict. It is worrying that research has indicated that advertising directed at young people produces an increased alcohol consumption. Imposing a levy on advertising, restricting advertising by industry, banning advertising completely or introducing regulatory controls on the drinks industry are options that have been instituted in different countries.

Alcohol education in schools has been shown to be ineffective unless accompanied by information about the social context in which drinking is likely to occur and training in coping strategies in such situations. Another important focus is primary care prevention, where the brief interventions described earlier can be optimally instituted. This is of proven effectiveness, and much under-utilised because of lack of training of primary carers in the techniques to equip them for this task.

Any realistic policy on prevention has to accept the drinks industry lobby, which in Britain provides 5% of total government income and spends £150.5 million on advertising. The number of outlets has increased with efforts to seek out new groups such as the young, women and family groups. In the US, billions of dollars are spent annually in advertising alcohol and to protect the industry against increasing controls or taxes.

The 'Health of the Nation' hints at remedial action whereas there is some evidence to react with greater confidence. For instance, as discussed earlier, increasing alcohol taxes, raising the minimum legal drinking age and increasing enforcement of drinking-driving laws are three areas where promising results have been obtained and that could have been incorporated into the document. The behavioural approach in training school-age children to resist social pressures may be another promising strategy.

Conclusion

The preoccupation with getting 'alcoholics better treatment' has faded. Drinking can be destructive prior to the individual ever becoming dependent. Reduction of alcohol problems requires intervention at an individual, community, national and international levels. A key to intervention is training as attitudes may change in response to education and confidence with increased skill (Glass-Crome, 1992; Tober &·Raistrick, 1990; Canadian Medical Association Journal, 1991; Rowland et al., 1987). Models of implementing treatment and service delivery have been refined by psychiatrists, psychologists, sociologists, historians and economists, who have underlined the worth of new approaches. In the alcohol problems field science and politics are fused, so that without a credible national alcohol policy progress will be stunted (Edwards et al., 1993, 1994; Glass, 1994).

Appendix: Questionnaires

Table 9A.1. *The WHO core screening instrument*

1. How often do you have a drink containing alcohol?				
NEVER	MONTHLY OR LESS	2–4 TIMES A MONTH	2–3 TIMES A WEEK	4 OR MORE TIMES A WEEK

2. How many drinks containing alcohol do you have on a typical day when you are drinking?

    1 OR 2   3 OR 4   5 OR 6   7–9   10 OR MORE

3. How often do you have 6 or more drinks on one occasion?

    NEVER   LESS THAN MONTHLY   MONTHLY   WEEKLY   DAILY OR ALMOST DAILY

4. How often during the last year have you found it difficult to get the thought of alcohol out of your mind?

    NEVER   LESS THAN MONTHLY   MONTHLY   WEEKLY   DAILY OR ALMOST DAILY

5. How often during the last year have you found that you were not able to stop drinking once you have started?

    NEVER   LESS THAN MONTHLY   MONTHLY   WEEKLY   DAILY OR ALMOST DAILY

6. How often during the last year have you been unable to remember what happened the night before because you had been drinking?

    NEVER   LESS THAN MONTHLY   MONTHLY   WEEKLY   DAILY OR ALMOST DAILY

7. How often during the last year have you needed a first drink in the morning to get yourself going after a heavy drinking session?

    NEVER   LESS THAN MONTHLY   MONTHLY   WEEKLY   DAILY OR ALMOST DAILY

8. How often during the last year have you had a feeling of guilt or remorse after drinking?

    NEVER   LESS THAN MONTHLY   MONTHLY   WEEKLY   DAILY OR ALMOST DAILY

9. Have you or someone else been injured as a result of your drinking?

    NO   YES, BUT NOT IN THE LAST YEAR   YES, DURING THE LAST YEAR

10. Has a relative or friend or a doctor or other health worker, been concerned about your drinking or suggested you cut down?

    NO   YES, BUT NOT IN THE LAST YEAR   YES, DURING THE LAST YEAR

Scoring for the WHO core screening instrument

Item 1:	Never	=0
	Monthly or less	=1
	2–4 times a month	=2
	2–3 times a week	=3
	4 or more times a week	=4
Item 2:	1–2 drinks	=0
	3–4 drinks	=1
	5–6 drinks	=2
	7–9 drinks	=3
	10+ drinks	=4
Item 3–8:	Never	=0

	Less than monthly	=1
	Monthly	=2
	Weekly	=3
	Daily or almost daily	=4
Items 9 & 10:	No	=0
	Yes, but not in the last year	=0
	Yes, during the last year	=4

The maximum possible score is 40.

Table 9A.2. *Severity of Alcohol Dependence Questionnaire (SADQ)*

AGE ....

SEX ....

First of all, we would like you to recall a recent month when you were drinking heavily in a way which, for you, was fairly typical of a heavy drinking period. Please fill in the month and the year.

MONTH .... YEAR ....

We would like to know more about your drinking during this time and during the other periods when your drinking was similar. We want to know how often you experienced certain feelings. Please reply to each statement by putting a circle around ALMOST NEVER or SOMETIMES or OFTEN or NEARLY ALWAYS after each question.

PLEASE ANSWER EVERY QUESTION

First we want to know about the physical symptoms that you have experienced first thing in the morning during these typical periods of heavy drinking.

1. During a heavy drinking period, I wake up feeling sweaty.
   ALMOST NEVER   SOMETIMES   OFTEN   NEARLY ALWAYS
2. During a heavy drinking period, my hands shake first thing in the morning.
   ALMOST NEVER   SOMETIMES   OFTEN   NEARLY ALWAYS
3. During a heavy drinking period, my whole body shakes violently first thing in the morning if I don't have a drink.
   ALMOST NEVER   SOMETIMES   OFTEN   NEARLY ALWAYS
4. During a heavy drinking period, I wake up absolutely drenched in sweat.
   ALMOST NEVER   SOMETIMES   OFTEN   NEARLY ALWAYS

The following statements refer to moods and states of mind you may have experienced first thing in the morning during these periods of heavy drinking.

5. When I'm drinking heavily, I dread waking up in the morning.
   ALMOST NEVER   SOMETIMES   OFTEN   NEARLY ALWAYS
6. During a heavy drinking period, I am frightened of meeting people first thing in the morning.
   ALMOST NEVER   SOMETIMES   OFTEN   NEARLY ALWAYS
7. During a heavy drinking period, I feel at the edge of despair when I awake.
   ALMOST NEVER   SOMETIMES   OFTEN   NEARLY ALWAYS
8. During a heavy drinking period, I feel very frightened when I awake.
   ALMOST NEVER   SOMETIMES   OFTEN   NEARLY ALWAYS

The following statements also refer to the recent peiod when your drinking was heavy, and to periods like it.

9. During a heavy drinking period, I like to have a morning drink.
   ALMOST NEVER   SOMETIMES   OFTEN   NEARLY ALWAYS
10. During a heavy drinking period, I always gulp my first few morning drinks down as quickly as possible.
    ALMOST NEVER   SOMETIMES   OFTEN   NEARLY ALWAYS
11. During a heavy drinking period, I drink in the morning to get rid of the shakes.
    ALMOST NEVER   SOMETIMES   OFTEN   NEARLY ALWAYS
12. During a heavy drinking period, I have a very strong craving for a drink when I awake.
    ALMOST NEVER   SOMETIMES   OFTEN   NEARLY ALWAYS

Again the following statement refers to the recent period of heavy drinking and the periods like it.

13. During a heavy drinking period, I drink more than a quarter of a bottle of spirits per day (four doubles or one bottle of wine or four pints of beer).
    ALMOST NEVER   SOMETIMES   OFTEN   NEARLY ALWAYS
14. During a heavy drinking period, I drink more than half a bottle of spirits per day (or two bottles of wine or eight pints of beer).
    ALMOST NEVER   SOMETIMES   OFTEN   NEARLY ALWAYS
15. During a heavy drinking period, I drink more than one bottle of spirits per day (or four bottles of wine or 15 pints of beer).
    ALMOST NEVER   SOMETIMES   OFTEN   NEARLY ALWAYS
16. During a heavy drinking period, I drink more than two bottles of spirits per day (or eight bottles of wine or 30 pints of beer).
    ALMOST NEVER   SOMETIMES   OFTEN   NEARLY ALWAYS

IMAGINE THE FOLLOWING SITUATION
1. You have been COMPLETELY off drink for a FEW WEEKS.
2. You then drink VERY HEAVILY for TWO DAYS.

HOW WOULD YOU FEEL THE MORNING AFTER THOSE TWO DAYS OF HEAVY DRINKING?
17. I would start to sweat.
    NOT AT ALL   SLIGHTLY   MODERATELY   QUITE A LOT
18. My hands would shake.
    NOT AT ALL   SLIGHTLY   MODERATELY   QUITE A LOT
19. My body would shake.
    NOT AT ALL   SLIGHTLY   MODERATELY   QUITE A LOT
20. I would be craving for a drink.
    NOT AT ALL   SLIGHTLY   MODERATELY   QUITE A LOT

10

Schizophrenia

ROBIN M. MURRAY

The concept of schizophrenia

The development of the concept

In the early nineteenth century many psychiatrists believed in the existence of a single unitary psychosis, 'Einheitpsychose', which could manifest itself in various forms (see Scharfetter, 1975). Then, in 1851, the French psychiatrist Falret delineated *folie circulaire* or manic depressive psychosis, and shortly thereafter his compatriot Morel applied the term *démence précoce* to a deteriorating psychosis in a patient whose withdrawal, bizarre mannerisms, and personal neglect had begun in adolescence. Hecker subsequently employed the term hebephrenia for a similar picture, and in 1874 Kahlbaum published a monograph on catatonia, which he described as a cyclical condition characterised by stereotyped movement, mannerisms, and occasional outbursts of intense excitement, automatic obedience, negativism, and stupor. Kahlbaum considered hebephrenia and catatonia quite distinct from one another and also from paranoia, a term that he reserved for those with primary systematised delusions (see the article by Altschule, 1976).

Emil Kraepelin (1896, 1919) brought hebephrenia, catatonia, and paranoia together into the single disease entity of dementia praecox, the characteristics of which included hallucinations, delusions, a decrease in attention towards the outside world, lack of curiosity, disorder of thought, lack of insight and judgement, emotional blunting, negativism and stereotypes. Kraepelin believed that the disease usually had its onset in early adult life (hence 'praecox') and generally, though not invariably, progressed to a pervasive impairment of cognitive and behavioural function (hence 'dementia').

The Swiss psychiatrist Eugene Bleuler (1911) did not regard dementia praecox as a disease *per se*, but spoke instead of 'the group of schizophrenias', a term he introduced because 'the disconnection or splitting of the psychic functions is an outstanding feature'. Bleuler distinguished primary symptoms – altered associations (thought disorder), affective blunting, ambivalence, and autism (a turning away from the external environment into a private world of fantasy) from secondary symptoms such as delusions and hallucinations, which he considered could occur in other illnesses. Unfortunately, Bleuler's primary symptoms were so difficult to define that they allowed clinicians a great deal of diagnostic latitude.

Table 10.1. *Schneider's first rank symptoms*

Auditory hallucinations of specific type
(a) Audible thoughts: voices repeating or anticipating the patient's thoughts out loud
(b) Two or more voices discussing the patient in the third person
(c) Voices commenting on the patient's behaviour

Thought interference of specific type
(a) Thought withdrawal
(b) Thought insertion
(c) Thought broadcasting so that thoughts are conveyed to others

Feeling, impulses or acts experienced as being under external control
Delusional perception (a form of primary delusion): an unshakeable belief arising in an unaccountable manner from some commonplace event

Schneider's criteria

The most influential attempt at a more precise definition of schizophrenia has been that of Kurt Schneider (1950), who regarded certain symptoms as being of *first rank* importance in differentiating schizophrenia from other conditions. Schneider made no theoretical claims for his first rank symptoms, but empirically considered that whenever any were found in the absence of organic disease or drug intoxication, one could make a diagnosis of schizophrenia. However, all of Schneider's first rank symptoms have the distinct quality that Jaspers referred to as 'non-understandable' (Table 10.1).

Wing and his colleagues (1974, 1978) have described first rank symptoms, and how to elucidate them, in detail. Thus, Wing (1978) states 'Typically thought insertion is described by the patient in terms of some causal idea, such as a radio set implanted in the brain, or rays directed from another planet, or telepathy . . .' Similarly, delusions of control are often elaborated thus: 'the patient says that someone else's words are coming out using his voice, or that his handwriting is not his own, or that he is a zombie or robot whose very movement is determined by some alien power'. Another symptom of discriminating power is delusional perception, in which a fully fledged delusion arises from some occurrence that others would regard as quite normal, e.g. a nurse passing an innocent remark about the weather conveyed to one patient the certainty that he was going to be murdered.

Schneider's criteria have been criticised as being both too narrow and insufficiently specific. Mellor (1970), for instance, studied chronically hospitalised patients who had been originally diagnosed as schizophrenic, and found that only 79% were known to have ever had any first rank symptoms. In the International Pilot Study on Schizophrenia (IPSS) carried out in nine countries, only 58% of 1202 acute patients with a hospital diagnosis of schizophrenia had one or more first rank symptoms (World Health Organization, 1973). The IPSS also demonstrated that first rank symptoms can occur in non-schizophrenic patients, especially those suffering from mania.

The frequency of different symptoms in the 306 most typical schizophrenic patients in the IPSS is shown in Table 10.2.

Table 10.2. *Frequency of symptoms in 306 concordant schizophrenics in the International Pilot Study on Schizophrenia (%)*

Lack of insight	97
Auditory hallucinations	74
Ideas of reference	70
Suspiciousness	66
Flatness of affect	66
Delusional mood	64
Delusions of persecution	64
Thought alienation	52
Thoughts spoken aloud	50

Acute and chronic symptoms

First rank symptoms are most obvious in the acute phase of schizophrenia and may be accompanied by other less specific but none the less bizarre delusions of, for example, a paranoid, religious, or sexual nature. Patients may also suffer perceptual abnormalities such as faces changing shape, experience odd smells or tastes (e.g. of blood or poison), have somatic hallucinations (e.g. of a sexual nature) or, less commonly, visual hallucinations. The onset of schizophrenia may also be characterised by delusional mood consisting of intense puzzlement with familiar surroundings seeming strange, relationships seeming changed, and a feeling that something inexplicable or sinister is going on.

Patients may show derailment of thought or the so-called 'knight's-move thinking', and illogical speech may deteriorate to the point where it becomes incoherent. There may be dislocation of words or, occasionally, the creation of new private words (neologisms), sometimes by the condensation of others, e.g. a patient whose initials were K.A.O. described his personal philosophy as Kaosophy. Schizophrenic patients may also give private idiosyncratic meanings to words that already exist. Sometimes speech becomes quite empty and devoid of meaning (poverty of content). Although all of these abnormalities are conventionally referred to as *formal thought disorder*, strictly speaking there are disorders of speech from which abnormality of thought is inferred.

Nayani & David (1995) have recently shown how the schizophrenic experiences appears to gradually 'colonise' the healthy parts of the mind. In particular, they describe how delusional explanations gradually become more complex and bizarre. In this way, one of the author's patients interpreted the ordinary anxiety-related experience of tightness of the throat as 'a penis being forced down my throat and suffocating me'.

Positive symptoms such as those emphasised by Schneider are easier to elicit and to measure reliably than negative symptoms, but the latter are more persistent and are probably of more serious prognostic importance. Negative symptoms include social withdrawal, emotional blunting, underactivity, lack of initiative and motivation, apathy, poverty of speech, and slowness of thought and action. These symptoms, which often occur together, are sometimes known as 'schizophrenic defect state' (Carpenter *et al.*, 1988). Although they tend to be most prominent in chronic patients, they can be exacerbated during acute episodes and improve during remission. The relative importance of positive and negative symptoms are discussed by David & Appleby (1992).

The classical subtypes

Attempts at subdividing schizophrenia on clinical grounds have not been very successful but many psychiatrists still find the classical subdivisions of hebephrenic, catatonic, and paranoid schizophrenia a convenient descriptive shorthand (Tsuang & Winokur, 1974). *Hebephrenia* is used to describe profoundly disturbed young patients with marked thought disorder. The term *catatonia* is applied to those with pronounced psychomotor abnormalities – stupor or excitement, posturing including waxy flexibility, stereotypes, negativism. Catatonic schizophrenia should be diagnosed with caution and always in the presence of other more typical symptoms, not only because it has become much less common in the industrialised world but also because catatonic symptoms may occur in both affective disorder and neurological conditions such as encephalitis lethargica.

Paranoid schizophrenia refers to those whose mental state is dominated by systematised delusions whether of persecution, grandiosity, fantastic or religious nature. Patients with paranoid schizophrenia are less likely to have pronounced thought disorder or to progress to a defect state, perhaps because they frequently have a later onset. Sometimes the term paraphrenia is used to describe those who develop this syndrome very late in life; it is more common in women and in the deaf whose handicap may render them particularly susceptible to ideas of reference and persecution.

Many regard the differences between these three classical subtypes as of a pathoplastic nature determined by age of onset. Patients can change their predominant symptomatology on successive admissions.

Nuclear and peripheral schizophrenia

Ways of classifying patients with functional psychosis who do not fit easily into the classical concepts of schizophrenia or affective disorder are discussed in detail in Chapter 11. Suffice it to say here that a great deal of controversy has focused on whether patients with both schizophrenia and affective symptoms should be considered within the limits of schizophrenia. Kasanin (1933) coined the term 'schizoaffective psychosis' for cases with a sudden onset and marked emotional turmoil, while Langfeldt (1939) distinguished between *process schizophrenia* (roughly equivalent to Kraepelin's dementia praecox) and *schizophreniform* illness with precipitating factors, a strong affective component, often disturbance of consciousness, and on the whole a good prognosis. Numerous other terms have been used, but the status of such individuals remains a persistent enigma. Because of the frequency of affective disorder in their families and their remitting course, many regard these patients as having a variant of affective disorder. Leonhard (1959) believes that they constitute a distinct third group of 'cycloid psychoses', while others consider them on a continuum between schizophrenia and affective disorders (see the papers by Procci, 1976; Pope & Lipinski, 1978; Crow, 1990).

Similar difficulties have been encountered with those patients on the borderline between schizophrenia and neurosis and personality disorder. In the rare cases in which *simple* schizophrenia is diagnosed, the diagnosis is based not so much on positive symptoms as on a gradual deterioration in personality with increasing emotional bluntness; occasional brief psychotic episodes are used to substantiate the diagnosis. A 'borderline syndrome' was proposed by Grinker and his colleagues (1968) to describe young patients without delusions who have repeated histrionic episodes and who show 'an ego alien quality to any transient psychotic-like behaviour'. The genetic studies of Rosenthal and Kety (p. 293) have suggested that borderline schizophrenia may be a real entity; their criteria are, however, quite different from those of Grinker.

Criticism of the concept

Criticism of the concept of schizophrenia developed in the 1960s with the 'antipsychiatrists' such as Thomas Szasz and R. D. Laing who regarded schizophrenia as a medical fiction invented for the needs of society, relatives, and psychiatrists rather than sufferers. Such arguments have been admirably dissected by Clare (1976). Criticism has also come from sociologists like Scheff (1974) who drew attention to the negative aspects of receiving a diagnosis of schizophrenia, and considered that many of the symptoms were a consequence of being labelled as mad. Certainly once an individual is diagnosed as schizophrenic his relations with family, employers, and doctors can be considerably altered, and the adverse effects of long-term hospitalisation are well established (Wing & Brown, 1970). It is easy to conceive how a social reaction might pressurise an individual into deviancy, but as Wing *et al.* (1974) states: 'it is difficult to imagine how a similar reaction would force him to adopt the central schizophrenic syndrome since this would need special coaching from an expert'.

Psychologists have also made assaults on the concept of schizophrenia. Rosenhan and colleagues (1973) managed to get themselves admitted to 12 American mental hospitals and diagnosed schizophrenic merely by declaring that they heard voices saying 'empty', 'hollow' and 'thud'. This study, which illustrated the dangers of both sloppy diagnostic practice and 'labelling', is a useful polemic against the practice of bad psychiatry. The issue of whether schizophrenic symptoms are qualitatively different from normal human behaviour has not been resolved. The Eysencks proposed a dimensional hypothesis for psychosis, as has Claridge (1972), who regards the schizophrenic predisposition as a continuously variable personality dimension.

The thesis of Mary Boyle (1990) is that schizophrenia did exist a century ago when it was a secondary consequence of viral and other neurological disorders, but although such neurological disorders have largely been eliminated, the concept is now erroneously applied to non-organic conditions.

Some psychiatrists react to such criticisms by totally denying their validity, and by reasserting a simplistic medical disease model of schizophrenia. However, this is less than satisfactory since there remains widespread confusion regarding the meaning, boundaries, and even value of the term schizophrenia. Some authorities define schizophrenia on the basis of symptomatology and some by characteristic course, while some consider it merely a syndrome and others regard it as a disease process not necessarily revealed in overt behaviour. The origin of the confusion is that we have failed to discover either the aetiology or pathogenesis of the condition(s) referred to under the term schizophrenia, and it is likely that our confusion will continue until the aetiology and pathogenesis are established.

Operational definitions

One response has been a proliferation of operational definitions of schizophrenia, most of them based on the classification systems outlined in Chapter 3. The longest established is the Present State Examination (PSE/CATEGO) system of Wing *et al.* (1974), in which the criteria are based mainly on Schneider's first rank symptoms.

The PSE/CATEGO system was used to investigate the fact that for many years the first admission rate for schizophrenia was considerably higher in the United States than in England and Wales. The suspicion that these differences were due to different diagnostic practices prompted a study in which patients in New York and London were interviewed by researchers using the PSE. The results were as expected; hospital psychiatrists in New York did diagnose schizophrenia more frequently than their counterparts in London but the project psychiatrists employing the PSE diagnosed the disorder in much the same proportions in each city (Cooper *et al.*, 1972).

A similar but wider study was carried out under the auspices of the World Health Organization (1973*a*). This International Pilot Study on Schizophrenia (IPSS) used the PSE to examine 1202 patients in nine countries. The three European and four developing countries had similar criteria for diagnosing schizophrenia, but once again the prevailing concept was broader in the United States, and also in Russia where categories such as sluggish and periodic schizophrenia were employed.

Since that time, a curious change has occurred. The predominantly European-based international concept of schizophrenia has remained relatively unchanged, becoming operationalised in ICD-10 (WHO, 1993). However, American psychiatrists have produced a series of stricter operational definitions with the paradoxical result that the American concept of schizophrenia is now narrower than that in use in Europe (Andreasen & Carpenter, 1993). The more important of these definitions have included the Research Diagnostic Criteria or RDC (Spitzer *et al.*, 1978*b*) and the DSM-III, DSM-IIIR and DSM-IV (American Psychiatric Association, 1980–1994). Like the PSE/CATEGO system, these definitions emphasise Schneiderian phenomenology but unlike it they incorporate a longitudinal component; thus DSM-IV demands the presence of active symptoms for one month (like ICD-10) and some signs of disturbance persisting for six months (unlike ICD-10).

Brockington *et al.* (1978), who compared ten different operational definitions of schizophrenia as applied to 119 psychotic patients, found that the number who qualified as schizophrenic on the various criteria ranged from 3 to 45! There were wide variations in the reliability, concordance and predictive powers of different criteria; thus Schneider's first rank symptoms were only weak predictors of future course while the RDC were relatively successful in identifying the poor prognosis group. The investigators concluded that 'inarticulate confusion' has been replaced 'by a babel of precise but differing formulations of the same concept'.

Thus, the situation is like that of the hungry visitor to the USA who has a bewildering choice of hamburgers from different fast food restaurants; each company's hamburger is highly *reliable* but slightly different from its rival's (e.g. McDonald's versus Burger King). However, the visitor cannot tell whether the hamburgers contain real meat or an artificial construct made of soya bean, i.e. have any *validity*. Similarly, there is no way of telling whether there is a biological entity at the core of any of the slightly different definitions of schizophrenia.

The current position

The current classification of the functional psychoses is extremely unsatisfactory, but there is no viable alternative to the use of the term schizophrenia. In the absence of evidence to the contrary, schizophrenia is best considered as a syndrome that may cover several different conditions. A relatively restrictive concept should be applied conservatively both in the interests of diagnostic homogeneity and because of the adverse consequences of labelling doubtful cases as schizophrenic. Schneider's first rank symptoms are included in most contemporary definitions but schizophrenia should not be diagnosed solely on the basis of first rank symptoms if other evidence points to an affective disorder. Furthermore, first rank symptoms may have less biological validity than other definitions (McGuffin *et al.*, 1984), and their transient presence does not necessarily imply a poor prognosis (Brockington *et al.*, 1978; Pope & Lipinski, 1978). Thus, the length of the symptoms and the degree of incapacity should also be taken into account in the diagnostic formulation, as should the presence of negative symptoms. The ICD-10 criteria represent a reasonable compromise but, given the range of currently available operational definitions and uncertainty about validity, some investigators advocate a 'polydiagnostic' approach in research; in the so-called OPCRIT system, clinical data are collected in sufficient detail for several definitions to be applied.

Differential diagnosis

The diagnosis should not be made simply on positive findings of schizophrenia, but must include an absence of features more characteristic of other syndromes. The conditions to be excluded include the following:

Drug-induced psychosis

Psychostimulant drugs such as amphetamine and cocaine can produce a psychosis mimicking schizophrenia (Davison, 1976). Indeed, the symptoms of amphetamine psychosis can be identical with those of paranoid schizophrenia (Connell, 1958). Amphetamine psychosis is most frequently observed in addicts who have consumed enormous quantities of the drug over prolonged periods, and usually resolves within a few days of ceasing the abuse.

Psychoses can also be induced by hallucinogens such as LSD, 'ecstasy', and phenylcyclidine (PCP or 'angel dust'). LSD tends to cause visual rather than auditory hallucinations while PCP, unlike other hallucinogens, can mimic negative symptoms. Debate continues over whether individuals who develop drug-related psychoses are constitutionally predisposed, and there is some evidence that patients who develop apparently genuine schizophrenia following drug abuse break down at an earlier state than those who have not taken drugs (Breakey *et al.*, 1974). Tsuang *et al.* (1982) contrasted patients with drug-associated psychosis whose illnesses lasted more and less than six months respectively. Those with the longer-lasting psychoses had more 'schizophrenic' symptoms, poorer premorbid personalities, and greater familial risks of psychosis. Clearly this group had more affinity to schizophrenia proper.

There is some limited evidence that heavy cannabis consumption is associated with an increased risk of later psychosis (Andreason *et al.*, 1987). McGuire *et al.* (1994) recently showed that the relatives of psychotic probands with a positive urine test for cannabis had a significantly higher morbid risk of schizophrenia than did relatives of probands with a negative urine test. One interpretation is that cannabis may precipitate psychosis in those carrying some susceptibility gene(s).

Alcoholic hallucinosis may also be mistaken for schizophrenia and once again there is dispute over whether this arises in those who have a genetic predisposition to schizophrenia (Cutting, 1978a).

Organic conditions

Distinction can usually be made from psychosis associated with gross cerebral pathology, infection or metabolic disorder because of the presence of clouding of consciousness, physical signs or laboratory abnormalities in such conditions (Lishman, 1987), but any newly presenting schizophrenic should receive a careful work-up including EEG and CT or, if available, MRI scan. In a small proportion (around 4–6%) definite organic pathology will be found (Davison & Bagley, 1969; Johnstone, 1994). The best established relationship is with temporal lobe epilepsy, which Slater *et al.* (1963) established may cause 'symptomatic schizophrenia' (Flor-Henry, 1976). Most puerperal psychoses are not schizophrenic, but a minority are, or later clearly become so (see Chapter 17).

Paranoid states

The exact classification of the paranoid states has long been a matter of controversy (Kendler, 1980; Post, 1982) and some authorities regard the differences between paranoid personality, paranoia, and paranoid schizophrenia as merely a matter of degree. Individuals with *paranoid personality* are generally rigid and inflexible, suspicious, and morbidly sensitive. They may be of rather dominant nature and their friendships of short duration. The so-called overvalued idea or *idée fixe* may be prominent. *Paranoia* (or '*delusional disorder*') is a relatively rare condition (Winokur, 1977) characterised by an intricate, complex, and elaborate delusional system without hallucinations. The delusions are systematised, firmly knit, and more or less isolated so that the rest of the personality remains relatively intact. Paranoia is rare before 30 years of age. Many paranoiacs are single, and few people bother with them provided they are not dangerous to themselves or others. But occasionally a paranoiac may consider that he or she has unique abilities and may seek political expression of his or her views.

In erotomania, also known as Clerambault's Syndrome (Enoch & Trethowan, 1979), an individual, usually female, presents ideas that she is loved by another person who does not make a direct avowal, but indicates his love in many indirect ways. The person cast in the role of lover is often of higher status, and is pestered by unwelcome letters or visits.

Morbid jealousy is characterised by delusions of marital infidelity and a search for evidence of adultery. Spouses may be followed or their underwear repeatedly examined for seminal stains. Improbable accusations may be succeeded by violence and occasional homicide of the wife or her supposed lover. Morbid jealousy may occur in paranoid states, schizophrenia, alcoholism or depressive psychosis (Shepherd, 1961).

In *folie à deux* a delusion is transmitted from one person to another so that the second comes to share the psychopathology of the first. Usually the two persons are living together, perhaps as husband and wife, or mother and daughter. The person to whom the delusions are transmitted is often passive and dependent, and usually recovers within a few months if the two are separated. *Folie à deux* and the other eponymous conditions have been well reviewed by Enoch & Trethowan (1979).

Other psychotic conditions

The boundaries between schizophrenia and affective disorder can be vague. One should be particularly aware of the intensifications of affect that may be an early symptom of schizophrenia, and of the occurrence of first rank symptoms and of over-inclusive thinking in manics. Even when the greatest care is taken, patients diagnosed on their initial hospitalisation as schizophrenic will sometimes need to be reclassified as having affective disorder and vice versa.

It may at times be difficult to differentiate between obsessive compulsive disorder and schizophrenia but a careful history should demonstrate that even the most bizarre obsessional thought does not have the quality of absolute certainty of a delusion.

Epidemiology

Schizophrenia typically presents in late adolescence or in early adult life; prepubertal children rarely manifest Schneiderian symptoms (Pilowsky & Murray, 1991). Males have an earlier onset than females – the mean age of first admission is about 22 years for men and 27 years for women (Castle & Murray, 1991). Female schizophrenics also tend to have milder illnesses with fewer negative symptoms and a better outcome than males, and as a result they are less likely to meet the strictest diagnostic criteria. Thus, Castle *et al.* (1993*a*) found in an incidence study in London that while the male:female ratio for broadly defined schizophrenia (e.g. according to ICD-9) was roughly equal, the ratio rose to over 2:1 for cases meeting the narrower DSM-III criteria.

Part of the reason for this is that the old DSM-III criteria excluded late-onset cases, and 38% of females but only 16% of males in this series had their first psychiatric contact with schizophrenia-like psychosis after age 45 (Castle *et al.*, 1993*a*). These late-onset cases showed more hallucinations and delusions and less thought disorder than early-onset cases (Howard *et al.*, 1993).

Social and economic differences

Most studies in developed countries suggest a life-time risk of schizophrenia of between 0.5% and 1%, the former being the average risk of narrowly defined schizophrenia (e.g. DSM-IV), the latter that of broader definitions (e.g. ICD-9).

In 1939, Faris & Dunham reported higher admission rates for schizophrenia in the central areas of lowest socio-economic status in Chicago than in the higher status suburbs. This pattern has been confirmed in other large cities in the United States and Europe. Two main explanations have been proposed. The first, 'the drift hypothesis', claims that schizophrenics and pre-schizophrenics are downwardly mobile, either because of their social and occupational incompetence, or because they actively seek out anonymity and isolation in the decaying areas of large cities. Goldberg & Morrison (1963) claimed support for 'the drift hypothesis' by finding that hospitalised schizophrenics were in lower status occupations than their fathers.

Until relatively recently, most authorities favoured 'the drift hypothesis' but there has been a revival of interest in the second theory. This 'social causation hypothesis' proposes that a poor social environment either causes schizophrenia or favours its onset in the predisposed by exposing them to factors such as poverty, poor nutrition and health care, or inadequate education. Recent studies from Sweden (Lewis *et al.*, 1992) and England (Takei *et al.*, 1995) suggest that the risk of schizophrenia may be greater amongst those born or brought up in urban areas. Similarly, Castle *et al.* (1993*b*) suggest that some factor(s) associated with birth/upbringing in poor urban areas may increase risk.

Geographic and temporal variations?

The question of whether the incidence of schizophrenia varies by time and place has been hotly debated. The 'recency' debate was initiated by Hare (1983), who noted that admissions to hospital for insanity greatly increased throughout the nineteenth century in the UK and USA. Hare postulated that this reflected an increase in the incidence of schizophrenia, only to be countered by Scull (1984) who claimed that the asylums were built simply because the newly industrialised society was less able to cope with the mentally ill than the largely agricultural society it replaced.

A new twist to this argument has been added by reports from Scotland, England, Denmark and Australia (see the paper by Gupta & Murray, 1991) that both first admissions and first contacts for schizophrenia have considerably declined over the last 25 years. In a mirror image of the 'recency' debate, protagonists (e.g. Der *et al.*, 1990) suggest that there has been a genuine decline while latter-day nosocomialists claim that the figures are simply an artefact of changes in diagnostic or treatment practices (Kendell *et al.*, 1993).

There is general agreement that schizophrenia is a universal phenomena though there remains argument as to whether its frequency and characteristics are the same in different countries. The World Health Organization (Jablensky *et al.*, 1992) attempted to resolve this issue by mounting a cross-national study of incidence. The study is frequently quoted as showing that there was no significant variation between countries in the incidence of nuclear schizophrenia as defined by the PSE/CATEGO system. However, it is more correct to say that the study had insufficient power to detect significant differences. Furthermore, when a 'broad' concept of schizophrenia was examined, the incidence varied fourfold.

Certainly, a well-replicated finding is that certain migrant groups have a higher than expected incidence of schizophrenia. As long ago as 1932, Odegaard found that schizophrenia occurred more commonly among Norwegians who emigrated to America than those who were left behind. The most recent, and best documented example is that of Afro-Caribbean people who migrated to the UK among whom high rates of schizophrenia have been reported frequently (Harrison *et al.*, 1988). Initially it was thought that these findings might be consequent upon underestimation of the number of immigrants in the population but studies using operational criteria for schizophrenia and population registers have replicated the earlier findings. Thus, a London study showed that the first contact rates of RDC and DSM-IIIR schizophrenia over a 20-year period were between 4 and 8 times greater among Afro-Caribbean than white individuals (Wessely *et al.*, 1991).

A number of studies (e.g. Susser *et al.*, 1994) have demonstrated that schizophrenia in less-developed countries tends to have a more acute onset and a more benign outcome than in more industrialised countries; the reason for this is unknown. It may be due to better family support or to easier integration into the rather simpler work environment in less-developed countries. However, another possibility is that acute remitting psychoses constitute a higher proportion of schizophrenia in the less-developed world.

Genetics

The evidence for a genetic predisposition to schizophrenia comes from three main sources:

Studies of relatives

The lifetime expectancy for schizophrenia, broadly diagnosed, in the general population is less than 1%, but much higher figures have been found in relatives of schizophrenic patients (Gottesman, 1991). Children, both of whose parents have had schizophrenia, have as much as a 46% chance of developing the condition, but where only one parent was affected the average risk is around 12%. Siblings of a person with schizophrenia have an average risk of 8%. The risk for parents is about 5%, this relatively low risk being explained by the fact that it is the healthier parents who tend to reproduce.

The figures given above relate to older studies using broad definitions of schizophrenia. In the early 1980s these studies were challenged by two groups who claimed that when operational definitions were used schizophrenia was not familial (Pope *et al.*, 1982; Abrams & Taylor, 1983). However, Kendler & Diehl (1993), who have reviewed seven recent studies with improved methodology, conclude that although criteria such as DSM-IIIR produced lower risks in relatives, the general population rates are also lower, and the risk to the first-degree relatives of schizophrenics remains about 10 times higher than that in the general population.

One of the most convincing of modern studies is that of Kendler *et al.* (1993*a*), who carried out a case-controlled epidemiological study in rural Ireland based on all schizophrenic patients on the Roscommon County Case Register (*n*=265) and a matched random sample from the electoral register (*n*=150). The lifetime risk of schizophrenia in the first-degree relatives of the schizophrenics was 6.5% compared to 0.5% in the relatives of the controls.

Studies of twins

The increased frequency of schizophrenia in the families of patients is compatible with transmission of the disorder either through genes or the family culture. The significance of twin studies lies in the fact that monozygotic (MZ) twins have exactly the same genes while dizygotic (DZ) twins share, on average, only half their genes. If, therefore, pairs of MZ twins share the same psychopathology more often than DZ twins, this can be taken as evidence of a genetic contribution to the disorder. Studies based on population registers or consecutive hospital admissions have consistently shown higher concordance rates (i.e. both twins schizophrenic) for MZ than DZ twins. The rates for MZ twins have ranged from 35% in Tienari's study to 58% in Gottesman & Shields', and for DZ twins from the 9% reported by Pollin to the 26% found by Fischer. Gottesman *et al.* (1982) pooled the available figures to give a concordance rate of 47% for 261 MZ co-twins and 14% for 329 DZ co-twins. The most recent figures, from the Norwegian twin register using DSM-IIIR criteria, give concordance rates of 48% for MZ and 4% for DZ twins (Onstead *et al.*, 1991).

It has been suggested that MZ twins might be more likely to be exposed to the same predisposing rearing factors than DZ twins but evidence against such an explanation is derived from studies of twins reared apart. Gottesman *et al.* (1982) collected from the literature 17 such pairs of whom 11 were concordant for schizophrenia, a remarkably high figure. Kendler & Robinette (1983) provide a useful review on twin studies, concluding that they are not systematically biased, and that heredity accounts for at least two-thirds of the variance in liability to schizophrenia.

Studies of adoptees

Since an adopted individual receives his or her genes from one family, but life experiences as a member of another, adoptive studies can be used to disentangle genetic and environmental effects. Heston & Denney (1968) followed up 47 adopted-away offspring of chronic schizophrenic mothers and a well-matched control group of 50 adoptees born to mothers without psychiatric disorder; all the children had been separated from their mothers by the age of two weeks. There were five schizophrenics among the offspring of the schizophrenic mothers, none in the control group.

A large Danish-American study (Rosenthal *et al.*, 1971) examined the frequency of schizophrenia among the adopted-away offspring of parents who were known to have been schizophrenic, and among a carefully matched control group of adoptees whose biological parents were free of psychiatric illness. Diagnoses were made in a 'blind' fashion from case abstracts. Subjects could be rated as having acute or chronic schizophrenia, borderline schizophrenia, or personality disorder, and all these diagnoses were included under the rubric 'schizophrenia spectrum disorder'. Of the index cases 32% received the latter label compared with 18% of control adoptees. Three of the index offspring were definitely schizophrenic whereas not one of the 67 controls was so diagnosed.

As part of the same collaboration, Kety *et al.* (1975) 'blindly' rated assessments of the biological and adoptive relatives of 33 schizophrenic adoptees. There was a significant concentration of definite schizophrenia in the former but not in the latter group; 21% of the biological relatives fell into the schizophrenia spectrum compared to 5% of the adoptive relatives. To exclude the possibility that very early environmental effects could have explained these findings, Kety *et al.* (1976) examined the paternal half-siblings of index cases and found that they also had an increased risk of schizophrenia. Since these paternal half-siblings separated early in life and share neither intra-uterine nor early maternal influences this further bolsters the case for genetic transmission.

One criticism of the Kety/Rosenthal studies was the vagueness of the conditions that they included in the schizophrenia spectrum. Kendler & Gruenberg (1984) re-examined the 'Kety' interviews and categorised them according to DSM-III definitions. Schizotypal personality was more frequent in the biological than the adoptive relatives, suggesting that it is genetically related to schizophrenia.

Recently, Kety *et al.* (1994) reported an extension of the Danish-American studies to a population outside Copenhagen. Once again, schizophrenia was more common in the biological relatives of schizophrenic adoptees (4.1%) than in the biological relatives of control adoptees (0.5%).

A large adoption study is also being carried out in Finland by Tienari (1991). Nine per cent of the offspring of schizophrenic mothers and 1% of the offspring of control mothers have developed a psychotic illness. This study suggests an interaction between genes and early social environment in that the risk of psychosis was greatest in those offspring of schizophrenic mothers adopted into poorly functioning families.

Genetic models

Almost all authorities regard the genetic contribution as the most important of the known aetiological factors with estimates of heritability of liability ranging from 50 to 85%. What is transmitted in families includes a predisposition to such features as poor psychosocial functioning, suspiciousness and oddness as well as to psychotic illness. Kendler & Diehl (1993) reviewed seven studies that examined schizotypal personality and paranoid personality disorder, and reported that these were consistently higher in relatives of schizophrenics than controls.

Genetic models can be divided into three broad categories: Single Major Locus (SML), polygenic, and genetic heterogeneity. Statistical analyses suggest that SML models, even allowing for incomplete penetrance, do not explain the available data very well.

The polygenic multifactorial model states that many genes each of small effect combine with a variety of environmental factors, and that schizophrenia results once a critical threshold of liability is passed (Gottesman & Shields, 1982). Such models provide a better statistical fit than SML models but do not exclude the possibility of one or two major genes operating against a polygenic background.

Advocates of genetic heterogeneity propose that schizophrenia can be divided into different conditions each with a different aetiology. One possibility is that there are genetic and environmental damage aetiologies and that these may be crudely reflected in 'familial' and 'sporadic' cases (Murray et al., 1985). Others have argued that this oversimplifies a complex pattern of findings (McGuffin et al., 1987).

Two main approaches are being used to try to clarify the situation. The first seeks to find evidence of abnormality in the relatives of patients. Abnormalities of P300 latency and amplitude have been found in both schizophrenics and their unaffected relatives. Indeed, two studies (Blackwood et al., 1991; Frangou et al., 1994) found a bimodal distribution in the P300 latency in the unaffected relatives in multiple affected families suggesting that some of the unaffected relatives are carriers of the schizophrenia genotype. The relatives of patients with schizophrenia have also been reported to be more likely than controls to have abnormal eye movements (Holzman, 1988) and poor performance of complex motor tasks (Manschreck et al., 1982) and cognitive tests such as the Wisconsin Card Sorting test (Pogue-Geile et al., 1991).

The second strategy arises from the success of molecular genetics in identifying the causal genes for many medical disorders, e.g. cystic fibrosis, Huntington's chorea. Consequently, researchers have been carrying out a systematic search of the entire human genome using known markers spread over the various chromosomes (e.g. Vallada et al., 1995). Other researchers have been examining genes that are suspected of possible involvement in schizophrenia; such 'candidate genes' include the family of dopamine receptor genes, the serotonin receptor family, and various genes involved in brain development.

So far, only one replicable finding has been reported, and that using a traditional HLA marker; seven studies have reported a modest association between *HLA-A9* and schizophrenia (Wright et al., 1995). The meaning of this 15 years after it was first reported remains quite unclear. Recently, Wright et al. (1995) have claimed that schizophrenics show a deficit of *HLA-DR4*; since *DR4* is associated with increased risk of rheumatoid arthritis, this may be the explanation for the repeated finding that the two illnesses occur together less commonly than expected.

Early environmental hazards

Recent years have seen considerable interest in the idea that early hazards to the developing brain may increase the later risk of schizophrenia:

Obstetric complications

Many studies have examined the frequency of pregnancy and birth complications (collectively termed obstetric complications or OCs) in schizophrenics. Some of these have relied upon maternal recall (e.g. Lewis et al., 1989) but birth certificates and midwives reports have also been used (e.g. McNeil & Kaij, 1978) to provide more robust data. In total seven out of eight studies that examined birth records and nine out of 13 studies that relied on maternal recall, found OCs to be more common in the histories of schizophrenic patients than control samples.

A history of OCs has been reported more frequently in those schizophrenics without a family history of the disease (Cantor-Graae et al., 1994) giving rise to a controversy over whether the resultant cases are non-genetic 'phenocopies' (Murray et al., 1985). Higher rates have also been noted particularly in males with early onset (McGrath & Murray, 1995) particularly those who have shown premorbid abnormalities, cognitive deficits and negative symptoms (Rifkin et al., 1994).

The OCs implicated have included low birth weight, prematurity and 'small for dates' status, pre-eclampsia, prolonged labour and asphyxia. Overall, OCs, as generally defined, only double the risk of schizophrenia in the OCs noted or recorded, and are presumably only proxy indicators for more important events causing neuronal damage. The direction of causality has also been questioned since a pre-existing neural defect could cause perinatal complications, and it is possible that the postulated neurodevelopmental abnormality underlying schizophrenia (*vide infra*) may contribute to the increased rates of OCs (see the paper by McGrath & Murray, 1995).

Prenatal viral infection

One of the most consistently replicated epidemiological features of schizophrenia is the small but significant excess of winter–spring births found in the Northern hemisphere and the reverse in the Southern hemisphere (Bradbury & Miller, 1985). Various theories have been put forward to explain this stubborn association, the most widely accepted postulating a teratogenic agent such as infection, diet, or temperature, which impairs foetal brain development.

Prenatal exposure to influenza has been the focus of much research. In particular, several studies have suggested that fetuses exposed during the second trimester to the 1957 A2 influenza pandemic have an increased risk of schizophrenia (e.g. Mednick et al., 1988; O'Callaghan et al., 1991). This link with second trimester influenza exposure holds true when the relationship between influenza epidemics and schizophrenic births is assessed over several decades (Sham et al., 1992). However, the association has not always been replicated (see the paper by McGrath & Murray, 1995).

Brain structure and function

In 1976 Johnstone et al. showed that compared with controls, chronic schizophrenics have enlarged cerebral ventricles, a finding subsequently confirmed by numerous computerised tomography (CT) and magnetic resonance imaging (MRI) studies. Lateral and third ventricular enlargement are the most consistent neuroanatomical changes found in schizophrenia but many MRI studies also show a decrease in the volume of the temporal lobe and certain temporal structures such as the hippocampus (Suddath et al., 1990).

Neuroimaging studies of schizophrenics during their first episodes show similar abnormalities, and studies following up patients for up to eight years have shown no general trend to progression. This suggests that the findings are not artefacts of treatment or chronicity but reflect a static lesion present at or before the onset of the psychosis.

Post-mortem studies have shown that schizophrenic patients have slightly smaller and lighter brains (Bruton et al., 1990), and more recently these and MRI studies have also shown generalised cortical grey matter volume decrements of the order of 5–10% (Harvey et al., 1993).

A succession of studies have reported abnormalities at the histological level; these range from disarray of pyramidal cells in the hippocampus through displaced pre-alpha cells in the parahippocampal gyrus to neurones lying deeper than normal in the frontal and temporal cortex. These cytoarchitectural abnormalities are of such a kind that they suggest dysgenesis rather than degeneration (Akbarian et al., 1993).

This notion of dysgenesis is also supported by evidence that minor physical abnormalities (MPAs) of, for example, eyes, ears and mouth, occur in excess in schizophrenia; these anomalies serve as 'fossilised' evidence of a deviant foetal development (see McGrath & Murray, 1995). Abnormalities of dermatoglyphics (finger and palm prints) are another pointer to deviant early development.

The above evidence, plus the literature on obstetric complications and prenatal influenza reviewed earlier, has given rise to the neurodevelopmental hypothesis (Lewis & Murray, 1987; Weinberger, 1987; Murray, 1994) which states that a substantial proportion of schizophrenic patients have experienced a disturbance of the orderly development of the brain, decades before the symptomatic phase of the illness begins.

What is the cause of these abnormalities? Brain growth is largely under genetic control, and Reveley et al. (1982; 1984), using CT, found a high heritability for ventricular size in normal twins. However, schizophrenic twins had larger ventricles than their MZ non-schizophrenic co-twins; Suddath et al. (1990), using MRI, confirmed this. One interpretation is that a genetic factor contributes to ventricular enlargement in both twins and that environmental damage may further increase ventricular size in the twin who goes on to develop schizophrenia.

Not surprisingly, a number of studies have attempted to relate structural brain abnormalities to the experience of obstetric complications (OCs). Certainly, there is evidence from perinatal medicine to support the link between OCs (e.g. prematurity) and enlarged ventricles in the general population. However, a review of the salient studies reveals an inconsistent picture (Jones et al., 1994b; McGrath & Murray, 1995).

The antecedents of schizophrenia

It is not possible to conclude from studies of already manifest schizophrenics whether any abnormal findings reflect the cause or result of the illness. Consequently, researchers have studied individuals at high risk of the condition such as the children of schizophrenics. The best known of these 'high risk' studies is that of Mednick et al. (1987) in Denmark. These authors chose 200 pre-adolescent and teenage offspring of schizophrenic mothers and matched them with 100 low-risk children; the average age of both groups was 15 years and they were followed up for six years. By that time 20 of the high-risk children had had a psychiatric breakdown; this 'sick' group were distinguished particularly by a history of obstetric complications, and on the original testing had shown more deviant autonomic responsivity.

Schulsinger *et al.* (1984) confirmed that it is particularly those high-risk offspring who have suffered obstetric complications who develop schizophrenia. The same group (Cannon *et al.*, 1993) subsequently reported that genetic predisposition and obstetric complications both contribute to abnormal cerebral structure with the former particularly affecting the cortex, and the latter particularly ventricular size.

Other characteristics claimed as occurring more frequently in high-risk children include deficits in attention (see the paper by MacCrimmon *et al.*, 1980), poor motor co-ordination, soft neurological signs, and disturbance of interpersonal relationships. Fish (1977) suggested that these were all manifestations of an underlying 'pandysmaturation'.

However, only a minority of schizophrenics have parents with schizophrenia, and therefore there is uncertainty over how far one can generalise from 'high risk' studies. Other approaches have, therefore, been used to elucidate the antecedents of schizophrenia. Firstly, researchers have interviewed the mothers of schizophrenic patients and asked them, retrospectively, about the child's development. For example, Foerster *et al.* (1991a,b) noted that mothers recalled their preschizophrenic children as having shown developmental problems particularly with reading, and an excess of schizoid and schizotypal traits.

Secondly, researchers have gone back to the clinic records of those adult schizophrenics who were seen earlier by child psychiatrists. Thus, Jones *et al.* (1994a) reported that such preschizophrenic children showed lower IQ and poor scholastic performance. Cannon *et al.* (1995) found a continuity between childhood and adult symptoms with those children who had shown most anxiety and oversensitivity being prone to develop passivity symptoms while those who had poor peer relationships tended to develop blunted affect.

A particular novel approach was employed by Walker & Lewine (1990), who obtained videotapes of children who subsequently became schizophrenic, and 'blindly' compared the videos with those of their growing siblings. The preschizophrenics were more likely to show behavioural and motor abnormalities such as clumsiness or odd movements.

A fourth approach avoids the biases intrinsic to all the above studies by following up unselected samples of children into adult life. Thus, Jones *et al.* (1994a) examined the life histories of 4746 children who had been born one week in 1946 in the UK, and contacted 19 times by the age of 43 years. The 30 children who went on to develop schizophrenia had slightly delayed motor milestones; at age four, they were more likely to play alone than the other children, and by age seven they already performed more poorly on cognitive tests; they were especially likely to have had language difficulties.

Thus, it is clear that a proportion of schizophrenics show deficits in motor, cognitive, and social performance long before they develop psychotic symptoms. What is not clear is (a) whether or not there exists a distinct subgroup only that is typified by childhood abnormality, and (b) whether the childhood deficits are an early manifestation of a neurodevelopmental lesion or whether they are independent risk factors for later schizophrenia.

Social factors

Many investigators have examined the question of whether the behaviour of mothers of schizophrenics may have a causal role. Certainly the mothers are more concerned, more protective, and possibly more intrusive than control mothers, but these attitudes are likely to have developed as a reaction to an abnormal child. Most well-conducted enquiries (see Hirsch & Leff, 1975) have suggested that the characterisation of the mothers of schizophrenics as 'schizophrenogenic' cannot be sustained.

Considerable effort has been devoted to studying family life after the onset of psychosis: Brown et al. (1972) demonstrated that schizophrenics are highly responsive to the quality of the emotional relationship between them and the relative with whom they live. These workers could predict relapse by using an index of the emotions shown by the relative that expressed the amount of critical comment, hostility, and emotional over-involvement of that relative; during the nine months after discharge from hospital 58% of patients from houses with high 'expressed emotion' (high EE) relapsed as against only 16% from low 'expressed emotion' homes. Vaughn & Leff (1976) almost exactly replicated these results. However, there is no evidence that high EE is of importance in contributing to onset of schizophrenia.

Current stress can precipitate schizophrenic illness. Brown & Birley (1968) studied acute onset schizophrenics, and charted the occurrence of life events for the preceding three months; the schizophrenic patients experienced a significantly higher frequency of such events during the three-week period prior to the onset of their symptoms than did a matched group of non-schizophrenic controls. This was true even of independent events that could not have been caused by the patient becoming ill. Brown et al. (1972) suggest that life events serve to trigger the florid onset and reappearance of symptoms 'in those who are predisposed and are experiencing tense and difficult situations'. Numerous other studies (e.g. Bebbington et al., 1993) have confirmed a role for adverse life events but most authorities regard social adversity as operating on already predisposed individuals to trigger onset or relapse, not as causal factors in their own right.

Psychology

The tradition of psychological research in schizophrenia stretches back to Kraepelin, who received his scientific training in Wundt's psychological laboratory. One classic line of research considered that in schizophrenia the ability to form normal abstract concepts is lost and instead concrete ones are formed. Certainly many schizophrenics appear to think in very concrete terms, as can be demonstrated by asking them to interpret a proverb. Another classic view suggested that schizophrenics have difficulty in maintaining the boundaries of concepts so that each concept spreads into others and thus becomes overinclusive.

Neuropsychologists have attempted to explain such findings in terms of the cognitive deficits found in patients with known damage to specific brain regions (see David & Cutting, 1994; Chua & Murray, 1995). Thus, studies have employed tests known to detect frontal lobe damage. For example, schizophrenics perform poorly on the Tower of London Test, which is a measure of planning ability, and on the Wisconsin Card Sort Test, which measures ability to alter cognitive set; they show deficits in such executive and conceptual functions as well as in initiating and monitoring their own actions.

Schizophrenics also perform poorly on tests of verbal fluency, which is normally associated with activation of the left frontal cortex. This accords with the view, first put forward by Kleist in 1930, that many of the speech abnormalities shown by schizophrenics are common to patients with left frontal damage. In a similar way, researchers have examined tests of temporal lobe functions such as memory, though here there is less consensus.

In general, the neuropsychological approach has been more successful in relating cognitive deficits to negative rather than positive symptoms. Furthermore, critics say that it is not surprising that schizophrenics do badly on neuropsychological batteries since they do badly at almost everything.

The alternative, experimental approach focuses on abnormalities of attention and preception, which are common in acute schizophrenia. McGhie & Chapman's patients (1961) described how once familiar objects become different and people may appear distorted in a terrifying manner; they also experienced being bombarded by stimuli, and these authors quote a patient as saying 'the sounds are coming through to me but I feel my mind cannot cope with everything. It's difficult to concentrate on any one sound. It's like trying to do two or three different things at one time'. McGhie & Chapman interpreted their findings in terms of Broadbent's 'filter theory' of input limitation, which suggests that some schizophrenics have a deficit in the filter mechanism that should limit sensory input to a level that the brain can deal with.

Gray *et al.* (1991), who were much influenced by Broadbent's 'filter theory', suggest that schizophrenics have a 'weakening of the influence of stores regularities' on their present actions. Such a theory predicts that patients will therefore do better than normals on tasks in which previous experience interferes with performance. One such task is 'latent inhibition' in which, as predicted, acute schizophrenics perform better than normal controls. Gray and his colleagues believe that a failure of latent inhibition, due to some dopaminergic abnormality, underlies many positive symptoms of schizophrenia.

Some of the most attractive explanatory models of schizophrenic symptoms have come from Frith (1992) who suggests that for normal social interaction it is necessary to have a 'theory of mind', i.e. some understanding of another person's point of view. He postulates that the schizophrenic is unable to discern the mental state of others accurately, and this inability to 'read the mind' of others leads to misjudgments and ultimately to paranoia.

Frith explains other symptoms in terms of a failure of internal monitoring. For example, we all use internal speech as we 'talk to ourselves' or think. He suggests that schizophrenics fail to recognise their inner speech as their own and instead misinterpret it as coming from some external source and therefore label it as 'voices'. Empirical support for this comes from McGuire *et al.* (1993) who found that when patients were experiencing auditory hallucinations, they showed activation of Broca's area on SPET imaging. McGuire and colleagues (1995) went on to show that although both normal and schizophrenic people activate Broca's area during inner speech, the normal subjects but not the schizophrenics contemporaneously use certain temporal lobe areas to determine that the speech is internal and not external.

Work implicating the temporal lobes in hallucinations and delusions goes back to Slater *et al.* (1963) who showed that patients with temporal lobe epilepsy had an increased risk of positive 'schizophreniform' symptoms. Barta *et al.* (1990) found that reduction of the volume of left anterior superior temporal gyrus (auditory association cortex) correlated with the severity of auditory hallucinations, while Shenton *et al* (1992) found that left superior temporal gyrus volume reduction was associated with thought disorder. These findings remain to be confirmed.

Neurochemistry

The dopamine hypothesis

The idea that there is a functional increase in dopaminergic transmission in the brains of schizophrenics is partly based on the evidence that amphetamine abuse (which increases synaptic dopamine) can produce ideas of reference, delusions of persecution, and auditory hallucinations (Connell, 1958). When large oral doses of amphetamines are given to normal subjects, psychosis invariably results within a few days (Griffith *et al.*, 1972); indeed intravenous amphetamine can produce the psychosis within a matter of hours. Furthermore, small doses of amphetamine exacerbate schizophrenic symptoms and schizophrenic patients are reportedly unable to differentiate an amphetamine psychosis from their usual symptoms.

The second strand of the dopamine hypothesis rests on the well-known tendency of the traditional antipsychotic drugs to cause parkinsonism. With the discovery that dopamine was deficient in Parkinson's disease, it appeared likely that the parkinsonian effects of the antipsychotics were due to their producing a functional dopamine deficiency. Carlsson & Lindquist (1963) then suggested that the antipsychotic effects were also due to the drugs blockading dopamine receptors. Johnstone *et al.* (1978) demonstrated this clinically by comparing the therapeutic efficacy of different isomers of fluphenthixol. Only one has dopamine-blocking activity and so only it should be antipsychotic; this proved to be the case. With the exception of clozapine, the potency of antipsychotics correlates closely with their dopamine D2 blocking potential (see Crow *et al.*, 1979).

If blocking dopamine receptors relieves schizophrenic symptoms, and drugs such as amphetamine and cocaine that flood the receptors with dopamine can cause psychosis, then could overactivity of central dopaminergic neurones underlie the symptomatology of schizophrenia? Unfortunately, conflicting results have come from post-mortem and more recently neuroimaging studies. One PET study (Wong *et al.*, 1986) showed elevated dopamine D2 receptors but a second (Farde *et al.*, 1990) did not. Thus, specific proof for the dopamine hypothesis has yet to emerge.

Other hypotheses

Dopamine dominated neurochemical thinking about schizophrenia for so long that other theories were neglected, but now other hypotheses are being developed not so much as alternatives but as adjuncts to the dopamine theory.

The first, the glutamate hypothesis, derives from evidence that phencyclidine (PCP), a glutamate agonist, induces a psychotic state closely akin to schizophrenia. Glutamic acid is an important excitatory neurotransmitter that can be toxic to neurones in excess; perhaps excitatory overstimulation may cause neuronal degeneration and secondary dopaminergic overactivity. One possibility is that this neurotoxicity may be produced by hypoxia or other insult to the developing brain; glutamate's activity is exerted via several receptor sites, amongst the most important are NMDA and kainate receptors. Kerwin *et al.* (1990) reported decreased binding of kainate in the temporal lobes of schizophrenic brains, and Harrison *et al.* (1991) suggest that this may be due to reduced gene expression reflected in reduced messenger RNA.

The second hypothesis implicates serotonergic abnormality, and stems from two sources. Firstly, many hallucinogenic drugs such as LSD have structural affinities to serotonin. One of the most intriguing is dimethyltryptamine (DMT), which was first isolated from the snuff used by Haitian natives to produce mystical states. When injected into human volunteers, DMT induces a short-lasting psychosis. Several groups reported DMT in the blood and urine of schizophrenics but subsequent results were contradictory (Murray *et al.*, 1979).

However, interest in serotonin has been reignited by the evidence that drugs such as clozapine and risperidone, which block S2 as well as D2 receptors, may have enhanced antipsychotic efficacy. A recent neuroendocrine challenge study (Abel *et al.*, 1996) has also suggested enhanced sensitivity of S2 receptors in drug-naive schizophrenics.

A third, and more recent, theory implicates the inhibitory transmitter GABA (gamma-aminobutyric acid). Busatto *et al.* (1995) have used SPET to show reduced GABA receptors in the left temporal lobe, and suggest that reduced inhibitory GABAergic tone contributes to temporal lobe malfunction and to positive symptoms.

Biology and nosology

Given that our present ways of classifying the psychoses are so unsatisfactory, biological studies have been used to try to develop a more satisfactory nosology. For example, on the basis that the genetic influence is the best-established aetiological fact, twin studies have been used to try to establish which operational definition produces the highest heritability (McGuffin *et al.*, 1984; Farmer *et al.*, 1987). The evidence is that a moderately broad definition appears more heritable than either an extremely broad or extremely narrow one.

Twin and family studies suggest that paranoid schizophrenia is the least heritable type. This may be related to its later onset. On the other hand, the relatives of patients with schizoaffective disorder have a high risk of psychosis themselves. The evidence, however, suggests that this risk is divided between schizophrenia and affective psychosis so this does not help to resolve the question of the status of schizoaffective disorder. Crow (1990) concludes that there is no genetic difference between schizophrenia and affective disorder, and speaks of a continuum of psychosis.

Murray *et al.* (1992) share Crow's dissatisfaction with the conventional 'Kraepelinian' distinction between schizophrenia and affective psychosis. However, they argue that the distinction has been made at the wrong point; they suggest that there exists a congenital or 'neurodevelopmental' form of schizophrenia that approximates to Kraepelin's original concept of dementia praecox, and a relapsing and remitting adult onset form that has much in common with affective psychosis.

Recent years have also seen attempts directly to relate physiological abnormalities to particular symptoms. Many of these take as their starting point the division of psychotic symptoms into the positive and the negative, which was popularised by Crow (1980). Dopamine receptor blocking drugs are more effective on the acute than the chronic symptoms of schizophrenia. This prompted Crow (1980) to suggest that only the acute positive symptoms (he calls them Type 1 schizophrenia) are a consequence of some disturbance of dopamine transmission, while he related the chronic negative symptoms (Type 2) to neurological abnormality.

Subsequently, Liddle (1987) carried out a factor analysis that subdivided the positive symptoms and has been replicated several times. Liddle's three factors are (a) psychomotor poverty, which essentially is another name for the negative symptom cluster; (b) disorganisation, which many liken to hebephrenia, and (c) reality distortion, i.e. delusions and hallucinations. Liddle used PET to show that psychomotor poverty was associated with decreased left frontal activity, disorganisation with increased cingulate activity on the right, and delusions and hallucinations with increased activity in the left hippocampal region.

Management

Anyone presenting schizophrenic symptoms for the first time deserves thorough investigation. First, given the serious personal implications of receiving a diagnosis of schizophrenia, it is vital to exclude conditions that may be mistaken for it. Secondly, a thorough exploration of the patient's psychological, social and physical status must be undertaken to elucidate possible aetiological or exacerbating factors. Thirdly, only after a comprehensive assessment of a patient's assets and liabilities can individually tailored treatment be instigated.

There are three essential principles of treatment. Antipsychotic drugs should be used to induce an initial remission, and in most cases to maintain that remission over prolonged periods. Secondly, psychological approaches should be used to enhance the patient's hold on reality. Thirdly, a variety of social measures should be used to provide a social and work environment to suit the patient's particular needs.

Antipsychotic drugs

Antipsychotic drugs have been studied in literally hundreds of double-blind trials, almost all of which indicate that they are superior to placebo in the treatment of both acute and chronic schizophrenia. A large number of such drugs are now available, whose pharmacology and clinical effects are described in detail in Chapter 24.

Traditional antipsychotics

The typical antipsychotic drugs all produce D2 dopamine blockade, and from the clinician's point of view, differ not so much in their efficacy as in (a) the amount of sedation that they produce, (b) their liability to produce extrapyramidal symptoms, and (c) occasional idiosyncratic toxic effects.

Sedation can be a desirable effect in the acutely disturbed patient, and for this reason many British psychiatrists prefer to commence treatment of such patients with chlorpromazine. It is usually necessary to reach at least 400 mg of chlorpromazine daily to achieve adequate effect, and occasionally the dose may be up to 800 or 1000 mg for a short time.

Haloperidol is the most widely prescribed antipsychotic in the USA, but has a high liability to produce extrapyramidal symptoms (EPS); partly for this reason the dosages used have been falling recently, and many authorities see no advantage in more than 15–20 mg per day. In a very excited aggressive patient, 10 mg intramuscularly may be necessary.

Thioridazine is another long-established drug that still has a place in the modern armamentarium. Although equally effective as haloperidol and chlorpromazine, it is less likely to produce extrapyramidal side-effects than either, since the drug itself has strong anticholinergic effects. Its use is somewhat limited by the occasional occurrence of retinal deposits and blindness if given in prolonged high (more than 800 mg) daily doses.

For those patients in whom sedation is not required, trifluoperazine is an effective drug.

The majority of patients begin to respond to traditional antipsychotic drugs within one to two weeks and most of the therapeutic gain occurs within the first six weeks of treatment. About two-thirds of patients will show significant improvement.

Atypical drugs

As noted in Chapter 24, the treatment of the remaining patients has been reinvigorated by the demonstration that a significant proportion of patients previously resistant to drug therapy will respond to clozapine. At present clozapine is licensed in the USA and UK only for such 'resistant' patients, but there is no doubt that it does produce remarkable improvement in some such patients (Kane et al., 1988; Meltzer, 1994).

Clozapine does not cause significant extrapyramidal side-effects (EPS). It is highly sedative and can also produce hypotensive episodes but these adverse effects can be minimised by starting at a low dose (e.g. 12.5 mg per day) and only slowly increasing it. Excessive salivation remains a problem, as is weight gain, and above 600 mg per day a significant number of patients have convulsions. However, the main reason for caution is that 3% of cases will develop neutropenia and 1% dangerous agranulocytosis. With weekly monitoring of the white blood cells, mandatory in most countries, these risks can be minimised.

The efficacy of clozapine has stimulated pharmaceutical companies into a race to produce other drugs with its benefits but not its dangers. Unfortunately, because of its complex effects on many different receptors, it has not been clear how to achieve this. Three main strategies are being adopted.

Firstly, 'smart D2 blockers' have preferential effects on mesolimbic and mesocortical dopaminergic pathways. Sulpiride is thought to act in this manner, perhaps thereby explaining its low propensity to EPS; it also causes little sedation. Secondly, a number of drugs with combined D2 and S2 blocking effects are being introduced. The first of these was risperidone, which appears as effective as traditional drugs, and has fewer EPS. It is now the most widely prescribed antipsychotic in the USA. Sertindole has even fewer EPS but ECG monitoring is advisable. Thirdly, drugs are being developed which, like clozapine, have a broad spectrum of effects at different receptors; ofanzapine is the first to become available.

Maintenance treatment

During the resolving phase of schizophrenia it is usually possible to reduce the dose of medication towards one-half of that necessary during the acute phase.Once patients have recovered from their psychotic episode, should they remain on antipsychotic medication? There have already been numerous controlled studies comparing the relapse rate of patients on placebo and on maintenance therapy, and in each one many more patients relapsed on placebo than on drugs. For example, Hogarty *et al*. (1974) followed up 374 schizophrenics for two years after discharge; 8% of placebo-treated patients relapsed compared with 48% of the drug maintenance group.

Since the greatest risk of relapse appears to be in the year following an overt psychotic episode, the great majority of schizophrenics should receive medication for this period. Then, they should be reassessed and only if they are symptom free, should the possibility of slowly decreasing the dosage be considered. In a minority, but only a minority, the antipsychotic can be gradually phased out over a period of many months without return of symptoms.

A major problem in maintenance therapy is ensuring that patients take their medication. Renton *et al*. (1963) reported that 46% of schizophrenic out-patients failed to take their tablets as prescribed and Hare & Willcox (1967) found that one-fifth of psychiatric in-patients did not take the medication given by the nursing staff. Van Putten *et al*. (1976) compared drug compliers with habitual defaulters and found that when the former decompensated they tended to develop dysphoric symptoms, while the latter were more likely to develop ego syntonic grandiose psychoses, which they preferred to relative drug-induced normality.

It is possible to check whether patients are taking some drugs (e.g. haloperidol) by measuring the plasma prolactin, but a simpler method of ensuring compliance is to use long-acting injectable preparations.

A variety of depot neuroleptics are now in common use – fluphenazine, flupenthixol, clopenthixol, haloperidol. In a double-blind trial of fluphenazine decanoate, Hirsch & Leff (1975) found that 66% of patients on placebo relapsed within nine months compared with only 8% on active drugs. The active injections significantly aided family relationships and decreased delusions and socially embarrassing behaviour.

Unfortunately, a minority of schizophrenics fail to respond significantly to all anti-psychotic drugs including clozapine. As yet there appears no proven way of predicting response except that individuals who have remained in an actively psychotic state without treatment for long periods are less likely to respond well. It may be that some of those who fail to respond do not absorb sufficient amounts of the drugs, or metabolise them in a different manner. Some clinicians have suggested that extremely high doses of antipsychotics might produce a remission in some previously resistant patients but there is little evidence in favour of this practice, and considerable evidence of its dangers. The addition of lithium or carbamazepine can be useful for patients who have mood swings or who are persistently aggressive

Side-effects

The most obvious side-effects of the antipsychotics are the extrapyramidal symptoms (EPS), parkinsonism, dystonia, and akathisia. They are most common with haloperidol and fluphenazine and least common with thioridazine and clozapine. Dystonic spasms usually affect the muscles of the neck, face and tongue and include torticollis and oculogyric crises. They tend to occur within a few days of treatment and are most frequent with high doses. Because they look so bizarre and dramatic, dystonic reactions are sometimes dismissed as 'hysteria'. However, it is important to recognise them because they are highly distressing and are rapidly relieved by IV procyclidine. Akathisia is sometimes known as the 'restless legs syndrome'; in it the patient has a great urge to move about and considerable difficulty in sitting still without fidgeting or rocking.

PET studies (Farde et al., 1992) have shown that such EPS occur when there are high levels of D2 dopamine blockade. Parkinsonian symptoms, dystonia, and akathisia can all usually be relieved by anticholinergic agents orally or occasionally in an emergency intravenously, but there is controversy over whether one should routinely administer these agents to all patients on antipsychotics. Certainly, immobility and mask-like faces may be misdiagnosed as worsening of negative symptoms. On the other hand, anticholinergic drugs may themselves cause side-effects including an atropine-like 'buzz' in some patients. Furthermore, not all patients develop side-effects on the neuroleptics and there have been reports that taking anticholinergics is actually associated with lowered blood levels of antipsychotics. It might therefore be more logical to treat EPS singly by lowering the dose of antipsychotic.

The most troublesome side-effect of antipsychotic medication is tardive dyskinesia (TD), which is characterised by slow irregular movements in the region of the mouth: grimacing, smacking of the lips, side to side movements of the chin and protrusion of the tongue. Approximately 5% of patients on chronic antipsychotic medication will develop TD each year (van Os et al., 1996a). The elderly and those with coexisting organic brain damage seem particularly susceptible. Stopping the medication does not necessarily lead to the disappearance of the dyskinesia and may sometimes make it worse. Some believe that long-term prescription of anticholingergics may increase the risk of TD.

Many antipsychotics also affect the autonomic nervous system and may cause postural hypotension, delayed ejaculation, difficulty in micturition, and constipation. Patients taking chlorpromazine become hypersensitive to sunlight and occasionally develop cholestatic jaundice, though fortunately the latter is rare. On the other hand, weight gain is a side-effect common to most antipsychotics and may be gross and disturbing to patients. Breast engorgement (due to elevation of prolactin) is also frequent though less than 5% of women complain of overt lactation; this however is a particular problem with sulpiride.

Social treatment

Suffering from schizophrenia can be seen as an extraordinary vulnerability, like walking a tightrope with the dual dangers of an under-stimulating environment leading to an exacerbation of negative symptoms on one side and over-stimulation leading to florid positive symptoms on the other. Wing & Brown (1970) studied chronic schizophrenics in three hospitals that differed in the length of time that patients spent doing nothing. The hospital with the most barren under-stimulating wards contained patients who were the most withdrawn, most silent, and most affectively blunted.

Paradoxically, too vigorous an attempt at rehabilitation led to excessive stimulation and the re-emergence of dormant delusions and hallucinations. Such relapse can be prevented by beginning with short periods of occupational therapy, then graduating the patient to an occupational training unit before going to work in sheltered employment or an industrial therapy unit. Over-stimulation may also result from over-enthusiastic milieu therapy; intense group meetings, searches for hidden meanings, and interpersonal confrontations constitute a toxic environment for schizophrenics with deficits in attention and information processing (van Putten & May, 1976).

As noted earlier, not only the family milieu but also the occurrence of independent life events can provoke the re-emergence of positive symptoms. Vaughan & Leff (1976) demonstrated that patients from homes with high 'expressed emotion' (EE) constitute a 'high risk' group, and a major effort should be made to ensure that such patients continue to receive medication and are exposed to as little 'high EE' as possible. This can be done by trying to alter the behaviour of 'high EE' relatives so as to diminish the degree of contention and disagreement in the patient's home (Anderson et al., 1980). An alternative is to ensure less exposure, for example by the patient attending a day hospital.

Rehabilitation

A wide range of facilities are necessary for effective rehabilitation. These should include occupational therapy units of graded complexity, a day hospital, an industrial therapy unit, sheltered workshops, good links with occupational retraining units, hostels, boarding houses, group houses and flats (Bennett, 1978).

Rehabilitation should proceed on both the social and domestic fronts. Thus, a severely handicapped patient may start simple occupational tasks for a few hours each day, then go to a supervised work unit where simple tasks are carried out for increasingly long periods. Thereafter, he or she may progress through a series of steps involving increasing responsibility, simulated industrial experience, a sheltered workshop and eventually return to normal employment.

Many patients will be discharged from a hospital ward to a hostel with nursing supervision, then a group home with less supervision, but may still need to attend a rehabilitation unit. Linn et al. (1975), who studied the effectiveness of different day centres in forestalling relapse, found that those that used intensive short-term treatments including group psychotherapy were less effective than those that relied on occupational therapy and a sustained non-threatening environment.

Community care

Inherent in the idea of community care is the belief that most schizophrenics can lead a happier and more productive life in the community than in the wards of a mental hospital. This belief, now backed up with considerable evidence, has been behind the long-standing drive both in Europe and America to reduce the size of mental hospitals and switch resources to community care. This approach has many advantages. Patients prefer it, and families are less disrupted when a spouse, parent, or child is away only for brief periods, and when care is given locally the family can continue to function as a unit despite one member being hospitalised (Muijen et al., 1992).

However, successful community care demands extensive community facilities and unfortunately the development of these facilities has rarely kept pace with the decrease in the number of psychiatric beds. Consequently, a series of reports in Britain (e.g. the Clunis Report, 1994) have been extremely critical of the way in which government policies have resulted in large numbers of chronic psychotic patients failing to receive adequate support in the community, with disturbing and occasionally violent consequences. Fortunately, considerable effort is now being put into addressing this scandal.

An effective registration and follow-up system is essential to ensure that patients do not drop out of the system. Case or care management systems are being developed in Europe and North America to ensure that this does not happen, and that the various agencies involved operate in a co-ordinated manner through a nominated key worker.

An important issue in community care is the effect that caring for a schizophrenic may have on the health and way of life of family members. Brown et al. (1966) found that the relatives of 19% of first admitted to 60% of previously admitted patients who were not in hospital five years later had one or more problems that the relatives attributed to the patients. The investigators considered that far from exaggerating their problems, the relatives in fact underestimated their hardships. The most frequent problems at home reported by relatives to Creer (1978) were patients' social withdrawal, doing nothing, lack of conversation, odd ideas and behaviour and restlessness. Many relatives were uncertain how to cope with schizophrenic behaviour, while others lived in a state of tension or even fear. Both Creer (1978) and Anderson et al. (1980) have outlined programmes whereby social workers and other professionals can help reduce the strain on relatives. Voluntary organisations such as the British National Schizophrenia Fellowship can also provide valuable understanding and companionship.

Combined drug and social therapy

Hogarty et al. (1974) studied the relationship between drug and social treatment in the after-care of 374 patients discharged from hospital. They demonstrated that social therapy had a differential effect on those at different stages of recovery. A combination of intensive social casework and vocational rehabilitation counselling improved adjustment and interpersonal relationships in relatively asymptomatic patients, while in patients with severe symptomatology this combination actually hastened relapse. Hogarty and his colleagues recommended that such treatment should be deferred until the patient is relatively asymptomatic.

There is some evidence that antipsychotics can provide some protection against such over-stimulation. Leff *et al.* (1973) looked at the proportion of patients experiencing life events in the five weeks preceding relapse on either placebo or phenothiazine. There was no increase over the expected number of life events among patients who relapsed on placebo, but among those who relapsed on active medication 89% had undergone a significant preceding life event. The result supports the view that antipsychotics raise the threshold of vulnerability to ordinary experiences so that a patient on medication requires a particularly stressful experience before he will relapse, while a schizophrenic not on medication can relapse without the additional stimulus of a significant life event. Antipsychotics also appear to decrease vulnerability to the over-arousing effects of living at home with hostile emotionally over-involved relatives (Vaughn & Leff, 1976).

Psychological treatment

A long-term supportive relationship is of great help both to patients and their relatives. In such a relationship the therapist may see him or herself as an 'ambassador of reality', giving understanding and advice and helping the patient to learn new techniques of adaptation. Surprisingly little is known of which approaches are most helpful to the schizophrenic. For instance, it is uncertain whether it is better to encourage a patient on recovery from an acute psychotic episode to integrate this period into his or her general life experience, or to deny and gloss over the psychotic episode.

In recent years more specific cognitive-behaviour techniques have attracted increasing attention as possible adjuncts to drug therapy. A variety of approaches are being explored. Some address symptoms directly; for example, attempt to provide, in a non-threatening and non-confrontational manner, alternative explanations of some delusional beliefs (Garety *et al.*, 1994; Kingdon *et al.*, 1994); others are directed at auditory hallucinations (e.g. Persaud & Marks, 1995). Most ambitious of all are those approaches that attempt to remedy the neuropsychological deficits that are found in many schizophrenics. First the particular deficits that trouble individual patients are identified, and then patients are taught techniques to help them overcome those deficits.

The various psychological interventions described above can produce considerable improvements in specific symptoms and performance on specific tasks but as yet it is unclear whether they can be sustained after the extra input ceases.

Outcome

Manfred Bleuler (1974), who followed up a cohort of 208 patients over a 22-year period, made the important observation that on average schizophrenics show little further deterioration after five years, but rather tend to improve. He pointed out that schizophrenia cannot be considered a progressive disease since 20 years after the event the proportion of recovered patients remains the same as five years after the onset. At five years about one-quarter of the schizophrenics who were alive were in hospital; thereafter, although individual patients were admitted or discharged, the percentage in hospital remained roughly similar.

There have been many studies of the factors that influence outcome in schizophrenia (Wing, 1982). There is unanimity that the outlook is bad if the illness leads to hospitalisation before the age of 15 years. This may be not only because earlier breakdown is indicative of more severe illness, but also because the younger patient has not had sufficient time to build up social and occupational skills to aid his rehabilitation. Other ominous features include low social class and low IQ. Women have a better prognosis than men (Van Os *et al.*, 1996*b*), and marriage appears to have a protective role against future relapse (Vaughn & Leff, 1976).

There is a high correlation between poor premorbid personality and bad outcome, and also, as Offord & Cross (1969) have suggested, between the latter and scholastic and other difficulties in childhood. A history of good adjustment in social, sexual, and occupational functioning indicates a more favourable prognosis, as do catatonic features, and a family history of affective disorder (Wittenborn *et al.*, 1977). The more acute the onset of psychosis and the more obvious the precipitants, the greater the chances of recovery, while not surprisingly, chronicity tends to predict chronicity. Lack of insight, emotional withdrawal, and blunting of affect are bad signs.

In a prospective follow-up study, Van Os *et al.* (1996*b*), examined and then followed up a large series of recent-onset psychotic patients for four years. Poor outcome was predicted by CT findings suggestive of cortical atrophy, while those patients who had suffered adverse life events had significantly better outcome.

Huber *et al.* (1980), who followed up 502 schizophrenic patients for 22 years, made the point that one should only make firm predictions when all the prognostic indicators point in the same direction. Indeed, Harding *et al.* (1987) recontacted a series of schizophrenics after several decades, and showed that even among patients who retrospectively met the DSM-III criteria for schizophrenia, and had appeared very ill, a surprising proportion were largely recovered and living independently. Thus, the only prediction one can usually give with certainty is that the outlook is uncertain.

11

Affective disorders

PETER McGUFFIN

Introduction

Depressive *symptoms* are frequent in psychiatric practice and are among the most common complaints in primary care (Chapter 19). They are also common in patients presenting to other hospital specialties and community surveys suggest that depressive *syndromes* are highly prevalent with many cases never coming to the attention of doctors or other health care professionals. One attempt to assess the risk of depression over a lifetime estimated that by age 65 seven out of ten women and four out of ten men could expect to have suffered from minor (but still possibly clinically significant) depression (Bebbington *et al.*, 1989). Not surprisingly the differentiation between 'normal' depressive symptoms and milder forms of depressive illness is often difficult and blurred. Only the more severe forms of depressive disorder give an appearance of a qualitative difference from normality.

By contrast, manic states, which are much less frequent than depression, seem to be distinct from normal experience. But even here it is possible to envisage a continuum between high spirits and frank elation. Given these blurred boundaries, it is understandable that the classification of affective disorders is problematic. Furthermore, although the concept of affective illness is often thought to be an ancient one, since descriptions of manic and melancholic states date back to classical Greece, this is probably a mistaken view. Berrios (1992) has pointed out that what is now called depression does not correspond closely with early notions of melancholia, and current thinking about what constitutes mania or depression dates back only as far as the late nineteenth century. Like most other psychiatric disorders, affective illnesses are defined purely in terms of their signs and symptoms. As yet there is no known pathophysiology and no reliable objective diagnostic tests. Consequently we must accept that modern definitions remain provisional and that they too will be subject to evolution and change.

Many of the separate components of affective disorder have been described in Chapter 1 but here we will begin by considering how the symptoms and signs cluster together and will examine the psychopathology of affective states.

Table 11.1. *Frequency of symptoms and signs in depressed patients presenting at a psychiatric hospital (unpublished data from the study by Bebbington et al., 1988)*

Symptoms	Freqeuncy (%)
Depressed mood	100
(variable)	(59)
(constant)	(41)
Anhedonia/loss of interest	72
Poor concentration	72
Lack of energy	72
Social withdrawal	65
Hopelessness	58
Weight loss	58
Sleep disturbance	
delayed sleep	52
early waking	32
Diminished libido	50
Self deprecation	45
Suicidal plans or acts	39
Guilt	32
Observed retardation	12
Delusions – agitation	4
– guilt	4
– persecution	3
– other	2
Auditory hallucinations	5

Psychopathology

Depressive states

Depression as a symptom in clinical practice is probably exceeded in frequency only by pain and the techniques for enquiring about both are rather similar. Thus it is important to know how long depression has been present, whether it is there all the time, whether anything relieves or exacerbates it and whether it shows any spontaneous variation in severity. One can gauge severity by asking the patient if it is the worst they have ever felt and what it makes them want to do (e.g. cry, 'hide away in a corner', or have thoughts of suicide). Typical severe depression is usually persistent, unresponsive to external events that might normally be expected to bring cheer, and shows a diurnal variation with exacerbations in the morning and perceptible lessening as the day goes on.

The relative frequencies of symptoms associated with depressive disorder are listed in Table 11.1. Among these, anhedonia, or the inability to experience pleasure, is usually prominent. The patient has a diminished enjoyment of both work and leisure pursuits and typically has a decreased appetite for food and a loss of libido. Loss of weight may follow and disturbed sleep with early morning waking is characteristic. Other patterns of sleep loss may also occur with difficulty falling asleep (or initial insomnia) or recurrent waking during the night (middle insomnia).

Lack of energy is a common symptom, together with lack of interest, poor concentration and difficulty sustaining attention. Patients with such symptoms often complain of difficulty in reading a newspaper article or following a television programme all the way through and sometimes complain of poor memory. Under these circumstances, testing usually reveals that recall of information is intact but registration of new material is inefficient and speed in thinking is reduced. On examination, slowness of movement may also be evident, described as psychomotor retardation. In severe cases lack of interest may show in poor self-care and an unkempt appearance. Typically, the patient has a sad and miserable facial expression but this is not always so even in some quite severe cases, where the patient may strive to appear normal (the brave face of so-called 'smiling depression'). In addition to assessing the subjective depth of the patient's low, or dysphoric, mood one should try to make an objective judgement based on appearance. Tearfulness at interview must be interpreted against the context of recent life happenings, the patient's cultural and social background and their gender. Sometimes in depressed patients the most visible shows of emotion are hostility or irritability rather than frank despair.

The content of thought usually includes poor self-regard, which may amount to feelings of worthlessness or guilt. The patient may spontaneously make self-depreciative remarks ('I am no good. I don't deserve help') and whether spontaneously mentioned or not it is mandatory in depressed patients to enquire fully about suicidal thoughts. Far from putting ideas into the patient's head that were not there before, enquiring about suicidal thoughts is often a comfort to the patient whose ideas about ending his or her life may have seemed to them to be evidence of going insane. A positive response to a question such as 'Have things seemed so bad that life is not worth going on with?' should lead to exploring whether a means of suicide has been considered. If so, one should find out what plans, if any, had been made to carry out an attempt and whether the patient thinks that it is likely that they will act upon such plans? In the same context, it is worth asking about whether the patient has any hope for the future. Believing that all is hopeless and there will be no escape from their current misery, if accompanied by suicidal ideas, usually indicates a high risk that the ideas will be acted upon.

Abnormal beliefs and perceptions in depression

In a minority of patients, abnormal ideas take on a quality of fixed beliefs, which may become of delusional intensity. Usually these can be seen as arising understandably out of a severely depressed mood (Jaspers, 1963) and hence can be described as mood congruent. These include delusions of worthlessness, which can be seen as an extreme form of a self-depreciation described earlier. Delusions of guilt or blame may result in severe worrying over real or imagined minor misdemeanours. In some cases delusions of guilt become more bizarre, such as in the man who believed he had become 'the worst devil created by Satan' or another who believed that he was responsible for the deaths of British soldiers killed in the 1991 Gulf War.

Persecutory beliefs may again be in keeping with the mood state, with the patient saying that he or she deserves to be tormented and punished. Similarly delusions of reference may include the belief that the patient is being marked out and talked about behind his or her back because of their wickedness. Delusions of poverty (i.e. that the patient is bankrupt or in great debt when in fact they are solvent) are rarer and in practice seem to occur most often in older patients. Also fairly rare, but striking when they are encountered, are nihilistic delusions where the patient believes that some part of the anatomy, usually internal, such as their brain or intestines has disappeared or has rotted away. An example was the case of a man who believed that all of his 'giblets' had been flushed away down the toilet pan.

Auditory hallucinations may occur as voices that are mood congruent in their content. For example, they may confirm that the patient is guilty of a crime and deserves persecution. or punishment. They are not usually either as vivid or as continuous as the typical derogatory voices heard by schizophrenics (Hamilton, 1985). Rarely tactile hallucinations can occur as 'funny sensations' on the skin or in the viscera, which may be interpreted as evidence that internal organs are disappearing. Unpleasant tastes or smells are occasionally described by severely depressed patients, who usually believe that they are emitting the smell themselves and again may interpret this as confirming that either their flesh or some internal organs are rotting.

Psychomotor disturbance may accompany severe depression, whether or not the patient also has delusions or hallucinations. Retardation is exhibited as marked slowness of both action and speech, so that there is a perceptible delay or latency in the patient's response to questions. In the most extreme cases retardation can progress to mutism and depressive stupor, in which the patient appears awake but lies motionless and mute, usually refusing to eat or drink, and sometimes being incontinent. The term agitation describes a different type of psychomotor disturbance, when the patient carries out a series of repetitive movements, usually with the facial appearance of obvious anguish and despair. The movements typically include the wringing of hands, rocking back and forth and pacing up and down. They can also include repetitive self-punitive movements such as banging the head against a wall, scratching flesh or pulling hair.

Other patterns of depression

Most of the variability in depressive disorders can simply be considered as on a continuum from severe to mild. However, at the milder end of the spectrum there may also be additional symptoms not typically associated with severe depression. Most prominent among these are symptoms of anxiety, which frequently overlap with and are difficult to disentangle from depressive features. Some patients with mild or only moderately severe depression also show 'reversed functional shift'. This means that instead of a classic 'endogenous' pattern of biological symptoms consisting of early morning wakening, decreased appetite and weight loss, the patient shows hypersomnia including a tendency to sleep through the day, an increase in appetite and weight gain. Other patients may show only psychological symptoms of depression with few or none of the biological features. Such patients have in the past been referred to as showing a reactive or neurotic pattern of depression, which was assumed to be more related to adversity and life's misfortunes than was depression with endogenous

313

features. As we shall discuss later in the section on aetiology, modern objective evidence does not support such a tidy dichotomy.

Mania

The typical manic patient looks and feel elated, but their exuberance and cheerfulness may turn to irritability as the episode wears on, or if others attempt to control and constrain their manic behaviour. Indeed, one fairly common finding in patients who have had multiple episodes of mania, is that irritability tends to become a more prominent component (Winokur *et al.*, 1969). The manic patient's subjective descriptions of elation varies and is frequently described as feeling 'high', 'on top of the world' or just 'very happy'. In most cases, particularly in first episode, the patient will not admit that anything is amiss but some acquire sufficient insight to detect when they are going 'over the top' or becoming 'too cheerful to be normal'.

It is of course not the mood changes as such that make manic states dangerous and disabling but rather it is the accompanying symptoms and behaviours that arise out of an expansive and heightened sense of well-being. In a manic state the patient typically feels full of energy, which manifests in over-activity and sometimes in recklessness. There is a decreased need for sleep and an increased appetite for sex. Typically there is also an increased appetite for food but the patient may not indulge in this because they are 'too busy to eat'.

Recklessness and lack of judgement frequently lead to lavish spending sprees, such as the university student who exceeded her credit card limited several times over within a week, or the man who thought the portable radios in his local electrical store such a good bargain that he bought 40.

Social disinhibition is a common feature, which may show as an over-familiarity with strangers or people in authority. Sometimes this may be fairly benign in effect, for example, walking into a room full of strangers and insisting on shaking hands with everyone. However, it often results in behaviour of a embarrassing or sexual nature. For example, a newly admitted woman in her late fifties announced in a ward round 'I love sex' and attempted to intimately fondle the consultant psychiatrist.

Speech in mania is typically rapid and increased in quantity. The patient's flow is difficult to interrupt and may be quite unstoppable. In normal conversation even the most habitually garrulous of individuals responds to non-verbal cues and attends to the hints that others wish to enter into the conversation. Manic patients with pressure of speech lose all sense of such conversational niceties. A usual accompaniment is flight of ideas, where thoughts move rapidly from one theme to another with tenuous but understandable connections. These may be based upon rhymes (or clang associations) or other irrelevant aspects of content. For example, asked to explain the proverb 'A stitch in times saves nine' a young women replied 'Its when you've got a cut and need a stitch. A stitch in time saves nine. Nine lives. Nine lives like a cat. I've got a little black cat actually'.

Not all patients show typical pressure of speech and flight of ideas but most during manic episodes will, if asked, report subjectively that their thoughts are going rapidly or 'crowding in' on their head. Lesser degrees of speech disorder, where speech is verbose, rapid and difficult to follow, even if not typical flight of ideas, is sometimes described as prolixity of speech.

Nearly all patients suffering from mania have an increased feeling of self-worth and importance. Their thought content consists of ambitious plans to which they see no obstacle and a self-assessment that exceeds realistic expectations. Although most patients are at least partially amenable to a firm but gentle persuasion not to act upon their beliefs, direct confrontation, as previously mentioned, may provoke an irritable outburst.

Abnormal beliefs and perceptions in mania

Grandiose delusions are the most common and take the form of a delusion of identity ('I am God') or of special powers or abilities ('I am better at mathematics than Einstein'). Persecutory beliefs and delusions of reference may also occur and tend to be congruent with the overall mood of grandiosity and expansiveness. In general, delusions in manic states are less persistent than those in schizophrenic illnesses but sometimes mood incongruent delusions such as delusions of passivity may occur. How such patients should be classified in controversial but most authorities (e.g. Goodwin & Jamison, 1990; American Psychiatric Association, 1994) currently allow that passivity and other Schneiderian first rank symptoms of schizophrenia can occur in manic states.

Many patients report that their perceptions are generally more vivid but in addition more obviously abnormal perceptions, particularly auditory hallucinations, may also occur in about a fifth of cases (Goodwin & Jamison, 1990). These usually take the form of voices, where the content is in keeping with the patient's prevailing persecutory or grandiose beliefs. Typically auditory hallucinations in mania are less persistent or continuous than in schizophrenia (Hamilton, 1985).

Mixed states

The co-occurrence of depressive and manic symptoms is not uncommon. For example, Winokur *et al.* reported that 68% of manic episodes were associated with some degree of depressive mood and Goodwin & Jamison (1990), in reviewing several clinical studies of mania, calculated that depression recurred in 72% of episodes. Mixed states are usually seen in a patient who is in the process of appearing to recover from a manic state but who may go on to develop a depressive state, or alternatively is seen in a patient with a depressive disorder who is about to swing into mania. Less commonly, however, both depressive and manic symptoms are persistent in the same patient at the same time, remaining evident for days or even weeks. The overall picture can be puzzling to both the clinician and the patient him or herself. Irritability with over-activity is a much more usual picture than frank elation but the mood is labile and can quickly turn to tearful despair. Persistent delusions are unusual but there may be a strange mixture of persecutory ideation, guilt and vague grandiosity. Mixed affective states, therefore, can present formidable diagnostic difficulties, particularly if the patient is being seen for the first time and when the clinician does not have the benefit of a previous history of mania or depression. Mixed states occurred in 16% of manic-depressive patients in one of the most carefully documented series

(Winokur *et al.*, 1969) but other studies (where the term is possibly used more loosely) describe mixed states occurring in up to two-thirds of patients (Goodwin & Jamison, 1990).

Classification

The recent history of the classification of affective disorders contains both controversy and confusion (Kendell, 1976), which has only been partially resolved in the current (10th edition) of the International Classification of Diseases (ICD-10) (World Health Organization 1992*a*) or the American Psychiatric Association's (1994) *Diagnostic and Statistical Manual*, 4th edition (DSM-IV). As discussed earlier, affective disorders are syndromes consisting of groups of signs and symptoms and cannot yet be considered as diseases with a well-understood aetiology and pathogenesis. Therefore, current classifications have to be thought of as a set of working hypotheses or conventions. They are designed to assist communication between clinicians, facilitate description and help predict outcome and response to treatment. They are nevertheless only conventions and cannot be thought of as immutable. Indeed, although there has been considerable convergence in the most recent additions of DSM and ICD, there are still some differences in the way affective disorders are divided, the terms that are used to describe the disorders and in the constituent items that make up the criteria.

The classifications of affective disorders in ICD-10 and DSM-IV are summarised in Table 11.2. The main difference between ICD-10 and DSM-IV is that ICD-10 exists in both a descriptive version for clinical use and a fully operational set of criteria for use in research, whereas DSM-IV, like its predecessor (DSM-III), gives operational criteria for all categories of disorder. (See Chapter 3 for discussion of operational versus descriptive diagnostic criteria). DSM-IV also allows for more sub-categories of affective disorder, with more 'specifiers' than ICD-10 for both clinical features and course of disorder.

Both classification systems contain main syndromes of mania and depression that are broadly similar. Indeed the definitions of mania are virtually identical, consisting of elevated, expansive or irritable mood together with three symptoms (four if the mood is only irritable) from a list including increased self-esteem/grandiosity, decreased need for sleep, pressure of talk, flight of ideas, distractibility, increased activity and reckless behaviour (e.g. sexual indiscretions or spending sprees). To fulfil the criteria for mania, the mood disorder has to be present for a week or the patient requires hospitalisation, but for hypomania a duration of only four days is required.

The classification schemes differ in their approach to depression. Whereas DSM-IV contains a single category of major depression, ICD-10 divides depressive episodes into mild, moderate and severe types. The terms used to describe depressive symptoms in the two classifications differ slightly but overall the list of symptoms in depressive disorders is virtually identical (Table 11.2) with only one symptom ('loss of confidence or self-esteem') present in ICD-10 but not in DSM-IV. Both ICD-10 and DSM contain exclusion criteria for a depressive episode that manic symptoms should not be present and the disorder should not result from a psychoactive drug or from a general medical conditions. In addition, DSM-IV

Table 11.2. *Comparison of ICD-10 and DSM-IV classification of affective disorders*

	ICD-10	DSM-IV
Main syndromes	Manic/hypomanic episode	Manic/hypomanic episode
	Depressive episode	Major depressive episode
	mild	Mixed episode
	moderate	
	severe	
Sub-categories	With/without psychotic symptoms (only in mania or *severe* depression)	With/without psychotic features
	Mood congruent/mood incongruent psychotic symptoms (only in mania)	Mood congruent/mood incongruent Psychotic features
		With/without catatonic features
		With/without postpartum onset
		With/without atypical features
Description of course	Single episode or recurrent	Single episode or recurrent, and, if recurrent, there are specifiers for recovery between episodes
		Rapid cycling and seasonal pattern

but not ICD-10, specifies that the symptoms should cause 'clinically significant distress or impairment' and that they should not be 'better accounted for by bereavement'.

ICD-10 contains two notable changes from its predecessor, ICD-9. The first is the separation between bipolar disorder, consisting of recurrent episodes of mania and depression (or less commonly mania alone) and unipolar disorder, consisting of recurrent episodes of depression. ICD-9 had followed Kraepleinian orthodoxy in lumping all severe affective disorders together under the heading of manic-depressive illness. The separation of manic-depression into bipolar and unipolar types was first suggested by Leonhard (1959) but was not accepted in any 'official' classification scheme until the publication of DSM-III (American Psychiatric Association, 1980), by which time considerable evidence from family studies and studies of treatment response had accumulated, supporting the utility of these categories. DSM-IV maintains the unipolar/bipolar division and in addition contains the category bipolar II for those patients who have episodes of depression and hypomania but no full-blown mania. The usefulness of this additional category is uncertain and it has not been included in ICD-10.

The second main difference between ICD-10 and ICD-9 is that the term depressive neurosis has now been abandoned in favour of the mild/moderate/severe typology. The abandonment of the neurotic depressive category again increases the similarity to DSM, where the term 'neurosis' has been entirely deleted since the third edition published in 1980 (American Psychiatric Association, 1980). Both ICD and DSM-IV classify a disorder with chronic 'low grade' depressive symptoms, which do not fulfil the criteria for depressive disorder as dysthymia. There has been some scepticism on the eastern side of the Atlantic as to whether this term, first introduced in DSM-III, is either useful or valid. The fact that it had

Table 11.3. *Symptoms of depressive disorder in ICD-10 and DSM-IV*

1. Depressed mood for 2 weeks
2. Loss of interest
3. Fatigue or decreased energy
4. Loss of confidence or self-esteem
5. Self-reproach or guilt
6. Recurrent thoughts of death, suicide or suicidal behaviour
7. Diminished concentration or indecisiveness
8. Agitation and retardation
9. Sleep disturbance (insomnia or hypersomnia)
10. Appetite and weight change (increase or decrease)

DSM-IV, Major depression: five symptoms including 1 or 2 (4 is not listed).
ICD-10, Severe depression: eight symptoms including 1 and 2 or 3.
Moderate depression: six symptoms including two of 1, 2, or 3.
Mild depression: four symptoms including two of 1 and 2 or 3.

been assigned the same code number (300.4) as depressive neurosis in ICD-9 was a particular source of confusion, since in practice probably the majority of patients with the diagnosis of depressive neurosis treated at British, or other European hospitals, would have fulfilled criteria not for dysthymia but for major depression. With ICD now becoming more DSM-like in nomenclature such terminological confusion should be avoidable.

Whether the traditional separation of depressive disorders into neurotic and endogenous types is now forever abolished remains to be seen. There has been a long debate between those who favour a continuum hypothesis between endogenous and neurotic depression and those supporting the existence of two entities (Kendell, 1976), with the continuum advocates now appearing to be in the ascendancy (Farmer & McGuffin, 1989). However, there remains, as we shall see later, evidence from genetic and other biological studies to suggest that recognising endogenous versus non-endogenous symptom patterns may have some utility. Furthermore, the majority of experienced clinicians would probably still regard the presence of endogenous features as useful when deciding to prescribe drug treatments or ECT. Despite this, there is also an increasing acceptance that depressive disorders can be viewed on a dimension of severity and this is reflected in the three categories of mild, moderate and severe in ICD-10. It follows that there is almost certainly a continuum between having 'normal' symptoms of depression and suffering from overt depressive disorder with no clear-cut line of demarcation.

Other classes and categories of depression

Both ICD-10 and DSM-IV classification allow that sub-categories of depression may occur depending, for example, on whether or not psychotic symptoms are present (Table 11.2). The notion of an endogenous sub-category also lives on in the ICD-10 category of severe depression with somatic symptoms (e.g. prominent sleep or appetite disturbance) and in DSM-IV melancholia. A less explicit feature of both systems is the distinction between primary and secondary depression but both ICD-10 and DSM-IV criteria imply that depressive disorder is a diagnosis applicable only when the syndrome is not a result of some other (non-affective) condition. The modern concept of primary versus secondary affective disorders is largely based on the views of the Washington University, St Louis School (Robins & Guze, 1972), who proposed that depression following alcohol or drug abuse, medical illness, personality disorder, schizophrenia, organic brain disease and a variety of other psychiatric disorders should be classified as 'secondary'. Only depressive disorders where mood disorder occurs first should be classified as 'primary'. Although this dichotomy has been widely used, particularly in North American, it has not been successfully validated by biological or treatment criteria (Grove et al., 1987).

Other attempts to delineate homogeneous sub-groups of depression have used multivariate statistical methods (Farmer & McGuffin, 1989). None of the proposed sub-categories have won general acceptance, but interestingly a study of over 400 American subjects in the community who reported depressive symptoms found that the commonest cluster of symptoms was nearly identical to the DSM-III category of major depression (Blazer et al., 1988). Other minor clusters derived by multivariate classification included a mixed anxiety–depression syndrome and a depressive syndrome associated with premenstrual symptoms in young women.

Epidemiology

From all that we have just considered it seems likely that different diagnostic criteria, even if they are superficially similar, will result in differences in the estimated frequency of depressive disorders in populations. Therefore research into the epidemiology of mood disorders has the same difficulty as studies of other common conditions such as obesity and hypertension, that is, where does the threshold between normality and disorder lie? However, there is an additional problem, that although it may be relatively straightforward to ensure that weighing machines or sphygmomanometers are calibrated in the same way, it may not be true that different psychiatric researchers elicit and describe signs and symptoms in a standard fashion. The general solution to this problem has been to use not only explicit diagnostic criteria but also to use standardised interviews for research.

As described in Chapter 4, several standardised interviews have been devised but in general the choice is between semi-structured interviews such as the Present State Examination (PSE) (Wing et al., 1974), its latest version incorporated in schedules for clinical assessment in neuropsychiatry (SCAN) (Wing et al., 1990), or more highly structured instruments such as the diagnostic interview schedule (DIS) and the composite international diagnostic interview (CIDI) (Robins et al., 1988). The PSE is designed for use by experienced clinicians while the DIS and CIDI can be used by trained lay interviewers. Although there are differences in the way symptoms are elicited, PSE and CIDI produce reassuringly similar results at the level of diagnostic classification (Farmer et al., 1987).

In their current forms, both CIDI and SCAN allow researchers to arrive at a range of diagnoses based on ICD-10 and DSM-IV. Unfortunately, the DIS and earlier versions of the

Table 11.4. *The prevalence of depressive disorder*

Criteria/ interview	Authors	Site	Total N	Period (months)	Prevalence (%)
CATEGO/PSE	Bebbington et al. (1989)	Camberwell, UK	800	1	7.1
	Henderson et al. (1979)	Canberra, Australia	765	1	6.1
DSM-III/DIS	Weissmann et al. (1988)	Baltimore, Durham, Los Angeles, New Haven & St Louis, USA	18 572	6	2.2
	Bland et al. (1988)	Edmunton, Canada	3258	6	3.2
	Joyce et al. (1990)	New Zealand	1498	6	5.3

PSE took rather different approaches to defining 'a case' of psychiatric disorder (Wing *et al.*, 1974). Whereas the PSE allows definition of 'caseness' using a quantitative scale called the 'Index of Definition' and then selecting a suitable cut-off between case and non-case, the DIS and other similar highly structured instruments in North American only allow case definition according to whether the criteria for certain categories (e.g. major depression) are fulfilled. The two approaches do not give exactly comparable results but, again reassuringly, the overall pattern of findings is rather similar. Results from recent studies in English-speaking countries are summarised in Table 11.3. Using the PSE, the one-month prevalences are as much as double the six-month prevalences obtained in surveys using the DIS and DSM-III criteria. Nevertheless, the range is fairly small from a low of 2.2% averaged over five centres in the epidemiologist catchment area (ECA) study, USA, to a high of 7.1% in Camberwell, UK.

Sex

Table 11.4 shows the prevalences of depression averaged for men and women. However, there is a consistent finding across the Western studies listed that depression is approximately twice as common in women as in men. This holds whether the period considered is one month or an entire lifetime. For example, Bebbington and colleagues (1989) found a one-month prevalence of 9.2% in women and 4.9% in men in the UK and in the USA, in the ECA study, Weissman and colleagues, found a lifetime prevalence of 7% in women and 2.6% in men.

Although this pattern is consistent for Western cultures, it is not always the case elsewhere. For example, Orley & Wing (1979) found lower male/female differences in the rates of depression in Uganda, and in Taiwan Hwu *et al.* (1989) found that the male/female ratio for a lifetime prevalence of major depression exceeded 2 in small towns and rural areas but was only 1.4 among urban dwellers. These findings suggest that social and cultural factors must contribute to the differing rates of depression in men and women. Jenkins (1985) tried to address this problem directly by studying a sample of British civil servants and carefully matching the sexes for a range of social variables. Taking a very broad perspective on psychiatric morbidity, which covered approximately a third of her sample, there was no overall difference between men and women, but women showed slightly more depressive symptoms including low mood. Although these findings suggest there is little difference between the sexes when social factors are controlled for, the subjects were all comparatively young (20–35 years) and the women were nearly all childless. The breadth of definition of depression alone does not seem to be a factor in reducing sex differences. For example, as noted earlier, Bebbington et al. (1989) estimated that the lifetime risk of minor depression to age 65 is 46% for men and 72% for women.

Social class

Although most studies in the UK focusing on women have found an association between depression and lower social class (e.g. those by Brown & Harris, 1978; Surtees et al., 1986), no association between social class and major depression was found in the United States in the ECA study. It has also often been suggested that depression is associated more with urban than with rural dwelling but the data are again inconsistent. For example, the ECA study was conducted in five sites in the USA. In one of these, Durham, North Carolina, depression was about twice as common in urban as in rural areas, whereas in St Louis, depression was actually more prevalent in the rural sample.

Ethnic factors

As shown in Table 11.4, the rates of depression in English-speaking countries are similar when the same methods of assessment are used. This seems to be true of other Western countries with, for example, one-month prevalences of depression at 7.4% in Athens, Greece (Mavreas & Bebbington, 1988) and 4.6% in Spain and Finland (Vazquez-Barquero et al., 1986; Lehtinen et al., 1990) in studies using the PSE. Most studies using the DIS have also found similar prevalence in different countries, with the exception of those by Hwu et al. (1989) who, using the DIS in Taiwan, found prevalence rates for major depression of about half those in the USA.

Cohort effects

Several studies have suggested an increase in incidence of depression among younger cohorts (Bebbington et al., 1989; Klerman & Weissman, 1989; Joyce et al., 1990), in addition there appears to be a increased lifetime prevalence of depression among younger groups. This is paradoxical, given that older subjects have lived through more of the period of risk for becoming depressed. A long-term follow-up in Sweden (Hagnell, 1986) suggests that this finding is not entirely due to older people simply forgetting past episodes of depression. There was a very marked increase in the rates of depression reported by young adults in the period 1957–1972 compared to 1947–1957. The differences were particularly striking for men, where there appeared to be a ten-fold difference. Although this might reflect a true increase in depressive disorders in recent years, other explanations need to be considered. In particular there may now be a greater willingness of younger cohorts to volunteer emotional symptoms but it is also possible that in the Swedish study, where operational criteria were not used, the breadth of diagnosis of depression simply increased.

Bipolar disorder

The lifetime prevalence of bipolar disorder in the USA as estimated by the ECA study is in the range 0.7 to 1.6% (Smith & Weissman, 1991). One-month prevalences of mania in studies using the PSE range from 0.08% (Vazquez-Barquero et al., 1986) to 0.8% (Bebbington et al., 1981). Thus overall, bipolar disorder is a much less common condition than severe or major depression. Unlike unipolar disorders there is no evidence of sex differences in the rates of bipolar disorder. The age of onset tends to be earlier than unipolar disorder, with a mean age of first onset of 21 years for bipolar disorder in the ECA study compared with 27 years for unipolar disorder. Epidemiological surveys suggest that ethnic differences exist, with particularly low rates being found in Taiwan (Hwu et al., 1989), where the lifetime risk was estimated at 0.7 to 0.16%. Hospital first admission rates and first contact in the UK vary between ethnic groups with particularly high admission rates for mania among Afro-Caribbeans (Van Os et al., 1994).

Studies particularly in the USA (Faris & Dunham, 1967; Weissman & Myers, 1978) suggest an association of bipolar disorder with social class. This is in the opposite direction to that sometimes suggested for unipolar disorder, in that patients with bipolar disorder tend to have *higher* soci-economic status than the population at large. The reasons for this association are unknown but the most popular speculations is that susceptibility to mania is associated with energy, drive and creativity rather than there being any stressors peculiar to those of higher social class that predispose to mania (Goodwin & Jamison, 1990).

Aetiology

The causation of affective disorders is complicated but in general terms can be considered to reflect an interplay between constitutional or biological factors (which are at least in part genetic) and reaction to environmental insults, which include both physical and psychosocial factors. Evidence on the causes of affective disorders come from a wide variety of sources.

Animal studies

As in other psychiatric disorders, researchers interested in the biological substrate of mood change are hampered by the lack of an animal model that will do justice to the complexity of human behaviour.

There is no really convincing animal model of mania. Nevertheless, several ingenious models of depression have been devised that have turned out to be useful in informing cognitive behavioural theories of depression and in providing ways to test the effectiveness of anti-depressant drugs.

Probably the best-known animal model of depression is the 'learned helplessness' paradigm put forward by Seligman (1976). In his original experiments, carried out on dogs, Seligman exposed the animals to recurrent aversive stimuli in the form of electric shocks from which they were unable to escape. Subsequently, the same animals were placed in a situation in which they were again given electric shocks but from which escape was possible. Unlike normal animals, which quickly learn to avoid the aversive stimuli, the dogs previously exposed to uncontrollable stress showed a marked impairment in learning to escape shocks. It was proposed that these dogs had learned to surrender to the inevitability of painful stimuli in a way that is analogous to the painful, hopeless despair of depressed humans. The paradigm has been criticised on the basis that in humans, how the environment is perceived and conceptualised, may be as important as the events that actually occur. Learned helplessness theory has subsequently been modified to take into account 'attributional style' (Abramson *et al.*, 1978).

Not surprisingly, the original learned helplessness model has also been criticised on ethical grounds. More recent animal work has mainly focused on rats. Although an inescapable shock paradigm is still used by some researchers, others have favoured less traumatic ways of producing a depressed-like state, such as exposing the laboratory animals to chronic, mild and unpredictable stress (Willner *et al.*, 1991). Components include change of cage mates, periods of food or water deprivation, tilting the cage and illumination at night. It has been argued that such measures provide a more realistic analogue of the sorts of stresses of daily life that might be relevant to depression in humans. Rats treated in this way, unlike normal animals, fail to increase their intake when a sweetener such as saccharin or sucrose is added to their drinking water. This has been put forward as an analogue of anhedonia (i.e. loss of interest or pleasure, one of the core features of depression as defined in ICD-10 and DSM-IV). An attraction of this simple measure is that it is easy to quantify and, interestingly, recovery of the normal pattern occurs when the animals are treated with tricyclic antidepressants (Willner *et al.*, 1991).

Other proposed animal models are based on studies of separation. This includes both separation of young animals from their mothers and mature animals from their peers. Both approaches produce a 'protest–despair' reaction that may be more analogous to grief reactions in humans than depression as such. Nevertheless, the behaviour is said to be preventable by treatment with imipramine (Suomi *et al.*, 1978). Separation models have been used mainly in primates but an alternative model may have more general applicability and can be used in rodents in manipulating the dominance hierarchy, after which animals with a reduced status are said to show behavioural alterations analogous to depression (Willner, 1990).

Genetics

Although in animal experiments it is implicit that environmental manipulation can produce a depressive-like response in any animal, strain differences have been demonstrated

Table 11.5. *Affective illness in the first-degree relatives of unipolar (UP) and bipolar (BP) probands (data from studies reviewed by McGuffin & Katz, 1986)*

Proband type	No. of studies	Relatives		
		Age-corrected[b] *n* at risk	Morbid risk[a] BP	(range) (%) UP
BP	12	3710	7.8(1.5–17.9)	–
		3648	–	11.4(0.5–22.4)
UP	7	2319	0.6(0.3–2.1)	9.1(5.9–18.4)

[a] Weighted means.
[b] Corrected denominator (*'Bezugsziffer'*) to allow for relatives who have not lived through the period of risk.

(Henn, 1996). In humans one of the most constant findings is that affective disorders tend to aggregate in families. Table 11.5 summarises the results of studies of the first degree relatives of index cases (or probands) suffering from unipolar or bipolar disorder. The rates are given as lifetime risks (i.e. the figures are age-corrected to take into account the probable proportion of relatives unaffected at the time of the studies but who will later become affected). Although in absolute terms the range of lifetime risks in first degree relatives is large, and this may reflect differences in diagnostic criteria, the overall pattern suggests that affective disorders are commoner in the relatives of affected probands than in the population at large. There are two other, more specific, findings to note. The first is that the overall risk of affective disorders is higher in the relatives of bipolar probands and the second is that relatives of bipolar probands have an increased risk of both unipolar and bipolar disorder, whereas in the relatives of probands with unipolar disorder there is only an excess of unipolar cases.

As in other disorders, two types of 'experiments of nature' have enabled researchers to decide whether the famiality of affective disorders is explicable purely in terms of shared genes, shared family environment or a combination of the two.

Twin studies of mood disorders (including unipolar and bipolar) are summarised in Table 11.6 and are consistent in showing higher monozygotic than dizygotic concordance. Monozygotic twins have all their genes in common whereas dizygotic twins share, on average, 50%. If we assume that environmental sharing is roughly the same for monozygotic and dizygotic twins (all of the studies in Table 11.6 looked only at same-sex dizygotic pairs) then higher monozygotic than dizygotic concordance strongly suggests a genetic component.

Only one study of twins (Bertelsen *et al.*, 1977) has included both unipolar and bipolar probands. The rate of affective disorder in the co-twins of probands with bipolar disorder was 79% for monozygous and 19% for dizygous pairs. With the probands of unipolar disorder the rate was 64% in monozygotic and 24% in dizygotic co-twins. The monozygotic/dizygotic ratio was therefore slightly higher for twins ascertained through bipolar probands, suggesting a stronger genetic effect, in keeping with family study results. There was a general tendency in the study for probands and co-twins to have the same type of

Table 11.6. *Twin concordance for disorders of mood (including unipolar and bipolar)*

Authors	n	MZ concordance (%)	n	DZ concordance (%)
Gershon *et al.* (1976)[a]	91	69	226	13
Bertelsen *et al.* 1977[b]	69	67	54	20
Torgersen (1986)[b]	37	51	65	20
McGuffin *et al.* (1991)	62	53	79	28

MZ, monozygotic; DZ, dizygotic.
[a] Combined figures from six earlier studies report pair-wise concordance.
[b] Systematic register-based studies reporting probandwise concordance.

disorder but the resemblance was incomplete in that in nine out of 55 monozygous pairs concordant for affective illness the proband showed one subtype of disorder while the co-twin showed the other.

Adoption studies have been less complete and extensive than in schizophrenia. One study, based mainly on health insurance records, in Sweden (Von Knorring *et al.*, 1983) found little evidence of either a genetic or family environmental component in affective illness. However, when another report, this time from Denmark, compared hospital records of the biological records of adoptees with affective illness with adopted relatives and relatives of match-control adoptees (Wender *et al.*, 1986), an 8-fold increase in unipolar depression in the biological relatives of adoptees with affective illness was found, as well as a 15-fold increase in the rate of suicide. In another study, which examined the parents of adoptees suffering from bipolar disorder, 28% of the biological parents had affective illness compared with 12% of adopting parents (Mendlewiez & Rainer, 1977). This study again suggested that the subtypes of affected disorder are not completely genetically distinct, as a majority of the affected biological parents of bipolar probands had unipolar rather than bipolar disorder.

Although, as we have already noted, a distinction between neurotic and endogenous patterns of depression no longer features in classifications such as DSM-IV and ICD-10, family studies have in general shown rather lower rates of severe depression in the relatives of probands with a neurotic pattern of symptoms. Twin studies also suggest that neurotic depression probably has a lower genetic component (McGuffin *et al.*, 1994).

Affective disorders rarely, if ever, follow a simple Mendelian pattern of transmission in families and it seems likely that depressive disorders are influenced by several, perhaps many, genes, each of which on their own have a small effect but in combination contribute a liability to the disorder. When further combined with environmental stressors, susceptible individuals will then push beyond the threshold for becoming affected. However, it is possible that, at least in those families where multiple members are affected over several generations, genes of major affect are operating. This hypothesis provides the basis for carrying out genetic linkage studies in which the co-segregation of the disorder and a variety of genetic markers is investigated. Recent advances in molecular genetics have resulted in the discovery of many DNA markers that can be precisely mapped to positions on the human genome (i.e. the 23 pairs of chromosomes), effectively providing reference points that may be used to map the position of genes contributing to diseases. The approach has been dramatically successful in simple Mendelian diseases such as cystic fibrosis and Huntington's disease. It is now feasible to apply the same sorts of technique to complex diseases including affective disorders, and linkage studies are the subject of intensive investigation, particularly bipolar disorder, where the possibility of genes of major affect seems the strongest (McGuffin et al., 1994).

Broadly, two strategies are being employed in attempts to locate and identify genes for affective disorders. The first is a systematic search employing DNA markers, roughly evenly distributed throughout the entire genome. This has resulted in initially promising findings, which now appear to have been false positives, but it should, in the long run detect major genes if they exist (McGuffin et al., 1994). Currently the most promising chromosomal region that may contain a gene for bipolar disorder is on chromosome 18 (Berrettini et al., 1994) but recent linkage findings on chromosome 12 are also of interest (Dawson et al., 1995). The second approach is to focus on so-called candidate genes, that is genes coding for proteins that might plausibly be involved in the pathogenesis of the disorder. These could include receptor proteins or enzymes involved in the synthesis or breakdown of neurotransmitters (Plomin et al., 1994). An association between variations in the serotonin transporter (SERT) gene and affective disorder has recently been reported by several studies (Craddock & Owen, 1996).

Techniques are currently under development using both genetic linkage and an allied but rather different, simpler technique, allelic association, to attempt to detect genes of comparatively small affect, so-called quantitative trait loci (QTL). Using QTL approaches it seems likely that eventually the genetic component of the aetiology of even milder unipolar type depression will be understood at a molecular level (Plomin et al., 1994).

Neurochemistry

The genetic evidence plus the certain knowledge that particular classes of drugs can alleviate depressive symptoms and even precipitate manic episodes while other drugs can produce a depressive-like syndrome, points to a neurochemical basis for affective disorders. However, because in life the brain is the most inaccessible or organs, progress has not been easy and even now, the precise neurochemistry of mood changes remains obscure. Essentially three lines of study have been pursued. First, and perhaps the most productive, have been studies of the effects and mechanisms of action of drugs that bring about mood change. Second, there have been studies of neurotransmitters and their metabolites in urine, blood and CSF as well as studies of neurotransmitter receptors in elements from peripheral blood such as lymphocytes or platelets, under the assumption that these may reflect what is also occurring in receptor populations in the brain. Third, there have been studies based on post-mortem brains, of patients suffering from affective disorders who have committed suicide.

Pharmacological studies provide the basis for the catecholamine hypothesis of depression, which stated quite simply that low mood is associated with low synaptic concentrations of adrenaline (Schildkraut, 1965). This was based on the idea that the catecholamine-depleting drug reserpine apparently caused depressive symptoms, while a variety of antidepressant drugs of the tricyclic group increase availability of noradrenaline by inhibiting presynaptic re-uptake. However, it became clear that some such drugs also inhibit re-uptake of serotonin or 5-hydroxy-tryptamine (5-HT) and that the precursor of 5-HT, L-tryptophan, had an antidepressant effect (Coppen, 1967). These observations led to the indoleamine hypothesis, that low synaptic concentrations of 5-HT bring about depression.

Although it has subsequently been found that the majority of effective antidepressant drugs have marked effects on indoleamine and catecholamine transmissions (Charney & Nelson, 1981), there is discrepancy between the time taken for synaptic NA or both HT concentrations to increase (almost immediate) and the delay seen in clinical practice before antidepressant effects become apparent (two–three weeks). A further problem is that studies of 5-HT or NA or their metabolites in the blood, urine or CSF of depressed patients have in the main failed to show any decrease (Charney & Nelson, 1981). Subsequently it has been proposed that the therapeutic effects of antidepressants depend on alterations in neuroreceptor density and sensitivity and there is considerable evidence from animal studies using both ligand binding methods to assess receptor number and affinity directly or by techniques looking at neuroreceptor gene expression as reflected in specific mRNA levels (Buckland *et al.*, 1992).

The situation is further complicated by finding that some drugs such as desipramine are selective for NA re-uptake and the development of a class of compounds such as fluoxetine and paroxetine, which are selective serotonin re-uptake inhibitors (SSRI). Both selective NA and 5-HT re-uptake inhibition are effective in ameliorating the symptoms of depression and although it may be postulated that different groups of patients are differentially responsive to different types of neurotransmitter re-uptake inhibition, there is no good evidence to support this. A more general hypothesis that unifies at the expense of being somewhat vague is that there is an overall dysregulation of neurotransmission in depression (Siever & Davies, 1985). This is likely to affect more than one neurotransmitter system, which antidepressants may favourably alter by a variety of mechanisms.

Receptor studies have concentrated on binding of various ligands to lymphocytes (or virally transformed lymphoblasts) and platelets. One of the more provocative findings was from the study of Wright *et al.* (1984), where bipolar patients and their ill relatives showed decreased numbers of beta-adrenoreceptors on lymphoblasts. Although this could not be replicated in subsequent studies (Berrettini *et al.*, 1987; Kay *et al.*, 1993) down-regulation of beta-adrenoreceptors with an agonist, isoprenaline, was less efficient in cells from bipolar patients than control lymphoblasts (Kay et al., 1993). Furthermore, incubation of the bipolar patients' lymphoblasts with lithium selectively enhanced their down-regulation by isoprenaline. Evidence of decreased binding to alpha-2-adrenoreceptors in platelets has come from a study (Piletz *et al.*, 1991) that also suggested a difference between patients and controls on internal membrane fluidity. This finding could suggest an abnormality of coupling of receptor cavity, since the patient/control differences were abolished by antidepressant treatment. It is not yet clear whether this phenomenon is related to the blunted response to stimulation of alpha-2 receptors in depressed patients, shown by neuroendocrine tests (see below). Serotinergic function has also been studied by receptor binding assays on platelets, with some results suggesting decreased binding in patients with depression compared to manic patients (Ellis *et al.*, 1991). This would fit with a general hypothesis of decreased serotinergic transmission in depression, or more specifically with the findings of a blunted prolactin response in depressed subjects following challenge with a serotonin releasing agent D-penfluoramine (O'Keane & Dinan, 1991).

Post-mortem studies of the brain of depressed subjects who have died by suicide have produced somewhat conflicting results relating to beta-adrenoreceptor binding. Two groups have reported increased numbers of binding sites in frontal cortex (Mann *et al.*, 1986; Biegon & Israeli, 1988) while a third (De Paermentier *et al.*, 1990) found decreased binding in most cortical areas with particular decreases in the frontal cortex of victims of violent suicide. Post-mortem studies of serotonin binding are also difficult to interpret overall. Lawrence *et al.* (1990) reported no difference in serotonin uptake sites between suicide victims or controls, but findings elsewhere had suggested either increased or decreased numbers of binding sites with the majority indicating an increase in serotonin receptors in frontal cortex (Ball & Whybrow, 1993).

Few investigators have focused attention specifically on the role of dopamine (DA) in depression and this is because drugs such as amphetamines and, even more potently, cocaine, which bring about the release of DA into synapses, do not appear to have a useful or consistent antidepressant effect. However, amphetamines have been implicated in the development of manic-type states as have other dopamine agonists including bromocriptine and L-dopa. The exact role of dopamine in the initiation of manic states is unclear but there is little doubt that a common mode of action of nearly all currently used drugs (with the exception of lithium) that are effective in alleviating manic symptoms is that they exert a post-synaptic blockade of dopamine receptors.

The suggestion that dopamine underactivity may play a role in depression is best supported by the observation that dopamine release appears to be a common feature in all highly rewarding or pleasurable activities. Thus, dopamine levels in the brain can be shown to be increased during sexual arousal and in association with administration of a wide variety of drugs used for 'kicks' such as alcohol, cocaine or opioids (Uhl *et al.*, 1993). Therefore, it may be that loss of interest and diminished capacity to experience pleasure, which forms a core feature of current concepts of depression, is related to an impairment in dopaminergic transmission.

Neuroendocrinology

Two early clinical observations have played an important role in stimulating research on the relationship between hormonal disturbance and affective disorders. First, was the existence of an obvious relationship between myxoedema and depressed mood. Patients with hypothyroidism, particularly in the early stages when physical signs are not prominent, can present with persistent mood changes that are easily mistaken for a primary depression. Mood changes are a prominent feature of Cushing's syndrome, again usually presenting with a depressive picture. Subjective mood change is also a common experience in patients taking corticosteroids in high doses. Some subjects experience depressive symptoms but others report a heightened sense of well-being that may amount to mild elation. Most work has therefore centred on the hypothalamic–pituitary–adrencortic and the hypothalamic–pituitary–thyroid systems, but other endocrine abnormalities have also been explored.

The hypothalamic–pituitary–adrenocortic (HPA) system

The finding that depression occurs in patients with adrenal tumours but is not found in association with Nelson's syndrome where there is elevated ACTH and low corticosteroid levels suggest that cortisol rather than ACTH levels are causally linked with depression (Kelly *et al.*, 1989). However, raised cortisol levels in depressed patients have been known to occur, since at least a quarter of a century ago, and were first interpreted as a non-specific reaction to stress. Better understanding of the physiology of the HPA system led to the development of more complex theories concerning increased HPA activity in depressive disorders. The essentials of the control of HPA activity are as follows: external stress that may be psychosocial or physical (e.g. infection) results in impulses conveyed via relevant brain areas to the hypothalamus, where corticotrophic releasing hormone (CRH) is produced. This permits the release of ACTH in the pituitary, which in turn stimulates secretion of mineralocorticoid and glucocorticoid steroids by the adrenal cortex. There is then a negative feedback mechanism to the hypothalamus, inhibiting further secretion of CRH together with additional negative feedbacks to higher centres and the pituitary directly.

Elevated levels of CRH in the cerebrospinal fluid has been demonstrated in depressed patients (Nemeroff *et al.*, 1984). CRH receptors have also been shown to be down-regulated in the brains of those dying of suicide, which would be in keeping with the theory that there is over-production of CRH in depression (Nemeroff *et al.*, 1988). Further evidence of HPA overactivity comes from studies using human CRH, which when given intravenously to depressed subjects results in a blunted ACTH response compared with controls. By contrast, cortisol response to CRH in depressed patients appears not to differ from controls. This has been interpreted as indicating a hypersensitive adrenocortex in depressed subjects, resulting from persistent exposure to high levels of ACTH (Holsboer *et al.*, 1987).

Much research has focused on the dexamethasone suppression test (DST) in depression, particularly in the subjects with an endogenous pattern of symptoms (Carroll *et al.*, 1981) and there was initial optimism that the DST might have a useful diagnostic role. The test depends on the fact that normal subjects show suppressed plasma cortisol levels throughout the following day after a dose of 1–2 mg of dexamethasone. A high proportion of severely depressed subjects showed an 'escape' from this suppression effect and continue to produce cortisol at normal or even slightly elevated levels. Although this phenomenon would then be in keeping with the hypothesis of HPA overactivity in depression, the DST shows only modest sensitivity (i.e. it 'misses' 20–30% of depressives) and incomplete specificity (i.e. the test is positive in as many as 10% of normal controls and an even higher proportion of non-depressed psychiatric patients). Furthermore, in subjects with recurrent depression an abnormal DST may occur in some but not in other episodes (Coryell *et al.*, 1990).

In summary, HPA overactivity undoubtedly occurs in depressive disorders. However, it is neither a constant feature nor one that is highly specific. The issue of whether HPA overactivity plays a causal role or whether it is a secondary manifestation of other neurochemical or other endocrine abnormalities remains unresolved but it has been argued that HPA changes are more likely to cause alterations in central monoamines than the other way round. This hypothesis derives from the well-established relationship between HPA overactivity and chronic stress (Dinan, 1994). It suggests that changes in monoamines are secondary and are perhaps mediated in depression-susceptible individuals by high levels of glucocorticoid receptors on central neurons.

The hypothalamic–pituitary–thyroid system

Here the control mechanisms are analogous to those in the HPA system. Thyrotrophin-releasing hormone (TRH), produced in the hypothalamus, permits secretion of thyroid-stimulating hormone (TSH) by the pituitary, which in turn stimulates release of thyroxin (T_4) and triiodothyronine (T_3) by the thyroid gland. Again, there are inhibitory feedback mechanisms to the hypothalamus as well as directly to the pituitary.

Small reductions in plasma concentrations of T_3 have been reported in depressed subjects (Rupprecht *et al.*, 1989). Similar modest changes have also been reported in fasting controls and in anorexia nervosa patients, so that slight reduction in T_3 may simply reflect loss of weight in depressed patients.

Although there is no convincing evidence of lowered basal TSH in depression, many studies have shown a reduced TSH response to TRH and there is also evidence of increased TRH production in depression (Checkley, 1992).

Antithyroid antibodies show raised titres in depressed patients compared with controls (Haggerty *et al.*, 1987). Furthermore, increased levels of thyroid antibodies are associated with depressive symptoms in the postpartum period even though there is no significant association between such symptoms and thyroid hormone or TSH levels (Harris *et al.*, 1992).

In summary, a number of mainly rather subtle changes in the hypothalamic–pituitary–thyroid system have been reported in affective disorders but it is not known to what extent any of these have a pathogenic role. The fairly consistent evidence of raised thyroid antibodies in association with depressive symptoms, independent of changes in hormonal level, is intriguing and warrants further investigation.

Other systems

Pituitary hormones other than ACTH and TSH have been the subject of less intensive scrutiny in affective disorders. Although there is little convincing evidence of abnormal growth hormone (GH) secretion in depression there is fairly consistent evidence of reduced GH responses to a variety of agents. Thus, the GH response to the alpha-2 agonist clonidine and the tricyclic compound desipramine has been reported as blunted in depressed patients. Although it is possible that these findings reflect a defect at alpha-2 receptors, a blunted GH response to clonidine or desipramine occurs in other psychiatric disorders (Checkley, 1992).

The release of prolactin by the pituitary is inhibited by dopamine. Therefore, the fact that prolactin levels have consistently been found to be normal in depressed subjects argues against any generalised abnormality of dopaminergic systems (see above). There is, however, some evidence of an increased response in prolactin release when a dopamine antagonist is given to patients with bipolar disorder (Joyce *et al.*, 1987). It is thought that prolactin release depends partially on stimulation of 5-HT1 receptors and one of the effects of antidepressants such as clomipramine, which affects 5-HT re-uptake, is to augment the prolactin response to the 5-HT precursor tryptophan. By contrast, the prolactin response to tryptophan is reduced in depressed subjects (Cowen & Charig, 1987). It has been argued that this, plus evidence of reduced neuroendocrine response to 5-HT-releasing agent (O'Keane & Dinan, 1991), and an absence of blunted response to 5-HT agonists, suggests an abnormality involving decreased 5-HT release rather than decreased receptor sensitivity (Cowen, 1993).

One of the circumstantial reasons for focusing on hypothalamic–pituitary activity in affective disorder is that diurnal variations are a constant feature of hormonal secretion and of mood in severe depression. More recently, there has been accumulating empirical evidence in favour of a longer cyclical phenomenon, that of seasonal affective disorder (SAD). This is characterised by a tendency towards depression, social withdrawal and increased sleep in winter months (Thompson & Isaacs, 1988). The existence of SAD has in turn led to interest in a possible role of melatonin in depression. This substance, secreted by the pineal gland, is known to have a role in the seasonal sexual activity of some mammals and bright light lowers melatonin blood levels in a variety of mammals, including humans. Although there is some evidence that exposure to bright light improves mood in patients with seasonal affective disorder (Thompson & Isaacs, 1988) there is little certain evidence that this is directly mediated by an overall suppression of melatonin levels.

Brain physiology and structure

Although there is no evidence of abnormalities in the electroencephalogram (EEG) during waking hours, much attention has been paid to 'sleep architecture' abnormalities as reflected in EEG patterns. The most consistent abnormality has been of a reduction in depressed subjects of the time between onset of sleep and first appearance of rapid eye movement (REM) sleep. This so-called reduced REM latency appears to be most strongly associated with an endogenous pattern of depressive symptoms and seems to be most pronounced in elderly subjects (Kupfer et al., 1983). Although REM latency decreases with age even in normal subjects, the decrease appears to be more marked in those with depression and it may be possible to discriminate between elderly depressed and demented patients in a reliable way, based purely upon EEG recordings made during sleep (Reynolds et al., 1988).

An important question, therefore, is the one that arises recurrently in studies of the biology of depression, as to whether the phenomenon of altered REM latency provides some clue about vulnerability to depression rather than being merely a secondary phenomenon that disappears once depression has been recovered from. Evidence that decreased REM latency may be a persistent trait comes from studies of patients in remission, some of whom, again particularly those who have had an endogenous pattern of symptoms, show a persistent reduction in REM sleep latency (Rush et al., 1986). Support for the idea that a decrease in REM latency may be an enduring trait rather than a transient state comes from family studies, in which it has been reported that the relatives of depressed patients are more likely than controls to show reduced REM latency and, furthermore, those relatives that show this alteration are the ones who themselves are most likely to suffer from depression (Giles et al., 1988).

The advent of computerised tomographic (CT) brain scanning and magnetic resonance imaging (MRI) has resulted in a renewal of interest in the possibility that structural brain abnormalities could be detected in affected disorders. The overall pattern of results is much less consistent than that for schizophrenia. Most authors carrying out CT or MRI brain scans in a careful manner have reported no change either in young bipolar patients (Johnstone *et al.*, 1989; Harvey *et al.*, 1994) or in a mixture of patients having bipolar or unipolar disorders (Weinberger *et al.*, 1982). A few have reported an increase in the size of lateral cerebral ventricles, most commonly associated with psychotic symptoms (Scott *et al.*, 1983) or mania (Nasrallah *et al.*, 1982; Andreasen *et al.*, 1990). Some authors have reported that cerebral ventricular enlargement is a feature of severe affective disorder in the elderly (Dolan *et al.*, 1985a; Abas *et al.*, 1990) but others have found no difference from age-matched controls (Jacoby & Levy, 1980).

To date, most attempts to use functional brain-imaging techniques in affective disorders have focused on cerebral blood changes. Again, there is unfortunately no consistent trend in the findings.

Several groups have reported a relative reduction in cerebral blood flow in frontal regions in depressed patients (Buchsbaum *et al.*, 1984b; Baxter *et al.*, 1989). These results suggest that 'hypofrontality' may be an abnormality of brain function that is common to both affective disorders and schizophrenia (see Chapter 4). However, other groups suggest that decreased cerebral blood flow in frontal areas is more specifically a feature of schizophrenia and cannot be demonstrated in unmedicated patients with unipolar depression (Gur *et al.*, 1983, 1984). A few groups have looked at subcortical regions but there is some consistency in finding a reduced metabolic rate of glucose in the caudate nucleus of depressed subjects (Baxter *et al.*, 1985; Buchsbaum *et al.*, 1986).

Clarification of these seemingly contrasting findings has come from more recent studies, where the relationship between types of depressive symptoms and patterns of regional blood flow in the brain have been examined (Bench *et al.*, 1993; Dolan *et al.*, 1992). Factor analysis of symptom ratings were performed and three factors were extracted. The first, loading mainly on anxiety, was correlated positively with blood flow in the posterior cingulate cortex and inferior parietal lobule. The second factor, loading on psychomotor retardation and low mood, correlated negatively with left prefrontal and left angular gyrus blood flow. The third, with a high loading on cognitive performance, correlated positively with left medial prefrontal cortical blood flow (Bench *et al.*, 1993). It was proposed that 'hypofrontality', specifically decreased left anterior medial prefrontal blood, characterises patients with so-called depressive pseudodementia (Dolan *et al.*, 1992). Such patients also exhibited increases in the blood flow to the cerebeller vermis.

Physical illness

There is a strong relationship between affective change, particularly depression, and the presence of debilitating physical disorders, and hospital in-patients on general wards have consistently been found to have high rates of affective disturbance (see Chapter 11). Although it is possible to conceptualise physical disorder as merely one type of adversity associated with an increased risk of depression (see below), some disorders appear to be more commonly associated with depression than others. The importance of recognising this is twofold. First, knowing that depression is a frequent accompaniment or aftermath is important in managing the physical disorder and second, the association with depression may give some clue as to the mechanisms involved in the aetiology of depression as a whole.

Among the acute infections, viral illnesses seem to be particularly prone to produce mood change as sequelae. Infectious mononucleosis is a classic cause of persistent low mood, usually accompanied by fatigue in young patients but a similar state is quite common after other acute conditions such as infectious hepatitis. The association between depressive symptoms, chronic fatigue and a wide variety of acute viral illnesses, including very common ones such as influenza, has recently become the subject of much research and considerable controversy. The latter centres on the extent to which post-viral fatigue, or chronic fatigue syndrome, can be explained partly or even entirely as a subform of affective disorder (see chapter 11). There is undoubtedly a high rate of depressive symptoms among patients presenting with chronic fatigue. But in recent studies only about one-third to one-half of patients fulfil criteria for depression disorder (Farmer *et al.*, 1995).

Less controversial is the association between mood change and brain disorders. Although euphoria is classically described as a feature of late-stage multiple sclerosis, associated with marked demyelination in prefrontal areas, depression is a more frequently encountered mood change (Lishman, 1987). Depressive disorders are also more frequently seen among patients with Parkinson's disease than in other disorders, not involving the central nervous system, producing a similar level of chronic disability (Mindham, 1970). Among the common neurological disorders, most recent interest has focused on the relationship between depression and stroke. It has long been recognised that depression is a common sequel to a stroke but recent work suggests that post-stroke depression is strongly associated with increased mortality (Morris *et al.*, 1993). There is no evidence as yet on whether antidepressant treatment improves long-term survival.

Intriguingly, the site of the lesion in strokes may provide an indication of the brain areas predominantly involved in affective disorders. A study using cerebral blood flow measures found that lesions in the left anterior and right posterior cortex were associated with depression (Yamaguchi *et al.*, 1992). Two other studies provide support for involvement of the left anterior hemisphere in post-stroke depression (Astrom *et al.*, 1993; Herrmann *et al.*, 1993).

Psychosocial adversity

The possible role of unpleasant happening or persistent social adversity in causing depression has long been a matter of interest but it is only comparatively recently that such factors have become the subject of systematic and scientific enquiry. To many the relationship between 'stress' and 'depression' seems obvious and hardly therefore even a subject that needs research. Certainly most members of the lay public or contributors to the popular media tend to explain depression or suicidal behaviour as a response to untoward events or stressful lifestyle rather than constitution or biological factors (see, for example, Manchip's (1994) discussion of media coverage of the death by suicide of the rock star Kurt Cobain).

Some of the reasons why it is more difficult than appears at first sight to show a relationship between life events and illness are discussed in Chapter 4. These include the fact that some events may be generated by the patient's own behaviour, and hence in turn influenced by the occurrence of a disorder such as depression, as well as the problem that people generally seek explanations for a state that they find themselves in. Thus a depressed patient in a search for meaning may attribute the onset of his or her disorder to a particular event whereas the same or similar events may be impinged upon others with no resultant mood disorder. A further and related problem is how to categorise and measure the severity of an event, given that the impact of the same event on different individuals may differ. There is a reasonable consensus (see Chapter 4) that semi-structured interview methods are superior to self-completed questionnaires in assessing life events and one of the widely used instruments is that derived by Brown & Harris (1978). Their life events and difficulty schedule (LEDS) is a semi-structured interview designed to detect the occurrence of life events over a recent period (usually the past six or 12 months). After interviewing a subject using the LEDS the re-searcher reports the result to a panel of raters, who are provided with no information about the patient's mental state. Ratings are made of the degree of threat of the event, whether it is independent, possibly independent or dependent on the subject's own actions, and of a number of other characteristics of the event such as whether it is 'self focused' (i.e. directly focused on the subject) or 'other focused'. There is now an overwhelming body of evidence both from Brown & Harris's own work and from a number of other studies (e.g. Bebbington et al., 1981, 1988; Brugha & Conroy, 1985; Roy et al., 1985) that there is an excess of events before the onset of the disorder in depressed subjects compared with controls. Studies using the LEDS have reported that it is threatening events that are predominantly associated with depression, but other workers using different terminologies (e.g. Paykel et al., 1969) have found that 'exit' events such as death of a loved one or departure by some other means such as divorce, or events that are in some other way undesirable, are most strongly associated with depression. The fact that independent events are associated with depression supports the view that the event has a causal role in the depression rather than the behaviour of the depressive causing the event. A causal role is also supported by the temporal relationship between life events and depression, with reported events showing a peak before rather than after the onset of the disorder (see, for example, Bebbington et al., 1988).

Brown & Harris (1978) have pointed out that persisting stressors, which they call chronic difficulties, are also found in excess before the onset of depression and have also looked in detail at more enduring psychosocial factors that can have a relationship with depression. Particularly influential has been their vulnerability model, where they have proposed, on the basis of their own studies in London, UK, that women with two or more young children at home, a lack of a confiding relationship and without employment outside the home, are particularly susceptible to develop depression after exposure to a threatening event. Much of the criticism of this hypothesis has centred on statistical arguments, which propose that the concept of vulnerability suggests that individuals characterised as vulnerable will show a proportionately greater response to life events than those who are not vulnerability. In practice most studies suggest that the effects of vulnerability factors and life events are additive rather than multiplicative (i.e. the increased risk of depression attributable to life events is about the same whether or not vulnerability factors are present) (Alloway & Be-bbington, 1987). Nevertheless, the presence of social support from relatives, friends or a spouse, with whom there is a caring intimate relationship, would certainly appear to have some buffering or protective effect against a depressive response to adversity (Champion, 1990).

The hypothesis that loss of parents during childhood increases the risk of depression in adult life has received much attention. Much of this derives from psychoanalytic theory and the notion that secure attachment to parents, particularly to the mother, is important in the development of mental health (Bowlby, 1951). Brown *et al.* (1977) proposed that loss of a mother, either by death or separation, before the age of 11 years, was associated with an increased risk of depression in adult life, and Brown & Harris (1978) incorporated maternal loss within their concept of vulnerability. However, a number of studies, including the largest control series (Birtchnel, 1972) have failed to find any convincing relationship between adult depression and the loss by death of parents during childhood.

Psychosocial adversity in the form of life events or chronic difficulties appear to be as strongly associated with an endogenous pattern or depressive symptoms as with a neurotic or 'reactive' pattern (Bebbington *et al.*, 1988). This would argue against the existence of two broad groups of depressive disorders, one largely resulting from psychosocial stresses and the other from constitutional or biological factors. Nevertheless, an earlier study did suggest that such an approach may have some utility. Pollitt (1972) categorised a series of depressed patients into those whose disorder had followed a physical illness or life stress and those where preceding stress 'was only a possibility'. Those patients whose illness arose in the absence of identifiable stressor had markedly higher rates of depressive disorder among the relatives than those patients whose depression followed stress. Subsequently other workers (Patrick *et al.*, 1978) failed to find an inverse relationship between presence of life events and degree of family loading for depression. A more detailed study examining a series of depressed patients and their first degree relatives using both the Present State Examination (PSE) and the LEDS produced similarly negative results (McGuffin *et al.*, 1988*a*). However, in addition two unexpected findings emerged. The first of these was that although there was a modest excess of life events in the currently depressed versus not depressed relatives of depressed patients, this was statistically non-significant and the size of the effect was certainly very much smaller than that usually seen in samples of patients and unrelated controls. Even more surprisingly, the first degree relatives of depressed patients reported threatening and (on the face of it) independent life events whether or not they themselves were depressed, at a rate that was roughly four times as high as in a sample of controls drawn from the general population. Taken together these findings might suggest that the relationship between life events and depression, which has now been reported by many studies, could, at least in part, be explained by a tendency to report both depressive symptoms and life events being familial. Recent twin studies on non-depressed subjects confirm that there is a familial component in the responses to life event questionnaires and that this may even receive a modest influence from genetic factors (Plomin, 1990; Kendler *et al.*, 1991; Thapar & McGuffin, 1996). Thus future research on psychosocial factors in depression should include a biological and genetic perspective as it now seems likely that the relationship between environmental stress and genetic predisposition appears more complex than at first sight it may have appeared.

Psychological theories and the role of personality

Psychoanalytic speculations about the origins of depression date back to Freud's writings of over a century ago and his theories were crystallised in a classic paper, 'Mourning and Melancholia' (Freud, 1917). Here he compared severe depression to a state of bereavement, noting that one of the key differences is that during normal grief, self-regard is usually unimpaired. Freud was, in fact, circumspect about the role of psychogenic factors in melancholia, acknowledging that the symptoms often 'suggest somatic rather than psychogenic affections'. He therefore confined his discussion to cases where the role of psychogenic factors seemed most likely. For Freud these were situations involving loss or rejection, where the melancholic patient identifies the lost object with his own ego by a process of introjection. He then turns the hostility generated by the loss into self-reproach and guilt. A more explicit formulation in terms of object relations theory was evolved by Klein (1934) who postulated that passage through a 'depressive position' is a necessary stage of normal development occurring in infancy. This occurs when the infant first reacts to separation from the mother and her breast with hostility and then realises that his destructive anger may have the consequence of damaging or even destroying the object of his love. Winnicot (1958) put forward the idea that a successful passage through the depressive position was necessary for the arrival at a 'stage of concern', where the child first develops the capacity to care for others and to recognise the effect upon them of his own emotion.

Although, in common with psychoanalytic theory as a whole, Freudian and post-Freudian explanations of depression do not generate testable hypotheses about the cause of depression, they are sometimes useful in interpreting the meaning of depressive symptoms in individual patients. In particular, the self-deprecation of a profoundly depressed patient expressing ideas of guilt and self-blame becomes more understandable when viewed as the angry and frustrated response to external events being turned inward on the self. Nevertheless, such insights into how patients' symptoms may evolve do not necessarily lead to therapeutic benefits. Dissatisfaction with the explanatory power and therapeutic utility of psychoanalytic theory led Beck (1976) to put forward his cognitive theory of depression (see also Chapter 25). Beck proposed that the depressed individual is characterised by a cognitive triad consisting of a negative view of self, current experiences and the future and that this influences the organisation of thought in a way that selectively attends to depressive ideas.

Beck considered that the cognitive triad of the depressed patient is maintained even in the face of contradictory evidence because of a style of thought, a 'schema' that the depressed individual acquires early in life, partly in response to childhood experience. This may lie dormant or inactive for a long period but is then evoked by adverse circumstances. Once activated, a negative cognitive schema overcomes the individual's capacity for voluntary control over his or her thoughts, and negative ideas and attitudes spring up in an autonomous or automatic way. The individual tends to make inferences in an arbitrary fashion, in a way that is unrelated to actual evidence and to over-generalise so that one unpleasant event or idea colours other unrelated experiences.

The notion of a fixed and maladaptive response-set in depression is also a feature of 'learned helplessness' theories of depression, which were discussed earlier. The reformulated theory of learned helplessness (Abramson et al., 1978) takes into account the attributional style of the depressed individual. That is, if someone experiences an unpleasant event over which they have no control, they will seek to interpret its occurrence. Characteristically, depressed subjects attribute the causes of events to factors external to themselves and tend to regard outcomes as non-contingent, i.e. independent of anything they actually do. Such attributions are associated with low self-esteem, in which the depressed individual feels that he or she has no control over the things that happen to him or her and hence develops a state of hopelessness and self-blame.

Low self-esteem was also a feature of Brown & Harris's (1978) original vulnerability model of depression and was later found by Brown and colleagues (1986) to be a strong predictor of depression following adversity in a study of women in Islington in North London. Bebbington (1985) has pointed out that there is a common theme of cognitive abnormalities running through the models of depression proposed by Beck, Brown & Harris and Abramson, all of which emphasise an inherent style of thinking, that is in a sense primitive and is assumed to be dependent upon early experience. Here at least there are echoes of psychoanalytic explanations. Recent attempts to refine cognitive theories of depression have looked more explicitly at anomalies of information processing (Teasdale, 1993). For example, a distinction is made between different types of meaning attached to ideas and events. Propositional meaning is to do with specific theories or constructs that the individual has about the world, whereas implicational meaning is to do with more general links between events, the personal implications for the individual and their emotional outcomes. Thus an information-processing model of depression sees the depressed subject as someone who has a negative recall bias (i.e. they preferentially recall unpleasant rather than pleasant stimuli), particularly when these are referring to the self. There is some experimental evidence to support this. For example, depressed patients are more likely than non-depressed controls to recall negative adjectives referring to themselves but, like controls, show the normal bias towards recalling positive adjectives when these are applied to someone else (Bradley & Mathews, 1983).

The extent to which depression is related to enduring and overt personality traits (as opposed to schemes that lie dormant and hidden from view) is controversial. The problem is difficult to resolve partly because questionnaires that purport to measure stable personality traits are partly confounded by emotional states. Thus, for example, neuroticism, N, or emotional instability as measured using the Eysenck Personality Questionnaire (EPQ) (Eysenck & Eysenck, 1975) shows an increase in scores in subjects when they are depressed (Kendell & DiScipio, 1968). Thus a study of relatives of depressed patients found the highest N scores in those relatives who themselves were depressed at the time of the study and the lowest levels in those who were neither currently depressed nor had a past history of depression. Relatives who were well at the time of the study but who had been depressed in the past, had intermediate scores (Katz & McGuffin, 1987).

While there is no doubt that people who have personality disorders generally have an increased risk of depression compared with those in the population at large, the majority of patients who present with depression do not have personalities that before the onset of their disorder, can be categorised as abnormal. As mentioned earlier, some authors distinguish between primary depression occurring when there is no pre-existent disorder and secondary depression occurring following some other disorder including personality disorder. Winokur (1975) has also put forward the notion of depression spectrum disorders, which cluster both in individuals and their families along with personality disorder and alcoholism. This he contrasts with 'pure' depression, which may arise either sporadically or as a result of a familial diathesis, but in either case is uncontaminated by abnormal premorbid personality.

Treatment

Mania

In the acute state it is nearly always necessary to admit the manic patient to hospital to protect them from the consequences of their own recklessness but it is also sometimes necessary for the protection of others. The main aim is to place the patient in secure and safe surroundings where their behaviour can be contained. Nursing the manic patient requires considerable skill that balances tact and non-confrontation with a firm setting of limits of what is acceptable behaviour.

Neuroleptic drugs with sedating properties are the mainstay of acute medical treatment. Haloperidol is the most widely used drug and in doses of 10 to 15 mg orally, three times daily, usually produces a satisfactory response. It may be necessary to start treatment by injection and a 'loading' dose of up to 30 mg intramuscularly may be given depending on the size and degree of disturbance of the patient. Rarely, severely disturbed patients may require a total daily dose of 100 mg. Droperidol is a related compound that is slightly more sedating and is therefore favoured by some clinicians as a mean of obtaining more rapid control of manic symptoms. It has the advantage of being available in an intravenous injection. Chlorpromazine is also effective in doses of up to 1000 mg per day but is somewhat more prone to cause drowsiness as well as producing other immediate side-effects such as postural hypotension. Some clinicians believe that chlorpromazine is less effective than haloperidol in rapidly dampening down overactivity but there is no controlled evidence to support this.

Lithium has a place in the acute control of mania and may be introduced if the patient is slow in responding to either haloperidol or chlorpromazine alone. Lithium has been shown to be effective in treating manic symptoms even when not combined with neuroleptics but has the disadvantage of requiring about five days before beneficial effects are seen. Although the usually quoted levels of lithium in the blood for effective maintenance treatment are between 0.4 and 1.0 mmol per litre, levels at the upper end of this range need to be aimed for if the treatment of acute mania is to be successful. One of the problems about starting lithium in the acutely ill patient is the potential delay in ensuring that the patient has adequate renal function (see below). This is not usually a problem in the young and physically fit but does limit the usefulness of lithium in the acute management of older patients.

There have been reports of severe extrapyramidal side-effects resulting from haloperidol and lithium given in combination and even rarer reports of death attributed to such a regime. However, there is little hard evidence that a lithium–haloperidol combination is any more toxic than a combination of lithium with any other neuroleptic and the chief guidelines for a safe approach to the drug treatment of mania are to aim for blood levels of lithium within therapeutic limits and to avoid 'heroic' high doses of neuroleptics.

One method of lowering the dosage requirement of neuroleptics in a severely disturbed and disruptive manic patient is to augment neuroleptic treatment with a benzodiazepine such as lorazepam for a limited period of not more than about 7–10 days. This may be given in quite high doses of up to 5 mg three times daily, at which level its sedating effect is useful.

In the rare patient who does not respond to such a regime it may be necessary to give electroconvulsive therapy (ECT). A course of bilateral ECT can have a dramatic effect in cutting short an episode of otherwise intractable mania. Clinical experience suggests that this is particularly effective when the treatments are more closely spaced than is customary in the treatment of depression. Thus in the treatment of a manic patient ECT may be given on alternate days or three times weekly.

While the aim in treating mania is to achieve a smooth recovery with remission of symptoms, a hazard to be aware of is a swing into depression. This may be quite rapid or may be heralded by the patient developing a mixed affective state, when manic and depressive symptoms co-occur. The most important practical point is to be aware that a depressed rather than normal mood is a possible outcome and to be vigilant for the first signs of this occurring. It is then better to reduce the dose of neuroleptics and attempt to titrate a balance between depressed symptoms and re-emergence of mania rather than immediately adding an antidepressant.

Having achieved a recovery from manic symptoms it is advisable to gradually tail off treatment with neuroleptics rather than to stop rapidly. Again, cautious titration against re-emergence of symptoms is the general rule. This can be done initially while the patient is still in hospital and then continued at an early out-patient follow up and discharge from hospital. A good guide to the rate at which neuroleptics can be reduced is the patient's subjective report of feeling sedated, as recovery is almost always accompanied by a marked decrease in tolerance to this particular action of the neuroleptics.

Depression

Psychotherapy

'Talking treatment' almost always forms a necessary component of the successful treatment of an episode of depression. In its simplest form (and sometimes its most potent) the doctor provides confident reassurance. The patient should be told unequivocally that he is going to get better and in this respect the therapist can usually look forward to reaping rewards since the majority of cases will, sooner or later, recover. It is important to accompany reassurance with acceptance and moral support. The depressed patient suffers not only from the primary effect of his symptoms but also from the secondary dismay of the situation in which he finds himself. This includes what may be perceived as the ignominy of having a psychiatric disorder as well as the fear of 'going mad'. It is usually reassuring to be told that the doctor has encountered the symptoms that the depressed patient describes in other patients and that the accompanying biological features together with self-depreciation, guilt or ideas of suicide are well-recognised features.

Of the specific therapies, cognitive behavioural therapy has been shown to be particularly effective and is dealt with in greater detail in Chapter 25. This form of psychotherapy derives largely from Beck's cognitive theories about the pathogenesis of depression (see above). The broad aims are to teach the patient how to challenge current thoughts about him or herself and the world and to turn these techniques to good use both in perceptions of the future and in the practical handling of future situations.

Another comparatively brief and focused form of psychotherapy that has gained a certain amount of recent attention is interpersonal therapy (IPT) as described by Klerman (1988).

Here the focus is upon the patient's relationship with others and the ways in which they habitually deal with everyday situations. The aims are again highly pragmatic and based upon competent handling of the 'here and now' rather than attempts to resolve past, deep-seated conflicts, frustrations or losses. In some respects Klerman's development of IPT has been viewed by experienced clinicians as an attempt to codify and refine some of the key elements that purveyors of successful 'talking treatments' have been practising for many years. Klerman's writings nevertheless provide a useful guide for the uninitiated and the elements of his approach, like cognitive behaviour therapy, lend themselves to scientific testing in a way that is difficult to achieve using traditional psychodynamic or insight-orientated approaches.

Drug treatment

Tricyclic antidepressants   For clinical purposes the tricyclic antidepressants can be broadly divided into two groups, those with sedative properties, such as amitriptyline, dothiepin and clomipramine, and those that are less sedative such as imipramine, nortripyline and lofepramine. Some tricyclic compounds such as protriptyline actually have mildly stimulating properties. The choice of drug is therefore influenced by whether or not sedation is desirable in a particular patient. Anxious or agitated patients may benefit from sedation as may those in whom sleep disturbance is a prominent symptom. Here it is useful to prescribe a sedative drug such as amitriptyline or dothiepin in a once-daily dose given at night.

Although sleep disturbance will usually show improvement in the first week after prescribing a sedative tricyclic antidepressant, other symptoms of depression often require two to three weeks before noticeable change is evident. In some patients the delay is even longer and it may take up to six weeks before definite beneficial responses are seen.

One of the key components of using tricyclic antidepressants effectively is making sure the patient is receiving an adequate dosage. In most patients this will mean at least 100 mg daily, but requirements may go as high as 250 mg per day. As a class the tricyclic antidepressants have a sufficiently long half-life that a once-daily dose can be given and this is most conveniently given at night whether or not sedation is required.

One way to ensure that the patient is receiving an adequate dose of antidepressants is to measure blood levels but as a routine practice this is no longer standard in most centres. Part of the rationale for measuring blood levels is that some tricyclic antidepressants such as nortriptyline have been shown to have a curvilinear dose response, so that for maximum response blood levels appear to be best kept within a 'therapeutic window' with either lower or higher levels proving less effective (Asberg, 1976). It has also been proposed that monitoring the orthostatic hypotensive response to tricyclics can serve as a surrogate for monitoring blood levels (Davis & Janowsky, 1974). It has been suggested that the dose of tricyclic antidepressant at which this side-effect begins to appear is just above that required for an adequate therapeutic response. Therefore, doses may be gradually increased until the patient exhibits orthostatic hypotension and then subsequently slightly lowered. In practice, in the majority of cases, it is possible to simply titrate the dose of tricyclic antidepressants against symptoms, balancing improvement against emerging side-effects.

Side-effects

The commonest problems are those resulting from antimuscarinic anticholinergic properties such as a dry mouth, blurring of vision, constipation or hesitancy in micturition. Tolerance to these symptoms usually develops and it is useful both to warn the patient in advance that such symptoms may occur and that they will improve over time. However, it is probably best to avoid tricyclic antidepressants altogether in patients with glaucoma, in whom an acute attack can be precipitated, or in men with prostatism, who may develop urinary retention.

The other troublesome and potentially more serious side-effects are those in the cardiovascular system. Postural hypotension has already been mentioned and can nearly always be abolished by simply lowering the dosage. Cardiac arrhythmia and conduction defects can occur, especially with older compounds such as amitriptyline. These are therefore contraindicated in patients who have had a recent myocardial infarction or a history of heart block. Some of the more recently developed tricyclics such as lofepramine appear to be much less cardiotoxic.

Other side-effects include weight gain, increased sweating, delayed ejaculation (hence low-dose clomipramine is sometimes used as a treatment for premature ejaculation) and lowering of the seizure threshold.

Atypical and non-tricyclic antidepressants   The so-called selective serotonin re-uptake inhibitors (SSRI) have been the most successful recently introduced class of compounds in the treatment of depression. They have comparatively few side-effects but are as effective as standard tricyclics in double-blind clinical trials (Song *et al.*, 1993). They include fluoxetine, paroxetine, fluvoxamine, sertraline and citalopram. They are non-sedative drugs with very low cardiotoxicity and therefore are safer than the tricyclics in overdose or with patients with heart disease. In contrast with the tricyclics, which tend to stimulate appetite, the SSRIs have a neutral or even slightly appetite suppressing effect. Nausea and vomiting are occasional side-effects and diarrhoea can also occur. Gastrointestinal side-effects are probably most common with fluvoxamine but are usually dose-related and usually improve on lowering the dose. Headaches may also be a problem and most commonly occur in patients with a history of migraine. Restlessness in the first week or two and an increase in anxiety may be reported but this does not usually persist. Most controversially, the SSRIs in general and fluoxetine, currently the most widely used drug, in particular, have been allegedly associated with violent behaviour and an increased risk of suicide. These claims are based upon uncontrolled reports and there is no hard evidence of higher rates of aggression or irritability in patients treated with SSRIs than with any other antidepressants (Harrison, 1994).

A controversy that is more deserving of attention is whether, given that they have comparable efficacy to the tricyclics but superior safety, SSRIs should replace tricyclics as the first line of treatment in depression. One of the few objections to the SSRIs is cost. Currently in the UK an SSRI is about 20–30 times as expensive as a tricyclic antidepressant. However, it has been argued that most of the failure to comply with tricyclic antidepressant treatment is because of their side-effects and that compliance with SSRIs is likely to be much superior. Therefore, given the costs of abandoned courses of treatment with tricyclics and secondary costs of treating health problems directly attributable to side-effects, the cost differential between using SSRIs and tricyclic antidepressants may be small. A simulated costing analysis suggested that if the problem was looked at in this way there is little to choose between the two classes of compounds despite the initially higher prescribing expenses when the SSRIs are used (Jonsson & Bebbington, 1993). Against this view is a finding from a metanalysis of clinical trials comparing SSRIs and tricyclics. The combined results from a total of 58 studies showed that not only were the two classes of compounds of equal efficacy, but also the patient drop-out rates were roughly the same. About a third of patients failed to complete drug trials whether or not they were taking SSRIs or tricyclics (Song et al., 1993).

From a theoretical viewpoint the specificity of action of drugs such as the SSRIs may appear attractive. The analogy would be with drugs used in other branches of medicine. For example, beta-blockers are used in the relief of cardiac symptoms, and it is known with reasonable certainty that the benefits result from blockade of beta-1 receptors in the heart while side-effects result from beta blockade elsewhere. However, in the case of depression much less is known about the pathophysiology of the disorder and it seems likely that a number of neurochemical mechanisms are involved. Therefore, although the specific inhibition of serotonin uptake is effective in the clinical relief of symptoms, in the majority of cases it is unlikely that this is the only specific mechanism that should be targeted (Rubin, 1994).

Before the introduction of SSRIs, a variety of other non-tricyclic drugs were developed in an attempt to obtain effectiveness that is at least comparable to standard drugs but with less antimuscarinic and cardiac side-effects. Those still in use include mianserin, trazodone and maprotiline, which have sedative properties, and viloxazine, which is less sedative. All are probably safer than tricyclics in patients with pre-existing heart disease but are not free of side-effects. In particular, mianserin can cause haematological abnormality (and so it is advisable to perform a full blood count at least monthly when using this drug). Maprotiline is associated with a risk of epileptic seizures and trazadone has an uncommon, but usually painful, side-effect of producing prolonged priapism.

Monoamine oxidase inhibitors (MAOIs) Monoamine oxidase inhibitors were the first effective antidepressants and were discovered by accident when isoniazid used in the treatment of tuberculosis was shown to inhibit monoamine oxidase and was observed to elevate mood. Currently available MAOIs include phenelzine, isocarboxazid and tranylcypramine. The main distinguishing feature is that tranylcypramine acts as a central CNS stimulant and gives some patients an amphetamine-like 'buzz'.

The MAOIs are used less frequently than tricyclics, partly because of doubts about their efficacy (MRC, 1965) but also because of their interactions with other drugs and with tyramine. Tyramine is found in many foods such as matured cheese, pickled herring, game and broad bean pods. It is also abundant in meat or yeast extracts such as 'Bovril', 'Oxo' and 'Marmite'. A tyramine response or 'cheese reaction' in patients taking MAOIs who eat such foods consists of a rapid and dangerous rise in blood pressure. Therefore, the patient needs to be warned of the potential reaction and it is usual to issue a treatment card listing the foods and drink to be avoided. MAOIs also interact with opioides such as pethidine and potentiate the effects of CNS depressants such as benzodiazepines, barbiturates and alcohol. Because of these problems, reversible MAOIs have been developed, of which the first to be made available is moclobemide. This is said to inhibit especially monoamine oxidase Type A. Moclobemide is much less likely than older MAOIs to potentiate the pressor effect of tyramine but it is nevertheless recommended that large amounts of tyramine-rich foods should be avoided in patients taking the drug. The manufacturers also advise the avoidance of sympathomimetics such as ephedrine. Because of its reversibility, it is possible to switch from moclobemide to a tricyclic antidepressant without a treatment-free period. This was a hazardous process with the older MAOIs because of the likelihood of hypertensive crises. It is nevertheless advisable not to start moclobemide for at least a week after tricyclic antidepressant has been stopped, or at least five weeks after stopping fluoxetine.

Drug choice and prediction of response   In general, patients with an 'endogenous' pattern of symptoms respond in a more predictable way to tricyclic antidepressants than patients with an absence of biological features or with atypical features such as hypersomnia and increased appetite. An exception to the rule of good response in patients with endogenous depression are those patients in whom delusions are prominent (Glassman *et al.*, 1975). Here it may be necessary to use a combination of an antidepressant and an antipsychotic. Recently there has been interest in the possibility that premorbid personality traits may be useful variables in predicting overall response (Joyce, 1994) but there is so far little evidence that personality measures are useful in deciding on which specific drug to use.

Choice of drug is often influenced by side-effect profile, e.g. the benefits or drawbacks of sedation or the need to avoid cardiotoxicity, but choice may also be influenced by the risk of the patient self-poisoning. Although recent evidence suggests that death by antidepressant drug overdose is less common in patients taking newer safer compounds such as SSRIs than in those taking the older tricyclics (Henry *et al.*, 1995), the overall risk of completed suicide does not differ between these two groups (Jick *et al.*, 1995).

Some advocates of treatment with MAOIs suggest that it is possible to define a particular profile where these drugs are likely to be beneficial. Such patients usually have a lack of biological or endogenous features and increased sleep and appetite (Nutt & Glue, 1989). Prominent anxiety symptoms, derealisation and depersonalisation and the occurrence of panic attacks are also said to be markers of a favourable response to MAOIs. Recent work also suggests that a contributor to the poor performance of drugs such as phenelzine in some clinical trials was that the dosages used were too low. Doses of at least 60 mg of phenelzine a day are needed if it is to be effective.

Electroconvulsive treatment (ECT)

Although it has attracted considerable criticism in popular media, there is overwhelming evidence that ECT is efficacious in the treatment of severe depressive disorder. ECT has been found to be more effective than tricyclics, MAOIs or placebo (MRC, 1965) and there have now been six controlled trials in the UK (Royal College of Psychiatrists, 1990*a*) comparing ECT with 'sham' ECT where an anaesthetic alone was given. Five of the six studies showed clear superiority of ECT over sham treatment. The negative study was one in which the

343

actual treatment consisted of a unilateral brief pulse stimulus, which is now agreed to be less effective than bilateral ECT.

The most common indications for ECT are persisting severe or moderately severe depressive symptoms despite an adequate course of antidepressant drugs for at least four (some would say six) weeks, or the presentation of severe depression where rapid treatment is needed. This is either because the patient presents a serious suicidal risk or when he is failing to eat or drink. Failure to eat or drink is a virtually constant feature of depressive stupor and here again ECT should be used as the first line of treatment. As we have noted, prominent delusions of guilt or persecution are usually associated with a poor response to tricyclics and it may therefore be justifiable to use ECT as the first line of treatment for such patients. The alternative of giving tricyclic antidepressants and antipsychotics in combination is arguably more hazardous in frail or elderly patients. Indeed there is some evidence that the presence of delusions is the most constant predictor of a good response to ECT (Johnstone *et al.*, 1980). A previous history of a good response to ECT, particularly where that history is also combined with poor initial response to antidepressant drugs, is an indication for progressing to ECT earlier rather than later.

ECT is always given under general anaesthetic with muscle relaxants and there is a consensus, as a result of recent trials, that bilateral is superior to unilateral ECT (Royal College of Psychiatrists, 1990*a*). Modern machines deliver a series of very brief (1–2 ms) direct current pulses at a rate of about 6–7 pulses per second. Fits lasting more than two minutes are associated with an increased likelihood of short-term memory loss. Although such an occurrence is uncommon, fits as long as this should be terminated by the anaesthetist with intravenous diazepam. The 'standard' course of treatment is 6–8 applications with two treatments being given per week. Some patients may require as many as 12–14 treatments but it is rare to see improvement beyond this stage if it has not already occurred.

Side-effects and precautions The most important risks of ECT are those associated with a short general anaesthetic. Therefore the usual precautions in checking that the patient has no cardio-respiratory disorder contraindicating a short general anaesthetic need to be taken. In addition, it is common practice to measure pseudocholinesterase to guard against the possibility of prolonged apnoea after muscle relaxant use. Severe complications of anaesthesia for ECT are in fact rare and lower than that following anaesthesia for surgical procedures. The death rate (with deaths usually being due to cardiovascular collapse) has been estimated at 1 in 10 000 (Scott, 1986).

Although there are no absolute contraindications to ECT, it is probably best avoided within the first four to six weeks following myocardial infarction. However, ECT is probably safer than tricyclic antidepressants in patients with severe coronary heart disease. Caution should be exercised in patients with a recent history of ventricular arrhythmias, either due to coronary heart disease or other causes. However, in practice the risk of ECT producing arrythmia is not high.

Fractures, dislocations and other traumatic injuries which, in the past, were hazards of unmodified ECT (i.e. ECT given without anaesthesia) are no longer a problem providing adequate muscle relaxation is given. This point, that providing muscle relaxation is the prime purpose of giving a general anaesthetic for ECT, although fundamental, is not always grasped by more junior anaesthetists in training.

Further details, including the mechanisms of action of ECT, are discussed in Chapter 24 but it is worth mentioning here that the side-effect that is most often complained of by the depressed patient, is of memory impairment. This is greater for bilateral than for unilateral ECT applied to the non-dominant hemisphere. Although some patients have a patchy memory loss for remote events even years before treatment, reversible and short-lived memory loss is the most common finding (Squire, 1986). Some patients do have continuing longer-term memory problems but these are usually associated with continuing affective or other symptoms or drug and alcohol abuse (Freeman *et al.*, 1980).

Treatment-resistant depression

Physical treatments bring about some improvement in nearly all patients and effect a satisfactory recovery with few or no remaining symptoms in 70–80% of patients after ECT and 60–70% after treatment with antidepressants. There remains a minority of patients, however, who show only slight improvement, transient improvement or no apparent response at all. Such patients, usually lumped together under the broad heading of 'treatment resistant' form an heterogeneous population. In assessing such cases it is always worth returning to first principles and asking, is the diagnosis correct? For example, in younger and middle-aged patients it is important to remember that schizophrenia can initially present with depressive symptoms (Chapter 10) and that up to a third of schizophrenics may receive a diagnosis of depression on their first contact with psychiatrists (Gottesman, 1991). In elderly patients the important differential diagnosis is between depression and dementia (Chapter 14).

It is essential to ensure that the patient with treatment-resistant depression really has received a course of 'standard' antidepressants in adequate dosage for an adequate length of time. Too often this has not occurred and the patient has received an inadequate dose or has failed to comply with medication or has been switched from one antidepressant to another within a short period after commencing treatment. Polypharmacy is also a hazard and it is not uncommon to come across patients who are 'unresponsive' to drug treatment who are taking several different sorts of tablets, each of which has been added on an ad hoc basis. These may include a daytime benzodiazepine for anxiety symptoms, a short-acting benzodiazepine at night to help with sleep, a low-dose neuroleptic plus an antidepressant (and sometimes even two antidepressants in low doses!). In such circumstances it is worth stopping all the medication (and this will usually require a gradual tailing off in the case of the benzodiazepines) and starting an antidepressant such as amitriptyline or, if a sedation is not required, imipramine. This should be given in does of up to 300 mg daily depending on tolerance of side-effects and should be continued for a period of six weeks.

If this still fails and the patient has features of endogenous depression with prominent biological symptoms, a course of ECT should be given. In the absence of such features it is probably preferable to change to another antidepressant and again ensure that an adequate dose is given for a period of at least six weeks. Which class of drug is prescribed may be influenced by the patient's symptom profile in that, as discussed earlier, prominence of anxiety, depersonalisation or atypical features have been suggested as markers of responsiveness to MAOIs. However, the new reversible MAOI, moclobimide, is currently being marketed as a general or 'broad spectrum' antidepressant rather than the one targeted on the group of patients for whom the older MAOIs have often been used. There is at least superficially pharmacological rationale for switching treatment for tricyclic antidepressants to an MAOI, since the two classes of drugs have different modes of action. More surprisingly, although both tricyclics and SSRIs inhibit presynaptic uptake of serotonin, there are definitely some patients whose illness shows a response to one class of drugs but not to the other (Amsterdam et al., 1994).

Combining tricyclic antidepressants and MAOIs is a potentially hazardous strategy but nevertheless some clinicians are convinced of its efficacy in those patients who have not responded to conventional treatments. Combinations of this type should be started while the patient is in hospital and where monitoring of blood pressure is possible. In practice combinations such as amitriptyline with phenelzine usually cause severe postural hypotension and doses need to be tailored to avoid this. The greatest potential hazard is from hypertensive crises, which are most likely to occur when an MAOI is combined with a drug having potent serotonin re-uptake inhibition. Therefore, tricyclics such as clomipramine are to be avoided in combination therapy, as is a mixture of SSRIs and MAOIs. Although the usefulness of tricyclic and MAOI combinations is supported by anecdotal evidence there is little controlled trial evidence of efficacy (Young et al., 1979).

Other types of combination therapy similarly lack solid scientific support but are less hazardous. In particular, in patients with unipolar depression who have shown some, but only partial, response to antidepressants, a more satisfactory recovery may be hastened by adding lithium (Dinan, 1993). L-tryptophan is a precursor of serotonin, which has been shown to have antidepressant properties in its own right. However, it is most commonly used to augment tricyclic antidepressant treatment, again in patients who have shown only a partial response to tricyclics alone. Unfortunately, as a result of reports of allergic reactions to L-tryptophan characterised by muscle aches and eosinophilia, L-tryptophan is currently only available in the UK on a 'named patient' basis.

Continuation and maintenance treatment

Terms such as prophylactic, maintenance and continuation treatment are used in a variety of different ways by different authors. Here the term 'continuation treatment' will be used to describe the continued prescription of a drug following an episode of affective disorder and 'maintenance treatment' to describe longer-term prescription of a drug after recovery with the aim of maintaining remission and preventing further episodes.

Bipolar disorder

After the first episode of mania, it is usual to reduce gradually the dosage of haloperidol, chlorpromazine or other antipsychotics with the aim of stopping treatment altogether. There is no evidence that routine continuation of antipsychotics after full recovery has any benefits.

However, in patients recovering from their second or third episode of affective disorder, at least one of which has been an attack of mania, maintenance therapy with lithium needs to be considered. It is not possible to lay down precise or absolute indications for long-term lithium therapy but the rule of thumb is that it must be considered when the patient is having a sufficient number of recurrences for these to interfere markedly with normal functioning. For example, if there have been two episodes requiring admission to hospital within two years, the risk of further episodes are obvious and the case for maintenance treatment is strong. More problematic is the patient who has had two such episodes over, say, five years. In every case the benefits and the problems associated with maintenance treatment need to be discussed with patients once they have sufficiently recovered from their acute episode. It is also advisable to involve the spouse or nearest relative in discussions.

Lithium is usually best given in the form of sustained release lithium carbonate. Before starting treatment it is important to check that the patient has adequate renal function and it is usually sufficient to carry out a test of blood urea, electrolytes and creatinine together with testing urine for albumin. Thyroid function should be normal as reflected in tests for T_3, T_4 and TSH levels. Although rare, lithium treatment has been associated with cardiac arrhythmias and it is therefore wise, particularly in the middle-aged or elderly, to obtain an ECG.

Serum lithium levels need to be checked at least weekly for a minimum of the first four weeks and thereafter three monthly once adequate and stable levels have been obtained. It is usual to obtain a sample of venous blood about 12 hours after the last dose and to aim for serum levels within the therapeutic range of 0.4–1.0 mmol per litre. The main hazard is of lithium toxicity, which commences with nausea, vomiting and diarrhoea and, if serum levels rise above 2.0 mmol per litre, results in gross tremor, confusion, ataxia and epileptic seizures, culminating, if untreated, in death. The early or gastrointestinal symptoms of toxicity are rare in patients whose blood levels are below 1.5 mmol per litre but a longer-term complication of renal impairment is a risk in patients maintained at blood levels at greater than 1.0 mmol per litre.

Within the therapeutic range, some patients develop a fine tremor but this is not usually problematic. A longer-term risk is of hypothyroidism. This occurs more often in women than men and it is usual to treat with L-thyroxin rather than to discontinue the lithium. A less common complication is the development of thirst and polyuria because of an effect of lithium on renal tubules causing a nephrogenic diabetes insipidus.

Maintenance therapy with lithium is most efficiently and effectively carried out by holding a lithium clinic or operating a lithium register within the general out-patient clinic. Once stabilised, patients can be seen routinely by an out-patient clinic nurse who checks lithium levels three monthly, and blood urea, creatinine and electrolytes plus thyroid function six monthly. There is overwhelming evidence that treatment with lithium reduces the relapse rate in bipolar disorder (Goodwin, 1994) but it does not abolish the prospect of further attacks. In particular, lithium is disappointing in patients with 'rapid cycling' bipolar disorder consisting of frequent brief episodes and swift swings between mania and depression. In most cases the implications of starting maintenance with lithium is that the patient will remain on it for life. This fact needs to be made clear to the patient at the beginning. Early studies (e.g. Baastrup et al., 1970) showed that changing from lithium to a placebo was associated with very high rates of relapse. A small double-blind, placebo-controlled, cross-over trial found that of 14 patients stabilised on lithium, seven showed overt relapses, and two showed re-emergence of symptoms. All nine cases of relapse were associated with the placebo phase of the trial and occurred within about two weeks of stopping lithium (Mander & Loudon, 1988). There is some evidence that recurrence risk of affective disorder is reduced if lithium is gradually discontinued rather than stopped abruptly and this may reflect a 'rebound' phenomenon (Faedda et al., 1993). In clinical practice, relapse of patients with bipolar disorder often appears to be associated with the unilateral decision on the part of the patient to stop taking lithium. This in turn is often associated with a lack of appreciation of the need to continue treatment and there is evidence that an educational programme designed to improve patients' knowledge also results in improved compliance (Peet & Harvey, 1991).

Even despite good compliance, many patients relapse. It is worth considering maintenance with carbamazepine, either in combination with lithium or as an alternative to it. Carbamazepine, although less effective than standard treatments in acute mania, has been reported to prolong remission (Watkins et al., 1987), with marginally poorer or equivalent effectiveness to lithium in preventing relapse in bipolar disorder (Lusznat et al., 1988). Some clinicians believe that it is more effective than lithium in preventing relapse in 'rapid cyclers'. Other anticonvulsants such as sodium valproate have also been shown to have antimanic effects and there are case reports of sodium valproate being successfully used either on its own or in combination with carbamazepine in the treatment and prevention of relapse of bipolar disorder patients refractory to more conventional treatments (Ketter et al., 1992).

Some patients who continue to have relapses despite lithium combined with carbamazepine may be stabilised over long periods by the addition of an antipsychotic in low doses. This can be given as chlorpromazine 25–100 mg at night or intramuscular flupenthixol decanoate 40 mg four-weekly. Although there is no evidence from clinical trials to support this approach, there is little doubt that it works in some patients where all else has failed to maintain stability.

Unipolar disorder

There is now very good evidence that continuation treatment with antidepressants for a period after recovery lowers the risk of relapse. This was first demonstrated in double-blind placebo controlled trials taking place over a period of six months (Mindham et al., 1973; Klerman et al.; 1974) but subsequent studies lasting up to a year showed a continuing benefit (Coppen et al., 1978). In early studies, and consequently in clinical practice, continuation therapy with psychiatric antidepressants used a considerably lower dose than that given during the active phase of treatment. However, more recent studies such as a large trial in the United States (Frank et al., 1990) not only showed that high doses for continuation therapy (e.g. imipramine 200 mg daily) were more effective but showed that there continues to be a benefit of active treatment over placebo in preventing relapse for a period of five years (Kupfer et al., 1992). This study investigated patients with recurrent unipolar depression who had had at least three episodes in the preceding two and a half years. In addition to comparing imipramine with placebo, comparisons were made of the effectiveness in preventing relapse of interpersonal therapy and cognitive therapy. Although psychotherapy proved superior to placebo alone it did not appear to confer any additional benefit on patients who were taking imipramine, and imipramine overall proved to be the most effective maintenance treatment. This contrasts somewhat with studies suggesting that although tricyclic antidepressants and cognitive behaviour therapy are approximately equally effective in the treatment of moderately severe depression, the subsequent relapse rate is lower in those treated with cognitive therapy (see Chapter 25).

A trial of continuation therapy in unipolar disorder in the UK comparing lithium with amitriptyline found that both were equally effective (Medical Research Council Drug Trial Subcommittee, 1981). However a trial in the United States comparing imipramine with lithium found that imipramine was superior in preventing relapse in unipolar depression and that little additional benefit was conferred by a combination of imipramine and lithium (Prien et al., 1984).

In summary, there appear to be clear benefits provided by continuation therapy for six to 12 months after a single episode of depression. In a patient who has had multiple incapacitating episodes of depression, maintenance therapy with antidepressants in full doses is likely to be worth carrying on for up to five years. At present it is unclear whether maintenance therapy over longer periods of time is beneficial but this question is one that needs addressing. Naturalistic studies in general practice (e.g. Kerr, 1994) suggest a rather haphazard picture concerning what actually happens to patients who have been treated with tricyclic antidepressants. Some continue to receive medication for many years with apparently no clear policy on the part of the prescribing doctor.

Course and outcome

Bipolar disorder

In general the age of onset of bipolar disorder is lower than that for unipolar depression and occurs in the twenties or early thirties. In contrast to schizophrenia there are no sex differences in age of onset (Winokur, 1975; Burke et al., 1990) but, like schizophrenia, onset in late middle-age or in the elderly is uncommon (see Chapter 14). Angst et al. (1973) found that 88% of cases had their onset before the age of 49.

According to Kraepelin (1921) the majority of manic episodes lasted for several months but nowadays chronic mania is virtually never seen and about a half of episodes of mania last a month or less (Coryell et al., 1989). The mean duration of episodes in modern studies is around 2–3 months (Winokur et al., 1969; Angst et al., 1973; Coryell et al., 1989).

Over half of patients with bipolar disorder begin their illness with an attack of mania rather than depression (Winokur et al., 1969; Dunner et al., 1976). Although Kraepelin (1921) maintained that 45% of patients presenting with mania would never have a further attack of affective illness, more recent studies suggest less favourable results. For example, in follow-ups at five years, Coryell et al. (1989) found that only 11% of patients originally presenting with mania had not had a further attack of mania or depression and in a follow-up of 393 patients lasting between one and 12 years Angst et al. (1973) found that less than 1% had only had one episode.

Another of Kraepelin's observations was that the time to relapse decreases over the first two or three episodes. This has been confirmed in other studies (Angst *et al.*, 1973; Dunner *et al.*, 1979). In some patients the course of the illness also tends to show a clustering effect with bouts of recurrences being interspersed with longer episodes of remission (Winokur, 1975).

An excess mortality in patients with bipolar disorder was a feature of some early studies and this appears to be due to a variety of physical causes, of which cardiovascular disorder was probably the most important. However, such excess mortality appears to be confined to patient samples identified before 1950 (Tsuang *et al.*, 1980) and is not a feature of more recent follow-up studies (e.g. Martin *et al.*, 1985). The risk of suicide, however, is high (Black *et al.*, 1987a) and although there have been suggestions that the risk of death by suicide is lower than for unipolar disorder, some studies (e.g. Morrison, 1982) suggest that the risk is higher while others found no differences (Perris, 1966; Tsuang, 1978). It is therefore probably best to assume that the overall risk of death by suicide is around 15% (Guze & Robins, 1970) whether or not the patient has unipolar or bipolar disorder.

Karaeplin's assertion that manic depressive illness has a better long-term outcome than schizophrenia is largely borne out by modern studies. However, the range of outcomes is wide and long-term deterioration is by no means rare. Tsuang *et al.* (1979) found that a quarter of patients continued to have incapacitating symptoms at a 40 year follow-up and McGlashan (1984) found that, 15 years after their initial episode, about a third of patients had more or less persistent and unremitting incapacity.

Unipolar disorder

It is difficult to make hard and fast divisions in describing the course and outcome of unipolar versus bipolar disorder, because even though the majority of patients with unipolar disorder will never have a manic episode, a substantial minority of between 4 and 20% (Akiskal, 1983; Lee & Murray, 1988; Coryell *et al.*, 1989) do eventually present with mania. There is a bigger variation in the age of onset for unipolar than for bipolar disorder, with the mean age of onset being later. In general, episodes of unipolar disorder tend to last longer than bipolar disorder but most episodes of severe depression do not persist for more than six months and the average recovery rate after one year from a survey of recent studies was 64% (Piccinelli & Wilkinson, 1994). The same review found that just over a quarter of patients had a recurrence of depression within a year of the index episode and 15% of patients had persistent depression with symptoms sustained throughout the follow-up period.

Medium-term follow-ups suggest that the great majority of patients, over 80%, have recovered after two years (Coryell *et al.*, 1987) but in those that have failed to recover by this stage there is thereafter only a very gradual improvement, so that at five years the recovery rate reaches 90% (Coryell *et al.*, 1989) and the remaining 10% having persistent and unremitting symptoms. Reported recurrence rates in medium-term follow-up studies have been high, with further episodes of between two and five years reported in 46–74% of cases (Piccinelli & Wilkinson, 1994).

There have now been four careful long-term follow-up studies of unipolar depression taking place over periods of greater than ten years (Angst, 1986; Kiloh *et al.*, 1988; Lee & Murray, 1988; Surtees & Barcley, 1994). One of these studies (Surtees & Barcley, 1994) focused on a selective group of patients whom the authors termed 'veteran depressives', who had already had multiple episodes of disorder. The other three studies were probably more representative but focused on the severe end of the spectrum, taking as their index case subjects who had in-patient treatment for their depression. In these studies the weighted average recovery rate, defined as a sustained recovery throughout the entire follow-up period, was 24% (Piccinelli & Wilkinson, 1994). The recovery rate was lowest in the London UK study of Lee & Murray (1988), highest in the Swiss study of Angst (1986) and intermediate in the Australian study of Kiloh *et al.* (1988). However, the range of recovery rates was fairly small (18–30%). Greater disparity was found between the UK and Australian studies when outcome was measured on a scale devised by Lee & Murray. This found that only 15% of the London series had an outcome characterised as 'very good' compared with 39% of patients in the Australian series. The study by Surtees & Barcley (1994) in Edinburgh, despite the selective nature of their sample, produced results that were more similar to the Australian findings with 34% of cases having an outcome classified as 'very good'. The London study also suggested a more troubled course in their subjects with 95% of those traced having had at least one recurrence, whereas in the Australian study (Kiloh *et al.*, 1988) the recurrence risk was only 63%. The weighted average for persistent depression throughout the entire follow-up period of ten years in the Swiss, Australian and London UK study was 12% (Piccinelli & Wilkinson, 1994).

Taken overall, therefore, the findings of long-term follow-up of hospital depressives go against the 'traditional' or Kraepelinian view that depression has a relatively benign prognosis. Indeed 34% of patients in the Lee & Murray (1988) study were categorised as having a very poor outcome, as were exactly the same proportion of patients in the Edinburgh follow-up (Surtees & Barcley, 1994) using the same operationalised outcome criteria.

12

Atypical psychosis

ANTHONY S. DAVID

Introduction

The term 'atypical psychosis' presupposes that there is such a thing as 'typical psychosis'. Modern diagnostic classification has been operationalised so that individual diagnoses follow reasonably explicit algorithms. These consist of various exclusion and inclusion criteria: essential features, features that *may* be present, diagnostic thresholds such as a minimum number of non-essential features, and other modifying factors such as length of illness and concomitant disability.

The diagnostic criteria for the 'typical' psychoses, that is schizophrenia and affective psychosis, are amply discussed in their respective chapters as are the problems and challenges of classification in psychiatry (see Chapters 3, 10 and 11).

An atypical case may be defined in several ways. First it may have some of the necessary features of the typical case but not enough to meet a predetermined threshold above which a diagnosis may be reached. Thus a few schizophrenic (or affective) symptoms are present but not enough to form the full syndrome. Second, the case may exhibit sufficient critical features to merit a diagnosis of more than one – supposedly mutually exclusive – condition. This may arise because of a true coincidence of two (or more) classical disorders in a single individual, or because atypical cases constitute a separate disorder that just happens to consist of many features common to other more familiar disorders. Third, an atypical case may have none of the features associated with typical cases.

Thus, schizoaffective disorder may be regarded as atypical because it is a little like schizophrenia; or a little like affective disorder; because it is *like* a combination of schizophrenia and affective disorder, or because it *is* a combination of schizophrenia and affective disorder or finally, because it is different to both schizophrenia and affective disorder.

This chapter will examine the mismatch between typical and atypical cases with respect to the various clinical dimensions that have been deemed to be significant over the years (Cutting, 1986), in the light of recent research.

Table 12.1. *Diagnostic criteria for schizoaffective disorders*

ICD-10 (WHO, 1992*a*)
Both definite schizophrenic and definite affective symptoms are prominent *simultaneously* (or within days or within the same episode).
May be manic or depressive types (must be prominent elevation of mood or prominent depression respectively), or mixed.

DSM-IV (APA, 1994)
A. An uninterrupted period of illness during which, at some time, there is either a Major Depressive Episode, a Manic Episode, or a Mixed Episode concurrent with symptoms that meet characteristic-symptom criteria for schizophrenia.
B. Delusions or hallucinations for at least two weeks in the absence of prominent mood symptoms.
C. Symptoms meet mood criteria 'for a substantial portion of the total duration' of the illness.
D. Not due to drugs or physical illness.

Bipolar and Depressive Types.

Phenomenology

Form

Mood-incongruent delusions are typical of schizophrenia while mood-congruent delusions are typical of affective psychosis. A psychosis may be considered atypical if both kinds of delusion are present with no principled rationale for adjudicating between the two implied diagnoses. The problem of mood-incongruent delusions in a setting of affective disturbance presents a classificatory conundrum. A thorough review by Kendler (1991) concluded that such cases were best seen as a subtype of affective disorder or a form of schizoaffective disorder on the basis of family history, outcome and other variables. If affective disorder is the starting point, the presence of mood-incongruent psychotic features clearly pulls a host of outcome variables (e.g. recurrence, occupational and residential status) in a less favourable direction (Tohen *et al.*, 1992). Significant elevation or depression of mood alongside hallucinations without clear affective valence (e.g. neutral commenting voices) is another uncomfortable juxtaposition or 'blending' that will lead to the diagnosis of schizoaffective psychosis. This term was proposed in 1933 by Kasanin on the basis of nine detailed case histories (republished in 1994). Modern-day diagnostic criteria are shown in Table 12.1.

Descriptive phenomenological studies suggest that plotting symptoms along an affective–schizophrenia continuum results in a uni-modal distribution (Kendell & Gourlay, 1970), supporting the notion of a 'unitary psychosis' (Crow, 1987) and by implication, schizoaffective symptomatology is typical. Tsuang (1991) excluded classically typical cases from a cohort of 510 patients hospitalised in Iowa during the 1930s and 1940s and carried out a similar phenomenological mapping with the remaining 310. Using logistic regression analysis, he found a non-normal distribution that could be subdivided into three overlapping groups, thought to represent in essence the two typical psychoses and a third, schizoaffective type accounting for 57 cases.

Very little data exist on the incidence and prevalence of schizoaffective disorder. Figures that are produced are exquisitely sensitive to diagnostic criteria and whether the overall scheme sets out with the *'zweiteilungs Prinzip* – two entities principle' so ensuring that atypical or intermediate forms become rare. Brockington & Leff (1979) came up with a range from 0.3 to 5.7 cases per 100 000 per year, about one-quarter that of schizophrenia and approximately that of mania. This corresponded to 8% of hospital admissions for psychosis. In the WHO 10 country study (Jablensky *et al.*, 1992) the schizoaffective category of ICD-9 was applied in only 3% of all schizophrenic disorders in developing countries and 8% in the developed countries.

Schizoaffective symptomatology itself has become prey to subdivision, such is the strength of our allegiance to older notions of madness and melancholia. The extremes of mood have led to the two subtypes mentioned in both the American Psychiatric Association and World Health Organization diagnostic systems. Empirical justification for this is lacking but goes back to work by Brockington and colleagues, who coined the terms schizomania and schizodepression (1980*a,b*). Their work, based on 32 manic and 76 depressive patients with schizophrenic or paranoid symptoms, suggested that schizomania was a non-persisting disorder in the majority of instances, and thus more akin to mania than schizophrenia, while schizodepression had an outcome intermediate between schizophrenia and affective disorder, with 30 receiving a final diagnosis of schizophrenia; episodes of mania were uncommon.

Like schizoaffective psychosis itself, arguments about the concept tend to recur in cycles over the years, generating strong expressions of affect, at times mixed with paranoia (Taylor, 1992*a*). The reason appears to be that many psychiatrists, particularly those brought up with early Kraepelinian notions, find it hard to relinquish the distinctiveness of the two major psychoses, especially their presumed aetiological distinctiveness. This implies separate major genes for the two disorders, as against polygenic or multifactorial aetiologies, or against Crow's recent formulation of a single 'psychosis gene' (1986).

The phenomenology of motor activity has often thrown up distinct psychotic disorders. *Catatonia* is the classical type described by Kahlbaum in 1874, and is generally regarded as a form of schizophrenia (see Chapter 10). However, catatonia is itself a heterogeneous condition with distinctive aetiologies (Johnson, 1993), from encephalitis lethargica to interpersonal crisis. Organic brain disease is a likely component in many cases, including forms of the neuroleptic malignant syndrome, where a sustained but reversible alteration in arousal occurs, pointing to brainstem dysfunction. In other cases a period of mute immobility gives way to manic excitement, during which the catatonia is explained in terms of a delusion. For example, the patient may say the world would have exploded if he or she moved, or that he or she was engrossed in a deep spiritual communion with God. Motor phenomena are a prominent feature of *cycloid psychosis*, to be discussed below.

Another group of psychotic disorders that may be distinguished on the basis of formal phenomenological properties are the delusional disorders (ICD-10 and DSM-IV, Table 12.2) formally known as paranoia.

The form of the psychopathology in delusional disorder is different from schizophrenia in that delusions dominate in the absence (or near absence) of hallucination and thought disorder. Such conditions are relatively uncommon accounting for 1–2% of psychiatric

Table 12.2. *Dignostic criteria for delusional disorder*

ICD-10 Persistent Delusional Disorders
–Delusions are the most conspicuous or only clinical characteristic (i.e. hallucinations may be present).
–Duration of three months or more.
–Not culturally accepted.
–No 'schizophrenic' symptoms such as delusions of control, thought broadcasting, etc.

DSM-IV
–Non-bizarre delusions (involving situations that occur in real life).
–Duration of one month or more.
–Criteria for schizophrenia not met (transient auditory and visual hallucination may be present and tactile and olfactory hallucinations may be prominent, if directly related to delusional theme).
–Transient mood alteration only.
–Social functioning not affected (other than as a direct consequence of delusion).

hospital admissions, with a lifetime morbidity risk of 1/20 to 1/10 that of schizophrenia (APA, 1994). When such disorders occur in late life (variably defined after 44 or 60 years), they may be called (late) paraphrenia (Chapter 14). Often such delusional disorders concern stable, specific, circumscribed beliefs, which may become more elaborate over time, hence their *content* may be used to distinguish one from another. From a clinical point of view, there are reasonable grounds for distinguishing delusional disorders from schizophrenia. Winokur (1977) retrieved the case notes of 93 patients with a diagnosis of paranoia from 21 000 admissions to the Psychiatric Hospital of the University of Iowa. Of these, 19 met his criteria for delusional disorder. As a group, they were more often male (70%), had a relatively late onset, and a chronic course over the 2.6-year follow-up, and only two were re-diagnosed.

Content

Content is traditionally regarded as less important in classical phenomenology than form (see Chapter 1). However, certain psychotic disorders have been distinguished in the past, primarily because of their content or subject matter, usually an intense, systematised and circumscribed delusion. Other delusions, though attracting curiosity (see Enoch & Trethowan, 1979), such as delusions of pregnancy (pseudocyesis), are almost always only one among many (Michael *et al.*, 1994). The most common themes for the beliefs of delusional disorder patients, according to Winokur (1977), are, in descending order of frequency, persecution, reference, jealousy and hypochondriasis, followed by miscellaneous. Delusions of reference have been shown to be the least specific for delusional disorder, occurring in all psychotic illnesses with delusions (Jorgensen & Jensen, 1994).

Classifying psychotic disorders by their content, though frowned upon, has proved to be valid in some cases, most notably the delusional misidentification syndromes (Förstl *et al.*, 1991; Fleminger & Burns, 1993). The most common of these is the Capgras delusion, named after the French psychiatrist who first described it in 1923. Here, the patient (usually elderly) believes that a familiar person has been replaced by a double or near double whom the patient recognises as an imposter, usually with sinister motives. Such cases resemble what neurologists call reduplicative paramnesias (after Pick), the first hint of their acquired, neuropsychiatric status, and may involve places and objects as well as people (Ellis & de Pauw, 1994). Modern neuroimaging studies have revealed a high proportion of brain lesions in such patients (affecting parietal and/or frontal regions). Fregoli syndrome is the mirror image of Capgras. The name derives from a once-famous Italian actor and mimic, and it denotes the patient's belief that a familiar person is impersonating others, perhaps by adopting a disguise; again, often for their own ends.

Cotard's syndrome also bears the name of the French psychiatrist who described it. Nihilistic delusions are the hallmark and are generally regarded as occurring in the severest form of depression. They appear under the list of atypical psychoses partly because they were described in the pre-Kraepelinian era as a distinct form of madness (Cotard, 1882/1974). The subject may believe his or her insides are rotten or their head is empty or even that they and the world do not exist. When taken to these extremes of irrationality it is easy to see them as more than 'just depression'. Cotard's syndrome is more often seen in the elderly, with or without overt cerebral pathology.

Another specific disorder for which diagnostic validity has been claimed is Monosymptomatic Hypochondriacal Psychosis (MHP) (Munro, 1988). This is a subgroup of delusional conditions in which the belief is centred around alteration or disease of a body part or system. This may include the conviction that one is emitting a foul odour. The belief in skin infestation (delusional parasitosis) is a common type and carries the eponym Ekbom's syndrome, after the Swedish physician who described seven cases in the late 1930s. It is often difficult to tease out whether there is a primary perceptual experience – such as itch or seeing innocent flakes of dead skin – or whether normal bodily sensations are misinterpreted and misattributed to some disease or malign influence by way of supporting evidence for the primary false belief. The difference between this and hypochondriasis *per se* is the implausibility of the misattribution and its fixity in the face of reassurance and contradictory evidence, but is only a matter of degree. As noted above, the DSM-IV specifies in the diagnostic criteria for Delusional Disorder, that the content of the delusion is 'nonbizarre'. The disorder may nevertheless shade into so-called over-valued ideas (see Chapter 1), which frequently involve bodily appearances (dysmorphophobia), such as the size of the nose or genitalia, and which trouble the plastic surgeon, urologist and dermatologist (Wessely & Lewis, 1989) long before the psychiatrist.

Munro's claim is that these disorders respond specifically to pimozide, a dopamine D2 receptor blocker. However, other neuroleptic drugs with less specific dopamine antagonist properties and even some antidepressants have been shown to be as effective in selected cases (Andrews *et al.*, 1986).

Delusional jealousy is an extreme case of the symptom of morbid jealousy, and is more properly thought of as a delusion of infidelity. There is little evidence to sustain its distinctiveness from other classifiable disorders except a suggested link with chronic alcohol abuse. The condition is characterised by increasing conviction of infidelity on the part of the subject's partner, again supported by or supporting delusional misattribution of innocent or chance events, as explicated by Shakespeare in *Othello* (Shepherd, 1961; Enoch &

Trethowan, 1979). One phenomenological curiosity that justifies its inclusion under the current heading of atypical content is that phenomenologists frequently cite delusions of infidelity as being occasionally true, and thus the exception to the definitional rule that delusions are false beliefs. Clinicians should also be aware of the propensity to violence against the supposedly unfaithful party by the patient.

Erotomania (described by another French psychiatrist, De Clerambault, in 1942) is a chronic delusional syndrome in which the patient falls in love with a virtual stranger and, more unreasonably, believes that this love is reciprocated. De Clerambault described primary (with acute onset) and secondary forms, the latter having other delusions and psychotic features. The patient is usually female and develops the delusion around a male, often of higher social standing or 'unattainable' in some other way – he may be a famous TV personality, a vicar or politician. Innocent remarks or acts are interpreted as confirming the patient's beliefs and may be construed as encouraging signs – essentially these are ideas or delusions of reference. There may be a prominent grandiose element at this stage (Rudden *et al.*, 1990). Frequently, a real or imagined slight turns the adoration into intense hatred. This may result in violent retribution, as in delusions of infidelity, especially in male patients. The modern phenomenon of 'stalking' of famous sport and entertainment personalities can be an example of this.

Course

Psychotic disorders that relapse and remit with some rapidity and regularity have long been considered 'atypical'. The term 'cycloid psychosis' was invented by Leonhard in 1961 as a new category of disorder. Perris was a strong proponent of this view and attempted to operationalise a definition, namely a psychotic episode (delusions and hallucinations) that resolves completely, during which there are mood swings, plus at least two of: confusion/perplexity; paranoid symptoms (e.g. mood-incongruent delusions of reference or influence); motility disturbances (hypo- or hyperkinesis); ecstasy; *Angst*, translated from the German as overwhelming fear of impending disaster or 'pananxiety'. Cutting and colleagues (1978) studied the prevalence and validity of the syndrome in patients admitted to the Maudsley Hospital. The diagnosis was applied to around 8% of psychotic admissions. The case-notes on 73 cases (90% female) were retrieved and compared to similar numbers of manic, depressive and schizophrenic cases plus 49 with a schizoaffective diagnosis. The cycloid group had a higher rate of relapse but a relatively good outcome. Their clinical diagnoses changed over subsequent admissions, more so than other groups, and overlapped most with schizoaffective disorder.

Brockington *et al.* (1982) studied a less highly selected group of 30 (12%) cases, extracted from 244 consecutive psychotic admissions to a number of hospitals. Using a battery of operational criteria, they showed that cycloid psychosis shares much of its phenomenology with schizophrenia but its course is clearly more benign, with recovery between episodes. Because of this they recommend viewing the disorder as a variant of manic depressive illness.

Schizoaffective disorders have repeatedly been found to run a long-term course that shows less deterioration than schizophrenia but more than affective disorder (e.g. Johnstone *et al.*,

1992). This holds regardless of whether or not depressives in the affective group have psychotic features. In a prospective study of 101 mixed psychotic patients diagnosed by Research Diagnostic Criteria (41 schizoaffective), Grossman *et al.* (1991) found that clinical and social outcome at both two and four to five-year follow-up time points was worst for schizophrenics and best for unipolar depressives. Again, differentiating the schizoaffective from bipolar manic patients on the one hand and schizophrenics on the other was difficult but an intermediate outcome was observed on most parameters. Similar findings emerged from an eight year follow-up of a small group of DSM-IIIR schizoaffectives in comparison to depressives – with and without mood-incongruent psychotic features – and patients with schizophrenia (Tsuang & Coryell, 1993). Likelihood of recovery was low (around 20% in the schizophrenic and schizoaffectives), significantly less than the other groups.

Atypical onset and duration

Acute onset appears atypical, against a backdrop of schizophrenic psychoses – whose stereotype is of a long prodrome and even premorbid decline in social functioning. Sudden onset combined with a short duration marks out a variation in course that forms the basis of classification for a number of Eurocentric schemes. An attempt has been made to bring these together under the heading of Acute and Transient Psychotic Disorders in the ICD-10 and Brief Psychotic Disorder in the DSM-IV. These encompass the 'reactive psychoses' or psychogenic psychosis of Scandinavian psychiatry; the hyper-acute *Bouffée délirante* of French psychiatry and, to some extent, cycloid psychosis from the German school. According to the ICD-10, 'acute' is defined as within two weeks, and abrupt, within 48 hours; duration must be under three months. The DSM-IV is more specific about duration, stipulating a period between one day and one month.

Brief, remitting psychoses have attracted interest through the extensive international studies carried out under the auspices of the World Health Organization. The familiar truism, that acute onset relates to brief duration, was confirmed (Leff *et al.*, 1992). Furthermore, these brief psychotic reactions were typical of the developing world, in fact they were ten times more common there in comparison to industrialised societies (Susser & Wanderling, 1994). Gender was another important factor: they were twice as common in females. Other studies have found a female excess in non-schizophrenic psychoses, including cycloid types, and also schizoaffective disorder, the latter being found in a catchment area study of first contact cases (the Camberwell Case Register), and therefore cannot be accounted for by selection factors related to chronicity (Castle *et al.*, 1994).

The *reactive* element survives in both systems as a qualifier, that is the presence of a precipitating stress is recorded. While Danish psychiatrist Erik Stromgren, in the 1970s, and others argued for the direct relationship between a psychological trauma, the onset and content of the psychotic disturbance (i.e. psychogenesis), this has not found general acceptance. First, life-events research has shown that many 'endogenous' psychoses, including schizophrenia, occur in the aftermath of a stressful life event (Norman & Malla, 1993) and second, a certain vulnerability has to be postulated to account for the reaction to stress being in this form. Finally, recurrence of the illness may occur despite the one-off nature of the original stress. Hence there is little evidence to support an aetiology separate from other 'typical' psychoses.

Duration of acute psychosis greater than one month (but less than six) strays into the 'Schizophreniform Disorder' category of the DSM-IV. The diagnosis was first suggested by Norwegian psychiatrist Langfeldt in 1926 as a means of separating schizophrenic patients with poor outcome from the remainder. Re-analysis of Langfeldt's original case summaries (Bergem *et al.*, 1990) has shown that, while there is general agreement on what constitutes typical poor outcome schizophrenia, most of the schizophreniform group met criteria for affective disorders with the rest attracting labels of schizoaffective, schizophrenic, schizophreniform and non-psychotic disorders.

An exhaustive review and meta-analysis of studies on schizophreniform disorder, as defined in the DSM-III original and revised editions, while different from Langfeldt's formulation, sheds important light on many of the questions raised above (Strakowski,1994). The temporal stability of the diagnosis was very poor, with around 30% recovering; the remainder went on to develop schizophrenia, affective or schizoaffective disorders over follow-up periods averaging 16 months. Neurological, endocrine and cognitive markers, did not reveal a distinct subtype but one useful trend could be discerned: the presence of biological or clinical 'markers' for schizophrenia, when found in the schizophreniform group, conferred a worse prognosis.

Should we be surprised at these conclusions? The arbitrariness of the one-month cut-off adopted by the DSM should not have raised hopes of providing a valid diagnostic entity separate from any others. Psychiatric syndromes may take time to reveal themselves in their true colours, if indeed they possess such purity in the first place. The utility of schizophreniform is that it allows the clinician to hedge. The data show that firm diagnostic pronouncements based on a one-month presentation are simply neither possible nor desirable and 'schizophreniform' provides an interim judgement. The situation is further complicated for the clinician who has to take into account the effects of early treatment interventions and also the possibility that the disorder was provoked by illicit drugs.

Cause

One time-honoured method of determining the nosological validity of new or atypical psychiatric illnesses is to look for the presence of similar illnesses in family members. Either they may be shown to breed true with other atypical cases, or rather they may show familial concordance with typical disorders. As a method of validation, it is flawed since it is known that even genetically identical individuals (MZ twins) display a range of discordant psychiatric morbidity. Nevertheless, family-genetic studies have yielded useful information. Maj *et al.* (1991), in Italy, reported equivalent elevations in the morbid risk for schizophrenia in relatives of schizophrenic and 21 DSM-IIIR schizoaffective (depressed type) subjects (8.8 and 8.7 respectively). Unfortunately, morbid risk for schizoaffective disorders was not recorded. Similarly, Tsuang (1991) found that relatives of the schizoaffective patients he extracted from a larger atypical group (described above), had an equally high chance of suffering from schizophrenia (6.6%) as relatives of a schizophrenic proband, and a risk of affective disorder, mid-way between relatives of the two typical psychoses (13%).

An epidemiological family study of 303 schizophrenic cases based in rural Ireland showed that 19 relatives met criteria for schizoaffective disorder and these were related to probands with psychotic and bipolar affective disorders (Kendler *et al.*, 1993*b*). When these schizoaffectives were combined with other non-schizophrenic and non-affective psychotic relatives, a relationship with schizophrenia and schizotypal personality disorder probands became significant. One of the largest of these studies, carried out recently in Mainz, Germany, included 115 individuals with RDC schizoaffective disorder (two-thirds female), and similar numbers of schizophrenics, bipolar and unipolar affectives plus alcoholic and general population controls (Maier *et al.*, 1993). The results showed that the lifetime morbid risks for each disorder was highest in relatives with that disorder, that is schizoaffective disorder was 3.9 times more likely in relatives of schizoaffective probands (risk for schizophrenia was 3.6); while morbid risk for schizophrenia was 5.2 times in relatives of schizophrenics; the risks for bipolar or schizoaffective disorders were between 1.2 to 2.3. However, bipolar disorder was 8.0 times higher in the relatives of the bipolar type of schizoaffective disorder and 7.0 times higher in the relatives of pure bipolars. Unipolar disorder seemed to be more related to schizophrenia than bipolar disorder.

In summary, the results of family studies in terms of delineating a subtype of psychotic illness distinct from classical schizophrenia or affective disorder are inconclusive. This probably reflects differences in diagnostic criteria and the dangers of defining schizoaffective disorder too narrowly. Again, a compromise solution similar to that of outcome studies might be that non-affective, non-schizophrenic (atypical) psychoses have genetic links with both (typical) disorders.

One last disorder may be considered a prime example of a psychosis with atypical cause, the *folie à deux* or Induced Delusional Disorder (ICD-10), Shared Psychotic Disorder (DSM-IV). This occurs when psychotic ideas (such as those occurring in delusional disorders or schizophrenia) become adopted by another person. The induction occurs because of the dominance exerted by the psychotic inducer over their submissive partner, and their insistence in the truth and importance of their beliefs. Furthermore, the couple (sometimes family), who may be related biologically or through marriage, live a life isolated from the wider world, which might have provided some reality testing. The induced disorder should disappear when the individuals are separated (Porter *et al.*, 1993).

Atypical response to treatment?

There is little justification for this heading. Schizomanic patients show a reasonable response to lithium, while schizodepressives show a weak response to neuroleptic drugs (Brockington *et al.*, 1978). The combination of lithium and neuroleptics appears to be superior to lithium alone in schizomanic patients (see Keck *et al.*, 1994 for review). When attempts to categorise the psychoses are abandoned and treatment decisions are made on a purely symptom-driven basis, the results are predictable. Manic symptoms respond to anti-manic agents including lithium; psychotic symptoms to neuroleptics and depressive symptoms to antidepressants (Johnstone *et al.*, 1988; Siris *et al.*, 1991). Other 'mood stabilising' agents are also of value especially when combined with neuroleptics (Simhand & Meszaros, 1992).

As newer antipsychotic agents are developed, some with atypical profiles and actions mediated by combinations of sub-sets of 5-HT and dopamine receptors, it is conceivable that specific disorders will show specific responses to specific drugs. Demonstrating such effects convincingly in clinical trials will present formidable logistic problems for researchers, given the vagaries of diagnostic criteria. Theoretically, it should be possible, and will feed back into diagnosis, hopefully leading to increasing and rational refinement.

Conclusion

Atypical cases are an irritant to any diagnostic classification that seeks order. International schools offering different perspectives have tried to demarcate such cases and provide them with appropriate labels, but, in the way of international initiatives, the result has been more Tower of Babel than Esperanto. A 'British School' is conspicuous by its absence (Shepherd, 1994), with British psychiatrists sitting on the sidelines, perhaps hoping this untidiness will disappear. Unfortunately, there is no way of dealing with atypical cases in a more principled manner since typical cases can only be defined tautologically – typical cases are those that possess typical features. The expectation of cleaving atypical cases on grounds of outcome – a crucial validator of typical cases – is almost bound to lead to disappointment since outcome is generally measured on a single dimension between schizophrenia (bad) and affective disorder (good), and anything else is bound to be 'somewhere in between'. In fact, there has been very little effort to find qualitative differences between typical and atypical psychoses in terms of biological markers (but see Hayashi *et al.*,1992), although a neuropsychological approach advanced by David & Cutting (1990) may yet find favour. Again, this is an understandable and sensible stance until proven markers of typical psychoses emerge. In the meantime, parsimony dictates we should proceed empirically (see e.g. Kendell, 1993), an approach that has been reasonably successful with respect to finding effective treatments. Similarly, as psychological research concentrates more on finding mechanisms that underlie symptoms, atypical cases, with their fluctuations, remissions and relapses, will provide excellent clinical material for hypothesis testing. Perhaps this will provide the basis of a British School.

13

Psychiatric manifestations of organic illness

R. J. McCLELLAND and A. B. WILSON

General considerations

Organic disorders are those psychiatric conditions where a recognised disturbance of cerebral function is the overriding cause. In the course of this chapter, we shall discuss the clinical presentation of cerebral dysfunction, the main physical illnesses that are responsible, relevant investigations, and guidelines for management.

The mental phenomena attributal to cerebral dysfunction reflect impairment of one or more psychological functions. Consciousness, orientation, attention and memory are vulnerable to most types of cerebral dysfunction. Other functions, perceptual, linguistic and motor, have more focal representation within the brain and their impairment has a closer connection with focal brain damage. Some functions of speech, thought, and mood are affected in both functional and organic psychoses, but these may be disturbed in a particular way in organic disorders. Mood change is a frequent accompaniment of organic lesions. The most distinctive features are lability and fluctuations in mood state.

Focal brain damage influences the clinical picture in a way characteristic for each cortical and subcortical area. One must consider not only the cortical site but also the site of the lesion. Subcortical areas of psychiatric interest include basal ganglia, brainstem, thalamus, hypothalamus, the limbic system, and the corpus callosum. The cerebellum has only a minor claim to our attention as a source of psychological dysfunction. Finally, the duration of cerebral dysfunction affects the clinical picture. One can therefore distinguish acute organic reactions, which include delirium, confusion, and toxic confusional states, from chronic organic reactions, covering general intellectual impairment (dementia) and focal disorders (e.g. Korsakoff's syndrome).

Impairments of psychological functions

History and behaviour

Organic pathology frequently presents with emotional and behavioural symptoms, the most common emotional change being depression. On the other hand, a functionally depressed patient with psychomotor retardation may perform poorly on psychometric testing (pseudodementia).

The organic mental state can be assessed in a systemic fashion, beginning with level of arousal and ending with the more complex higher functioning. If a patient has a problem with language, it may be difficult to assess verbal reasoning. Similarly a patient with an attention deficit will miss the information needed to assess memory. Thus an organic mental state assessment performed without attending to the hierarchical nature of cognition may draw erroneous conclusions.

The history should be directed towards four major areas of enquiry:

1. the possibility of organic change (e.g. amnesia or a dysphasia);
2. a functional psychiatric syndrome mimicking organic pathology;
3. premorbid behaviour and level of functioning;
4. general medical condition.

Levels of arousal

The characteristic feature of acute organic reactions is clouding of consciousness. This refers to a reduction in level of awareness. Any disturbance of this elementary function will affect higher-level functioning. Arousal refers to activation of the cortex by ascending activating systems and should be distinguished from the actual content of consciousness (Teasdale & Jennett, 1974). The activating system originates in the brainstem reticular formation and extends to the cortex via the diffuse or non-specific thalamic projection system. Any damage to this system will have widespread effects rendering the patient difficult to arouse. A small lesion in the reticular formation will lead to a total disruption of its function and a coma state will ensue. The same result may be caused by drug intoxication or metabolic disturbance causing alteration in both cortical and reticular function.

Damage to the reticular system above the brainstem results in one of four patterns of arousal deficit: akinetic mutism (apathetic state); akinetic mutism (alert/coma vigil); persistent vegetative state (decorticate state); locked-in syndrome.

In akinetic mutism (apathetic state), a lesion in the midbrain/subthalamic region disconnects the reticulocortical pathways. Reticular activity remaining intact innervates the extraoccular nerves and the patient opens his or her eyes and appears alert. However the cortex does not receive the 'input necessary to produce voluntary speech or movement' and the patient remains in the coma-like state. While the condition was first described in a patient with a third ventricle cyst, the most common cause is occlusion of the small vessels entering the brainstem. If the lesion affects the septal area, anterior hypothalamus or cingulate gyri, the patient is again akinetic and mute but in this instance is more alert. During periods of arousal, patients may exhibit an intensely violent outburst termed septal rage, making their management difficult. The common causes of such a lesion are rupture of the anterior communicating artery or a deep frontal tumour (Plum & Posner, 1980).

In akinetic mutism (alert/coma vigil), there is bilateral decortication, which causes bilateral hemiplegia and clinically differentiates the condition from akinetic mutism (apathetic state).

The term persistent vegetative state describes a state where there are extensive lesions at a cortical and a subcortical level, such as occur following a serious head injury.

The locked-in syndrome occurs with a lesion at the level at the pons. This disconnects the corticospinal tracts leaving the patient unable to speak or swallow, quadriplegic, but fully conscious and aware of their surroundings (Jennet & Plum, 1972).

Level of consciousness

This refers to the level of awareness, of one's surroundings. It may fluctuate, for example, becoming worse at night, and may range from slight dulling through to coma. Mild forms are inferred from daytime drowsiness and lapses in concentration.

Attention and perception

Attention refers to the ability to attend to specific stimuli without being distracted. This contrasts with alertness, which is a more basic arousal process. The alert but inattentive patient will be attracted to any novel sound or movement in the environment. Vigilance (concentration) is a term that refers to the ability to sustain attention over a period of time. This may be impaired in both organic and functional disorders. The concept is applied in two quite different clinical states (Mesulam, 1981). In the first, the patient is clinically inattentive because of an arousal problem due to general cerebral dysfunction, as in acute organic reactions or dementia, or focal lesions (frontal, right parietal, and brainstem). The dysfunction shows itself in distractibility and slowness. In the second, inattention is specific to stimuli that are lateralised to the side of the body opposite to a unilateral brain lesion. In the extreme, the patient is unaware of people approaching on the inattentive side; this is referred to as neglect (Black, 1976).

Traditional tests of attention include serial sevens (subtracting seven serially from 100 allowing one mistake in one minute) and digit span (correct immediate repetition of six or more digits forwards).

The most common cause of decreased attention is diffuse brain dysfunction due to metabolic disturbance, drug intoxication, systemic infection or extensive bilateral cortical damage. Inattention characterised by indifference and perseveration is found in patients with bilateral lesions of the frontal lobes of the limbic system, (e.g. Korsakoff syndrome). They have great difficulty shifting from one category to another, which is the basis of the Wisconsin card sorting test. Right hemisphere lesions have a more pronounced effect on attention, possibly due to the reticulocortical fibres being denser to the right hemisphere.

Perception

The two classical disorders of perception are agnosia (perception without meaning) and hallucinations (perception without an object). Agnosia can be visual, auditory of tactile. Visual agnosia may be specific for objects (object agnosia), faces (prosopagnosia), global appreciation of pictures with preserved perception of detail (simultanagnosia), failure of acknowledgement of hemiplegia (anosognosia) or spatial context (visuospatial agnosia).

Agnosia is a disorder of the meaning that we attach to our perceptions. Object agnosia can be of two types – aperceptional (where a subject with a right hemisphere lesion fails to discriminate between physically similar items) and associational (where a subject with a left hemisphere lesion only fails on semantic classification). Prosopagnosia is a rare disorder in which the subject fails to recognise previously familiar faces. This deficit requires bilateral occipital lesions. Simultanagnosia is produced by a left temporo-occipital lesion and is a failure in the temporal integration of a visual array. Anosognosia is almost invariably the result of a right parietal lesion and is usually seen in the immediate aftermath of a stroke when the subject denies his left hemiplegia. The appreciation of the spatial context of a visual stimulus is a complex act. It requires an intact right parieto-occipital region and can be tested for by asking the subject to draw a clock, copy simple geometrical patterns, and construct a star with matches.

The hallucinations of an acute organic reaction are characteristically visual. However, illusions and misinterpretations are more typical perceptual abnormalities. Visual hallucinations also appear after focal damage to three focal regions: right parieto-occipital, temporal, and the cerebellar peduncles. Auditory hallucinations are likely to be non-verbal and to have a connection with background noise. Tactile hallucinations, classically associated with cocaine abuse, can occur in other organic disorders.

Language

Brown (1977) has defined speech as 'one form of action through which language is realised'. Its integrity must be established early in the organic mental state assessment as its function is critical to most cognitive functioning. Subsequent parts of an examination must be interpreted with some caution in aphasic patients. Knowing the patient's dominance for language is important in assessing an aphasia syndrome. Ninety per cent of the population are strongly left-hemisphere dominant for language. Left-handed individuals have a different pattern for cerebral dominance. Eighty per cent of left-handed individuals, especially those with a family history of sinistrality, have a pattern of mixed dominance with some degree of language representation on both hemispheres (Albert, 1981). Whereas language is remarkably resistant to cerebral dysfunction except in specific areas of the left hemisphere, the speed, rhythm, and pragmatic functions of speech are all vulnerable to a variety of insults. The study of right-handed individuals has resulted in a generally accepted schema of cortical localisation of language (Gloning, 1977).

With lesions in the posterior language area (Broadmans area 44), or Wernicke's area, speech is fluent but marred by paraphasias[1] and often devoid of meaning. The core feature of Wernicke's aphasia is a severe disturbance of auditory comprehension, so that the person is unable to monitor the output of his or her speech, and thus is unaware of personal difficulties. The more severe the deficit in auditory comprehension, the more the underlying lesion involves the posterior portion of the superior temporal gyrus. If single word comprehension is intact and there is loss of comprehension of complex material the lesion is more likely to involve the parietal lobe. In an extreme example the output becomes

---

[1] Paraphrasia: easily flowing speech that is remarkably empty of content and contains many abnormal words.

incomprehensible, and is termed jargon aphasia; this can be confused with the thought disorder found in schizophrenia. Behavioural disorder is common as the patient is unaware of his or her problem and can become euphoric, or develop a paranoid reaction.

A lesion in the anterior speech area produces a non-fluent dysarthric effortful type of dysphasia. The patient utters high content words, verbs and nouns, in a telegraphic and agrammatical fashion. Lesions restricted to Broca's area alone (area 44) produce a transient dysarthria and dysprosody[2] and not the full clinical picture (Benson, 1973). The emotional change associated with a Broca's aphasia is characterised by frustration, agitation and depression (Benson, 1973).

The most common type of aphasia seen in the clinical setting is a global aphasia, due to an occlusion of the internal carotid artery with damage to both the anterior and posterior speech areas. It is characterised by absent or reduced spontaneous speech. Comprehension is reduced to recognition of the patient's name or a few selected objects.

When the two speech areas become disconnected from each other a conduction aphasia develops. This can result from a lesion to the arcuate fasiculus, a long tract of fibres between the anterior and posterior areas, or a lesion that damages the insula and white matter underlying the auditory cortex. The result is an aphasia characterised by good comprehension and spontaneous speech being halting in nature. Repetition is, however, severely affected, demonstrating that repetition and prepositional speech (everyday descriptive language), are distinct psycholinguistic processes (Damasio & Damasio, 1980).

Anomic aphasia, where the difficulty is in word finding and naming objects is produced by lesions of the dominant hemisphere. By itself it has poor localising value. However, a severe form of anomic aphasia results from a lesion to the second or third gyri of the temporal lobe. Whether this area represents a true 'word dictionary', or part of a critical pathway is unclear.

A combined syndrome of alexia, agraphie and anomic aphasia localises the lesion to the left parietotemporal area.

Transcortical aphasia is characterised by intact repetition but comprehension and spontaneous speech are affected (the opposite to a conduction aphasia) (Robens & Kertesz, 1983). It is caused by extensive crescent shaped infarcts between the territories of the middle and anterior cerebral arteries the most common causes of which are: anoxia (as in cardiac arrest), occlusion or stenosis of the carotid artery, carbon monoxide poisoning and dementia. Here the lesion spares both anterior and posterior speech areas with an intact perisylvian cortex. The patient is able to repeat long sentences and may become echolalic, repeating everything that is said, but has difficulty formulating speech.

Subcortical damage with lesions to the thalamus, putamen/caudate or internal capsule will result in dysarthria, mild anomia, comprehension deficits, yet good repetition skills (Naeser et al., 1982). The mechanism by which these aphasias result is unclear, since it is the cortex that is responsible for language. One possibility is that subcortical damage results in disruption of the metabolism of the overlying cortex.

In dementia speech becomes circumstantial, with perseveration, circumlocutions and redundant phrases (Critchley, 1964). In the late stages of the disease there is little spontaneous speech and echolalia is often seen. In the final decorticate state, the patients become mute.

---

[2] Dysprosody: interruption of speech melody, with speech inflection and rhythm being disturbed.

Memory

This is a general term for a mental process that allows the individual to store experiences and perceptions and recall on demand. Memory processes can be divided into three stages:

1. registration, temporary or short term;
2. storage and permanent, or long term storage; storage is an active process requiring repetition and rehearsal;
3. retrieving a memory (also an active process).

Each of these stages has a distinct neuroanatomic substate and requires the integrity of the earlier steps.

Clinically, memory is divided into three basic types on the timespan between the presentation of the material and retrieval. Immediate memory refers to the recall of a memory trace after an interval of a few seconds, such as that used in digit span. The entire process can be performed by the language cortex surrounding the sylvian fissure (patients with a transcortical aphasia can perform well on digit span). The mechanism by which these short-term memories are maintained is unknown, but is thought to involve reverberating circuits and is a distinct property of the cortical sensory, motor, and integrative areas. Recent memory or working memory is the capacity to remember day-to-day events and requires the ability to store and retrieve new information, for example a name and address recalled after five minutes (Parkin, 1982). Remote memory is traditionally used to refer to the recollection of early events and historical events.

Careful attention to memory testing can detect the presence of an organic brain syndrome before the development of frank neurological findings. Anterograde amnesia (new information that cannot be retained) and retrograde amnesia (old information that can no longer be retrieved) are the most common initial symptoms of early organic brain damage. Different organic processes differ in the type of memory disturbance that results, from the severe deficit in relative isolation in Korsakoff's syndrome to a general cognitive impairment seen in dementia. Performance on memory testing requires patient co-operation and attention, therefore depressed or anxious patients often have apparent difficulties on memory testing and can present a difficult diagnostic problem. Accurate assessment of remote memory requires the information to be verifiable from someone other than the patient, as many patients with readily demonstrable memory deficits will deny their problem and produce confabulated answers. Historical facts such as who is the prime minister and the dates of World War II can be used to screen memory deficits.

The ability to orientate with respect to person, time and place depends on being able to continually update memory and is a sensitive and reliable pointer to an organic disorder (Hinton & Withers, 1971). Mistakes in place, year, and month are more significant than failure to give day or week or exact date (Cutting, 1980).

Some aspects of memory can be correlated with neuroanatomic structures (Warrington & Weiskrantz, 1982). The hippocampi, the mamilliary bodies, and the dorsal medial nuclei of the thalami are essential subcortical links for storage and retrieval of verbal and non-verbal data. These structures act as a 'relay station' to process and retrieve information from a neocortical level. Damage results in the individual being unable to store new information (anterograde amnesia) or retrieve information from the recent past (retrograde amnesia).

Such patients perform well on tests that do not require new learning ability. The syndrome has a number of causes: herpes simplex encephalitis, bilateral hippocampal infarction. Wernicke/Korsakoff syndrome, ill-judged temporal lobectomy in the presence of contralateral disease, carcinomatous encephalopathy.

In the Wernicke/Korsakoff syndrome, the patient often goes through an acute encephalopathy (Wernicke's encephalopathy), due to vitamin B1 deficiency and the underlying lesions involve bilateral destruction of the mamilliary bodies and the dorsal medial nuclei of the thalami (Victor *et al.*, 1981).When damage is restricted to the thalamus and mamilliary bodies the problem is in the retrieval of data, rather than its storage. This can be illustrated by representing the amnesic patient with previous material that he or she has not been able to recall in a 'multiple choice' format. If the patient is able to select the right answer, the material has been stored but the patient has difficulty with the retrieval process. Patients with hippocampal and temporal lobe damage have difficulty with storage and retrieval.

Transient global amnesia is a self-limiting defect of ongoing memorising associated with a short retrograde amnesia (Heathfield *et al.*, 1973). The episode lasts several hours only and is usually the manifestation of vascular disease in the posterior cerebral region causing a transient ischaemia of both medial temporal lobes. It clears spontaneously leaving only amnesia for the incident itself.

Remote memories are stored in the appropriate association cortex (i.e. visual memory on the visual cortex) (Rose, 1993). However, large areas of cortex can be lost without a clinically evident loss of remote memory. The pattern of amnesia found in dementia involves several different mechanisms. Initially degeneration in the hippocampal area causes difficulty in recent memory acquisition, immediate memory becomes affected by loss of the basic association cortex, especially around the sylvian fissure. As more widespread degeneration occurs throughout the cortex, there occurs patchy loss of remote memory.

Ganser's syndrome, or the syndrome of approximate answers, in which patients give answers so consistently close to the correct answer indicating that they know more than they are indicating, was originally described in prisoners. The syndrome is uncommon and can include clouding of consciousness, hallucinations, and somatic conversion symptoms. The aetiology of the syndrome is unclear and there maybe an organic component. However, most are instances of malingering or an hysterical dissociative state.

Very rarely an amnesic state is part of a frank malingering condition. In such a case there will be gross inconsistencies on formal testing and often the presence of other unexplained symptoms.

Constructional ability

This is defined as the capacity to draw or construct two- or three-dimensional figures (Mack & Levine, 1981). It is high-level non-verbal cognitive function that involves the integration of the frontal, occipital and parietal lobes. Because of the extensive cortical representation, constructional impairment is an early and sensitive indicator of organic disease, and in some patients may be the only indicator of underlying organic disorder. It is rare for the patient to complain voluntarily of constructional difficulties and it therefore should be assessed routinely. Simple testing of constructional impairment involves both the reproduction of simple line drawings and the drawing freehand of figures from memory, typically a clock or a house. The parietal lobes are the principal cortical areas involved in visual–motor integration, necessary for constructional tasks. The side of the lesion influences the type of constructional impairment, with right (nondominant) parietal lobe lesions, producing more severe deficits than left (dominant) hemisphere lesions. Also in right-sided lesions, the patient tends to lose the basic outline, orientation and spatial relationships of the drawing. With left-sided lesions the external configuration is maintained but there is loss of internal detail. The most common causes are: dementia, metabolic or toxic disturbance, and a focal parietal lobe lesion.

Higher cognitive functioning

This relies on the basic building blocks of memory, language and attention. The integration of these functions includes manipulation of learned material, arithmetic computation and abstract thinking. Loss of abstract thinking, usually tested by proverb interpretation, has been assumed to be a frontal lobe sign. However, with more detailed testing, concreteness of reply is more associated with posterior than frontal lesions. Verbal reasoning and abstraction are lateralised to the dominant hemisphere. Dyscalculia can be caused by lesions in either hemisphere, although dominant hemisphere lesions, particularly in parietal lobe, tend to be more severe, occurring as a component of Gerstmann's syndrome[3].

Thought

Thinking is disordered in all forms of cerebral dysfunction. Paradoxically it is probably least affected in left anterior hemisphere lesions where there is gross aphasia. The form of organic thinking varies according to chronicity and site of lesion. In acute organic reactions it resembles schizophrenia with neologisms, tangentiality, and distractibility (Cummings et al., 1980). In chronic organic reactions it is concrete, stereotyped, and impoverished. In right hemisphere lesions, there is a loss of the richness of imagery and in subcortical lesions there may be a dreamy, oneiroid state (delusional mood). The content of thought, particularly in chronic disorders, is meagre. There may be loosely held paranoid delusions that have some basis in reality.

Apraxia

Apraxia (Hecaen, 1981) is the inability to carry out purposeful movements in the presence of normal strength and co-ordination of the muscles and normal comprehension of the act. The two major types are ideomotor and ideational. In the former an individual gesture (e.g. blowing a kiss) is disordered; in the latter there is disruption to the logical and harmonious succession of separate elements in an act, the elements themselves being normal (e.g. lighting a cigarette). The lesion responsible for both of these is in the posterior half of the left hemisphere, parietal or temporal. The other forms of apraxia that have been described are

---

[3] Gerstmann's Syndrome: classic but controversial syndrome consisting of four major components: finger agnosia, right/left disorientation, dysgraphia and dyscalcalia.

probably composite impairments of several psychological functions. These include constructional and dressing apraxia (with visuospatial agnosia from right parietal lesions), unilateral left-sided ideomotor apraxia (associated damage to the corpus callosum producing a disconnection syndrome), and facial and oral apraxia (closely linked with Broca's aphasia).

There are several miscellaneous motor disorders, perseveration (repetition of own movements), echopraxia (repetition of others' movements) and catatonia, which may have an organic basis but may form part of a functional psychosis.

The effects of focal damage

Occipital lobe damage

This is least likely to have psychiatric sequelae. Visual hallucinations may occur, but these take the form of simple patterns and distortions. Subjects are usually unaware of their cortical blindness (Anton's syndrome) and the disorder falls within the category of denial of illness.

Parietal lobe symptoms

These usually first come to the attention of neurologists. Perceptual disorders from right-sided and language disorders from left-sided lesions are the rule. This does not do justice to the complexity of parietal disorders, carefully documented by Critchley (1953). Sequelae with a psychiatric component include confusional states from right parietal infarction (Mesulam *et al.*, 1976), anosognosia (denial of hemiplegia) and other abnormal attitudes to a hemiplegia (Cutting, 1978*b*), reduplicative paramnesia (maintaining that one is simultaneously in hospital and at home: Benson *et al.* (1976) and possibly Capgras syndrome (Christodoulou, 1977).

Temporal lobe dysfunction

This is a powerful generator of psychiatric disorder. It forms part of the limbic system, the cortical and subcortical representation of autonomic pathways and also contains the secondary auditory association areas. Memory circuits reside in the medial portion. It also acts as a tertiary association area, integrating information from all modalities. Damage may therefore produce mood change (ictal fear), auditory hallucinations, amnesia and qualitative distortions of memory (*déjà vu*), and complex visual hallucinations affecting size (e.g. Lilliputian hallucinations) or body image (e.g. autoscopic hallucinations, seeing oneself looking at oneself). Temporal lobe dysfunction is implicated in the development of schizophrenia (Flor-Henry, 1969) and can lead to particular kinds of personality change (Bear & Fedio, 1977).

Frontal lobe dysfunction

This also has a special link with psychiatric disorder. Although the functions of the frontal lobe are not well understood (Jouandet & Gazzaniga, 1979), the effect of damage is well documented. Personality change, loss of general intellectual abilities, mood change, and disorders of thinking may all follow (Petrie, 1952). The most common features are apathy or euphoria, irritability and social inappropriateness. The behavioural consequences of frontal lobe disorder differ depending on the locus of the lesion. Basal–orbital lesions result in disinhibited behaviour with irritability and lack of concern. Lesions to the dorsal–lateral area produce apathy, reduced drive and impaired planning.

Subcortical damage

Disease of the basal ganglia has been dealt with in the section on movement disorder. The brainstem contains the reticular activating system, the nexus of nerve cells that mediate arousal. Damage to this area produces one of several varieties of stupor or mutism. There are three syndromes of thalamic damage – anterolateral producing involuntary movements, posterolateral producing disturbances of sensation and pain, and medial producing vegetative and psychiatric disorder. The Kleine–Levin syndrome (Carpenter *et al.*, 1982) is an example of the last. This consists of periodic somnolence in young males, who show excessive eating, disturbed sexual behaviour, and oneirophrenia when awakened from their sleep. The hypothalamus has a role in the regulation of vegetative functions and tumours in this area have produced a syndrome indistinguishable from anorexia nervosa. The limbic system comprises cingulate gyrus, hippocampus, mamilliary bodies, amygdala, thalamus, and associated fibres. Its functions concern emotion, motivation and memory. Damage to any part of it will have an effect on these functions. Amnesia, emotional disturbance, and impaired drive will result. The most dramatic combination of these phenomena is the Kluver–Bucy syndrome (Cummings & Duchen, 1981) with emotional blunting, agnosia, unrestrained exploring, prominent oral tendencies, hypersexuality, and altered dietary habits.

Clinical syndromes

Acute organic reaction

The final common clinical pathway for all causes of general cerebral dysfunction is remarkably similar, namely clouding of consciousness to a greater or lesser degree, inattention, amnesia, muddled thoughts, lability of mood, and fleeting hallucinations and delusions. The terms delirium, confusion, and hallucinosis merely emphasise the relative prominence respectively of clouding of consciousness, muddled thinking or hallucinations (Strub, 1982). Delirium is an acute organic reaction in which the clinical picture is dominated by impairment of consciousness along with intrusive abnormalities derived from the fields of perception and affect (Lishman, 1987). Lipowski (1978) has added disorders of wakefulness and psychomotor behaviour to this definition.

Chronic organic reaction

The effect of a chronic pathogen on brain function is to alter the mental phenomena from positive (liability of mood, florid thought disorder, and hallucinations) to negative (apathy, poverty of thought content, amnesia). In most cases it will be correct to describe the whole mental state as dementia. In other cases one specific dysfunction will predominate; these focal disorders have been covered earlier. The causes of dementia will now be considered. It can usually be subdivided into presenile and senile depending on whether it develops before the age of 65. However, this age-related division is gradually losing favour to presumed differences in underlying pathology. The chief causes of presenile dementia are Alzheimer's disease, Pick's disease, frontal lobe dementia, Creutzfeldt–Jakob disease, multi-infarct dementia, Lewy body disease, communicating hydrocephalus, myxoedema, alcohol, and drugs. Head injury, cerebral tumour, metabolic disorders, toxins, and vitamin deficiency are other rarer causes, but dementia is not usually the presenting feature.

Hallucinosis

This is given the status of a syndrome by both Bonhoeffer and Lipowski. The clinical picture is dominated by auditory hallucinations, as in alcoholic hallucinosis. Although DSM-IIIR includes the diagnostic category of organic hallucinosis, the clinical symptoms that differentiate the disorder from a functional disorder have not been defined (Cutting, 1978b).

Dementia

This has three meanings. It is sometimes used for any chronic organic reaction. This is inappropriate as there exist chronic disorders with selective mental impairment (e.g. amnesia). It is sometimes used to mean a specific disease, usually senile dementia. This is also inappropriate because there are several forms of dementia, each with a different prognosis and response to treatment. It is best to regard dementia as a clinical syndrome of global intellectual decline and when referring to disease entities to qualify this (e.g. senile, Alzheimer's).

Amnesic syndrome

Although a variety of focal deficits may dominate the clinical picture, an isolated disorder of memory is sometimes given the status of a separate amnesic syndrome.

Organic personality change

There are several facets to the relationship between cerebral dysfunction and depressive illness. Brain damage increases the likelihood of a depressive condition (Ross & Rush, 1981).

Within a group of depressed patients, particularly elderly subjects, a significant proportion will show cerebral atrophy (Jacoby *et al.*, 1981). The issue is complicated by the fact that depression impairs attention and memory even in the absence of pathological evidence of cerebral dysfunction (McAllister, 1981), referred to as pseudodementia (Caine, 1981). Some manic disorders develop out of cerebral dysfunction, which Krauthammer & Klerman (1978) called secondary mania. The likelihood of schizophrenic illness is increased by acute (Cutting, 1980) or chronic cerebral dysfunction (Davison & Bagley, 1969). Left-sided temporal lobe dysfunction particularly has such an effect (Flor-Henry, 1969). Personality change is a consequence of most forms of cerebral dysfunction, more so if the disorder is chronic and more so with frontal (Petrie, 1952) and temporal lesions (Bear & Fedio, 1977).

Movement disorder

Chorea (involuntary movements of mouth and tongue can occur following multiple subcortical infarcts); Wilson's disease (chorea, cirrhosis and dementia) due to an inherited deficiency of the copper-carrying protein caeruloplasmin and Huntington's disease (an autosomal dominant genetic disorder).

Athetoid movements are writhing in nature and involve proximal muscles. They are mainly seen as an accompaniment of cerebral palsy.

Hemiballismus is a violent throwing movement of one side of the body, usually the result of vascular damage.

Tremor at rest not attributable to anxiety or thyroid disease may arise as a benign essential tremor, a familial condition, or a symptom of Parkinson's disease.

Disturbance of the flow of movement forms the central part of Parkinson's disease. The cause may be a previous encephalitis, vascular disease, antipsychotic medication, or, most often, idiopathic primary degeneration of dopamine containing neurones. Slowness of movement and of mental faculties (bradyphrenia: Wilson *et al.*, 1980), tremor, increased tone and disturbances in the initiation and changing of movements are the main features. Psychiatric manifestations (Sroka *et al.*, 1981) may be the consequence of treatment or of the disease itself. These include bradyphrenia, an increased risk of depressive illness, and an increased incidence of dementia. In addition, anticholinergics (benzhexol), L-dopa and amantidine all have a tendency to induce an acute organic reaction with vivid visual hallucination. Oro-buccal-facial dyskinesia (tardive dyskinesia) is a long-term side-effect of neuroleptics (Marsden & Jenner, 1980).

Neuropsychiatric consequences of neurological disease

Epilepsy

An epileptic seizure may be defined as an abnormal paroxysmal discharge of cerebral neurones that leads to an observable alteration in movement or behaviour or a subjective experience. The motor and sensory alterations are an important part of the definition and electroencephalographic evidence of abnormal discharges in isolation does

Table 3.1. *Classification of seizures*

I Partial Seizures
(A) Simple (consciousness not impaired)
    with motor signs or somatosensory symptoms
    with autonomic symptoms
    with psychic (dysphasia, cognitive impairment, mood change, illusions, hallucinations)
(B) Complex (consciousness impaired)
    simple at onset followed by impairment of consciousnes, with or without automtisms.
    with impairment of consciousness at onset, with or without automatisms
(C) Partial seizure evolving to generalised seizure
    simple partial seizure evolving to secondary generalised seizure
    complex partial seizure evolving to secondary generalised seizure
    simple partial seizure evolving to complex partial seizure, then to generalised seizure

II Generalised Seizures
(A) Absence seizures
(B) Myoclonic seizures
(C) Clonic seizures
(D) Tonic seizures
(E) Tonic–clonic seizures
(F) Atonic seizures

III Unclassified epileptic seizures

---

not constitute a seizure or a diagnosis of epilepsy. Epilepsy is the state of continuing tendency to recurrent seizures. Epidemiological studies suggest an overall prevalence in the range four to ten per thousand (Zielinsky, 1982). However, there are clear age differences in prevalence and for the adult population Hopkins (1981) has estimated the prevalence to be two per thousand.

While the classification of the epilepsies and epileptic seizures is often a source of confusion, probably the most pragmatic classification of individual seizure types is that produced by the International League Against Epilepsy (Porter, 1993) (Table 13.1). The main emphasis in this classification is placed on a behavioural description of the seizure. Two main types are recognised, partial and generalised. On the basis of symptomatology, partial seizures can be regarded as simple, complex or secondarily generalised. Simple partial seizures include motor movements, sensory disturbance, autonomic disturbance or disturbance of mental function, excluding consciousness itself (for example, dysphasia, amnesia, affective disturbance, illusions, and hallucinations). Central to complex partial seizures is impairment of consciousness manifested as impaired awareness and impaired responsiveness. Seizures that have generalised tonic-clonic features but are preceded by either simple or complex disturbances are regarded as secondarily generalised seizures. Seizures that are generalised from the outset (showing bilateral bisynchronous disturbances of body movement such as tonic–clonic, myoclonic or atonic features) are considered generalised seizures.

The classification of the epilepsies takes into account the electrophysiological as well as the clinical behavioural manifestations. The current classification was proposed by the International League Against Epilepsy, in which two major groups are defined: the generalised epilepsies and the partial epilepsies. Generalised epilepsies can be divided into those that are clearly secondary to underlying brain pathology and called either secondary, symptomatic or lesionary. This distinguishes them from those generalised epilepsies that appear to have no obvious underlying pathology associated with them and are referred to as primary or asymptomatic epilepsies. The other main group are the partial epilepsies, which are secondary or symptomatic in type.

Psychological problems are more common in people with epilepsy, compared with the general population, and epilepsy occurs more frequently in people with mental illness. While these relationships can only be fully explained by considering specific psychiatric disorders and specific types of epilepsy, several general links can be discerned. First, the onset of epilepsy is both a psychological as well as a physical event. The physical antecedents of epilepsy may have a direct causative role in mental impairment, cognitive or conative. The stress of epilepsy and its effects on lifestyle, personal and family, may have far-reaching psychological consequences. Anticonvulsants can affect cognition and psychomotor speed, even at dosage levels within the therapeutic range. Second, many people with psychiatric problems are at increased risk of seizure disorder particularly those in whom there are underlying or associated coarse changes in brain structure. Finally, the similarity of some of the phenomena of epilepsy and some psychiatric disorders may lead to diagnostic confusion that may be compounded by the fact that some patients may simulate attacks.

The relationship between epilepsy and psychiatric disorder can best be understood by considering separately those states that occur in close temporal proximity to the seizure itself and those that are unrelated.

Peri-ictal psychiatric disorders

The importance of this group is that the phenomena of seizure-related activity may be misinterpreted as symptoms of functional psychiatric disorder. During the hours and occasionally days before a fit, patients may complain of prodromal mood changes such as depression or irritability. A variety of psychical phenomena have been observed during the course of a partial seizure (Fenton, 1981). During and following generalised seizures and many partial seizures, attention, awareness, and responsiveness are grossly impaired. Within the present classification of seizures, the following categories of mental impairments have been recognised. In simple partial seizures, abnormalities of perceptions, such as hallucinations or illusions may occur in any or several sensory modalities. Mood change may occur, most commonly fear and anxiety. A third group of psychiatric phenomena are related to disturbances of memory, the most familiar being distortions of memory in which an abnormal sense of familiarity of unfamiliarly are prominent features. Ictal dysphasic attacks resulting from a left hemisphere discharge have also been reported. In complex partial seizures, awareness is reduced and in some clouding of consciousness and confusion may be the only sign.

Automatisms are most commonly found in temporal lobe epilepsy, occurring in up to 45% of cases. Automatisms may appear in the course of a seizure or during the post-ictal confusional state. The relationship between epilepsy and automatism has been reviewed by Fenton (1980). Three phases have been recognised. During the first phase normal activity ceases; the second is characterised by repetitive stereotyped activity; while in the third phase behaviour is complex and semi-purposeful. The attack is usually brief and rarely lasts more than an hour, while amnesia for the event is usually complete. While the prevalence of epilepsy is higher in prisons and borstals, Gunn & Fenton (1971) have shown that it is extremely rare for crime to be committed during a seizure or in the post-ictal period.

Chronic states

Patients with epilepsy may have chronic cognitive impairments. In children this may be manifest as reduced attention, learning difficulty, specific reading retardation, intellectual retardation, or intellectual decline. In community studies of people with epilepsy, about 10% have been shown to be intellectually disadvantaged (Pond et al., 1981). Conversely, the prevalence of epilepsy among intellectually disadvantaged children is much higher than that found in the general population. This ranges from 3 to 6% for children in the community, while for the severely intellectually impaired, the incidence can be as high as 30%. When multiple physical handicaps accompany severe intellectual impairment, the incidence can be as high as 60% (Corbett, 1981). The strong relationship between prevalence of epilepsy and severity of intellectual impairment points to a common origin in underlying brain damage. More rarely, however, severe and uncontrolled epilepsy may itself lead directly to intellectual deterioration (for example infantile spasms, Lennox–Gastaut syndrome, status epilepticus). It also appears that milder degrees of intellectual impairment may result from frequent and poorly controlled seizures that begin early in life (Dikmen et al., 1977). The type of epilepsy is another important variable; cognitive impairment has been more frequently observed in association with epilepsy arising from the left temporal lobe and in primary generalised epilepsy, in which there are frequent interictal generalised discharges (Stores, 1981).

While it has been recognised that antiepileptic drugs in the toxic range lead to marked impairment of cognitive function, more recent studies have shown that even drugs within the therapeutic range may lead to clinically detectable psychomotor slowing and intellectual deterioration (Corbett et al., 1985; Dodrill & Temkin, 1989). The newer anticonvulsants are less problematic in this respect. Medication may also play a significant part in the development of behaviour disorders (Werry, 1968), and in some contributes to the development of hyperkinesis (Ounsted & Lindsay, 1981). Neurotic disorders, such as anxiety states, social withdrawal and behaviour disorders are also over-represented in children with epilepsy.

Epilepsy rarely occurs as an isolated problem and the effects of other variables need to be taken into consideration before concluding that seizures are a direct cause of psychological disturbance. Some of these variables are related to the epilepsy, such as the presence of underlying brain damage and anticonvulsant medication (Goodman & Graham, 1996). Constitutional predisposition and psychosocial factors are of considerable importance just as they are in those without epilepsy. There is a high incidence of social rejection and broken homes among children with epilepsy and also a high incidence of physical handicap and intellectual, language, and education difficulties. A significant association has been observed between the presence of psychomotor attacks, parental social class and evidence of emotional disturbance in the mother. Emotional distress was more commonly observed in

376

the mothers of epileptic children compared with mothers of children with other chronic handicaps; overprotection was common, and unnecessary restrictions frequently placed on the child's activities. It is likely that these attitudes lead to excessive passivity in the child and Hartlage *et al.* (1972) have suggested that epileptic children are more dependent on their parents than non-epileptic children with physical impairments. Stores & Piran (1978) observed increased emotional dependency, particularly in children with temporal lobe epilepsy. As Stores (1981) has noted, teachers and parents often have low expectations of children with epilepsy and tend to underestimate their intellectual potential. Such low expectations are often transmitted to the child and lead to underachievement. The effects of these processes on the developing child and the resulting boredom probably contribute to the increased prevalence of conduct disorder in childhood and adolescence.

In the case of adults, the same factors lead to problems in personality development. Although the generalised description of the epileptic personality as 'languid, spiritless, slow and sticky' has not stood the test of more careful and systematic enquiry (Tizard, 1962), it is probable that a small percentage of patients with chronic epilepsy do share some of these traits. Bear & Fedio (1977), in a study of temporal lobe epilepsy, observed a distinctive pattern of traits including dependency, obsessionality, emotionality and irritability. In a small group of patients with temporal lobe epilepsy, Waxman & Geschwind (1975) noted a symptom cluster of hyposexuality, religiosity, and hypergraphia, and suggested that these may be concomitants of abnormal limbic activity. In considering such personality and behavioural difficulties, however, the contributions and interactions of underlying brain damage, medication and the many psychological and social difficulties, all need to be considered (Fenton, 1981; Sorensen *et al.*, 1989). The relative importance of each factor will vary from individual to individual.

Anxiety and depressive symptoms are a common accompaniment of epilepsy beginning in adult life. Although probably no more common in epilepsy overall than that observed with other chronic physical disorders. Edeh & Toone (1987) found a higher prevalence associated with partial compared with generalised epilepsy. Apart from the natural fears that are frequently expressed about epilepsy, the patient will often have to come to terms with alterations in his or her work and social life. One particular problem that epilepsy brings is the threat of loss of control, a threat also for family and peers (Betts, 1993). The phenomenon of complex partial seizures can sometimes be confused with panic attacks (Laidlaw & Khin-Maung-Zaw, 1993). Suicide in epilepsy has been shown to be about four times as common as in the general population. While increased risk has been associated with temporal lobe epilepsy (Barraclough, 1981), other risk factors include impulsive and explosive personality, psychotic disturbance, and ready access to drugs (Mendez *et al.*, 1989).

The inter-ictal psychoses are a group of psychiatric disorders occurring as discrete illnesses during the inter-ictal period, each with its counterpart among the functional psychoses. The relation between the inter-ictal psychosis and the epileptic process is uncertain and controversial, each running a course largely independent of the other (Toone, 1981). As indicated above, depressive symptoms are common in epilepsy for many reasons. It is less clear, however, whether depressive psychosis occurs more commonly among patients with epilepsy (Toone, 1981; Perez & Trimble, 1980).

There is more conclusive evidence of an association between epilepsy and schizophrenia. As such they constitute an important paradigm for schizophrenia. The first clear delineation of a syndrome closely resembling schizophrenia occurring in epilepsy was reported by Hill (1953). The schizophrenia-like psychoses of epilepsy appear to be more commonly found in focal temporal lobe epilepsy. This view was first proposed by Slater *et al.* in 1963 and substantiated by more recent studies (Perex & Trimble 1980; Perez *et al.*, 1985). Flor-Henry (1969) reported an association between schizophrenia-like psychosis and left temporal lobe foci, again supported by recent evidence (Marshall *et al.*, 1993). Precise estimates of the prevalence of inter-ictal epileptic psychoses have been difficult to achieve, and critics of the reported association between psychosis and epilepsy have highlighted the biased nature of the sample of patients in which the association has been found (Stevens & Hermann, 1981). Studies based on neurological clinic attendance have reported the prevalence of psychotic illness among patients with epilepsy in general to be around 4% (Small & Small, 1967). Age of onset of epilepsy again emerges as an important variable. In one large series, in which the average age of onset of temporal lobe epilepsy was 22 years, the prevalence of psychosis was 2% (Currie *et al.*, 1971) compared with 8% in a group whose seizures began in childhood (Ounsted & Lindsay, 1981). A common origin for both conditions in focal brain damage seems likely. In a recent re-analysis of the Maudsley temporal lobectomy series, the schizophrenia-like psychoses were significantly associated with mesial temporal lobe pathology arising in the foetal and perinatal period (Roberts *et al.*, 1990). A family history of psychosis is usually lacking and premorbid personality normal. There appears to be general agreement that the psychosis usually follows the onset of epilepsy with an interval of between 10 and 25 years.

More controversial is the evidence of a relationship between seizure activity and psychotic symptomatology. Slater *et al.* (1963) reported six cases in which psychotic symptoms arose at a time when seizure frequency was decreasing. In assessing the relationship between the emergence of the psychosis and seizure frequency, the contribution of anticonvulsant medication must be considered (Reynolds, 1968). Finally, differentiation needs to be made between the inter-ictal psychosis and the paranoid hallucinatory psychoses which may occur as a post-ictal event. In the latter, there is usually some evidence of cognitive impairment and confusion and the onset is typically heralded by a series of seizures. The course of the post-ictal psychosis is usually brief in contrast to the inter-ictal psychosis, which often runs a chronic or fluctuating course lasting several weeks or months.

The prognosis for seizure control has been transformed in recent years by the advances in anticonvulsant medication. An overall remission rate of about 70% can be anticipated – reduced in the presence of known aetiology, partial seizures and where there is EEG evidence of epileptic activity (Annegers *et al.*, 1979; Shafer *et al.*, 1988). Recent evidence suggests that treatment of a single seizure reduces the risk of epilepsy developing at all. The modern anticonvulsants, carbamazepine and sodium valproate, are generally well tolerated with low side-effects when used within the therapeutic range. To these have been added three recent newcomers – lamotrigine, vigabatrin and gabapentin. When used in combination with established drugs, these new drugs have been shown to give significantly improved seizure control in those with intractable epilepsy.

It is beyond the scope of this chapter to give detail on the management (biopsychosocial) of the patient with epilepsy and interested readers are referred to authorative reviews such as *A Textbook of Epilepsy* (Laidlaw *et al.*, 1993).

Head injury

The extent to which psychiatric disability after head injury results from brain damage remains an issue of considerable practical and theoretical interest, particularly since head injury should in theory prove ideal for an improved understanding of the relationship between cerebral disorder and psychiatric disability. Post-traumatic brain lesions are in the main non-progressive and uncomplicated while the clinical outcomes that result can embrace most of what is found in psychiatric symptomatology (Goodman & Graham, 1996; Lishman, 1968).

Head injury has been described as the 'silent epidemic' of our time, attributed in major part to the fast pace of modern lifestyle and compounded by the advances in technology that increase the probability of survival following injury (Adamovich *et al.*, 1984). It is a major health problem for young adults and accounts for approximately 15% of all deaths among young adults in the UK (Jennet & MacMillan, 1981). Similar findings from the United States indicate that head injury is the major cause of death in adults under 35 years of age (Adamovich *et al.*, 1984). Probably the most reliable guide to incidence is attendance rates at accident and emergence departments. In Scotland, 18 attendances for every 1000 of the population each year result from head injury (Strong *et al.*, 1978).

The incidence rates belie the enormity of the problem, since the survivors from severe closed head injury are predominately adolescents and young adults with relatively normal life expectancies and constitute a major burden on families and on services. While psychosocial adjustment is only one aspect of outcome, quality of life is greatly affected by such issues, as time since the injury increases.

Physical impairments such as spasticity or isolated cranial nerve lesions usually improve over a period of several months and are infrequent causes of major handicaps for either the patient or his family. Mental impairments (personality change, chronic affective disturbance, intellectual deterioration, memory impairment, impaired concentration, dysphasia) are often more enduring and contribute most to chronic disability and handicap (Jennet & Bond, 1975). Mental and physical impairments often coexist, compounding the total disability. In evaluating the outcome of head injury, one must consider not only the patient but also the effects on his or her family, and here again it is the mental impairments that are often more stressful.

As Lishman (1973) has commented it is most unlikely that the large range of mental and physical impairments that have been observed in the post-head injury period share a common aetiology, even though all will have appeared to have taken origin from the common event.

Dementia

Following severe closed head injury, intellectual impairment, memory deficits, and personality change are found in a substantial proportion. The degree of dementia appears to be related to severity of injury, and long-term prognosis is worse following open head injury and when the period of post-traumatic amnesia is longer than 24 hours. There is some improvement over a period of months. This is in part the consequence of re-education of intact brain tissue, but it is probable that motivational disturbances and emotional responses to injury and impairment make substantial contributions to the overall disability in the early stages (Lishman, 1973). There is general agreement that the more severe the initial head injury, the greater the cognitive impairment. However, as Lishman (1973) has pointed out, the size of the correlations between such measures of initial injury as post-traumatic amnesia (PTA) and outcome are often small. Other factors besides the severity of the injury affect outcome. Brain damage is rarely homogenous, and localised lesions can have very different effects. Considering cognitive impairments in general, damage to the hemisphere dominant for speech has more severe effects than comparable damage to the non-dominant. Following focal penetrating injuries, deficits may be quite discrete, for example dysphasia or hemiparesis. With closed head injuries, which are the most usual type in civilian life, global impairments are more usual (Lishman, 1973).

Neurosis and personality change

An altered and idiosyncratic reaction to persons and situations is undoubtedly one of the most distressing problems for the patient's family, and for those involved in his/her subsequent care and management. In one five-year follow-up study of severe head injury, most patients were found to have evidence of severe personality change (Brooks et al., 1986). There is substantial evidence for a neurological basis for such changes, with damage to the frontal and temporal lobes being major contributory factors. The frontal lobe syndrome, characterised by disinhibition, euphoria, lack of tact, and childishness, is now well recognised as a late sequel to frontal lobe damage. Following injury to the temporal lobe, aspects of the frontal lobe syndrome may be observed, together with irritability and increased aggressiveness. Damage to central and basal frontal areas is typically accompanied by loss of spontaneity and lack of vitality. Accompanying this wide range of personality changes there is usually some loss of insight and awareness.

Depression, anxiety, irritability, and obsessional traits are frequently observed following head injury of all types. These may be better regarded as symptoms of a neurotic reaction than personality change and are among the most common of the psychiatric sequelae of head injury (Lishman, 1973). However, the commonly held view of a simple double dissociation between severe brain damage and organic symptoms on the one hand and mild brain damage and neurotic symptoms on the other is an over-simplification. Frequently patients with severe organic brain damage exhibit neurotic symptoms, although it is often difficult to disentangle these from the more florid aspects of behaviour and thinking which may dominate the clinical picture (McKinely et al., 1983; Fedoroff et al., 1992). In all grades of head injury the importance of psychological mechanisms must not be overlooked. The high incidence of depressive and anxiety states following spinal cord injuries, burns and chronic physical illness fully demonstrates the importance of non-organic factors in symptom formation (Judd et al., 1989). Therefore, in the evaluation of individual cases the contributions of personality, vulnerability and the stressfulness of the head injury need to be assessed, giving due consideration to the full social context of the event and its consequences.

Psychosis

Psychotic reactions have been reported more commonly than expected in the late post-traumatic period. In part these may be the result of non-specific effects of stress precipitating a specific reaction in those individuals who are constitutionally vulnerable. Depressive psychosis is definitely more common than schizophreniform. However, some patients develop schizophreniform reactions in the absence of any constitutional loading and damage to the temporal lobe seems to be of specific aetiological importance (Davison & Bagley, 1969).

Post-concussional syndrome

A particular constellation of symptoms appears after mild head injury, defined as injury in which consciousness is lost only briefly, if at all, or in which the post-traumatic amnesia (PTA) is brief. In most studies the boundary between minor and major head injuries is a PTA of 24 hours. The prevalence of minor head injuries is much higher, yet it is with this group that the greatest controversies remain regarding the chronicity of symptoms and the relevance of psychological and physical factors in their causation. A wide range of symptoms are frequently observed following minor head injury. These include somatic symptoms, particularly headache, dizziness, hearing difficulty, and fatigue, and psychological symptoms, such as impaired concentration, memory difficulties, irritability, anxiety and depression. Most patients have several symptoms during the 48 hours following injury and even at six weeks as many as 50% still have symptoms. (McClelland, 1985). Lewin (1968) has suggested that these early post-traumatic symptoms are the direct result of the organic insult itself and an indicator of the time course of the recovery process. Several studies support such an organic basis for at least some of the immediate post-head-injury symptomatology. Oppenheimer (1968), in a study of post-mortem material, found diffuse microscopic lesions in a high proportion of human brains after mild head injury (capillary haemorrhages and severing of nerve fibres). Such lesions were visible many months after injury and were attributed to surface shearing, contusion, stretching and tearing of small blood vessels, and stretching and tearing of nerve fibres. Taylor & Bell (1966) in a study of 70 patients with post-concussional symptoms found slowing of the cerebral circulation and observed a positive relationship between improvement of symptoms and return of cerebral circulation time to normal. More recent neurophysiological studies provide additional evidence for brainstem and cortical dysfunction and damage following mild head injury (Montgomery et al., 1991; Jenkins et al., 1986).

Greater controversy surrounds the persistence of symptoms and the relation between chronic symptoms and severity of injury. In some patients it is possible that subtle neurological changes persist, leading to chronic residual symptoms. In support of a chronic neural deficit is the evidence provided by the cumulative effects of repeated minor head injuries such as occur in boxers (Gronwall & Wrightson, 1975). A polar opposite view was given by Miller (1961), who argued that most of the chronic symptoms following minor head injury can be considered 'accident neurosis' and 'invariably resolve' once compensation is obtained. However, Kelly (1975) and others have present strong evidence against this view, showing that a majority of patients with symptoms return to work before compensation is settled. Similar symptoms are common in patients not receiving compensation. Nevertheless, it seems likely that psychological mechanisms are important in the development of chronic symptomatology. Pilowsky (1985) has demonstrated that accidents are often more traumatic psychologically and emotionally than appears at first sight, and it is paradoxical that the accident experience is often least discussed and worked through by those responsible for patient management.

The balance of organic and psychological factors in the aetiology of chronic head injury sequelae in individual cases can only be established by a careful analysis of the facts. The persistence of several symptoms from the time of injury and evidence of neurophysiological dysfunction suggest an organic basis for a patient's symptoms while the late development of new symptoms and negative neurophysiological findings point to a likely psychological origin.

Social impairment and handicap

The full impact of brain injury and resulting impairments is manifested in social adjustment. Livingston (1986), in a study of patients with severe closed head injury, reported high levels of dependency. Almost half were considered by relatives incapable of being left in charge of the home and over 20% required someone to look after them. The studies of both Oddy *et al.* (1978) and Thomsen (1974) highlight the social isolation and social dislocation resulting from severe closed head injury.

Another dimension of social outcome is family stress and burden. Brooks *et al*'s (1986) study of patients with severe head injury revealed a high burden of care in the great majority. In the same series, Livingston (1986) reported high scores of the General Health Questionnaire among the principal carers, with many families complaining of being stressed.

A major factor affecting long-term outcome and family burden is service provision. Several studies report major deficiencies in the provision of care (Panting & Merry, 1972; Thomsen, 1974; Oddy *et al.*, 1978; Livingston, 1986).

Newson-Smith (1983) has commented on the lack of services, lack of community and hospital provision and lack of clear planning for the young brain-damaged adult. Livingston (1986) has stressed the priority needs for services for the families of the brain-damaged individual. There is a need for and yet a marked shortage of specialist rehabilitation services for patients with head injuries and their relatives, services that integrate both the physical and psychological aspect of management (Gloag, 1984 and Lancet, 1990).

The Royal College of Psychiatrists (1991a) has provided proposals for the development of Brain Injury Rehabilitation services within the UK, which takes advantage of the existing network of community-orientated mental health services. A comprehensive analysis of current concepts of rehabilitation and the principles that should guide rehabilitation services is given by Wood & Eames (1989).

Sleep disorders

Sleep has been defined as a recurring state of inactivity accompanied by loss of awareness and a decrease in responsiveness to the environment (Fenton, 1975). Although not strictly classifiable as psychiatric manifestations of organic illness, sleep disorders are usually regarded as the province of the neuropsychiatrist.

Incidence and classification

Problems with sleep are common and from community surveys about one in seven of the population have frequent problems with initiating sleep, maintaining sleep or early morning waking (Karacan *et al.*, 1983). For many sleep disorders, there is associated increase in day-time sleepiness and an increased risk of accidents at work and driving. In a recent community study, 10% of subjects were classified as excessively tired and over 1% attributed accidents and other mishaps to this problem (Martikainen *et al.*, 1992). Parkes (1993) has suggested that the disabilities caused by severe day-time sleepiness is comparable to that of severe epilepsy.

Sleep disorder can be categorised into four main groups (Karacan *et al.*, 1973):

1. First, primary sleep disorders in which disturbance of sleep is the predominant symptom. The largest category within this group is insomnia, characterised by disturbances of sleep induction, maintenance of quality of sleep (Disorders of Initiating and Monitoring Sleep – DIMS). Second is a group characterised by excessive daytime sleepiness and consisting of two major subgroups, narcolepsy and the hypersomnias (Disorders Of Excessive Somnolence – DOES) (Thorpy, 1988).
2. Secondary sleep disorders in which sleep impairment is secondary to some other disorder. This may be functional, for example, psychiatric illness, chronic alcoholism, metabolic and nutritional disorders, or structural brain disease.
3. The parasomnias, characterised by behavioural phenomena that arise during sleep but are inappropriate to the sleeping state. These include sleep talking, night terrors, sleep walking, nocturnal enuresis, and bruxism.
4. Disorders modified by sleep. These include ischaemic heart disease, migraine, duodenal ulceration, bronchial asthma, neuromuscular disorders, and epilepsy.

In this chapter only the primary sleep disorders will be dealt with.

Insomnia

This may be defined as the inability to fall asleep or maintain adequate sleep (Solomon, 1956). It is the most common sleep disorder. Although the term implies lack of sleep this is unusual, and most patients present with such symptoms as unrefreshing sleep, abbreviated sleep or sleep punctuated by abnormal restlessness and interruptions (Luce & Segal, 1969). There is considerable heterogeneity of both complaints and of EEG signs of sleep disturbance. Many patients complaining of insomnia underestimate the amount of sleep obtained and overestimate their sleep disturbance (de la Pena, 1978). Some clinicians and researchers question the existence of primary insomnia as a distinct entity (Karacan *et al.*, 1973). Nevertheless, some patients show certain qualitative differences from normal, such as an intermingling of alpha and delta EEG activity during sleep, and a high variability in sleep patterns from one night to the next. Other studies have indicated that groups of insomniacs have significantly delayed sleep onset and decreased sleep efficiency (Karacan *et al.*, 1973). Some exhibit EEG signs of disturbed sleep induction, sleep maintenance or sleep quality in keeping with their subjective complaints (Frankel *et al.*, 1976). While the causes of primary insomnia remain poorly understood, high levels of arousal would appear to be an important mechanism for some. Studies of personality variables associated with primary insomnia show wide variations, although high rates of neurosis and depression are common (Beutler *et al.*, 1978).

Narcolepsy

Although the term narcolepsy was first coined by Gelineau in 1880, it was not until the development of electroencephalography, and especially sleep polygraphy during the last 30 years, that a full understanding of the nature of the underlying disorder became possible (Karacan & Howell, 1988). Present estimates of prevalence suggest that 0.03-0.06% of the population are affected by this condition. The main symptom of the narcoleptic syndrome is a sleep attack consisting of irresistible sleep, characteristically of short duration, ranging from 30 seconds to 15 minutes. Attacks may occur singly or in clusters ranging in frequency from 1 to 200 attacks daily. They are typically facilitated by situations in which the patient is passive such as watching television. The second most frequent symptom is the cataplectic attack consisting of a sudden loss of muscle tone associated with an inability to move. These attacks are usually provoked by emotion, particularly strong emotion accompanied by activity or intended movement. Consciousness during the attack is usually normal and the duration of attacks ranges from a few seconds to a few minutes. Patients may have one or two attacks in their lifetime while others have as many as 100 attacks daily. Cataplexy occurs in approximately 70% of cases of narcolepsy. A third symptom, sleep paralysis, is a state resembling cataplexy but occurring while the patient is either falling asleep or awakening. Attacks may last from one to ten minutes and occur in approximately 25% of cases (Yoss & Daly, 1960). The fourth component of the narcoleptic syndrome is hypnagogic hallucinations consisting of visual, auditory or somatosensory hallucinations occurring during the period of falling asleep. These may last from one to 15 minutes and have been reported to occur in approximately 25% of cases of the narcolepsy syndrome (Yoss & Daly, 1960).

Two additional symptoms frequently observed in the narcolepsy syndrome are obesity and automatic behaviour. The latter occurs typically when the patient tries to continue his activity in spite of drowsiness.

Two forms of narcolepsy are commonly recognised, idiopathic and symptomatic. The symptomatic narcolepsies are in most cases the consequence of brain concussion, encephalitis or a tumour of the mesodiencephalic region. While idiopathic narcolepsy runs in families, and the transmission pattern is strongly associated with the human leucocyte antigens (HLA) DR2 and DQRV1, present evidence argues for genetic heterogenicity (Ditta *et al.*, 1992; Matsuki *et al.*, 1992). The idiopathic form of narcolepsy typically begins around puberty or shortly after, although several years may elapse before the full clinical picture manifests itself. The first symptoms to appear are usually narcoleptic attacks. Our understanding of the mechanism underlying narcolepsy and its main symptoms have been based primarily on polygraphic findings, particularly since the discovery of REM sleep and the differentiation of the two forms of sleep, REM and non-REM sleep. It would appear that in isolated narcolepsy the sleep attacks are accompanied by non-REM sleep due to the facilitation of the non-REM sleep system. Narcoleptic attacks occurring in patients with narcolepsy–cataplexy are frequently accompanied by REM sleep signs and often by sleep onset REM periods (Derment et al., 1972). Present evidence suggests that all symptoms of narcolepsy–cataplexy are manifestations of dissociated or undissociated REM sleep (Passouant et al., 1967).

A high level of psychopathology has been found in patients with narcolepsy, although this is thought to arise mostly as a reaction to the disorder and its effects in daily living and is not of aetiological significance.

The diagnosis of narcolepsy should not present formidable difficulties provided a careful analysis of the symptoms has been made. A narcoleptic attack involves irresistible sleep of short duration and is not a state of unconsciousness. The coexistence of cataplexy greatly assists the diagnosis and according to Kales et al. (1982) removes the need for sleep laboratory investigation.

Primary or functional hypersomnia

According to Roth (1980) primary or functional hypersomnia is the next most common disorder after narcolepsy among patients with excessive daytime sleepiness. Unlike narcoleptic attacks, the hypersomnia is characterised by *prolonged* periods of daytime sleepiness. In some forms of the disorder there is also long night-sleep with sleep drunkenness on awakening. There is frequently a positive family history.

Recent studies suggest that *sleep-induced apnoea* is a major cause and according to Guilleminault & Dement (1988) is the most common cause of excessive daytime sleepiness in the absence of cataplexy. Apnoea is defined as the cessation of air exchanged at the nose and mouth lasting at least ten seconds, and the sleep-induced apnoea syndrome is usually defined as the occurrence of more than 5–10 second apnoea per hour of sleep (Lancet, 1985). Respiratory irregularities are more common among men than women and this probably accounts for the fact that the syndrome shows a male/female sex ratio of approximately 10 to 1 (Guilleminault & Dement, 1988).

Three subtypes of the disorder have been recognised. In one there is some obstruction in the respiratory tract, while in the second there is a central disturbance of respiratory control mechanisms. In a third form excessive airway resistance and a central disturbance of respiratory control coexist (Ancoli-Israel et al., 1987).

Although the most common presenting complaint is excessive daytime sleepiness, some patients present with insomnia. This is particularly the case with the central type of sleep apnoea. Guilleminault & Dement (1988) found that 19 out of 30 patients were overweight (body weight 20 per cent more than expected). Four of these overweight patients had the 'Pickwickian Syndrome'. All 30 patients had abnormal respiration during sleep, with an average of approximately 400 sleep apnoeas during an eight-hour polygraphic recording. In some forms of hypersomnia the duration of sleepiness lasts for several days or even weeks. The Kleine–Levin syndrome consists of long attacks of hypersomnia associated with marked hunger and over-eating occurring exclusively in males usually in the age range 15–25 (Critchley, 1962). During the attacks there may be marked changes in the patient's mental state ranging from mood disturbance with irritability to disorientation and impairment of memory. In view of the experimental evidence of the importance of the hypothalamus in sleep and appetitive behaviour, it has been suggested that some disorder of hypothalamic function exists (Oswald, 1962).

Hypersomnia may result from overt brain disease (the symptomatic or secondary hypersomnias), the most frequent causes being inflammatory diseases of the brain, brain trauma, tumours and vascular disorders. An example is Von Ecomomo's encephalitis lethargica.

Dementia

Alzheimer's disease

This is by far the most common type of dementia. It is identical to parenchymatous senile dementia (Schneck et al., 1982). Three clinical phases can be recognised: subjective cognitive deficits, objective confusion, and severe dementia with disorientation and the negative symptoms outlined above. Investigations that should rule out most causes of reversible dementia are liver enzymes, electrolytes, full blood count, urinalysis, chest X-ray, serology for syphilis, thyroid function, serum B12 and folate, CT scan and more recently MRI-scanning. There are three characteristic neuropathological features – neurofibrillary tangles, senile plaques, and granulovacuolar bodies. The parietal and temporal lobes (particularly posterior hippocampus) are mainly affected. Biochemical abnormalities include a reduction in choline acetyltransferase and acetylcholinesterase, findings that suggest that a pharmacological treatment may be available some day. The aetiology is still unknown. Most authorities incline to the view that it represents some form of accelerated ageing; the three most plausible candidates for a specific cause are slow virus, toxin (particularly aluminium), and immunological dysfunction. More recent work has focused on the apolipoprotein-E gene on chromosome 19, which is a risk factor for late-onset familial and sporadic Alzheimer's disease and the amyloid precursor protein on chromosome 21, a risk factor for early familial AD, the hope being that a clinical marker will allow prophylactic treatment (Hardy & Allsop, 1991).

Non Alzheimer's dementia

Pick's disease

Pick's disease (Wechsler et al., 1982) is another variety of parenchymatous dementia. It is rarer than Alzheimer's disease and differs from the latter in pathology and clinical presentation. The main brunt of the damage is to the frontal and lateral temporal lobes, unlike Alzheimer's disease where parietal and medial temporal lobes are first affected. The characteristic pathology is the Pick cell balloon-like changes with argyrophilic inclusions. Clinically, a frontal-lobe syndrome with social, emotional, and motivational change supervenes early. Language is also affected but constructional and mathematical ability is relatively spared.

Frontal lobe dementia

This has become increasingly recognised as a form of cerebral atrophy distinct from Alzheimer's disease, and which is more common than previously supposed (Neary, 1990). This disorder occurs at an earlier age than Alzheimer's disease and approximately half the patients have a positive family history of early dementia. Patients present with striking change in personality and social conduct followed by progressive impairment in speech but with preservation of visuo-spatial ability. A biopsy reveals atrophy of the frontal and temporal lobes with loss of large cortical neurones and cortical spongiform change. Neuropsychology confirms a 'frontal lobe' syndrome, with serotyped behaviour and hyper-oral tendencies.

Lewy body disease

This is a syndrome of dementia and rigidity in which Lewy bodies are found in midline cerebral nuclei (Byrne *et al.*, 1989). Initially patients are often thought to have Parkinson's disease because of akinesia and rigidity. However, this is accompanied by a fluctuating mental state with hallucinations, behavioural changes and a sub-acute confusional state. The pathology shows Lewy bodies not only in the substantia nigra but widespread throughout the cerebral cortex. The Lewy bodies themselves are simply degraded intracellular proteins and are therefore aetiologically non-specific. This has lead to sceptism about Lewy body disease as a distinct disease entity.

Subcortical dementia

With more sophisticated testing of patients with predominately cortical, as opposed to subcortical disorders such as Parkinson's disease, Huntington's chorea and progressive supra-nuclear palsy, there has emerged distinct neuropsychological differences (Brown & Marsden, 1988). Cortical dementia is characterised by insidious amnesia and linguistic errors in its early stages; in contrast subcortical dementia begins with slowness of cognitive processing (bradyphrenia) and an amnesia where storage is intact but recall is impaired (Cummings & Benson, 1988).

Creutzfeldt–Jakob disease

This is a rare, rapidly progressive dementia with more pyramidal and extra-pyramidal involvement than in any other dementia (Lishman, 1987). Myolclonus, cerebellar ataxia and spinal cord disease supervene. The characteristic pathology is status spongiosus cavities in the cortex. A transmissible disease until recently the cause was thought to be a slow virus, however irradiation of infected material that should stop viral transmission has been shown to have no effect. When a chemical was added that would neutralise a protein, transmission was stopped.

In the inherited form of CJD a gene mutation on chromosome 20 creates an abnormal protein. This is a mutated form of a small protein involved in neurotransmission and is termed a prion. Contact with a prion triggers a reaction in normal versions of the protein, transforming them into more prions. It is assumed that in sporadic CJD a sporadic event creates a prion (Hardy, 1989), which in turn generates a cascade. That it is also transmissible is illustrated by Kuru (a dementia in cannibals in New Guinea who eat the infected brains of their ancestors) and through transplantation of infected material such as corneas. Episodes of transmission also took place from infected growth hormone.

The possibility that bovine spongiform encephalopathy (BSE) might transmit to humans has been acknowledged since the disease was first recognised in British cattle. A new variant of Creutzfeldt–Jakob disease has been identified and although there is no direct evidence to date, the most likely explanation is that the affected individuals had been exposed to BSE (Almond, 1995).

Multi-infarct dementia

This (previously known as arteriosclerotic dementia) is probably the second most common form after Alzheimer's disease. It is caused by the accumulation of cortical and subcortical infarcts, nearly always related to hypertension. Clinically, its characteristic feature is a step-wise progression with a history of small strokes. A variety of multi-infarct dementia known as Binswanger's disease (or subacute arteriosclerotic encephalopathy) has been rediscovered (Loizou et al., 1981). It can only be distinguished reliably by CT scan, where areas of 'low attenuation' (darker than normal indicating white matter damage, possibly demyelination) appear around the enlarged ventricles.

Communicating hydrocephalus

Also known as normal pressure hydrocephalus this is a treatable form of dementia in which the absorption of cerebrospinal fluid is disturbed due to some inflammatory or traumatic incident in earlier life. The pressure, unlike that in congenital forms, is normal or even lower than normal. A triad of dementia, ataxia and incontinence are described (Pujal et al., 1989). Recently reports of depressive and paranoid presentations have appeared, the psychiatric symptoms preceding the other signs (Silverstein et al., 1991).

Myxoedema, alcohol and a variety of drugs

These are relatively common treatable causes of dementia. The prevalence of alcoholic dementia is considerable and probably rising, and should always be suspected as a likely cause of presenile dementia. The range of drugs that can produce a dementia is only just being realised. For example, phenytoin in therapeutic doses produces a chronic impairment in cognitive function.

Cerebrovascular disease

Diseases of the blood vessels supplying the brain or within the brain can result in stroke (haemorrhage or infarct). Of these predisposing diseases, hypertension and atherosclerosis make up the large majority of cases. Emboli from the heart, rare inflammatory disorders (for example, systemic lupus erythematosus) and congenital aneurysms account for most of the minority. Occlusion to a vessel results in infarction; rupture of the vessel, usually at a weak spot where there is a hypertensive microaneurysm, leads to haemorrhage, which may be predominantly into the brain tissue (cerebral haemorrhage) or into the subarachnoic space (subarachnoid haemorrhage).

The psychiatric sequelae of such events depend on the nature, extent, and site of the damage. Acute haemorrhage into cerebral tissue is a neurological emergency and carries a considerable mortality. Chronic recurrent or small acute infarctions to neurologically 'silent' areas of the brain are most likely to present to psychiatrists, the former as multi-infarct dementia, the latter as an acute psychosis. Right parietal infarcts are particularly prone to present in this last way (Mesulam et al., 1976) and, according to Levine & Finklestein (1982), the onset of psychosis may be delayed. Most strokes present to general physicians and neurologists and we rarely encounter the bizarre acute neuropsychological sequelae such as anosognosia. The rehabilitation of a patient with a stroke is also rarely supervised by a psychiatrist. Nevertheless a sophisticated approach is needed to untangle the complex interaction between psychosocial and organic factors in producing depression, apathy and other affective changes.

Cerebral tumours

Although psychiatrists are occasionally criticised by their neurological colleagues for having missed a brain tumour, the index of suspicion amongst psychiatrists is probably as high as it need be. Tumours rarely present solely with psychiatric symptoms and even if they do they may be inoperable. A slow growing glioma or meningioma should be on one's differential diagnosis of the cause of presenile dementia; subcortical tumours, particularly limbic and those compressing the hypothalamus, may produce schizophrenic, affectiform, and organic personality syndromes.

Infections

HIV disease

The HIV-1 specific DNA was isolated in the brains of AIDS patients in 1985 (Wallack et al., 1991). From that time several neuropsychiatric syndromes have been identified. Various terms have been used to describe the dementing illness associated with HIV infection, including HIV encephalitis, subacute encephalopathy, and the AIDS dementia complex (ADC). Symptoms of dementia may result from opportunistic infections and malignancies, causing cognitive deficit through the direct destruction of brain tissue. Also an acute confusional state can arise from systemic and metabolic disturbance. It is important to differentiate between the irreversible ADC and potentially reversible dementia. In ADC, amnesias, aphasias and agnosias occur late in the dementing process. Such focal syndromes often result from CNS toxoplasmosis or from CNS lymphomas. The cognitive decline in ADC is usually very gradual, typically taking place over a number of months whilst changes due to opportunistic infections takes place over a period of days. Delirium is often the result of the severe medical complications of HIV infection and presents with acute cognitive impairment, agitation and psychosis. It is indistinguishable from delirium caused by any other acute medical cause.

Painful neuropathies occur very frequently in HIV subjects. These are distal, symmetrical and characterised by a painful, burning paraesthesia. There is evidence for cognitive change in individuals who are HIV positive, but who are medically asymptomatic (Malouf *et al.*, 1990). Some early studies suggested that these patients may develop an insidious dementia process, without ever developing the other clinical features of AIDS. However, more recent studies using larger numbers of patients have found definite cognitive impairment only in patients with clearly advanced disease.

Acquired immune deficiency syndrome dementia presents with cognitive, motor and behavioural disturbance (Goethe *et al.*, 1989). The early symptoms are poor concentration and memory, clumsiness, difficulties with gait and fine hand co-ordination. Eventually psychomotor slowing evolves into mutism, ataxia, paraparesis and an eventual vegetative state. CT scanning reveals cerebral atrophy and MRI scans detect multifocal patches and diffuse white matter abnormalities (Everall *et al.*, 1991).

Syphilis

Despite the historical importance of syphilis as a major cause of psychiatric disability and as a powerful influence on our diagnostic concepts, it rarely figures in neuropsychiatric practice these days. Luxon *et al.* (1979) reported a series referred to a neurological clinic in Britain; of 17 cases, only three had cerebral parenchymatous neurosyphilis, and of these, two were untreatable dementia and one had an acute organic reaction. Most cases were picked up through pupillary abnormalities.

Meningitis

Meningococcal or pneumococcal bacterial meningitis is usually a dramatic medical event and if promptly treated has no neuropsychiatric sequelae. Tuberculous meningitis has a more insidious onset and has been known to present with psychological features. It also leaves psychiatric sequelae in the form of an amnesic syndrome. Viral meningitis may present with a combination of physical symptoms (headache, generalised aches and pain, visual changes) and psychiatric complaints (muzzy head, poor concentration, apathy) and may be diagnosed as depression.

Encephalitis

A viral infection of the brain itself will inevitably produce psychiatric symptoms. The absence or paucity of medical or neurological symptoms and signs (fits, paralysis, fever, headaches) will determine whether the patient is referred to a psychiatrist. Equally inevitably some such patients will be diagnosed as schizophrenic (Wilson, 1976). There are some psychiatrists, of course, who believe many cases of schizophrenia are viral in origin. The pandemic of encephalitis lethargica after the First World War gave rise to a number of bizarre neuropsychiatric syndromes. Obsessive-compulsive neuroses, affectiform, and schizophreniform disorders and personality change were all seen. Rail *et al.* (1981) have reported a recent series of neurological and psychiatric disorders, as a result of sporadic encephalitis in earlier life. Bilateral temporal lobe encephalitis, from herpes simplex, can present acutely as the Kluver-Bucy syndrome and persist chronically as a dense amnesic syndrome. There is some doubt about the condition of benign myalgic encephalomyelitis. This occurs as sporadic outbreaks of a febrile illness with lethargy, muscular pain, transient neurological signs (such as an extensor plantar), and mood and cognitive abnormalities. Some authorities regard these incidents as examples of mass hysteria (Royal Free disease).

Cerebral malaria

Cerebral malaria (Toro & Roman, 1978), typhoid, typhus, brucellosis, cholera, and cysticercosis can all produce acute organic reactions (Cutting, 1983). In children, who have a lower threshold, mumps, measles, and chickenpox may produce short-lived organic reactions.

Miscellaneous neurological diseases

Those neurological diseases with predominant motor dysfunction have been dealt with earlier in this chapter. Disseminated sclerosis (multiple sclerosis), Friedreich's ataxia, myasthenia gravis, and muscular dystrophy are four relatively common disorders, each illustrating a different facet of neuropsychiatry. In established disseminated sclerosis with permanent neurological deficit there are nearly always associated cortical plaques, which cause cognitive impairment and the mood change typical of a frontal lobe syndrome. In Friedreich's ataxia the characteristic cerebellar and spinal degeneration is often associated with cerebral atrophy and dementia. In myasthenia gravis, the psychiatric component lies with the differential diagnosis: the weakness is often mistaken for depression or neurasthenia in the early stages. In muscular dystrophy the psychiatric sequelae are psychosocial and not organic.

Neuropsychiatric effects of systemic disease

Heart disease

Heart failure, infective endocarditis, and emboli from rheumatic heart disease may cause an acute organic reaction. Open-heart surgery is the most likely operation to cause a post-operative psychosis. Cardiogenic dementia, although denied by Emerson *et al.* (1981), is regarded by many as a definite entity. Recurrent cardiac dysrhythmia with resulting anoxia is the proposed pathogenesis.

Liver disease

Considerable interest was shown in the neuropsychiatric complications of liver disease in the 1950s (Davidson & Summerskill, 1956). Little has been added to our knowledge since then (Jones *et al.*, 1989). The links between liver disease and neuro-psychiatry are several: acute hepatic failure, chronic hepatic encephalopathy, the interaction of alcoholic cirrhosis with alcoholic neuropsychiatric disorders, and the added effects of an extensive portal–systemic collateral circulation.

Endocrine disease

Thyroid

Thyrotoxicosis is responsible for three types of psychiatric disorder (Bauer & Whybrow, 1986). Thyrotoxic crisis is the first; this is an acute organic reaction that before the advent of medical treatment for the condition often led to death. An apathetic type of organic reaction is also recognised; this is a chronic affective disorder. Thirdly, there is an anxiety state that forms part of the clinical presentation. Myxoedema is a cause of presenile dementia, an affective disorder that is identical with endogenous depression from non-organic causes, and a schizophreniform disorder, sometimes known as myxoedema madness.

Parathyroid

Hyper- and hypoparathyroidism both lead to psychiatric disorders. In the former, the hypercalcaemia is responsible for an acute or chronic organic reaction, depending on the speed with which the calcium has risen. The hypocalcaemia of the latter is more likely to present as tetany and enter into the differential diagnosis of hysterical overbreathing.

Pituitary

Hypopituitarism from tumour or infarct, will present as an acute organic reaction or as coma.

Growth hormone

Acromegaly leads to the distortion of the face, hands, and feet. The change in body image is a possible psychological factor in the genesis of psychiatric disorder. Little is known of the effect on cerebral function.

Adrenal

Cushing's disease is associated with depressive illness, which remits with effective treatment. Addison's disease is more likely to produce delirium or dementia.

Insulin

Diabetes mellitus may be a source of chronic neuropsychiatric disability for a variety of reasons: cerebrovascular and renal disease are more common, recurrent hyper- and hypoglycaemic episodes may impair cerebral function, there may be neuronal damage, and encephalopathy directly attributable to the diabetic process (de Jong, 1977). An insulinoma will produce hypoglycaemic episodes that may present as fits, brief confusional states or transient affective disturbance.

Vitamin deficiency

Deficiency of four vitamins, B_1 (thiamine), B_6 (nicotinic acid), B_{12}, and folic acid, may lead to psychiatric disorders. Thiamine deficiency leads to cerebral beri beri (general cognitive impairment), Wernicke's encephalopathy and, if still unrecognised, to Korsakoff's syndrome. Nicotinic acid deficiency causes pellagra (a triad of dementia, dermatitis, and diarrhoea), the scourge of the Southern United States until the cause was discovered in the 1930s. B_{12} deficiency, pernicious anaemia, is a cause of presenile dementia. Folic acid deficiency is associated with dementia but is almost certainly an effect rather than a cause.

Renal and electrolyte disorder

Uraemia, particularly with a urea level above 40 mmol, causes an acute organic reaction in one-third of cases. Hyponatraemia and hypokalaemia are causes of a chronic organic reaction, characterised by lethargy, apathy, and depression. Acidosis produces delirium, alkalosis, hyperventilation, and tetany. Renal dialysis may relieve the uraemic mental state but may produce one of its own, dialysis dementia (thought to be due to excess aluminium in the dialysate) (Parkinson *et al.*, 1979).

Alcohol, drugs, toxic substances

Alcohol is dealt with more fully elsewhere. The neuropsychiatric complications (Patterson, 1992) comprise the effects of acute intoxication (memory blackouts, pathological intoxication), withdrawal (simple withdrawal state, delirium tremens), chronic consumption with or without nutritional deficiency (psychological deterioration, alcoholic dementia. Wernicke's encephalopathy, Korsakoff's syndrome) and affective and schizophreniform disorders (secondary depression, secondary mania, alcoholic hallucinosis, alcoholic paranoia, morbid jealousy). Drugs, illicit or legitimately prescribed, are responsible for a considerable neuropsychiatric morbidity. Legitimate drugs were the most common cause of an acute organic reaction in a London hospital in the late 1970s (Cutting, 1980). They feature high up on the list of surveys of the causes of presenile dementia. They must also be regarded as frequent causes of affective disorder, for example depression from antihypertensives or anxiety from intermittent benzodiazepine withdrawal. Illicit drugs such as barbiturates, LSD, cannabis, amphetamines and opiates may cause all forms of psychiatric disorder;

textbooks on drug abuse should be consulted. Heavy metals (lead, mercury, manganese, arsenic and thallium) are all causes of acute and chronic organic reactions.

Miscellaneous causes of metabolic disorder

Cancer

There is a high incidence of psychiatric disorder in patients with cancer (Levine *et al.*, 1978). Much of this is neuropsychiatric rather than psychosocial in origin, due mostly to metabolic effects of the tumour.

Porphyria

The most common form in Britain, the acute intermittent type, produces the whole range of psychiatric syndromes. It is rare but one should suspect the diagnosis in atypical psychosis with abdominal pain and neuropathy.

Anoxia

There are four varieties of anoxia: anoxic deficient oxygenation of the blood, e.g. chronic bronchitis); anaemic (deficient oxygen carrying power, e.g. carbon monoxide poisoning); stagnant (reduction of blood flow, e.g. heart failure); and metabolic or toxic (impaired utilization of oxygen by tissues, e.g. hypoglycaemia). Acute anoxia may induce euphoria but severe forms that recover may leave the patient with a cerebral infarction in the boundary or watershed zone between anterior, middle, and posterior cerebral arteries (parieto-occipital).

Systemic lupus erythematosus (SLE)

Although SLE is an inflammatory vascular disease, the effect on cerebral function is not solely through infarct or haemorrhage. There is manufacture of antibrain antibodies and the resulting psychiatric disorder, which may be acute or chronic, reflects a breakdown in blood–brain barrier and the development of an allergic, auto-immune encephalitis (Hay *et al.*, 1994).

Investigations

Investigations are directed toward establishing the organic nature of the clinical picture and then searching for a cause. They may be clinical, psychological or laboratory-based (electrophysiological and radiological).

Clinical

The chief consideration here is to recognise the symptoms and signs of an organic mental state. Some of these are shared by the functional psychoses and one should develop discriminators. Disorientation, clouding of consciousness, and the fluctuating character of the visual phenomena are particularly useful for this purpose. Memory and attention deficits, although classically disturbed in organic states, are notoriously misleading.

The history and physical examination may uncover obvious causes, or at least limit the range of possibilities. The circumstances at onset, sex, age, and background should also be of assistance. An elderly widow found alone in her flat and a young man brought into a casualty department by friends should suggest different orders of likelihood of organic disorder. A history from an informant is crucial to establish dementia, trauma, epilepsy, alcohol abuse, and drugtaking. Physical examination may reveal signs of endocrine disease, fever, trauma, alcohol abuse, or drugtaking.

Psychological

Because organic and functional states are so easily mistaken clinically, psychological tests have been developed in the hope of distinguishing between them. The Wechsler Deterioration Indices are perhaps the most widely used measures of organic impairment. 'In general, the gradual falling off of ability in later age may be considered as an indication of normal decline; a marked and disabling loss, at any age, as a sign of definite impairment' (Wechsler, 1958). One major problem, however, is the assessment of previous cognitive level. It was noted that the age curves of the subtests in the Wechsler Adult Intelligence Scale (WAIS) decline at different rates so that deterioration could be assessed by comparing 'slowly' declining abilities using Hold Tests (information, vocabulary, object assembly, and picture completion) with abilities that declined 'quickly' using Don't Hold Tests (Digit Span, Similarities, Digit Symbol and Block Design). Experience with the WAIS suggests that verbal abilities are more resistant to impairment than performance and that a discrepancy of greater than 20 points between the two scales is a statistically significant indication of organic impairment. The National Adult Reading Test (a verbal task), which is independent of the WAIS, can be used to assess premorbid intellectual level. Results should be interpreted in conjunction with other psychological measures of brain damage.

Available evidence suggests that performance on verbal learning tests is significantly impaired by brain damage. Two useful and frequently used tests are the Modified Word Learning Test and the Paired Associate Learning Test. Perceptual and motor-perceptual assessment techniques have also been used to diagnose organic disorders. Among the most useful and best standardised are the Minnesota Percepto-Diagnostic Test, the Benton Visual Retention Test, Graham-Kendall Memory for Designs Test, the Trail Making Test, and the Halstead Category Test (Lezac, 1983).

As some intellectual functions appear to be localised within one of the cerebral hemispheres, use has been made of the fact that some psychological tests focus on these specific skills to localise areas of brain damage. In general, verbal capacity is better than performance in patients with right hemisphere lesions and it is generally assumed that marked discrepancies between verbal and performance on the WAIS in favour of verbal capacity is not only characteristic of diffuse cerebral pathology but may also be indicative of pathology in the right hemisphere. The reverse pattern (Performance IQ greater than Variable IQ) differentially characterises left hemisphere disturbance. The Halstead Category

395

Test, in which the subject is presented with a series of pictures projected on to a screen and asked to press one of four possible levers according to four possible concepts linking the pictures (colour, shape, etc.), is thought to be particularly sensitive to frontal lobe dysfunction. The Rey-Osterreth Test, which involves copying and recall of a design, is differentially sensitive to right temporal lesions, while tests such as visual naming and word fluency assess dominant (usually left fronto-temporal function). Psychological tests are usually inappropriate if there is any significant element of impairment of consciousness. It is useful to discuss the clinical problem with a neuropsychologist.

Laboratory-based tests

A biochemical screen is justified in all cases, even if the cause is known, because electrolyte imbalance may complicate and exacerbate other conditions. Further investigations will be suggested by the information already obtained. In a study of consecutive psychotic patients admitted to a public mental hospital in North America (Hall *et al.*, 1980) 45% of those with either a functional or organic mental state had a physical illness picked up on biochemical screen.

Radiological

Radiological investigations comprise CT and MRI scanning. The advent of CT and MRI scans has revolutionised neurology and organic psychiatry. CT can identify enlarged ventricles and cortical atrophy, and localise focal abnormalities that might be infarct, tumour or demyelination. The MRI scan is particularly useful in posterior fossa lesions.

Electrophysiological

Electroencephalography is of particular value in the diagnosis and classification of epilepsy. It is also employed in the investigation of sleep disorders where the facilities of an all-night sleep laboratory are usually required. The EEG has been largely superseded by CT and MRI in the diagnosis of organic brain disease. Nevertheless it provides a useful screen for suspected organic disorder and can usually differentiate between intracerebral and extracerebral disease and focal and diffuse intracerebral pathology (Fenton & Standage, 1993).

Management

The chief considerations in the management of organic reactions are to recognise the clinical picture and to carry out a systematic search for a cause. Treatment is primarily a matter of alleviating the condition that has been identified. In many cases, however, other considerations apply, either because the underlying condition is not amenable to specific therapy (e.g. inoperable cancer) or because disturbed behaviour disrupts investigation and specific treatment, or constitutes a hazard to the patient and his attendants. While the major causes of organic reactions have been covered in the course of this chapter, it is, however,

Table 13.2. *Likely causes of delirium and dementia (% of cases)*

Delirium	%	Dementia (presenile)	%
Alcohol	19	Unknown	57
Drugs	16	Cerebrovascular	11
Carcinoma	14	Tumour	9
Epilepsy	8	Normal pressure hydrocephalus	6
Pneumonia	7	Creutzfeldt–Jakob	4
Renal failure	6	Huntington's chorea	4
Head injury	5	Head injury	1
Heart failure	4	Encephalitis	
Endocrine disease	4		
Systemic infections	3		
Liver failure	1		
Respiratory failure	1		
Brain tumour	1		

useful to bear in mind the likely causes of the two common syndromes, delirium and dementia. The circumstances at onset, age, sex, and background of the patient will obviously affect these. A series of 74 cases of delirium seen in the general wards of hospital (Cutting, 1980) and 84 cases of presenile dementia (Marsden & Harrison, 1972) admitted to a neurological hospital give some idea of priorities (Table 13.2).

Specific treatment, if appropriate, should follow correct diagnosis of clinical picture and cause. In the case of acute organic reactions some general recommendations to nurses may improve the task of management. Delirium tends to be worse under conditions of sensory and social isolation, and so nursing in an open ward, installing a radio beside the bed and encouraging nurses to talk to the patient can improve the mental state. The administration of sedative drugs should be as sparing as possible as they may aggravate the underlying physical cause. The choice of drug, if essential, should be determined by the range of side-effects that are most compatible with the underlying condition. For example, phenothiazines should be avoided in delirium tremens because they are epileptogenic and the condition already carries a risk of fits. Phenothiazines with only mild extrapyramidal side-effects – promazine, thioridazine – or benzodiazepines are recommended.

In chronic reactions management is a more complex matter. Remedial causes should be tackled, but the chief consideration is usually to achieve the best social welfare for the patient and his or her attendants. Deterioration may result from causes other than progression of the condition itself. Intercurrent illness (pneumonia), adverse social circumstances or an unnecessary drug regime may impair the quality of life. Social work support both in choosing the best living conditions (home, warden-supervised flat, hospital) and in supporting relations is essential. In non-dementing forms there have been attempts by psychologists to improve the functioning of sound areas of the brain, for example the right hemisphere in patients with aphasia. Brain function therapy (Powell, 1981) may be the first choice in the future, but at the moment one awaits evaluation of its efficacy.

14

The psychiatry of old age

E. JANE BYRNE and A. BURNS

Introduction

The psychiatry of old age, like the population it serves, has expanded in the last ten years. Demographic changes, more detailed research data on illnesses affecting elderly people and their service needs, have contributed to this growth.

Demographic changes in the population aged 65 years and above

Fertility and mortality rates are the determinants of population age structure. The reduction in fertility rates in the UK in the later half of this century is well established; what has only recently been acknowledged is the effect on population age structure of the decline in the mortality of the very old (Murphy, 1990; Preston et al., 1989). Population projections of 1976 (based on OPCS data), which probably underestimated the decline in mortality rates of the old, differ by a factor of 50% from revised projections made in 1991 (Grundy, 1992). Table 14.1 shows these revised projections derived from OPCS data by Grundy, (1992) expressed as percentage of the total (elderly) population of England and Wales. Grundy (1992) also described other important changes affecting the population of old people – the cohort with marked female preponderance (due to World War II) is now being replaced by a cohort who are more likely to have married and in whom the sex differential is less marked. These 'new' cohorts of old people are more likely to have children but less likely to live with them. Old people's attitudes to care have changed, with more old people preferring to receive care from statutory agencies rather than from family or friends.

Socio-economic factors and the health of old people

The link between adverse social circumstances and health at all ages (and the old in particular) is well established. In recent years both governments sources (DHSS, 1985) and academics (e.g. Johnson et al., 1989) have taken the view that the elderly in Britain are (in general) no longer poor. The evidence to the contrary has been summarised by Laczko (1990)

398

Table 14.1. *Numbers of elderly people in 1981 and projected for 1991–2001 in 1991 (1989 base) as % of numbers projected in 1976 (1974 base), England and Wales*

	Year		
Age group	1981	1991	2001
65–71	102	104	106
75–84	103	115	116
85+	109	130	156
65+	103	108	114

Source: Grundy (1992). Reproduced with permission from John Wiley.

and by Hedstrom & Ringen (1987). Epidemiological studies of mental and physical health in old people continue to show an association with poverty and other adverse social factors (Ebrahim *et al.*, 1988; Evans *et al.*, 1991; de Figueiredo & Boerstler, 1992).

Psychogeriatric services

United Kingdom

From reviews of early psychogeriatric services in the UK (MacMillan, 1967; Arie, 1970; Jolley & Arie, 1978) to recent overviews of current practice and organisation of services (Tym, 1991; Dening, 1992; Jolley & Arie, 1992) the principle of care in the community for old people with mental illness is paramount. Services differ in their style and organisation but the common theme is community outreach, performed by a multidisciplinary team, usually with the consultant psychogeriatrician as the 'nucleus of the service' (Jolley & Arie, 1992).

In the UK, the Royal College of Psychiatrists (1989) suggested that one old age psychiatry specialist would serve a population of 22 000 elderly people (65 years +). However, it is now recognised that this is a heavy burden for one consultant and more recent recommendations suggest that services should aim to support elderly populations of about 15 000. For this population the recommended 'plant' is 22.5 acute beds, 45 continuing-care beds and 45 day-hospital places (RCP & RCPsych, 1989).

Resources in such facilities vary around the country (UK) (Shulman & Arie, 1991; Dening, 1992), and many services report inadequate resources. In such circumstances some services have developed, with the philosophy articulated by Lennon & Jolley (1991) 'the best service that could be offered within the constraints of existing facilities was the only meaningful aim possible'. Alongside this internal rationing, continuing advocacy on behalf of the services, with health authorities, government, the public and other bodies is recognised as an important role for psychogeriatricians (Jolley & Arie, 1992). Useful reviews of the services in Europe and elsewhere in the world can be found by Jolley & Arie, 1992 and Bleeker, 1994).

Europe

Elsewhere in Europe the trend towards community care and away from residential care is similar to that in the UK. This has been determined by both economic and ideological factors (Condou, 1989). The most dramatic example has been seen in Italy, where from 1978 by law all long-stay psychiatric hospitals were closed, to be replaced by care in the community. Whilst this has led to worthwhile developments in community services, the most disabled have suffered from a lack of residential care (Bleeker, 1994).

There are great differences across Europe in the types of services for older people with mental health problems. For example, Nijkamp *et al.* (1990) reviewed the use of residential care facilities for older people in the European Community (European Union) and found that the population who used such facilities varied widely, from 1.58% to 10.12%. These differences could not be explained simply on the basis of the level of economic development of a country or its welfare provision, as some developed welfare states such as Belgium and West Germany (3.6%, 4.76% respectively) had much lower use of residential services than others such as the Netherlands (10–12%).

North America

In Canada a 'UK' model has developed in many areas (Shulman *et al.*, 1986). In the USA the majority of elderly people are treated in the community but there is great variation in the type, provision and quality of services for the elderly with mental health problems. (Office of Technology Assessment United State Congress, 1990). There are developments in community outreach (Jolley & Arie, 1992) and home care (Cohen, 1991) but nursing homes form part of the care for the most disabled, especially those with dementia (Rovner *et al.*, 1990).

Rest of the world

Care of the elderly with mental health problems shows great variability elsewhere in the world. By and large, ageing populations and economic development go hand in hand, although having adequate economic resources does not necessarily mean they are distributed on the basis of need. Nigeria is a rapidly developing nation but still has a relatively 'young' population. Osonstokun *et al.* (1992) have reported very low rates of Alzheimer's disease in post-mortem series. Japan has an ageing population with low birth rate and increased longevity. Sociological changes in household composition, with fewer generations living together, has led to a great shift towards residential care for the elderly Japanese population. There has also, however, been an increase in the provision of day care and home care (Hasegawa & Imai, 1994).

Development of psychogeriatric services in the UK

The development of psychogeriatric services has taken place in the context of changes in provision and organisation of social services, primary health care services and the growth of the private and, to a lesser extent, the voluntary sectors.

Changes in social services

The Community Care Act 1900 seeks to 'promote the development of a mixed market economy in the provision of community care' (Dobson & Culhane, 1991). Local authorities have responsibility for the provision of social services; the new act gives them lead responsibility in the six key objects of the Act (Department of Health, 1989), which include assessment of need and case management, and the development of domiciliary and other services to enable people to live in their own homes. Local authorities are encouraged not only to provide services but also to develop a purchaser role with the private and voluntary sectors. The need for multi-disciplinary assessment and service provision is acknowledged by the Act. Local Authorities have always differed in their levels of provision of social services. It remains to be seen whether the new Act will lead to a more uniform provision of care.

Changes in primary health care

The market economy has also been introduced into the National Health Service. General practitioners have the option to become fund-holders (Secretaries of State, 1989), that is to review and administer a budget for primary health care for the population that they service. Fund-holders have the choice of purchasing services from whom they please. Some psychogeriatric services, in common with other services, may find that their facilities are not purchased by some fund-holding general practices. Health screening for the over 75s (Health Departments of Great Britain, 1989) is another recent task for primary health care, and includes screening for cognitive disorders. There is potential for early identification of dementia and other mental health problems although there is good evidence that general practitioners had become more sensitive to such problems in elderly patients (Cooper, 1991) before the introduction of health screening.

Functions of a psychogeriatric service

These have been summarised by Jolley & Arie (1992). There is now general consensus on the value of home assessment in psychogeriatrics (Arie & Jolley, 1982; Dening, 1992). Where psychogeriatricians differ is in whether or not non-medical team members should undertake this initial assessment. The Community team at Guy's Hospital, London (Coles et al., 1991; Collighan et al., 1993) have presented evidence in favour of non-medical initial assessment, arguing that these team members are as effective as doctors in delineating mental health problems. Others have argued that the assumption of an assessment role for non-medical members of the multi-disciplinary team detracts from their service role (Woff et al., 1988; Jolley & Arie, 1992; Jolley, 1993). The composition of the multi-disciplinary team varies from service to service (Dening, 1992).

Among the professions who regularly contribute to such teams are nurses, social workers, occupational therapists, physiotherapists, clinical psychologists and speech therapists. Other professions who may be part of the team are health visitors, pharmacists, chiropodists, continence advisors. Perhaps more important than the composition of the team is the individual who is flexible in role irrespective of their professional background (MacDonald, 1991b).

Collaboration and advocacy

The philosophy of community outreach, which underlies psychogeriatric services, entails close collaboration with other health providers, social services independent sector, in terms of service delivery and with administrations, local authorities, health authorities and government in terms of service planning. The two roles often overlap and are not mutually exclusive. Important aspects of collaboration and advocacy are summarised in Table 14.2. The need for close collaboration and advocacy has perhaps never been more apparent than at present. There is a danger that change for change's sake may worsen rather than help some of the most vulnerable members of society. Rationing of resources is now somewhat more overt than covert (Dening, 1992) but to avoid the 'Desiderative Fallacy – the supposition that because a situation arises which appears to need certain resources, therefore those resources must somewhere be available' (Arie, 1977) there is an urgent need for even more glasnost.

Dementia

Introduction

Dementia is defined as 'an acquired global impairment of intellect, memory and personality, but without impairment of consciousness' (Lishman, 1987). Most people would accept that the definition assumes that dementia is progressive, irreversible and of long duration (current diagnostic criteria suggesting six months). Until the 1950s, nosology in psychiatry of old age was somewhat primitive. The neuropathological basis for the major forms of dementia had been described half a century before by pathologists/clinicians such as Alois Alzheimer, but disorders in the elderly were all too often assumed to be secondary to atherosclerosis and attracted diagnostic and therapeutic nihilism. Roth, in his seminal work on patients in Graylingwell Hospital, West Sussex, England (Roth, 1955) used a longitudinal method of investigation to validate clinical distinctions between five groups of patients – senile psychosis (equivalent to senile dementia, primary degenerative dementia, Alzheimer's Disease), arteriosclerotic dementia, paraphrenia, depression and confusional states. The case notes of 450 patients over 60 years of age admitted to Graylingwell Hospital between the years 1934/36 and 1948/49 were examined. Each case was assigned to one of the five categories. A follow-up study determined the status of the patients at six months and again at two years after admission. Clear differences in mortality were demonstrated at both follow-up intervals in the five groups. At six months, patients with a diagnosis of senile psychosis had the highest mortality (58% were dead). After two years the patterns were broadly similar to those at six months with the exception that, in the arteriosclerotic dementia category, the death rate had risen dramatically to 93%. The mortality rate in senile psychosis had gone up to 82%. It was found that women had a significantly lower mortality across all diagnostic groups (except confusional sates). For the first time, it was shown that different diagnostic groupings had differential survival, suggesting that these groupings were distinct diagnostic entities.

Alzheimer's disease is the major form of dementia seen in the elderly, vascular dementia is

Table 14.2. *Collaboration and advocacy in psychogeriatrics*

Primary health care	Joint role in care of individual patients
	Liaison role performed by some psychogeriatricians
	Collaboration in service development
Other medical specialties	Liaison in DGH
	Planning
	Education
Social services	Team membership
	Assessment
	Planning
	Education
Independent sector	Outreach
	Liaison
	Service delivery
	Planning
	Education
Government/Public/Media	Advocacy
	Liaison
	Education
Information technology	Planning
	Education
Other professional bodies	Advocacy
	Education
	Planning

the second commonest and other types of dementia include that associated with Lewy bodies (Lewy body dementia, cortical Lewy body disease, demential or senile dementia of Lewy body type, Byrne *et al.*, 1991; McKeith *et al.*, 1992) and dementia of frontal lobe type (Neary *et al.*, 1988). Reversible causes of dementia account for around 5% of cases, but this varies according to the population under study. An exhaustive list appears in Table 14.3.

Research in the primary dementias, subsequent to Roth's 1955 paper, developed in two ways. First, the work of the Newcastle group in the 1960s documented the association between clinical and pathological findings (senile plaques, see neuropathology section) in the primary degenerative dementias (Blessed *et al.*, 1968; Tomlinson *et al.*, 1970). A significant correlation (0.74) was found between senile plaques and the clinical features of dementia during life (measured by the Blessed Dementia Scale, which incorporated tests of cognitive function i.e. orientation, memory and concentration changes in behaviour and changes in personality). Such an association was expected, as it included both demented and non-demented subjects but the correlation was still positive (but less so) when only demented subjects were included. Subsequent studies showed the association to be positive between clinical dementia and the formation of tangles. Neurochemical changes in Alzheimer's disease were documented in the 1979s, the first being deficits in the cholinergic system (Bowen *et al.*, 1976; Whitehouse *et al.*, 1982). These deficits have been found consistently and form the basis of the current neurotransmitter-based replacement therapies. These neurochemical changes have also been correlated with the clinical features of the dementia

Table 14.3. *Causes of dementia*

Primary cerebral degenerations
Alzheimer's disease
Vascular (multi-infarct) dementia
Pick's disease
Huntington's disease
Parkinson's disease
Cortical Lewy Body disease
Progressive supranuclear palsy
Prion dementias
Gerstmann–Straussler syndrome
Dementia of frontal lobe type
Cerebellar degenerations
Focal cerebral atrophy
Dementia in association with motor neurone disease

Cerebral lesions
Tumours (primary or secondary)
Subdural haematoma
Communicating hydrocephalus (normal pressure hydrocephalus) and non-communicating
hydrocephalus
Dementia pugilistica
Anoxic brain damage
Neurosyphilis/inflammatory disease
Sarcoidosis
Limbic encephalitis
Cranial arteritis
Systemic lupus erythematosis
Subacute sclerosing panencephalitis
HIV
Neurocysticercosis

Toxins
Alcohol
Drugs
Metals (e.g. lead, mercury, manganese, bismuth)
Industrial agents (tri- and perchlorethylene, toluene)

Endocrine disorders
Hyper, hypothyroidism
Hyper, hypoparathyroidism
Cushing's syndrome
Addison's disease

Systemic disorders
Porphyria
Vitamin B_{12} deficiency
Folic acid deficiency
Hepatic encephalopathy
Renal failure
Whipple's disease
Lymphoma
Distant effects of cancer

Table 14.3. *(cont.)*

Very rare
Membranous lipodystrophy
Mitochondrial encephalomyopathy
Idiopathic basal ganglia calcification
Cerebrotendinous xanthomatosis
Metachromic leucodystrophy
Marachiafava–Bignani disease
Myotonic dystrophy
Adult polysaccharidoses
Adult Schilder's disease
Hereditary dentatorubral pallidoluysian atrophy
Late onset Hallervorden–Spatz disease

Reproduced with permission from Burns, A. Howard, R. and Pettit, W. (1995) *Alzheimer's Disease: A Medical Companion*. Blackwell Scientific Publications, Oxford.

syndrome (Perry *et al.*, 1978). Second, the heterogeneity of Alzheimer's disease was examined from a clinical perspective. McDonald (1969) was among the first to show that certain features in the clinical syndrome, notably age and the presence of apraxia, were related to survival – patients who were younger and had performed poorly on tests of parietal lobe function, and a much reduced survival compared to those without these signs. A number of clinical features have been documented as being indicative of possible subtypes (Burns & Levy,1992) and neuropathological, neurochemical and genetic subtypes have also been described.

Currently, excitement surrounds the molecular biology of Alzheimer's disease and the findings of recent genetic studies. These are very important developments that cannot be underestimated, but at the same time attention should be paid to the clinical manifestations of the dementia syndrome in Alzheimer's disease.

Epidemiology

Dementia is a syndrome of ageing, the proportion of subjects being affected rising rapidly with increasing age. There are excellent recent reviews to which the reader is directed (Jorm, 1990; Jagger & Lindesay, 1993; Livingston, 1994). The study of the epidemiology of dementia is fraught with methodological pitfalls – in particular the way in which the syndrome is diagnosed and the population from which a sample is drawn. Some early studies used a psychiatrist's clinical diagnosis, whereas it is now universal practice to use standard diagnostic criteria and recognised assessment instruments. Personal interview by the research team has become the norm and inspection of case-notes for diagnostic purposes would not be acceptable in most studies. With regard to the population to be examined, a large sample will be more representative of the general population but there will be fewer resources to examine individual cases. Samples based on hospital referrals will have a higher prevalence of dementia than others based in the community. Also, because of the strong

Table 14.4. *Prevalence of dementia (from Hofman et al. 1991)*

Age range	Percentage prevalence
65–69	1.4
70–74	4.1
75–79	5.7
80–84	13.0
85–89	21.6
90–94	32.2
95–99	34.7

association between dementia and ageing, the age range of the population under study must be made explicit, as samples including a disproportionate number of older individuals will produce much higher rates of dementia – it is now standard to describe in detail the age structure of the population when reporting results.

Jorm (1990) has estimated that, regardless of baseline, the prevalence of dementia doubles every 5.1 years. Recent UK studies include those by Copeland *et al.* (1987), Livingston *et al.* (1990) and O'Connor *et al.* (1989). A recent analysis of European studies combined the prevalence rates from 12 reports that satisfied strict comparability criteria consistent with contemporary views of the epidemiology of dementia (Hofman *et al.*, 1991). Briefly, these included studies using recognised diagnostic instruments, inclusion of patients both in and out of institutions and studies of at least 300 subjects. The rates for different age groups are shown in Table 14.4.

Prevalence was higher in men than women in the 65–74 group but commoner in women thereafter. The incidence of dementia (number of new cases per year) is approximately 1%. Morgan *et al.* (1993) described the incidence as 3.7% over four years and Copeland *et al.* (1992) found it to be 0.92% over one year. In a recent study of over 85-year-olds, Skoog *et al.* (1993) showed that 30% had significant dementia. It was found that 47% of these had vascular dementia, a proportion higher than previously suggested. Rocca *et al* (1991) reviewed European studies on the prevalence of vascular dementia and found that the prevalence increased with age, ranging from 1.5% in women aged 75–79, to 4.8% for men in the same age group and 2.8% for women in the 80–89 age group, to 16.3% for men in the 80–89 age group. Men, generally, were more often affected than women.

Alzheimer's disease

Aetiology

The cause of Alzheimer's disease is currently unknown, although many risk factors have been implicated. Only three have been proven – increased risk with increasing age, a family history of dementia and suffering from Down's syndrome.

The *genetic component* of Alzheimer's disease is well documented. About 30% of late onset cases have a positive family history of dementia of some description. There have been a number of families reported in the literature as autosomal dominant but more recently molecular genetic studies have revealed definite mutations. It was reported in 1987 (St George Hislop *et al.*) that there was linkage between familial Alzheimer's disease (FAD) and markers on the long arm of chromosome 21. The search on this chromosome was prompted by the known association between Alzheimer's disease and Down's syndrome, of which the most common form is trisomy 21. Around the same time it was found that the gene encoding for APP (amyloid precursor protein) was also on chromosome 21 and, for a short time, it was considered that the two might be the same. However, there was no linkage found between affected individuals and the APP gene in some families (for review, see Clark & Goate, 1993).

However, direct screening of the APP gene in FAD was carried out and three single point mutations were found on codon 717 (valine to isoleucine, phenylalanine glycine). A double mutation has been found in a Swedish family at codon 670–671 and two Dutch families have been described with a form of cerebral angiopathy and associated cerebral haemorrhage who have mutations at 692 and 693 (clinically they are unlike Alzheimer's disease).

A large number of genetic markers have been identified in the Human Genome Project and it has been possible to link these to Alzheimer's disease in some families. It has been found that, in some, early-onset FAD was linked to markers on chromosome 14 and it is estimated that three-quarters are explicable in terms of an, as yet, unidentified mutation in this region with 25% associated with the chromosome 21 mutation. Late-onset Alzheimer's disease has been found to be associated with a marker on chromosome 19. Patients who are homozygous for the E4 allele at the apolipoprotein locus (a lipoprotein connected with neuronal metabolism and repair) have a 76% chance of developing Alzheimer's disease. The risk for those who are heterozygous is about 25%. The importance of these genetic studies is that they prove the relevance of the amyloid protein in the genesis of Alzheimer's disease and thus facilitate further molecular biological studies. They can begin to point to areas that may indicate potential areas of treatment. In families where a genetic abnormality is found it offers pre-disease screening although there are considerable ethical problems with this approach. Finally, it offers the chance to look at very early manifestations of Alzheimer's disease in those unfortunate individuals who carry the defective gene but have not as yet developed the disease.

Epidemiology has shown beyond doubt that age is strongly associated with Alzheimer's disease. The old notion that the disorder was merely an extension of normal ageing has been laid to rest by the finding of the genetic abnormality. Patients with Down's syndrome (most of whom have an additional copy of chromosome 21) invariably develop plaques and tangles by the age of 35. Other risk factors that have been shown to be associated with Alzheimer's disease include head injury (of interest as amylkoid is deposited in the brain within 24 hours after head injury), sex (women affected more than men), race (suggestions have been made that certain ethnic groups have higher prevalence of Alzheimer's disease), education (evidence suggests that the 'use it or lose it' saying may have a basis in fact), smoking appears to be protective of Alzheimer's disease (in those with a family history) and aluminium (there is evidence that aluminium is neurotoxic but no absolute evidence that it is a causal factor). For a review of risk factors see Van Duijn *et al.* (1991).

Neuropathology and neurochemistry of Alzheimer's disease

In Alzheimer's disease the brain, macroscopically, shows evidence of generalised atrophy with widened sulci and increased ventricular size. Regional atrophy is usually apparent, affecting particularly the frontal, parietal and temporal lobes. Microscopically, there is neuronal loss affecting large neurons in the neocortex and cholinergic neurons in the basal nuclei. Synaptic density is decreased by up to 50%. Senile plaques and neurofibrillary tangles are the hallmarks of Alzheimer's disease. Senile plaques are also seen in normal ageing and are extra-cellular structures consisting of a core of B-amyloid (also called A4 protein) surrounded by dystrophic neurites. The amyloid core consists of filaments of 41–43 amino acid protein. Neurofibrillary tangles are not specific to Alzheimer's disease and can occur in other neurodegenerative disorders such as Parkinson's disease. They are inclusion bodies, i.e. are intracellular and consist of paired helical filaments with the characteristic double-helix pattern. Senile plaques are seen in normal ageing. Lewy bodies occur inside the cells and consist of a central core with radially arranged dendritic processes. They are found in the limbic system and the cingulate cortex and brainstem. Other neuropathological features described in association with Alzheimer's disease are Hirano bodies and granulovacuolar degeneration (for review of neuropathology, see Lantos & Cairs, 1994).

The main neurochemical abnormalities identified have been deficiencies in cholinergic neurotransmission evidenced by defects in synaptosomal acetylcholine, and low levels of associated enzymes such as acetylcholinesterase and especially choline acetyl transferase (the enzyme catalysing synthesis of acetylcholine from acetyl co-enzyme a and choline). This is particularly so in the ascending projections from the basal forebrain nuclei such as the nucleus basalis of Meynert. Post-synaptic receptors appear to be intact whereas pre-synaptic receptors are affected. Abnormalities of noradrenaline and dopamine, serotonin and glutamate and GABA have also been described.

Two proteins that have been the focus of much interest are β-amyloid and tau protein. β-amyloid, as we have noted, is found at the core of the senile plaque. It is a starch-like substance of some 40 amino acids in length and is derived from a larger molecule, the amyloid precursor protein (APP), which, as has been discussed earlier, is encoded by a gene on chromosome 21. The two metabolic pathways of amyloid metabolism are the lysosomal pathway involving cellular lysosomes and a secretase pathway, which cleaves the molecule in half at a site incompatible for amyloid production. Tau protein is the major constituent of paired helical filaments. Tau appears to be abnormally phosphorylated in Alzheimer's disease. Tangles are less specific to Alzheimer's disease and it may be that there is an interaction of tau and APP resulting in the neuropathological features of Alzheimer's disease. Both proteins may be amenable to alteration by drugs, leading to the possibility of therapeutic intervention aimed at altering the basic molecular abnormalities in the disorder.

Clinical features

These were well documented by Alzheimer in his original report (Alzheimer, 1907), which emphasised that behavioural disturbances and psychiatric symptoms such as delusions and hallucinations (i.e. non-cognitive features) occurred, as well as cognitive deficits such as amnesia, aphasia, apraxia and agnosia. Alzheimer's disease was defined in terms of cognitive loss with other factors deemed secondary and therefore of secondary importance. This is still the prevailing concept but in recent years non-cognitive features have been established as being of importance. The reasons for this include: increasing understanding of stress and strain on carers, which in a large part is due to non-cognitive features; the effectiveness of existing treatments on non-cognitive features; the importance of non-cognitive features in the diagnosis of Alzheimer's disease (whether in terms of early diagnosis or differential diagnosis) and the fact that Alzheimer's disease, in which the neuropathological changes are well documented, may serve as a basis for the understanding of so-called 'functional' psychiatric disorders.

The most common symptom of Alzheimer's disease, and usually the presenting problem, is that of memory loss (amnesia). Indeed its absence should call into question the diagnosis. It is often reported by relatives and carers as being manifest by forgetting a birthday or anniversary (in someone with previous impeccable recall) and when it is particularly marked causes intense frustration in carers who often have to repeat themselves constantly. In Alzheimer's disease, the onset is characteristically gradual and the decline smooth without fluctuation.

During progression of the disorder, other focal cortical signs such as aphasia, apraxia and agnosia may occur. Aphasia can be expressed or receptive (usually a combination of the two). Apraxia is most often manifest by an inability to dress (clothes may be put on in the wrong order) or problems with eating (inability to use a knife and fork). Agnosia can be of several varieties but is often manifest by an inability to recognise a familiar face such as that of a spouse or a child. Occasionally this can be the presenting sign (often particularly distressing for carers) and finger agnosia can occasionally be seen as part of the Gerstmann syndrome (indicative of dominant parietal lobe dysfunction and consisting of a quartet of signs – finger agnosia, dycalculia, dysgraphia and right/left disorientation). These so-called 'instrumental' signs have been associated with early onset Alzheimer's disease (Constantinidis, 1978; Seltzer & Sherwin, 1983), poor prognosis (McDonald, 1969) and accelerated cognitive decline (Yesavage et al., 1993).

Non-cognitive features have begun to be investigated extensively (for reviews see Wragg & Jeste, 1989; Cummings & Victoroff, 1991; Hope & Patel, 1993). These can be divided into two main types – psychiatric symptoms and behavioural disturbances. The former consist of experiences complained of spontaneously by the patient (although the history can often come through the relatives). Examples are: delusions, paranoid ideation, affective symptoms (both elevated and depressed), hallucinations (mainly auditory/visual), misidentification (misidentification of patient's image in a mirror, misidentification of others in the house, belief that other people are living in the house and the misidentification of television images leading to a belief that they are occurring in three-dimensional space). Behavioural disturbances are features observed by others, examples being aggression, wandering behaviour, eating disorders, sleep disturbances and sexual disinhibition.

The proportion of patients with Alzheimer's disease affected by such symptoms varies widely. Approximate estimates appear in Table 14.5, based on work by Burns et al. (1990). Along with these early changes, relatives invariably report changes in personality and subtle

Table 14.5. *Proportion of demented patients with non-cognitive features (%)*

Delusions	15–20
Paranoid ideas	20
Visual hallucination	15
Auditory hallucination	10–15
Depression	20–60
Mania	5
Misidentifications	10–25
Aggression	20
Wandering	20
Sexual disinhibition	10

alterations in emotional responsiveness. These are encompassed in the Blessed Scale (Blessed *et al.*, 1968), where changes in personality were described thus:

Increased rigidity
Increased egocentricity
Impairment of regard for feelings of others
Coarsening of affect
Impairment of emotional control
Hilarity in inappropriate situations
Diminished emotional responsiveness
Sexual misdemeanour
Hobbies relinquished
Diminished initiative/growing apathy
Purposeless hyperactivity

Neurological signs are important in the investigation of Alzheimer's disease. Focal neurological signs may indicate the presence of vascular disease and extrapyramidal signs the presence of Lewy bodies. In primary dementia, primitive reflexes have been documented in both normal ageing and primary degenerative dementia (Burns *et al.*, 1991; Franssen, 1993) in rates of between 5% and 80%. The grasp reflex (the involuntary grasping of the hand following a palmar stimulus) is present in between 5% and 20%, the palmomental reflex (contraction of the mentalis muscle consequent on stimulation of the ipsilateral palm) in 2%–60% and the snout reflex (pouting of the lips after a stimulus to the middle of the upper lip) is the commonest, being present in between 25% and 80%. The snout reflex is particularly associated with age and is the reflex most often found in normal ageing. Biological brain changes have been associated with neurological signs, both in terms of CT scan appearance (Burns *et al.*, 1991) and neuropathological changes (Forstl *et al.*, 1992). They have also been associated with a poorer prognosis.

Other types of dementia

Vascular dementia (multi-infarct dementia) is due to vascular disease of the brain. Multi-infarct dementia has been the preferred term for some years, based on the assumption that only infarcted tissue could produce a dementia syndrome. This had a basis in the early neuropathological studies in the 1960s and was emphasised by the seminal work by Hachinski and colleagues (1975), when the ischaemic score was introduced. This consisted of a number of ratings taken from a standard textbook of psychiatry, which were considered to be indicative of vascular disease (Alois Alzheimer has described these in 1895). They were amalgamated into a score and it was shown, using measures of cerebral blood flow, that a group of patients with dementia could be divided into two – those who scored highly and were presumed to have vascular dementia, and another group of those who did not and were presumed to have a primary dementia. Each feature was weighted. A total score of 4 or less was indicative of a primary degenerative dementia, 7 or above a vascular dementia and between 4 and 7 a mixed type of dementia. Subsequent validation studies have emphasised the importance of some features over others; specifically, focal neurological signs and symptoms, history of strokes and hypertension are considered most important. The score does not take into consideration newer imaging techniques, which are now powerful diagnostic tools. The features (with scores) are:

Abrupt onset	2
Stepwise deterioration	1
Fluctuating course	2
Nocturnal confusion	1
Preserved personality	1
Depression	1
Somatic complaints	1
Emotional incontinence	1
Hypertension	1
History of strokes	2
Associated arteriosclerosis	1
Focal neurological signs	2
Focal neurological symptoms	2

Classically, vascular dementia presents with an acute onset and stepwise deterioration with episodes of confusion occurring after minor strokes.

In more recent years, *dementia of Lewy body type* has been described, which is characterised by the presence of Lewy bodies in the neocortex. These are neuronal inclusion bodies that are associated with degeneration of the neuron. Lewy bodies are a pathological hallmark of Parkinson's disease, where they are often confined to the basal ganglia. It is said that there is a characteristic clinical presentation of Lewy body disease and diagnostic criteria have been suggested. These include (Byrne *et al.*, 1991; McKeith *et al.*, 1992):

fluctuating cognitive impairment – affecting memory, language, visuo-spatial skills, praxis and reasoning;
at least one of the following:
   (a) visual or auditory hallucinations;
   (b) extra-pyramidal signs either mild or as an exaggerated response to neuroleptics;

411

(c) falls or loss of consciousness; a progressive illness with fluctuations lasting for months and;

The absence of other factors that could account for the fluctuation and in particular the absence of factors associated with vascular disease.

Identification of this particular type of dementia is of importance as it has been shown that these patients are particularly sensitive to neuroleptics. Great caution should be exercised in their prescription in this group of patients.

In the elderly, it is estimated that up to 10% of patients will have a potentially reversible lesion. Metabolic or endocrinological causes seem to be more common in younger patients and structural brain lesions can occur in all age groups. Table 14.7 outlines a list of possible causes of a dementia syndrome. Reviews of reversible dementia include those by Byrne, 1987; Philpot & Burns, 1989.

Management

Investigations

An individual presenting with a dementia syndrome should first have a full history, mental state and physical examination, and second have physical investigations (these are outlined in Table 14.6). This will reveal the cause of the dementia in the vast majority of cases. Physical examination should pay particular attention to the central nervous system. Blood tests should include a full blood count, ESR, urea and electrolytes, liver function tests, blood glucose, syphilis serology, thyroid function tests, vitamin B_{12} and folate levels and, if indicated, a test for HIV infection. Urine culture, chest X-ray and EEG should also be performed. The EEG can be useful in excluding patients with delirium – a frankly abnormal EEG with relatively minor dementia is suggestive of some form of encephalopathy whereas advanced dementia with a relatively normal EEG is more likely to be due to Alzheimer's disease.

Neuroimaging has a place to play. CT scan is useful in excluding structural brain lesions that may be the cause of dementia syndrome, such as brain tumours, haematomata and normal pressure hydrocephalus.

Magnetic resonance imaging gives a much better picture of cerebral anatomy and is better at detecting white matter changes. Single photon emission tomography gives a measure of regional cerebral blood flow that can be helpful in looking at dementias affecting particular brain regions such as the frontal lobe. Positron emission tomography, which measures brain metabolism directly, remains primarily a research tool.

Treatment

Management of Alzheimer's disease consists of combining investigations and appropriate treatment towards the victim and attention to the family situation, support for carers both in

Table 14.6. *Investigations of suspected Alzheimer's disease*

History:	Present illness, family history of mental illness
Mental state:	Cognitive function (AMTS, MMSE, CAMCOG)
	Assessment of psychiatric symptoms, behavioural changes and personality changes. Physical (especially neurological) examination
Blood tests:	FBC ESR, urea and electrolytes, LFTs, glucose, syphilis serology, thyroid function tests, vitamin B_{12} and folate (red cell serum), HIV

Urine Culture
Chest X-ray
Electrocardiogram
Electroencephalogram
Computed tomography scan of the head

Other Investigations:
  Lumbar puncture
  Single photon emission tomography
  Magnetic resonance imaging
  Positron emission tomography
  Magnetic resonance spectroscopy
  Brain electrical activity mapping

AMTS, Abbreviated Mental Test Score; MMSE, Mini Mental State Examination; CAMCOG, Cognitive section of CAMDEX (Roth *et al.*, 1986). Reproduced with permission from Burns, A., Howard, R. and Pettit, W. (1995) *Alzheimer's Disease: A Medical Companion*, Blackwell Scientific Publications, Oxford.

terms of practical interventions (attendance at a day centre, respite care, sitting services) and more general support in the form of carers' groups and contact with the Alzheimer's Disease Society. Investigation and treatment of physical illness is important, as this can often worsen an individual's mental state and early intervention against physical disabilities may avert an inappropriate admission. There is currently no effective treatment for the disorder, although drugs directed against the known neurochemical abnormalities have been the most consistently studied. The judicious use of medication can be helpful, with thioridazine or haloperidol being the most useful neuroleptic sedatives (the former tends to induce postural hypotension and the latter has a higher incidence of extrapyramidal side-effects). Depression should be treated with antidepressants and sleep disturbance with chlormethiazole or a short-acting benzodiazepine.

   Treatments aimed at reversing the cognitive deficit are experimental at present, although physostigmine has been used with some success and recent publicity surrounds the possible introduction of tetrahydroaminoacridine (tacrine or THA). This has been shown in several studies to have a beneficial effect on cognitive function, producing an improvement over six months of the same magnitude as the deterioration that would have been expected of the same time interval. Between a quarter and a half of patients improve. However, side-effects, notably hepatic toxicity, will limit routine use. For the future, it is likely that treatments aimed at reversing the more basic biological abnormalities will be successful.

Delirium

Delirium in old people is common in hospital populations, has high morbidity and mortality yet is often unrecognised. Delirium has many definitions, both descriptive (e.g. Lishman, 1987) and operational (e.g. DSM-IIIR; American Psychiatric Association, 1987). Most agree that it is a *syndrome* of acute disturbance of brain function (with both cognitive, i.e. memory impairment, and non-cognitive, i.e. hallucination, (deficits), which has many different causes. While delirium has been recognised as a syndrome for several centuries (Lipowski, 1990) there is continuing debate as to its definition.

DSM-IIIR differs fundamentally from DSM-III in that it relegates reduced level of consciousness to a secondary feature and considers disordered attention and disorganised thinking to be primary features. ICD-10 (WHO, 1992) includes 'impairment of consciousness and attention' as one of five factors that must be present for a diagnosis of delirium (the others are global disturbance of cognition, psychomotor disturbance, disturbance of the sleep–wake cycle and emotional disturbances). Attempts have been made to operationalise the diagnostic criteria for delirium (Johnson *et al.*, 1990 for DSM-IIIR) and several diagnostic instruments have been devised (e.g. Trzepacz *et al.*, 1988), which include observations of the variation of clinical features over time. Lipowski (1990) has suggested that the level of psychomotor activity (hyperalert/hyperactive or hypoalert/hypoactive) is not only a defining characteristic of sub-types of delirium but also a powerful reason for the lack of recognition of the syndrome, the hypoactive patient being more likely to be overlooked. Liptzin & Levkoff (1992) have shown that sub-types can be identified in old people in hospital. In their study they found that 15% were hyperalert, 19% were hypoalert and 52% showed mixed picture (probably reflecting fluctuation in clinical features) and that the hyperalert type had the best outcome in terms of morbidity – shorter length of stay and lower mortality, although these findings were not statistically significant.

Epidemiology of delirium

Community

There are very few data on the prevalence of delirium in the community. Folstein *et al.* (1991) found a prevalence of 1.08% in community residents aged 55 years or more. In nursing homes the prevalence is about 6% (Rovner *et al.*, 1986; Bienenfeld & Wheeler, 1989).

Hospital

In hospital the prevalence of delirium on medical wards (general medicine and geriatric medicine) is between 15 and 25%, on surgical wards 26–61% (Levkoff *et al.*, 1991) and psychiatry of old age wards about 13% (Kaponen *et al.*, 1989).

Aetiology of delirium

A number of factors have been identified that may predispose to delirium, such as age and pre-existing dementia (Lipowski, 1990), and others such as sensory impairment may

Table 14.7. *The commonest causes of acute delirium in old people*

Very common	
Heart failure	– left ventricular failure
	– congestive cardiac failure
Infection	– urinary
	– respiratory
Carcinomatosis	
Common	
Cerebrovascular	– transient ischaemia
	– drugs
Drugs	– anticholinergic (e.g. tricyclic antidepressants, benzhexol)
	– interactions
	– withdrawal (alcohol, benzodiazepines)
Metabolic	– hypoglycaemia
	– disorders of fluid and electrolyte balance
	– renal or hepatic failure
Anoxia	– respiratory, anaemia, reduced cerebral perfusion

Sources: Royal College of Physicians, 1981; Lipowski, 1992.

act as maintaining factors (Beresin, 1988). Risk factors for the development of delirium in elderly surgical patients include age, previous alcohol or drug abuse and prolonged operations (Whittaker, 1989). Several authors have provided extensive reviews of the causes of delirium in old age (e.g. Beresin, 1988; Liston, 1982), but such lists are all inclusive and may not indicate which are the commonest causes.

Table 14.7 lists these common causes. Recent prospective studies of delirium in elderly hospital in-patients (Francis *et al.*, 1990; Jitapunkul *et al.*, 1992; Kaponen & Riekkinen, 1993) confirm the consensus findings of the RCP (1981) and the observations of Lipowski (1992) (the sources for the list shown in Table 14.7). Francis *et al.* (1990) emphasised the high frequency of comorbidity in the aetiology of delirium in old age.

Clinical course and outcome

Prospective studies of delirium in old people in hospital have found mean durations of 19.5 days and 21.6 days (Thomas *et al.*, 1988; Kaponen & Reikkinen, 1993). In some patients, in these studies, delirium lasted for more than one month. Although DSM-IIIR criteria do not specify duration as a defining characteristic in the notes, relating to the criteria the following statement is found 'it is rare for delirium to persist for more than a month'. Mori & Yamadori (1987) found delirium to persist for three months or more in 6% of their series of patients with right middle cerebral artery strokes. Further studies will clarify the situation but long-lasting delirium may be much commoner than previously supposed. Most studies have shown that delirious patients (aged 65 years or more) have significantly longer hospital stays than do non-delirious patients (Thomas *et al.*, 1988; Francis *et al.*, 1990) although Jitapunkul *et al.* (1992) found no differences between such groups.

Mortality rates in all studies are high, in the range 15%–30% (Lipowski, 1992), perhaps not surprising in view of the close association of delirium with serious physical illness (Francis *et al.*, 1990), but nevertheless an observation worth repeating and perhaps justifying the statement that delirium is a medical emergency. It is possible that quantitative electroencephalography (QEEG) may prove to be a useful technique in the detection and monitoring of delirium in old people (Leuchter & Jacobsen, 1991).

Management of delirium

The two basic principles of management of delirium are to identify and treat the underlying cause and to treat or manage the behavioural and psychiatric symptoms of the disorder (Lindesay *et al.*, 1990; Fairweather, 1991). There has, however, been little systematic assessment of the latter approach (MacDonald *et al.*, 1989). Neuroleptic drugs may be indicated in cases of severe agitation or distressing psychiatric symptoms (persecutory delusions) and haloperidol has been advocated as the drug of choice by some (Lipowski, 1989; Taylor & Lewis, 1993). Care must be exercised in its use as it has a long half-life in the elderly of up to 60 hours and is a powerful inducer of extrapyramidal symptoms. Doses of 2 mg have been suggested (Fairweather, 1991) but effective benefit has been observed by us from even smaller doses, 0.5–1 mg.

Manipulation of the environment in which the delirious patient is nursed is 'prescribed' by many. There is no experimental data on which to base these 'prescriptions'. For example, keeping the patient's room lit for the full 24 hours to minimise the effects of illusions and hallucinations is clinically effective but may disrupt biological clocks, adding to the problems caused by disruption of the sleep–wake cycle. 'Prescribing' isolation in a side-ward is usually to reduce the level of disruption that may be caused by delirious patients, rather than the stated aim of avoiding over-stimulation, and often leads to neglect (MacDonald et al., 1989; Lindesay *et al.*, 1990).

Affective disorders

Depression

Depression in old age is one of the commonest problems encountered in psychogeriatrics, yet, as with younger patients, there is still continuing debate as to its nosology, aetiology, treatment and outcome. The nosological problem in psychiatry, with two major and often incompatible nosological systems (DSM-IIIR; APA, 1987 and ICD10–WHO, 1992*a*), is not confined to depression, but is well illustrated by it. Broadly speaking, the debate focuses on the definitions of major depression (severe depression, depressive illness) and, especially in regard to the latter, the definition of caseness. Some have argued quite persuasively that the expression of depression in old age is very inadequately defined by both systems, both in earlier versions (Blazer *et al.*, 1987) and in the current system (Caine *et al.*, 1994), as much of what is called depression consists of affective symptoms that do not reach caseness (as defined by DSM-IIIR) and which are frequently comorbid with other psychiatric disorders, especially anxiety. The frequency of the comorbidity of depression in

Table 14.8. *Recent community epidemiological studies of depression in old people (65 years)*

Study	*n*	Screening instrument/ diagnostic system	Location	Prevalence of significance
Copeland *et al.*, 1987	1070	CMS Agecat	Urban UK	11.5% (including 3% psychotic depression)
Morgan *et al.*, 1987	1042	SAD	Urban UK	10% (65–74 year) 9.5% (75+)
ECA (Weissman *et al.*, 1988; Johnson *et al.*, 1992)	4701	DIS/DSM-III	5 communities USA	23% (+6% 'cases')
Lindesay *et al.*, 1989	983	CARe/Catego	Urban UK	13.5% (including 4.3% severe)
Livingston *et al.*, 1990	932	CARE	Urban UK	15.9%
Fuhrer *et al.*, 1992	4050	CES-D	Urban & rural France	13.4%

ECA, National Institutes of Mental Health – epidemiological catchment area; GMS, geriatric mental state schedule; Agecat, computer-derived diagnostic system linked to GMS; DIS, diagnostic interview schedule; CARE, comprehensive assessment & referral examination; Catego, a computer diagnostic classification system; CES-D, Centre for Epidemiological Studies – depression scale; SAD, symptoms of anxiety and depression scale.

old age with anxiety has led to renewed interest in the concept of generalised neurotic disorder (Larkin *et al.*, 1992).

Epidemiology of depression in old age

Community studies

Both in North America and in Europe, recent epidemiological studies of old people have shown that depressive symptoms are much commoner than cases of depression. Some of there studies are summarised in Table 14.8. All used interviews or depressive symptom rating scales, some of which are linked to diagnostic systems; only one (ECA) applied DSM-III diagnosis. The prevalence rates shown in Table 14.8 are those for the prevalence of the total sample who scored above threshold on the various depression symptom rating scales.

In validation studies of these depression symptom rating scales, some groups were able to define more tightly severity or caseness – in these instances percentages are in brackets. Despite the varying methods and types of populations surveyed there is a degree of consistency between these studies; 10–15% of old people living in the community have depressive symptoms but only about 3% have severe depression.

Depression in other settings

Much higher rates of depressive symptoms are reported in hospital in-patients and in old people living in residential homes or nursing homes. Recent studies of depression in Part III homes (reviewed by Ames, 1991) reported prevalence rates of 34–75%. In general medical wards and orthopaedic wards, 30–40% of patients aged over 65 years have depressive symptoms (Cooper, 1987; Pitt, 1991; Shamash *et al.*, 1992). A high prevalence of DSM-IIIR major depression (20.3%) has been found in Geriatric Day Hospital patients (Turrina *et al.*, 1992). Benbow (1987) has stressed the importance of psychogeriatric liaison with other medical specialties; these prevalence figures can only reinforce this case. There is a need for studies on the effects of intervention in such cases.

Depressive symptoms in old age

There is now good evidence to support the contention that 'depression is depression at any age' (Baldwin, 1991). Studies such as that of Musetti *et al.* (1989) have found no difference in the types of frequency of symptoms of major depression between community residents aged less than 65 years or those aged greater than 65 years.

Aetiology

Predisposing factors

Genetics Whilst there is some genetic contribution to the aetiology of major affective disorder with onset in old age, this is much weaker than that shown in patients with onset below 60 years of age. Musetti *et al.* (1989) found family history of affective disorder in 45.6% of patients whose illness began before 40 years of age, 35.5% of these with onset before 60 years of age and 28.6% of these with onset after 60 years of age. Baldwin (1990) did not find any significant difference between early onset cases (<60 years) and late onset cases(>60 years) in the frequency of a family history of affective disorder (21% and 23% respectively). Both of these studies, however, support the notion that a family history is common in late-onset affective disorder.

Biological factors The evidence as to whether the ageing process intrinsically predisposes to late-onset affective disorder is equivocal. Epidemiological studies that show that the prevalence of major affective illness declines with age would suggest that it does not. Reviews of neurotransmitter changes in depression in relation to ageing have reached opposite conclusions, one in favour of age-related changes (Philpot, 1986), another arguing that such changes as there are are protective (Futen *et al.*, 1989). Depressive symptoms are commoner in older people and their aetiological relationship with the ageing process – both in biological and psychological terms – is only just beginning to be addressed (see below).

Depression is very common in association with some diseases that are more prevalent in old age, such as Parkinson's disease (Baldwin & Byrne, 1989) and stroke (House, 1987), although in neither is the aetiological relationship with age understood. There is some evidence that structural brain changes may be significant in late-life depression. Recent reviews of CT scan changes (MacDonald, 1992*b*) and MRI scan changes (Baldwin, 1993) reach similar conclusions. Older depressive patients have more, albeit mild, cerebral atrophy than age-matched controls and a greater incidence of white matter lesions and other evidence of putative cerebrovascular changes. Both reviews advocate caution in the interpretation of such findings, however, as many of the studies had an in-built selection bias towards those with severe depression and, to a lesser extent, comorbid brain disease. Baldwin (1993) suggests that the bringing together of neuro-imaging techniques (to examine structure) and dynamic imaging (i.e. single photon omission computed tomography to examine function) is more likely to enhance understanding than either approach on its own. However, as many authors have pointed out, depression in old age may be overlooked either because it is seen as an 'understandable' consequence of senescence or because it arises in association with physical ill health (Epstein, 1976; Pitt, 1986; Baldwin, 1991). Newmann et al. (1991), in a careful appraisal of the experience of depressive symptoms in older women, suggested that 'older persons may be at decreased risk for depression in its classical form, although at increased risk for a quieter more unconventional form'. This quieter form was given the name of depletion syndrome of the elderly (Fogel & Fretwell, 1985) and is characterised by social withdrawal and disengagement rather than by a feeling of despair and emotional distress. Where depression in old age arises with physical illness it is important to obtain a history of change from the patient and relatives, and to look for features such as loss of pleasure and depressive thoughts (feelings of guilt, worthlessness). More classical features of depression, such as sleep disturbance and fatigue, are often less reliable in the context of physical illness (Cohen-Cole & Stoudemire, 1987; Baldwin, 1991).

Treatment of major depression

Physical treatment

Antidepressants and ECT may safely and effectively be used in the treatment of depressive illness in old age (Benbow, 1989; Baldwin, 1991). There is still uncertainty as to the dosage and type of antidepressant and the duration of treatment (Flint, 1992). Some have reported that effectiveness of low dosage (e.g. amitriptyline, 10 mg daily as a starting dose increasing to 30 mg daily) (Davies et al., 1973). As there are very little data on dosage in the literature, one pragmatic approach is to consider the overall well-being of the individual; frail thin patients will probably require very small doses, whereas fit well-nourished patients may tolerate full dosages. Which type of antidepressant is also controversial. Beaumont (1989) recommended that tricyclic antidepressants should no longer be the treatment of first choice for depression, because of their toxicity. Whilst Baldwin (1991) suggested this has probably been 'exaggerated', Katona (1994) advocated the newer antidepressant drugs as first choice therapy. He rightly points out that there are almost no placebo-controlled data for the new generation of antidepressants, including the SSRIs and meclobomide in the elderly.

The duration of treatment is not yet firmly established. Reviewing the available evidence, Flint (1992) concluded that six months treatment was not enough and that elderly patients may benefit from a much longer period of treatment. The Old Age Depression Interest Group study (OADIG, 1993) supports the view; continued treatment with dothiepin for two years reduced the risk of relapse by two and-a-half times that of the placebo group in elderly patients with major depression.

Antidepressants alone may be insufficient treatment in some patients. Those with delusions or other psychotic features have a better outcome if treated with a combination of antidepressants and neuroleptics or with ECT (Baldwin, 1988). 'Treatment resistant' depression is variously defined, as depression not responding to antidepressants after one and four weeks lithium augmentation therapy; providing lithium in addition to antidepressants is at least as effective as in younger patients, with about two-thirds of elderly patients showing benefit (Finch & Katona, 1989).

Electro-convulsive therapy (ECT) is both safe and effective in elderly patients (Benbow, 1989; Godber *et al.*, 1987) and the indications for its use are well-established. These old people with features of major depression and with prominent anxiety have a good response to ECT (Fraser & Glass, 1980; Salzman, 1983; Benbow, 1991). Non-physical treatments may also be effective in depression in old age. Ong *et al.* (1987) found that a support group reduced the risk of relapse or re-admission in elderly depressives. Jarvik *et al.* (1982) found that group psychotherapy (dynamic or cognitive) for elderly depressives was more effective than placebo but less effective than the group treated with antidepressants. Baldwin (1991) suggests that psychotherapy will be more effective if combined with antidepressants or when used in adequately treated patients. Cognitive (Yost *et al.*, 1986) and family therapy (Benbow, 1988) may also be used with benefit in older people.

Outcome

The results of initial treatment of a depressive episode in old age are good, with about 70% improving (Baldwin & Jolley, 1986). Murphy's (1983) prospective study had a less favourable outcome, with only 35% having a favourable outcome at one year. Baldwin & Jolley (1986) have suggested that these findings are due to differences in treatment; in particular, ECT was used less frequently in Murphy's (1983) series.

The longer-term outcome is less good. Some 40% who either have a poor recovery with residual symptoms or remain continuously ill (Baldwin, 1991). Major depression in old age carries an increased risk of mortality from vascular disease (Murphy *et al.*, 1988). Adverse prognostic factors are: the presence of brain 'pathology' (such as cerebro-vascular disease) (Jacoby, 1981); a slow or incomplete recovery (Godber *et al.*, 1987): and adverse life events before onset (Murphy, 1983).

Mania

The true prevalence of manic illness in old age has not been established. In hospital populations, about 5% of admission of elderly patients per year have manic illness (Yassa *et al.*, 1988). There is some evidence that an increased inception rate for mania is associated with increasing age (Eagles & Whally, 1985), although Broadhead & Jacoby (1990) found the mean age of onset of manic episodes in a group of manic patients to be bimodal, with a peak at 37 years and another at 73 years.

Aetiology

As with depression, in old age genetic factors in mania are probably less important than in younger cohorts (Stone, 1989). Onset of manic illness in old age may, in 8–12% of cases, be linked to cerebral organic disease (Jacoby, 1991). Krauthammer & Klermann (1978) coined the term 'secondary mania' to describe such cases. There is still debate as to whether such individuals lack a genetic predisposition. For example, Starkstein & Robinson (1989) found a positive family history of affective disorder in patients developing mania after stroke and Broadhead & Jacoby (1990) reported a previous history of affective disorder in two patients developing mania after stroke. Amongst elderly manic patients most series report a high prevalence of cerebral organic disease, between 24% and 43% (Stone, 1989; Broadhead & Jacoby, 1990). Shulman & Post (1980) also reported such high figures for elderly manic men (61%) but not for the elderly manic women (10%). The results of the relatively few studies of cerebral blood flow (CBF) and cerebral metabolic rate of glucose (CMR glu) in mania in younger patients are intriguing in this respect. Both CBF and CMR glu are increased in mania and are reduced in the depressed phase of bipolar illness (Joyce, 1991), although others report no such changes (Gustafson et al., 1981; Silfverskiold & Risberg, 1989). Whether such functional changes relate to the observed structural changes in late-onset mania remains to be established, but such studies might clarify the aetiological significance of cerebral disease.

Clinical features

Early studies, such as that of Post (1965), suggest that mania in late life often has a prominent admixture of depressive features. The only prospective study (Broadhead & Jacoby, 1990) compared the clinical features of the young-onset and late-onset mania and found no differences between them. The late-onset manias were, however, more likely that the early-onset manias to have a depressed phase during their index admission. Occasionally, manic symptoms in late life may herald the onset of dementia, especially of the frontal lobe type (Gustafson, 1987) but in established Alzheimer's disease they are uncommon. Burns et al. (1990) found that they occurred in only 3.5% of their series of 178 patients.

Treatment

Lithium is a safe and effective treatment for both the acute illness and for prophylaxis in elderly manic patients (Foster et al., 1990). There are, however, quite substantial differences between psychiatrists in the dosage, duration of treatment and monitoring of serum levels of lithium, renal function and thyroid function (Bramble, 1992), which may relate in part to clinicians' perception of the safety of lithium. In one retrospective series of elderly manic patients admitted to hospital, half received lithium prophylaxis whilst half did not, and no significant difference in outcome between the two groups was found (Stone, 1989). Neuroleptics are also effective in the acute phase alone or in combination with lithium (Jacoby, 1991).

Outcome

The outcome of the index admission for mania in old age is good but there is little data for the longer-term outcome. Shulmann & Post (1980) found that the majority of elderly manic patients suffered from recurrent affective illness.

Late paraphrenia

Clinical features

Late paraphrenia is a comparatively rare disorder, accounting for about 10% of psychiatric problems in the elderly. The incidence described by Holden (1987) was in keeping with the rest of the literature, suggesting an incidence of about 20 per 1 000 000. The term was introduced by Roth (1955) to denote elderly patients in whom persecutory delusions (usually systematised) were associated with auditory hallucinations and occurred with preservation of personality and no affective change. Since then, there have been two lines of thought. First, there are those who consider late paraphrenia as merely an expression of schizophrenia occurring in the elderly and there is no justification for a separate diagnostic category (Grahame, 1984). Second, some researchers have investigated the condition to find it a heterogeneous disorder and merely a convenient descriptive label to cover a number of other diagnoses such as early dementia with prominent psychotic features, atypical affective disorder and an extreme form of personality type characterised by paranoid beliefs. Post (1966) divided late paraphrenia into three main types. First, a group in whom paranoid ideas were circumscribed, simple and directed at particular neighbours or people of importance to the individual. Second, individuals where the experiences had extended and persecution was perceived to be from many individuals, often manifest by intrusive interference such as shining lights through the window or the installation of machinery aimed at torturing the patient. Often, auditory hallucinations accompanied the persecutory ideas. Third, was a group of individuals with symptoms indistinguishable from schizophrenia and showing first rank symptoms. Subsequent work has shown that this latter group has less cerebral atrophy, and possibly less organic pathology, than individuals without first rank symptoms (Howard et al., 1991). There is evidence that patients with late paraphrenia have cognitive deficits, as shown by global measures of cognitive function (the mental test score and digit copying test) and while some did show a deterioration over a four year follow-up, a few achieved a diagnosis of dementia (Hymas et al., 1989).

There is a nosological debate as to how late paraphrenia should be categorised. The original description by Post (1966) was of 'persistent persecutory states', which encompassed those elderly patients in whom paranoid symptoms were prominent. The diagnosis of late paraphrenia has been essentially disallowed by ICD-10, which will now be diagnosed under paranoid schizophrenia or persistent delusional disorder. Unfortunately, this last category excludes prominent hallucinations, which are experienced by a significant proportion of individuals with late paraphrenia. In the USA, such patients are now diagnosed as having late-onset schizophrenia, since the arbitrary upper age limit for the onset of schizophrenia in DSM-III (45 years) was removed in DSM-IIIR.

Aetiology

Premorbid personality has long been associated with the development of late paraphrenia and often it is hard to ascertain whether a new illness has supervened or if the condition is merely an extension of the existing personality with exacerbation of eccentricity, suspiciousness and social isolation. There has been little systematic investigation of the genetics of late paraphrenia. The contribution of organic brain lesions has been emphasised by a number of studies, which have shown changes on CT scanning (enlarged cerebral ventricles, white matter, cerebral infarctions and cortical atrophy: Naguib & Levy, 1987; Rabins et al., 1987; Burns et al., 1989; Miller et al., 1991).

Holden (1987) showed that individuals with a diagnosis of late paraphrenia and cerebral organic factors had a poorer prognosis than their non-organic counterparts. Other factors associated with late paraphrenia include: social isolation, sensory impairment (deafness more than visual impairment) and being female. The features often associated with late paraphrenia are captured best by a brief and yet often typical case. The patient is usually an elderly woman who has either never married or has married late and often has no children, she leads a relatively isolated life, has few close friends, has moved house often on a number of occasions to escape her persecutors. Aided by helpful social workers and housing officials, she is generally in good physical health, does not have past psychiatric history but has sensory deficits, usually hearing loss, often compounded by poor vision.

Management

With regard to investigations, these should follow conventional lines, paying particular attention to physical illness, bearing in mind the particular association between late paraphrenia and cerebral organic pathology. Treatment is as with any psychotic illness and consists of maintenance of a good relationship with the individual (usually fostered extremely well by the CPN service) and standard doses of neuroleptics. There is evidence that patients with cerebral organic lesions respond less well to neuroleptics, although compliance may be a particular problem in this group. The prognosis of late paraphrenia is obviously dependent on any underlying physical or cerebral organic lesion found but in the absence of that survival seems to be little different to that of the general population.

Neurosis

There is now increasing evidence that neurosis at all ages is a unitary syndrome with changing symptoms over time (Tyrer, 1985b; Lindesay, 1991a,b; Larkin et al., 1992) at least in the case of depression and anxiety. Obsessive-compulsive disorder is the exception, being less common in old age (Myers et al., 1984) and being relatively constant over time.Others have argued against the unitary theory (Roth et al., 1972). Prevalence rates of neurosis in old age, however, are usually reported by symptom type or nosological category (e.g. DSM-IIIR). Lindesay & Banerjee (1993) have shown that the diagnostic system used in epidemiological studies of phobic disorders greatly influences the observed prevalence rates; a similar effect was shown by Kay et al. (1985) for depression.

Table 14.9. *Per cent prevalence of neurotic disorders in community surveys of people ages 65 years or more*

Study	Generalised anxiety	Panic disorder	Agrophobia	Social phobia	Specific phobia	Total phobia	Depression	Obsessional-compulsive
Lindesay et al. (1989)	3.7	0	7.8	1.3	2.1	10	13.5	0
Copeland et al. (1992)	1.1	–	–	–	–	0.7	8.5	0
Regier et al. (1993)	5.5	0.1	–	–	–	4.8	1.8	0.8

Community studies

The results of three large epidemiological surveys are shown in Table 14.9. There are great differences in reported rates of all neurotic disorders except panic disorder, which was rarely found in any of the studies. These differences are partly due to the different survey instruments used, but may also represent observer differences or geographical differences. Whilst neurotic disorders in the youngest members of the elderly population are more common in females than in males, this gender difference tends to narrow in the very old, largely as a result of the decreasing rates of neurotic disorder in older women, whilst those for men remain relatively stable across the age range (Nilsson & Pearson, 1984). Longitudinal community surveys of depressive neurosis in the UK (Copeland et al., 1992) and Singapore (Kua, 1993) show high mortality rates (23.2% and 16.1% respectively) and changing symptom patterns over the follow-up period. Recovery occurs in only about 19% for neurosis overall (Larkin et al., 1992).

These recent community studies do not comment on the age of onset of neurosis.Others have done so and found that in between 5% (Kay et al., 1964) and 24% (Bergmann, 1971) of neurosis in older people the onset was in old age. Some symptom types amongst neurotic disorders may be more likely to begin in old age. Bergmann (1971) found that nearly half of anxiety disorders began in old age and Lindesay (1991a,b) found that a third of phobic disorder began in old age. Community surveys almost always reveal higher morbidity for neurotic disorders that is shown in hospital admission rates or in consultations in primary care (Lindesay, 1991a,b).

Goldberg & Huxley (1980) showed that anxiety disorders in the elderly do not easily pass through the pathways to psychiatric care. It is not clear why this is so but for anxiety disorders Jarvik & Russell (1979) suggested that the elderly may 'freeze' rather than display the classical fight or flight anxiety reaction and thus the true nature of their condition may not be recognised. Larkin et al. (1992) suggested that 'ageism' on the part of clinicians may influence attitudes to neurotic disorders in old age (including unwarranted pessimism) and thus might be supposed to reduce the likelihood of psychiatric referral. The significant proportions of sub-cases who subsequently develop neurotic disorders at a case level found in surveys such as those of Copeland et al. (1992) suggest that intervention might not only be warranted but might also be effective.

Treatment

Freud, whose case reports include no one over the age of 50 (Clare, 1985) has unduly and adversely influenced the attitude of therapists towards psychological therapy for old people, with a few notable exceptions. Butler has long advocated a psychotherapeutic approach for the treatment of neurotic disorders and psychological reactions to adverse life events, such as loss, in older people (Butler, 1968). Yost et al. (1986) have outlined adaptations of Beck et al's (1979) model of cognitive therapy for older people. Morris & Morris (1991) reviewed the studies of behavioural and cognitive therapy in old people with depression and concluded that, where used appropriately, these therapies are beneficial.

Suicide and deliberate self-harm in the elderly

Suicide

As in younger cohorts, suicide in the elderly is associated with mental illness, especially affective disorders and with male gender (Lindesay, 1991a,b; Pritchard, 1992). Suicide rates increase with increasing age in most studies from the developed world (reviewed by Pritchard, 1992).

Deliberate self-harm

Deliberate self-harm (DSH) is less common in older people than in younger people. In one study in Wales, 5.4% of all cases of DSH seen in a district general hospital, over a 12-year period, were aged 65 years or more (Pierce, 1987), the majority of whom were depressed (93%) and female (male to female ratio 1:1.5).

In Canada, Dyck *et al.* (1988) found that the prevalence of 'suicide attempts' was not associated with increasing age in men and decreased with increasing age for women. This study was a survey of psychiatric disorders in 3258 residents and contained few old people (11% aged 65 years or more).

Alcohol abuse

Prevalence

There have been several recent community surveys of alcohol abuse in elderly people, reporting prevalence rates ranging from 0.01% (Livingston & King, 1993) to 3.6% of men and 3.2% of women (Iliffe *et al.*, 1991). The range of prevalence rates can probably be attributed to the methods of case identification, and the differing socio-economic status of the populations studied (high socio-economic status populations tending to have higher prevalence rates).

Clinical picture

It is now established that alcohol abuse in old age is composed of two groups: Group I, the graduate alcoholic, the majority of whom have features of the alcohol dependence syndrome and have been drinking for many years. They tend to present with physical problems and the sexes are equally represented. Group II, elderly people who began to abuse alcohol in old age and rarely have symptoms of the alcohol dependence syndrome. They present with falls, self-neglect and intermittent confusional states. They are usually female and are often isolated and suffer from chronic ill-health (Rosin & Glatt, 1971; Jolley & Hodgson, 1985).

Management

Some elderly alcoholics are in contact with the Alcohol Treatment Services but they are a small minority (Glatt *et al.*, 1978). There are few data on management of Group II alcoholic abusers. Jolley & Hodgson (1985) suggested that hospital admissions might be used to 'break the circle of alcohol use' with a careful assessment of social, psychological and physical problems and appropriate treatment of each as the basis for successful management. They also advocated the use of vitamins and tranquillizers. Perhaps the most important factor is to recognise these patients in the first place, which is not always easy.

Other psychiatric disorders of old age

Senile self-neglect (Diogenes syndrome)

Such patients are characterised by reclusiveness and breakdown of self-care, to the extent that they may pose an environmental health hazard; not infrequently they hoard rubbish and reject help from relatives or statutory services. The condition is not necessarily associated with poverty; many patients have a lot of money, perhaps reflecting the high intelligence or professional background of such patients.

Men and women are equally affected, and occasional cases of '*Diogenes à deux*' in married couples have been described (MacMillan & Shaw, 1966; Cole *et al.*, 1992). The condition is not common; an annual incidence of 0.5 per 1000 of the population aged over 60 years was reported by MacMillan & Shaw (1966). Such people form a heterogenous group, both in their symptom profile and their mode of presentation. Post (1982) considers that many are personality disordered, the rest suffering from dementia or paraphrenia. The contact with medical services is rarely initiated by the patients themselves but often by neighbours, although at the time of referral many are mentally ill or disabled and mortality is high (MacMillan & Shaw, 1966; Clark *et al.*, 1975). Not infrequently the environmental hazards are the cause of contact with medical services.

Charles Bonnet syndrome

De Morsier (1938) used this eponym to describe a syndrome of complex visual hallucinosis in mentally normal, but unusually visually impaired, old people. Podoll *et al* (1990) have proposed an operational definition that briefly requires the presence of visual hallucinations in clear consciousness and in the absence of cerebral pathology or psychosis and visual impairment as a usual but not necessary concomitant. The authors found a prevalence of 1–2% of psychiatric elderly out-patients, very similar to the 1.3–1.8% reported by Berrios & Brook (1984) in a similar population.

Characteristically the visual hallucinations begin suddenly, last for only brief periods (seconds or minutes) and are commoner in the evening or at night. They are vivid; about a third are simple (patterns). When complex, human forms predominate over inanimate objects. Insight is maintained (Fuchs & Lauter, 1992). Some authors have attempted to widen the boundaries of the syndrome to include those who subsequently develop cerebral cortical pathology, such as cerebrovascular disease (Brabbins, 1992). Charles Bonnet syndrome has been reported as the presenting feature of Alzheimer's disease (Crystal *et al.*, 1988) and stroke (Ball, 1991). Even in cases as defined by Podoll *et al.* (1990), mild abnormalities in the EEG were found.

Treatment is of the visual impairment where possible, for example removal of cataracts, can be successful (Siatowsky *et al.*, 1990). Visual hallucinations in a 65-year-old woman with depression were successfully treated by episodic blindfolding (Naik & Jones, 1993).

The future

Psychogeriatricians worldwide face a future that is both uncertain and exciting. Uncertain because of increasing restraints on resource allocation, exciting because this in itself offers a new challenge for service development. Exciting also with the growth of the specialty and the research into disease of old age. No longer is there any justification for the therapeutic nihilism which so often was associated with the treatment of the mental disorders of old age. The specialist in the psychiatry of old age has the means to alleviate distress and the hope, in the not impossibly distant future, of even more effective treatment for some of the commonest mental health problems of old age, depression and dementia.

15

The psychiatry of learning disability

W. I. FRASER

Introduction

Terminology and definitions

In recent years, the debate over how to refer to mental impairment from early life has come to a conclusion in England. The Department of Health has replaced the term 'mental handicap' with the term 'learning disability'. The American Association of Mental Retardation (AAMR) has decided the term 'mental retardation' is here to stay. It will be used in this chapter interchangeably with learning disability (LD). The AAMR no longer use terms such as 'mild, moderately, severely and profoundly' but in this chapter the distinction between mild LD (IQ 50–70) and moderate, severe, profound LD (IQ 0–50) will be made.

There is no single 'correct' definition of learning disability (mental retardation). We need several different ones depending on the purposes to be served. The most carefully conceptualised and consensually agreed is that of the AAMR (1993):

> 'Mental retardation refers to substantial limitations in present functioning; characterised by significant sub-average intellectual functioning existing concurrently with related limitations in two or more of the following applicable skill areas: communication, health care, home living, social skills, community use, self direction, health and safety, functional academics, leisure and work; manifest before the age of 18 years'.

This definition departs from the previous definitions by regarding mental retardation as a *state* that can change (rather than a stable trait). Functioning is impaired in specific ways beginning in childhood. In this state, limitations in intelligence (IQ 70–75 or below) and adaptive skills coexist, and, with appropriate supports, this person will function better.

Thus the concept with which the clinician has to work is an administrative one, in which low intelligence is a necessary but insufficient criterion. This chapter will concentrate on the elucidation of clinical states but before doing so, will briefly consider the epidemiology and aetiology of learning disability. The reader is referred to Fryers (1992) for a more extensive account of epidemiological aspects and to Fraser & Minns (1992) for details of aetiologies.

Table 15.1. *Mean prevalence of learning disability (per 1000)*

Age (years)	Severe (IQ 0–50)	Overall (IQ 0–70)
7	2.4	7–19
11–18	3.8	21.2

From multiple surveys in the United Kingdom (Hallas *et al.*, 1982)

Epidemiology

The *incidence* of handicapping disorders usually are expressed as cases per 1000 live births in a particular year, but accurate rates for incidence of disorders are extremely difficult to establish. Only where a condition can be clearly recognised at birth, e.g. Down's syndrome, it is possible to be definite about an incidence rate. The *prevalence* of a handicapping disorder is a measure of the number of people found to have that disorder within a given population in a defined period : the age specific prevalence rate is the prevalence of a particular age. Knowledge of administrative prevalence, i.e. reliable information about the number of people with learning disabilities needing services, is necessary to service planning. Knowledge of true prevalence will inform administrative prevalence.

The prevalence of learning disability varies according to age (see Table 15.1); at ages 15–19 years for moderate/severe learning disability the administrative prevalence is 3.8/1000 general population (Kushlick & Blunden, 1974). The administrative prevalence for mild learning disability has been estimated at 8.7/1000 (Koller *et al.*, 1983). However, there is a large social class effect, with up to nine times more learning-disabled individuals in social class 5 than social class 1.

Causes of learning disabilities (mental retardation)

Although there remain many disorders causing learning disability whose cause is not known, the number is shrinking. Table 15.2 indicates current known causes. The most common disorder is still Down's anomaly; the next most common is fragile-X (FXMR), with a prevalence in Caucasian populations cited at 1 per 1250 males and 1 per 2000 females (Webb & Bundey, 1991), but more recently estimated at 1 per 1000 males and 1 per 700 females or even lower (Reiss, personal communication). The next commonest after FXMR are likely to be disorders caused by a single gene (15%). Some monogenic disorders present as treatable metabolic disorders, e.g. phenylketonuria. Perinatal injuries are considered by Weatherall to comprise 7%, but it is difficult to estimate how many of such children are prenatally vulnerable. For about 20% of learning disabled people, still no cause can be found.

In moderate/severe LD, aetiology can be established in 50–80% of cases, with chromosomal and genetic causes predominating (Craft *et al.*, 1987, p. 83). Over 500 recognised

Table 15.2. *Causes of severe handicap in children under 16 years*

Down's syndrome	32%[*]
Overall chromosome abnormalities	26.5–50%
Monogenic, e.g. PKU, tuberous sclerosis	15%[*]
Cerebral palsy	6.5–7%[*]
Birth injury	2.0
Infective/post infective or immunological causes	2.0
Nutritional or metabolic causes	2.0
Psychiatric syndromes	4.0
Cerebral anoxia	1.5
Cultural–familial causes	1.0
Heredofamilial degenerative diseases of CNS	1.5
Epilepsy	1.0
Recognised syndromes of unknown aetiology	1.5
Other conditions	3.0
Learning disability (not elsewhere classified)	4.0
No known cause	20–34.5[*]

Compiled from Corbett *et al* (1975); Craft *et al.* (1987) and [*]Weatherall (1983)

syndromes involving a genetic disorder have now been isolated (Thapar *et al.*, 1994).

In mild learning disability, aetiological factors include social deprivation, nutritional, education, lead poisoning, smoking and material alcohol consumption in pregnancy. Mild LD cannot simply be explained as consisting of those who are at the lower end of the normal distribution curve. For example, studies show that 3–11% have chromosomal abnormalities (Gostavson *et al.*, 1991). However, there is overwhelming evidence for family resemblances in respect to IQ scores throughout the normal range – about 50% of the variation in the population is explicable by additive genetic effects (Thapar *et al* ., 1994). It is assumed that the same pattern of genetic and environmental influences applies to people whose IQ scores are within the 50–70 range. It seems likely that as with other continuously distributed measures of behaviour, the effects of genes on IQ are accounted for by several, perhaps many, loci. Research has recently begun attempting to identify the so-called quantitive trait loci (QTL) responsible for variation in intelligence (Plomin *et al.*, 1996).

The role of adverse obstetric factors in contributing to the *causation* of mild learning disability is significant. Hagberg *et al.* (1981), in a population study of mild learning disability in Gotheburg, found 25% had prenatal and 20% perinatal adverse factors. Rao (1990) showed a large number of adverse perinatal factors in a population of children with mild learning disability.

Up to 59% of children with mild learning disability will present with behavioural problems by the age of 21 years (Koller *et al.*, 1983). Many reviews have indicated that psychiatric disorder is more frequent in people with LD than in the general population. Most estimates for the prevalence of serious psychiatric disorders in the severely mentally handicapped (including most personality disorders and psychosis) vary enormously and range from 8% to 15%; when minor emotional disorders are included, estimates reach over 50% of the eligible population. It is notable that much prominence is placed in the new AAMR definition on the emotional needs of people with learning disabilities.

Distinguishing behaviour disturbance and psychiatric disorder

The psychiatrist is initially presented with an individual who is causing management problems. Behaviours are labelled 'disturbed' and reacted to as such because (1) the disturbed person reacts in an idiosyncratic or inappropriate manner given their age and level of development, i.e. the behaviour is difficult to understand; (2) their actions flout the smooth functioning and norms of the relevant social groups. Of course, the norms of contact between social groups vary and people have individual perception of behaviour disturbance with different threshold – what is acceptable in a longstay hospital is less so in a middle-class suburb. It should also be acknowledged that such behaviours have a long-term negative effect on interactions with the disturbed person.

The term 'challenging behaviour' has recently been introduced and one definition of *severe challenging behaviour* is: behaviour of such an intensity, frequency and duration that the physical safety of the person or others is in serious jeopardy, or behaviour that is likely to seriously limit or deny access to a use of ordinary facilities (Emerson *et al.*, 1987). Challenging behaviour is a final common path with many causes and contributory factors: psychiatric disorder is one of them. Dual diagnosis (mental illness and learning disability combined) is a useful term but also encourages oversimplification.

Behaviour disturbance in people with LD stems from an interplay of two types of factor: *environmentally independent factors*, such as stage of development, preservation of homeostasis, habitual state of arousal of the individual, organic or functional mental illness; and *environmentally dependent factors*, such as aberrant behaviours that have been inadvertently reinforced, and aberrant, failed communication attempts. Behaviour disturbances can further be caused by major emotional universal needs in handicapped people (e.g. security, friendship) being unmet (Baumeister, 1989).

Behaviour disturbance *by itself* is thus insufficient to warrant a psychiatric diagnosis. Reiss (1993) has suggested some guidelines to help the clinician:

1. Diagnose patterns of symptomatology, i.e. is this behaviour disturbance part of a correlated pattern of symptoms that is recognisable as a psychiatric disorder?
2. Diagnose changes in behaviour. With the exception of personality disorder, a psychological disorder should have a recognisable onset and represent change in behaviour from premorbid periods.
3. Consider the impact of intellectual handicaps on the expression of symptomatology. '*Diagnostic overshadowing*' (Reiss *et al.*, 1982) is when the presence of intellectual disability decreases the diagnostic significance of an accompanying mental health disorder.
4. Accept the aetiology of the behaviour disturbance may be ambiguous, especially in the more severely handicapped.

In view of the above guidelines, the following basic questions should be asked:

Has the behaviour changed recently?
Could the behaviour be caused by physical illness?
Is the living environment suitable?
Are there opportunities to develop satisfactory relationships?
Are there difficulties in holding attention?
Are there any communication problems?
Are there any sensory impairments?
What difficulties are there with cognitive and emotional development?
And finally, is there an underlying mental illness?

The assessment of the above in an unstructured clinical interview often requires to be supplemented by standardised checklists (of which there are many). The reasons include cross-validation of the interview and more precise measurement of outcome, clinical audit and research.

Checklists and inventories approaches have, of course, their limitations. There is no substitute for direct observation in the natural environment accompanied by structured questioning about the function of the behaviours, e.g. the Motivation Analysis of Self Injurious Behaviour (Durand & Crimmins, 1988), and direct observation under either purely ethological or evocative conditions e.g. Iwata *et al.*, 1982).

The psychiatrist should start with basic skills in pen-and-pencil event recording. Repp & Felce (1990) have developed a system that allows for the recording of up to 45 incidents on a portable computer. This allows the environment/behaviour to be analysed and judgements made as to which variable is independent and dependent, and may shed light on whether, for instance, a stereotyped movement is environmentally independent.

The US Department of Health and Human Services's comprehensive critique of 45 instruments (Aman, 1991), assessing psychopathology and behaviour problems in persons with mental retardation, is the standard reference manual and 'the shopper's guide' to behaviour checklists. The commonest questionnaire is the Adaptive Behaviour Schedule (Nihira *et al.*, 1974); the Aberrant Behaviour Checklist (Aman *et al.*, 1985) is particularly sensitive and can be used for quite subtle medication monitoring; the Psychosocial Behaviour Scale (Espie *et al.*, 1988) is particularly good at detecting hysterical behaviours and pseudo fits. These scales consist of five or six factors that include: aggression to others, communicative breakdown, self-aggression, mood disturbance, antisocial conduct, and mannerisms and stereotypes. They are relatively insensitive to frequency, intensity and severity of behaviours, although the Behaviour Disturbance Scale (Leudar *et al.*, 1987) is rather more sensitive to severity of disturbance. For psychiatric disorders, the most useful are Diagnostic Assessment for the Severely Handicapped (Matson *et al.*, 1991); Psycho-pathology Instrument for Mentally Retarded Adults (Senatore *et al.*, 1985); the Reiss Screen (Reiss, 1988) and the Psychiatric Assessment Development Schedule for Adults with Disabilities (PAS–ADD) (Moss *et al.*, 1993).

A developmental perspective to assessment

Information gathering should be developmentally based whether the subject is child or adult. The clinician must ask: what does the history of this person's developmental history tell us? Do we need further explanations to account for this behaviour beyond developmental arrest? Quite often the behaviour is appropriate to the subject's mental and emotional age.

Developmental assessments such as the Griffith's Developmental Tests for babies and young children should be sought; particular attention being paid to the profiles of motor, social and language development often expressed as Developmental Quotients (DQs). There must be close questioning about reciprocal social interaction in infancy, especially between mother and infant, such as ability to 'take turns' in communication, lack of gaze, lack of interest in other people as people, abnormal seeking of comfort in the first year against the background of impairments in social behaviour; whether there was a restricted repertoire of movements, activities and interests; and when mannerisms and stereotypes appeared or disappeared. Questions about sleep problems and about the child's temperament, activity output and attention span may suggest attention deficit disorder and hyperkinesis, oppositional defiant disorder and conduct disorder. Questioning should also specifically be about the child's difficulties with visuo-spatial organisation, tactile perception, psychomotor and non-verbal problem-solving skills and abilities, and contrasted with strengths and weaknesses in linguistic skills such as rote verbal learning and high verbal output; crucial evidence to help explain, over the course of development, subsequent emotional disturbances. Such developmentally originating disorders are common antecedents to challenging behaviour in adult life. The important contribution of autistic spectrum disorders to adult challenging beheaviour warrants special attention (see later).

Three assessment instruments for children with LD are recommended because of their good standardisation: Reiss Scales for Children's Dual Diagnosis for screening purposes (Reiss, 1993); the Aberrant Behaviour Checklist (Aman et al., 1985); and the Developmentally Delayed Children's Behaviour Checklist (DDBCCL) (Einfield & Tonge, 1991) – the latter is particularly useful as it has two forms: one for administration by parents and another by such caregivers as teachers, and they can be compared, and clear sensitivity/specificity information is provided. Einfield & Tonge also addressed the issue of the applicability of DSM-III criteria in learning disability, particularly in children. Not only is there a lack of external validation of DSM-III criteria for severely mentally handicapped children, but the inter-rater reliability of psychiatric diagnosis in the group has never been systematically examined.

Clarifying the autistic spectrum

Common abnormal behaviours in children with LD include autistic behaviours. These have been classified in DSM-IV and ICD-10 under the clumsy term Pervasive Developmental Disorder. Autistic Disorder (Childhood Autism ICD-10) is a subtype of Pervasive Developmental Disorder but is the principal one. There is a general consensus that

Autistic Disorder encompasses three diagnostic pillars, the 'Triad' of Wing & Gould 1979), namely : delay and deviance in social relationships, *communication disorder* and *repetitive behaviours*. The original criterion of onset before 36 months is no longer essential. Wing (1991) has argued convincingly that Asperger syndrome, a disorder characterised by social impairment, narrow interests, repetitive routines, speech and language peculiarities, non-verbal communication problems and motor clumsiness (Gillberg & Gillberg, 1989) is in the spectrum of autism. Such people use language freely but fail to make adjustments to social contents or the needs of listeners, and wish to be sociable but fail to make relationships (Tantum, 1991). Although such people are commonly not by definition mentally retarded, many retarded people show this syndrome, too. The notion of Asperger syndrome as a high-level autism is importance because (a) it suggest that 'Autistic Spectrum Disorders' is a valid concept; (b) such disorders are more common than before realised; and (c) where autism usually leads to problems that present early to the child health services and later to the learning disability services; patients with Asperger syndrome often do not present for psychiatric consultation (to the generic services) until adult life.

Such developmental diagnoses as autism are clinical diagnoses, and require a thorough family history, family assessment neuropsychiatric examination, and a rating scale administered by a trained rater during observation, for example, the Autism Behaviour Checklist (ABC), (Krug *et al.*, 1988), a 57-item questionnaire of simple statements. This incorporates rating scores in a system qualifying the data obtained. A score of 67 is selected as a high probability cut-off for the classification of autism. The range between 54 and 67 includes individuals who are either high-functioning austistics or have certain behavioural characteristics commonly associated with autism: these may be severely learning disabled, deaf, blind, severely emotionally disturbed or brain damaged. Such scales should not be taken in isolation. Sevin *et al.* (1991) have compared three diagnostic instruments: the Childhood Autism Rating Scales (CARS), the Real Life Rating Scale (RLRS) and the Autistic Behaviour Checklist. Of the three, the ABC seems least reliable, particularly with adult groups. The recently developed Autism Diagnostic Interview (ADI), with a complementary instrument – the autism Diagnostic Observation Schedule (ADOS), is a particularly detailed and searching tool for the differential diagnosis of Pervasive Developmental Disorders. It is not a standardised question respondent-based interview but is an investigator-based approach in which an experienced and specially trained interviewer obtains detailed descriptions of actual behaviours, present before and current (Le Couteur *et al.*, 1989). Pragmatic language assessments, cognitive tests, an IQ test and an intensive review of the child's medical history are also important. A complete learning disability screen includes chromosome analysis (involving DNA analysis for Fragile-X Mental Retardation: FXMR), EEG and brain-imaging examinations.

Parents will be anxious to know the cause – autism is now regarded as a behaviourally defined syndrome of neurological impairment with a major genetic component and a wide variety of underlying medical contributory factors: fragile-X mental retardation, neurofibromatosis, rubella. The final common path is cognitive – a relative or absolute absence of a Theory of Mind (ability to make inferences about others' mental states) (Baron-Cohen, 1989).

In the developmental disorders, a Learning Rate Prognosis should be attempted. This is the hardest aspect to be definite about, as development occurs in spurts and plateaux. Promising approaches to estimating learning potential include the Zone of Proximal Development (ZPD) defined by Vygotsky (1978) as the distance between active developmental level and probable development, as determined through problem solving under adult guidance or in collaboration with a more capable peer. While Vygotsky's work was sadly curtailed by his death, there is a renewed interest in measures of potential based on social interaction. Some extremely hyperactive (ADDH) children reach ultimately normal social and academic functioning, but in the case of the autistic spectrum disorders, the absence of useful language by the age of five years is a very poor prognostic feature.

Delayed, strange and inappropriate language

Slow language development is expected in learning disability. However, children with uncomplicated LD do their best to obey the maxims of conversation (that is, they try to take turns and be co-operative in conversation, make their intentions known and be as clear as they can). People with autistic spectrum disorders – children and adults – whatever the cause, infringe many aspects of language. Whilst straightforward children with LD are simply *slow* in their acquisition of syntax, people with autism and psychosis sometimes violate the rules of syntax, phonology, prosody and pragmatics. Most of all, their language seems *inappropriate*. Bishop & Adams (1989) have made a start in disentangling the concept of inappropriacy in speech, broadly dichotomising it into due to linguistic difficulties and due to social and cognition difficulties. If people with LD are inappropriate, it is mostly due to social cognition deficits. They are also inappropriate to a variable extent because of their linguistic difficulties. Rapin & Allen (1983) introduced the term 'semantic pragmatic deficit syndrome' as part of a subcategorsation of developmental language disorder in children. Such children's language is structurally well-formed but they have difficulty including meaning relevant to the conversational situation. The differentiating factor between semantic pragmatic disorder and autism is the *severity* of the disturbance and also the *pattern* of symptoms. Bishop differentiates autism, Asperger syndrome and semantic disorder – autistic children have persistent deficits in both the social and language impairment. Children with Asperger syndrome have no appreciable language problems but present themselves as socially inept, and those with semantic pragmatic problems present early language delay with persistent communication disorders. Bishop (1989) points out that diagnosis of autism will be made before the age of five years, but Asperger problems will not be diagnosed until much later, because of the overtly milder communicative disturbance and because parents may have some autistic traits (Berney, 1992).

One example of the distorted directions in which development can go is the non-verbal learning disability syndrome described by Rourke (1988). Thirty-six per cent of one cohort of 1000 children born before 33 weeks gestation in 1979–82 now show IQ verbal performance bias greater than 15 points (Reynolds, personal communication), indicating the likelihood of severe non-verbal learning deficit.

In Rourke's model, it is suggested that a constellation of learning disabilities emerges in children who suffer from disordered functioning of systems in the right cerebral hemisphere or from some lack of access to such systems, due to white matter destruction, e.g.

peri-ventricular haemorrhage or hypoxic ischaemic insults. Deficient performance in early infancy in non-dominant hemispheric functioning, e.g. visuospatial organisational ability, leads to extreme difficulties in dealing with novel and complex environmental situations, while automated rote language skills become increasingly well-developed and a clumsy, awkward verbose personality who is resistant to change is the consequence; explaining many developmental manifestations of what Rourke called non-verbal learning disabilities and exemplified in the hydrocephalic child's 'cocktail party speech' (inconsequential and prolix) and Asperger syndrome.

Evidence from communication about mental states

People with learning difficulties may not stand out because of their appearance, but their communication will almost always distinguish them. The careful analysis of their communicative patterns can reveal a good deal about their mental state. How does the person with LD greet the interviewer? (e.g. the characteristic greeting posture of the person with fragile-X: a formal awkwardly extended hand with lowered and averted head) (Wolff *et al.*, 1989). How does the speaker initiate verbal activity, gain/regain attention, request, give feedback, signal topic change, distress, surprise, agreement? Does he or she take turns? How does the person with LD link together his ideas and thoughts (coherence)? How informative is he or she? Can the person with LD locate and spontaneously 'repair' trouble spots in the conversation (e.g. repeat himself when he realises he is unclear)? Can he work with the listener to accomplish acceptable opening and closing routines (e.g. I should like to say the following . . . I must stop now)? (Bryan, 1989; Lesser & Milroy, 1993).

By close attention to these questions, the clinician can appreciate the difficulties the person with LD faces even though he or she may have superficially good grammar and vocabulary. The distinction between developmental disorder and superadded mental illness is crucial. Too often in the past, high-functioning autistics were considered 'psychotic'. If the clinician does detect incoherence, he/she should proceed to use a standardised measure such as Andreasen's Scale for the Assessment of Thought, Language and Communication (Andreasen, 1986).

Pathogenesis of psychiatric disorders

A memorable phrase for the lifestyle of people with learning disabilities is 'the management of a spoiled identity'. Rutter describes a chain of constraining environmental events set off by a single negative factor – a genetic defect, an event in the womb or in infancy. Brain damage, perhaps due to genetic vulnerability, may cause both the mental handicap and psychiatric disorders. Neuroepileptic conditions are associated with a five-fold increase in psychiatric disorders of childhood compared with normal children (Rutter *et al.*, 1970). Early childhood for such children may be accompanied by a series of hospital admissions and separations, and may be an experience of absence of function through accompanying severe physical disability or sensory impairment. Communication difficulties may arise through a variety of causes, from profound mental handicap to developmental language disorder; poor attention-span leading to an inability to acquire the prerequisites of learning; non-verbal learning disability leading to unadventuressness and environments that are unstimulating; low intelligence leading to poor coping mechanisms and vulnerability to exploitation; family difficulties, parental ill-health and discord leading to inadequate discipline and chaotic rearing. Failure to acquire social, interpersonal and recreational skills may impair relationships and predispose to physical ill-health, low self-esteem from repeated failure, true or perceived repeated rejections from the family, a dysmorphic unattractive appearance, and to subsequent labelling: being placed in insensitive unsuitable school settings and thereafter to unemployment and loneliness. In short, brain dysfunction interacts with an inflexible environment to cause a high rate of psychiatric disorders.

Schizophrenia

The lifetime risk of schizophrenia in those with a learning disability is 3% compared with 1% in the non-handicapped population (Turner, 1989). There are problems of 'diagnostic overshadowing' in differentiating between the symptoms of learning disability and those associated with the symptoms of schizophrenia, i.e. amotivation, slowness of thought and action, poverty of speech and emotional blunting (Murray, 1986), and the differentiation of schizophrenia from depression in people who are non-verbal is extremely difficult. There is no defined constellation of symptoms of schizophrenia without words. It is not possible to diagnose schizophrenia in individuals with an IQ less than 40 (Reid, 1983). As stated above, a careful developmental history will separate autistic spectrum disorders from schizophrenia. Reid (1980) has reported that the natural history is the same as in the non-disabled, and Meadows et al. (1991), comparing 25 patients with mild mental handicap and schizophrenia with 26 schizophrenics of normal intelligence, have demonstrated that the clinical phenomena elicited were the same in both study groups but persecutory delusions and formal thought disorder were less common in the dual diagnosis group. This is unsurprising as Frith (1992) has suggested that sophisticated symbolic capacity is required for delusions to occur. In people with LD, schizophrenia usually presents as withdrawal, fearfulness, sleep disturbance and hallucinations without complex delusional systems (Heaton-Ward, 1977; Eaton & Menolascino, 1982).

Affective disorder

Affective disorder is amongst the commonest psychiatric diagnosis in this group (Sovner & Hurley, 1983; Szymanski & Biederman, 1984). For those functioning in the mild/moderate range, standard diagnostic criteria can be used (Sovner & Hurley, 1983), aided by modified standard depression inventories (Kazdin et al., 1983). In the more severely disabled, a diagnosis can be made, even in the absence of language development, on behavioural and vegetative changes, which may require more prolonged study of behaviour, levels of motor activity, weight and sleep patterns. States of severe depression can occur in people with learning disability and vigilance must be exercised, particularly for depression in autistic spectrum disorder (Wing & Wing, 1976). Depression usually presents in adults with a deterioration in social skills. Suicide is virtually non-existent in the most severely handicapped. Manic depressive illness is rather easier than schizophrenia to diagnose and features increased motor output and talkativeness, vocalisation, aggression and sleeplessness; also depression, decreased activity, or conversely wandering, poor appetite, sleeplessness or hypersomnolence. Tyrer & Shakour (1990) used a technique known as spectral analysis, which is akin to Fournier analysis, and aims to discover periodicities in a series that on visual inspection does not appear to show any cyclised change; or a periodogram to define a definite pattern of mood swings and behaviour from longitudinal accounts of behaviour, weight and sleep patterns.

Neurotic disorders

With the resettlement of people with a learning disability into the community, it might be thought that more anxiety states will occur as these people, with often multiple handicaps, try to preserve dignity in everyday life. In Day's (1983) study of admissions to a mental handicap hospital over a five year period, 28% were diagnosed as 'neurotic'. Everyday situations, e.g. visiting a post office, may be stressful, and minor upsets or unanticipated situations may induce a state of agitation. They cannot be trained for every eventuality. Individuals with autistic spectrum disorders are thought to be particularly anxious, living as they do in an often kaleidoscopic cacophonous world, unable to make sense of many of the stimuli staring in upon them, and the more able people with Asperger syndrome might be envisaged to be living apprehensively, as if every day they half expected to be made redundant by lunchtime. In a study of institutionalised learning disabled people, a prevalence of 3.5% was reported for obsessive-compulsive disorders Vitiello et al., 1989).

Phobic states are widespread amongst the learning disabled, and may be situational specific and well-circumscribed, or protean, as in avoidant personality disorder, which is common in mild LD. Phobias are particularly prevalent in phenylketonuria that is untreated or where treatment was terminated in childhood (Tuinier & Verhoeven, 1993).

Conversion and dissociative hysteria features are common, and sometimes grotesque in people with learning disability. This is a function of increased suggestibility and secondary gain being readily available.

Personality disorder

Reid and Ballinger (1987) in their survey of hospitalised mild/moderately handicapped adults reported 56% as having features of abnormal personality, and in 22% this was felt to be of a severity to suggest a personality disorder, and Day (1985) found personality disorder to be the commonest psychiatric diagnosis in the learning-disabled amongst first admission psychiatric patients. In the more severely disabled, to diagnose personality disorder using current DSM-IIIR or ICD-10 typologies is not possible.

Personalities associated with particular phenotypes

Fragile-X

Fragile-X syndrome has been named after the fragile state at the long arm of the X chromosome (Xq 27.3), which can be seen with cytogenetic testing in folic acid-deficient medium in 2–60% of the cells in affected males (de Vries *et al.*, 1994). Most affected males have, as main clinical features, intellectual disability, macroorchidism and large everted ears. The facial features are less marked in females and children. In families with the fragile-X syndrome, both males and females have to be studied for their carrier status as there are 'normal transmitting males' to complicate the chromosome inheritance. A minority of individuals with autistic spectrum disorder have fragile-X syndrome, and some people with fragile-X do demonstrate typical autism. The typical behavioural profile of the person with fragile-X is, however, of social anxiety rather than social indifference; speech and language abnormalities, stereotyped behaviour and self-injury are common. This can be considered as a 'growing gene defect', going through a premutation stage that does not seem to be associated with obvious gene dysfunction. While the full mutation more than 200 CCG triplet trinucleotide repeats is necessary for intellectual disability, there is a suggestion that premutation and the fragile-X genetic defect in female heterozytes confer increasing vulnerability to some form of adult psychopathology, including schizotypal features (for a review, see Turk, 1992*b*).

Prader-Willi and Angelman syndromes

These are disorders where genomic imprinting plays an important part, that is, whether the child has Prader–Willi or Angelman syndrome depends on the parent at origin of the chromosome bearing a specific defect, a micro deletion of the long arm of chromosome 15 (male chromosome microdeletion for Prader–Willi syndrome). There is considerable variability in the extent and severity of the clinical manifestations of this disorder; there are some common behavioural and personality problems. In addition to disturbed behaviours due to hyperphagia, and related to dysfunction in endorphinergic systems (Lehnert *et al.*, 1990), psychosocial adjustments and relationships are often impaired, partly because of sensitivity about physical appearance and also feelings of worthlessness and inferiority (Berg & Gosse, 1990). In questionnaire surveys, the following characteristics have also been noted: skin picking, belligerence, stubbornness, irritability and impulsiveness (Greenswag, 1987), and psychotic episodes (Curfs *et al.*, 1991). The Angelman or Happy Puppet syndrome (female chromosome microdeletion) has a very different phenotype, viz. indiscriminant smiling and jerky athetoid movements (Summers *et al.*, 1995).

The study of behavioural phenotypes is an expanding and potentially important area for psychiatry, and phenotypes have been delineated for Lesch-Nyhan's syndrome (Goldstein *et al.*, 1985), Down's (Gath & Gumley, 1986), Rett's syndrome (Rett Syndrome Workshop, 1988), Cornelia de Lange syndrome (Ireland *et al.*, 1991) *inter alia*. Many of these syndromes are rare. The prevalence of Prader-Willi is 12 per 100 000 and of Rett's is 2.5 per 100 000.

Differential diagnosis

In more-disabled individuals it can be difficult to distinguish personality factors from the long-term consequences of psychotic illnesses. The operational definitions of some personality disorders include symptoms that may be difficult to identify as separate from the features of a learning disability, e.g. inadequacy, passivity (again diagnostic overshadowing occurs – a characteristic of LD is the individual's need for external reinforcers).

Organic psychoses

The effects of organic cerebral diseases are more pronounced in people with learning. disabilities than in the general population.

Acute organic brain syndromes

An important cause of acute confusional states in the learning disabled are drug side-effects. Not only are they susceptible to the unpredictable dosage and side-effects of anticonvulsants, antidepressants and tranquillizers – but face the added hazards of frequent polypharmacy. People with learning disability are one of the most highly medicated populations in our society.

Chronic organic brain syndromes

People with Down's syndrome who survive into middle age are prone to develop Alzheimer neuropathology that is not universally manifested as a frank clinical disease. The appearance of brain dysfunction in people with Down's syndrome in middle life is complicated by the increased likelihood of pseudo-dementia due to hypothyroidism. By the age of 50, only 40% of people with Down's can confidently be said to be euthyroid. Regular screening of thyroid-stimulating hormone, thyroid antibodies, thyroglobulin and microsomal antibodies are necessary.

The cognitive deterioration and changes in personality are often subtle and hard to detect. Franceschi *et al.* (1990) reported that the prevalence of clinical dementia in a mildly handicapped Down's group increased from 0% in the 20–29 age group to 55% in the 40–55 age group. Acknowledging the unrepresentative nature of their sample, the authors still felt that this was an underestimate of the true prevalence, with difficulty in detecting early clinical signs as the main source of error.

Withdrawal from conversation, loss of interest in activities, increased mental rigidity and irritability, occasionally inappropriate mischievousness, deterioration in gait – shuffling and loss of co-ordinated walking pattern – were found by Lott (1982) in a detailed study of individuals with early onset dementia. (However, whether gait could be attributed only to dementia or the possible effects of atlanto-axial subluxation (Cooke, 1984), which may present as a gait problem, and even paralysis due to sudden exercise causing abrupt flexion and extension of the neck remains uncertain). Urinary and faecal incontinence are later manifestations of the dementia. At this time, patients may show moderate or severe cortical atrophy on CT scans. Most of the research in this area is based on cross-sectional descriptive data, and there is a need for longitudinal prospective studies to determine the relationship between such variables as clinical decline and neuropathological changes.

Individuals with moderate and severe mental retardation who survive into old age tend to be the higher functioning individuals in good health (Moss, 1991).

Epilepsy

Epilepsy is common among the learning disabled and the prevalence rate increases with the severity of brain damage and the degree of intellectual handicap (Corbett *et al.*, 1975). As mentioned earlier, Rutter *et al.* (1970) demonstrate that there was an association between epilepsy and psychiatric disorder, although the nature of this relationship remains unclear. Studies have produced contradictory results with regard to the relationship between temporal lobe epilepsy and psychoses, and although bipolar affective disorders do not seem to be associated with epilepsy, there is some evidence that depressive disorders are more common in epileptic patients. Deb & Hunter (1991*a,b*) found no support for the belief that people with LD and epilepsy were more behaviourally difficult or that personality disorder was related to epilepsy.

Treatment issues

The techniques available

In the management of an emotionally disturbed person with learning disability, an Individual Programme Plan (IPP) will contain a variety of psychological approaches (for review of non-medical treatments see Fraser & Rao, 1991). These include sensitive disclosure of diagnosis (Bicknell, 1983), which has resulted in guidelines to paediatric staff aimed at reducing the family's hopelessness and encouraging a realistic attitude of relative optimism; psychodynamic psychotherapy (Frankish, 1989); behaviour/cognitive therapies for specific syndromes such as phobias (Lindsay, 1991); and anger management approaches such as the Novaco technique (1975), which incorporates at various stages cognition, expectations,and appraisal of situations in which the client has shown unreasonable anger, and is taught alternative social skills to address anger-evoking problems. For self-injurious behaviour (SIB), a range of extinction procedures, positive reinforcement, differential Reinforcement of Other Behaviours, (DRO) (see Zarkowska & Clements, 1988), and Gentle Teaching involving interrupting aggressive and self-injurious behaviours, and redirecting the subject to certain tasks, which are socially reinforced. The technique claims to enhance 'bonding' (McGee *et al.*, 1987). There are specific therapies like Permission/Limited Information/Specific Suggestion/Intensive Therapy (PLISSIT) (Anon, 1976) in the management of inappropriate sexual behaviour. Augmentive manual communication techniques such as Makaton (a simplified British Sign Language) (Walker & Armfield, 1981) can circumvent communication breakdown and alleviate maladaptive styles of communication such as self-injurious behaviour.

Medication

A major concern in medication of mental illness in persons with mental retardation is the major effects of psychopharmacological agents on functions of people with retardation and mental illness. It is unlikely that biological dysfunction and effective psychopharmacological treatment are specific for nosological entities (Tuinier & Verhoeven, 1993). Learning disability is moving to treatment based on specific clinical features rather than on psychiatric diagnosis. The use of drugs simply to control behaviour disturbance is therefore being frequently challenged in the US Courts, and firmer guidelines are now being developed by the National Institutes of Mental Health and Association for Retarded Citizens, and in the UK by the Royal College of Psychiatrists. Whilst the prescription of the major tranquillizers for mentally ill people with learning disability is warranted, medication has to take account of the multiple additional handicaps these people have (cardiac, renal and metabolic); the medical histories are likely to be incomplete and informants not present or capable. We do not know the idiosyncrancies of side-effects of medication on the protean disorders and phenotypes. People with learning disability seldom complain about side-effects.

Prescriptive guidelines

The Royal College of Psychiatrists' Learning Disability Section has accepted the guidelines for the use of psychotropic medication in individuals with developmental disability devised by Einfeld (1990). Accordingly, these guidelines form the basis of regular audit in most clinical teams. They involve particular scrutiny of the notes for descriptions of the behaviours and setting out the case for a choice of one medication over others; what other treatments coincide with this; describing what inter-disciplinary consultation there is about addressing the target symptoms, and what specific assessment instruments (e.g. Reiss Screen) are being used to validate neuropsychiatric diagnosis and to measure real improvement as distinct from anecdotal improvement; what the review dates are and when they are reached; the reasons for further continuation or cessation of medication and plans to deal with withdrawal effects.

Consent issues

Where there may be mental incapacity, for safe practice the following points are axiomatic: 1) the ability to consent should be assessed objectively by specific questions to demonstrate lies, ignorance, linguistic incompetence; 2) an independent third party should be present to check for influence in decision-making; 3) a person should be allowed enough time to answer; 4) language used should be easily understood; 5) acceptance of the next-of-kin is desirable; 6) sometimes a guardian, court-appointed depending on the national or State laws, should be consulted. There are batteries of tests for suggestibility; if there is real doubt, then the firmness and confidence with which the subject completes progressive matrices and a state anxiety inventory should be completed. People with learning disabilities often are compliant to save 'face'. In addition to suggestibility and voluntariness, there is understanding of the risks of a treatment. Further problems are how much can parents and guardians consent – in most countries, they cannot. Often treatment is started on the basis of a double negative – the patients does not disagree. Implicit consent is for meals, clothes and toileting. In the past this included taking tablets; this assumption of agreement on behalf of people with learning disability is now becoming an issue. Where the person is unconscious and the treatment is lifesaving and not to act would constitute negligence, the doctrine of necessity prevails. The use of antipsychotic medication to control aggressive behaviour is accepted by AAMR (1993) as occasionally necessary.

The significance risk of fatal cardiac effects when high doses have been used for people of normal intellect, apply even more to people with learning disability, as they are likely to receive such IM or depot doses when they are 'monitoring' or agitated – times that will increase drug absorption. Deaths have been reported (Goldberg, 1993). There is some evidence that psychotropic medication may reduce aggression and stereotyped behaviours such as overactivity and self-injurious behaviour (Aman *et al.*, 1985) but learning speed may also be reduced. The conventional medications, chlorpromazine, thioridazine and haloperidol, may be beneficial in very low dosage when combined with behavioural interventions (Aman, 1987). There is evidence that neuroleptics that are primarily dopamine D2 receptor blockers, such as haloperidol, are, however, less useful than D1 blockers, e.g. zuclophenthixol, or D1–D2 blockers, e.g. fluphenazine, for self-injurious behaviour (Goldstein *et al.*, 1985). When there are indications of clinical depression, dietary increases in serotonin and combined dietary serotonin increase (e.g. with banana, kiwi fruit supplements) combined with medication, namely 5-HT receptor agonists (Gedye, 1990) have been used successfully to reduce aggression that may be due to depression. Serotonergic mechanisms are implicated in some self-aggression and self-mutilative behaviours in people with LD, and there are several papers, e.g. Sovner et al. (1993), Markowitz (1990), using fluoxetine successfully. Dietary supplements have also been successfully used in the form of folate therapy in young people with FXMR (Webb *et al.*, 1986; Turk., 1992*b*), and vitamin B6 and magnesium supplements (Rimland, 1993) with an improvement in concentration and restlessness, but not in conduct disorders. In attention deficit disorder, additive restrictions, e.g. the very restricted 'few food' diet have now been shown to be effective (Graham, 1993), and where there is a clear indication of phasic behaviour and aggression, it is worth trying lithium (Tyrer *et al.*, 1984). In children with attention deficit disorder with hyperkinesis (ADDH), stimulants such as amphetamines, methylphenidate or pemoline have shown benefit. Methylphenidate is not usually prescribed under the age of seven years. In younger children, anecdotal evidence suggests that dexamphetamine sulphate is preferable. In ADDH with epilepsy, anticonvulsants such as vigabatrin may improve attention and concentration (McGuire *et al.*, 1992), and lamotrigine, mood.

A recent review (Tuinier & Verhoeven, 1993) found no firm conclusion on the use of opiate antagonists in the treatment of self-injurious behaviour can yet be made. Most assessments with naltrexone showed improvement but were single case-studies.

In conclusion

The coexistence of mental retardation and mental illness in the same individual presents unique diagnostic and treatment challenges. There has also been definitional confusion in the past and traditional classification has not been adequate to deal with people with such atypical development and lack of communication.

Behaviour disturbance in people with LD has multiple origins, with psychiatric disorder being just one possibility. Professionals have conceptualised 'challenging behaviour' restrictively from their own discipline's typologies, practices and perspectives. Clear distinctions are necessary between behaviour disturbance and psychiatric disorder, and rigorous guidelines are needed in the use of psychotropic medication, which should be used only in combination with psychosocial interventions. In each prescription, a rational *behavioural* pharmacotherapy must be attempted.

16

Sexual disorders

M. J. CROWE

Introduction

Sex is a powerful influence in the lives of most people, and in those who suffer from psychiatric disorders it often plays a central role. There are five areas in which sexual problems are likely to interact with psychiatry: the first is that of sexual dysfunction, the second is alternative sexuality, the third is gender dysphoria, the fourth is the choice of inappropriate sexual objects and illegal sexual activities and the fifth is the aftermath of traumatic sexual experience.

The sexual urge is one of the most compelling in the field of biology, and in most animals sexual reproduction is the only method of propagating the species. It is not therefore surprising that because of its strength this urge sometimes becomes attached to inappropriate objects, or that in the case of dysfunction its lack of fulfilment can lead to feelings of global inadequacy.

The biological basis of sex has been well reviewed by Bancroft (1989). The sexual experience is essentially psychosomatic, involving cognition, emotions, the endocrines (including testicles and ovaries), an arousal centre in the limbic system, spinal arousal centres, the cardiovascular system generally, the genital nerve and blood supply, the male genital tract, the vagina and the uterus. Thus there are a large number of steps in the cycle that may go wrong, and it would be surprising if some problems did not arise in such a complicated series of responses.

In males the presence of testosterone is needed for the 'spontaneous' expression of sexual behaviour (Bancroft & Wu, 1983). Men seem to have a more biologically determined sex drive, whereas women seem to be more susceptible to the effects of social learning in their sexuality (Udry et al., 1986). However, there is a great deal of individual variability in the level of sexual interest in both men and women.

Other influences on sexuality are social and cultural. An example of the social factors is the great increase in pre-marital sex in most western societies in the past 30 years, and the institutionalisation of non-marital cohabitation. On the cultural side, there are persisting differences, for example, between Asian immigrant groups in whom pre-marital sex is still quite rare and Afro-Caribbeans in whom it is common.

In the past four decades there has been a great increase in permissiveness about sex, and a parallel increase in the amount of help available to those with sexual dysfunctions. At the same time a reduction has occurred in the disapproval shown in both forensic and clinical settings to those who show variant sexual desires or behaviour (Gagnon, 1975). By the same token, however, this openness about sex has led to a greater consciousness of the quality of the sexual experience and to worries about not meeting the high standards of sexual performance continually set, either explicitly or implicitly, by the media. There is also a good deal of anxiety among some patients about the shape or size of their sexual organs, and urologists are often approached to perform surgical corrections on genitalia that may not in fact be far from average in size or shape. Sexual matters are probably destined always to be the subject of political and moral attention, and any account of the clinical aspects of sexual function must also be set in the context of the rules and attitudes prevailing at the time.

Sexual dysfunctions

Although the typical couple presenting sexual dysfunction is a married heterosexual one, it is increasingly common for couples who are not married to enter treatment, and at times one also sees couples who are homosexual (male or female) and unattached individuals. Much of what is written in the present chapter will be orientated to the typical heterosexual coupe, but may in most cases be read as applying equally to the more atypical couples or to individuals.

Classification

Sexual problems can be broadly divided into those of interest (desire), arousal and orgasm. Following the classification of Kaplan (1974), Hawton (1985) has devised the schema shown in Table 16.1. In addition, Masters & Johnson (1970) have distinguished between those dysfunctions that are primary (present since the first attempt at intercourse) or secondary (following a period of normal function), and between those that are total (present in all circumstances) or situational (present only under certain conditions). The other frequently used division, into functional and organic problems, is less helpful, since in most problems there are both organic and psychological aspects that are hard to disentangle and must both be taken into account in a comprehensive treatment programme.

The human sexual response

Masters & Johnson (1966) distinguished four stages of the physiological response cycle: (1) excitement, (2) plateau, (3) orgasm and (4) resolution. The first two of these involve vasocongestion of the corpora cavernosa and corpus spongiosum in the male (leading to erection) and the clitoris and vaginal walls in the female (leading to swelling and lubrication of the vagina and erection of the clitoris). In both sexes these responses are mediated by a combination of psychological and sensory stimuli, and involve the parasympathetic nervous

447

Table 16.1. *Classification of sexual dysfunctions*

Aspect of sexuality affected	Women	Men
Interest	Impaired sexual interest	Impaired sexual interest
Arousal	Impaired sexual arousal	Erectile dysfunction or impotence
Orgasm	Orgasmic dysfunction	Premature ejaculation Delayed ejaculation Ejaculatory pain
Other types of dysfunction	Vaginismus Dyspareunia Sexual phobias	Dyspareunia Sexual phobias

system. They are not, however, blocked by atropine, and therefore probably have a different transmitter from acetylcholine; this may be VIP (vasoactive intestinal polypeptide), which is found in erectile tissue, and which can lead to erection when injected intracavernosally. There also appears to be a second mechanism involving the blocking of inhibitory alpha-adrenergic impulses, and it has been shown by Brindley (1983) that intracavernosal injection of phenoxybenzamine, an alpha-1-adrenergic blocker, can produce an erection in males. The physiology of sexual arousal is still incompletely understood, but the information we have has led to effective forms of pharmacological treatment for erectile dysfunction (see below).

The physiology of orgasm is even less well understood. In males the reflex that leads to ejaculation is usually triggered by rubbing the penis or by thrusting during intercourse. It is a two-stage process. The semen in the first stage is pooled in the prostatic urethra. In nocturnal emissions it is then slowly emitted from the urethra, whereas in ejaculation it is forcefully expelled by 8–10 rhythmic contractions of the muscles of the pelvic floor. The reflex is probably co-ordinated in the sexual centre in the hypothalamus, and the sense of pleasure accompanying orgasm is also appreciated cerebrally.

Orgasm in the female is probably very similar in nature, and it is similarly caused either by clitoral stimulation or by the thrusting of sexual intercourse. The sensation of pleasure is often also accompanied by rhythmic contractions of the pelvic floor, and in some women there is said to be an additional 'ejaculation' of a fluid from the urethra similar to prostatic fluid (elicited by stimulation of the 'G' or Grafenberg, spot on the anterior vaginal wall).

The prevalence of sexual dysfunctions

It has been estimated that between one-fifth and one-third of a normal population complains of sexual dissatisfaction or dysfunction (Frenken, 1976; Frank *et al.*, 1978). The frequency of some disorders increases markedly with age: for example Kinsey *et al.* (1948) found the prevalence of impotence to be 0.8% at age 30, 6.7% at age 50 and 55% at age 74. More recent surveys, with less good methodology, have estimated that premature ejaculation occurs in at least 10% of married men (Sanders, 1987) and that anorgasmia during intercourse is present in 42% of women (Sanders, 1985), although only 10% were totally anorgasmic in the survey by Kinsey *et al.* (1953). The uncertainties of this kind of survey are compounded by the difficulty in defining the problems in a simple and understandable way and in deciding at what level of severity to make the cut-off point in deciding whether a problem is present. They can therefore be accepted only as rough approximations at best.

There has been a change in the nature of problems presenting in sexual dysfunction clinics. Whereas Masters & Johnson (1970) found the most common female problem to be anorgasmia, Bancroft & Coles (1976) found that loss of sexual interest was the most common female problem, and this continues to be the picture in most clinics today.

Factors contributing to sexual problems

The sexual relationship is, as previously stated, a complex one, and the factors responsible for problems are not only quite numerous but in most cases multiple causes are present. They can be fairly crudely divided, however, into three categories: (1) physical factors, (2) individual psychological factors and (3) relationship factors.

1. Physical factors
   a) *Endocrine factors.* In males the absence of testosterone leads to loss of sexual interest rather than impotence (Bancroft, 1989). The same effect may result from pituitary damage, for example by tumours or meningitis. In women the level of sexual interest may vary with the menstrual cycle in various patterns: the most frequently found is a peak during the postmenstrual phase, but in some women a peak is also found in the premenstrual phase, and in others there is no peak as such (Warner & Bancroft, 1988).
   b) *Neurological factors.* Many conditions affect sexual function. Injuries or other lesions of the lumbar spine will usually be associated with impotence in the male and lack of arousal in the female. Thoracic lesions cause similar problems, but with these 'reflex' erections may occur, and ejaculation is possible, though this may cause a dangerous rise in blood pressure.

   Multiple sclerosis is often associated with impotence, especially when bladder function is disturbed. Other spinal conditions such as subacute combined degeneration may cause sexual dysfunction.

   Diabetes is associated with impotence and lack of arousal, partly because of autonomic neuropathy and partly because of vascular changes to the arterioles of the penis and vagina. There are also in many diabetics psychogenic aspects connected with invalidism and depression. The incidence of impotence in male diabetics is more than four times higher than that in the general population, but it is of course far from universal in this group.

   In those suffering from chronic brain syndrome, loss of desire is often found (Fairbairn *et al.*, 1982). In epilepsy there is often a reduction of sexual desire in both sexes, and this has been attributed party to the condition itself and partly to the anti-androgenic effects of some anticonvulsants.
   c) *Vascular problems.* In patients in whom the arterial supply of the penis is reduced (for instance, after pelvic injuries or where the aorta is blocked) there is often a loss of erectile capability. Damage to the arterioles by diabetes (see above) can cause

449

Table 16.2. *Medications and other substances that may affect sexual function and desire*

1   Antidepressants
MAOI: impotence/delayed ejaculation
Tricyclics, noradrenaline uptake inhibitors: impotence and rapid ejaculation
SSRI and 5-HT uptake inhibitors: mainly delayed ejaculation
Antidepressants can increase sex drive
2   Anithypertensives
Betablockers can contribute to impotence.
Ganglion blockers, reserpine and methyldopa can cause impotence. Most recently introduced antihypertensives do not affect potency.
3   Diuretics
Most thiazide diuretics can contribute to impotence
4   Tranquillizers
Most benzodiazepines can contribute to impotence and may reduce sex drive
Most antipsychotics can contribute to low sex drive (some such as benperidol are used to lower unwanted sex drives)
5   Antiparkinsonians
Both bromocriptine and L-dopa can cause disinhibition and appear to increase sex drive, but it is probably not a direct effect.
6   Drugs of addiction
All such drugs lower sex drive when the patient is addicted. Heroin is probably the most likely to do so even without addiction, and there are unsubstantiated claims that cannabis can enhance sexual experience
7   Alcohol
This can produce disinhibition and probably aids sexual experience in small doses, but it has several negative effects:
reduces testosterone levels
increases blood pressure
reduces genital sensitivity
in long-term use can damage nerves
makes the drinker clumsy and demanding
partner finds the drinker unattractive

impotence. The venous drainage of the corpora cavernosa may be too effective, either through fistulae or as a result of abnormal veins in the pelvic region. This can lead to inability to sustain erection, or to impotence. Surgical correction is possible, but not always very successful (Rossman *et al.*, 1990).

Hypertension predisposes to atheroma, and is associated both for this reason and through other less understood mechanisms with an increased incidence of impotence; in addition some of the drugs used to treat the condition can cause impotence (see Table 16.2).

d) *The effects of medication.* Many drugs, both prescribed and unprescribed, can contribute to sexual dysfunctions. The list in Table 16.2 is not exhaustive, but gives the most commonly encountered ones.

e) *Local pelvic conditions.* These are mostly involved in the causation of dyspareunia in women. Local infections of the vagina such as herpes genitalis, candidiasis and urethritis can all cause pain during intercourse. Deeper pelvic conditions such as salpingitis, tumours and cysts can also cause dyspareunia. Hysterectomy has a variable effect on sexuality, but some women report interference with orgasm, and others lose sexual interest.

In men, the effects of prostatectomy are quite complex, and between 5 and 20% of men have erectile problems after the operation (Bancroft, 1989). There is also a high incidence of retrograde ejaculation in this group.

f) *The effects of ageing.* In both sexes there is a delay in genital vasocongestion in response to sexual stimulation with increasing age. Erection and lubrication are slower to develop, and may be more easily lost during sexual activity.

In males, there is a steady reduction in the preferred frequency of sexual release, and an increased tolerance for frustration. It is not clear whether this is due to the slight decrease in free testosterone with age or to more subtle psychological or physical aspects of ageing. Individual variations are quite extreme, and some men are sexually active into their eighties, while others stop in their late forties.

In women, there is a decrease in sexual interest with age, most marked between the ages of 50 and 60. At the menopause there is in some women a degree of atrophy of the vaginal walls, leading to thinning, shrinkage and reduction of lubrication. This can be corrected by hormone replacement therapy.

Age is, however, no bar to sexual therapy, and many older couples are well-motivated and achieve good outcomes in treatment.

2. Psychological factors
   a) *Stress.* This is a pervasive cause of sexual problems, perhaps affecting interest somewhat more than function as such. Stress at work, the difficulties of unemployment, the responsibilities of looking after young children or interpersonal conflict can all contribute to sexual problems. The presence of marital relationship problems is one of the most damaging types of stress, since the source of the stress and the sexual partner is one and the same person.

   b) *Psychiatric problems.* Most psychiatric conditions can lead to a reduced interest in sex. This is most obviously the case in depression, in which loss of libido is a common symptom. In most anxiety states, in agoraphobia and obsessive compulsive disorder, sexual problems are quite common. In schizophrenia sexual interest may be maintained, but the disturbance of interpersonal relationships inhibits sexual activity. In hypomania the libido may be increased, and some such patients may have a more active sex life than usual, but again the approach is often off-putting to potential partners and sexual activity may be reduced.

   Alcohol has a complicated effect on sexuality. It reduces inhibition, and may be a short-term mild aphrodisiac. In more regular use, however, it can reduce testosterone levels, may cause neuropathy, raises blood pressure and reduces genital sensitivity. All these reduce interest and responsiveness, and in addition the intoxicated partner may be both demanding and clumsy, thus reducing the other partner's interest in sex. Unfortunately, giving up alcohol does not usually restore sexual function, at least in the short term.

   Drugs of addiction tend to produce a low level of interest in sex, parallel to the loss of interest in anything other than the addiction itself. There is little to be done to improve an addict's sexual relationship until he or she can control the addiction.

c) *Pregnancy and childbirth.* Couples usually reduce their sexual activity in late pregnancy. After the birth most couples return to their previous level of sex, but in some this remains low. In most cases there is no demonstrable physical cause for this, but there are many other possible factors. The woman may centre her satisfaction on the baby at the expense of sex, she may be continually worried about the baby's welfare, she may be very short of sleep, she may resent the man's lack of help with baby care or the man because of his impatience may put her off sex.

d) *Past traumatic sexual experience.* Many women, and some men, have experienced child sexual abuse (CSA) or rape. In women the prevalence of severe or prolonged past CSA is at least 7% (Fritz *et al.*, 1981) and the incidence of past CSA in women under treatment for sexual dysfunction can be as high as 80% (Jehu, 1988). There may be disturbances of sexual function in such abuse survivors, but the usual pattern is of low sex interest accompanied by aversions to specific activities that formed part of the abuse. Other consequences of sexual abuse are described in a later section.

e) *Poor self-image.* This can be associated with past CSA, but is also found in other circumstances such as in those who have been brought up in institutions or in patients with personality disorders. It is often associated with a low sex drive, and with a general inhibition of enjoyment.

f) *Deviation in one partner.* This can often be compatible with an apparently normal sexual and general relationship, and it is only when the presence of the deviation is discovered that the problems begin in the relationship. In some cases the deviant impulse acts as a drive in competition with that for heterosexual intercourse, while in others the activities only occur when the deviant partner is depressed or otherwise below his or her optimal function. In therapy it may be possible to achieve a compromise, for example for the couple to agree that normal sex takes place on certain nights while the other activities are carried out by mutual consent on other occasions.

3. Relationship factors

A number of relationship factors can contribute to sexual dysfunctions (Crowe & Ridley, 1990). In turn, the sexual dysfunction may affect the general relationship, so that a kind of vicious circle can build up in which both problems become perpetuated. Some particular patterns are more common than others in contributing to sexual problems, as will be outlined below.

a) *Excessive politeness and consideration.* In such couples it is not unusual for the presenting problem to be that of non-consummation, either due to vaginismus or primary impotence. Both partners have a strong ambivalence towards sexual intercourse, and both seem very reluctant to cause or to receive any form of discomfort. They seldom have arguments, and it is often useful in therapy to help them to communicate more openly about their disagreements or resentments, in addition to more conventional sex therapy techniques such as sensate focus and the use of dilators.

b) *Continual hostilities.* Here the couple have very few periods in which there is sufficient peace between them to allow sexual activities to take place. One of Masters &

Johnson's (1970) most clear findings was that couples who experienced much marital distress were more difficult than others to treat for their sexual problems.

c) *Inequalities of dominance or assertiveness.* This can often be associated with inequalities of sexual desire. The more dominant or outspoken partner, whether male or female, is characteristically the more sexually interested, while the other partner may harbour a number of resentments that he or she never expresses. The arguments may centre around sex and its lack of frequency, but in some of these couples the non-dominant partner may be so good at avoiding arguments that they hardly ever occur, and the problem is put down by both of them to some 'illness' on the part of the uninterested partner. The remedy may lie in couple therapy techniques such as encouraging arguments or setting timetables rather than in more conventional sex therapy (Crowe & Ridley, 1990).

d) *Protective relationships.* In these sex seems to have a low priority. Here we are dealing with those relationships in which one partner might be depressed, anorexic, alcoholic or physically ill. The other partner may have taken a protective approach to the 'sick' one, out of proportion to the degree of handicap, and a relationship is formed rather similar to that of a nurse and a patient, or a parent and a child. In many of these couples sex is not an issue, and the goal of increasing sexual activity should not be imposed in therapy if the couple have not asked for it. However, where sex is desired, it may be necessary in therapy to try to equalise the 'balance' between them before expecting any improvement in their sex life.

e) *Inability to close the bedroom door.* Some couples find that sexual frustration builds up because they have not found a good way to exclude children from the bedroom, and therefore cannot find an opportunity for sex. The same problem may occur, especially in Asian immigrants, in finding an acceptable way to spend time as a couple away from the extended family with whom they are living. In both cases the therapist may need to work in a fairly practical way to help them to change ingrained attitudes and to find some privacy as a couple by drawing an appropriate boundary around their relationship.

f) *The influence of extramarital affairs on the sexual problems.* This situation may present the therapist with both ethical and practical dilemmas. The extramarital affair may have the effect of diluting both the emotional and sexual bonds that stabilise the relationship. However, the involved partner may be unwilling to let the outside relationship go, and the 'innocent' partner may be reluctant to forgive the other or to work on their sexual relationship, whose problems may have been part of the reason for the affair in the first instance. Therapists have to tread a careful path in such cases to help both partners without being censorious or too permissive.

Assessment

Initial assessment should include a full account of the presenting sexual problem, both from the patient and (if available) the partner. Sexual development should be covered, as should the sexual and general aspects of the relationship, and attempts to treat the problem so far. Specific points such as the presence of morning erections and sexual preferences should be recorded. In addition the presence of other psychiatric conditions, especially anxiety or depression, and any physical illnesses, with special reference to diabetes, hypertension or neurological illnesses, should be excluded. Individual problems with self-esteem and problems in the relationship should be explored.

The question of whether to pursue physical investigations in cases of impotence at this stage is debatable, with some clinicians carrying out nocturnal penile tumescence measurement, Doppler probes, penile–brachial blood pressure estimation and cavernosograms, and others leaving these investigations until after a trial of psychosexual therapy and a trial injection of papaverine. In our clinic we take the latter course, only referring the patient for these further investigations if there is an indication for urological treatment.

In cases of low sexual interest in males it is of use, where there is a question of testicular or pituitary failure, to investigate hormonal status, using testosterone, sex hormone binding globulin, luteinising hormone, follicle stimulating hormone and prolactin levels to give a composite picture of the patient's endocrine status. In the great majority of cases, however, the results are all normal and other causes for the problem must be sought.

Similar considerations apply to referral for gynaecological opinion, and in cases of dyspareunia we only refer those cases where there is no resolution of the pain following a course of psychosexual therapy and relaxation.

The components of sexual therapy

Psychosexual therapy consists of four main components. These are the behavioural component, the educational component, the psychotherapeutic component and relationship work.

1. Behavioural component

Masters & Johnson (1970) in their pioneering book outlined the programme for treatment of couples with sexual dysfunctions that most therapists use today, with additions and variations, as the basis of their work. The treatment is brief, symptom-focused and directed mainly at reducing performance anxiety and improving communication. Common to the treatment of all dysfunctions is the Sensate Focus homework technique. This involves an initial ban on intercourse, and on touching genitals or breasts. Instead the couple take turns in caressing each other, increasing tactile communication and giving non-orgasmic physical pleasure. At the next therapy session they discuss the experience and any problems that may have occurred. Paradoxically some couples break the ban on intercourse, and although this may not solve the problem permanently it can increase their morale and improve motivation. For many couples the use of relaxation exercises (Jacobson, 1938) is a helpful adjunct to sensate focus. They then progress to touching genitals and breasts, and after that begin to use specific techniques according to the particular dysfunction complained of.

For premature ejaculation, Semans' (1956) stop–start technique is used, in which the erect penis is stimulated, stopping short of the 'moment of inevitability', and thus inhibiting the urge to ejaculate: it is used first by the man, then by his partner and eventually intravaginally as part of the process of intercourse.

For erectile impotence Masters & Johnson recommended sensate focus followed by gradual intromission of the erect or semi-erect penis into the vagina with the woman on top or the couple side by side. The man should avoid 'spectatoring' and think relaxing thoughts.

For anorgasmia the couple are encouraged to practise clitoral stimulation using fingers, water spray or a vibrator. Most women find it easier to achieve orgasm this way than during intercourse, and after therapy the couple are asked to consider incorporating these techniques into their normal sex life.

For couples where the female partner has vaginismus (perhaps exacerbated by the male, see above) the use of gradual dilatation and vaginal muscle relaxation using either fingers or graded dilators is recommended, followed by slow progression to penile penetration, usually with the woman on top.

In couples with delayed or absent ejaculation the technique of penile 'superstimulation' is advocated, and the prognosis for this problem is much better if ejaculation is possible in masturbation rather than where the problem is 'total'.

2. Educational component

It is sometimes surprising to find quite marked levels of ignorance of sexual function, even amongst well-educated people. It may be necessary in this situation to discuss basic sexual anatomy and physiology with them, perhaps using slides or videotapes. This has the advantage of giving a common language to be used in further therapy, although in the great majority of couples it is not in fact needed.

3. Psychotherapeutic component

There are several approaches involving the application of methods derived from psychodynamic therapy to sexual dysfunctions. The Institute of Psychosexual Medicine (Tunnadine et al., 1981) has developed an approach based on the work of Balint in which interpretations of the meaning of the dysfunction are made by the GP or Family Planning doctor during vaginal examination. The conflicts thus exposed can often be rapidly resolved, with an improvement in the dysfunction.

Kaplan (1974) extended the Masters & Johnson approach, adding two components: the first was to give the clients an understanding of patterns of behaviour and their dynamic significance, and the second was to give deeper developmental insight where necessary. In some cases this entailed taking one partner into brief individual psychotherapy before returning to conjoint work.

Similar approaches are used by hypnotherapists (Fromm et al., 1970) to reach the subconscious factors inhibiting sexual expression. Again these may be combined with conjoint therapy to treat the combination of the 'turn-off' mechanism and the sexual dysfunction itself.

In cognitive therapy the individual is encouraged to alter assumptions and cognitions that are causing psychological problems including sexual dysfunctions (Beck, 1979). In some cases there is a history of sexual abuse or other adverse sexual experience in the past, and in these cases it is helpful to use a cognitive approach as in post-traumatic stress disorder, usually with the disturbed partner alone, as a preliminary to couple therapy (Douglas *et al.*, 1989).

4. Relationship work

For most couples with sexual dysfunctions it is useful to see the couple together, both to reinforce the need for co-operation in homework and to deal with aspects of communication and non-sexual relating that are contributing to the dysfunction. Hawton (1985) states that marital discord is the most common factor in the causation of sexual dysfunctions, and advocates the use of reciprocity negotiation (Stuart, 1980) to improve marital interaction and to help co-operation on sexual tasks. In this approach couples are encouraged to convert their complaints to wishes for future mutually rewarding behaviour, and sex can be brought into the exchange in a similar way to any other form of interaction.

More detailed couple therapy techniques can be helpful in sexual dysfunctions, especially those involving motivation (Crowe & Ridley, 1990). There are many couples where the unmotivated partner is quite unassertive and spends a good deal of the time they are together avoiding conflict and placating the more dominant partner. The more motivated partner (whether male or female) is often more open, and able to express emotion and to withstand conflict. In therapy it may be useful to engineer a conflict (preferably on a trivial or everyday topic) and to help the unassertive partner to keep his or her end up, while not antagonising the other. They will often thereby learn how to avoid some of the typical repetitive sequences of interaction that contribute to sexual withdrawal.

In those cases where there is a reluctant female partner and a male who is not only keen on sex but also pressurises her to comply, the 'negotiated timetable' (Crowe & Ridley, 1986) can be a very useful approach. In this, the couple are asked to plan their sexual activities for a particular day of the week, with a ban on sex on the other days. The plan has to be adhered to by both partners, and is often able to take the heat out of the sexual conflict. Both partners gain, the woman by the reduction of pressure on the 'non-sex' days and the man by knowing that he will be rewarded with sex on one day each week (or more if this was the agreement).

If these methods fail to resolve the problem the therapist can resort to a 'paradoxical' approach in which the couple are asked to continue the problematic interaction, for example the conflict over sexual frequency, but with a 'systemic' reason for doing so, such as the avoidance of further conflict or boredom. In some stuck cases this paradoxical injunction can unlock the impasse and produce improvement (Crowe & Ridley, 1990).

Mechanical and pharmacological treatments

A number of methods are available in the management of sexual dysfunctions when psychosexual therapy is ineffective.

The vibrator is now fairly widely used to produce orgasm in anorgasmic women (see above) and is also of assistance to men who suffer from delayed ejaculation (sometimes with the addition of yohimbine 30 mg by mouth half an hour before the attempt). A commercial vibratory body massager such as those made by Carmen or Wahl is usually satisfactory, but in more difficult cases a Ling vibrator will produce a more powerful stimulus.

Penile rings and vacuum devices (Cooper, 1974, 1987) are useful in some cases of erectile impotence. The vacuum device, when placed over the penis, will draw blood passively into the corpora cavernosa, and this can then be retained by means of a ring round the base of the penis. The tumescence produced may be sufficient to allow intercourse, but the penis is swollen rather than erect, and the method is not universally accepted. Rings alone or simple elastic bands may be used for those who can obtain a partial erection that is subsequently lost.

Intracavernosal injections may be used to produce 'pharmacologically induced penile erections' (PIPE). Wagner & Brindley (1980) used alpha-adrenergic blockers to produce this effect, but the approach of Virag (1982) has been more influential. He used the smooth muscle relaxant papaverine to produce erections, and until recently the most common treatment has been to use papaverine alone (between 8 mg and 120 mg) or in combination with phentolamine (2 mg) to give an erection lasting between 30 and 120 minutes. The patient has to learn the technique of self-injection, and since each patient has his own specific dose response it may be necessary to give two to three test doses before the optimum dose is found. The great majority of impotent patients can obtain erections in this way, but it is not acceptable to all patients, or indeed to their partners (Crowe & Qureshi, 1991), and there is a small risk of iatrogenic priapism if the dose is exceeded. If this occurs the patient is advised to attend the treatment clinic or accident department for decompression of the corpora by the removal of 50 ml of blood and the injection of an antidote (metaraminol 2 mg or phenylephrine 3 mg) intracavernosally. The use of prostaglandin E (Coverject) as an alternative has the advantage of being fully approved by the Committee on the Safety of Medicines, and not carrying the risk of priapism, but can cause quite severe pain in 30% of patients, and is highly expensive.

Yohimbine by mouth is fairly widely used as a treatment for erectile impotence, and appears to act centrally by an alpha-2 adrenergic blocking effect. Like papaverine it is not fully approved for use with patients, but clinically between 15 mg and 40 mg daily in divided doses can facilitate the erectile process. Controlled trials have shown a significant advantage for yohimbine over placebo in cases of situational impotence (Riley et al., 1989). However, some patients find the side-effects (mainly headache and nausea) intolerable. It should not be given to hypertensive patients without consultation with their medical advisors, as it can cause a rise in blood pressure.

In cases of premature ejaculation clomipramine (25 mg–50 mg by mouth one hour before intercourse) can help to delay ejaculation: however the effect is not a major one, and it is unpredictable which patient will respond. It is also found that the SSRI (specific serotonin re-uptake inhibitor) antidepressants have the same effect, but it is better to use the stop–start approach as the mainstay of treatment and to give medication only in those cases where psychosexual therapy is not controlling the problem.

The prescription of hormones is still somewhat controversial. In men with clearly demonstrable reduction in testosterone there is a need for replacement therapy, and this is best given parenterally in a long-acting preparation (since testosterone is metabolised by the liver after absorption from the gut). In cases with proven high prolactin levels it is reasonable to give testosterone or bromocriptine. However, androgens have no significant effect in enhancing erection, and they have a marginal effect in increasing libido, and this tends to reduce with time (as the natural testosterone production is suppressed by negative feedback). Their use has to be offset against the known risks of heart disease and prostatic carcinoma from androgens.

For women, however, the prescription of hormone replacement therapy can reverse the atrophic vaginitis that follows the menopause, and the risks appear to be outweighed by the general benefits to the health of the patient.

Surgical management

In cases of impotence unresponsive to other methods of treatment there are two surgical procedures that may be considered. If there is excessive venous outflow from the corpora, operations can be done to reduce this: they are however not uniformly successful, and even when they are the patients do not always make use of their new abilities in sexual activity. The other surgical approach is the implantation of Teflon rods or inflatable tubes into the corpora cavernosa. This can only be recommended with considerable caution, because of the significant technical failure rate and the irreversible loss of natural erectile function.

Successes and failures

These have been reviewed by Crowe & Jones (1992). Masters & Johnson, in their uncontrolled series, made some fairly ambitious claims. These have not been borne out in subsequent trials. For example, Hawton *et al.* (1986) found a 60% improvement rate in premature ejaculation as opposed to the 98% of Masters & Johnson. In vaginismus, however, we can accept that, as in Masters & Johnson's series, almost all cases can be helped to have a much more normal sexual life with complete penetration.

The treatment of impotence by psychosexual therapy seems to produce rather less than 50% improvement, but with the use of yohimbine, papaverine and prostaglandin E this total may be raised much higher, depending more on the acceptability of treatment than its effectiveness.

Controlled trials of therapy have not yet been done on the treatment of motivational sexual problems by the use of couple therapy (see above), but encouraging results have been found in pilot studies (Crowe & Ridley, 1986, 1990).

Alternative sexuality

I have used this term to cover many forms of sexual activity that differ from the conventional heterosexual mode but which in today's ethical climate are considered to be acceptable. Thus, male and female homosexuality, transvestism and transsexualism come into this category, as do many of the harmless forms of variation such as mild sado-masochism, fetishism and bondage.

Homosexuality

This variation from the norm is one of the most common. In the pioneering work of Kinsey (Kinsey *et al.*, 1948, 1953) it was shown that there is a spectrum from the totally heterosexual (Group 0) to the exclusively homosexual (Group 6), and that there are many individuals who do not fit the extreme categories but have had varying degrees of experience with members of both sexes. In both men and women there was a small minority who were exclusively homosexual (4% of men and 1% of women) but those who had had at least one homosexual experience, leading to orgasm, since adolescence comprised 37% of men and 18% of women. Subsequent surveys have on the whole arrived at lower estimates of homosexuality, perhaps due to better methodology (Johnson *et al.*, 1992). However, the greater numbers of bisexuals compared to exclusive homosexuals has been confirmed.

Historically attitudes to homosexuality have varied greatly. In ancient Greece and Rome male–male relationships were tolerated and even commended, although in most cases the men were also expected to father children. In most Western countries until the 1960s male homosexuality was considered a sin and in many also a crime. In many African and Asian societies today there is scant tolerance of it, but in most Western countries it is tolerated, and in some countries homosexual marriages can be solemnised. In the period between about 1945 and 1970 in this country and the USA, when its criminalisation was being questioned but before it was defined as a legitimate alternative way of life, male homosexuality was considered to be a psychiatric condition, and treatment was given, in the form of dynamic or behavioural psychotherapy.

Controversy still rages over the cause of homosexuality, and the 'illness' hypothesis still holds a number of adherents, perhaps especially among the parents of young men and women who have recently declared their homosexual orientation. The postulated causes divide themselves broadly into medical (mainly genetic), developmental (Freudian or other early environmental) and current influences (the idea that it results from contact with other homosexuals).

There is no agreement about the putative causes. Recent work by Hamer *et al.* (1993) has suggested that there might be a linkage between a gene on the X chromosome and male homosexuality. In view of the contradictory evidence from twin studies (Heston & Shields, 1968; Bancroft, 1989) this finding should be interpreted with great caution, and other evidence of biological differences between heterosexual and homosexual individuals is similarly inconclusive. For example, the levels of testosterone do not reliably distinguish heterosexual and homosexual males (Meyer-Bahlburg, 1977). However, the complete failure of behaviour therapy to re-orientate exclusive homosexuals (Bancroft, 1974) seems to offer some support for a lasting sexual orientation factor in such individuals which might be shown eventually to be biological.

Other possible theories include the effects of upbringing, with a weak or absent father and a dominant mother who encourages behaviour appropriate to the opposite gender. Another possibility is that low self-esteem may lead to such fear of heterosexual encounters that the individual chooses an easier path and becomes homosexual. The concept of environmental pressure to become homosexual is probably of more relevance to those who are potentially bisexual than to the exclusively homosexual. While there are well authenticated anecdotal examples of this occurring, it would be difficult to demonstrate that it was the only or even the main cause of altered sexual orientation in general. It remains, therefore, of only speculative explanatory value.

It is not unusual for those with a primarily homosexual orientation to express a wish for a change. The wish may arise from family pressure, from a wish to conform or from a wish to avoid the disadvantages of the gay life-style. If the person is totally homosexual in orientation and fantasy, a change to heterosexuality is very unlikely, regardless of the method used. However, if there has been any heterosexual interest or experience, the possibility of change of orientation is possible, and some combination of orgasmic conditioning, covert sensitisation and self-control techniques can be effective, but the person will remain essentially bisexual and will continue to have the potential to respond homosexually if the situation arises. In the majority of cases, however, it is best for the therapist to encourage the homosexual or bisexual individual to adjust to the status quo and accept his or her orientation.

Transvestism and transsexualism

The sexual significance of cross-dressing is complex, and it has at least four distinct forms (Bancroft, 1989).

1. Fetishistic transvestism is usually found in males who wear female clothes (usually underclothes) in order to achieve sexual pleasure. This behaviour is very similar to other types of fetishism, and the cross-dressing is usually restricted to the sexual situation, whether in intercourse or in masturbation.
2. The transsexual. This person (male or female) believes that he (or she) is really a woman (or man) who has been born into the wrong body. They cross-dress in order to feel comfortable and 'right', and usually try to be accepted as a member of the opposite sex. They are very likely to wish for hormone therapy and surgical sex reassignment, in order to be consistent with their 'psychological' gender (see below).
3. The double-role transvestite. This is usually a man who spends most of his time as a normal heterosexual male but at times has a strong but non-sexual urge to dress and pass as a woman.
4. The homosexual transvestite. This is a man or woman who is attracted to members of the same sex and who cross-dresses partly as a means of attracting partners and partly as a kind of caricature.

There is no genetic or hormonal cause that has been identified to account for either transvestism or transsexualism. However, some findings have suggested raised androgen levels in some female to male transsexuals (Sipova & Starka, 1977), and many male to female transsexuals are reported to have low sex drive (Hoenig & Kenna, 1979). The significance of these findings is uncertain, and it is probable that they are irrelevant to the majority of transsexuals.

Early childhood influences are often cited as factors in transsexualism, but are probably important in only a minority. They include (in feminine boys) overprotection by mother, an absent or rejecting father and encouragement by parents of feminine behaviour or interests. Most female to male transsexuals have been 'tomboys' in childhood, but less is known about other antecedents. Sometimes there may be a specific illness such as a paranoid psychosis or a depression that leads the patient for the first time to seek gender reassignment, and in these cases the resulting adjustment, if reassignment is offered, is often very poor.

The management of transsexualism has been reviewed by Christie Brown (1990). In many cases the surgical and hormonal reassignment process, which must be entered into only after a fairly prolonged period of counselling and a period of two years living as a member of the opposite sex without any surgical intervention, is often quite successful. However, a large number of social and legal hurdles (including changing name and identity) have to be overcome, and it must be emphasised that gender reassignment is not the simple process that many would-be transsexuals imagine it to be.

Other variations of sexual preference

Fetishism

This involves the arousal of sexual feelings by different parts of the body (e.g. by feet or ankles), by articles of clothing or footwear or by a specific material such as leather or rubber. In some cases the fetish is the only thing that produces arousal while in others the fetish is used as an adjunct to more 'normal' sexual activities.

It is generally believed that fetishism arises from specific conditioning of sexual responses to particular stimuli (Bancroft, 1989): however, there is probably a general predisposition to being aroused by unusual stimuli, which determines that a fetishist remains attracted to this fetish rather than (as in most males) allowing his sexual preferences to evolve and mature with experience. Rachman & Hodgson (1968) were able to condition erections to unusual objects such as boots, but these experimental subjects did not go on to become fetishists. As with other sexual variations the exact cause of the behaviour remains obscure.

Sado-masochism

This involves the arousal of sexual feelings in response to the inflicting of pain (sadism) or the experience of pain (masochism). It can include bondage, and some people are aroused both by inflicting and experiencing pain. While fetishism is almost exclusively a male preoccupation, the milder forms of sado-masochism attract both males and females: however, involvement in the more serious sado-masochistic activities including physical injury or extreme domination is more restricted to males. There is obviously a danger of serious injury or even death in sadistic activities, and there is a fine line at times between the harmless seeking for sexual pleasure in this way and the situation where it becomes unwelcome or frankly dangerous for (usually) the female partner. Among male homosexuals, too, the sado-masochistic elements of sexual arousal can lead to dangerous activities and injury or death.

461

Sexual offences

These can be divided into those that take place without the consent of the other party (i.e. rape, other sexual assaults, exhibitionism and voyeurism), those where the other party is under age (16 years for heterosexuals and 18 years for male homosexual behaviour); and those in which the behaviour itself is prohibited (e.g. bestiality and incest).

Rape

Heterosexual rape is clearly a common form of sexual assault, although the exact figures are not known. Much legal and other expertise has been directed to the dividing line between legitimate sexual intercourse and 'date rape' in which the man assumes a degree of consent that the woman feels she has not given. This is not, however, the only reason why the figures for rape are not well known, and there must be a considerable measure of under-reporting because of the reluctance of women to go through the legal process.

The characteristics of convicted rapists have been studied, and the majority of these are single and below the age of 24. Rape seems to correlate with other forms of aggression in some groups, and in others to be associated with a fear of rejection by women and a low self-esteem. The presence of attitudes in society that assume that women are 'fair game' have been blamed for the prevalence of coercive sexual behaviour by men. In particular, during war rape is documented to be quite a frequent occurrence, and some appalling examples have been reported from Bosnia.

The victim of rape is, like the perpetrator, more likely to come from the lower socio-economic groups, and in the USA black women are more likely that the rest of the population to have been raped, although no class, age or racial group is immune. The response of rape victims to the experience varies, but in one study (Becker et al., 1986) it was reported that 51% were significantly depressed and 59% showed sexual problems afterwards. There is conflicting evidence as to whether rape by a stranger is more or less traumatic than rape by someone known to the victim (Bancroft, 1989).

Paedophilia

This may involve sexual activities with either girls or boys, and at least 90% of those who abuse children are male. In some cases the abuser is unknown to the child, but it is probable that in a majority the abuser is a friend, acquaintance or family member. In a majority of convictions involving paedophiles no actual penetration has taken place, and indecent assault is a more common charge than rape or illegal intercourse. Men who are attracted sexually to children are a heterogeneous group, some being apparently stable and happily married while others have poorer adjustment and have had childhoods characterised by emotional deprivation and few friends (Bancroft, 1989).

Child sexual abuse within the family

This is much more likely to be perpetrated by men than by women, and the abuser is often a father, stepfather, elder brother, uncle, grandfather or other relative. In contrast to non-family abuse, the activity is likely to continue for a considerable time, and the betrayal of parental responsibility and the secrecy involved make it usually more damaging for the child. Families often break up under the stress of disclosure of sexual abuse, and the legal process is often emotionally damaging both to the victim, the perpetrator and the family as a whole.

The motivation for CSA within the family is probably quite varied, and not all incest perpetrators are paedophiles in a more general way. Some appear to do it in response to sexual problems within the marriage, others as a misplaced way of showing affection, and others again in the context of wider paedophilic desires. It has been reported that incest families have been characterised by frequent crises, sexual promiscuity and a higher than average number of children. The mother is often away from home because of employment or illness, with unsatisfactory child-care arrangements being made.

Exhibitionism

Indecent exposure is a specific crime in the UK but not in all countries. Rooth (1971) has reviewed the subject. Some perpetrators appear to be almost courting detection, such as those who practise it from their houses or cars, whilst others are careful not to be recognised. Some masturbate openly during the exposure, whilst others do so afterwards or not at all. As with rape, there appears to be a preoccupation with taking control of or insulting the female victim, if only to produce the reaction of shock. The typical offender is thought to be sexually lacking in confidence, and it has been suggested that there may be an unexpressed anger towards women in many cases.

Voyeurism

Again predominantly a male deviation, this is more an offence of the younger, single man (Gebhard et al., 1965), and the activity does not in most cases lead to sexual assault. It is often accompanied by masturbating, and can be seen as a publicly expressed version of the very common private activity of masturbating to pornographic pictures of women in magazines.

Obscene telephone calls

A recent form of sexual deviation that has features in common with exhibitionism and voyeurism, and can sometimes be carried out by the same individuals. There is a similar feeling of power over the 'unknown' victim, and in many cases the caller masturbates while talking to the victim.

Management

The management of sexual offenders is not an easy task. Many of them are unwilling to accept treatment unless they are already in prison or on probation, and even then their motivation is often suspect. However, in some cases there is sufficient motivation for out-patient or in-patient treatment, and in these cases there is a number of options. In the first instance it may be possible to suggest orgasmic conditioning. In this home-based self-treatment the patient is encouraged to masturbate with whatever fantasy (usually a deviant one) is able to stimulate the activity, and before achieving orgasm to switch the fantasy (perhaps with the aid of magazines or videotapes) to a more acceptable one. This is not a particularly powerful procedure, but may help some offenders.

In aversion therapy the patient imagines the deviant activity and then experiences an unpleasant sensation such as an electric shock to the forearm, or (in self-aversion) stings himself on the wrist with an elastic band pulled tight and released. This can be useful in some milder cases of deviation, but has not yet been subjected to controlled evaluation. A more acceptable approach, covert sensitisation, involves a similar procedure, but the unpleasant event is replaced by imagining an unpleasant consequence such as arrest, humiliation or adverse publicity. The offender is encouraged to carry out the covert sensitisation as homework as well as in the clinic.

Other approaches include group and individual therapy of a dynamic type, to explore and explain the underlying conflicts involved in the behaviour and thus to get it under control. No assessment of efficacy is available.

In extreme cases, where the behaviour is unable to be controlled by the therapies above, it is possible to administer cyproterone acetate by mouth. This has the effect of reducing all sexual drive, and not only the deviant impulses. However, in some cases this is an acceptable price to pay for freedom from unwanted and dangerous impulses, and the patient can sometimes be managed in the community with the aid of cyproterone where otherwise a custodial sentence would be the only viable alternative.

Sexual abuse and its consequences

Much has been discovered recently about the incidence of sexual abuse within and outside families. In adult females the prevalence of previous intrafamilial abuse up to age 13 in Los Angeles and San Francisco is 12–17% (Wyatt & Peters, 1986) and in the UK the incidence is estimated to be about 4 or 5% (Baker & Duncan, 1985). There is a much larger number of women who report having encountered 'non-touch' abuse in childhood, which may simply consist of being shown erotic materials or experiencing exhibitionism.

The consequences of intrafamilial abuse are very difficult to assess, in that some patients make inconsistent reports and in none of the cases is it certain that the symptoms reported have been caused by the abuse itself. However, in a review of a number of surveys (Jehu, 1988) it appears that in various psychiatric populations there is a higher than expected prevalence of prior sexual abuse. These include multiple personality and sexual dysfunctions (both above 80%), anorexia-bulimia (51%), drug abuse (44%) and psychogenic pelvic pain (36%). In addition there are many cases of past sexual abuse among patients who repeatedly attempt suicide and among those who mutilate themselves. Commonly, persons who have experienced abuse have more specific sequelae of the abuse including flashbacks, nightmares, phobias and avoidances. There is also likely to be low self-esteem, guilt and depression. The increased prevalence of prior abuse in the patients who suffer from the above symptoms or behaviour patterns provides suggestive evidence for a causal connection, but it is not yet fully proven that this is the case (Mullen *et al.*, 1993).

The traumatic after-effects of sexual abuse are experienced by both men and women, and when the victim is male there is not only the pattern of behaviour experienced by female victims but also the increased possibility that the victim may himself become an abuser of others. Women too may become perpetrators of sexual abuse, and there also seems to be a tendency for women who have been abused to marry or cohabit with men who themselves abuse the children of the relationship.

The treatment of post-abuse cases is very similar to that of any other patients with similar symptoms, and depends on the pattern of symptoms found. In some cases antidepressants may be helpful, whilst in others shorter- or longer-term psychotherapy may be the treatment of choice. In many the problem of past sexual abuse may be seen as a post-traumatic stress disorder to be treated by a cognitive approach similar to that used in survivors of disasters or victims of violent crime (Jehu, 1991). For those with sexual dysfunctions a combination of individual and conjoint treatment probably offers the best hope of improvement (Douglas *et al.*, 1989). In some cases the problems are so severe that the only possible treatment approach is medium- to long-term psychiatric admission.

Little is known about the ultimate outcome in these cases in terms of adjustment, but individual case reports suggest that some people who have survived abuse can be very well adjusted in later life. However, others have a poorer outcome, some commit suicide, some become chronically psychiatrically ill and others become abusers themselves (see above), thus repeating a 'cycle of abuse' into the next generation.

Conclusions

Sexual disorders are of importance in many areas of psychiatry, from the sexual dysfunctions themselves through the deviations to the consequences of sexual traumas in earlier life. Sex is an integral part of most intimate relationships, and sexual function can be disturbed in most types of psychiatric disorder. There are now a number of sexual problems that can be effectively treated by a range of approaches from the psychotherapeutic to the pharmacological and surgical. In the present cultural climate in which sexual matters can be openly discussed there is a great opportunity to research the area and produce further advances in the understanding and treatment of these important and common problems.

17

Mental illness in childbearing women

R. KUMAR, R. J. McIVOR and A. DAVIES

Introduction

Mental illness may adversely affect obstetric outcome and childbirth can precipitate or exacerbate mental illness. Childbearing women who are also mentally ill have very special needs, which are poorly recognised and incompletely met. The evidence for and against these generalisations is reviewed in this chapter, which begins with a short survey of psychological and social influences on obstetric outcome. We examine how pregnancy may affect psychological adjustment and review screening and management procedures. There are three conditions that are believed, to a greater or lesser extent, to have their origins in the reproductive process: the maternity blues, postnatal depression and postpartum psychosis. We shall examine the boundaries between these conditions and the nosological status of the two clinical disorders, postnatal depression and post-partum psychosis, with special reference to hypotheses about their aetiologies. The chapter ends with a survey of services and provisions for the detection and prevention of psychiatric disorders in childbearing women.

Psychological and social influences on obstetric outcome

Spontaneous abortion

It is very difficult to obtain accurate statistics about the frequency of miscarriage and it is estimated that up to 20% of diagnosed pregnancies do not progress beyond 20 weeks (Iles, 1989; Stirtzinger & Robinson, 1989). Given that the vast majority of spontaneous abortions, be they single or recurrent, are caused by sporadic chromosomal abnormalities or anatomical defects (Stirrat, 1990), it seems more likely that spontaneous abortion may cause psychological disturbance rather than vice versa (Osler et al., 1992). Methodological limitations of earlier research (e.g. Weil & Tupper, 1960; Kaij et al., 1969) restrict the significance of the reported links between stressful life events, personality characteristics and pregnancy loss. Leppert & Pahlka (1984) found that about 16% of a series of women who miscarried had levels of emotional distress and depression that were comparable in intensity and duration with emotional reactions to stillbirth or to the death of an adult. Friedman & Gath (1989) found that nearly half their sample of women admitted to hospital for a D and C after miscarriage were psychiatric 'cases', mainly depression – a rate four times greater than for women in the general population. Similarly, Thapar & Thapar (1992) found that women who had a miscarriage scored significantly higher on the depressive sub-scale of the General Health Questionnaire up to six weeks after the event when compared to control antenatal attenders. These findings underline the importance of recognising the distress that miscarriage brings, and the need for adequate treatment provision, be it at a specialist clinic (Turner et al., 1991) or in the community (Prettyman & Cordle, 1992).

Stillbirth

In the past it was common practice for a stillbirth to be treated as a non-event – the dead baby was delivered under drapes and parents neither saw nor held it, and the body was disposed of by the hospital on their behalf. A series of influential papers (Bourne, 1968; Lewis, 1976; Lewis & Page, 1978) began to change professional attitudes and practices and the expectations of parents by showing how denial of a life led to distorted mourning with consequent problems for the mother, the surviving family and any future babies.

The active management of stillbirth or perinatal death is primarily in the hands of obstetricians, midwives and primary health care workers. Savage (1988) has listed the following essential features of good practice:

1. Honesty with the bereaved parents.
2. Active involvement of parents in decisions about the funeral, keeping mementos, counselling and making contact with voluntary organisations.
3. Clear delineation of medical, paediatric, obstetric and midwifery responsibilities.
4. Consultant to be responsible for seeing parents and supervising staff – and for ensuring continuity of care.
5. Recognition of shock and denial phases of grief and opportunity for parents to change their initial decision.

Epidemiological and longitudinal studies (Kendell et al., 1981; O'Hara & Zekoski, 1988) have demonstrated associations between stillbirth and a raised risk of both psychotic and non-psychotic affective disorder. Psychiatrists can therefore exert an influence in two ways, firstly advising on and shaping the first tier of service, and secondly by accepting referrals where more intensive and specialised care is needed. It should be noted, however, that although a foetus of under 24 weeks gestation may be considered legally non-viable, it is a baby in the parent's eyes and therefore the management of early or late miscarriage should be sensitive to the needs, wishes and experiences of parents (see the Polkinghome Report, HMSO, 1989, which addresses issues about the disposal of the miscarried foetus, and the use of foetal material for research or therapeutic purposes).

Termination of pregnancy

In 1991, in England and Wales, nearly 20% of pregnancies were terminated under the terms of the Abortion Act, 1967 (CSO, 1992). The Act requires that two doctors must recommend that 'continuance of the pregnancy would involve risk of injury to the physical or mental health of the pregnant woman or any existing children of her family, greater than if the pregnancy were terminated'. Assessment of such risk takes account of the pregnant woman's actual and reasonably foreseeable environment. There are no *absolute* psychiatric indications for abortion and it is very unusual nowadays in Britain for a psychiatrist to be one of the two doctors recommending termination. Prior to the Abortion Act it was necessary for doctors to assert that to continue with a given pregnancy would almost certainly result in a mother becoming a 'physical or mental wreck' (BMJ, 1938) and expert psychiatric evidence, e.g. about suicide risk, was required in the comparatively rare instances when an abortion was contemplated on legal grounds.

The incidence of psychiatric disorders such as depression following therapeutic abortion is much less than that after live birth (Greer *et al.*, 1976; Ashton, 1980) and there may indeed be some resolution of psychological problems related to unwanted pregnancy in an unstable relationship (Brody *et al.*, 1971; McCance *et al.*, 1973). In contrast with postpartum psychosis, the occurrence of post-abortion psychosis is very rare (Brewer, 1977). In women who are determined not to have a baby but who are denied a termination, there are risks associated with subsequent criminal abortion, suicide (Whitlock & Edwards, 1968), depression (Hook, 1963; Pare & Raven, 1970) and conduct problems in the children (Forssman & Thuwe, 1966; Dytrych *et al.*, 1975). Women who repeatedly seek terminations and those who have abortions because of suspected foetal abnormalities (Donnai *et al.*, 1981; Iles, 1989; Iles & Gath, 1993) may be at greater risk of becoming depressed, but overall there is little evidence that there are significant long-term psychological sequelae in the majority of women following abortion (Zolese & Blacker, 1992; Clare & Tyrrell, 1994). The need for support and counselling, especially for vulnerable women, is underlined by a report (Kumar & Robson, 1978) of a reawakening of feelings of guilt and self-blame many years after a termination in the context of a subsequent pregnancy.

Failure to attend antenatal clinics

Although there is no simple relationship between pregnancy outcome and attendance for antenatal care (Hall & Chng, 1982), very late or non-attendance is associated with increased complications and a raised mortality risk (Ryan *et al.*, 1980). Factors associated with late or poor compliance with antenatal care include multiparity, ethnic minority group, lower socio-economic group, unplanned pregnancy, unstable marital and family relationships, insecure occupational status and a history of drug misuse. Many of these factors are also found in conjunction with mental illness (see Brown & Harris, 1978) and, therefore, it seems reasonable to argue that psychiatric disorder may also play a part in late attendance for antenatal care. It may be especially important to follow-up such women after delivery.

Impact of pregnancy on pre-existing mental illness

Pregnancy and psychosis

Some clues about the impact of pregnancy on rates of mental illness can be gleaned from large-scale epidemiological research and from studies of case-registers (e.g. Paffenbarger & McCabe, 1966; Pugh et al., 1963; Kendell et al., 1976, 1981). Overall, there appears to be a slight but significant reduction in rates of contact with psychiatric services and admissions during pregnancy compared with periods before and after childbirth, and studies of selected women with histories of bipolar and schizo-affective disorder suggest that pregnancy is usually a time of quiescence or remission (Marks et al., 1992).

Pregnancy and non-psychotic disorders

There is little evidence of any exacerbation of pre-existing affective disturbance during pregnancy (see reviews by Kumar, 1982; O'Hara & Zekoski, 1988; Marks et al., 1992). The risk of suicide during pregnancy is very low indeed, with a standardised mortality ratio of 0.05 (Appleby, 1991; Kendell, 1991b).

Pregnancy may herald the onset of obsessive-compulsive disorder (OCD) (Pollitt, 1957; Ingram, 1961), or may cause it to worsen (Brandt & MacKenzie, 1987). Neziroglu et al. (1992) found that in their group, 39% (n = 23) of OCD mothers had onset of illness during pregnancy. More than any other life event, pregnancy may hasten the onset of OCD (Stein et al., 1993). In contrast, there is limited, but conflicting evidence that panic disorder and related symptoms may improve during pregnancy (Klein, 1993, 1994; George et al., 1987; Cowley & Roy-Byrne, 1989). In a retrospective postal survey Villeponteaux et al. (1992) found that 14 of their 22 pregnant women with pre-existing panic disorder noted an improvement during the gestation period. Little is known about the effect of pregnancy on hypochondriacal symptoms, illness behaviour or beliefs. Savron et al. (1989) measured self-rated illness attitudes during each trimester in 26 pregnant women. As pregnancy progressed, childbearing women expressed more hypochondriacal fears and beliefs and conviction of disease than did normal controls. Such attitudes can obviously influence the sense of well-being of women, but their influence on the mother–baby relationship is not known.

Pregnancy only rarely precipitates the onset of an eating disorder, but it remains a difficult time for sufferers, particularly those with anorexia nervosa (Fahy & O'Donoghue, 1991). The weight gained in early pregnancy may exaggerate distortion of body image, as well as confronting aspects of sexuality, interpersonal relationships, mothering ability and issues of control (Franko & Walton, 1993). Most anorexic women will experience a worsening of their psychological health in the early stages of pregnancy, and may become more restrictive in their eating pattern. After delivery, many rapidly return to their pre-pregnancy weight (Stewart et al., 1987). With bulimic patients, bingeing and purging behaviour tends to regress during pregnancy itself, only to return, often more disturbed, in the postpartum period (Lacey & Smith, 1987). Women with eating disorders appear to have an excess of obstetric complications, including hypertension, difficult labours, miscarriage

469

and increased perinatal mortality (Fahy & Morrison, 1993). Babies may be born prematurely, have abnormal Apgar scores, and be of low birth weight. Indeed, bulimic behaviour or strict dieting may be a cause of teratogenicity in the foetus. Finally, sufferers may not be adequately able to look after or feed the baby, who may fail to thrive (Stein *et al.*, 1994).

Adverse effects of prescribed psychotropic drugs in pregnancy

One of the main sources of risk of harm to unborn infants of mentally ill women is from the ingestion of drugs, and the problem for psychiatrists is how to balance the mother's need for treatment against the potential threat to the developing foetus. It should be noted that the dose requirements for drugs may increase as pregnancy progresses because of changes in metabolic activity, fluid volume and absorption rates (Wisner *et al.*, 1993). For example, the lithium dose may need to be increased by 30–50% in the second trimester because of an increase in lithium clearance (Weinstein, 1980).

Lithium is believed to be associated with cardiac malformations if exposure is in the first trimester (Schou *et al.*, 1973; Weinstein, 1977), though recently these conclusions have been challenged (Jacobson et al., 1992; Cohen *et al.*, 1994). Until further studies have been reported, the use of lithium in the first trimester is best avoided. There are reports of stigmata and of developmental delays (Jones *et al.*, 1989) associated with carbamazepine exposure, mainly in early pregnancy. Neuroleptics, e.g. phenothiazines and butyrophenones, produce toxic effects in newborn infants medicated *in utero* (Hammond & Toseland, 1970; Hill *et al.*, 1966; O'Connor *et al.*, 1981) but Slone *et al.* (1977) did not find any evidence of teratogenicity. No information is yet available on the effects of the newer antipsychotic agents, such as risperidone or clozapine, on the developing foetus.

Initial reports of teratogenic effects of tricyclic antidepressants (McBride, 1972) have proved to be largely unfounded (Wisner & Perel, 1988). There are case reports of convulsions in newborn infants exposed to tricyclics *in utero* (Cowe *et al.*, 1982; Shrand, 1982) and it is therefore important to monitor neonates in such circumstances. In a preliminary report, Misri & Sivertz (1991) found that on follow-up, a group of women taking antidepressants during pregnancy did not experience an increase in labour complications or foetal abnormalities, nor were there any adverse effects in the breast-fed infants of those women. Short-term withdrawal effects were, however, present in the neonate. Monoamine oxidase inhibitors are not recommended during pregnancy. As with the newer antipsychotics, there is no information available on newer antidepressants such as the serotonin specific re-uptake inhibitors (SSRIs). Following exposure to benzodiazepines, dysmorphic features, growth retardation and CNS defects have been reported (Laegreid *et al.*, 1989) and follow-up studies are underway.

As far as possible, drugs of any type should not be prescribed in pregnancy. From the limited information available, one can conclude that it is relatively safe to prescribe tricyclic antidepressants and the older neuroleptics in later pregnancy. Recent evidence indicates that the use of lithium during pregnancy may not be as unsafe as once thought. However, as with carbamazepine, SSRIs and the more novel neuroleptics, its use should be avoided until more information is available.

Adverse effects of alcohol, and non-prescribed drug abuse in pregnancy

Alcohol and drug abuse during pregnancy and in the puerperium represent major public health and social problems. Pregnancy provides a powerful motivator for abstinence, but although attitudes to alcohol use appear to be improving (Ihlen *et al.*, 1993), those who are most addicted, and therefore most at risk, are least likely to give up. The situation is complicated because this vulnerable group is more likely to be socially disadvantaged, unsupported, report more adverse life events, and have a history of childhood and adult abuse (Closser & Blow, 1993); they are also likely to abuse more than one substance. Engaging these women represents a major challenge to the health professional. It is essential that indirect causes contributing both to the perpetuation of the abuse and to adverse psychological outcome are addressed, such as adverse psychosocial factors or psychiatric disorders (Raskin, 1993).

ECT and pregnancy

There are no scientifically controlled studies examining the impact of ECT on either the pregnant mother or the developing foetus, and the literature regarding this subject is limited to review articles (e.g. Impastato *et al.*, 1964; Brockington & Kumar, 1982) and case reports (e.g. Varan *et al.*, 1985; Yellowlees & Page, 1990). This work suggests that ECT does not carry an excess risk of adverse effects for either party. Indications for ECT during pregnancy are identical to those for non-pregnant patients and it is most commonly used for treatment of severe depressive illness.

The practical administration of ECT to pregnant women has been the subject of discussion and some authors have proposed their own guidelines (Remick & Maurice, 1978). Relative contraindications to ECT specific to pregnancy include risk factors for the precipitation of premature labour, such as cervical incompetence, and antepartum haemorrhage. It is therefore suggested that the obstetric team are involved in the management of all such patients, and that in addition to standard measures, external fetal heart monitoring is used during and for a short time after each treatment.

Psychiatric problems associated with the puerperium

Classification and chaos

The three main conditions associated with childbirth are the maternity blues, postnatal depression and postpartum psychosis, and it is surprising how often these names are inappropriately used – a floridly psychotic woman may sometimes be described as a 'bad case of the blues' and someone who is depressed may be referred to as a case of postpartum psychosis. There are two reasons for such confusion, one related to psychiatry in general and the other specific to mental illness related to childbirth. As with other psychiatric conditions, the criteria distinguishing, for example, severe postnatal depression with suicidal ideation

471

from postpartum psychosis have not been well described. There is a tendency to use the terms 'maternal', 'postnatal', 'puerperal' and 'postpartum' interchangeably, without clearly defining their meaning in terms of length of time after delivery. These factors, together with the lack of a pathognomonic symptom or syndrome, has led to a move away from regarding these disorders as etiologically linked with childbirth in modern classification systems (see ICD-10 [WHO, 1992a] and DSM-IV [APA, 1994]). Consequently it has become virtually impossible (see Meltzer & Kumar, 1985) accurately to identify 'cases' unless, as in Edinburgh, there is both an obstetric and a psychiatric case register available (Kendell et al., 1987).

Postpartum psychosis

The vast majority of cases present as affective illnesses, conprising either bipolar disorder (manic-depressive psychosis) or schizo-affective disorder. Schizophrenia presenting de novo in the puerperium is very rare. Postpartum psychosis has an incidence of 1:500 to 1:1000 live births. The risk of relapse following subsequent pregnancies is remarkably high, ranging from 20–50% (Schopf et al., 1984; Dean et al., 1989; Marks et al., 1992). Marks et al. (1992) have extended this finding to show that the primary clinical factor underlying the risk of recurrence is the time that has elapsed since the last episode of illness. Postnatal psychosis has much in common with other affective psychoses unrelated to childbirth in terms of symptom profile, previous history of manic-depressive illness, subsequent psychiatric morbidity and family history, and thus in the present state of knowledge cannot be considered to be a separate diagnostic entity.

Epidemiological surveys (Paffenbarger, 1964; Kendell et al., 1987) have shown the risk of mental hospital admission is raised significantly in the first three months postpartum compared with the two years before delivery. Kendell et al. (1987) have further demonstrated that for primiparous women the risk of developing a psychotic illness in the first month after delivery is raised by a factor of 35. Such a relative risk, which is one order of magnitude higher than the risk, for example, of becoming depressed following bereavement, suggests that childbirth plays a key role in provoking psychosis. This supposition is strengthened by the observation that the interval between birth and onset of illness is typically very short, most beginning within two weeks of delivery (Brockington et al., 1982). Further support comes from transcultural and historical surveys (see Kumar, 1994; Rehman et al., 1990) which show that neither the incidence of psychotic breakdown postpartum nor its manifestations have changed across time and culture.

It is tempting to speculate that the mechanism by which childbirth precipitates psychotic illness is related to the sudden fluctuations in hormone levels that occur following labour, and it has been proposed that psychosis may be triggered by the effects of postpartum oestrogen withdrawal on central dopaminergic function (Cookson, 1985). The observation that some sufferers are prone to relapse of their illness around the time of resumption of menstruation (Brockington et al., 1988) provides some clinical evidence in support of the oestrogen hypothesis for puerperal psychosis. In addition, Wieck et al. (1991), in a study of women at high risk of developing postpartum psychosis, have demonstrated enhanced dopaminergic sensitivity on the fourth day postpartum compared to a normal control group.

Clinically, symptom profiles vary. Insomnia is often the first reported symptom together with overactivity. Evolution of the condition is rapid and symptoms such as lability of mood, delusions and hallucinations follow quickly, often with accompanying behavioural problems. Suicidal and infanticidal ideation must be particularly looked for. While some authors (Brockington *et al.*, 1982) have emphasised the high prevalence of symptoms such as confusion and perplexity there is not sufficient evidence to suggest a pattern of symptoms unique to this disorder.

As a general rule women suffering from postpartum psychosis require admission to hospital, although a community-based service geared towards the management of severe postnatal mental illness in the patient's home has been described in Nottingham, UK (Oates, 1988). Mother and baby are usually admitted together either to a general psychiatric ward in which one or more rooms are set aside for this purpose, or to a specialised mother and baby unit. Where neither facility is available it may be necessary to admit the mother alone and make other provision for the care of the baby, either with other family members or social services.

All contact between mother and baby is initially supervised by the nursing staff. This is a matter of constant review and, as a patient's condition improves, contact with her baby increases accordingly. Physical treatment is dictated by the clinical picture, and neuroleptics, antidepressants, mood stabilisers and ECT are all used as appropriate. Some treatments, such as the use of lithium carbonate, will influence breastfeeding (Buist *et al.*, 1990). ECT has the reputation of being a particularly effective treatment for postpartum psychosis, particularly when symptoms such as confusion and perplexity form part of the clinical picture, although there are no controlled trials comparing the efficacy of ECT with other physical treatments.

The prognosis for postpartum psychosis is good and patients generally respond well to treatment. Illness relapse is, however, well recognised in the weeks or months after initial recovery and, as mentioned, this may be related to the onset of menstruation. Consequently, such patients merit careful follow-up and close liaison with general practitioners and health visitors.

Because of the high rate of recurrence following subsequent pregnancies, prophylactic treatment may be important. This is an area that has received little systematic attention, although there have been reports suggesting that lithium given immediately after delivery may protect against relapse (e.g. Stewart *et al.*, 1991). The use of neuroleptic and antidepressant drugs in the prevention of postpartum psychosis has not been evaluated to date.

Speculation regarding the role of falling levels of sex steroids in the precipitation of postpartum psychosis has led some workers to examine the utility of both oestrogen and progesterone in the prevention of this conditions (e.g. Schmidt, 1943; Bower & Altschule, 1956). The most promising report is that of Hamilton & Sichel (1992) who, in an uncontrolled study, reported no cases of relapse in a series of 50 women described as being at high risk, who were administered a combination of oestrone and conjugated oestrogens for 14 days after delivery. While it should be stressed that administration of sex steroids is not part of routine clinical practice, these findings merit further scientific exploration.

Postnatal depression

Following the seminal study by Pitt (1968) describing the onset of depression in the six weeks following childbirth in women who were not depressed antenatally, there was a plethora of confirmatory studies (see reviews by O'Hara & Zekoski, 1988; Kumar, 1994), placing the prevalence of depression in the first six weeks postpartum at between 10 and 15%. However, two controlled comparisons – one (Cooper et al., 1988) contrasting rates of postnatal depression with a general population survey (Surtees et al., 1983) and the other comparing a cohort of childbearing women with an approximately matched cohort of non-childbearing best friends (O'Hara et al., 1990) – challenged the concept of postnatal depression, because the rates were not raised above those in controls or in the general population. Recently, Cox et al. (1993) have shown that the risk of depression is about three times higher in childbearing women than in control subjects, but only in the first month. This finding requires replication, but it re-opens the question of whether there are depressions that are specifically postnatal. The answer may come from examining the aetiological factors that associate with depression of earlier (first month) as opposed to later postnatal onset. Several investigators (see review by O'Hara & Zekoski, 1988) have reported that a history of depressive disorders confers a higher risk of recurrence of depression following childbirth and Marks et al. (1992) showed that in comparison with women with no previous psychiatric history the risk is raised about threefold.

Links with severe dysphoria (Kendell et al., 1981; Hannah et al., 1993) and with emotional lability and even elation (Glover et al., 1994) highlight the importance of searching for physiological factors that might be implicated in the transition from blues to depression. Follow-through by Harris et al (1994) of their sample of mothers showed no association between salivary progesterone concentration at any time and the development of depression 35–40 days postpartum, thus undermining unsubstantiated claims by Dalton (1980) that postnatal depression is a progesterone insufficiency syndrome. There have been no studies as yet to test speculations about the role of oestrogen in postnatal depression (Studd & Smith, 1994), but there is some indirect evidence to implicate oestrogen in the pathogenesis of the illness following the finding that it is superior than placebo in treating postnatal depression (Henderson et al., 1991).

Initial investigations into the role of thyroid hormone dysfunction in postnatal depression (Hayslip et al., 1988; Harris et al., 1989 and Pop et al., 1991) suggested weak associations between depressive symptoms and measures of thyroid dysfunction. In a later report, Harris et al. (1992) described an overall increase in depressive symptoms in thyroid-antibody positive women followed for up to eight months postpartum. There are, therefore, several clues indicating that part, at least, of the aetiology of early-onset postnatal depression may have an endocrine flavour. In contrast, the depressions that develop later may have an aetiological profile that resembles that seen in the context of depression more generally (Brown & Harris, 1978; Paykel et al., 1980) – i.e. a combination of social adversity and life stress, on top of a cluster of vulnerability factors. The importance of such distinctions lies in the possibility that the early onset of depression may respond better to certain kinds of therapeutic interventions than to others, e.g. hormones (Henderson et al., 1991; Harris, 1994) versus psychological treatments (e.g. Holden et al., 1989).

The diagnosis and treatment of postnatal depression mainly occurs in the primary care setting, and only 2–3% of severe or treatment resistant cases are referred to psychiatrists. The midwife, health visitor and GP are in an ideal position to assess and diagnose, but research shows that up to 50% of cases go undetected (Sharp, 1992). The clinical picture is similar in many ways to other types of depression, but there are several features that should alert the clinician to the possibility of depression. The woman may be unable to care effectively for her baby, expressing difficulty in handling or feeding. She may be excessively concerned about the baby's health, or feel guilty that she is not coping. Despite the increase in psychiatric morbidity in the puerperium, the suicide rate in the first year postpartum is one sixth of what one would expect in an age- and sex-matched non-pregnant population (Appleby, 1991).

Since depression in the postnatal period shares many of the clinical features of depression occurring at other times, treatment options retain a similar framework (Elliott, 1989). Reassurance and supportive counselling are often all that is required, and these do not have to be provided by a doctor to be effective (Holden et al., 1989). Self-help and support groups encourage mutual support and advice concerning mothering and childcare, as well as more specific issues in dealing with depression. If the depression is associated with social circumstances such as marital or housing difficulties, these issues should be tackled.

Anti-depressant medication may be indicated, and the criteria for prescribing are the same as for non-puerperal depression. Breast feeding can usually be continued (Buist et al., 1990). Inappropriate use of benzodiazepines should be avoided. Adequate doses should be used, and treatment continued for the appropriate length of time. For severe, psychotic depression, neuroleptics or ECT may be indicated.

Demonstrations of adverse effects of maternal postnatal depression on childrens' cognitive and social development (Cogill et al., 1986; Murray, 1992; Kumar & Hipwell, 1994; Cummings & Davies, 1994) highlight the need for early detection and effective intervention.

Minor transitory mood disturbance (the 'maternity blues')

The term 'maternity blues' is somewhat misleading, since women in the immediate postpartum period may experience mild 'highs' as well as mild depressive swings (Hannah et al., 1993; Glover et al., 1994). The term 'minor transitory mood disturbance' may reflect a more accurate clinical picture. The condition is very common indeed, with anywhere between 50 to 75% of postpartum women experiencing a short-lived dysphoric reaction in the first week following delivery. It can thus be considered to be a statistically normal phenomenon. O'Hara et al. (1991) found a link between a greater fall in pre- to postnatal plasma oestriol concentration and the blues but no such association with oestradiol or progesterone. Harris et al. (1994) have found a similar link between the blues and the fall in progesterone concentration. Other investigations (Okano & Nomura, 1992) report association between high blues scores and concurrent plasma cortisol concentrations.

Transient postpartum mood disturbances do not require any specific treatment apart from reassurance and explanation. It is important that they be distinguished from the prodromal features of puerperal psychosis, which often commence during the same time period. If they persist for longer than two weeks then a diagnosis of depression should be considered.

Services for childbearing women with psychiatric disorders

The conclusions of a recent British survey of services for mentally ill mothers and their infants (Working Party, Royal College of Psychiatrists, 1992*b*) included the observation that 'there were few comprehensive services, large deficits in in-patient provision and designated hospital facilities, as well as a lack of specific consultant-led teams with specialist knowledge of the impact of mental illness on the baby and older siblings, as well as on the infant's father'. The forgoing review shows that it is possible to estimate from community surveys, the approximate proportion of women who will have either concurrent psychiatric disorders, or histories of such disorders that are in remission as they conceive and go through pregnancy. Similarly, rates of onset of psychotic and non-psychotic postpartum disorder are well established and, therefore, it is relatively easy to see whether the process of screening is functioning adequately in any given district, where the birth rate is known.

It is surprising that in most districts there is no systematic screening of antenatal populations for current mental illness or for risk (Royal College of Psychiatrists, 1992*b*). There are a few districts in Britain where clinicians have recognised that childbearing women who are mentally ill have special needs and that there is much to be gained from being proactive rather than having to react to crises. There are reports of screening measures (Riley, 1986; Appleby *et al.*, 1989; Oates, 1989) but the methods still lack sensitivity and specificity (Appleby *et al.*, 1994). Nevertheless, there is an awareness that much can be achieved to promote mental health and to prevent problems postnatally, because uniquely, the fact of pregnancy is an easy identifier, the subjects are in repeated contact with health professionals, and finally there is likely to be a higher degree of focused motivation in childbearing women.

Hospital based services for mentally ill mothers are relevant only for the small minority of severely ill women and in Britain, there is a tradition of admitting mentally ill mothers jointly with their infants (see review by Kumar, 1992). Outside the UK, Australia, Canada and New Zealand, it is the norm to separate infants from their mentally ill mothers for most or all of the period of admission. There have been no studies to compare outcome – e.g. in terms of rate of maternal recovery, the mother–infant relationship, risk to the infant, or of child development. Very few women would prefer to be separated from their infants despite being severely mentally ill at the time. There is a clear need to examine different models of care in terms of short- and long-term costs, benefits and disadvantages to mother and baby and also to plan services in a way that effectively meets a clearly defined need.

PART III

PSYCHIATRY IN SPECIAL SETTINGS

18

Social and transcultural psychiatry

PAUL BEBBINGTON

Introduction

Social psychiatry is the study of the social causes, concomitants and consequences of psychiatric disorder, and of the effectiveness of social management, interventions and treatments in psychiatry. For its scientific bases, it depends on the disciplines of epidemiology, sociology, psychology and cultural anthropology. The methods of the subject come from epidemiology, while the other disciplines provide its conceptual basis.

The subject comprises a series of topics. These include the *social epidemiology of mental disorder* – issues like the sociodemographic correlates of affective illness, the relationship between immigration and mental health, the change in incidence and prevalence of particular conditions over time, and the mental health consequences of unemployment. Epidemiology in turn depends on the definition of cases of disorder, and many social psychiatrists have been involved in the development of case-finding instruments (see Chapter 4).

Another important area of research in social psychiatry is connected with the concept of *psychosocial stress*. This underlies many of the more specific ideas in social psychiatry, such as life events or expressed emotion, which have both been very fruitful lines of enquiry. Role conflict is another type of stress, albeit less extensively studied. The social environment may also cause trouble by being impoverished rather than overstimulating, an idea that directed the early studies of institutionalism. Positive aspects of the environment include the support provided by effective social networks.

Research in social psychiatry has been successful in generating ideas for social treatments and strategies of management. Examples include the use of structured environments to combat the worst effects of institutionalism, and interventions with relatives to modify overstressful family environments. These treatments have in turn been evaluated in order to establish their effectiveness.

Evaluation research is becoming an increasingly important arena for social psychiatrists, and techniques of evaluation are growing in sophistication. As the name implies, evaluative research is unusual in relying inevitably on overt value judgements – judgements about the correct aims of a psychiatric service. Provided these are overt, people are able to contest them if they want to, but once they have been chosen it becomes possible to measure the achievements of a service against its aims. This topic is dealt with elsewhere in this volume (Chapter 20).

Because publicly funded services are answerable to a collective, they are guided by implicit or explicit collective principles. Chief among these is that members of the community have equal access, and that funds are used to provide the services that optimise individual and collective benefit. The provision of one type of treatment or services takes up resources that cannot then be used for different treatment or services. This is the concept of *opportunity cost* that forms the ethical basis of economic evaluation, another important and growing area of social psychiatry.

Transcultural psychiatry relies on concepts that are essentially similar to those of social psychiatry, but uses them to compare the form and frequency of mental illness between societies (Leff, 1981). Thus differences in social class or family structure might be related to patterns of mental illness; an example is the way in which the benign outcome of schizophrenia in India can be linked with the predominance of low expressed emotion family attitudes, although not with the extended configuration of families (Kuipers & Bebbington, 1988).

The value of transcultural psychiatry lies not in its exotic appeal but in the way it throws light on general attributes of psychiatric disorder. The study of illness patterns across cultures illuminates the nature of illness in an absolute sense, by establishing the utility of identifying a common core of features, and an outer margin whose characteristics are much more of a cultural product. This is illustrated most clearly by depressive disorder (Bebbington, 1993), and a good example is provided by Kleinman's (1986) studies of neurasthenia in China.

In the past much thought has been bestowed on the so-called culture-bound syndromes (Yap, 1967). In my view, the more culture-bound they are, the less interest they can have for psychiatry, and the more for social anthropology. They are perhaps better regarded as evidence of the pathoplastic effect of culture – fuller examination always reveals similarities with Western psychiatric concepts.

The twentieth century has seen a great unifying of cultures. In the process, cultures change, and these changes have an impact on the individuals experiencing them. This process of *acculturation* is another form of psychosocial stress. It is quite hard to study empirically, but is of particular relevance for immigrant groups. Societal modernisation is another form of acculturation.

Epidemiology

What distinguishes epidemiology from other applications of the survey method is the concept of disease, the choice of a particular way of ordering clinical material to define the dependent variable. Hence, epidemiology is the study of the distribution of diseases in populations.

It has four main functions, which concern the nature of the condition studied, its impact on communities, its implications for the provision and delivery of services, and its impact on individuals:

- Epidemiology is a key element in the recognition of syndromes, the completion of the clinical picture, and the identification of potential causes.
- It provides an idea of the burden of a condition on whole populations and the way this has changed and will change with the passage of time.
- It forms the basis for operational analyses of health services.
- Finally, it permits the establishment of individual risks, and the individual consequences of suffering from the disorder.

When studying given disorders, epidemiologists are faced with three major tasks. The first is to enumerate the size and characteristics of the population under review, the second is to define the disorder sufficiently precisely to be able to count its frequency, the third is to specify, preferably on a theoretical basis, which subgroups of the population will be likely to yield disproportionate numbers of cases (MacMahon & Pugh, 1970).

The ratio of cases to unit population is known as a *rate*. This is most commonly expressed either as a percentage or the number of cases per hundred thousand, according to its magnitude. More than one type of rate is used in epidemiology, depending on the purpose of the investigation.

It is generally argued that, when considering possible causal factors, the appropriate rate is the *incidence* – the number of new cases appearing in a defined population at risk during a given period of time, usually one year. This is because a rate based on an onset at least allows the identification of pre-existing conditions to serve as potential causes. It is then possible to calculate the *relative risk* of new cases appearing in otherwise comparable subgroups of the population distinguished by the presence of the supposedly causal factors.

In some publications, the term incidence is erroneously and misleadingly applied to an *attack rate*. While incidence is the rate of *new* cases, attack rates include new episodes in people who have already previously experienced an onset. This can be useful in examining the potential causes of episodes, although there is always the problem that people who have already experienced an episode are in consequence no longer ordinary members of the population. In conditions like depressive disorder, this may be an important point.

Another useful rate, the *prevalence*, measures the number of cases in a defined population on a given day, or during a given period of time. The *period prevalence* includes cases that appear for the first time during the period in question, together with those with an earlier onset that are still active at some time during the period. The *point prevalence* contains those cases that are active on a given day. Prevalence is more useful for studying the course of disorders and the need for various forms of treatment and service within the population. Nevertheless, it can still provide ideas for hypotheses about potential causal influences, and when linked to modern statistical techniques can be used as the basis of plausible explanatory models.

Lifetime prevalence is the proportion of the population that is suffering or has suffered from the disease. Robins and her colleagues (1984) have discussed the epidemiological advantages and disadvantages of lifetime prevalence compared with period prevalence. It identifies a larger number of affected cases and is less likely to be affected by the duration of episodes. Moreover, it allows calculation of annual first episode rates by excluding persons who are not at risk of a first episode. On the other hand, lifetime prevalence is likely to be reduced artificially by mortality in older persons if the disorder carries an increased death rate (as schizophrenia and severe affective disorders do), and in particular by errors of recall (Bromet *et al.*, 1986). Where differences between demographic groups relate more to the frequency of episodes than to the initial emergence of disorder, they will be obscured by the use of lifetime prevalence. Negative findings must therefore be interpreted cautiously. Because individuals in the general population are of all ages and have therefore lived through varying degrees of the period of risk, it is possible to use this measure as a first indication of changes in risk in succeeding cohorts. Thus if people with later birth dates are more prone to develop depressive disorders, their lifetime prevalence may actually be higher than that of older members of the same population. However, as these conditions have a variable age of onset and fluctuating course, estimates of lifetime prevalence do not provide a definitive basis for comparison.

It is sometimes more useful to estimate the risk that subjects will suffer from the condition at some point during their lifetime, the *morbid risk*. Since cross-sectional surveys can only gather information about episodes of depression up to the date of interview, the data have to be manipulated to create a notional lifetime risk. There are several well-established techniques for doing this (Thompson & Weissman, 1981). Morbid risk permits comparison across groups with different age structures and different mortality-for-age rates.

Specifying the two components of a rate – *cases* in the numerator and *population* in the denominator – and identifying factors on the basis of which to compare rates of disorder in subgroups of the population comprise the *epidemiological method*.

Social science and psychiatry

Not all ideas from the social sciences have been suitable for adoption by social psychiatrists, who have in any case sometimes been unimaginative in their choice. In other instances, social ideas have been developed specifically for use in psychiatry. The consequence is that the conceptual basis of social psychiatry may appear to lack coherence. Like a good shopping list, however, there is little doubt of its utility.

Social class

It is clear that in virtually every society resources are not equally accessible to all members. This variation lies at the core of the sociological concept of class. Class is defined in relation to power, prestige and wealth. Although these three indicators do not always go together, they often do. They may be distributed more or less continuously, but people tend to see themselves as belonging to relatively discrete groups defined by their access to resources. Consciousness of membership of a particular class tends to reinforce its cohesiveness, and it is this that makes class membership so significant for developing the attitudes, beliefs and lifestyle of individuals. It also means that class is likely to be an important factor in the development and treatment of mental illness.

Social class poses a number of problems of interpretation for sociologists. The function of social class is held to be stabilising – if people know their place, they know how to behave towards each other, and society is thereby stabilised. However, this raises the need to explain how classes themselves are maintained, and also how in certain circumstances they are revised. Sociologists also have to explain social mobility, that is the movement of certain individuals up or down the social scale, and how mobility can be accommodated without changing the basic class structure. Another phenomenon requiring explanation is how class structure can vary between societies and still be regarded as reflecting the same process and serving the same function: how is it that social class can be fairly fluid in Western Europe, and so rigid in India that mobility is almost eliminated? How is it that the rigid structure of the caste system, which ought to be inherently unstable, has managed to survive changes of dynasty and changes of religion? Different schools of though offer different explanations. However, from a psychiatric point of view, the important influence of class is on the individual's beliefs and behaviour, rather than on society as a whole.

For practical purposes social class has been assessed in may ways, using a variety of identifiers. In the US, income has been used, while the British are more reticent about such information. Other yardsticks have included education, area of domicile and, above all, occupation. In Britain, social class means occupational class. The Registrar General's office has provided more than one categorisation of this type, but these are invariably 'armchair' judgements, guesses at what most people would infer from a given occupation about the social prestige of the individual. Others have made empirical studies, allowing people in the general population to attribute prestige to different occupations. An example is the 36-class scale of Goldthorpe & Hope (1974). These empirical scales probably represent the best methods of classifying people in socio-economic terms, although they are culture- and time-bound and thus require appropriate revision.

Illness behaviour and the sick role

Becoming ill is not a simple or unitary process, and neither is the behaviour that accompanies it. When people become aware that there is something wrong with them physically – pain, discomfort, or loss of function – they respond in a whole range of ways. These possible responses have been called illness behaviour (Mechanic, 1962).

Illness behaviour has a clear social dimension – the way people respond to the possibility of illness is constrained by society's beliefs about illness. These beliefs vary from culture to culture, although in Western societies the pattern is broadly similar. The interaction of beliefs and behaviour result in the elaboration of the sick role (Sigerist, 1932; Parsons, 1951).

It is possible to distinguish this special role because the behaviours that go with it are only provisionally *legitimised*, to use the sociologists' jargon. If people behave in the way appropriate to sickness when they are not sick, their actions are regarded as *deviant*. It is only when those around them ascribe the status of sickness to them that the behaviour becomes legitimate. Individuals must appear to be adequately sick before it is acceptable for them to spend the day in bed – if they were not seen as sick, friends and relatives would quickly lose patience with them.

The sick role involves exemption from ordinary duties, commensurate with the degree of illness. Wage-earners may stay off work, others may be relieved of child care or cooking. The sick become the focus of the duties of others, who have an obligation to look after them and to take over their responsibilities if necessary. However, although ascribing the status of sickness does legitimise appropriate illness behaviour, it does so only partly. The sick are always teetering on the edge of deviance. For this reason, they do acquire one important new duty, the duty to get well, that is, to take any action that will serve that aim. This may involve staying off work, resting in bed, going to see the doctor, taking medicine as prescribed or even going into hospital. It is acceptable for people to adopt the sick role as long as they give every appearance of doing so only temporarily.

The first problem about illness behaviour is that pain and discomfort are quite common, at least in mild or moderate degree, and there is a long-standing and usually appropriate tradition of putting up with it. This means that illness behaviour is not seen as an appropriate set of responses to the mere presence of discomfort and people must exercise judgement about when to behave as though they were ill. Individuals obviously differ in how they do this, and there is a range of acceptable responses. Outside this range lies abnormal illness behaviour (Pilowsky, 1988). This may result from an abnormal reluctance or eagerness to adopt, or to relinquish, the sick role. Usually in psychiatry and in medicine, we may be concerned with an abnormal eagerness to adopt the sick role and therefore to claim the exemptions it sanctions. However, in, say, an X-ray screening programme for tuberculosis, the medical team is more likely to be concerned with reluctance to adopt the sick role, like putting up with a cough and not coming forward for an X-ray.

Illness behaviour may be abnormal for a variety of reasons, and a number of psychiatric conditions can be interpreted in this way. In *hypochondriasis*, because of a fear of illness, the patient may have a very low threshold for entering the sick role. In *hysteria* and *malingering*, the patient may also have a reluctance to leave it, because of the advantages it brings (secondary gain) (See also Chapter 6).

Doctors have an important function in validating the sick role. Although minor and temporary adoptions of the sick role can be sanctioned by relatives or employers, or in some cases by paramedical staff, more serious adoptions need the approval of a doctor. This is at its most formalised and obvious in the case of a 'sick note', but a little thought will confirm that it occurs in more subtle and informal ways.

Doctors also have a role in shaping illness behaviour, in which they act both as the agents and the originators of general social beliefs. An interesting example includes the way psychiatrists punish histrionic behaviour and 'acting out', and reinforce introspective self-descriptions.

Illness behaviour, the sick role and the process of diagnosis are all intertwined. The doctor is much more likely to sanction the sick role when the patient's illness behaviour, which of course includes the description of symptoms, matches one of the patterns that permit at least a possible diagnosis. When doctors fail to diagnose, they may well withhold the necessary approval, putting the patient in an uncomfortable and marginal position. The failure to diagnose may arise from the doctor's lack of expertise or from the state of the medical profession's knowledge – as time goes by, the allowable patterns (that is, recognisable diseases) change and generally increase in number.

Some illnesses do not get better. Those who suffer from such conditions may not be very popular, but they are usually tolerated. They are finally relieved of the obligation to get better whilst remaining the responsibility of others, but at the cost of being a little less than full citizens. Public attitudes towards deafness and blindness illustrate this clearly, but it is perhaps most apparent in long-standing psychiatric disorder.

It is useful for psychiatrists to be aware of the concepts of illness behaviour and the sick role – it can give an added dimension to the understanding of patients, although it puts the physician in the odd position of being at the same time both on the inside and on the outside of a social system. It is of particular relevance for liaison psychiatry (see Chapter 21).

The concept of the sick role implies that social recognition of illness changes the behaviour of the sick. This idea also lies behind the application of *labelling theory* to illness (Lemert, 1951; Scheff, 1974). This was originally developed as an explanation for deviance and can crudely be conveyed as the consequences of 'giving a dog a bad name'. As used in psychiatry, in its strong form it suggests that people's behaviour is wholly constrained by the ascription of a label, in its weaker form, that labelling makes a considerable difference to the behaviour of the labelled person. In both forms, the label is seen as a source of disadvantage, preventing sufferers from full participation in their social world. The concept is central to the arguments of the antipsychiatry movement of the 1960s and 1970s, for instance Szasz's (1961) critique of the concept of schizophrenia. The finding of significant pathological abnormalities in the brains of those with schizophrenia has at least defused the strong form of labelling theory (Chapter 10): however any disorder identified solely from the self-reports and behaviour of sufferers because there is no identifiable pathology is easy game.

An acknowledgement of the appropriateness of the sick role actually has potential advantages for people suffering from psychiatric disorders like schizophrenia. This is because it absolves them from some of the responsibility of their actions and allows carers to interpret their behaviour in a different light. Hence, labelling in order to sanction the sick role is an essential part of the psycho-educational component of psychosocial interventions with families in schizophrenia and other mental disorders (e.g. Kuipers *et al.*, 1992). Despite the success of these programmes, there are still those who are wary of the way they use labelling (Hatfield *et al.*, 1987).

Life events and their measurement

The study of life events exemplifies both the methods and the inherent problems of the social sciences. The topic of social sciences is humanity and its systems of meaning. It has been argued for over a century and a half that this makes for an absolute distinction between the methods of the physical sciences (explanation) and those of the social sciences (interpretation). According to this account, the former proceed by reproducible experimentation, the latter by an intuitive process of understanding that has no absolute point of reference. This view had several unfortunate consequences, for instance the rejection of much of the potential subject matter of psychology by extreme behaviourists. Nowadays, it appears simplistic, and the difficulty of achieving consensus over measurement is acknowledged in both types of science. The assessment of life events combines the process of interpretation with the sort of empirical investigation typical of the physical sciences.

Most studies involve the evaluation of the response of sufferers to a wide range of potential life events. This inevitably brings up issues of measurement, since, once life event stress is considered as a whole, it becomes clear that events are not equivalent. There must therefore be some way of assessing the likely impact of a given event on a subject. This depends on a large number of variables, relating both to the nature of the event and to the subject's prior experiences. Inevitably, each person's experience of events is unique and is responsible for a unique susceptibility.

General statements can nevertheless be made about relative impact. The death of a child will always vastly outweigh a child moving out of the home to go to college or to get married. However, most events are like the last examples rather than the first, and distinguishing their relative severity is difficult and heavily dependent on context. It might seem an obvious strategy to ask subjects how they were actually affected by the events they experienced. However, this leads to two types of potential bias. First, subjects unfortunately share their research hypotheses with the researcher: it is characteristic of human beings that they seek to impose meaning to their lives in terms of their experiences. The second bias is that the effects of mental illness itself may distort subjects' assessments of their experiences. However, if we decline to accept a respondent's own judgements, we are faced with the difficulty of arriving at our own.

There have been two basic attempts to deal with this problem. One was to define events by constructing a list of event types. This is the so called 'inventory approach', associated with the names of Holmes & Rahe (1967). A history is then elicited from respondents by presenting them with the list, either on paper or verbally, and asking them to identify events experienced within a given period. The disadvantage of this method is that it largely delegates to the respondent the judgement of deciding whether an experience matches up with an event category, leading to what Dohrenwend and his colleagues (1993) called the problem of *intracategory variability*.

The authors of the inventory approach dealt with the problem of the differential impact of events by using a *rating sample* to ascribe values to each event category. The scores of the rating sample were then averaged to give a stress rating for the event. The effect of this was to give a crude rating completely divorced from the specific circumstances that might surround given events in the individual case. It was certainly one way of discounting the subjective evaluation of individual experience.

Event inventories are still used in psychiatric research although the method is an insensitive one. The alternative technique, of a semistructured interview based around role areas, offers a considerable improvement (Brown, 1974; Brown & Harris, 1978). People using this approach have relied heavily on the development of the Life Events and Difficulty Schedule (LEDS) by Brown and his colleagues, although it is sometimes modified to suit local circumstances (e.g. Day *et al.*, 1987). Potential life events are identified by the interviewer and then presented to a panel of raters, who ascribe a severity rating to the elicited events. As the interviewer is able to provide a considerable amount of context, so the individual circumstances of the event can be taken into account, in a way that is not feasible using an inventory approach. Thus, some degree of individuality of response is retained, while the subjects' evaluation is removed from consideration. This represents a reasonable compromise between pure subjectivity and the crudeness of evaluating events merely be categorising them.

A further problem concerns the choice of dimensions along which to rate impact. There was dispute between those who thought impact was best denoted by the amount of *change* following an event, and those who felt that the degree of *stress* was a more crucial attribute. Most life event research has involved depressive disorders and it was found empirically that the most predictive dimension was stressfulness (Mueller *et al.*, 1977), although this raises more conceptual difficulties than focusing on the measurement of mere change. The LEDS relies on measures of *threat*, although events can also be rated according to the degree of loss they connote.

However, other important issues apart from the dimensions of impact must be considered in evaluating the causal relationship between events and any kind of psychiatric disorder. Thus, it is not always possible to be absolutely sure that the temporal requirements for a causal inference have been made. Plainly, for an event to be responsible for the onset or relapse of psychiatric disorder, it must precede it. However, onset and relapse can both be difficult to define and date, so we may not be sure that they occurred after the identified event. The event may have come about because of changes in the subject's behaviour that were themselves the result of impending relapse.

In response to this problem, Brown and his colleagues have developed the concept of *independence* (Brown & Harris, 1978). This is a measure of the extent to which events are independent of illness-related behaviour on the part of the subject. This rating has become increasingly complex over the years since it was introduced, so that it now includes categories like events that involve the subject's physiology or those that depend on the subject's compliance with an external situation, intentional acts or negligence. However, most of the existing life event research using the LEDS depends on a threefold division of events into *independent*, *possibly independent*, and *dependent*. Independent events are basically those that are in logical terms very unlikely to have been brought about by impending breakdown, while possibly independent events are those where such a relationship cannot be ruled out, but where there is no actual evidence that the event was brought about by changed behaviour.

Social networks and social support

Social relationships obviously vary in quality and intensity, so there is a real problem in deciding what is to be covered by the intuitively understandable concept of *social support*. This forms a bridge between explanations of differing purpose, operating at very different levels. It can be seen in terms of its function for individuals, that is, in meeting their needs. It also has a function for society through its role in maintaining relationships. It can be analysed in terms of the behaviour of others towards the subject. It also enters the study of the subject's own behaviour, that is, in seeking support, when it becomes an aspect of coping. Finally, its effects as a reinforcer may be examined.

This complexity makes it difficult to determine the qualities of social support relevant to mental health research. Psychologists have defined behavioural, affective and cognitive aspects of the concept (Hinde, 1979), whereas those with a sociological orientation have focused more on the function of social support for the individual and the structures within which it is offered (Weiss, 1974). It is not easy to integrate these viewpoints, and this is one reason for the variety of measures that have been used to research it.

One of the first investigators to give attention to both the structure and function of social relationships was Charles H. Cooley (1909), with his formulation of the *primary group*. Primary group membership involves people in intimate association and co-operation (i.e. behaviour), but such groups are primary particularly in the sense of their importance in forming the social nature and ideals of the individual. This emphasises the cognitive function of the system. People also interact with those who are not members of their primary group: the totality of those with whom they interact forms their *social network*.

Both the structure and function of social networks might influence the risk of psychiatric disorder. Structure includes such items as size of primary group, size of secondary group, whether other members of the network know and interact with each other, whether members of the primary group are members also of the subject's household and so on. The potential functions of social relationships are many. Weiss (1974) specified six that might characterise satisfactory relationships: attachment, social integration, reassurance of worth, opportunity for nurturing others, reliable and practical help, and guidance in difficult situations. However, for practical purposes, the number of conceptual headings can be reduced. Several workers concur in distinguishing between practical help and emotional support, that is, the instrumental and expressive, or the behavioural and the affective. Kahn & Antonucci (1980) are probably right to broaden description to the three headings of 'affect' (someone saying they like you), 'affirmation' (someone saying they are of like mind) and 'aid' (helping and advising).

Although a number of workers have reported deficiencies in the size of the social networks of patients, most work has concentrated on the perceived function of relationships. The problem for research workers is that the structural characteristics of social networks, though determined by self-report, are relatively objective, but the extent to which they are reported as fulfilling their functions is very much a matter of the subject's perceptions. As a result, the measurement of such variables poses problems comparable to those of life event research, and few have so far really made a serious attempt to circumvent them.

Research workers have generally chosen to assess practical or emotional support or both. The role of 'affirmation' has not often been distinguished, although it may form part of other measures, for instance Brown's concept of intimate confiding. Ideally, all three of Kahn & Antonucci's (1980) aspects should be measured, and their contribution discerned empirically. In most cases researchers have decided intuitively that it is the emotional support of close relationships that is likely to be important in preserving psychological well-being and staving off the effects of misfortune. Other research workers have looked further afield, by seeking to use involvement in more organised aspects of the community (churchgoing, membership of clubs, etc.) as a crude measure of social integration, which might be taken to indicate the availability of all three of Kahn & Antonucci's (1980) triad. Brown & Harris (1978), in contrast, saw the availability of an extremely close and confiding relationship as the crucially important factor. This group have now, however, moved to assessment of a broader range of relationships (O'Connor & Brown, 1984).

Until very recently research workers have examined the effect of routine social support. However, it is likely that if social support has an affect in moderating the impact of acute psychosocial stress, it is because it is both available and drawn on at the time of crises. The assessment of *crisis social support* in the context of specific life events is recent (Brown *et al.*, 1986). Routine social support may appear to moderate psychosocial stress through its association with actual levels of crisis support, or with some other factor such as self-esteem. Crisis support is very difficult to measure except retrospectively. Veiel (1985) has provided a useful review of the conceptual issues in social support research.

Assessing the social consequences of psychiatric disorder

Psychiatric disorders characteristically impair social performance. This term has several meanings (Wykes & Hurry, 1991). *Social role performance* is a measure of how individuals cope in the major role areas of work, relationships, home-care and self-management. While there are many instruments for measuring social role performance, there is actually quite good consensus about how it should be done: the areas covered should be jointly of broad coverage, and be assessed individually rather than globally. Performance in role has to be measured against group expectations, and this has always caused problems for researchers. Adopting a high threshold for identifying impairment increases the cross-cultural applicability of the definition. Using instruments of this sort permits a fair degree of precision in describing the social consequences of relatively mild psychiatric disorders.

The adoption of even higher threshold for identifying abnormality reduces the cultural component of measure still further, and is of use in assessing people with several and long-standing disorder. This is characteristic of social behaviour schedules, which measure social behaviour so basic to the normal functioning of human beings that they transcend role expectations and thus, to a large extent, culture.

It is important to assess the social consequences of psychiatric disorder because they cannot readily be predicted from its symptomatic characteristics. Thus, social role performance associated with depressive disorder takes longer to improve than depressive symptoms (Weissman & Paykel, 1974), and much of the management of long-term psychosis is concerned not with symptoms but with the associated impairment of social behaviour.

The social consequences and concomitants of psychiatric disorder can be approached in another way, by anatomising the causes of social disablement in a manner borrowed from rehabilitation in physical medicine. The causes can be divided into *impairments*, *disadvantages* and *self-attitudes*. Impairments are abnormalities of biological or psychological function. In schizophrenia, these may be the result of hallucinations, delusions, impaired concentration, loss of motivation, social anxiety and so on, in other words, both positive and negative symptoms. If impairments of this type are persistent, they are sometimes called 'intrinsic', the implication being that they probably have a biological basis.

The second potential cause of social disablement is environmental disadvantage – things like poverty, poor educational or training opportunities, and isolation. These disadvantages are likely to be compounded by negative social attitudes, sometimes termed 'secondary deviance' (Lemert, 1951). The picture is complicated because the causal relationship between disadvantage and impairment is usually reciprocal. Thus, stigma may increase isolation and hence social anxiety and the loss of social skills.

To this stew of disablement must be added the third ingredient, that is, the maladaptive attitudinal and behavioural changes that result from it and then add to it further.

This terminology may at first appear confusing. This is because it represents an attempt at a difficult task, that is, to bring clarity to the complex interplay between its elements. This is actually its strength: it is crucial to the rational consideration of the appropriate components of individual packages of social treatment for disablement.

Health economics and psychiatry

The costs of psychiatric services can only be ignored for short periods – in the end, all health services are cost-limited. The cost of care is particularly at issue in Britain at present because of new policies towards the organisation and objectives of the National Health Service. Thus, the White Paper *Working for Patients* (HMSO, 1989) required District Health Authorities to buy care according to need, to buy quality care, and to get value for money. This sets out clearly a trade-off between quality and cost; in particular that standards of care must be stipulated, and its effects evaluated. Although clinicians sometimes cavil at this approach, it embodies the central ethical principle of economic evaluation: that resources out not to be consumed in a given activity if they would generate greater benefit elsewhere. In order to pursue this utilitarian objective, we need to consider both benefits and costs. It is only because economic evaluation does this that it can appraise opportunity costs: more cost here equals less benefit there (McGuire & Drummond, 1993).

The simplest form of economic analysis actually ignores benefit. *Cost minimisation* seeks merely to reduce costs irrespective of the consequences. *Cost-effectiveness* is a type of economic analysis that relates a monetary cost to an outcome identified and measured in non-monetary terms. It requires comparison between the costs of two different methods of achieving an outcome. This looks seductively simple for drug treatments, although less so than at first appears (Jönsson & Bebbington, 1994). It becomes very difficult where treatments are social: the style of service delivery inevitably becomes intertwined with specific expertise in a way that is difficult to tease out.

When outcomes are measured in monetary terms, the evaluation is referred to as *cost-benefit analysis*. There have been very few of these in psychiatry because of the sheer difficulty of attributing monetary value to many aspects of outcome. This is compounded by the fact that attributes that would sometimes be regarded as costs, for instance in-patient treatment, may also be invoked as outcomes, for example, the reduced need for admission. Finally, *cost utility analysis* attempts to place a value on concepts that are inherently difficult to measure, like quality of life. They have been used in physical medicine to evaluate procedures like kidney or heart transplants, but are very difficult to carry out in psychiatry.

Selected topics in social and transcultural psychiatry

Community psychiatric surveys

The necessary process of standardising case definitions involves two elements: the first is the standardisation of the collection of the necessary clinical information, the *database*, and the second is the standardisation of the *rules* for deriving a diagnosis from this material.

The first real attempts at standardisation were in studies from Canada and the USA in the 1950s (Srole *et al.*, 1962; Leighton *et al.*, 1963). Self-report schedules were used to provide a standard coverage of possible symptoms, and subjects were then divided into groups according to their degree of impairment. There was no attempt to classify symptoms, although in follow-up studies algorithms have been created to do this (Murphy *et al.*, 1989).

The next phase involved the development of standardised instruments for eliciting and classifying psychiatric phenomena. The two instruments that have been used most widely for psychiatric community surveys are the British 9th edition of the *Present State Examination* (PSE – Wing *et al.*, 1974), and the American *Diagnostic Interview Schedule* (DIS – Robins *et al.*, 1985). These instruments take somewhat different approaches to the problem of case-finding. The former is based on the principles of the psychiatric interview, using cross-examination to elicit a description of experiences corresponding to defined symptoms. It is thus best suited to use by trained clinicians. The DIS, on the other hand, was constructed for use by lay interviewers. While for the originators of the PSE, clinical judgement was a requisite, for those of the DIS it thus became a problem. To circumvent it, the instrument has an absolute structure that interviewers must follow.

Both instruments have been used widely in psychiatric community surveys, but those involving the DIS have employed lay interviewers and covered larger samples. Being specifically linked with the DSM-IIIR classification, the DIS provides a wide range of diagnoses; however, there must be greater reservations about the validity of the results than those derived from the PSE (Romanoski *et al.*, 1992).

The DIS was used in the five population surveys of the Epidemiologic Catchment Area (ECA) programme (Eaton & Kessler, 1985), which between them covered around 20 000 people. The results have now been extensively published (Robins & Regier, 1991). It has also been used in population surveys in Puerto Rico, Edmonton, Taiwan, Christchurch, Munich, Seoul, and Beirut. The findings have been surprisingly consistent, particularly for the relatively common affective disorders (see Bebbington, 1990, for a review).

The 9th edition of the PSE has also been used extensively, in 15 surveys worldwide. Again there have been consistent results for depressive disorders and anxiety states. The differences between the surveys are of the degree that might actually mean something in terms of the social and cultural characteristics of the areas in which they were carried out. This situation can be contrasted with the early history of psychiatric surveys, when much larger discrepancies were almost certainly methodological. It is of interest that the highest rates for these conditions come from economically disadvantaged countries or from those undergoing rapid economic and cultural transition (Ghubash *et al.*, 1992). It is also possible that overall rates of psychiatric disorder are higher in Mediterranean countries than in Northern European cultures, mainly because of a greater frequency of anxiety states (Mavreas & Bebbington, 1988).

The findings of the DIS and PSE surveys suggest that rates of all types of psychiatric disorder in industrialised countries probably lie between 10 and 20%, and that the prevalence of major depressive disorder is around 2–3%. However, the very careful study by Romanoski and his colleagues (1992), based on a re-examination of subjects from the Baltimore ECA survey by trained clinicians, suggests that the true prevalence of major depressive disorder might have been as low as 1%. Getting these figures right is obviously of great importance for mental health service planning.

Recently, the Department of Health in Britain has mounted a very large, nationwide survey of psychiatric disorder involving around 10 000 subjects (Jenkins & Meltzer, 1994). This has used good sampling methods and its results are awaited with interest. Another development is the attempt to measure the needs for psychiatric treatment directly in surveys in south London and Derry (Bebbington et al., 1996), rather than estimating them indirectly from the prevalence of disorder. This has involved the development of a Needs for Care Assessment suitable for use in community surveys.

Despite the reservations that must even now still exist about the findings of psychiatric community surveys, they provide a rich source of information about the impact of social attributes on prevalence. These are too extensive for a brief review but can be found in the references alluded to.

Cohort effects

Although most authors are ready to accept that lifetime prevalence and age of onset may differ according to demographic status, they are often treated as fixed in relation to time. However, they may not be, and a number of authors claim to have discovered cohort effects indicating an increasing frequency of affective disorders with succeeding generations (e.g. Klerman et al., 1985; Gershon et al., 1987; Lavori et al., 1987).

If these postulated cohort effects are genuine, they are very interesting. It would be difficult to argue that they arise from changes in gene frequency over so short a time, and the explanation must therefore be environmental, and probably social. Gershon (1989) has, however, suggested that the cohort effect for affective disorders is more marked in the relatives of those with affective disorders than in the general population, implying a gene–environment interaction.

The American authorities place considerable weight on these findings. In fact, they must be treated with caution. It is very difficult to model separate age, period and cohort effects statistically, because fixing any two of these factors constrains the third. Wickramaratne and his colleagues (1989) have attempted this task by making certain assumptions about potential period and cohort effects in the ECA data set. The model of best fit for females required only age and cohort effects, while for males, it required age, period of cohort effects. Other reservations compound these statistical difficulties (Bebbington, 1991), of which the most important is probably the failure of recall – older folk may appear to have a lower lifetime prevalence because they are unable to remember episodes occurring many years ago. An excellent account of the potential pitfalls in studies of this type is provided by Klerman & Weissman (1989).

Social class and psychiatric disorder

There are different ways in which social class might directly influence the incidence and prevalence of psychiatric disorder. First, as it flags access to resources, those of lower social class have less access, and are thereby more likely to be exposed to misfortune.

However, the reality is likely to be more subtle than this. Class shapes individual beliefs, the perceptions of circumstances and coping responses, and these are the mechanisms whereby it is most likely to influence the origins of psychiatric disorder.

Studies of the social class distribution of schizophrenic patients have consistently shown that they are over-represented among the lower classes (by a factor of five in the ECA surveys – Robins & Regier, 1991). Since the classic work of Faris & Dunham (1939), showing high rates of schizophrenia in the culturally and economically impoverished central areas of Chicago, there has been a controversy over the reasons for this distribution. Some authorities have attributed high rates of schizophrenia primarily to the poor socio-economic conditions experienced by members of the lower class (Kohn, 1973), while others have explained the class distribution as the result of the downward social drift consequent upon the effects of the illness or of its prodromal features (Goldberg & Morrison, 1963). These are the *breeder hypothesis* and the *drift hypothesis*, respectively.

Alternative theories have included those that suggest that failure to achieve an expected social class may produce stresses that cause illness (Turner & Wagenfeld, 1967) and that doctors employ different diagnostic and therapeutic practices towards the lower-class sick (Hollingshead & Redlich, 1958). The controversy is by no means settled, but as far as schizophrenia is concerned, most work strongly supports the social drift hypothesis (Hare *et al.*, 1972; Eaton, 1980).

The relationship between social class and the frequency of affective disorders is more complex. Because bipolar disorder is relatively rare, investigations have usually relied on treated cases. Most people with this condition are likely at some point to come to treatment, and the bias involved in using referred samples is probably not great. In some studies (e.g. Noreik & Odegaard, 1966; Bagley, 1973) bipolar disorder appears to cluster in the higher social classes, and it was claimed that this was because of a genetic link with creativity. Bipolar disorder appears to be particularly common in creative artists (Andreasen, 1987). However, a number of other researchers have found no social class variation at all in bipolar disorder (Der & Bebbington, 1987). Severe unipolar disorder also seems to be fairly uniform in its distribution (Faris & Dunham, 1939; Der & Bebbington, 1987; Bebbington, 1988).

The use of referred series for analysis is much more problematic for depression of mild or moderate severity, since social class may well affect the likelihood that sufferers gain access to specialist services (e.g. Srole *et al.*, 1962), although the effect is probably small once the severity of disorder is controlled for (Hurry *et al.*, 1980). Nevertheless it is probably best to use general population surveys to establish the link between social class and moderate depression.

The received opinion is that moderate depression is commoner in the lower social classes. This is probably right, although several surveys report no relationship. The link is probably stronger in urban areas. In Britain, surveys from London and Edinburgh suggested the rate of depressive disorder may be from two to three times higher in working class subjects (Brown & Harris, 1978; Surtees *et al.*, 1983; Harris *et al.*, 1986). However, the ECA surveys found little difference in the prevalence of affective disorder in relation to socio-economic status (Robins & Regier, 1991). There is no satisfactory explanation for this discrepancy with the prevailing tenor of the literature, although in view of the size and quality of the ECA project, one is required.

Although psychosocial adversity, as indicated by life events or chronic difficulties, is commoner in working-class subjects, this is insufficient to account for the difference in prevalence of depression (Bebbington *et al.*, 1991). At an epidemiological level, working-class people are more likely to develop depression in response to an event, that is, they are more vulnerable to its effects, and this probably reflects differences in coping resources (Bebbington *et al.*, 1986).

Life events and psychiatric disorder

The large majority of studies of life events have related them to the onset of cases of affective disorder, usually relatively mild. This raises a conceptual problem neglected by researchers. The idea of the stress connoted by life events derives from common human knowledge of states of distress. However, these states of distress shade into the more extreme conditions that conform to the concept of depressive disorders. Some argue that the relationship between stressful life events and depressive disorder is therefore a tautology. A less extreme view is that the relationship, while to an extent empirical, is just not very interesting. It is not very unlikely that stressful life events will cause distress and that distress may be so extreme as to qualify as depressive disorder. The theory that stressful life events cause depression thus has relatively low information content.

Some authors have responded to this by employing the life event–depression link as an entry-point for more interesting relationships: thus Brown & Harris (1978) used it to develop a model of vulnerability based on particular social statuses and circumstances, while Bebbington and his colleagues (Bebbington *et al.*, 1988; McGuffin *et al.*, 1988*a,b*) adapted it to investigate the tendency of depression to run in families.

Life-event theories of aetiology become more interesting when they are applied to psychiatric disorders with characteristics rather different from what we would see as normal distress responses, for instance schizophrenia (Bebbington *et al.*, 1993; Norman & Malla, 1993). This is of particular significance because for a long time schizophrenia was regarded as a condition relatively immune to psychosocial influence.

However, the research linking life events and schizophrenia is inconclusive (Bebbington *et al.*, 1995). The lack of robustness in the findings might justify the conclusion that social factors were relatively unimportant in schizophrenic relapse. However, this must be set against the expressed emotion (EE) studies, which suggest a large and robust effect for another sort of social factor. It is possible that the relatively abrupt changes represented by life events may be less important in producing relapse than the more persistent stress of living with a high EE family member. Another possibility is that people with schizophrenia are unnaturally *sensitive* to life events, so that relapse can be brought about by events that on the surface would seem incapable of provoking much emotional response. This would certainly tie in with the experience of many clinicians, who are very concerned to protect people with long-standing schizophrenia from even minor changes in their daily routines.

The effects of life events on episodes of bipolar illness have not been studied exhaustively. Firm conclusions are difficult because of varying methodology, but stressful life events probably do operate as precipitating factors in some subjects with bipolar affective disorders, particularly in first episodes. It remains to be seen whether there is any difference between those patients from whom psychosocial events contribute to onset and those for whom they appear to have no significant role.

The psychiatric condition regarded as organic *par excellence* is dementia. Orrell & Bebbington (1995) have compared the frequency of life events before admission and before deterioration in dementia patients, dementia controls living in the community, and fit elderly people matched for age and sex. Specific scales were developed to measure the changes in routine and the social environment brought about by events. Their results supported their initial hypothesis, that it is the social disruptiveness of change rather than the threat implied by life events that is associated with cognitive deterioration in dementia. On the other hand, depression in these demented subjects was much more associated with stress than with change in routine and environment.

Refining the relationship between life events and depression

The relationship between life events and depression has been confirmed in innumerable studies, good, bad and indifferent, in clinical and general populations, in mild, severe and psychotic cases. Whatever the conceptual reservations about this finding, there is no doubt about its clinical utility. The social circumstances and precipitants of depression must be evaluated carefully in any proper clinical assessment, and should shape the approach to management.

The best life-event research in depression has attempted to go beyond the basic relations and to explore the context that moderate the impact of events. Much of this work has been carried out by Brown and his colleagues in London. Thus, in the 1970s, they argued that the impact of life events was reduced for people who were able to call on good social support (Brown & Harris, 1978). The nature of this social support became the focus of later work developing the idea of 'very close relationships' (O'Connor & Brown, 1984). In general, good social support is associated with a reduced rate of depression, although the causal direction can not be guaranteed. Some studies suggest that poor support is linked to depression because unsupported people respond particularly badly to stress (the *buffering theory* of social support). Others are more in accord with the view that the link between poor support and depression is direct (Alloway & Bebbington, 1987).

Events clearly derive their meaning from previous experiences. These may have a general effect on resilience, as, for example, the claim that early loss of a parent increases the tendency to respond to events by becoming clinically depressed (Brown *et al.*, 1977). However, cognitive theories of depression suggest that events are more likely to have a drastic effect if they key into some specific attribute of prior experience. This idea lies behind further elaborations by Brown and his colleagues (1987) of the context of events. They argue that events will have an especially powerful effect if they have a specific resonance with *commitments*, long-standing *difficulties* or *role conflict*. These are termed *matching events* and seem to be strongly related to the development of depression. The authors have thus increased explanatory power by specifying event context more precisely.

If events are linked to depression, they may equally be associated with recovery. Although to clinicians this might appear naive, one obvious proposal is that pleasant events should cheer depressed subjects up. There is little evidence for this, but more refined links between events and recovery have some empirical support. Thus, Tennant and his colleagues (1981*b*) showed recovery was hastened by events that specifically neutralised the consequences of the adverse events linked to the original development of depression. More recently, Brown and his colleagues (1992) have defined categories of 'fresh start' events, which provide hope for the future, and 'anchoring' events, which convey a sense of security. The former appear to have particular significance in recovery from depression but not from anxiety (again this ties in with cognitive theories of depression). Anchoring events, in contrast, are associated with recovery from anxiety but not from depression. Thus, the social determinants of recovery also confirm the importance of specifying the context within which events occur.

Integrated theories of depressive disorder

Enough is known to say that depressive disorder has no single cause. Moreover, the factors identified as having a causal role are common in the general population. Thus, susceptibility is the central issue – why, when so many people are exposed to these factors, do relatively few develop this disorder? If individual factors are neither necessary nor sufficient, what *combinations* of factors are sufficient?

An enormous amount of research has been devoted to the aetiology of depressive illness. Consistent findings have emerged in the course of genetic, epidemiological and social investigations, and there have been numerous attempts to integrate them within bio-psychosocial models of depression (e.g. Akiskal *et al.*, 1975; Depue *et al.*, 1979). Such models are best tested through studies that establish data at the biological, psychological and social level from the same samples.

There have been very few of these. Perhaps the first to integrate biological and social factors was conducted by Calloway, Dolan and their colleagues (Calloway *et al.*, 1984*a,b*; Dolan *et al.*, 1985*b*; Calloway & Dolan, 1989). Neuroendocrine and psychosocial factors were evaluated in 72 depressed patients. A family history was also canvassed, although only by enquiry from the probands. There was a roughly even spread between endogenous and neurotic forms of depression.

There were no differences between the patients with and without a family history in terms of their experience of antecedent life events. Nor were there differences between suppressors and non-suppressors on the dexamethazone suppression test. However, urinary cortisol in the 24 hours before the test was *raised* in those with life events or difficulties. This measure may represent a reactive neuroendocrine change, while the resetting of the system, as indicated by the DST, is not stress-related. The results relating to the hypothalmic–pituitary–thyroid axis were very hard to interpret and must await further research.

The Camberwell Collaborative Depression Study (Bebbington *et al.*, 1988; McGuffin *et al.*, 1988*a,b*) also examined social and familial factors in the same set of subjects. The probands were selected because they had recently experienced episodes of depression with a defined onset, and interviews were sought with all first-degree relatives aged over 18. The authors initially postulated that depressive disorders could be separated into mild forms, and severe forms of the sort typically associated with 'endogenous' symptoms. Mild disorders were thought likely to be responses to psychosocial adversity, while severe types would be less socially reactive and more commonly associated with a family history. Because of shared family culture, where probands with depressions related to adversity had affected family members, the illness in the relatives was also expected to be adversity-related.

The actual findings did not confirm these predictions: an excess of life events preceded mild and severe depression alike; mild and severe depression were both familial; and a relationship with adversity in the proband's illness did not predict an equivalent relationship in unaffected relatives. The results were thus very much in favour of a unitary view of depression.

However, the situation was complex; the findings relating to severe depression were suggestive of the action of a major factor (perhaps genetic), while mild depression could be interpreted as resulting from the action of several minor factors (Bebbington et al., 1991). Moreover, although high life event rates in probands were associated with high rates in other family members, the latter appeared relatively immune to their effects (McGuffin et al., 1988b); a more plausible model is thus that the familiality of depression results from both genetic inheritance and a common culture that means some families have eventful lifestyles, but also appear to be more effective in coping with crises.

The work of Kendler and his colleagues (1991) is of particular interest as it involves the study of social and psychological factors in 827 female twin pairs. However, assessments were based on relatively simple self-report measures of life events, coping and depression, and must therefore be treated with caution. Factor analysis yielded three coping factors: turning to others and problem-solving, which were both associated with good mental health; and denial, which was positively related to anxiety and depression. The first two factors protected subjects from developing anxiety or depression in response to life events, while denial tended to raise the level of anxiety following events. The authors fitted structural equation models to the data. It was possible to explain twin resemblance in turning to others and problem-solving entirely by genetic factors. In contrast, twin resemblance for denial could best be explained by familial–environmental factors. Thus, genes may affect the vulnerability to affective disorders in part by influencing coping behaviour.

Expressed emotion and relapse in schizophrenia

The origins of the measure of expressed emotion (EE) have been reviewed extensively (Leff & Vaughn, 1985; Kuipers & Bebbington, 1988, 1990; Kavanagh, 1992). It was developed over a period of a decade, following the observation that returning to a family home was not always associated with a good outcome in severe mental illness (Brown et al., 1958) and the speculation that this might be due to social aspects of the home environment.

EE is rated from an audiotape of an interview with a carer (the Camberwell Family Interview, CFI – Brown & Rutter, 1966). This has a semi-structured format that allows a flexible use of standard questions and probes, and encourages the interviewer to listen to information as it emerges. It covers the onset of problems, focuses on the pre-month prior to interview, and encompasses other aspects of relationships, such as irritability and tension. The interviewer enquires after symptoms and coping responses, and probes for recent examples if the carer is reticent or vague. The interviewer also establishes a time-budget for a typical week. This allows an evaluation of the amount of time that the patient and the carer spend together.

The definitive ratings are then made from the audiotape of the interview, based on the content, but more importantly, the non-verbal aspects of speech like pitch and emphasis. This is intended to allow the rating of emotional aspects of communication regardless of specific contents. High EE is conventionally defined either as criticism exceeding a cut-off of six critical comments, or a moderate amount of emotional involvement, or any degree of hostility. The consequences is that EE is probably a dimorphic rating, since hostility and criticism are clearly related to each other, but less so to over-involvement

The literature using EE as a measure predictive of relapse in schizophrenia has relied on similar research designs. Typically, a sample of patients is followed up following recovery from an episode of florid symptoms of schizophrenia. When they are well on the way to recovery, commonly at the point of discharge, carers are interviewed with the Camberwell Family Interview to establish levels of EE. Patients are then followed up for at least nine months, and evaluated for signs of relapse. The definition of relapse has typically varied, in some cases being based on symptomatic criteria, and in others merely on readmission to hospital. Patients are divided into high and low EE groups, usually on the basis that at least one relative in the immediate family is rated as high EE.

There are now at least 27 prospective studies of the role of expressed emotion as a risk factor for relapse in schizophrenia, although more are in progress. An aggregate analysis of 25 or these studies, covering 1346 patients, has recently been carried out (Bebbington & Kuipers, 1994). Data on individual cases were obtained from the original authors of 17 of the studies.

The overall relapse rate for high EE cases was 50%, whereas that in low EE cases was 21%. This result was overwhelmingly significant. Multivariate analyses confirmed that this strong association was unaffected by the location of the study. Although the outcome in terms of relapse was better overall in females, the degree of association between relapse and high EE is virtually identical in the two genders. The effect of EE calculated from these data was actually stronger than that of medication, and virtually identical in the medicated and non-medicated groups. Medication and EE were thus independently related to relapse, confirming that EE status has no bearing on the decision to prescribe medication.

The amount of face-to-face contact was found to be of importance: the strength of association between high EE and relapse was greater where contact is high, while living in high contact with a low EE relative was if anything protective.

The acknowledgement that the family atmosphere pays a role in relapse in schizophrenia has now led to several intervention studies (e.g. Falloon et al., 1982; Leff et al., 1982). These have been successful in some; but not in all, cases (Lam, 1991). This indicates that family atmosphere can be modified to reduce relapse rates, but that this is probably dependent upon the techniques and expertise deployed by the therapists. The changes leading to a reduction in EE seem to be a sufficient but not a necessary component of intervention. These studies thus provide good evidence that the elements of family atmosphere detected by the EE measure are causally related to relapse in schizophrenia. Interestingly, clinical staff have levels of EE similar to those of relatives (Moore et al., 1992) and this too may have adverse consequences for the patient.

Immigration and mental health

On the face of it, immigration looks like the sort of natural experiment that social psychiatrists dream about. Immigrants leave one society and enter another, in the process exposing themselves to stresses of considerable magnitude. One would expect therefore that the rate of psychiatric disorder would consequently be raised. In some immigrant groups, this is true. However, the immigration paradigm may be more of a snare than an opportunity.

This is because all immigrations differ, and interpretation becomes correspondingly complicated. First, the immigrants carry with them their own genetic and cultural inheritance, and this may itself lead to a susceptibility to psychiatric breakdown different from that of the indigenous inhabitants. Culture may increase exposure to physical influences, for instance if it encourages religious or recreational use of drugs.

Secondly, they are a self-selected group, perhaps because they had the energy to seek economic advancement, perhaps because the conditions for immigration were such that more rootless people found it easy to go abroad. In the first but not the second example the immigrant group would be selected for good mental health. Some immigrants arrive as refugees and have often had extremely bad experiences beforehand. They may thus have high rates of post-traumatic stress disorder. Some are obliged to leave considerable assets behind them in exchange for impoverishment, prejudice and an inability to find work or use skills. This is true of Vietnamese groups in south London, who are also isolated by language barriers.

Economic migrants may also face difficulties, but often bring resources and skills with them that they are able to build on. In many cases, *chain migration* means they come to areas inhabited by people from their own country or even village, with the consequent availability of social support. The act of immigration is in itself a stress and can provoke the development if illness.

Once the dust of the move has settled, the immigrants have to adapt to a greater or lesser degree to the host culture, and this may be variably successful, usually dependent on the amount of difference between hosts and guests. This process may be interfered with by racism, in many cases based on colour. This process of acculturation is a long-drawn-out stress. Immigrants are often economically disadvantaged. There may be secondary effects like disruption of social supports and family ties, and the provocation of family conflict. Changes in physical environment potentially expose immigrants to novel micro-organisms and other physical agents.

These various possibilities can be teased out by establishing rates of disorder in the home society, in the immigrant group, and in the native members of the host society, and relating these to social disadvantage, the experience of racism, the timing of breakdown, and to problems over acculturation. Unfortunately, few studies have taken account of these aspects and in consequence interpretation is often difficult or impossible.

Thus, using immigration as a test bed for social theories of psychiatric disorder is less easy than at first sight, and requires quite sophisticated measures of a range of potential influences. Nevertheless, the existence of sizeable immigrant minorities may have considerable public health significance, and be worth researching in its own right.

Britain has seen a considerable influx of immigrants from various parts of the world since the last war, although immigration is now very limited indeed. There are quite large populations of people whose families originated from the Caribbean or South Asia. Although some South Asian groups are particularly disadvantaged, in general they are well-established: they have retained much of their culture, often sustained by their religious affiliation. Their style of adaptation has been described as *parallel accommodation*. There is no evidence that people of South Asian origin in Britain have increased rates of psychiatric disorder of any type.

In contrast, adaptation to British society among people of Afro-Caribbean origin has taken the form of *assimilation*, but because of prejudice and disadvantage, this has not been wholly successful. Despite this, Afro-Caribbean people have rates of minor psychiatric disorder similar to those of the white British-born (Bebbington *et al.*, 1981*a*). However, several studies concur in suggesting that this group has a much higher incidence of psychotic disorder than white Britons. Preliminary evidence suggests that the rate of psychosis in the Caribbean is no higher than in the white British, thus ruling out explanations in terms of genetic or cultural inheritance and possibly also of the recreational use of cannabis. Moreover, since the rates seem to be particularly high in the second generation, that is, in people born in Britain (McGovern & Cope, 1987; Harrison *et al.*, 1988), the origins of psychosis may lie in increasing social disadvantage. However, it is possible that the incidence of psychosis has peaked and is now declining in Afro-Caribbean groups (Glover *et al.*, 1994). If so, the excess of cases of psychosis may be a cohort effect – one suggestion is that this might be mediated by exposure of Afro-Caribbean mothers to a novel infectious agent at the time of immigration.

Cultural change and psychiatric disorder

It is possible to perceive similarities in the 'traditional' cultures of the world, but these are generally outweighed by their differences. This makes it very dangerous to generalise widely from the very few and localised psychiatric surveys that have been carried out in such societies. Nevertheless, there is a major experience that is shared by many traditional societies, and that is the *process of change*. The rate of change in economically underdeveloped countries can be staggeringly fast. Developments that took 200 years in the West are being telescoped into 50 or even 20 years in some non-Western countries. This makes the cultural environment unpredictable and may have a major effect on the frequency of psychiatric problems.

The changes affect all areas of the life of the community but may be uneven in what they affect. Along with changes in economic and social stratification, diversification, and specialisation of human activities, there is a progressive alteration in traditional norms of interpersonal interaction, group values, and the external environment. These changes can be described in terms of the processes of urbanisation, modernisation, acculturation, social change, and more wide-reaching cultural change.

Urbanisation is one of the clearest manifestations of social change affecting less-developed countries. The cities of the Third World are outstripping their old-established counterparts in the West. This comes about partly from high birth rates, but largely because of migration from rural areas. The consequences are an inevitable disruption of social ties.

Modernisation has a number of different aspects – political, economic, industrial, social and cultural. Political modernisation involves the development of key institutions like political parties, legislatures and the instruments of government. Social and cultural modernisation often leads to changed patterns of life, a decline of traditional authority, increased literacy, secularisation, and nationalism. Economic modernisation is associated with an increasing division of labour, the use of industrial management techniques, improved technology, and the growth of commercial facilities (Abercrombie *et al.*, 1988).

Acculturation has been described by Leighton (1959) as: 'The process in which the customs, knowledge, attitudes, values and material objects of one cultural way of life become adopted, in whole or in part, by people of another'. These days, more emphasis is given to the *reciprocal* influence of cultures in collision (Abercrombie *et al.*, 1988), although one culture is usually dominant in the sense that it changes less. The term has largely been used to describe the experience of immigrants, who are usually in a minority and enter a culture that in consequence is inevitably more powerful than their own. However, the process can be seen in most parts of the world as a consequence of Western cultural imperialism. Because of opportunities for economic exploitation, some parts of the world are particularly open to Western influences.

One of the crucial elements is the rapidity with which these changes come about. In some cases, the consequence can be widespread disruption of society: customs, communication, authority systems, cooperation, and shared values.

It is possible to study these changes both at the societal and the individual level. At the societal level, the measures of overall change can be correlated with changes in rates of mental illness. Ideally, this requires either comparison between societies changing at different rates or, better still, comparison of the same society at different points in time. At the individual level, it is possible to evaluate the change from traditional patterns in the attitudes and activities of individual subjects, and relate these to the likelihood of psychiatric disorder. It is also possible to identify locations within given societies where the process of change may differ and to see if the inhabitants of these different areas vary in their risk of mental illness.

In fact, there have been very few studies of the process of social change. Lin and his colleagues (1953, 1989) conducted community psychiatric surveys in Taiwan, 15 years apart. In the intervening period, Taiwan moved from being a relatively underdeveloped country into one of the 'Tiger' economies of the Pacific Rim. This spectacular change can hardly be over-emphasised. The authors have provided data both for manic-depressive illness and for neurotic disorder. There was a spectacular increase in neurotic disorder, which was not parallelled by any increase in manic-depressive illness. The prima facie implication is that the disruptions of development influence milder affective conditions preferentially, and quite drastically. However, the survey was carried out by lay interviewers, and psychiatric diagnoses were made secondarily. This must cause one to pause before accepting that results really do represent a striking increase.

Bahar (1989; Bahar *et al.*, 1992) carried out a community survey of minor psychiatric morbidity in Palembang, Indonesia. He was able to divide the population up according to area of residence. These areas differed in socio-economic development, a difference that he measured with a broad range of indicators, such as the frequency of television sets, electricity, telephones, and running water in the households. Bahar's expectation was that the process of economic development would increase psychopathology. However, the prevalence of minor psychiatric morbidity was *less* in areas with more access to Western facilities. In the higher echelons of Palembang society, the rate of psychiatric disorder did tend to increase again. On the basis of these results, Bahar hypothesised that, up to a point, the good effects of improvements in material resources outweigh the bad effects of societal disruption arising for urbanisation and modernisation.

Finally, Ghubash and her colleagues (1994) conducted a community psychiatric survey in Dubai, an oil-rich state, which in the last quarter of a century has seen spectacular changes in lifestyles accompanying the dissemination of oil riches. Virtually no section of the national population of Dubai is exposed to material disadvantage. The authors first hypothesised that it would be the rapidity of change that was associated with increased rates of psychiatric disorder. They developed an acculturation scale specifically to evaluate the change in attitudes and behaviours as their subjects moved from the traditional lifestyle of Dubai to a more modern and liberal culture.

The prevalence of psychiatric disorder was generally high in Dubai females, but this did not seem to differ much in relation to the modernity of their attitudes and behaviour. Subjects did have high rates of morbidity if they lived in an area of Dubai characterised by the most Western lifestyle. However, the most interesting finding was of significantly greater frequency of disorder in women whose behaviour seemed more modern than their attitudes. These women were obviously in a position of some conflict. The authors tried to evaluate conflict directly using an Ease Index, indicating how much at ease subjects felt with their changing society. Although those least at ease had the highest psychiatric morbidity, the differences were small and non-significant.

19

Psychiatry in general practice

GREG WILKINSON

Introduction

While the importance of psychiatry in general practice has long been acknowledged, an appropriate level of integration between the two clinical disciplines has been slow to develop. The theoretical and practical underpinning of the subject is substantial (Williams & Clare, 1979; Cooper & Eastwood, 1992; Pullen *et al.*, 1994) and, as a result of international political impetus towards efficiency and effectiveness in primary health care, a more rapid pace of change is becoming apparent.

A large number of investigations have documented the hitherto unsuspected, large volume of mental illness in communities worldwide (Wilkinson, 1985; Gater *et al.*,1991); the central role of GPs in the detection, identification and treatment of psychiatric disorders; and, as a corollary, they have lent support to the growth of a novel style of service based on GP/psychiatrist attachments in primary care settings.

Empirical studies of mental health and disorder in general practice led to a significant conclusion:

> 'that the cardinal requirement for improvement of the mental health services in this country is not a large expansion and proliferation of psychiatric agencies, but rather a strengthening of the family doctor in his therapeutic role'.
>
> (Shepherd *et al.*, 1966).

In the United States a similar verdict has been reached (National Institute of Mental Health, 1980), and the World Health Organization has endorsed the principle:

> 'The crucial question is not how the general practitioner can fit into the mental health services but rather how the psychiatrist can collaborate most effectively with primary care medical services and reinforce the effectiveness of the primary physician as a member of the health team'
>
> (World Health Organization, 1973).

Figure 19.1. *Goldberg and Huxley's model*

Level 1   Psychiatric morbidity in the community
First filter: Decision to consult GP
Level 2   Psychiatric morbidity in general practice
Second filter: Recognition by GP
Level 3   'Conspicuous' psychiatric morbidity in general practice
Third filter: Decision to refer to psychiatric service
Level 4   Psychiatric out-patients
Fourth filter: Decision to admit
Level 5   Psychiatric in-patients

Epidemiology of mental disorders in primary care settings

Goldberg & Huxley (1980) constructed a simple model of levels and filters on the 'pathways to psychiatric care' (Figure 19.1). Level 1 refers to all psychiatric disorders in the population, which pass into level 2 when the patient decides to consult a general practitioner. At level 3, a general practitioner correctly recognises a proportion of the people consulting with psychiatric morbidity. Of people with psychiatric disorders, 90–95% are treated at level 3 by the general practitioner. The rest, a minority, pass through subsequent filters into levels 4 and 5.

Prevalence of psychiatric illness in general practice

In the classic study, Shepherd *et al.*, (1966) found that 14% of a general practitioner's patients consulted their doctor at least once in a 12-month period for a condition diagnosed entirely or largely as psychiatric in nature. Two-thirds of the mental disorders found in the primary care setting are accounted for by depressive, anxiety and somatoform disorders. Behaviour and stress disorders account for a third of diagnoses. A minority (7%) of diagnoses are for psychotic disorders and dementias.

Multi-axial systems of classification appear most appropriate in this setting. Current classifications (e.g. DSM-IV and ICD-10, and that produced by the World Organization of National Colleges, Academies, and Academic Associations of General Practitioners/Family Physicians) appear to be largely inadequate for use in primary care (Mann *et al.*, 1981*a*; Jenkins *et al.*, 1988) and have had little impact in practice.

Chronicity

Over half the patients identified by general practitioners as having psychiatric illness have chronic conditions, defined as those continuously present for at least one year, or recurring with sufficient frequency to cause continuous disability or to require continuous prophylactic treatment (Shepherd *et al.*, 1966). Thus about 8% of patients seen in a primary care setting suffer from chronic mental disorders with some degree of functional impairment.

Within this group of disorders, affective disorders are commonest, but psychotic, anxiety and personality disorders contribute the greatest proportion of severe disability.

Diagnostic practices

The GP has a continuous relationship with patients and their families, which results in a different perspective of illness and diagnosis than is usually the case in hospital practice. As an illustration, Mann *et al.* (1981*a*) found differences between the diagnoses made by general practitioners and psychiatrists in neurotic illness: (i) psychiatrists diagnosed more people as suffering from depression than GPs, finding such cases from among those classed as anxious by the GPs; and (ii) psychiatrists diagnosed an anxiety state in many cases classified by the GPs as physical disorders of psychogenic origin and insomnia.

Ability of GPs to detect psychiatric illness

Surveys from general practice indicate considerable inter-practice variability in rates of diagnosis: within practices, there exists individual practitioner variability, in overall illness episode and patient consultation rates, in attitudes among doctors to the recognition and management of psychiatric disorders, and in doctors' rates of identification of psychiatric morbidity.

Demographic characteristics of patients that are associated with increased likelihood of a doctor detecting psychiatric illness are: unemployment, female sex, and marriage ending in separation, divorce, or death (Marks *et al.*, 1979). Variations in two attributes account for much of the wide variation among GPs in their ability to detect psychiatric illness: these are, 'interest and concern', and 'conservatism'. The way in which a doctor interviews patients is important, and there are interactions between types of interview style and the doctor's personality.

Family practice trainees who are self-confident and outgoing, of high academic ability, with directive techniques and realistic concepts of psychiatry, tend to make more accurate psychiatric assessments (Goldberg *et al.*, 1980). Doctors who give greater emphasis to psychiatric questions during their interviews tend more frequently to assess their patients as psychiatrically ill but do not tend to be more accurate in their assessments.

Therapeutic practices

The majority of psychotropic drugs and 'psychotherapy/listening' provided to adults in general practice is given in visits during which no diagnosis of mental disorder is recorded. A common characteristic of consultations leading to the prescription of a psychotropic drug is the focus of patient and doctor on both physical and emotional issues. This occurs more frequently that either diagnosis of psychiatric disorder or the presentation of symptoms classes as psychosocial.

505

Most general practitioners consider the treatment of mental illness to be an integral part of their work, and the majority of doctors use a combination of drugs and psychological methods. However, a substantial percentage of people with psychiatric illness in general practice receive little or no treatment other than consultation. About a quarter of those patients identified as having psychiatric illness are treated by listening and counselling and about a third receive psychotropic medication, while about half receive no specific treatment.

There has been general criticism from psychiatrists that the psychotropic drug-prescribing practices of general practitioners are poor. Tyrer (1978) analysed the current drug treatment of all patients referred from general practice to a psychiatric out-patient clinic over four years. Half of the drugs were considered to be incorrectly prescribed on pharmacological grounds, the main errors being unnecessarily prolonged regular treatment, incorrect dosage (particularly common with antidepressants), and poly-pharmacy with drugs of similar pharmacological action.

Of general practice patients beginning a new course of psychotropic drug treatment, and characterised by extensive physical and psychological morbidity, about one in five are still receiving psychotropic drugs six months later. Such prolonged treatment is associated with increased age, previous psychotropic drug use, higher levels of psychological morbidity at the inception of treatment and, in women, social problems as perceived by general practitioners. In addition, there is substantial physical morbidity in patients receiving psychotropic drugs, and these drugs are commonly prescribed for patients with known physical illness.

Treatment of depressive illness in general practice

The costs associated with specialist treatment of new episodes of depressive illness presenting in general practice are not commensurate with their clinical superiority over routine GP care. Comparative clinical efficacy, patient satisfaction and cost of three specialist treatments for depressive illness with routine care have been studied by Scott & Freeman (1992). Patients meeting DSM-III criteria for a major depressive episode were randomly allocated to either: amitriptyline prescribed by a psychiatrist (who was permitted by protocol only to talk about/monitor medication); cognitive behaviour therapy by a clinical psychologist; counselling and case work by a social worker; or routine care by a GP. Marked improvement in depressive symptoms occurred in all treatment groups over 16 weeks. Clinical advantages of specialist treatments over routine GP care were small, but specialist treatment involved at least four times as much therapist contact and cost at least twice as much as routine GP care. Psychological treatments, especially social work counselling, were most positively evaluated by patients.

Treatment adherence in primary care

The main factors contributing to treatment non-adherence are psychotropic drug side-effects; negative attitudes to medication; and inadequate doctor–patient communication. Johnson (1981) illustrates some of the problems associated with 'the adequate drug treatment of any condition' in a study of compliance in patients with a new depressive illness.

Within one week of the initial GP consultation, 16% had stopped medication; 41% had done so within two weeks, 59% within three weeks, and 69% within four weeks. About one-third claimed a remission of their symptoms within this period. When recovered patients were excluded from consideration, at four to six weeks following the initial consultation, 57% of patients who were still depressed at this time had defaulted from their drug treatment.

Educating GPs about suicide is of doubtful preventive value

The much-vaunted anti-suicidal effects of an educational programme for general practitioners on Gotland (a small island of 56000 inhabitants off the Swedish mainland) have been interpreted over-optimistically and cannot be generalised to other settings (Rutz *et al.*, 1989*a*,*b*; Rutz *et al.*, 1992*a*,*b*).

During 1983–4 16 of the 18 permanently employed general practitioners on Gotland took part in a programme comprising 20 hours of lectures, discussions, and videotape presentations in two two-day sessions covering aspects of depression. There were fewer than expected suicides during the period studied. The results lack credibility. Suicide rates on Gotland were falling before the study began. Recorded numbers of suicides were small (the suicide rate was lowest in 1985 and rose again in 1986). Puzzlingly, suicide data were presented differently and inconsistently in the relevant publications, rendering independent assessment difficult. The point is this:

> 'Evaluation of teaching GPs about suicide prevention would require enormous sample sizes with huge numbers of GPs over long periods of time and is quite unlikely to show any statistical difference unless there is an enormous difference in the efficacy of different methods. So, please, can we now have a moratorium on this idea that practitioners can prevent suicide?'
>
> (MacDonald, 1992*a*).

Nursing care

The role of trained psychiatric nurses in the care of patients with mental disorder in primary care settings, though ill-defined and rarely researched (Marks, 1985), is likely to increase greatly. The community psychiatric nurse (CPN) maintains links with the psychiatric services in the district. Many have close links with the GP surgery or health centre; others only come in on request. Their key role should be to support the severely mentally ill, as new community care policies come into force replacing long-term stay in psychiatric hospitals. However, many CPNs wish to broaden their role and work more closely with GPs, receiving direct referrals for assessment from the doctor. The evidence suggests that CPNs tend to treat patients with neurotic, personality and behavioural problems in primary care rather than reduce demands made on traditional services.

Suitably trained general practice 'practice nurses' may have a useful role in the management of patients with a psychiatric disorder presenting in general practice (Wilkinson *et al.*, 1993). Their main functions in treating patients with depressive disorders include: assessment of depression; monitoring clinical progress; enhancing treatment compliance; promoting social change and education of the patient and carers.

Counselling

Counselling – provided by a new profession of counsellors – appears to be growing rapidly in general practice, but its impact on the outcome of psychiatric illness remains largely unknown.

Brief counselling by GPs can be an effective alternative to prescribing psychotropic drugs (Catalan *et al.*, 1984). Patients with new episodes of minor affective disorder were selected by their general practitioner as suitable for anxiolytic medication. Half were allocated randomly to a drug-group (anxiolytic medication), and half to a non-drug group (brief counselling). Psychiatric and social assessments were made one month and seven months later. Anxiolytic medication consisted of minor tranquillizers of the doctor's choice for up to two weeks. Thereafter the doctor was free to prescribe further anxiolytic medication for as long as necessary. Brief counselling, given by the doctor, included explanation of the nature of any symptoms and why they had occurred; exploration of underlying personal or other problems, and ways of dealing with them; and reasons for not prescribing drugs. Before treatment, the two groups were similar on all the main variables measured. Subsequently, improvements were similar and parallel in the two groups.

Psychotherapies

Psychotherapies are increasingly being used in general practice settings, but the evidence that they are effective remains controversial (Blackburn *et al.*, 1981; Brodaty & Andrews, 1983; Robson *et al.*, 1984; Teasdale *et al.*, 1984). Patients in psychotherapy receive far more therapeutic attention than those in treatment-as-usual groups, and this factor rather than specific effects of the psychotherapies may be responsible for the majority of differences observed. Psychotherapies are generally too complex and time-consuming to become widely available in nationalised health services.

Care of people with long-term mental illness

Caring for people with chronic mental disorder in general practice requires a long-term commitment. The management objectives include:

- identification of all patients with chronic mental disorder in the practice population;
- assessment of their medical and social needs and the needs of their relatives;
- early recognition of relapse;
- provision of cost-effective care that is responsive to patients' changing needs;
- reduction of stress in the patient and family;
- education of patients, relatives and voluntary carers in the long-term treatment plan, in association with members of the primary care team;
- establishment of communication between all involved in the patient's care;
- continuous evaluation of the effectiveness of care provided;
- prevention of disability, self-injury, stress, institutionalisation in the community, relapse, therapeutic non-compliance, and the breakdown of family and social supports.

These objectives might be promoted by the wider use of primary care case-registers and the adoption of the principles and practice of shared-care between generalists and specialists in the treatment of patients with chronic mental disorder (Essex *et al.*, 1990). Developments in psychotropic drugs apart, the main medical options for improving the treatment of patients with chronic mental disorders in primary care are in improving psychiatrist/general practitioner liaison-consultation attachment schemes; the therapeutic role of community psychiatric nurses and other mental health professionals; and in the family-based management of psychiatric disorder.

Referral and consultation

Referral and consultation patterns vary widely depending on local factors and service features. For example, Tantum & Burns (1979) compared a Boston neighbourhood health centre with a mental health service in London. Patients with severe but long-standing psychiatric illness, or patients with transient emotional problems, were likely to be treated by a general practitioner in London and by non-medical health specialists in Boston. These patients received more overall care, more specialist, non-medical care, but made as many visits to the medical practitioner, other than a psychiatrist, in Boston as they did in London. Psychiatrists saw more acutely ill patients for a shorter time than non-medical specialists in both places. In both Boston and London, there was a highly selective referral process that resulted in psychiatrists from both areas seeing approximately the same proportion of the population of their catchment areas.

Patients with psychotic disorders, severe depression, alcoholism or violence are the most frequently referred groups by GPs to mental health services. In a third of cases the reason for referral is that a patient's disorder is beyond treatment in general practice, usually because the patient is in acute crisis or is considered to require treatment that could not be given in general practice. In another third the general practitioner wants a second opinion on the diagnosis and treatment of a patient who is either not improving or is deteriorating. In the rest, the general practitioner has been requested by patient, relative, or health or social services personnel to refer the patient to the psychiatric services, or another member of the patient's family is already being treated by a psychiatrist and it is considered beneficial that the patient should also attend; or the doctor wishes to enlist the support of a psychiatrist in helping a patient with legal or administrative problems.

Over half the cases referred to psychiatrists are thought by the general practitioners to have benefitted from referral to the psychiatric services, and about a quarter are not thought to have benefited (Robertson, 1979).

GP/psychiatrist liaison–consultation

In 1984, Strathdee & Williams reported that one in five consultant psychiatrists in England and Wales spend some time working in a primary care setting, and the figure is probably higher now. In 1988, Pullen & Yellowlees found the percentage in Scotland to be 56%.

There are three main models of such liaison–consultation but there are few examples of empirical evaluation of them (Horder, 1988; Creed & Marks, 1989):

1. Shifted out-patient clinic
   a traditional out-patient clinic is conducted by a psychiatrist in the GP surgery of health centre (the commonest model, by far).
2. Consultation model
   a GP selects specific patients for discussion with a psychiatrist who advises on diagnosis and treatment. The GP then treats the patient.
3. Liaison–attachment model
   the general practice and psychiatric teams work together, sharing attitudes, knowledge and skills.

Psychiatric clinics conducted in general practice tend to be strongly preferred by patients, mainly because of ease of access and relative absence of stigma (Tyrer, 1984). The patients seen encompass the entire range of psychiatric disorders, and most are treated at the clinic or by other members of the primary care team. Tyrer et al. (1984) reported that such clinics lead to an increase in the number of psychiatric out-patients seen, a fall in the number of new referrals, and a 20% fall in the number of admissions to psychiatric hospital. A day hospital opened simultaneously in the area and may have accounted for some of the drop in admission.

Referral from GPs to mental health workers in general practice

Increasing numbers of patients with a wide variety of mainly neurotic, personality, relational, sexual, and habit disorders, as well as long-term mental illnesses, are being referred by GPs to paramedical mental health professionals in general practice (Wilkinson, 1989). There is now an increasing move of personnel from the mental health sector to attach themselves to primary care settings. There may be a psychiatrist, a psychologist or a psychiatric social worker who visits the practice for an occasional session, but more often there will be regular visits from a community psychiatric nurse or counsellor.

Kendrick et al. (1993) have described the distribution of mental health professionals working in 1880 general practices in England and Wales. No mental health professional was on site in 726 practices: one was reported by 515, two by 205, three by 71, four by 19, and five by six practices. The number of practices reporting the presence on site of each type of professional were 528 for community psychiatric nurses, 266 for practice counsellors, 177 for clinical psychologists, 132 for psychiatrists, 96 for psychiatric social workers, and 45 for psychotherapists. Mental health professionals tend to cluster together in larger, training practices running stress, bereavement, or other mental health clinics.

Outcome of mental disorder in primary care settings

Few studies of the outcome of mental disorders have been conducted in general practice. Initial estimate of the severity of psychiatric morbidity and a rating of the quality of the social life at the time of follow-up tend to be the main factors that significantly predict outcome of the patient's psychiatric condition (Mann *et al.*, 1981*a*; Catalan *et al.*, 1984). Social measures predict a pattern of illness characterised by a rapid recovery after the initial assessment, and patients who report continuous psychiatric morbidity tend to be older, physically ill, and to have received psychotropic drugs.

Discussion

There are demonstrable differences, which are largely unaccounted for, in the abilities of general practitioners to recognise, treat, and refer patients with mental disorders appropriately. Though there are indications that training can improve attitudes, knowledge and skills, the effects of these differences among general practitioners on patient care and outcome are virtually unknown. It is not clearly established that the increased recognition of mental disorders by general practitioners is associated with improvements in their management of such disorders and in the outcome for patients.

It is difficult to identify specific mental disorders for which general practitioners' current clinical practices are most effective. Problems in the classification of mental disorders in general practice make it difficult to identify mental disorders reliably and validly, and general practitioners' clinical practices are diverse. The most pressing areas for study in this context are anxiety and depression, chronic mental disorder, and drug- and alcohol-related morbidity.

There is little evidence that clinicians and research workers are beginning to focus on longitudinal studies relevant to the causes, courses and outcomes of psychiatric disorders presenting in general practice. Simple questions remain largely unanswered: what are the effects of illness labelling in general practice; to what extent does counselling affect the course of mood disorders; and, what is the optimal management for patients with a somatic presentation of affective illness?

The main focus of future research should be on efforts to improve general practitioners' treatment practices for patients with mental disorders, rather than on increasing referral of patients to mental health specialists (Wilkinson & Williams, 1985). A wider use of medical audit to monitor process and outcome of care by primary health care teams is likely to directly improve patient care (Crossley et al., 1992).

Mental health is a public health issue

It is clear that the extent of psychiatric morbidity in general practice is beyond the capacity of even the most perfect collaboration between GPs and psychiatrists and has become, in essence, of public health and economic concern (Croft-Jeffreys & Wilkinson, 1989).

From this perspective, three main issues have become apparent from research findings:

1. Promotion of mental health, and prevention and management of mental illness in general practice, require resources beyond those available to mental health specialists.

2. General practitioners require specialist advice and help to promote mental health and manage mental illness more effectively
3. Mental health and mental illness in general practice are not exclusively medical concerns and require an approach encompassing multidisciplinary organisation and team-work.

Acknowledgements

I am grateful to Dr Ben Green, Consultant Psychiatrist, Halton Hospital, and Dr Ian Pullen, Consultant Psychiatrist, Dingleton Hospital, for reading and providing helpful comments on an earlier draft.

20

Community psychiatry and service evaluation

GERALDINE STRATHDEE and GRAHAM
THORNICROFT

Introduction

Now . . . the question may properly be asked, whether . . . we cannot recur, in some
degree, to the system of home care and home treatment; whether, in fact, the same care,
interest, and money which are now employed upon the inmates of our lunatic asylums,
might not produce even more successful and beneficial results if made to support the
efforts of parents and relations in their humble dwellings.

(Stallard, 1870).

The time for debate about whether locally based forms of care should supplant
traditional institutions is over . . . we should formulate and co-ordinate clear mental
health targets and strategies at each level to achieve their implementation over the next
decade.
(Prince Charles' address to the Annual Meeting of the Royal College of Psychiatrists at
Brighton in 1991).

This chapter focuses upon such targets and strategies, to give the reader an understanding of
the scientific basis for developing community mental health services. First, the historical
background and current context of these developments are reviewed. Second, the common
infrastructures that have been found necessary internationally for the planning, implementation and organisation of community care are described. Third, the emerging consensus on
the *core service components* necessary in any comprehensive mental health service are
described. Throughout these sections the focus is on the methods used and the findings in
evaluations of these developments; this area presents perhaps more methodological
difficulties in evaluation than in many other areas of medical enquiry. Finally, the likely
directions of future services development and research endeavour for the remainder of the
1990s are discussed.

The definition of community psychiatry

The term community psychiatry has been used to describe a vast range of models
and practices used in contemporary psychiatry. The concept ambiguously implies both care
in and by the community, and so has united supporters of the former (libertarian radicals)

and the latter (fiscal radicals). It may imply merely a change in the locus of care from the hospital to the community setting, or more comprehensively to the methods and financing of care delivery (Goldman *et al.*, 1983*a*). Sabshin's view (1966) was that the nature of the care is more important than locality, and proposed that

> community psychiatry involves the utilisation of the techniques, methods, theories of social psychiatry and other behavioural sciences to investigate and to meet the mental health needs of a functionally or geographically defined population over a significant period of time, and the feeding back of information to modify the central body of social psychiatric and other behavioural science knowledge.

In this text community psychiatry is defined as:

> the network of services which offer continuing treatment, accommodation, occupation and social support and which together help people with mental health problems to regain their normal social roles.

The key elements of any properly functioning community psychiatry service, then, are continuity over time, integration between elements or nodes of the network, the recognition of a real or potential host 'natural' community, the view that home treatment is often preferable to institutional care, the acceptance of a need for some acute and highly staffed treatment setting, and a concern that such provisions are acceptable to service users and their neighbours.

The policy framework

Over the past four decades mental health policies in Europe and the USA have resulted in the uneven development of community psychiatric services, which form partial alternatives to institutional care. The organisation and funding of health care systems, and local geography and health service history, have been fundamental in influencing the diversity of models of community service developments (Mechanic, 1987; Ramon, 1988; Klein, 1991).

International Community Psychiatry developments

Of an estimated 1.7–2.4 million chronically mentally ill persons in the United States (Goldman *et al.*, 1983*b*), only 116 000 remained within state mental hospitals by 1983 (Bachrach, 1986). The United States community programmes have influenced much of the service development in Europe, despite differences in the organisation of health care systems. Present United States government policy is embodied in the National Plan for the Chronically Mentally Ill, which was a consequence of a wide-ranging review of policy (General Accounting Office, 1977) demonstrating that community based facilities, developed in line with plans to introduce a national network of comprehensive community mental health centres, had in fact been implemented 'in the absence of a planned, well-managed and systematic approach'.

Far reaching policy changes have been introduced more rapidly in Italy than in Britain and the United States (Mollica, 1983), and allow limited comparisons to be made. Law 180, enacted in 1978, formalised and accelerated this pre-existing trend in the care of the mentally ill (Tansella *et al.*, 1987). In contrast to the policies in the USA and Britain, the major provisions set out that no new patients be admitted to the large state hospitals, nor should there be any re-admissions after 1st January 1982. No new psychiatric wards or hospitals were to be built. Psychiatric wards in general hospitals were not to exceed 15 beds and must be affiliated to community mental health centres. Community-based facilities would be responsible for a specified geographical area, staffed by existing mental health personnel (Mosher, 1983). In essence, the legislative reforms reversed the previous order of priorities accorded to hospital and community forms of service provision (Tansella, 1986).

In Scandinavia, the dominant model in the organisation of psychiatric care has been the creation of geographically defined areas, known as sectors. A series of political, legal and organisational changes influenced the development of the services. In Sweden, two factors were particularly significant. Firstly, in 1967 the responsibility for mental health services was decentralised from federal to local government with the aim of integrating with other health care services (Goldie & Freden, 1991). Secondly, in 1973 the National Board of Health and Welfare outlined a plan that gave the primary care services increased responsibility for minor psychiatric morbidity, with the psychiatric services to provide in-patient and out-patient care for the more seriously ill (Lindholm, 1983). Similarly decentralisation and the creation of sectors was embodied in a law passed in 1978 in Finland. There was even greater emphasis on the role of primary care with the idea that psychiatric out-patients should be treated by primary care staff in health services centres with advice and consultation available from specialists in polyclinics and hospitals.

In Britain in 1961 Enoch Powell, then the Minister of Health, announced that the mental hospital population should be halved by 1975, and that most of those psychiatric in-patients remaining would be treated in units in district general hospitals (Holloway, 1990). The trend to develop district services, which presented an opportunity to bring psychiatry back into the mainstream of medicine, was welcomed by psychiatrists in particular (Carse *et al.*, 1958; Leyberg, 1959). There was an extension of the out-patient clinic services in general hospitals (Gillis & Egert, 1973), polyclinics or health centres within urban areas and the development of occasional day places and hostels (Foucault, 1971; Walsh, 1987).

In Britain, the decline in numbers of psychiatric in-patients has continued at an even rate since 1954 (Thornicroft, 1988). The 1975 Government White Paper (DHSS, 1975) set a target of 47900 in-patient psychiatric beds after the completion of the programme of closure of psychiatric hospitals (Thornicroft & Bebbington, 1989). Eighty-four per cent of this planned reduction in long-stay psychiatric beds has now taken place. The average number of psychiatric beds occupied each day in 1985 in England and Wales, for example was 64800 (Audit Commission, 1986). Only the final sixth of long-stay patients remain to be relocated. Alongside this attrition, there has been a corresponding increase in the annual number of admission: from 78 586 in 1955 to 185 514 in 1981 (House of Commons Social Services Committee, 1985).

Mental health policy in Britain has evolved rapidly since 1975. Several reports have been published, of which the most influential include Social Services Committee, 1985; Audit

Commission, 1986; Griffiths, 1988; Murphy 1988; Secretaries of State, 1989 to the current statutory framework (House of Commons, 1990). This now requires local social service and health authorities to draw up jointly agreed community care plans that clearly indicate the local implementation of needs-based individual care plans for the chronic and severely mentally ill.

Case and care management

If deinstitutionalisation has been the giant of *policy* shaping the development of community mental health services, case management has been the giant of *practice*. Its roots lie in social case work and within the mental health field the central co-ordinating function was first formally recognised in the USA by the Community Mental Health Centres Act of 1963, and its 1975 amendments, which explicitly required the centres to link with other agencies providing care for long-term patients. Despite this, community based services for the long-term mentally ill in the USA have too often been fragmented (Braun *et al.*, 1981; Kiesler, 1982). Methods of drawing together the components of care were therefore developed, especially in federally funded initiatives such as the Community Support Program (Tessler & Goldman, 1982).

The principles most often described at the root of the care management concept are outlined in Table 20.1. Continuity here refers both cross-sectionally, to a comprehensive range of services for long-term mental illness, and longitudinally, to emphasise the need for enduring and possibly indefinite care for a substantial proportion of this group (Anthony *et al.*, 1988). In Britain, usage of the concept gained currency rapidly after 1985, when the House of Commons Social Services Committee Report on Community Care recommended that 'the Government give high priority to encouraging and monitoring the developing use of keyworkers (House of Commons, 1985). Sir Roy Griffiths took up the idea, under a different name, in 1988 in specifying that 'no person should be discharged without a clear package of care devised and without being the responsibility of the named care worker' (Griffiths, 1988).

The provisions of the 1990 National Health Service and Community Care Act (House of Commons, 1990) aim to fulfil a number of important objectives (Table 20.1). The Act makes the following statutory requirements of case managers:

> where it appears to a local authority that any person for whom they may provide or arrange for the provision of community care services may be in need of any such services, the authority (a) shall carry out an assessment of his needs for those services and (b) having regard to the results of that assessment, shall then decide whether his needs call for the provision by them of any such services.

Health and the nation targets

A related policy initiative in 1992 was the publication of national mental health targets within the framework of *The Health of The Nation* (Department of Health, 1993*a*). The targets set were:

Table 20.1. *Key objectives of NHS and Community Care Act, 1990*

To promote the development of domiciliary, day and respite services to enable people to live in their own homes wherever feasible and sensible.
To ensure that service providers make practical support for carers a high priority.
To make proper assessment of need and good case management the cornerstone of high-quality care.
To promote the development of a flourishing independent sector alongside good quality public sevices.
To clarify the responsibilities of agencies and so make it easier to hold them to account for their performance.
To secure better value for taxpayers' money by introducing a new funding structure for social care.

- To improve significantly the health and social functioning of mentally ill people.
- To reduce the overall suicide rate by at least 15% by the year 2000 (from 11.1 per 100 000 population in 1990 to no more than 9.4).
- To reduce the suicide rate of severely mentally ill people by at least 33% by the year 2000 (from the estimate of 25% in 1990 to no more than 19%).

These targets can be expected to increasingly inform service purchasing decisions, provider plans and service evaluation during this decade.

Seven steps to community services

We propose that establishing community mental health services can be seen as a process of seven steps (Table 20.2).

Step 1: Agreeing the guiding principles of community psychiatric services

Having identified the individuals for whom the service is to be provided and assessed their range of needs, users and providers can form a helpful alliance in developing a range of core service components. A surprising consensus can be found among clinicians, planners and user organisations in their formulations of the essential principles that should underpin such community services. Those outlined below represent the views of such disparate groups as MIND (1983), the Department of Health (1985), the Royal College of Psychiatrists and the National Institute of Mental Health (1987).

Services should be local and accessible and to the greatest extent possible delivered in the individual's usual environment.
Services should be comprehensive and address the diversity of needs of the individual.
Services should be flexible by being available whenever and for whatever duration. There should be a range of complementary models that provide individuals with choice and vary, depending on need, at any point in time.

Table 20.2. *Seven steps to establishing a community service*

1. Agreeing the guiding principles
2. Setting sector boundaries
3. Estimating population needs
4. Information infra-structure
5. Target priority groups
6. Assessing needs of individual patients
7. Delivering the service components

Services should be consumer-orientated that is based on the needs of the user rather than those of providers.

Services should empower clients by using and adapting treatment techniques that enable clients to enhance their self-help skills and retain the fullest possible control over their own lives.

Services should be racially and culturally appropriate and include use of culturally appropriate needs assessment tools, representation on planning groups, cross-cultural training for staff, use of indigenous workers and bilingual staff, identification and provision of alternative basic facilities.

Services should focus on strengths. They should be built on the skills and strengths of clients and help them maintain a sense of identity, dignity and self-esteem. Patients should be discouraged from adopting the sick-role and the service from developing an environment organised around permanent illness with lowered expectations.

Services should be normalised and incorporate natural supports by being in the least restrictive, most natural setting possible. The natural work, education, leisure and support facilities in the community should be used in preference to specialised developments.

Services should meet special needs with particular attention being paid to those with physical disabilities, mental retardation, the homeless or imprisoned.

Services should be accountable to the consumers and carers and evaluated to ensure their continuing appropriateness and acceptability and effectiveness on agreed parameters.

Step 2: Setting sector boundaries

The first step in service developments is to establish the boundary conditions, usually in terms of sectors. The term sector now generally refers to a delineated geographic area, with a defined catchment population. Internationally the concept of the sector permeates community service development. The first sectors formed in France in 1947, and by 1961 the country had over 300. In America, the Kennedy Community Mental Health Centres Act of 1963 introduced the principle of a catchment area for each CMHC, and by 1975, 40% of the population had services based on the notion. In Europe throughout the 1970s, sector development grew but with sizes varying between countries (Lindholm, 1983). West Germany has sector sizes in the range of 250 000, Netherlands around 300 000, while the areas for the Scandinavian countries are smaller, with Denmark averaging 60–120 000, Finland 100 000, Norway 40 000, and Sweden 25–50 000. Of all countries, however, Italy has most comprehensively adapted the concept by virtue of Law 178 (1978), which established sectors in the range of 50–2000 000 population.

In Britain, as in many European Countries, sectorisation is regarded as an essential prerequisite to the development of effective community services (Strathdee & Thronicroft, 1992). A recent study (Johnson & Thornicroft, 1993) indicates that 81% of districts nationally have divided their catchment area into sectors. The division of a district into sectors is influenced by: geographical considerations such as the rural or urban nature of the area, the presence of a river or other natural structure which impairs access; the need to achieve co-terminosity with either a social services boundary or general practice location; division of the total district into areas of equal numbers of population. It could be argued that a division of resources, based on a knowledge and understanding of the degree of psychiatric morbidity and social deprivation at the local level would form a more rational basis for the creation of sectors and their teams (Strathdee & Thornicroft, 1992).

Research has concentrated almost exclusively on ascertaining if sectorisation would facilitate the development of community alternatives to in-patient hospital treatment. In Nottingham, Tyrer *et al* (1989) found the following reductions: number of admissions (5%), duration of admissions (4%), use of in-patient beds (38%). One Swedish study (Hansson, 1989) found a decrease in: number of admissions (20%), bed days used (40%), and compulsory admissions (25%). Another (Lindholm, 1983) found similar, but non-significant trends.

Step 3: Estimation of population needs

Scaling services to local needs

There is considerable debate about the numbers of psychiatric treatment and care places that are necessary (Wing, 1971, 1989). The 1975 British White Paper suggests targets for 50 District General Hospital beds per 100 000 of the population, together with 35 for the elderly severely mentally infirm and 17 for the 'new' long-stay patients. More recently, the House of Commons Social Services Committee report on Community Care (1985) noted that 'a smaller number of in-patients beds is now thought necessary for general psychiatric services', and a Royal College of Psychiatrists working party has specified this as 44 acute beds for a population of 100 000 (Hirsch, 1988).

The most important proposed change will be better co-ordinated between primary care, secondary care and social care, with all three components focused on community facilities. There are a number of different population scales on which health care services are currently provided:

for 500 000 people upwards:	Regional Secure Unit, specialist child services
150 000–300 000 population:	acute beds, intensive care beds, social services
35 000–75 000 population:	sector community mental health teams
fewer than 20 000 people:	primary care

Table 20.3. *Estimated illness prevalence in a population of 500 000*

Shizophrenia	1000–2500
($\frac{1}{3}$ to $\frac{1}{2}$ in contact with services)	
Affective psychosis	500–2500
Depression	10 000–25 000
Anxiety	8000–30 000

Department of Health (1993)

Table 20.4. *Estimated annual mental health patient contacts in a population of 500 000*

Psychiatrists	10 000
Admissions	2000–2500
Mental illness treated in general practice	30 000–40 000

Table 20.5. *Proposed range of district acute and continuing care general adult psychatric places for 250 000 population*

Type of provision	Range of places
24-hour staffed residences	40–150
Day staffed residences	30–120
Acute psychiatric care	50–150
Unstaffed group homes	48–80
Adult placement schemes	0–15
Local secure places	5–10
Respite facilities	0–5
Regional secure unit	1–10

Many mental health purchasing authorities have responsibility for a population of about a half of a million, and Tables 20.3–20.5 show the likely number of people suffering from mental illness, the number of professional contacts, and the estimated needs for treatment and care services.

In an ideal world, having established sectors, the development of appropriate and adequate services would then be based on a systematic assessment of the needs of the identified population of mentally ill and services developed based on an aggregation of this estimated need. However, information infrastructures are as yet remarkably primitive and the whole process of planning is relatively pragmatic. Three methods are commonly used as proxy, each with their own limitations (Shapiro *et al.*, 1985). First, there are estimates derived from past service utilisation rates (Goldberg & Huxley, 1980, 1992; Goldman, 1981). Second, there are calculations based on the relationships of mental health disorders to age, sex, ethnic group, marital status, economic status and other social variables (Thornicroft, 1991). Finally, needs are often defined by a focus on the seriously impaired chronically mentally ill (Thornicroft & Strathdee, 1991).

Social and demographic factors are closely associated with the measured rates of psychiatric disorder. The age structure of the population has useful pointers to service needs.

Over-representation in the 20–29 age range will predict a higher rate of population at risk of developing psychotic disorders. The association between psychiatric disorders and social class (particularly for schizophrenia and depression) is one of the most consistent findings in psychiatric epidemiology. The Jarman combined index of social deprivation is highly correlated with psychiatric admission rates for all Health Districts of the South East Thames Region, and may be used to estimate the degree of excess morbidity (Jarman, 1983, 1984; Hirsch, 1988; Thornicroft, 1991).

Ethnicity also has a powerful influence on service utilisation, with non-white ethnic groups having a higher risk than their white neighbours of being admitted to psychiatric hospital (Moodley & Thornicroft, 1988), increased risk of compulsory admission (Ineichen *et al.*, 1984), and a very substantially raised risk of being diagnosed as suffering from schizophrenia (Harrison *et al.*, 1988).

Step 4: Information infrastructure

Having collected the general epidemiological information identified above, some services have moved on to set up a clear, systematic and continuing method of collecting clinical and social need and service usage data as required. The most comprehensive method to elicit, code and store these data is the case register (Wing, 1989). Although such systems were formerly labour intensive, the recent availability of on-site micro and mini computers has made their more widespread use a practical option. The most fundamental question in setting up a register is defining the patient group to be registered. Classically this has been a health service only definition and has depended, in turn, on the mission statement and objectives of the overall service. Since, in any year, one-quarter of the general adult population will suffer from some form of mental health problem (Goldberg & Huxley, 1980), mental health services must define which subgroups from within this vast reservoir of suffering they can target as being the highest priorities to help. In many areas mental health teams have been concerned to focus their resource on those with the most severe and disabling mental health difficulties. Three of the most practical working definitions are those of Goldman (1981), McLean & Liebowicz (1989) and Merson *et al.* (1992), which predominantly relate to service utilisation patterns.

Step 5: Target priority groups

We propose a simple principle: Highest priority to the most disabled. As an example of this in practice, we have developed a form of triage into high, medium and low support categories of patients suitable for the general adult community mental health team (Table 20.6).

Step 6: Assessing the needs of individual patients

Mental health depends not only on health-related care, but on the provision of a wide range of services that address the diverse needs of patients. Table 20.6 identified many of these and is adapted from the American National Institute of Mental Health's document

Table 20.6. *Guidelines for high priority patients target groups*

High support group	Individual with severe social dysfunction (e.g. social isloation, unemployment, and/or difficulty with skills of daily living) as a consequence of severe or persistent mental illness or disorder. In particular, individuals with the following difficulties will be identified for high levels of support:
	  current or recent danger to self or others
	  severe behavioural difficulties
	  high risk of relapse
	  history of poor engagement with mental health services
	  little contact with other providers of care, e.g. GP or social services
	  precarious housing (e.g. bed & breakfast)
	  carers who experience particular difficulty in coping with a relative suffering from mental illness

Medium support group	Individuals with a lesser degree of social dysfunction arising from mental illness or disorder, e.g. those able to work at least part-time and/or to maintain at least one enduring relationship.
	This group will also include the following individuals:
	  those likely to recognise and to seek help in response to, signs of relapse
	  those receiving appropriate services from other agencies

Low support group	Individuals who, following assessment, have been found to have specific and limited mental health-related needs that do not require extensive, multi-disciplinary input. In general, such individuals are likely to respond to brief or low-intensity intervention. For example:
	  adjustment reaction or bereavement
	  personality disorder/difficulties
	Identify those at risk of:
	  in-patient admission
	  suicide (Health of the Nation)
	  challenging/forensic behaviours

Toward a model plan for a comprehensive community-based mental health system (1987). In this section, Stevens & Gabbay's (1991) working definition of need will be used, that is 'the ability to benefit in some way from health (and social) care'.

The issue of how best to make such an assessment has taxed both researchers and clinicians alike, not least because their requirements differ. An ideal assessment tool for use in a routine clinical setting would be one that is brief, takes little time to administer, does not require the use of personnel additional to that of the usual clinical team, is valid and reliable in different settings and across gender and cultures and, above all, which can be used as an integral part of routine clinical work, rather than as a time-consuming extra. MacDonald (1991a) suggests that in addition they should be sensitive to change, their potential inter-rater and test–retest reliability high and that they logically inform clinical management (Hillier *et al.*, 1991). Individual needs should be assessed along a range of functional domains, such as those included in the recently developed Camberwell Assessment of Need (CAN) (Table 20.7).

Table 20.7. *Problem areas covered by the Camberwell Assessment of Need*

Accommodation
Occupation
Specific psychotic symptoms
Psychological distress
Information about condition and treatment
Non-prescribed drugs
Food and meals
Household skills
Self-care and presentation
Safety to self
Safety to others
Money
Childcare
Physical health
Alcohol
Basic education
Company
Telephone
Public transport
Benefits

Step 7: Delivering the service components

Tansella (1989) counsels 'what is important in community care is not only the number and characteristics of various services but the way in which they are arranged and integrated'. Mechanisms must be found that enable effective service delivery, the three principles of which have been enunciated by Paumelle, an early proponent of community care in France (Walsh, 1987; Strathdee, 1991). First, *continuity of care* should be ensured. This, Paumelle believed, could best be achieved by ensuring that persons and families were dealt with at all stages and at all levels of illness by the same team. In turn, this meant assigning such teams and their associated structures such as beds and clinics to populations of manageable size. Given the range of needs of individuals with mental health problems, *coordination of care* was cited as the second fundamental principle. Only by the introduction of multidisciplinary and interagency teams could the range of treatments necessary to overcome the impairment and disability of the mentally ill be delivered. *Integration of care* was regarded as the third essential based on the promise (WHO, 1983) that in any community, first contact for individuals in distress is often not with the psychiatric specialist team, but rather persons in key positions of responsibility in the community such as teachers, police, public health nurses, community nurses, social workers and general practitioners. The specialist team must therefore integrate its efforts with those of the non-specialists, as well as taking the lead in educating and counselling non-specialists.

Table 20.8. *Ten core components of a comprehensive mental health service*

1. Establish care registers
2. Crisis response services
3. Hospital and community places
4. Assertive outreach and care management services
5. Day care
6. Assessment and consultation services
7. Carer and community education and support
8. Primary care liaison
9. Physical and dental care
10. User advocacy and community alliances

The ten core components of a comprehensive mental health service

The development of community services has had two consistent themes: that services should be directed to meeting individual needs and that the traditional inherited service systems dominated by large institutions should be replaced with a more balanced and flexible range of alternative services (Hunter & Wistow, 1987). This section focuses on the ten components of community services. The categories delineated are not mutually exclusive, and as in any local settings, the organisation and form of services should be built on local information and circumstances (Table 20.8).

1. Establish case registers

Only a proportion of the severely mentally ill come into contact with the psychiatric services and a sizeable proportion of these lose contact. Murray Parkes *et al.* (1962), following up a cohort of schizophrenic patients discharged from London mental hospitals, found that although almost three-quarters had seen their GP in the year after discharge, less than 60% had attended hospital out-patient clinics. Similarly, Pantellis *et al.* (1988) in the South Camden Schizophrenia Study identified that only three-fifths of the known individuals with schizophrenia in the area were in contact with the psychiatric services. Lee & Murray (1988), studying the long-term outcome of a group of depressed patients, found that over half had lost contact with the hospital services; those out of contact included some of the most severely ill. Johnstone *et al.* (1984), following a cohort of discharged schizophrenics similar to that of the Murray Parkes group, found that 245 were seeing *only* their GP in a five-year follow-up period.

As indicated above, the establishment of care registers is easier. The ethical, moral and confidentiality issues before setting up a register should be addressed at the local level. The user advocacy group MIND has identified appropriate safeguards in its recent policy paper (MIND, 1990). The further routine collection of clinical contact data also allows for detailed service evaluation, to show, for example, patterns of service use by diagnosis (Der &

Bebbington, 1987; Tansella & Williams, 1989), social class (Wiersma *et al.*, 1983); and geographical mobility (Lesage & Tansella, 1989). Further, the use of standardised coding and diagnostic systems allows comparisons of service use within local areas (Giel & Horn, 1982), within regions (Torre & Marinoni, 1985), and between countries (Horn *et al.*, 1986; Sytema *et al.*, 1989). Such data can therefore indicate how variations in treated morbidity occur with local socio-demographic characteristics, with the nature and extent of local service provision, and with the service trends at the national level. Two important further information issues are the compilation and widespread circulation of accurate and updated street lists naming the responsible team for each address, and a well indexed directory of services to allow agencies to cross-refer. The use of registers is now likely to become very much more important as services are required by the Department of Health to identify and offer continuing support and supervision to the patients at risk of harm to themselves and others.

2. Crisis response services

The aim of the services should be to enable the client, family members, and others to cope with the emergency while maintaining the client's status as a functioning community member to the greatest extent. The services should be available on a 24-hour, seven-day basis, manned by experienced mental health professionals and known to providers, families, clients, and the community (Johnson & Thornicroft, 1993). Immediate psychiatric consultation should be available for rapid evaluation, diagnosis, and chemotherapeutic interventions as indicated.

Indeed adequate, early treatment, associated with client, family, and staff education and training can prevent the onset of many crises (Birchwood *et al.*, 1989). Falloon & Pederson (1985), for example, claimed reductions in family disruption, physical and mental disorders, and perceived burden after structured family interventions. Because of the episodic nature of the illness, however, there will be instances that require acute care and rapid response crisis stabilisation services.

The traditional provision of crisis intervention has been through consultation at the local general practitioners surgery (Murray Parkes *et al.*, 1962), domiciliary consultation (Littlejohns, 1986; Fry & Sandler, 1988; Sutherby *et al.*, 1991) and, in many districts, accident and emergency departments of general hospitals. With the development of community services this has been extended by a range of options that include 24-hour telephone helpline; walk-in emergency clinics (Lim, 1983; Haw & Lanceley, 1987); community mental health centres facilities and mobile outreach crisis intervention teams (Boardman, 1987); community crisis residential beds for temporary respite care outside the normal residential environment when needed; and in-patient beds in a variety of settings such as the psychiatric units of a district general hospital. In reviewing the community care experience of the USA, Bachrach (1984) has cautioned that the decrease in beds has led to excessive use of emergency services by young psychotic patients who use no other facilities. The system to open access of British primary care services may result in primary care teams having an increasing role to play in this regard (Kendrick *et al.*, 1991).

3. Hospital and community places

For modern day mental health services to work, a wide range of hospital and community beds or places are necessary and interrelated. These should range from secure facilities for mentally disordered offenders, through well-staffed units in hospital and the community for those with challenging behaviours, acute hospital beds and a range of community beds for crisis diversion, quarter- and half-way hostel purposes and respite facilities to residential and permanent accommodation.

Acute treatment facilities should be available to provide assessment by a multi-disciplinary team; investigation facilities to exclude an organic basis for a mental health disorder; supportive counselling and psychotherapeutic treatment; mechanisms for the provision and monitoring of medication to ensure education, maximal therapeutic effectiveness and a range of residential facilities. The location of such services has been the subject of major debate. Particular attention has been paid to the question of the role of the hospital and the appropriateness of alternative facilities, including hospital hostels, home-based teams and pre-admission facilities. Tyrer (1985a), in proposing his 'Hive' model, advocated that the hospital base should form the core of a system with closely co-ordinated sub-units of care such as day hospitals, community clinics, or mental health centres located in areas of greatest morbidity.

The practices covered by the term 'respite care' are of increasing importance in mental health service provision. Such respite care provides relatively brief planned periods of residential care, usually of between one week and one month, during which the patient may be fully reassessed, treatment can be modified, the family can benefit from relief of the burden of care, and when the patient may be given temporary sanctuary from the demands of everyday life, which may include an emotionally charged atmosphere at home. To date, respite care has been most fully developed for people with learning difficulties (Gerard, 1990),with physical disabilities (Robinson, 1984) and for the elderly (Harper, 1988). While there is evidence of substantial benefits for patients and their carers, within mental illness services, respite services are as yet poorly developed and await full evaluation.

The success of community-based services is crucially related to the nature and availability of accommodation with appropriate levels of support. Within the British context, Wing & Furlong (1986) have described a tenfold typology of sheltered housing for people with severe psychiatric disorders. The level of least supervision is that of unsupervised housing, where the individual lives alone or with family or friends and contact with psychiatric services is through non-residential staff. A variation of this arrangement is to afford a degree of administrative protection, for example from eviction for arrears of rent. At the next level, supervised housing provides regular domiciliary supervision by a mental health practitioner to sustain standards of hygiene, nutrition, and household maintenance. In group homes, which may be arranged in clusters, several residents with psychiatric disorders share the same house, which may be supervised by a residential landlady, with support from visiting staff.

In supervised hostels, residents may each have a bedroom and share communal facilities, with residential staff offering close daily supervision (Goldberg, 1986). A higher level of supervision is required for residents more disabled by psychiatric or physical conditions: the hostel model can be supplemented with night nursing staff, the provision of meals, and the supervision of budgeting. For those with severe challenging behaviours, an intensive supervision hostel (either hospital based as a hostel-ward, or in a well-staffed community place) may be needed, characterised by high staffing levels, a structured regime, a perimeter area, and the rapid availability of extra staff (Garety & Morris, 1984). Finally, a form of basis nursing unit will be necessary for people who are incontinent, immobile or disoriented.

To ensure the success of community housing provisions, liaison with community members and caring agencies is essential. Horder (1990) has defined practical guidelines for the functioning of community hostels. She states that they should be within easy access of shops, sports facilities, cinemas, day centres, workshops and pubs; a clear plan for medical cover should be formulated before the admission of residents; there should be detailed discussion with all staff members, especially GPs, if they are to be involved and agreement about spheres of responsibility, emergency work, prescribing and communication to be reached. Aside from permanent housing, homeless individuals who are mentally ill will require additional living situations with varying degrees of supervision and structure, including emergency shelters (Fischer & Breakey, 1986).

Mental illness rates in the homeless are in the range 41–93%, with alcohol dependency in over 60%, and chronic medical and dental problems in over 40% of this group (Morrisey & Levine, 1987, Bassuk et al., 1984; Kroll et al., 1986). These individuals characteristically have restricted social support networks, little contact with psychiatric services, lower re-admission rates than their domiciled counterparts, and little likelihood of referral to long-term care facilities (Appleby & Desai, 1985). Local psychiatric facilities clearly do not serve these homeless mentally ill at all adequately (Lamb, 1984). Even so, it is important to avoid over-generalisations about the homeless mentally ill, who have been shown to demonstrate considerable variations between the sites of detailed studies (Bachrach, 1992), for example as to proportion of such people who originated in the local area.

4. Assertive outreach and care management services

Since the early 1960s a number of studies have compared acute home-based care with hospital care (Pasamanick et al., 1967; Langsley et al., 1969; Polak & Kirby, 1976; Test & Stein, 1980; Fenton et al., 1982; Pai & Kapur, 1982; Hoult & Reynolds, 1984; Marks et al., 1988; Dean & Gadd, 1990). Despite differences in the models and evaluative methodologies used, these studies confirm a decrease in hospital admissions, improvement in clinical outcome and social functioning and greater patient satisfaction from acute home-orientated care. Indeed these findings have recently been replicated in the Daily Living Programme at the Maudsley Hospital (Muijen et al., 1992).

Reviews of the community-orientated approach to continuing care (Braun et al., 1998l; Kiesler, 1982) have shown that outcome from assertive outreach programmes is in no published case worse than for standard hospital-based treatment, and is often better. To date, however, these studies have not indicated which subgroups among the seriously mentally ill may be most and least likely to benefit from these forms of care (Mosher, 1983; Tantam, 1985). Further, they have often used service usage indices as the major outcome variables. With the exception of these few studies, however, most work describing community forms of psychiatric care has been very methodologically weak. Such evaluations should fulfil the following scientific criteria: random allocation to experimental and control programmes, clear patients characterisation, validated diagnoses, clearly described treatment programmes, outcomes measured with properly validated instruments.

In practice case management for the long-term mentally ill has developed into a range of techniques that can be described along 12 different axes (Table 20.2) (Thornicroft, 1991), which aim to ensure that patients with long-term psychiatric disorders receive consistent and continuing services for as long as they are required (Torrey, 1986), and that services do not inappropriately focus on patients with less severe conditions (Patmore & Weaver, 1991).

The direct caregiver variants of case management emphasise the staff–patient relationship as the key component through which effective care is channelled, in the tradition of social case-work. Brokerage models, however, give the case manager a central, distant co-ordinating function without any necessary direct contact with the patient. There is considerable consensus about the range of tasks that case management can offer at the individual level, and which are summarised in Table 20.3 (Intagliata, 1982; Challis, 1986; Renshaw et al., 1988).

5. Day care

Day hospitals were begun in Britain in 1946 after their establishment in the Soviet Union a decade earlier. They provide a service than can compare favourably with standard in-patient treatment for those in acute relapse (Dick et al., 1985). Unless, however, day hospitals are especially orientated to the needs of the chronic mentally ill such patients are more likely to attend Social Services day centres, which are less well staffed, and more oriented towards support than treatment. Day-care facilities vary enormously and in a comprehensive review Holloway (1988) defines five possible functions of the day hospital: an alternative to admission for the acutely ill; provision of support, supervision and monitoring in the transition between hospital and home; source of long-term structure and support for those with chronic handicaps; site for brief intensive therapy for those with personality difficulties, severe neurotic disorders and those who require short-term focused rehabilitation; an information, training and communication resource.

6. Assessment and consultation services

Until the past few decades the majority of consultation services were conducted in hospital out-patient settings. Evaluation of these services indicates dissatisfaction with communication patterns (Pullen & Yellowlees, 1989), and with clinical and referrer outcome (Kaeser & Cooper, 1971; Strathdee, 1990). Two innovations in community provisions have begun to redress these deficiencies. First, there has been an evolution of out-patient clinics from hospital sites and the establishment of consultation clinics in primary care settings. Nineteen per cent of all consultant general adult psychiatrists in England and Wales (Strathdee & Williams, 1984) and a half of Scottish psychiatrists work in this way. The evidence indicates that these clinics enhance continuity of care, particularly when the psychiatric team work in an integrated manner with their primary care colleagues. Additional advantages are that patients prefer the accessibility and non-stigmatising setting of their local surgery; the GPs enhance their knowledge of psychiatric disorders and treatment techniques; and the psychiatric team have increased access to community resources and are better placed to intervene at an earlier stage in the development of illness and relapse (Tyrer, 1984; Mitchell, 1985; Hansen, 1987; Creed & Marks, 1989; Joseph *et al.*, 1990).

Second, a growing number of community mental health centres have been established. Kingdon's survey (1989) indicates that they have been developed in 18% of districts with plans afoot in another 40%. The American community mental health centres attempted to provide five services: in-patient, out-patient, partial hospitalisation, emergency services, consultation and education. In the UK those described have functioned more as a resource for crisis intervention, co-ordinating multi-disciplinary teams, and as consultation services (Ovretweit, 1986).

7. Carer and community education and support

Much caring for the mentally ill is done by relatives, although not all carers are blood relatives or spouses by any means: some of the most successful caring relationships are made by friends, landladies or home helps (Kuipers & Bebbington, 1991). People with schizophrenic illnesses show a severe reduction in regular social contact, down from a norm of perhaps 30 people to only four or five. In this situation, carers share the problems and difficulties of relatives.

The process of daily care for relatives who have severe social and behavioural disturbance takes place at the cost of disruption to family routine, resulting physical and psychological morbidity to the health of the other family members, and costs to the economic viability of the family unit. A recent survey of carers of this group found that practical help was often forthcoming (e.g. housing, financial advice), but that emotional help was always deficient.

There should be assistance to families that provides education on the nature of the illness, consultation and supportive counselling on handling daily problems and intermittent crisis situations, appropriate involvement in the treatment planning process, respite care and referrals to family support groups and advocacy organisations such as the National or local Mental Health Associations. In addition, in order to facilitate community integration and acceptance, practical support and education should be available to landlords, employers, educationalists, community agencies and others.

By itself, education does not change EE attitudes or outcome. Indeed, it leads to very small changes in the amount of knowledge carers have about psychotic illnesses. The best way of offering it has not been established. Varying styles have been tried in the experimental studies: one-day workshops, with several families at a time (Anderson *et al.*, 1986): didactic sessions at home, with or without written information and relatives' groups with a didactic structure.

The content of this education has not been standard either, but it usually consists of some relatively straightforward attempt by the professionals to explain what we know, and what we do not know about these illnesses, to discuss issues of diagnosis, cause, and pharmaceutical and social treatments, and to examine ways relatives can influence outcome (MacCarthy *et al.*, 1989).

8. Primary care liaison

In Britain these elements must be considered in the light of two important aspects of our health care system. Firstly, there is a powerful primary care tier of care. General practitioners play a major role in the care of those with both acute and chronic psychological disorders (Shepherd et al., 1966; Goldberg & Blackwell, 1970; Sharp & Morrell, 1989; Paykel, 1990). For many patients with severe, long-term disorders the general practitioner is indeed the only source of continuing care (Murray Parkes et al., 1962; Johnstone et al., 1984; Brown et al., 1988; Lee & Murray, 1988; Pantellis et al., 1988). As Jones concluded: 'unless attention is given to finding administrative solutions to the repeated official exhortations (DHSS, 1975, 1978, 1981; Griffiths, 1988) for collaboration and co-operation with GPs we will fail to provide the mix of services needed'. Second, there is no unitary core agency responsible for assuring the delivery and co-ordination of all mental health services. Given the nature of the involvement of health, social and the range of non-statutory agencies, the organisation of services is therefore fundamental to their ability to fulfil the principles of delivery.

Ninety-eight per cent of the British population is registered with a GP, and of these 60% will consult at least once a year. The average GP has 2010 patients on his or her personal list and over the course of any two-year period can expect to see 90% of the entire registered population (Sharp & Morrell, 1989). On an average working day, 750 000 people visit their GP. Between one-fifth and one-quarter of all consultations to the average GP's daily surgeries are undertaken by individuals who have a mental health component either as the sole, or a major component of their problems (Shepherd et al., 1966). In the average consultation time of six minutes, just under a half of these problems are recognised by the doctors (Goldberg & Bridges, 1988). While the majority of mental health disorders fall within the less severe or 'neurotic' areas, of those individuals identified as having a mental health disorder, one-tenth have a chronic disorder defined as continually present for one year, or requiring prophylactic treatment (Regier et al., 1985). The primary care team has always dealt with the majority of mental health morbidity within the team. Only one in 20 are referred on for specialist care. General practice consultations are in a ratio of 10:1 for psychiatric out-patient attendances and 100:1 for psychiatric admissions.

Clinical psychologists working in primary care are significantly more likely than CPNs or practice counsellors to be referred patients with the following disorders, which are usually treated with behaviour therapy: psychosexual problems, eating disorders, phobias and obsessive-compulsive disorders. Patients report a high degree of satisfaction with behavioural treatment, and, as with other professionals involved in counselling, result in decreased drug prescribing. One study indicated that 28% of the psychologist's salary could be found from drug savings alone. Where psychologists have used their specialist training in cognitive therapy to treat depression, studies have found a significantly greater improvement compared to GP treatment alone, but no difference three months after completion of treatment. It has been suggested that the most important role for clinical psychologists is to provide education and consultative liaison for the GP and consultation for self-help or other voluntary sector organisations.

The attachment of community psychiatric nurses to particular general practices has followed two general models. In those services where the nurses are hospital-based and work as members of the secondary care team, 80% of their referrals are from psychiatrists with individuals with severe and continuing mental health disorders forming a considerable proportion of their workload. In the second model, that of the nurses, although employed by secondary care services, being attached to a particular general practice, the referral pattern shifts, with 80% of their referrals coming direct from GPs. In the latter model the caseloads are characteristically large, composed of patients with neurotic and adjustments disorders, with large numbers of patients receiving care from the CPN as the sole involved discipline. Although the caseloads of both the hospital-based and primary-care based CPNs remain similar in terms of the numbers of individuals with schizophrenia, the mean time in contact with psychotic patients is a third of the time spent with non-psychotic patients and almost entirely limited to the administration of injections. Research evidence indicates that CPNs trained in psychosocial interventions with the families of individuals with schizophrenia produce significantly greater improvement in negative symptoms, social adjustment and family satisfaction compared with controls (Brooker et al., 1992).

In a study in 1992, Sibbald and her colleagues identified that one in 20 practices in England and Wales consider themselves to have a counsellor working on site. In 1992, half of the employed counsellors had specialist training in counselling, but the employing GPs were unaware of the qualification of the counsellors in their practices in one-fifth of instances. Counsellors are referred a wide variety of problems ranging from family and relationship difficulties to drug and alcohol abuse and psychiatric illness. The introduction of counsellors into primary care has been demonstrated to reduce psychotropic drug prescribing, GP consultation rates and referrals to psychiatrists, as well as providing patient and GP satisfaction.

The development of registers of vulnerable individuals can form a practical focused first step to the development of good liaison between primary and secondary care services. Such initiatives are facilitated by practices having computerised age/sex registers with repeat prescribing lists and by local mental health services having care programme approach or other comprehensive registers. Without registers of the most vulnerable individuals, GPs may be unaware of the needs or existence of this client group until they present in crisis. Having identified such individuals, the joint development of practice policies in optimal care offers a useful strategy for the organisation of practices to maximise care of this client group (Strathdee & Phelan, 1993).

9. Physical health and dental care

Patients treated in the community are often the most severely ill and vulnerable who have significant requirements for physical, as well as psychiatric care (Brugha et al., 1989). In a study of 145 long-term users of hospital and social services day psychiatric facilities, Brugha et al. (1989) found that 41% suffered medical problems potentially requiring care. Therefore it is important to liaise with the providers of medical care, most often the primary care doctors. This aspect of need is advantaged when services are located in the general hospital.

10. User advocacy and community alliances

The importance of advocacy and user involvement at all levels with services have been increasingly acknowledged (Brandon & Brandon, 1987; World Psychiatric Association, 1989). Bassett *et al.* (1991) define four categories of involvement. At the individual clinical level, active participation can include having access to documentation and involvement in goal-setting and reviews. Involvement of users at all stages of the planning process may facilitate alliances between professionals and their clients and ensure more effective implementation of the services. User participation in the monitoring and management of the service and in training and education are also important areas. Users' charters emphasise the rights of patients to privacy, consultation, information and choice. Mechanisms to inform individuals and their families of their legal rights are the responsibility of the services.

Over the past 10 years there has been an increasing research interest in the views of individuals using general health and hospital services. Studies in the area have revealed some interesting findings and a detailed picture of a user perspective on health care is gradually being built up. Individuals using hospital and related services for physical disorders are, on the whole, satisfied with the care they receive (Locker & Dunt, 1978) although there is greater scepticism about the beneficial value of prescribed drugs (Calnan, 1988) and the uptake with alternative therapies may indicate a level of dissatisfaction with more traditional services (Sharma, 1990). In the area of mental health, the need to consult widely with users is increasingly recognised and relevant methodologies are being developed (Kingsley & Towell, 1989; McIver, 1991; Brandon, 1991; Beerforth *et al.*, 1990). However, little work has been done that specifically addresses the ascertainment of users' views on the provision of primary care mental health services. Pertinent evidence has emerged from the recent survey of 516 users, the National MIND/Roehampton Institute People First, which found some clear messages about primary care (Pilgrim & Rogers, 1993; Rogers *et al.*, 1993). These can be summarised as follows:

- GPs are the most important gatekeepers to health and welfare services for psychiatric patients.
- A majority of patients (73.8%) found their GPs to be helpful and to have a positive attitude (62.5%). Both these votes of confidence were greater than those expressed about psychiatrists.
- Dissatisfaction with GPs centred on the overuse of drugs at the expense of referral for counselling or other specialist help and complaints about insufficient information about both problem and definition and treatment. Particular concern was expressed about the tendency of GPs to see users only as 'mental' cases, i.e. the respondents felt that they received poor *physical* care.
- Satisfaction with good primary care focused on the accessibility of the service compared to specialist services and the flexibility of help offered. The tendency of GPs to pathologise behaviour less than psychiatrists and their ways were also positively valued, as was being seen outside a hospital context. GPs were liked because they provided continuity of care (cf. rotating hospital doctors) and because they were sources of access to material and social resources.

Conclusion

The widespread transformation of mental health care systems, as in the last 20 years in both the US and Europe, is no new phenomenon. Such rapid system changes were common in the last quarter of the nineteenth century when our predecessors established the psychiatric institutions. The challenge for clinicians and researchers at the end of the twentieth century is, in this cycle of transformation, to measure accurately the effects of patient interventions and service changes in order to produce, as we have defined community psychiatry, a 'network of services that together demonstrably help people with mental health problems to regain their normal social roles'.

21
Liaison psychiatry

G.G. LLOYD

Introduction

Psychological factors play an important role in medical and surgical practice. Clinicians from all specialties need to be able to manage patients whose physical complaints are accompanied by psychiatric disorder but they often require the assistance of psychiatrists to assess and manage the more complicated problems. Collaboration has been facilitated by the establishment of psychiatric departments within general hospitals, thus enabling psychiatrists to become more familiar with the type of psychiatric problems that develop in medical and surgical patients.

Liaison psychiatry, the interface between psychiatry and other branches of medicine, covers the whole range of psychiatric illness and the principles of diagnosis and treatment are similar to those employed in the more familiar setting of a psychiatric hospital. The term denotes a style and location of practice where the psychiatrist has particular skills to contribute to the care of the physically ill and those patients whose psychiatric illness presents with somatic complaints (Lloyd, 1991). Some prefer the term 'consultation-liaison psychiatry' to emphasise two distinct styles of practice. In this context consultation is essentially a patient-orientated process, the psychiatrist assessing and advising on treatment in response to a specific request from another specialist. Liaison, in contrast, has a broader aim in which psychiatry is considered to have a preventive as well as therapeutic role. This role requires the psychiatrist to develop closer links with a particular clinical team, mediating between patients and staff to maintain communication, reduce conflicts and prevent the deterioration of clinical care (Lipowski, 1974). These two styles are not mutually incompatible; many psychiatrists who predominantly provide a consultation service nevertheless establish closer links with certain units with whom they work in a liaison capacity.

Psychosomatic medicine

Liaison psychiatry has evolved from psychosomatic medicine. Johan Heinroth introduced the term 'psychosomatic' in 1818 to describe the aetiology of insomnia

(Margetts, 1950) but its roots can be traced back much further in medical history (Ackernecht, 1982). The psychosomatic movement reached the heights of its influence between 1930 and 1950 in the United States, when much attention was given to attributing psychological causation to a number of physical illnesses. Few attempts were made to confirm these psychosomatic theories and some of the more speculative hypotheses discredited psychiatry in the eyes of other clinicians. Despite these difficulties, psychiatric units were established in general hospitals to provide a service for patients who were primarily under the care of medical or surgical specialists. Liaison psychiatry has expanded particularly in the United States (Lipowski, 1979) but in Britain its recognition has been less evident. There have been important research contributions and reports of clinical collaboration from some hospitals but throughout the country psychiatric expertise has not been readily available on general wards. Few psychiatrists have been able to devote a substantial proportion of their time to liaison work and services have grown haphazardly. However, where close links are established with particular units the referral rate for a psychiatric opinion increases considerably (Brown & Cooper, 1987), suggesting that there is a large unmet need for psychiatric involvement in the management of medical patients.

The association between psychiatric and physical morbidity

Several studies of hospital and community populations have provided empirical evidence of an association between psychiatric and physical illness. Furthermore, psychiatric disorder is associated with a high utilisation of medical facilities. Consequently the prevalence of psychiatric morbidity among general hospital patients is higher than in the general population. Rates vary widely according to the criteria used (Mayou & Hawton, 1986). Some rating scales and research interviews overestimate psychiatric morbidity because of their inclusion of somatic items that are due to physical rather than psychiatric illness.

A number of mechanisms explain the links between psychiatric and physical morbidity (Lloyd, 1991) and some of these are considered below.

Stressful life events

The importance of life events in the genesis of illness has been studied frequently in recent years. The most convincing findings have concerned the role of life events in precipitating episodes of depression; their relevance to physical illness is less well established but there are several reports of their significance (Creed, 1985).

The tendency for episodes of illness to occur in clusters was demonstrated by Hinkle & Wolff (1957). These authors found great individual differences in susceptibility, the most vulnerable being prone to all forms of illness, major and minor, physical and psychiatric. They proposed that episodes of illness occur at times when a person is exposed to stressful events with which he has difficulty in coping and this has become known as the 'cluster theory' of illness.

Subsequent investigators have used standardised methods to measure life events.

535

Connolly (1976) found an excess of life events during a three-week period before illness in men suffering an acute myocardial infarction compared to controls. Similarly, Creed (1981) has demonstrated an excess of life events prior to appendicitis. However, in this study, patients who underwent appendicectomy but had no pathological evidence of acute appendicitis, had experienced more life events that were considered severely threatening than those with an acutely inflamed appendix. This observation suggests life events may have a greater effect on illness behaviour than they do on the development of organic pathology. Other conditions that have been reported to be influenced by life events include viral infections, recurrent breast cancer and multiple sclerosis.

A study by Murphy & Brown (1980) throws some light on the nature of the link between life events and onset of organic illness. Among a large sample of women aged 18–65, life events were only related to illness in those who had an associated psychiatric disorder. The psychiatric disorder, predominantly depression, invariably preceded the onset of organic disorder, prompting the authors to suggest that the causal link between life events and organic illness is mediated by the psychiatric condition.

The effects of mental illness and behaviour on physical health

Alcoholism and drug dependence have well-known adverse effects on physical health and are responsible for many admissions to general hospitals. There is also evidence that other forms of psychiatric illness, particularly affective disorders, carry increased risks of physical morbidity and mortality.

The mortality rate of psychiatric patients has been shown repeatedly to be higher than that of the general population. Malzberg (1937), for example, found that among in-patients suffering from involutional melancholia the mortality rate increased sixfold. Diseases of the heart constituted the leading cause, being responsible for 40% of all deaths. Subsequent studies, using information from various sources, confirmed the increased mortality of patients with psychiatric illness although its magnitude has been falling. The incidence of myocardial infarction appears to be especially increased in those who have experienced symptoms of phobic anxiety (Haines et al., 1987) or depression (Appels, 1990).

These observations can be explained by several factors, particularly differences in diet, exercise, smoking, alcohol and drug consumption, and exposure to infection, but it remains possible that mental illness might affect physical health more directly. In a cohort of male college students followed prospectively by Vaillant (1979), those with poor ratings of mental health in young adult life were more likely to become chronically physically ill or to die prematurely. The relationship between previous mental health and subsequent physical health remained significant even when the effects on alcohol, smoking, obesity and ancestral longevity were excluded.

In addition to mental illness, a number of other psychological precursors have been postulated. Hopelessness, for example, was found by Schmale & Iker (1966) to be associated with malignancy in women awaiting cone biopsy of the cervix while Engel (1967) has proposed that a similar affective state the 'giving-up, given-up complex', is often a setting for the development of illness.In women awaiting biopsy of breast lumps, Greer & Morris (1975) have found suppression of feelings of anger to be significantly associated with the development of cancer.

Personality traits

Personality traits extend the role of psychological precursors of illness. Interpretation of most research in the area is hampered by its retrospective nature and firm conclusions cannot be drawn for many illnesses. The most convincing research concerns Type A behaviour, which has been assessed prospectively in a study of ischaemic heart disease. This behaviour is characterised by ambition, hostility, competitiveness and a chronic state of time urgency (Friedman & Rosenman, 1959) and can be assessed reliably by means of a standardised interview. As part of the Western Collaborative Group Study, Type A behaviour was measured in a group of over 3000 Californian men who were originally free of evidence of coronary disease. Subjects were examined at intervals for a total of eight-and-a-half years and the rates of myocardial infarction, and other forms of ischaemic heart disease, were significantly higher in Type A subjects compared with Type Bs (Rosenman *et al.*, 1975). Further research has shown that Type A characteristics can be modified by cognitive therapy; this approach significantly reduces the re-infarction rate in patients who have already suffered a myocardial infarction (Friedman *et al.*, 1986).

Not all other studies have confirmed the original findings of the Californian Group. Certain aspects of Type A behaviour may be more relevant than others and there is evidence that hostility is particularly involved in the development of coronary disease (Johnston, 1993).

Physical illness causing organic mental reactions

Pathological factors in the brain, or acting on the brain from a distant focus, often give rise to psychiatric disorders with characteristic clinical features. Many physical illnesses, particularly in the elderly, initially manifest themselves entirely through disturbance of mental functioning. The acute presentation, now referred to as delirium, includes impairment of consciousness, psychomotor retardation, muddled thinking, amnesia and perceptual abnormalities, particularly in the visual modality; in chronic reactions, in addition to amnesia, there are changes in personality, and a decline in general intelligence. The disturbance of cerebral function may be widespread or circumscribed and Lipowski (1978) has proposed a classification that incorporates aetiological as well as phenomenological considerations. According to this classification, delirium and dementia are global disorders of cognition resulting from diffuse brain dysfunction. Other syndromes, such as hallucination, the amnesic syndrome, organic personality change and those resembling functional disorders, involve a more limited disturbance of mental function and are typically associated with focal brain lesions.

The physical illness causing these reactions are numerous (Taylor & Lewis, 1993) and can frequently be elicited during the history-taking and clinical examination, but laboratory and radiological tests are often necessary to establish the precise aetiology. Rapid diagnosis and treatment of the underlying illness are required to restore mental function to normal;

antipsychotic medication may also be required if there is behavioural disturbance. When treatment is delayed, permanent brain damage may result and the clinical features become irreversible. This subject is discussed in detail in Chapter 15.

Anxiety and affective disorders may also result from metabolic disturbance or structural brain disease. It is well established that an anxiety disorder can be the presenting feature of hyperthyroidism, hypoglycaemia or phaeochromocytoma. Similarly, affective disorders, either depression or mania, can result from various neurological, endocrine, collagen or malignant diseases. These organic anxiety or affective disorders should be suspected if there is no previous personal or family psychiatric history, if they develop for the first time in middle or late life and if there is no discernible psychosocial precipitant

The emotional impact of physical illness

Physical illness can cause psychiatric morbidity by virtue of its emotional impact as well as by its toxic effect on the brain. The psychological reactions to illness vary widely in their nature and severity, with no clear division between normal and abnormal (Lloyd, 1991). There is no consensus regarding their classification or their relationship to primary psychiatric illness. Indeed it has been claimed that the psychiatrist's traditional diagnostic models are not applicable to the common problems that confront the physician (Strain, 1981). For practical purposes it is usual to regard the reaction as morbid if it interferes with the patient's adjustment to or recovery from the illness, or if the reaction itself is a source of distress to the patient.

Many different influences determine the psychological response, including premorbid personality, the severity of the illness, the treatment environment and the social circumstances at the time of onset (Lloyd, 1991). The response is not specific to the type of illness, similar reactions being seen in patients with AIDS, cancer, heart disease and neurological disease.

Adjustment disorders

The most frequent psychological reaction is an adjustment disorder with either anxiety, depression or a combination of both. The symptoms develop within a short time of the awareness of being ill, sometimes within two or three days. Their duration closely parallels the progress of the underlying physical illness and they tend to subside within a few weeks when physical recover occurs (Lloyd & Cawley, 1983). Their content is intimately related to the impact of the illness. Patients are preoccupied with the effects of illness on their future lifestyle, earning capacity and family relationships. They may be concerned with possibility of long-term invalidism and in the case of terminal illness they may be preoccupied with death and the process of dying.

Psychotropic medication is not usually required. The emotional distress can be alleviated by explanation, support and reassurance. In many patients the emotional symptoms result from inadequate understanding of their illness and a poor relationship with medical or nursing staff. Improved communication on behalf of the therapeutic team goes a long way towards relieving this distress. Some hospitals now provide special counselling services to help patients cope with the problems of malignant disease and HIV infection.

Anxiety disorders

Anxiety symptoms occasionally persist long after acute physical symptoms have subsided. They may be generalised and free-floating but are more likely to be linked to specific aspects of the illness. Phobic anxiety disorders are well-recognised reactions to various treatments. For example, some insulin-dependent diabetics may develop a needle phobia that interferes with daily insulin injections and leads to poor glycaemic control. Conditioned phobic reactions can also occur during radiotherapy or chemotherapy, which can produce unpleasant side-effects such as anorexia, nausea, vomiting and hair loss. Patients come to associate the treatment with these undesired effects and may develop an anticipatory anxiety that is itself associated with nausea and vomiting. Devlen *et al.* (1987) observed that conditioned responses to chemotherapy occurred in 32 out of 120 patients being treated for lymphoma. In some cases the anticipatory anxiety is so severe that further chemotherapy or radiotherapy is avoided. Behaviour therapy is then required to overcome the problem and allow further treatment to continue.

Post-traumatic stress disorder (PTSD) occurs in people who have been involved in trauma of an exceptionally threatening nature that would be expected to cause distress to virtually everybody. In general hospitals it is seen in patients who have sustained multiple injuries or burns as a result of road traffic accidents, assault, terrorist activity or natural disasters. There is usually a delay of several weeks between the trauma and the onset of symptoms. The characteristic features include recurrent intrusive memories (flashbacks) of the trauma, disturbed sleep, nightmares, tension, irritability, emotional numbing and avoidance of situations that evoke memories of the original incident. The risk of developing PTSD continues after discharge from hospital, so it is important to enquire about the relevant symptoms when reviewing patients who have been exposed to trauma. Mayou *et al.* (1993) studied patients who had been involved in serious road traffic accidents and observed that PTSD developed in 10% during the subsequent 12 months. The symptoms of PTSD overlapped with those of phobic travel anxiety, which often led to changes in driving behaviour.

Most hospitals now have emergency plans that have been devised to manage victims of major disasters. These plans should include immediate psychological help to provide counselling and other appropriate therapy to alleviate the acute psychological distress and prevent the subsequent development of PTSD. In established cases of PTSD there is a proven role for antidepressant medication, either tricyclics or monoamine oxidase inhibitors (Davidson, 1992). Cognitive and behavioural techniques also appear to be effective.

Depressive disorders

Depressive illness can be precipitated by any major physical illness. Several studies have reported on its prevalence in patients with cancer, lymphoma, heart disease, diabetes and various neurological disorders. The reported rates vary considerably but at a conservative estimate depressive illness develops in at least a fifth of these patients during the 12 months following the diagnosis of serious physical disorders. In establishing the diagnosis of depression, greater significance than usual has to be given to the psychological symptoms, particulary anhedonia and loss of interest in external affairs; the somatic symptoms of depression, such as anorexia, weight loss and fatigue, may be misleading from a diagnostic viewpoint because they can all be related to the physical disorder rather than to accompanying emotional symptoms.

Depression contributes significantly to the disability of the physically ill. It can lead to marital, sexual and interpersonal tensions, delay return to work and preclude the resumption of leisure activities. Depression also contributes to the increased risk of suicide. It often remains undetected and untreated or may be regarded as an inevitable consequence of illness. However, the importance of diagnosing and treating depression in these patients is well established. Antidepressant medication should be prescribed if symptoms warrant it (Series, 1992). Tricyclic antidepressants are poorly tolerated by physically ill patients and they may be completely contraindicated in some cases, for example, in the presence of prostatism, glaucoma or second- or third-degree atrioventricular block. Newer drugs, particularly the selective serotonin re-uptake inhibitors, may be more acceptable. The initial dose should be smaller than is used with physically healthy patients. Particular caution should be observed in the presence of hepatic or renal impairment because of delayed metabolism or excretion. Monitoring of plasma drug levels is helpful in adjusting dosage.

Various forms of psychological therapy can also alleviate symptoms of depression. Brief, problem-orientated treatment using cognitive-behavioural techniques is eminently suitable for physically ill patients and has been shown to reduce the severity of anxiety and depression in women with breast cancer (Greer *et al.*, 1992). There are also reports that psychotherapy influences the course of malignant disease and increases survival (Spiegel *et al.*, 1989). For patients who have experienced a recent myocardial infarction a home-based exercise rehabilitation programme can significantly reduce symptoms of anxiety and depression (Lewin *et al.*, 1992).

Acute transient psychoses

An acute psychotic disorder with no disturbance of cognitive function occasionally develops in association with physical illness. It usually occurs after admission to hospital, particularly in intensive care units or isolation rooms, settings that patients find most threatening. The sudden emotional impact of acute illness with disruption to the patient's familiar routine and environment is probably the crucial factor in precipitating a psychosis of this type (Cutting, 1980).

The characteristic feature is an acute delusional system. The patient believes the nursing or medical staff are planning to harm him and he may retaliate by attacking members of staff or insist on leaving hospital immediately. Hallucinations and thought disorder do not usually occur. This type of psychosis has to be distinguished from acute delirium, acute schizophrenia and an affective psychosis. The prognosis is inevitably good, complete recovery occurring within a few days. However, careful management is required while the patient is psychotic. Neuroleptic medication, for example haloperidol 5–20 mg orally or intramuscularly, is needed to control disruptive and aggressive behaviour. Whenever possible the patient should be moved from an area of high technology to the less intimidating environment of a general ward and discharged home as soon as the medical condition permits.

Elaboration of physical symptoms

Symptoms of illness sometimes appear exaggerated or prolonged when objective evidence suggests that recovery has occurred. The patient is more incapacitated functionally than would be expected. Return to work and resumption of other daily activities are delayed; there are persistent symptoms similar to those of the original illness but for which no satisfactory physical explanation can be found.

This pattern of behaviour develops in patients who are dissatisfied with the results of medical treatment and in those who believe, rightly or wrongly, that their illness or injuries are due to someone else's negligence. Legal action involving claims for compensation is thought to prolong the disability further. It is also reinforced by changes in the behaviour of relatives and friends. They often become over-protective, reversing previous dominance hierarchies and rewarding the patient's invalidism and need for attention (Tarsh & Royston, 1985).

In cases that involve litigation it is important to establish liability and to agree on compensation as soon as possible to prevent further entrenchment in the sick role. Active rehabilitation should be planned for patients with extensive functional disability. This needs to include family therapy when relatives' attitudes are contributing to the illness behaviour. Unfortunately the legal process is slow and causes great frustration to those involved in accidents, the majority of whom do not appear to be exaggerating their disability (Mayou, 1995).

Disability may also be prolonged through poor compliance with treatment. This occurs in several chronic illnesses such as diabetes and renal failure, when patients find it difficult to adhere to dietary restrictions, regular treatment and blood monitoring. Compliance is especially poor among adolescents who resent restrictions that distinguish them from their peer group.

Drug-induced disease

Many psychiatrically ill patients develop physical pathology as a result of their drug treatment. The phenothiazines and butyrophenones are notorious for causing extra-pyramidal symptoms including parkinsonism, akathisia, acute dystonia and tardive dyskinesia. Cholestatic jaundice, postural hypotension, photo-sensitive skin rashes, retinal pigmentation, and lenticular opacities can all result from long-term phenothiazine administration. Clozapine, recently introduced for the treatment of resistant schizophrenia, may cause leucopenia or fatal agranulocytosis; epilepsy and hypersalivation are other unpleasant complications. Tricyclic antidepressants can give rise to cardiac arrhythmias, postural hypotension, acute glaucoma, and retention of urine. Lithium carbonate can lead to hypothyroidism, diabetes insipidus, and extra-pyramidal disorders.

The reverse also occurs. Various psychiatric syndromes are induced by drugs used to treat physical illness and Davison (1981) has reviewed these under the collective heading of toxic psychosis. The adverse reactions have been grouped into several categories: behaviour change (particularly irritability and aggression), acute confusion, affective reactions, paranoid and schizophrenia-like psychoses, hallucinatory states, dementia and neuro-psychiatric states. They are non-specific in that a single drug, for example levodopa, may induce mania, depression, acute confusion, dementia or paranoid psychoses (McClelland, 1981). Among the drugs commonly incriminated are digitalis, atropine-like drugs, methyl-dopa, reserpine, beta blockers, levodopa, corticosteroids, and anticonvulsants.

Somatic presentation of psychiatric illness

A substantial proportion of patients who consult their physicians and surgeons are suffering from a psychiatric rather than physical illness. The presenting symptoms, however, are physical and the distinction of psychiatric from physical morbidity can pose considerable difficulties. The psychiatric disorder is masked by the facade of physical complaints: emotional symptoms seldom are volunteered and have to be uncovered by direct questioning. This presentation of psychiatric illness is usually referred to as somatisation and several factors are thought to influence it. The stigma that still surrounds the mentally ill is undoubtedly important, as is the belief that doctors are more interested in physical than psychological complaints. Many people are relatively unaware of their emotional feelings but are more perceptive of the bodily changes that accompany psychiatric illness. The elderly, lower social groups, and immigrants from developing countries are particularly likely to present with physical symptoms when psychiatrically ill. Leff (1981) has shown that Western languages permit greater expression and differentiation of emotional states than do those of traditional cultures where distress is more likely to be expressed in somatic terms. Even in Western culture, it has been claimed that the ability to perceive and articulate discrete affective changes is probably a recent development (Katon *et al.*, 1982).

Patterns of physical symptoms

(a) Pain

Pain is common in psychiatric illness and is often the presenting feature, with the head, chest, and abdomen being the most common sites. Bond (1978) has contrasted the characteristics of psychogenic pain with pain of largely physical origin. Psychogenic pain tends to be indefinite in nature with no clear-cut onset; it is poorly localised and may vary with changes in the patient's mood; furthermore it may be relieved by alcohol and psychotropic medication. A premorbid history of neurotic traits or mental illness is often present. Pain may be due to increased muscle tension or an exaggerated perception of the normal aches and pains that everyone experiences.

The most common psychiatric diagnoses associated with pain are affective, anxiety and personality disorders. In depressive illness, preoccupation with pain may so dominate the clinical picture that the patient may not appear depressed and will not admit to feeling depressed. Lascelles (1966) has illustrated this phenomenon in facial pain, which may respond well to a monoamine oxidase inhibitor or tricyclic antidepressant (Feinmann *et al.*, 1984).

(b) Fatigue

There has been an increased awareness of the psychiatric accompaniments of chronic fatigue during the last decade and an explosion of new cases presenting in medical and psychiatric practice (Lewis & Wesseley, 1992). The characteristic features include extreme fatigue after physical or mental exertion, poor concentration, reduced exercise tolerance, muscle tenderness and sleep disturbance that often involves hypersomnia. This syndrome may follow a viral illness such as influenza, glandular fever or hepatitis and the term myalgic encephalomyelitis is used by those who favour a viral aetiology. However, in the great majority who present with chronic fatigue there is no convincing history of viral infection nor any laboratory evidence of infections (Fukuda *et al.*, 1994).

The terms chronic fatigue syndrome or neurasthenia are more appropriate because they make no assumptions about aetiology. There is considerable overlap with patients suffering from a primary depressive illness. Up to 80% of patients fulfil operational criteria for psychiatric disorder, most having a diagnosis of major depression (Kendell, 1991). However, there is a striking resistance to any implication that they are psychiatrically ill and many patients cling tenaciously to the belief that their symptoms have a viral aetiology. This attitude appears to worsen the prognosis (Sharpe *et al.*, 1992a), perhaps because it encourages excessive bed-rest and avoidance of exercise, an approach that many doctors regard as contributing to invalidism.

(c) Neurological symptoms

At least a fifth of patients presenting to neurological out-patient clinics have no neurological disorder but they complain of symptoms that prove to be due to psychiatric disorder (Schiffer, 1983). The commonest symptoms are headache, dizziness, pain and disturbance of higher cortical functions. The majority prove to have an anxiety or depressive illness and respond well to conventional treatment with behaviour therapy or psychotropic medication.

Dissociative symptoms are uncommon in contemporary neurological practice but they give rise to major diagnostic difficulties. They have been defined as symptoms that lead to distortion or loss of neurological function that cannot be adequately explained by organic disease (Marsden, 1986). Psychiatrists usually want to establish that the symptoms are due to psychological factors, either an unresolved emotional conflict, recent severe stress or an associated psychiatric illness. It is assumed that the symptoms are not produced intentionally, as in malingering, but result from unconscious motives. However, this distinction is often not clear-cut and the patient's degree of insight varies from time to time.

Careful neurological examination usually enables motor weakness, sensory loss or gait disturbance to be recognised as being due to dissociative mechanisms. Pseudo-seizures are more difficult to evaluate because they are episodic and may coexist with genuine epilepsy (Fenton, 1986). A description from a reliable informant is important but it is essential for the clinician to witness an attack before making a firm diagnosis. Dissociative, or psychogenic amnesia, also creates diagnostic difficulties and may be mistaken for delirium, transient global amnesia or other causes of acute memory impairment. In dissociative amnesia the loss of memory usually develops suddenly in close relation to a markedly stressful event. The amnesia is patchy, predominantly involving emotionally charged memories. Characteristically there is a loss of personal identity so the patient cannot recall his name, age, address, occupation or family details. Recovery usually occurs within a few days but in some cases the amnesia persists and is accompanied by an apparently purposeful wandering away from home or place of work. During this episode, known as dissociative fugue, a new name and identity may be assumed.

(d) Cardio-respiratory symptoms

Symptoms of psychological origin that focus attention on the chest are chiefly due to autonomic arousal associated with anxiety. Palpitations, central chest or left mammary pain, breathlessness, tiredness, decreased exercise tolerance, and irritability are the most common complaints.

Chest pain not due to ischaemic heart disease, sometimes referred to as atypical chest pain, is a common reason for cardiological consultations (Mayou, 1989). These patients are usually younger than those with angina; the pain is located in the left chest, is described as aching or stabbing in character and may be associated with localised or diffuse tenderness over the anterior chest wall. Other somatic symptoms are prominent including breathlessness, reduced exercise tolerance, faintness and excessive sweating. Psychiatric disorder is common in these patients, more so than in those with definite ischaemic heart disease. Anxiety, panic attacks and depression are the commonest diagnoses made if the patients are assessed from a psychiatric viewpoint.

Breathing difficulties are often closely associated with cardiac symptoms and themselves give rise to a number of diffuse complaints. Burns & Howell (1969) described patients attending a respiratory medicine clinic whose symptoms of breathlessness were disproportionately severe in relation to their pulmonary disease. Many were found to be suffering from a psychiatric illness, either depression, anxiety or hysterical reaction, and successful treatment of the psychiatric disorder was associated with complete or partial resolution of breathlessness. The common respiratory symptoms were hyperventilation attacks or an unpleasant sense of pressure on the chest, giving rise to a respiratory dysrhythmia. In a later paper Burns & Nicols (1972) identified a number of factors influencing the localisation of symptoms to the chest in depression; these included previous and current organic chest disease, an excessively health-conscious personality, a family history of severe respiratory disease, and recent bereavement. Lum (1981) has drawn attention to the frequency and protean manifestations of hyperventilation. In extreme form the resulting hypocapnia leads to tetany and coma but less severe degrees cause more subtle symptoms that may overshadow the respiratory complaints. Dizziness, paraesthesia, excessive fatigue, palpitations, and chest pain are among the most common symptoms but diagnostic attention can be attracted to virtually any organ in the body. Bass & Garnder (1985) have shown that approximately half of a group of patients with hyperventilation have a psychiatric disorder; panic attacks and phobic disorders are especially common. Various psychological treatments for breathlessness have yielded encouraging results and there is clearly a place for collaborative research in this area.

(e) Gastrointestinal symptoms

Loss of appetite is a characteristic symptom of affective disorders, particularly depression. Together with weight loss, abdominal pain, and disturbance of bowel function it draws attention to the gastrointestinal tract and a variety of organic illnesses may be suspected.

Non-ulcer dyspepsia is the latest in a succession of terms used to describe unexplained upper abdominal pain. Stressful life events, neurotic personality traits and affective symptoms have all been implicated as aetiological factors among those attending hospital clinics (Lloyd, 1992). Similar claims have been made in relation to the irritable bowel syndrome (IBS), the commonest condition seen in gastroenterology clinics. Creed & Guthrie (1987) estimated that 40–50% of patients attending hospital clinics with IBS have a psychiatric disorder. Lower figures have been reported in community samples and it is not clear whether psychiatric symptoms are an integral part of IBS or whether they influence the decision to seek medical treatment. Persistent vomiting as an isolated symptom is also considered psychogenic in origin. Hill (1968) found several potentially important psychological factors including an excess of hostile family relationships, parental loss in childhood, and family history of vomiting. However, overt depression was not common in his series of patients. In young women the symptom may be a manifestation of bulimia nervosa in which case it usually follows bouts of gross over-eating. This syndrome shares much of the psychopathology of anorexia nervosa.

(f) Dermatological symptoms and body image disturbance

Psychiatric illness presents to the dermatologist chiefly in the guise of itching, burning, excessive redness, hair loss, and hirsutism, the most frequently affected body areas being the face, scalp and genitalia (Cotterill, 1981). Depression was the most common psychiatric diagnosis in Cotterill's patients and could usually be managed by supportive psychotherapy and antidepressant medication. Occasionally a skin complaint is the presenting feature of a more sinister, psychotic illness in which the classical symptom is a delusion of infestation with skin parasites. This delusion may be part of a more widespread psychiatric disturbance such as toxic psychosis, schizophrenia or depressive psychosis. In other cases the delusion is the only evidence of psychopathology, and the personality remains otherwise preserved. Psychiatric classification of this type of symptom is unsatisfactory but some regard it as a mono-symptomatic hypochondriacal psychosis (Munro, 1980b). The single hypochondriacal delusion can remain unchanged for many years and response to treatment has been regarded as poor but a more optimistic view now prevails after reports of an encouraging response to pimozide.

Dermatitis artefacta is another unusual condition heralding psychiatric disorder. There are bizarre, often necrotic lesions with sharp geometrical outlines; they are seldom distributed symmetrically but occur in sites accessible to the patient's dominant hand. Sneddon & Sneddon (1975) have reported a series of 43 patients, some of whom continued to produce lesions for several years. A wide variety of psychiatric illnesses, personality problems, and social difficulties were apparent and the dermatitis artefacta was only one incident in a long history.

Cotterill (1981) reported disturbed body image to be commonly associated with depression in dermatological patients. A concern with generalised body size and shape is an essential feature of anorexia nervosa but patients are occasionally seen whose presenting complaint concerns the appearance of a particular feature such as their nose, chin or legs. The term dysmorphophobia has been used to describe this phenomenon when the objective appearance is within normal limits. In many cases dysmorphophobia coexists with affective disorder, obsessive-compulsive disorder or social phobia (Phillips *et al.*, 1993). The problem has usually been present for many years by the time patients are referred with a request for cosmetic surgery. Their lives are greatly restricted and it is common for a wide range of social and personal difficulties to be attributed to the alleged deformity. The results of surgery are unsatisfactory if expectations are unrealistic or if a psychiatric disorder is undetected and not treated. Patients requesting cosmetic surgery should therefore be evaluated carefully from a social and psychological perspective before a decision to operate is taken.

(g) Genito-urinary symptoms

Menstrual irregularities are often emotionally determined and complete amenorrhoea is another cardinal feature of anorexia nervosa. Many patients attending gynaecological departments are therefore found to be suffering from a psychiatric illness rather than gynaecological pathology.

Sexual symptoms, particularly impotence and inability to achieve orgasm, may result from a depressive illness or anxiety state while other genital symptoms convince the patient he has venereal disease. Pain in the penis, pruritis or the complaint of smells emanating from the genitalia are typical symptoms with which psychiatric illness presents to a genito-urinary medicine department. Recurrent urinary symptoms including dysuria, frequency, urgency and feeling of incomplete bladder emptying have also been attributed to psychological factors although recent research has cast doubt on this assumption (Nazareth & King, 1993).

Psychiatric disorders associated with somatisation

It is important to establish the underlying psychiatric disorder associated with somatisation. This enables a plan of management to be devised and the prognosis to be estimated. Although any psychiatric disorder may present with somatic symptoms it is unusual for somatisation to result from mania, schizophrenia or organic disorders. In these conditions the clinical picture is dominated by a variety of psychological abnormalities that make the diagnosis of psychiatric illness readily apparent.

The psychiatric disorders associated with somatisation can be divided into acute and chronic groups according to their duration and to whether their time of onset can be determined with reasonable confidence. They are listed in Table 21.1.

Table 21.1. *Psychiatric disorders in somatising patients*

Acute	Chronic
Adjustment disorder	Somatisation disorder
Depressive disorder	Hypochondriacal disorder
Phobic anxiety disorder	Somatoform autonomic
Panic disorder	dysfunction
Generalised anxiety disorder	Somatoform pain disorder
Dissociative disorder	Neurasthenia

Adjustment, depressive and anxiety disorders

These are the conditions most commonly diagnosed in somatising patients. The characteristic psychological symptoms can be elicited by direct enquiry and the conditions respond to the conventional psychological or pharmacological treatments that would be used for non-somatising patients. Treatment is more likely to be successful if the patient's perception of the illness is modified so that symptoms come to be attributed to psychological factors rather than to organic disease. This is discussed further in the section on management.

Dissociative disorder

This term is used by ICD-10 to describe those conditions previously diagnosed as conversion or dissociative hysteria. Although hysteria has been omitted from contemporary classification systems because of controversy surrounding its various meanings, it is still widely used as a diagnostic category in clinical practice.

Dissociative disorders present with symptoms that suggest lesions in the motor or sensory pathways of the voluntary nervous system, but the distortion of neurological function cannot be adequately explained by organic disease. A psychological assessment usually uncovers evidence to link the symptoms with recent severe stress, emotional conflict or associated psychiatric disorder.

Somatoform disorders

The characteristic features of this group of disorders are defined by ICD-10 as repeated presentations of physical complaints together with persistent requests for medical investigations despite repeated negative findings and medical reassurance that the symptoms have no physical basis. The glossary adds that the degree of understanding that can be achieved about the cause of the symptoms is often disappointing and frustrating for patient and doctor.

Somatisation disorder has many similarities to Briquet's syndrome and St Louis hysteria. It is much commoner in women and its main features are multiple recurrent symptoms involving any organ or part of the body. By the time the condition is diagnosed the patient has a long history of contact with various specialists, many negative investigations and unrewarding operations, particularly hysterectomy and cholecystectomy.

Hypochondriacal disorder reflects a persistent preoccupation with having a serious physical illness, for example cancer or AIDs. The nature of the complaint is constant but its intensity fluctuates; it does not have the fixed quality of somatic delusions seen in psychotic depression. A variety of the condition, body dysmorphic disorder, involves a preoccupation with disfigurement and insistent requests for cosmetic surgery.

The symptoms of somatoform autonomic dysfunction are usually located to the chest, gut or urinary tract. Clinical examples include cardiac neurosis, psychogenic hyperventilation, non-ulcer dyspepsia and irritable bowel syndrome. Some of these conditions involve disturbance of physical function but not to the extent to affect the vital function of the relevant organ.

Somatoform pain disorder is a chronic condition in which pain occurs in association with psychological conflict. The pain cannot be adequately attributed to physical pathology or physiological disturbance; it does not conform to nerve root or peripheral nerve distribution and it varies in intensity in response to changes in psychological stress.

Neurasthenia

This is the ICD-10 category that includes chronic fatigue syndrome. There are persistent and disabling complaints of exhaustion and prolonged fatigue after mild physical or mental exertion. This fatigue is accompanied by various other symptoms, notably dizziness, muscular aches, tension headaches, anhedonia and sleep disturbance (usually hypersomnia). Fatigue that follows a definite infectious illness should not be diagnosed as neurasthenia.

Managing chronic somatisation

A central theme in managing patients who are chronic somatisers is to help them change the way they perceive their symptoms. This process of re-attribution depends on the interviewing and communicating skills of the doctor; these skills can be readily acquired if properly taught (Goldberg et al., 1989). Certain general strategies should be adopted so that the doctor is seen as consistent and flexible (Bass & Benjamin, 1993). By the time the patient is recognised as a somatiser, several physical examinations and laboratory investigations will have been carried out. These results should be summarised and the patient given clear information about their relevance. Limits should be set on further investigations. Psychosocial factors should be identified and discussed, together with reasons for linking them with the presenting symptoms. Drug therapy plays a minor role in management. Patients should not be given medication for illnesses they do not have; antidepressants may be required for specific episodes of depression and for psychogenic pain. It is important to identify factors that perpetuate the somatic symptoms and illness behaviour and to modify them whenever possible. Relatives and friends often reinforce symptoms and preoccupation with disease; they need to be seen with the patient so that their attitudes are modified in a way likely to reduce illness behaviour.

Psychological techniques derived from cognitive and behaviour therapy are being adopted successfully by liaison psychiatrists (Sharpe *et al.*, 1992*b*). Klimes *et al.* (1990) have demonstrated the efficacy of this approach in reducing symptoms and functional disability in patients with non-cardiac chest pain. Patients were discouraged from seeking reassurance, for example by checking their pulse repeatedly, and their beliefs about organic disease were challenged by presenting contradictory evidence. They were taught to control pain using relaxation, respiratory control and distracting techniques and to engage in graded exercise to overcome avoidance behaviour. Similarly, cognitive behaviour therapy can reduce the functional impairment associated with chronic fatigue (Sharpe *et al.*, 1996).

Dynamic psychotherapy may also be effective for some somatising patients. Guthrie *et al* (1993) have shown that brief psychotherapy conducted over a period of 12 weeks led to an improvement in both physical and psychological symptoms in patients with refractory irritable bowel syndrome.

Factitious disorders

These are divided into two broad groups according to the clinical presentation and social background of the patients. In the commonest type, signs of disease are fabricated in a subtle and deceitful manner. Superficial ulcerating wounds may be produced (dermatitis artefacta) or repeated self-bleeding induced to give the clinical features and laboratory abnormalities of iron-deficiency anaemia. Other presentations include self-induced pyrexia, hyperthyroidism and hypoglycaemia. These patients are usually young unmarried women, often working as nurses or in other occupations allied to medicine. Their motives are usually obscure; some are considered to have unresolved conflicts of dependency, hostility and sexuality but their predominant characteristic is a need to gain access to the sick role and to be the centre of medical attention. The diagnosis is difficult to establish. It is often not considered until many expensive investigations have been undertaken and even then it may be dismissed because there is no obvious gain to the patient. Doctors are also reluctant to resort to the subterfuge needed to establish the diagnosis and to confront the patient with their opinion that the illness is self-induced.

The other main type of factitious disorder, Munchausen's syndrome, is seen in men with a history of poor social adjustment or psychopathic traits. They present repeatedly to hospital casualty departments with symptoms that suggest a medical or surgical emergency demanding immediate attention. Their history may be sufficiently convincing to persuade an inexperienced clinician to arrange emergency surgery; many of these patients accumulate several laparotomy scars, which should alert the clinician to the nature of the problem. Once the patient is recognised and confronted an angry scene develops; it usually terminates with the patient marching out indignantly, only to present later at a neighbouring hospital, often under another name.

Factitious disorders are distinguished from somatoform and dissociative disorders by the fact that symptoms and signs are under voluntary control. They differ from malingering in that there is no obvious benefit such as avoiding criminal prosecution or obtaining financial rewarded. Management of patients with factitious disorders is usually unsatisfactory. They are extremely resistant to any form of psychological intervention. An improvement in the pattern of behaviour is more likely to result from personal maturation and altered life circumstances than from psychiatric treatment (Sneddon & Sneddon, 1975).

Future developments in liaison psychiatry

There is substantial evidence that attitudes towards psychological problems in medical patients are changing in a favourable direction (Creed, 1992). Physicians are increasingly aware of the importance of psychological factors in influencing the course of physical illness and of the large numbers of psychiatrically ill patients who consult them with functional somatic symptoms in their out-patient clinics. There is a desire for more collaboration with psychiatrists in managing these clinical problems. Demand has increased with the emergence of HIV infection (King, 1993) and the development of new techniques to treat advanced disease, for example heart and liver transplantation (Mai, 1993; Collis & Lloyd, 1992).

The time seems right for an expansion of liaison psychiatry beyond the rudimentary services that currently exist in many hospitals. The tasks facing the liaison psychiatrist are formidable; in addition to acquiring the relevant clinical skills they are expected to teach physicians how to improve emotional care of their patients and to overcome prejudice about psychiatric referral (Creed, 1992). Limited manpower has prevented the expansion of liaison psychiatry to meet the needs that have already been identified. Only by increasing the number of consultant and training posts will the tasks facing the liaison psychiatrist be discharged and needs of the patients met.

Now that psychiatric units have been established in general hospitals, opportunities exist for closer collaboration with physicians and surgeons along the lines that child psychiatrists have established with paediatricians. However, these opportunities may be undermined by the move towards developing community facilities unless purchasers of psychiatric services can be convinced that liaison psychiatry is an essential component of comprehensive medical and psychiatric care.

A report on the psychological care of medical patients (RCP & RCPsych., 1995) has emphasised the importance of a readily available liaison psychiatry team, which should include a consultant psychiatrist, one or more trainee psychiatrists, two clinical nurse specialists, a social worker and a clinical psychologist. An adequate service requires at least five weekly consultant sessions; a large hospital with several specialised units requires a full-time consultant liaison psychiatrist. Few hospitals currently possess such multi-disciplinary teams. The future development of liaison psychiatry may depend on its funding being provided by the medical directorates whose patients benefit from improved psychological care rather than by community mental health budgets.

22

Suicide and self-harm

LOUIS APPLEBY

Suicide is the deliberate act of self-destruction. It is ultimately an individual action but results from a combination of psychological processes, social circumstances and cultural influences. It has been estimated that there are approximately 350–400 000 suicides annually throughout the world.

Epidemiology

International comparisons

In many countries suicide is the cause of a small but significant proportion of total mortality, although rates vary widely. The variation arises in part because of inconsistent practices in the recording of cause of death, influenced by legal, moral and cultural taboos. In addition, differences in crude national rates reflect the different age composition of developing and developed countries, but it also seems certain that reported patterns of cross-national variation reflect genuine differences.

In general, rates are higher in Europe and countries whose population is European in origin, such as the USA, Canada, Australia and New Zealand, than in the developing world. Within Europe, rates are highest in the north and east – Hungary has recorded a rate of over 60 per 100 000, five times the rate in the UK. Moslem countries report low figures, and Egypt has even reported a figure of almost zero (WHO, annual publication).

Despite these differences, certain common trends are evident. In many countries of the world the suicide rate has been increasing steadily for several decades; mainly because of a rise in suicide among young men (WHO, annual publication).

Rates

In the last two decades the annual suicide rate in the UK has been around 10–12 per 100 000 population. This includes 2–3 deaths per 100 000 recorded as resulting from an 'external cause, cause undetermined'; these are usually suicides but, as in the case of open verdicts at coroner's inquest, the evidence for this has been considered insufficiently conclusive. In addition, it is generally thought that some 'accidental' deaths, e.g. single-person car accidents, are suicides – certainly there is evidence that psychiatric patients have a high rate of accidental death (King & Barraclough, 1990), some of which may be by self-inflicted injuries.

The suicide rate in the UK has fluctuated throughout the twentieth century, although it fell, particularly in men, during both world wars. Rises were recorded during the early 1930s, a time of high unemployment, and the late 1950s, one of relative prosperity. The rate fell in the mid-1960s after the relatively non-toxic natural gas was introduced into the domestic gas supply (Kreitman, 1976) but in the 1970s and 1980s rose gradually. In recent years there have been over 5000 suicides and deaths from cause undetermined annually in the UK. This represents 1% of total mortality. However, in young adults suicide is one of the three principal causes of death (the others are road traffic accident and malignant disease).

In the USA the rate in recent years has been around 13 per 100 000 but the pattern through the century has been similar. There are approximately 30 000 suicides nationally each year.

A number of demographic characteristics influence the suicide rate:

Age

In general, the suicide rate increases with age. This is true of both sexes, though the increase is more gradual in women. In the UK the rate in men rises rapidly from around five per 100 000 in 15–19-year-olds to around 13 per 100 000 in those aged 20–24. The rate is then reasonably stable at 15–18 per 100 000 until the early seventies. In women the rate in late teens is around two per 100 000, and the peak of six per 100 000 occurs in late middle age and later.

The effect of age has changed dramatically during the last three decades. In this time, the suicide rate in men in their late teens and early twenties has doubled, most of the increase occurring since 1980, while there has been a 30% fall among over-65s, a change of equivalent numerical size. The reason for former change is unknown, although possible factors including rising rates of alcohol and drug misuse, divorce and unemployment, and increasing use of dangerous methods of self-harm. A rise among young people is a common finding around the world but the late-life fall in the UK is unusual.

Sex

Suicide is considerably more common in men. As the figures above show, the rate in men is around three times higher than that in women across all age groups. The sex difference is maximal in young adults and the elderly.

Social class and employment

The suicide rate varies according to social class, with the highest rate being found in the lowest classes (social class V in the UK), followed by the highest (professional) classes. The lowest rate is found between these, in skilled workers (social class III). Unemployment is a risk factor (Sainsbury, 1955), as are certain forms of employment such as medicine and farming. The risk among university students has been reported to be high (Hawton *et al.*, 1978), though recent evidence disputes this (Hawton *et al.*, 1995).

Race and immigration

The suicide rates of immigrant ethnic minorities often reflect the rate in their country of origin. Thus in the UK, the suicide rate is lower among Afro-Caribbeans and higher in Eastern European immigrants than it is in the indigenous population (Soni Releigh & Balarajan, 1992). In the USA and Canada, high rates have been reported in native North Americans. Specific racial subgroups, such as young Asian women in the UK, appear to be at high risk (Soni Raleigh *et al.*, 1990).

Marital status, children and living circumstances

Suicide is more common in people who are single, separated or divorced, or widowed. Recent widowhood is thought to be an important risk factor in the elderly but one study (Kreitman, 1988) of marital status and male suicide found that bereavement had most effect on relatively young adults while divorce was associated with the greatest risk in the elderly. Part of this risk is presumably related to living alone, which appears to be independently associated with suicide.

Although depression in women has been linked to the presence of children in the home, and is common after childbirth, the influence of children on potential suicides seems to be protective. A study in the UK found the rate in the first postnatal year to be only one-sixth of the rate in the general female population (Appleby, 1991), and a Norwegian study found an inverse relationship with the number of children in the family (Hoyer & Lund, 1993).

The relative rates of suicide in urban and rural populations has varied. In the late 1980s in the UK the suicide rate was highest in rural regions such as East Anglia and South-west, but most recent figures show the highest rate in the North-west, a more urban region. Socially and economically poor parts of cities also tend to show high rates.

Psychiatric, behavioural and medical history

A history of mental illness is one of the most important of all risk factors. A study of Swedish conscripts, i.e. age and sex uniform, found it to be the most powerful predictor of suicide over the next 13 years, leading to an 11-fold increase in risk (Allebeck & Allgulander, 1990). Most studies have identified depression as the most frequent mental disorder, and it has been shown that most, if not all, suicides have suffered from some form of psychiatric disorder before death (Robins *et al.*, 1959; Barraclough *et al.*, 1974). However, the recent rise in suicide by young people may break this established pattern as most young suicides do not visit their general practitioners before death (Vassilas & Morgan, 1993), although there is also evidence that GP attendance does increase to some extent prior to suicide, even in young males (Appleby *et al.*, 1996).

Other psychiatric diagnoses associated with suicide are alcohol dependence (Robins *et al.*, 1959; Kessel & Grossman, 1965; Barraclough *et al.*, 1974), drug misuse (Fowler *et al.*, 1986) and personality disorder (Ovenstone & Kreitman, 1974). There is a strong association with previous non-fatal self-harm, criminality, and chronic physical illness (Robins *et al.*, 1959; Barraclough *et al.*, 1974).

Biological factors

A family history of suicide increases the individual's risk of suicide (Tsuang, 1983; Shafii *et al.*, 1985), a finding that may be explained by observational learning as well as genetic predisposition. However, the genetic explanation is supported by twin studies that have shown an increased concordance for monozygotes (Roy, 1990), and a study of Danish adoptees who have committed suicide, which found a high rate of suicide in their biological but not adoptive parents (Schulsinger *et al.*, 1979; Wender *et al.*, 1986).

What is inherited is unknown. The most consistent findings from biochemical studies of the cerebrospinal fluid of suicides are of reduced 5-HIAA, reflecting reduced serotonin metabolism in the brain (Traskman *et al.*, 1981). This may be related to impulsive or violent suicidal behaviour independent of psychiatric diagnosis (Asberg *et al.*, 1976; Oreland *et al.*, 1981).

Seasonality

Just as the prevalence of depression shows seasonal variation, with higher rates in winter months, the suicide rate also follows a seasonal pattern. In the UK the rate is highest between April and June, and most countries – including those in the Southern hemisphere – show a similar rise in spring.

Method

In the UK in the 1970s the most frequent method of suicide was self-poisoning by drug overdose. Since then, however, the commonest methods have been hanging and self-poisoning with car exhaust fumes (McClure, 1987), each of which now accounts for 25–30% of self-inflicted deaths (OPCS, 1995). In women, drug overdose remains the principal method, accounting for around 50% of deaths, the main substances used being analgesics and psychotropic drugs. In the USA, firearms are the commonest means of suicide in males (Tsuang *et al.*, 1992). Certain methods are associated with specific groups, e.g. self-burning in Asian women (Soni Raleigh *et al.*, 1990).

Suicide by psychiatric patients

Suicide is the most serious consequence of psychiatric illness and most major psychiatric disorders carry a high suicide risk. In the UK approximately 50% of all suicides have history of contact with psychiatric services, although the figure appears to be less in young adults (Vassilas & Morgan, 1993). The exact risk has been estimated in cohort studies such as those of Rorsmann (1973) who found a rate of 1.4% in the five years following out-patient attendance, and of Martin *et al.* (1985) who found the rate of 'unnatural mortality' in out-patients to be three times as high as in the general population. Using a similar approach, Pokorny (1966) calculated the rate to be 165 per 100 000 person-years at risk, 16 times the general population rate. However, the risk is not uniform over time, and has been found to be raised over 30-fold in the six months since last hospital discharge (Temoche *et al.*, 1964; King & Barraclough, 1990).

Risk factors

A number of demographic and social characteristics increase the suicide risk further in psychiatric patients. In general these are similar to risk factors in the population as a whole. Studies have found an association with male sex, low social class, being single, divorced or widowed, and living alone. However, most studies have found young rather than older males to be at risk. King & Barraclough (1990) found the relative risk of suicide following hospital discharge to be 39 in men aged 35–44, and four in men over 75 years.

The most consistently reported clinical risk factor is a history of parasuicide, which is found in 50% of psychiatric suicides (Rorsmann, 1973; Myers & Neal, 1978; Roy, 1982*a*). The most recent admission is twice as likely to have followed self-harm (Flood & Seager, 1968), or to have required detention under mental health legislation (Dennehy *et al.*, 1996), and there is a tendency for the previous self-harm to have been violent or particularly dangerous (Rorsmann 1973; Myers & Neal, 1978). Additional behavioural risk factors are addiction to alcohol or drugs, and antisocial personality (Martin *et al.*, 1985). At least some of these associations may be with mental illness in general rather than with suicide by the mentally ill – one recent study found conventional population risk factors did not distinguish suicides in people with mental illness once age, sex and diagnosis had been controlled (Dennehy *et al.*, 1996). The characteristics of suicide in specific syndromes are as follows:

Schizophrenia

Most estimates of the suicide rate in schizophrenia are in the region of 5–10%, slightly less than in major affective disorders, although one Swedish study found schizophrenia to be the diagnosis most at risk (Allebeck & Allgulander, 1990). The same Swedish group also studied a cohort of discharged in-patients with schizophrenia and found the rate of suicide over the next ten years to be 3.9%. The standardised mortality ratio was raised in both sexes, at 9.9 in men and 17.5 in women (Allebeck & Wistedt, 1986).

A number of mental state features have been related to suicide, particularly depressed mood (Drake *et al.*, 1984; Roy, 1982*a*; Cohen *et al.*, 1990), suicidal ideas (Roy, 1982*b*; Drake *et al.*, 1984), and hallucinations with a suicidal content (Roy, 1982*b*; Crammer, 1984; Sims & O'Brien, 1979). A past history of depression has also been linked to later suicide (Cohen *et al.*, 1990), underlining the importance of low mood, even when the primary diagnosis is not affective disorder. However, this is not a universal view. One study found that the relationship with depression *per se* disappeared once multivariate analysis had controlled for the symptom of hopelessness (Drake & Cotton, 1986). Another found no link to depression and concluded that most schizophrenic suicides were impulsive rather than mood-related (Allebeck *et al.*, 1987).

Only one study has reported a relationship between suicide and aspects of insight, namely an awareness of the effects of the illness, and fear of further mental disintegration (Drake *et al.*, 1984). However, several have found risk to be greatest during the period of clinical recovery (see below).

Affective disorders

The long-term risk of suicide in primary affective disorder has been estimated at 15% (Guze & Robins, 1970), this widely-quoted figure being based on the varying results of early studies. More recent long-term follow-up studies have reported lower rates, however – 8.5% in the case of in-patients with depression (Berglund & Nilsson, 1987), and 3.6% in a cohort of affective, including schizo-affective, disorders (Fawcett *et al.*, 1987, 1990). A number of clinical features seem to be linked to suicide, and these appear to vary with time, early (within one year) deaths being associated with anxiety, panic, insomnia, anhedonia, poor concentration and alcohol abuse, while longer-term risk is associated with hopelessness (Beck *et al.*, 1985; Fawcett *et al.*, 1990).

Alcoholism

The long-term suicide rate in alcoholics who have been in-patients has been calculated to be 6.7% (Berglund & Nilsson, 1987), though this represents less than half of total mortality. Once again, a past history of depression is the most important clinical risk factor (Berglund, 1984), and recent loss of a relationship, usually by separation, has been described in one-third of suicides (Murphy *et al.*, 1979). Similarly, interpersonal loss or conflict has been reported as preceding many suicides by substance (including alcohol) abusers (Rich *et al.*, 1988).

Neurosis

When neurotic disorder is severe enough to require admission, the suicide rate appears to be as high as in major mental illness. One follow-up of in-patients found the relative risk to be 6.8 (Sims & Prior, 1978) when neurotic depression was included. Most later studies of anxiety-related disorders, excluding depression, have confirmed an elevated rate of suicide, and this has been attributed primarily to the risks in patients with panic attacks or disorder (Coryell *et al.*, 1986). The long-term risk of suicide in anorexia nervosa appears to be high, 7% in one recent follow-up study (Ratnasuriya *et al.*, 1991).

Timing

Duration of illness

Most of the research evidence points to a maximum risk during the first few years of an illness: several studies have found a mean illness duration of less than four years (Flood & Seager, 1968; Goh *et al.*, 1989; Cohen *et al.*, 1990). However, this is not a universal finding, possibly because of differences between patient samples, and no time can be regarded as characteristic. One study of suicide in schizophrenia reported a sex difference, longer histories being found in women (Roy, 1982*b*).

Episode

The beginning of an acute relapse and the recovery period represent the times of maximum risk during an episode of illness (Copas *et al.*, 1971; Gale *et al.*, 1980). Eighteen per cent of in-patient suicides have been reported to occur within a week of entering hospital (Crammar, 1984); 18% of discharged suicides within one week of leaving (Roy, 1982*a*). Thirty to fifty per cent of psychiatric suicides occur within 1–3 months of discharge (Flood & Seager, 1968; Roy, 1982*a*; Goldacre *et al.*, 1993; Dennehy *et al.*, 1996). The majority die within a month of their last appointment with a psychiatrist (Roy *et al.*, 1982*a*) or general practitioner (Myers & Neal, 1978).

Method

Violent methods of suicide are more common among psychiatric suicides than the general population, accounting for 70–90% of deaths (Roy, 1982*a*; Langley & Bayatti, 1984; Goh *et al.*, 1989; Morgan & Priest, 1991). Similarly, studies of suicide by jumping from a height have found a preponderance of severe psychiatric illness (Sims & O'Brien, 1979; Pounder, 1985; Cantor *et al.*, 1989). However, in non-psychotic disorders such as sociopathy and alcohol or drug dependence, overdose remains a common method (Ovenstone & Kreitman, 1974).

Psychiatric services

Location

The increased risk of suicide at the beginning and end of an episode of illness raises the question of how the current development of community-based care, with delayed and shorter admissions, will affect the suicide risk in psychiatric patients. In Sweden, shortened admissions have been blamed for a rise in suicide soon after discharge (Perris *et al.*, 1980) but the direct evidence is conflicting (Flood & Seager, 1968; Roy, 1982*a*). Rapid institutionalisation in Italy did not coincide with a rise in suicide (Williams *et al.*, 1986). One study in the UK, although finding no overall change in suicide after a community psychiatric service began, believed the risk in the elderly had declined (Walk, 1967).

Aspects of care

There is little evidence relating suicide or suicide prevention to individual components of psychiatric care (Dennehy *et al.*, 1996), although one study reported no effect of social case-work or day care (Roy, 1982*b*). Inadequate treatment, particularly of depression, increases the risk (Myers & Neal, 1978; Rorsmann, 1973; Modestin, 1985) but many suicides are receiving suitable prophylaxis or treatment (Wilkinson & Bacon, 1984; Schou & Weeke, 1988). The fact that relatively toxic drugs such as tricyclic antidepressants are sometimes used as the means of suicide implies that newer, less toxic alternatives should be used in depression. However, suicides by people who are on antidepressants do not appear to be associated with older tricylics (Isacsson *et al.*, 1994).

Poor relationships with staff (Flood & Seager, 1968; Virkkunen, 1976; Morgan & Priest, 1984), inadequate staff numbers or morale (Kahnne, 1968; Coser, 1976; Crammer, 1984), and inadequate ward design or location (Sims & O'Brien, 1979; Crammer, 1984) have been linked to hospital suicides.

Parasuicide

In this section the terms parasuicide and deliberate self-harm (DSH) will be used interchangeably to refer to non-fatal acts of self-poisoning or self-injury. These terms are preferred to 'attempted suicide' because many self-harming patients do not wish to die, or are too distressed or impulsive to have formed a clear intent.

Epidemiology and risk factors

It is estimated that there are 100 000 episodes of self-harm annually in the UK, while in the USA the figure is believed to be at least 250 000. Many Western countries experienced a rapid rise in parasuicide in the 1960s and early 1970s, although the rate in the UK appears to have fallen since then (Platt *et al.*, 1988).

Many of the risk factors for parasuicide reflect its close link with social and interpersonal adversity, and many are also associated with completed suicide. However, the population at maximum risk differs, being middle-aged and elderly men in the case of suicide and young women in the case of parasuicide. In both sexes the peak incidence comes between the late teens and early thirties (Platt *et al.*, 1988). In women the rates are approximately twice as high as in men (Morgan *et al.*, 1975; Platt *et al.*, 1988).

There is a strong association with low social class and unemployment (Platt & Kreitman, 1984, 1985), and with being single or divorced (Bancroft *et al.*, 1975). A high rate of life events is found in the six months before a parasuicidal act (Paykel, 1975), and difficulties in interpersonal relationships are particularly common (Bancroft & Marzack, 1977; Morgan *et al.*, 1975).

Many patients who harm themselves have experienced significant neurotic symptoms before the act (Newson-Smith & Hirsch, 1979*a*) and many have recently consumed alcohol (Morgan *et al.*, 1975). However, few have severe psychiatric illness, and the commonest diagnoses are neurotic depression, personality disorder and alcoholism. Between 10–30% have no psychiatric diagnosis (Morgan *et al.*, 1975; Kreitman, 1977; Urwin & Gibbons, 1979). Impulsive and hostile behaviours are common, including towards doctors and health staff. A history of physical or sexual abuse in childhood is often obtained.

Method

In the UK, approximately 90% of episodes of parasuicide are overdoses of drugs, often psychotropic drugs and analgesics (Morgan *et al.*, 1975). Paracetamol is now the most commonly used drug in overdose in the UK (Hawton & Fagg, 1992a) and is particularly common in self-poisoning by adolescents (Hawton & Fagg, 1992b). More violent methods are associated with suicidal intent, although it cannot be assumed that those who take relatively harmless overdoses have no wish to die. The commonest form of self-injury is self-laceration, usually of the forearms, using glass or a razor-blade. This method tends to be used by young patients at times of mounting anxiety following an emotional, often interpersonal, crisis. Many report feelings of depersonalisation at the time of cutting, and relief of tension afterwards.

Risks of suicide and parasuicide repetition

Approximately 1% of parasuicides kill themselves in the following year, and the long-term risk is increased up to 25-fold (Hawton & Fagg, 1988). Suicide following self-harm is said to be associated with the same risk factors as suicide in the general population – male sex, living alone, unemployment, psychiatric illness or personality disorder, alcohol or substance abuse – and with older age, previous self-harm and suicidal intent at the time of the parasuicidal act. In young people there is a particular association with substance abuse (Hawton et al., 1993).

In the three months after parasuicide, 15–25% of patients will repeat the self-harm (Buglass & Horton, 1974; Morgan et al., 1976; Bancroft & Marzack, 1977). Repetition can be seen as the effect of stressful life events on individuals who are cognitively vulnerable and who have developed a maladaptive pattern of stress-induced behaviour and service contact (Appleby & Warner, 1993). Repetition is associated with several factors common in self-harm:

(a) demographic – male sex, low social class or unemployment, living alone, being divorced or separated;
(b) psychiatric – previous psychiatric contact, drug or alcohol abuse, previous self-harm;
(c) behavioural – past violence, criminality

Many of these features are also thought to be the characteristics of the young people in whom suicide has recently become more common. This suggests that suicide has become more common in a group who were previously at risk of repeated deliberate self-harm, perhaps because the preferred method of self-harm has changed from drug overdose to the more dangerous carbon monoxide poisoning.

Suicide prevention

Protective factors in populations

Certain population characteristics appear to counterbalance risk factors, acting protectively without altering the risk factors themselves. For example, low rates are found in countries where alcohol is banned, and where the prevailing religion is Islam or Catholicism. In the UK, the reported male suicide rate fell during both world wars, an echo of the French social scientist Emile Durkheim's finding that fewer suicides occurred in the mid-1800s in those countries experiencing revolution (Durkheim, 1951). Durkheim postulated that vulnerable individuals were more likely to commit suicide when the cohesive forces in a society broke down, a condition he termed *anomie*. Conversely, when a society was held together more strongly, as in facing a common foe, the rate would fall. A similar explanation has been put forward to account for the stable suicide rate in Northern Ireland despite its civil war (Curran, 1988).

Therapeutic strategies depend on translating such population effects into individual cases. One epidemiological study reported a low rate of suicide in postnatal women despite their high rate of morbidity and suggested that cognitive factors such as self-worth might be protective and might become the focus of a cognitive intervention in other settings (Appleby, 1991).

One important requirement of suicide prevention is the identification of high-risk individuals. After GPs on the Swedish island of Gotland were trained to recognise and treat depression, a localised fall in the suicide rate was found, which was not evident nationally (Rutz *et al.*, 1989*b*). However, without further training, the low rate was not sustained (Rutz *et al.*, 1992*a*). Although these are important findings, there are doubts about their broader applicability, for instance to heavily populated urban areas. There is also conflicting evidence that young suicides have a lower rate of GP attendance before death (Vassilas & Morgan, 1993; Appleby *et al.*, 1996).

An alternative public health approach is to prevent access to the most common methods of suicide. For example, the present common use of self-poisoning from car exhausts suggests the need to detoxify exhaust fumes through the widespread use of catalytic converters (Lester, 1989).

Assessment of risk in the individual

Because the risk factors for suicide are common in the population, predicting which high risk individuals will commit suicide is difficult, both clinically and statistically (Pokorny, 1983). When faced with a potentially suicidal patient, it is important to examine the following:

Demographic and clinical risk factors

As described above.

Mental state

Delusions or hallucinations with suicidal content indicate serious risk. When depression is present, its severity and persistence should be estimated, as well as the key cognitions of worthlessness and hopelessness (Beck *et al.*, 1985).

Suicidal thoughts

The persistence, intensity and detail of thoughts about suicide and death should be established. Important details are the degree of planning, the lethality of the proposed method, 'rehearsal' actions such as counting out tablets, and reasons for not proceeding.

Intent

Many suicides have indicated their intention to someone, often a relative, friend or doctor (Robins *et al.*, 1959; Barraclough *et al.*, 1974). Statements of intent may also be a feature of suicide, occurring in patients diagnosed as sociopathic, or dependent on drugs or alcohol (Ovenstone & Kreitman, 1974). This is important, as such patients are often dismissed in clinical practice as 'manipulative' or 'attention seeking' (Lewis & Appleby, 1988).

Suicidal acts

When a suicidal act has occurred, assessment should be made of (a) antecedents – planning, precipitating factors that may be unresolved, actions taken to prevent discovery, 'final' actions such as making a will or leaving a note; (b) the attempt itself – lethality, expectation that it would be fatal; (c) attitude to the attempt – embarrassment, regret over its failure.

Management of suicidal or self-harming patients

Although acutely suicidal and self-harming patients are a heterogeneous group, there are treatment approaches common to all. Young self-harming patients, however, particularly those who repeat the act, may require a different approach.

General principles

The features of good general psychiatric care can also be expected to reduce the risk of suicide, e.g. early detection and prompt treatment of depression and relapsing psychosis, and satisfactory after-care. The degree of supervision provided should be compatible with the immediate risk of suicide. In those cases at highest risk, admission to hospital is necessary, sometimes under a compulsory order – most mental health legislation allows the detention of suicidal patients. Close nursing observations is then essential. For less suicidal individuals, other treatment locations may be suitable if support is available, e.g. family living at home, and if there is an agreed plan, including contact with services, for times of crisis. One pilot study suggested that having easy access to services (by telephone) might lower the risk of self-harm without producing an increase in demand for help (Morgan *et al.*, 1993).

Specific treatment approaches in deliberate self-harm

Brief out-patient counselling has been shown to benefit female parasuicides and those with relationship problems (Hawton *et al.*, 1987) but without improving the risk of repetition. In one small study, cognitively based problem-solving led to a non-significant reduction in repetition of self-harm (Salkovskis *et al.*, 1990). However, a form of psychotherapy based on cognitive-behavioural methods has been able to reduce repetition over one year, when used intensively in vulnerable (borderline) individuals (Linehan *et al.*, 1991).

Services for self-harming individuals

Most intervention studies in deliberate self-harm have assumed that the appropriate treatment is a combination of emotional support, problem-solving advice, and regular follow-up, and have focused on the organisation of services providing such treatment. All studies agree that both initial assessment of suicide risk and further follow-up can be satisfactorily carried out by staff other than psychiatrists. After suitable training, social workers (Newsom-Smith & Hirsch, 1979*b*) and nurses (Catalan *et al.*, 1980) can perform skilled assessments of parasuicides. The benefits of counselling (with female patients and in relationship problems) do not differ whether it is administered by psychiatrists, general practitioners or non-medical staff, at a clinic or at the patient's home (Hawton *et al.*, 1981, 1987).

Better outcome, measured by further episodes of self-harm, has been found in those parasuicidal patients who receive (or accept) psychiatric assessment and continuing contact (Greer & Bagley, 1971; Kennedy, 1971). However, more specific studies of intervention have not demonstrated that the repetition of parasuicide can be prevented in the short-term despite effectiveness in resolving social problems (Chowdury *et al.*, 1973; Gibbons *et al.*, 1978).

The benefit of suicide services, such as the Samaritans in the UK, has not been proved. Although they provide valuable support to people in crisis, and many dissuade individuals from killing themselves, there is no clear evidence that their impact is sufficient to reduce suicide rates (Jennings *et al.*, 1978).

In summary, there are few research findings to guide clinical practice towards specific preventive interventions. Clinical services should aim to identify and closely supervise certain high-risk groups while recognising that suicide prevention requires a public health policy directed at the social risk factors and likely methods.

23

Forensic psychiatry

PAMELA J. TAYLOR

Introduction

One indication of the coming of age of a specialty is its development of sub-specialities. In England there is a continued shortage of forensic psychiatrists, but there is a sufficiently well-established network of services that a need is emerging for people who can specialise in such areas as the forensic psychiatry of mental retardation, forensic psychotherapy, or child and adolescent forensic psychiatry. English service development has followed from repeated, national, multidisciplinary reviews of need for services (Ministry of Health, 1961; Department of Health and Social Security, 1974; Home Office, Department of Health and Social Security, 1974, 1975; Department of Health, Home Office, 1992). The resultant remit for forensic psychiatry is perhaps broader than in many other parts of the world. The principles of practice, however, have more in common than not across international boundaries, and differences tend to be organisational, for example in details of legislation or in what tasks are undertaken specifically within forensic psychiatric services. Thus, in most countries, psychiatry has or is developing systems for:

1. assessing and treating those who have a mental disorder but who are also offenders – whether or not they become the subjects of criminal proceedings;
2. the assessment and management of risk in people with a mental disorder;
3. providing the courts with advice pertinent to judgement of criminal responsibility, and disposal if convicted;
4. research into links between mental development or disorder and crime;
5. the assessment and treatment of the problems created by criminal victimisation (and other comparable situations, such as major accident or disaster);
6. provision of advice to courts or statutory bodies relevant to restitution, reparation and compensation for victims, and victim witness competence;
7. open debate on controversial and ethical issues in the field; these include the ethics of compulsory treatment, or of not providing such treatment; the place and satisfactory management of institutions and of security; potential conflicts of duty – between primary duty to the patient (the usual medical position) and primary duty to others if the risks

from the mental disorder are predominantly to others; the obscenities of medical involvement in capital punishment;
8. specialist training in these matters.

Britain differs from some other countries, and particularly the USA, in requiring extended (3–4 years) of specialist training once general professional training in psychiatry is complete. This is set out in more detail by Gunn (1986) and in the handbook of the training accreditation body (Joint Committee on Higher Psychiatric Training, 1995).

Victims of crime

An area, still gaining recognition, but that is fundamental to good forensic psychiatric practice, is an understanding of the effect of being a victim of crime or other serious trauma. For some people this can be a contributory factor to becoming a criminal (see below). Already, however, most professionals working in this field accept the importance of considering potential victims when assessing risk from an offender patient. When trying to estimate the true amount of crime in any community (as opposed merely to recorded crime and/or various levels of activity in the criminal justice system) it has long been accepted that community surveys of victimisation rates provide the only way of approaching the real picture (e.g. in England and Wales, Mayhew et al., 1993; in the USA, Reiss & Roth, 1993).

Within quite restrictive limits, victims of crime or disaster may claim compensation for their injury, including psychological injury (Gunn, 1996). In some jurisdictions forensic clinicians have put much, if not most, emphasis in the work on civil compensation. In Great Britain awards to victims are generally not very high. This is most true for crime victims, and particularly if made directly from a criminal court or from the statutory body, the Criminal Injuries Compensation Board. Awards are made mainly in respect of calculable financial losses, excluding legal costs (Miers, 1978; Newburn, 1989). USA schemes are perhaps more generous (McGillis & Smith, 1983), but in the USA too there is a sense that a victim of crime is often more 'used' than helped by the criminal justice system, and even politicians (Elias, 1993). The primary victim of a crime is usually construed as the state, and, although sensitivity in these matters is improving, the person actually injured in some way may never even be informed if and when the case comes to court (Shapland et al., 1985). Unlike the alleged offender, the person alleging injury has no right, in the UK at least, to legal representation, nor to confidentiality during the trial with respect to antecedent history.

Witness competence, including victim witness competence, may be decided by the Court, certainly in England, without calling specific evidence. Although most work on the assessment of individuals for witness competency decisions has been done with children (e.g. Dent & Stephenson, 1979; Wehrspann et al., 1987), an approach of relevance to adults with learning disability has also been described (Gudjonsson & Gunn, 1982), while much of Gudjonsson's work on interrogative suggestibility could also apply (Gudjonsson & Clark, 1986; Gudjonsson, 1987). Courts could be made more aware of the possibilities for objective assessment of victim and witness competence. Many victims may simply need information and support if they are to handle their witness role effectively. The USA appears to be the leader in both victim witness (Schneider & Schneider, 1981) and the more strident victim advocacy schemes (Du Bow & Becker, 1976).

Court work apart, it is increasingly apparent that there is an important role for forensic psychiatrists, and others, in the management and treatment of the psychiatric disorders that arise in a substantial proportion of people who have been victims. In many cases the more acute anxiety and distress states following a major trauma, principally now subsumed under the diagnosis of post-traumatic stress disorder (PTSD), may be self-limiting. It is still far from clear whether psychiatry or psychology has anything specific to offer in such circumstances, but full awareness of the longer-term impact of trauma is still emerging. Data on Vietnam veterans have demonstrated the range of risk from trauma experienced as an adult. In one large study of 8000 veterans and 7000 controls (Centers for Disease Control 1988), 15% of the veterans qualified for a research diagnosis of PTSD, but other anxiety states were also prominent, as was depression, and 14% were abusing alcohol. Men who had entered military service were 65% more likely than the rest of the population to die subsequently by suicide and 49% more likely in a road accident. Alcohol abuse, road accidents, and even some suicide acts may put more people at risk than the subject, but some Vietnam veterans studies have also shown that severe PTSD may be correlated with criminal violence (Wilson & Zigelbaum, 1983; Solursh, 1988, 1989). Men in these samples generally did not have a pre-combat history of antisocial or violent tendencies. McFall et al. (1991) made very similar observations about violence that had not attracted the attentions of the criminal justice system in a sample of veterans seeking help for substance abuse. Collins & Bailey (1990) examined a large (1140) sample of recently imprisoned non-veteran men. They demonstrated not only that PTSD was followed by violence, but also that the more symptoms of PTSD rated the more likely it was that the man had been arrested for homicide, rape or serious assault. Evidence is accumulating for an hypothesis that repetitive serious violence may, in effect, be a sign of one form of chronic PTSD. Hodge (1992) has suggested that the forms of personality disorder that are of particular relevance in work with offender patients may be variants of chronic PTSD. The World Health Organization gave first recognition in 1992 to a form of enduring personality change after catastrophic experience as a class of disorder in ICD-10.

Childhood experience of violent abuse, sexual abuse or both has also been implicated not only with the subsequent emergence of psychiatric disorder, but also with criminality (e.g. Burgess et al., 1987, Widom, 1989, 1991). It is, however, hard to separate out the direct effects of abuse from the impact of the environment in which it occurs (Mullen et al., 1993a). West (e.g. 1982) and Farrington (e.g. 1978, 1979, 1986, 1991) in prospective, longitudinal study of Camberwell boys, have linked indicators of environmental deprivation with both subsequent antisocial behaviour and social dysfunction. A rather more outgoing personality with capacity to relate to peers seems to be the additional factor that relates to delinquency persistent beyond the age of 30, while loners from similar backgrounds suffered similar levels of dysfunction but without the antisocial activities (Farrington & West, 1993). Although individuals undoubtedly vary in their inherent strengths and weaknesses (e.g. see Thomas & Chess, 1984), organic brain damage resulting from abuse or deprivation may be as disruptive as emotional damage, and not uncommon. Lewis (1992) reviewed the complex extent of such interactions. It is unfortunate that many such traumatised or disadvantaged people do not present to services until they are well into the pathway of self- and other-destructive disorders. Maden *et al.* (1993), in their survey of the treatment and security needs of English special hospital patients, were particularly impressed with the similarities in the presentations and needs of the patients, regardless of ICD-9 (WHO, 1978) diagnosis. One probable factor accounting for this was the very high rate of histories of early childhood deprivation and abuse among the patients.

Many who suffer even severe or prolonged traumas show remarkable resilience and recovery, but the range and frequency of disorder after trauma means a need for systematic study and service. Forensic psychiatry has simply been that branch of psychiatry that deals with patients and problems at the interface of legal and health care systems, but it seems increasingly important to include in the main tasks the prevention and treatment of disorders associated with victimisation, and indeed prevention of some cases of victimisation (Gunn & Taylor, 1993*a,b*).

The nature, range and distribution of crime

Psychiatrists, even forensic psychiatrists, often develop a very distorted impression of crime, partly because of the bias in cases for which their help is likely to be sought, but also because of the considerable difficulties in defining crime.

Crime, at its simplest, covers just those activities that are expressly against the law. In general, acts that are designated criminal are harmful or threatening to an individual or to society as a whole, but the opposite is not necessarily true. Not all antisocial, not even all harmful conduct is proscribed in law, and certainly not all is prosecuted. Smith & Hogan (1988), whose discussion of the nature and definition of crime goes far beyond anything that can be attempted here, suggest that within the construct is generally some concept of a public wrong and of a moral wrong, although neither in itself is sufficient to constitute crime. They suggest an increasing tendency to prohibit acts on grounds of social expediency rather than immorality. They cite two relevant illustrations of this, in society's treatment of suicide and homosexuality. In England and Wales after 3rd August 1961 it became lawful to kill oneself and after 17 July 1967 it became lawful for men of 21 or over to have homosexual relations in private. Before those dates those acts were crimes, after they were not, but the acts themselves had not changed. Smith & Hogan also draw attention to a related characteristic of the law, its tendency to take a binary approach to matters. Psychiatrists, who are trained to deal in probabilities and continuities, often find this particularly troublesome, and this difference in approaches can lead to difficulties in working with lawyers or the courts. What psychiatrist or psychologist has not found him or herself struggling to give an honest account of the probabilities than an important element of the mental state was extant at the time of an offence in question, only to become the butt of legal derision, 'Come doctor, was the patient hallucinating, yes or no?'.

Another way of construing crime is as deviance, that is acts or omissions that lie outside the common practice. Maguire *et al.*, (1994) explored this in introducing their splendid collection of essays covering criminology from a British perspective. They have described criminology as the only highly developed social science that explicitly takes a social problem as its defining subject matter. This, however, may leave it exceptionally vulnerable to manipulation or misinterpretation, not least by political forces. The discipline is divided. In one school there are those who contend that in accepting designated 'crime' as the focus of interest, criminology is gravely compromised as a science by handing the agenda for the work to the government of the day; in the other camp are those who argue that the alternative academic-led 'sociology of deviance' tends to be a distraction from issues that are consistently damaging to individuals and society by emphasising the study of relatively marginal issues such as popular youth culture or football hooliganism. Maguire and co-workers take 'rigorous scholarship, respect for evidence and clarity of analysis and exposition' as the way through, acknowledging that while reduction of harm caused by crime is an important issue so is the acknowledging of the accountability of the system formally established to control crime.

Dilemmas of definition face psychiatrists in this field too. Two of the common difficulties for psychiatrists, or perhaps more accurately those who would seek help from them, lie in the areas of sexual problems and substance abuse. There is confusion over the division between mental disorder based concepts of sexual deviancies, such as transvestism or fetishism, which are not illegal, legally based concepts of crime (e.g. rape), which do not constitute recognised mental disorder and behaviours that are equally at home in either system, such as exhibitionism. Further, even professional clinicians seem unable to keep moral judgements about a piece of behaviour out of their work. Sowers & Daley (1993) and Mosher & Yanagisko (1991), for example, particularly considering drug use, have suggested that it is this intrusion of morality that has been a key factor in shifting intervention responsibility for such problems away from medicine and on to law enforcement agencies. They have described the legal solution as a manifest failure in the USA, problematic use of illegal drugs now being surpassed only by anxiety disorders in prevalence (Robins & Regier, 1991). It is also worth emphasising that Epidemiologic Catchment Area studies show that substance-abuse disorders are the mental disorders most commonly associated with self-reported violence to others (Swanson et al., 1990). Of particular interest for England and Wales, where compulsory treatment for substance abuse per se is expressly forbidden in law, Sowers & Daley review work that shows that a number of compulsory treatment programmes in the USA are demonstrably effective in reducing abuse and consequent damage, whether or not the individuals were initially motivated for treatment. Given all these difficulties, it is a step in the right direction, that, when considering the planning and delivery of health and personal social services, the English Department of Health and Home Office Report (1992; 'The Reed Report') put the broadest possible construction on the prospective clientele – 'mentally disordered offenders and others requiring similar services'. From a medical perspective the wisest approach to defining 'crime' or 'offending' and even 'disorder' must indeed be flexible, albeit always explicit for the circumstances.

Problems with identification of crime

Only a small proportion of all crime, even taking the strict legal definition, is ever 'cleared up'; undetected crime is often ominously referred to by criminologists as the 'dark figure'. Estimates of crime rates have improved since the introduction of victim-centered population surveys. Many victims do not report their experiences to police, although this varies considerably with the nature of the crime, and with the consequences of reporting. In England, where car insurance in mandatory and house contents insurance quite common, crimes such as car theft and burglary have a high report rate; such a report is generally required in order to be able to make a claim. By contrast, except at extremes, the reporting of physical or sexual assault is relatively low. The relationship between non-violent and violent crimes is in the opposite direction for detection, with homicide having the best clear-up rate. The reporting of violent crime is complicated by many factors; these include the fear, and to some extent the reality, that the victim has a hard time in the criminal justice system, and the fact that assailants are often known to their victims. In the USA, the National Crime Survey (victim report data) noted over 6 million violent victimisations in 1990, while the Uniform Crime Reports (recording events that the police have classified as crimes) counted just over 2 million (Reiss & Roth, 1993). The discrepancies in the UK, and doubtless in other jurisdictions too, are of a similar order.

Common ground in recognising and understanding crime

In spite of all the factors mitigating against it, the possession of a criminal record is not unusual. In England and Wales nearly 40% of men will have been convicted of at least one standard list (non-traffic) offence by the age of 50, but only 12% of women (Farrington, 1981). Rates are lower in some countries, such as Sweden, (Stattin et al., 1989) and higher in others, such as the USA, (Blumstein & Cohen, 1987). There are some international differences too in the patterns of crime. Violence, for example, dominates the figures in the USA, and a quick glance at criminal homicide rates shows that it has long been among the world leaders in this regard (Schipkowensky, 1973; Coid, 1983). Reiss & Roth (1993) show the Bahamas as having an annual rate of 11 homicides per 100 000 population, with the USA as equal second, with over 8 per 100 000. Canada and most European countries have rates under 2 per 100 000, with England and Wales at half that.

Psychiatrists tend to see proportionately more violent offenders than other groups, perhaps because, of all classes of offence, violence seems most likely to be related to psychiatric disorder (see below). Overall, however, non-violent offending is much more common. Of the nearly 4 million crimes recorded in England and Wales in 1988 (Home Office, 1989) 4.3% were of violence against the person, and 0.7% sexual offence. Criminal damage to property accounted for a further 16% of offences, a little of this, such as arson, possibly posing a threat to life. Under 1% lay in drug offences, but the rest – nearly 80% – was theft in one form or another, including fraud. There is a tendency for adults to specialise in crime, following violent careers or property-driven careers (Blumstein et al., 1986; Farrington et al., 1988). Blackburn (1993) has described attempts to classify offenders by crime, although he is more inclined, on the basis of research evidence, to emphasise the heterogeneity of personal attributes within and between the classes. Certainly most lengthy criminal careers will contain at least one violent offence, and prediction of violent behaviour from arrest records is poor (Monahan, 1988).

The sex and age distribution of crime, and evidence on predisposing factors, make common ground on crime within and between nations. Men are disproportionately represented in all crime statistics compared with women, unless the crime can, by definition, only be committed by women (infanticide and soliciting), where the offences are related to child rearing or sexual mores, and where the link between mental disorder and violence leaves women particularly vulnerable. d'Orbán (1993) summarises the male:female ratios for offending, in decreasing order from 82:1 for sex offences, through 26:1 for burglary and 9:1 for violence to 3:1 for theft and handling stolen goods. Häfner & Böker (1973/82), within their substantial sample of people who had a mental disorder and had attempted or completed homicide, found that the ratio of men to women was about 3:1, but for one small but important subgroup – depressive homicides – this ratio was reversed.

People of 60 and over constitute the most rapidly growing section of the population in many western countries, and there are hints that there are some concomitant rises in elderly offending (e.g. Feinberg, 1984). Nevertheless, crime is mainly a youthful activity. Criminologically speaking, old age arrives in the fourth decade. Greenberg (1983) has cautioned against overstating this effect, nevertheless, as Farrington (1993) points out, a peak of recorded criminal activity in the teenage years is seen remarkably consistently across different countries and different time periods. He summarises the pertinent Home Office figures for England and Wales for 1987, when indictable (serious) offenses among males increased from 0.9 per 100 at age 10 to a peak of 7.9 at age 15, before decreasing to 6.0 at age 20 and 3.0 at age 25–29. Federal Bureau of Investigation (1988) figures for arrest rates in the USA in 1986 showed comparable trends. Women show a similar peak, but the offending rates decline more slowly (e.g. Home Office, 1988 in England; Pollak, 1950 in the USA). Among people who offend when over 60, importance of alcohol has been consistently emphasised (Moberg, 1953; Keller & Vedder, 1968; Epstein et al., 1970; Shichor, 1984; Taylor & Parrott, 1988).

There is much concern about an apparent over-representation of people from ethnic minorities at each point of contact with the criminal justice system. For England and Wales the report in 1993 of the Royal Commission on Criminal Justice (comparable to a President's Commission in the USA) could only conclude that 'there should be further research to establish the extent to which members of the ethnic minority communities suffer discrimination within the criminal justice system'. As part of the extensive research programme the Commission established within the two years of its work, a critical review of work on ethnic minorities and the criminal justice system was completed by Fitzgerald (1993). She considered the evidence variously for real over-representation of ethnic minorities among offenders and for different treatment at stop and arrest; cautioning, charging and prosecution; bail remand and level of court of trial; outcome of trial and sentencing. She pointed out that, from what is known about the aetiology of crime, there are good reasons for expecting that real crime rates for indigenous whites and Afro-Caribbeans would differ because of other demographic factors. Afro-Caribbean men and women, are, on average, a younger group in the general population than their white peers, and therefore more likely to fall within the peak age groups for offending. Afro-Caribbean men are also more likely to suffer the adverse socio-economic factors particularly associated with offending, including high levels of unemployment, low educational attainment and residence in high crime areas. Evidence on treatment in the criminal justice system is inconsistent, with a hint that earlier

P.J. TAYLOR

studies may have been more likely to find discrimination than some of the later ones. One thing that is clear is that there are no simple relationships between ethnic status and offending or its treatment. Reiss & Roth (1993), in their review of the situation with respect to violence in the USA, provide a rather different emphasis, which is less often remarked, but very important. The overall 1990 violent victimisation rate as reported to the National Crime Survey was 39.7 for black Americans, 37.3 for Hispanics but just 28.2 for whites. Homicide is the leading cause of death for African Americans between the ages of 15 and 34 (United States Department of Health and Human Services, 1991). Research expenditure by the USA, however, on violence per year of potential life lost is $31. For cancer it is $794 and for AIDS $697 (Reiss & Roth, 1993). This strange balance in priorities seems unlikely to be confined to the USA.

Farrington (1988, 1993) has presented a list of the 16 key long-term cohort studies which provide the basis for much of the current knowledge about the origins of crime. They include four from the UK (Douglas & Wadsworth (e.g. Wadsworth, 1979); Miller & Kolvin (e.g. Miller et al., 1985); Rutter & Quinton (e.g. Rutter, 1981); West & Farrington (e.g. 1977, Farrington & West 1993)); four from elsewhere in Europe (in Sweden, Janson (1984) and Wikstrom (1987) as well as Magnusson (e.g. Stattin et al., 1989); in Denmark, Mednick (e.g. Mednick & Christiansen, 1977)); in Finland, Pulkkinen (e.g. 1988); one from French-speaking Canada (e.g. LeBlanc & Frechett, 1989) and one from New Zealand (e.g. Moffitt & Silva, 1988); and six from the USA (Elliott & Huizinga (e.g. Elliott et al., 1989); Glueck & Glueck (e.g. 1968); McCord & McCord (e.g. McCord, 1977, 1978, 1988); Robins (e.g. 1966, 1978); Werner (e.g. 1987); and Wolfgang & Figlio (e.g. Wolfgang et al., 1987)). The smallest sample size from this group was 369 (in Finland) and most exceeded 1000. In each case the subjects were studied prospectively, the shortest follow-up being for five years with some still ongoing after more than 30 years, and they were studied on many measures including self-report. There is consistency in findings that, as a group, offenders differ from non-offenders in being of significantly lower intelligence, albeit well within the average range as measured by IQ tests; having long-standing personality difficulties, especially impulsivity; low income and large-size family; parents who have problems of their own, including criminality, and often with harsh and inconsistent practices in discipline; adverse peer influences; poor socio-economic status and from geographical areas of deprivation.

Associations between mental disorder and crime

Both crime and mental disorder are common, and some association therefore likely by chance. The assumption of a special link between them, however, is very long-standing, particularly between violence and mental disorder. Monahan (1992) has provided a brief overview of the history, the extent to which the current media and popular fiction continue to reinforce this perception, and a useful introduction to some of the realities. There have long existed very powerful accounts of individual cases describing a clear association, even causation between mental illness and violence in those cases, and the account of the McNaughton trial by West & Walk (1977) is one of these. His case led to the McNaughton rules, which are the basis of the insanity defence in common law jurisdictions to this day. It is

570

only since the 1980s, however, that a satisfactory picture of the extent and nature of the relationships has begun to emerge. Up to a point, popular fears have been confirmed, in that there does appear to be a greater than chance risk of violence, but equally it seems likely that effective treatment and management of individual cases could almost eliminate this small but important segment of violent crime. Three research approaches have been crucial – the cross-sectional general community survey, the comparative study of illness and criminal careers, and phenomenological work.

Until 1990, almost all efforts to look at quantitive associations between mental disorder and crime had been on highly selected populations. Monahan & Steadman (1983) showed that there were studies that illustrated true disorder rates within selected criminal samples, and true offending rates within selected samples of people with a mental disorder, but none that could directly consider true crime–true disorder links. Studies of unlawful homicides formed a near exception. There is a high clear-up rate for homicide, and therefore the samples for any given geographical area might be regarded as more or less complete. There is, however, still bias in reporting of national statistics in that deaths by dangerous driving, or corporate negligence in industry or transport systems, are among the figures not included under the category of unlawful homicide; among unlawful homicides, the mentally ill are disproportionately represented (e.g. Taylor & Gunn, 1984; Wilcox, 1985). Wessely & Taylor (1991) updated discussion of the problems and biases in research into crime and mental disorder.

In 1990, data from a large community sample, unselected for violence or mental disorder – the Epidemiological Catchment Area studies in the USA – confirmed a significant association between self-reported violence and mental disorder (Swanson et al., 1990). Although being young, male and of low socio-economic status were significant associates of violence, mental disorder accounted for significant additional variance. More than half of the violent sample (55.5%) met criteria for at least one DSM-III diagnosis (American Psychiatric Association, 1980) other than personality disorder, compared with just under 20% of the non-violent respondents. Both affective disorders and schizophrenia were three times commoner among the violent than the non-violent; substance abuse or multiple diagnoses accounted for even stronger associations with violence. Link et al. (1992) focused their attentions on a New York community sample supplemented with an identified patient sample. They counted official arrest records, self-reported arrests and seriously violent episodes. Each of the patient groups – first contact, repeat contact and former contact patients – showed consistently higher percentages of incidents than never-treated community residents. Further analysis of the sample, however, revealed that arrest rates for non-violent crimes were remarkably similar between the groups. They differed only in violence.

Among the career studies Hodgins (1992) reported on the widest range of mental disorder. She conducted a 30 year follow-up of a Swedish sample of discharged psychiatric patients drawn from a birth cohort of over 7000 men and 7000 women. For the women, only substance abuse and major mental disorder (almost invariably schizophrenia) were significantly correlated with a record of at least one criminal office; for the men this was also true, but mental handicap was also correlated. Over the 30 years the people with a mental disorder had committed at least as many offences as those without, the highest rates, however, were for men with a major mental disorder or substance abuse and for women with substance abuse. Violent offences were four times more likely among the men with schizophrenia than those without disorder, and over 27 times more likely in the comparable comparison for the women; intellectual handicap was also associated with violence, but again substance abuse proved an ever higher risk factor. The other striking finding was that the patterns of onset of offending varied with disorder group. The most important was that the men with major mental disorder showed two peaks, one between 15 and 18 (most of the men without mental disorder were well established on their offending careers by then) and a later one between 21 and 30. A re-examination of the data confirmed that once the late onset group started their offending, their rate of violence exceeded that of the early start groups; the early onset men had many more convictions for non-violent crime. While the commonest age of onset of illness for the men was probably in the late teens, it only became well-established during the mid- to late-twenties, when violent offending became prominent (Taylor & Hodgins, 1994). The onset of schizophrenia tends to be later in women than men, and it is interesting that the women with mental disorder in this cohort showed only the later peak of onset of offending.

Psychosis and violence

The other mental disorder–offending career studies focus almost exclusively on schizophrenia and offending, and provide perhaps the most convincing evidence of a direct relationship between schizophrenia and crime. Lindqvist & Allebeck (1990) followed a different Swedish cohort of people with schizophrenia, for 15 years after their discharge from Stockholm hospitals. They could not make comparisons of the onset of careers, but they were able to show differences in the progression of the offending career between people with and without schizophrenia. Officially recorded criminal violence was four times commoner among the men with schizophrenia than those without. For the women the rate of all offending was higher among those with schizophrenia.

In a study of pre-trial prisoners in England (Taylor, 1993), interview accounts were collated with a range of previous health, social and criminal records. It was thus possible to compare the onset of any violence to other people (not just that appearing on criminal records) against the onset of illness in the subgroups of 40 men with schizophrenia and 21 with affective psychosis who had also been violent. In nearly 90% of cases in the group with schizophrenia and over 80% of those with an affective psychosis, the violence had post-dated the onset of the illness. By contrast, onset of non-violent offending was evenly distributed around onset of illness.

Among all twins seen in the Bethlem Royal and Maudsley hospital between 1948 and 1988, of whom at least one of each pair had a functional psychosis, Coid and her colleagues (1993) found that offending was a significantly greater problem for the men with schizophrenia, and post-dated first psychiatric contact in nearly 60% of cases. Offending was rated solely from official criminal records and, in the report, treated as a unitary phenomenon. Coid has since re-analysed the data and found that for 12 of the 14 men and both of the women with schizophrenia who had been violent, the violence clearly post-dated the onset of illness (see Taylor & Hodgins, 1994).

A study by Wessely *et al.* (1994) again relied solely on official criminal records for offending history and hospital records for psychiatric history, but is of importance because it is from a cohort of all people making a contact with psychiatric services in one London Borough, and not of people selected for schizophrenia or for offending. Four hundred and ninety-one 'cases' of schizophrenia and 383 'controls' – the next adjacent case with a hospital record but without a diagnosis of schizophrenia – formed the sample. Any specific effect of schizophrenia on career might thus be separated from the more general effect of mental disorder. More or less in line with the Swedish study, the rate of all offending was elevated for the women with schizophrenia, but only the violent offending for the men. Unemployment, ethnic group, substance abuse and low social class accounted for much of the variance, but schizophrenia made a significant additional difference. Even after adjustment for time at risk – which here meant time at liberty in the community – the criminal careers for people with schizophrenia began later and ended earlier than those of the controls.

The remaining strand of evidence linking mental illness to violence, lies in phenomenology, although this is an area that has been remarkably under-researched. Aside from a few anecdotal accounts linking specific symptoms to particular pieces of behaviour, most of the relevant data come from the German case record study of Häfner & Böker (1973), two separate studies of men in prison in England awaiting trial on criminal charges, which included extensive interview work (Robertson & Taylor, 1985; Taylor, 1985), and further analysis from the New York community survey described earlier (Link & Stueve, 1994). Delusions as potentially dangerous symptoms seem to cut across diagnostic boundaries. Delusions are very common among people with schizophrenia, but Häfner & Böker showed that homicidal offenders with schizophrenia were more likely to be delusional than their non-violent schizophrenic peers. Taylor (1985) showed that up to 40% of offenders with a psychotic illness (and none of those without) specified a delusion, without necessarily recognising it as such, as the trigger to their offence. This was significantly more likely for a seriously violent offence than a trivial one. Almost all had contemporaneous delusions, but a direct link with offending could not be established for the others. In the second pre-trial series it was even possible to show a gradient from the more purely delusional forms of a psychotic illness, associated with the most serious violence, to the forms almost without positive symptoms at all, which were generally associated with the most trivial of offending (Taylor *et al.*, 1993*a–d*). Delusions of passivity and delusions of religious or paranormal influence were significantly associated with violent actions. The Link & Stueve (1994) finding that 'threat/control-override' symptoms (i.e. passivity, thought insertion and persecution) were the most important clinical predictors of violence among patients, fits with this. In an interview study of general psychiatric patients using the Maudsley Assessment of Delusions Schedule (MADS) (Taylor *et al.*, 1994), it was shown that acting on delusions is very common indeed (60% of deluded patients over one 28-day period). Even in this sample over this short time-scale over 10% of the patients had acted violently at least once (Buchanan *et al.*, 1993; Wessely *et al.*, 1993).

The association between hallucinations and violent actions is far less clear. Experience with ill offenders suggests that auditory hallucinations are rarely implicated (Häfner & Böker, 1973; Taylor, 1985), but hallucinations of taste or smell, particularly in conjunction with delusions of being poisoned, should perhaps raise alarm (Mowat, 1966; Mawson, 1985).

A number of studies of hospital in-patients have focused on auditory command hallucinations. No positive association with violence to self or others has been found. Hellerstein *et al.* (1987), however, in recording an absence of association, noted that patients with hallucinations were more likely to have been secluded or under special nursing than those without.

Organic brain damage and violence

Clearly localised brain damage is rarely implicated in association with violence. There is a substantial literature on the greater likelihood of finding evidence of non-specific brain damage among violent, particularly repetitively violent, offenders. Most of this work has, however, lacked scientific rigour, for example, soft EEG signs were not rated blind to behaviour state (Kligman & Goldberg, 1975). Few studies have included multiple measures, an exception showing best correlation between psychometric testing and MRI (Chesterman *et al.*, 1994). Only one study (Milstein, 1988) has attempted to correlate repeated measures of brain dysfunction over time with change in behaviour – showing change on both counts, but with no predictable directional correlation. Systematic study of a particular problem has often exploded previous hypotheses. Epilepsy, for example, may be slightly more commonly associated with some kinds of offending than would be expected by chance, but even the very small statistical relationship that exists is more likely to be explained by indirect associations or common etiological factors (Gunn, 1977). An epileptic fit is very rarely a direct cause of violence (Gunn & Fenton, 1971). Another example is provided by the story of the XYY chromosome abnormality. For many years it was confidently asserted, on the basis of small samples identified in prisons, that such men were exceptionally violence-prone. Theilgaard (1984) showed that, although violent cases occur, violence is not characteristic of the condition and, among aggressive or violent cases, social explanations for the behaviour are often evident.

For a more extended discussion of organic brain disorders, mental handicap, learning disabilities and offending see Taylor *et al.* (1993*b*).

Substance abuse and offending

In many societies, use of drugs may in itself constitute an offence, regardless of effect. In others it may be the supply of the drug that is illegal, or the age at which it is consumed, or the circumstances in which the effects become manifest. Drunkenness in Britain, for example, only becomes an offence in a public place, or in association with certain other behaviours including indecency or disorderliness. Substance abuse, however, has also been shown to have an association with crime more generally and with violence in cross-sectional and longitudinal epidemiological studies as described above. The nature of the relationships are, however, far from clear, and probably multifactorial. Possibilities include intoxication with the substance as a direct precipitator of crime; the substance as a facilitator for offending arising from associated social relations or desires; the substance as a precipitant of a psychiatric disorder, which may in turn trigger offending; crime as a practical solution to financing the habit; substance abuse and offending being linked by some common aetiological factor; or some combination of the possibilities. Psychiatric consequences of substance abuse and the legal constraints on use are dealt with more fully in Chapter 8; a more extended discussion of other important links with offending is provided by Taylor *et al.*, 1993*d*).

Personality disorders and offending

A most sensitive and difficult subject for discussion is that of personality disorder. First, there is the question of whether personality disorders are true mental disorders, then, if so,whether any are associated with a propensity for offending but not solely defined by it, and thirdly whether such conditions are treatable. The law has been drawn into dealing with people who fall into these categories. The effect can be to facilitate their rejection. Within psychiatry the arguments about the nature of disorder shown by people often crudely referred to as 'psychopaths' tend to turn on whether the heterogeneity of symptoms and signs cluster as multiple diagnoses or just one. Coid (1992) is one proponent of the school that emphasises comorbidity, while Tyrer (1992) represents those who favour a broader diagnostic conceptualisation,which tends to show better reliability in application. He argues for subsuming the borderline, narcissistic, sadistic, schizotypal, antisocial, histrionic and impulsive personality disorders under the single collective of 'flamboyant personality disorders'. Disorders of deception, self-deception and dissociation, including multiple personality disorder, perhaps also belong among personality disorders of interest to those working with offenders or violent people (Mullen *et al.*, 1993*b*).

An alternative to struggling with diagnostic categories, preferred by psychologists, is to measure traits, clusters of traits and interpersonal styles. Blackburn (1988, 1992, 1993) is one impressive proponent of this approach. He has developed a scale for the assessment of personality in a multiply disordered offender population – the Special Hospitals Assessment of Personality and Socialisation Schedule (SHAPS) (Blackburn, 1982, 1987, 1993). Another well-recognised system is the Hare Psychopathy Checklist (Hare, 1991; Hare *et al.*, 1990, 1991). Blackburn's scale suggests two core factors – *belligerence*, which measures impulsivity and hostility versus conformity, and *withdrawal*, which measures shyness and poor self-esteem versus sociability and confidence. Hare's scale leads to two core dimensions – one of *selfish, callous and remorseless use of others*, and the other a dimension of *socially deviant lifestyle*. Even within the more widely used and reliable systems for measuring 'psychopathy' its association with offending thus tends to be too much intrinsic to the rating to allow confident assertions on the relationship between the disorder and crime. Hare & Hart (1993) are among those that none-the-less attempt this. Perhaps it is anxiety about subscribing to this possible confusion that deters psychiatrists from offering help to this group of people, but it is likely that Reid (1985) came closer to the truth: 'the most pervasive reason for our failure to deal effectively with anti-social behaviour lies in the collective anger that the public, and to some extent, mental health professionals, feel toward antisocial people'. Maier (1990) mused further: 'could it be that after all these Freudian years, psychiatrists have denied the hatred they feel for psychopaths and criminals, and thus have been unable to treat psychopaths adequately because their conceptual base for treatment has been distorted by unconscious, denied feelings from the start?' Similarly Dubin (1989) emphasised that the principal problem for the therapist in treating such patients is to recognise the strength and variety of the counter-transference.

Treatment for people with a personality disorder is, in fact, far from hopeless. A reading of evaluative studies is bedevilled by the fact that much reporting stops short at descriptions of a particular model or regime, or, if it goes further, the treatment groups are poorly defined or outcome measures are very limited – to re-offending or re-hospitalisation without context. Taken together, treatment studies are certainly not describing the effects of an easily standardised intervention on an homogenous group of people with meaningful outcome measures. Dolan & Coid (1993) have provided a useful overview. Gunn *et al.* (1993*a*) offer guiding principles for treatment, as, more formally, does the Australian and New Zealand College of Psychiatry as part of the Quality Assurance Project (1991*a,b*).

Sexual disorders and sex offending

In principle, sexual disorders and sexual offending are different entities. Sexual offending is simply a breech of societal code, and thus wholly dependent on the mores of society at any given time for definition. Sexual disorders are defined within the International Classification of Diseases (World Health Organization, 1992*a*), and fall into three main groups – the paraphilias, the dysfunctions and others, mainly to do with distress about orientation or body image. It is the paraphilias that are most likely to overlap with offending, but by no means all paraphilias constitute offences. It would be easy to overstate the role of psychiatry for sex offenders, but in practice they are offered little. Most effort to help sex offenders seems to take place through people working in the criminal justice system; in the community this tends to be by the probation service, albeit sometimes with psychiatric input (e.g. Cook *et al.*, 1991), in the prison service by non-clinical psychologists. Thornton & Hogue (1993) have described, and begun to evaluate, the large-scale provision of pro- grammes for imprisoned sex offenders in England, which have features in common with elements of penal programmes in parts of North America (Grubin & Prentky, 1993; Porporino & Baylis, 1993). Some states in the USA have legislated to eliminate hospital- based treatment for the most seriously violent and repetitive sexual offenders, notionally in the interests of community safety, but in a litigious society it may well be merely the therapist who benefits by being relieved of a difficult responsibility. Society is more likely to accept people with unchanged deviance from prison, even when their problems may have been complicated by anger following abuse while resident. The fact that prisons are attempting to offer more therapy suggests that indeed the withdrawal of health services for such problems has not been to the advantage of offender or community.

Blackburn (1993) gives a useful introduction to the psychology of sexual deviation and offending. West *et al.* (1993) have offered an eclectic approach to the contributions that psychiatry may make to assessment and treatment. Assessment must include evaluation of arousal behaviour, of social skills, gender role behaviour and the possibility of cognitive distortions. Very often goals in treatment have to be towards acceptable modification of behaviour rather than radical change. Homosexual paedophiles may, for example, be more successful in shaping their interest toward adult men than attempting complete reorientation even if they wished it. Libido-suppressing drugs may be useful enablers of treatment in some cases, but rarely a total solution. Many sex offenders will refuse such medication, even if they recognise risks to themselves as well as to others if they cannot control their sex drive, but some find immense relief. There is acceptable evidence of efficacy (e.g. Freund, 1980). Psychological and social treatments are generally worthwhile in themselves or in conjunction with antilibidinals, although evaluation on more than an individual case basis is rare.

Laws as they affect people with mental disorder

People with a mental disorder are generally subject to all the laws of the society in which they live, but, in most societies, they may be subject to additional legal constraints that apply to no one else. They may also be excused certain kinds of responsibility, for example, being technically relieved of guilt for a criminal offence. Underlying this special treatment are two principles, the protection of society, often known as 'the police powers doctrine', and the 'parens patriae' or 'benevolent paternalism' doctrine, which reflects society's perception of its obligations. Each could bring the doctor into conflict with his more usual and expected relationship with his patient, in which confidentiality and freedom of choice of treatment are presumed.

Compulsory detention in hospital of a patient with mental disorder

Any law permitting compulsory detention in hospital must include a definition of the disorders to which it applies, and of the special features in a patient that might single him out for such confinement. It must have well-defined procedures for the process of detention, including safeguards against unnecessary breach of the patient's autonomy. These will include checks at the time of admission, and also regular reviews in the event of continuing detention. There is no substitute for reading the relevant legislation if a psychiatrist has to invoke the law for any patient, but the following attempts to show the sort of arrangements possible, using as an illustration the principal current legislation for people with mental disorder in England and Wales, the Mental Health Act 1983 (MHA 1983).

The first section of the Act provides the definitions of mental disorder. 'Mental illness' as one sub-category is limited only by the exclusion of 'suffering by reason only of promiscuity or other immoral conduct, sexual deviancy or dependence on alcohol or drugs'. The other three categories in the legislation are mental impairment, severe mental impairment and psychopathic disorder. As in so much other legislation, the use of words in common usage, or terminology which can have another meaning in another context, can cause confusion. These terms are merely figures of legal convenience, and cannot be taken to imply diagnosis. Each is generally reflective of a very complex clinical situation. England and Wales are unusual for making powers of detention explicit for people with a primary personality disorder; some other legislation, for example in Scotland, does not preclude the possibility but avoids terminology like 'psychopathic disorder'.

Compulsory admission to hospital under Part II of the MHA 1983

Civil provisions In addition to fitting the definition of a mental disorder, the essential conditions of detention are that it should be in the interests of the patient's own health and safety, or with a view to the protection of others. This is sufficient for mental illness or severe mental impairment, but in the other two categories a statement that treatment is likely to alleviate or prevent a deterioration in the condition is also necessary. The concept of 'treatability' in this context has proved difficult, but a 1994 High Court ruling (*Canons Park Mental Health Review Tribunal*) has brought much greater clarity. Lord Justices Roch, Kennedy and Nowse endorsed the guidance in the MHA 1983, which includes nursing, habilitation, rehabilitation and care under medical supervision within the legal definition of treatment, but added some helpful points. Detention in hospital simply as an attempt to coerce into group therapy would not be acceptable; alleviation or stabilisation of the disorder need not, however, be immediate, and indeed some initial deterioration might be expected and acceptable, for example, reflecting increased anger at being detained.

Detention procedures differ according to whether the issue is emergency admission to hospital, emergency detention of a person who first entered hospital voluntarily, admission for assessment or admission for treatment. Procedures necessary for legal detention are more stringent for the longer detention periods.

Emergency provisions allow for maximum flexibility in the process – *one* doctor *and* a family member *or* social worker for admission, one doctor *or* one approved nurse only for retention in hospital. They allow for a maximum of 72 hours detention, or just 6 hours in the case of nurse-mandated retention. Use of emergency provisions is discouraged, because there is no right of appeal against them under the Act; they are audited to some extent by the special health authority (the Mental Health Act Commission) set up by the MHA 1983 to oversee the application of the Act. Emergencies may happen in all sorts of circumstance; the Act also gives police powers to take a person from a public place to a 'place of safety' (not necessarily a hospital) for assessment by a doctor and a social worker. If necessary, magistrates (a lower court) may issue a warrant allowing entry to the home of the person with suspected mental disorder, to enable assessment.

Admission explicitly for assessment means that the patient can be detained for up to 28 days, with mental disorder unspecified. Admission for treatment requires specification of the mental disorder, but detention may last for up to six months and be renewable. In either case, however, *two* doctors, from different employing authorities, must have seen the patient and recommended the admission. One of them must be 'approved by the Secretary of State as having special experience in the diagnosis or treatment of mental disorder'. In addition an approved social worker must have seen the patient and applied for admission, having also seen the patient's nearest relative (defined in the Act), and been satisfied, from a knowledge of pertinent resources, that there is no equally satisfactory but less restrictive provision for the patient. Compulsory admission is finally valid when, and only when, the hospital managers have formally accepted the applications. The patient and his relatives have rights of appeal in every period of detention (or its renewal) to the hospital managers, whose role is (Nov. 1996) under review, *and* to a mental health review tribunal. The latter is a truly independent body chaired by a lawyer, and including a specialist doctor and a social worker or lay person. Detainees *must* be referred to a tribunal at the end of six months and thereafter once in every three years if there would otherwise have been no hearing in that time.

Even though each jurisdiction, even within Britain, differs in the detail of its legal procedures for detention, the principles are similar in attempting to balance the range of patient interests, the occasionally conflicting interests of the patient and the community, and safeguarding the assessing and treating professionals. It is perhaps illustrative of this point that, regardless of jurisdiction, changes in the law seem to change the mechanisms by which people are detained rather than the fact of detention. In England and Wales, for example, introduction of the MHA 1983 was effective, as planned, in reducing emergency admissions, but a parallel rise was seen in the much longer-term detention for treatment (Webster et al., 1987). In the USA, the Group for Advancement of Psychiatry (1994) cites a number of studies showing similar effects from changing the type of detention. A 263% increase in the number of criminal commitments to psychiatric hospitals was shown, for example, after the introduction of a restrictive civil commitment procedure in Wisconsin (Roche Report, 1978). Further, lawyers and doctors may differ in their readiness to detain. Lebuffe and colleagues (1979) studied two places in the USA that had demographically similar populations, but differed in legal process for detention. Where two medical signatures were required the civil commitment rate was 6.5 per 10 000 population, half that where a judicial order was required (12.3 per 10 000).

Detention in hospital for people concerned in criminal proceedings or under sentence

Most jurisdictions, in recognising that people who commit criminal offence may have a serious mental disorder, make provision for their diversion from the criminal justice system (CJS) to hospital. As for any other contact with people with a mental disorder, most of the assessment and treatment is done with the person as a voluntary patient. In the British mental health acts, however, there is provision for compulsory transfer to hospital at each stage of the process if necessary. A lower (magistrates') or a higher (Crown) Court may remand an individual to a hospital for assessment pre-trial, and a lower court for treatment pre-sentence on the evidence of one doctor; a higher Court may so remand for treatment at any stage on the evidence of two doctors, or, after conviction, make an interim treatment order for up to six months. Both lower and higher Courts may, on conviction of a person for an imprisonable offence, make a hospital order on the evidence of two doctors; in England and Wales, a lower court, by definition dealing in matters of disposal with less serious offences, may make such an order without recording a conviction, a practice for acknowledging the impaired responsibility of a person with serious mental disorder that is perhaps underused; a higher Court, if it appears that 'it is necessary for the protection of the public from serious harm so to do', may add restrictions on discharge, removing the powers of decision in this regard from the medical profession to rest with the Secretary of State at the Home Office (a justice minister). Oral evidence from one of the doctors is required in the Court, but the restrictions may be imposed regardless of the medical view.

Once charged with a crime, a person may be remanded to prison to await trial, sentencing or both. This does not invariably reflect the seriousness of offence; not having a fixed home, a common problem for people with a serious mental disorder, is one of the commonest reasons for pre-trial remand. Courts consider lack of a home, a mental disorder or both may decrease likelihood of return to court (Gibbens et al., 1977). The rates of serious mental disorder among pre-trial prisoners are high (e.g. Taylor & Gunn, 1984; Torrey et al., 1992). Although

579

the process of law does tend to select out those people who should be in the health care system by the sentencing stage, mistakes are made, and some people become sick after imprisonment. Consequently the rates of mental health need among sentenced prisoners are far from negligible (e.g. Gunn *et al.*, 1991). In the mental health acts of the UK, provision is made for transfer of prisoners to hospital. The rules differ slightly according to whether the prisoner is pre-trial or under sentence, but in either case two medical recommendations are required, one by a doctor with special experience of mental disorder. The Home Office issues a warrant for transfer if the minister is persuaded. Almost invariably such transfers are accompanied by restrictions on discharge, in the case of fixed-term sentences enduring until the earliest release date, and for indefinite sentences also being indefinite. Leave or discharge from the hospital in these cases has to be approved by the Home Secretary. In these circumstances there is still no review tribunal that can order release in any real sense; in England and Wales the effect of a Mental Health Review Tribunal (MHRT) order that such detention in hospital is no longer valid means that the individual must be taken back to prison. This sometimes happens.

Compulsory treatment in hospital

In most circumstances, giving a form of physical treatment, including the administration of drugs, without the explicit consent of the patient would constitute battery. Failure to obtain valid consent by virtue of not having provided sufficient information on which a decision about treatment could be based could constitute negligence. For these purposes, in England and Wales sufficient information would be that regarded as adequate by the body of professional opinion (*Sidaway*). The nature of mental disorder, however, means that a number of patients will not be able to understand their illness nor the implications of treatment, however well explained, and thus not be able to give valid consent to the treatment. Most countries make provisions to protect patients and psychiatrists alike in these circumstances.

In those jurisdictions in which the legal system has its origins in the Napoleonic code (e.g. France, Bulgaria, Denmark) there has been a tendency toward all-or-nothing concepts of competency. Once a person is deemed by reason of a mental disorder to be incompetent to take one sort of decision or responsibility, there follows a presumption of incompetence in other areas too, generally throughout the rest of life. Reform is, however, now progressing or projected in most West European countries (Schulte, 1989). Most common law countries, including the UK and the USA, make no such presumptions. Not even compulsory detention in hospital for treatment necessarily implies that the individual concerned is incapable of taking decisions about individual treatments, nor on the grounds of the detention order alone that he can be compelled to accept such treatments. The basic common law principle that every person's body is inviolate is subject to modification, however, by a number of exceptions, the principal one being the 'doctrine of necessity'. This states that the doctor is entitled, and probably has a duty, to carry out such emergency treatment as is necessary to preserve the life, health and well-being of a patient, notwithstanding that he is unable to give or withhold his consent through gross incapacity, including unconsciousness. This position continues to evolve. There may be circumstances where, if in advance and while capable of making the decision, a person has indicated that he does not want certain things to happen, which must be respected. An example of this in practice in Britain is that if an adult Jehovah's witness has indicated on religious and personal grounds a wish not to have a blood transfusion, in any circumstances that wish will be respected.

In the UK, the most recent mental health legislation is the principal vehicle for the authorisation of treatment for mental disorder when there is any doubt about the patient's capacity to consent to it. These Acts, however, add nothing with respect to treatments for physical disorder for those who cannot give consent. Here, the 'doctrine of necessity', described above, has been extended in some other ways. The landmark case in England was *Re F.*, about the sterilisation of a mentally incapacitated young woman. The Law Lords ruled that the lawfulness of operating on or otherwise treating a mentally incapacitated person depends on whether such treatment is in the patient's best interests. The standard to be applied in determining the patient's best interests are drawn from *Bolam* and from *Sidaway*, that is that they should be accepted as proper by a responsible and competent body of professional opinion. For most forms of treatment, a clinical decision taken in this context should suffice, but in the case of non-therapeutic interventions, such as sterilisation, it would be strongly recommended that an application be made to the Court for this to be determined in advance. A more extended account of these and other areas for decision-making by mentally incapacitated adults is contained in a very useful book prepared by the Law Commission (1991). Although writing from primary experience in the UK, it includes extensive references to situations elsewhere in the world, where the courts are more likely to be involved.

Specifically for the treatment of mental disorder in England and Wales, the MHA 1983 recognises three classes of consent: treatment requiring consent *and* a second opinion, treatment requiring consent *or* a second opinion, and treatment not requiring consent. This is use of the term 'consent' in strict legal terminology. The last category does not offer licence to ride roughshod over a patient's wishes. Treatment 'not requiring consent' principally covers nursing, habilitation and rehabilitation for detained patients when given under the direction of the responsible medical officer, although specific psychological treatments would fall within this category too. Similar arrangements are detailed in the Mental Health (Scotland) Act 1984 and the Mental Health (Northern Ireland) Order 1986 (and summarised by Gunn et al., 1993b).

The treatments that require consent *and* a second opinion are psychosurgery, and *surgically implanted* hormones for the control of sexual drive. Here the procedures apply to all patients, not just the compulsorily detained, and require first an assessment to confirm that the patient is capable of giving consent and is consenting. If so, a further assessment follows, requiring multidisciplinary involvement, to certify that the treatment is likely to confer an advantage in the particular case. The consent *or* second opinion rules apply to detained patients only, and exclusively to ECT or psychotropic medication. Either the responsible medical officer (patient's consultant/specialist attending) must be able to sign a form confirming that the patient is capable of consent and consenting, *or* a doctor appointed by the Mental Health Act Commission (MHAC) for the purpose, after reviewing the treatment plan and consulting with the responsible medical officer (RMO), a nurse and someone from at least one other discipline in the clinical team, must confirm in writing that the treatment may proceed. Good practice dictates that the status of the patient's understanding of treatment and consent to it must be kept under constant review; the legal requirement is that renewal of consent is formally recorded at every renewal of detention. The legislation is fairly pragmatic, in allowing for three months' medication before the formal consent procedures are necessary, and in allowing for immediate or urgent treatment before the legal procedures are completed. This means that a course of ECT might be started, but it is vary rarely necessary to invoke this provision. One of the tasks of the MHAC is to ensure that procedures are being followed correctly, and, as well as hearing any patients' complaints, the Commission makes regular, routine visits to all hospitals with detained patients. In Britain, prison 'hospitals' are not recognised for these purposes, so specific treatments can only be given without consent in a bona fide emergency, under common law.

British law thus leaves a great deal of responsibility with doctors for deciding on treatment that is ethical and legal. Models for good practice are essential. One simple word 'INFORM' may act as a useful *aide-mémoire*, for important elements (Taylor, 1983). This stands for:

Informed psychiatrist (one who is not as fully informed as possible of the problem and the range of options for treatment cannot convey adequate information);
Non-technical presentation to the patient;
Familiarity with the patient and his range of problems, the context of the target problem may influence solutions;
Other informant present, e.g. family, primary nurse;
Repetition of information – few people can absorb everything at once;
Moral obligation to the patient (no threats to the non-compliant!).

Appelbaum & Roth (1984), leading American thinkers and researchers in this field, proposed a series of discussions with the patient that would be almost therapeutic in themselves.

Other forms of coercion into treatment

Most people who need treatment for mental disorder do not need to be in hospital, even for essential treatment, providing that there is some way of ensuring that treatment continues. The majority of those treated as out-patients are fully capable of voluntary co-operation; it may be appropriate to respect treatment refusal by some patients. On 1st April 1996, the Mental Health (Patients in the Community) Act 1995 was implemented with the few others in mind, to have the effect of amending existing mental health legislation throughout Britain. It is hard to see how this law could have much to offer beyond pre-existing provisions if these were used to the full. The civil provision of guardianship under the MHA 1983, or its companion, the guardianship order for those convicted of a criminal offence in the criminal courts, both of which remain, give powers:

(a) to require the patient to reside at a place specified by the authority or person named as guardian;
(b) to require the patient to attend at places and at times so specified for the purpose of medical treatment, occupation, education or training;

(c) to require access to the patient to be given, at any place where the patient is residing, to any registered medical practitioner, approved social worker or other person so specified.

Perhaps one of the clauses (section 1(4)) of the new Act is most revealing. It specifies that 'A supervision application may be made in respect of a patient only on the grounds that . . . c) his being subject to after-care under supervision is likely to help to secure that he receives the after care services to be so provided'.

The provisions stop short only in not specifying the treatment, and in not making immediate re-hospitalisation on failure of compliance an inevitable legal sanction. If compulsory admission were necessary, then use of one of the other sections of the MHA 1983 (described on pp. 577–8) would also be necessary. Only where an offence has been committed, and a Crown Court has judged that it is necessary for the protection of the public from serious harm and imposed a restriction order, does the law for England and Wales allow for immediate re-admission to hospital without such procedures, in the event of a breach of conditions for community residence. In this event an MHRT must be convened as soon as possible to review the detention.

Provisions for commitment to out-patient treatment in the USA are generally very little different in practice (Miller, 1992). While re-hospitalisation is probably still the major remedy for non-compliance, a majority of states now require judicial hearings before this is extended, and non-compliance with treatment or even clinical deterioration is no longer sufficient justification. Geller's (1990) guidance on the indications for out-patient commitment is particularly useful, reminding practitioners that, notwithstanding a coercive element in treatment, the patient must have enough competency to understand the stipulations and capacity to comply with the treatment plan if such an order is to be feasible. In many ways this is most reminiscent of the English probation order with a condition of treatment. This is another option for the offender patient. It is a contract between the patient/client, the psychiatrist and the probation officer for community supervision and treatment. All sanctions, in the event of non-compliance, are, however, against the patient. A health service model perhaps has more potential for emphasising professional responsibility. Returning to Geller, commitments to be extracted from the services would include:

If the patient discontinues treatment, there would be ample opportunity to take corrective action before the patient or anyone else is injured.

There is a mechanism whereby failure to follow the treatment plan will result in prompt hospitalisation.

The prospective clinic is willing to be responsible for the patient and is able to deliver the ordered treatments.

The patient will be living in a setting that includes people who can bring the patient's behavioural changes to the attention of the clinic.

Other aspects of law in relation to people with a mental disorder

Apart from involvement in criminal proceedings, dealt with below, almost all the other issues on which the law specifically affects the person with mental disorder are to do with competency. The Law Commission Consultation Paper (1991) is a good introduction to incapacity to make contracts, wills, marriage and divorce, to engage in lawful sexual intercourse, to take part in jury service, to vote, or to give evidence in court and its consequences. Since then, for England and Wales, the Royal Commission on Criminal Justice (1993), in its main report and in some of the research commissioned to inform the work (Clare & Gudjonsson, 1992; Gudjonsson et al., 1993), has added further clarification on who constitutes a vulnerable adult with respect to witness statements, and, above all, in confessions to crime. The Commission added specific recommendations about extending the range of the Police and Criminal Evidence Act 1984 (PACE) to the mentally disordered as a group and not solely those with a mental handicap.

Additional details of the application of law to people with a mental disorder in Britain and the Republic of Ireland can be found in the paper by Gunn et al. (1993b), and further international comparison in Harding (1993).

Specialist service provision

The criminal justice system deals with people who have been accused or convicted of having committed a crime, while the health services deal with people who are sick. In most jurisdictions the two systems are run by different government departments. Although there are usually legal provisions, some described above, for allowing a flow of cases between them, flexibility in dealing with people who have multiple problems tends to be a characteristic of rare individuals in the systems rather than inherent in the services. The danger is ever apparent of one system using the other as a depository for its unloved failures rather than as part of a coherent plan to maximise effective and efficient management. Some of the landmarks in services specially designed for mentally disordered offenders have been characterised as much by their capacity to isolate them, and to a worrying extent also the professional staff that work in them, than by great advances in treatment. Allderidge (1974, 1979) described recurring patterns in the history of abuse and rejection of the 'criminally insane' in England, while reports continue to surface worldwide of exceptionally deprived or brutalising conditions in supposedly specialist hospitals, and also in prisons (Gunn et al., 1993c). From time to time, however, there is an important coming together of interested parties and resultant coherent planning. In England, the Butler Committee (Home Office, DHSS 1975) was one such occasion. The development of a network of medium secure units followed, which have provided the focus for specialist consulting and community forensic psychiatry services as well as in-patient work. They have provided a model that has been copied in other parts of the world, including Norway and New Zealand. In 1990, the Justice and Health Departments came together again, resulting in the Reed Report (Department of Health, Home Office 1992). It affirmed as government policy for England and Wales that mentally disordered offenders needing care and treatment should receive it from health and personal social services rather than in custodial care, and set out five guiding principles. These are the patients that should be cared for:

(i) with regard to their needs as individuals;

(ii) as far as possible, in the community, rather than in institutional settings;

(iii) under no greater conditions of security than is justified by the degrees of danger they present to themselves or to others;

(iv) in such a way as to maximise rehabilitation and their chances of sustaining an independent life;

(v) as near as possible to their own homes or families if they have them.

Dean (1992) subsequently criticised the lack of urgency in ministerial response to the report. An interim injection of capital monies will not go far towards meeting the needs outlined. All effective services depend on a substantial and skilled workforce, particularly as more and more emphasis is given to community work.

Specialist health services for the mentally disordered offender

Secure hospital services

For England and Wales there are three hospitals designated under the NHS Act 1977 to provide for patients 'requiring . . . special security on account of their dangerous, violent or criminal propensities'. One to the north-west of the country (Ashworth Hospital), one in the East Midlands (Rampton Hospital), and one to the south-west of London (Broadmoor Hospital), they provide between them up to 1700 beds. About two-thirds of the patients have a psychotic illness, almost invariably schizophrenia, about one-quarter have a severe primary personality disorder, the majority of these patients having a history of serious and often prolonged physical or sexual abuse in childhood. The remaining patients fall into a mentally impaired category under the MHA 1983; their numbers are falling, and should continue to do so. The number of women detained in special hospitals is also falling. A census in 1990 of the views of the hospitals' medical staff for each of the patients (Taylor et al., 1991), a slightly later, independent survey of a 20% service-wide sample of the patients, their records and staff views (Maden et al., 1993), and a similar survey, complete but of the resident patients from one health region only (Shaw et al., 1994), all agreed that at any one time only around half of the patients truly require conditions of high security. Most of the rest were rated as needing medium security, but in many cases for longer than the two years to which most purpose-built medium security units will make a commitment. A survey of sentenced prisoners (Gunn et al., 1991), however, had suggested a shortfall in bed provision at all levels in the health service, in the case of high security provision more or less accounting for the beds that would be freed if medium secure provisions were increased elsewhere, but confirming a further need for medium secure beds. The NHS provides about 35 high security beds per million population for England and Wales, but only 20 medium secure beds. A one-day census of health service provision for England and Wales towards the end of 1993 showed no medium secure bed unaccounted for, but people still awaiting placement (Coid, 1993).

The main differences between English high and medium security hospital services lie in the extent to which they rely on physical security. The special hospitals visibly put an emphasis on strong perimeter security, including high walls. There are also electronically controlled gate houses where any patient movements out of the hospitals are double-checked, visitors are screened and staff exchange identity tags for keys. Internally too the physical security is high, with repeated locked barriers to free movement. Until 1992, all patients were routinely locked into their rooms or dormitories for 10–12 hours overnight, with minimal prospect of egress or therapeutic action. Thus they were, effectively, secluded, regardless of mental state or behaviour, and the hospitals functioned as hospitals only by day, and more or less as prisons by night. This practice has been eliminated, with recognisable hospital care available round the clock as monies and staff became available. Previously heavy reliance on seclusion of patients at all times for control of dangerous or very disturbed behaviour is changing too, but unlikely to be eliminated entirely among intensive care or admission cases until further breakthroughs in psychiatric treatment. The risk of violence to staff and other psychiatrists is high (e.g. Maden *et al.*, 1993). People are admitted because of the risk they pose, often even in other secure conditions. In the medium secure units, security depends less on the buildings and more on the skills and numbers of clinical staff sharing detailed knowledge on each individual patient; the overall nurse:patient ratio is at least 2:1, still much higher than in the special hospitals.

The problems of the special hospitals, and similar high security hospitals elsewhere in the world, are often blamed simply on their size (in England 500–600 beds each), at a time when large institutions have gone out of fashion. Their geographical and professional isolation is probably more important. The issue of size is not as easily resolved as might first seem. Most of the patients stay in a special hospital for a long time – the average length of stay is 8.5 years – and have complex, multiple problems. They require a lot of physical space and a wide range of facilities, to an extent not provided in other in-patient units. The theoretical and practical difficulties inherent in setting up new services of this kind have been well documented (Snowden, 1985; Stocking, 1985). By contrast, it is possible to minimise professional isolation, which is effective in recruiting and retaining high calibre staff in large state hospitals or prison services (Knesper, 1978 and Metzner, 1992 respectively), in turn ensuring a steady flow of new ideas and evolution of practice. Individualisation of treatment planning for each patient is the other key factor likely to maximise positive outcome and minimise institutionalisation. This appears to be as true for prisons (where the preferred terminology is sentence planning) (e.g. Lösel, 1993; Porporino & Baylis, 1993) as for specialist institutions for young people (e.g. Bailey, 1993; Garrido & Redondo, 1993), and general psychiatric hospitals (e.g. Wing, 1993).

Community care and treatment

As with any other branch of psychiatry, safe and congenial community living is the principal aim of treatment for the mentally disordered offender, and treatment in the community should in most cases be the longest phase of treatment. Successful management in the community depends first on the development of a sense of security, founded in reality, for the patient, support staff and all others who come into contact with the patient and secondly on the patient's wish to live in the community and capacity to comply with the necessary requirements for doing so. For the patient to feel secure, there must be satisfactory accommodation, adequate finance for basic needs and the skills to manage monies; the sense that even if symptoms remain or return they are not intrusive and can be controlled; the knowledge that even if there is a crisis there are people to turn to for immediate help, and that the system for getting to them can be mastered. If all these elements are in place, the psychiatrist and co-workers can also feel fairly secure. They must, however, not only see the patient regularly, but also continue checks on his social context, and regularly reconfirm that the conditions and specific treatment fit with the patient's needs.

For a number of the most demanding patients, professional staff, even at the most senior levels, may need systems of support and advice for themselves. Some patients will remain extremely dependent and demanding in spite of all efforts to wean them away from intensive levels of care. An occasional independent review of management in these circumstances is good practice, to ensure that the clinical team does not become inappropriately fixed in its practice. If maintenance of the presenting state of the patient is a valid objective, then staff who might otherwise become disillusioned at lack of change may be reassured and remotivated, and high continuing resource input explicitly defended. If a possible innovation has been missed, this can be remedied.

Lest anyone thinks that treatment in the community for people with a serious mental disorder that predisposes them to violent and erratic behaviour is straightforward or well done, the Report of the Inquiry into the Care and Treatment of Christopher Clunis (Ritchie et al., 1994) makes salutary reading. As Mr Clunis' illness got worse, so his care and treatment also deteriorated. A number of individuals struggled to offer him a service, but therein lies one of the principal problems. The individuals were functioning more or less in isolation, were not in receipt of all relevant information at all material times, and did not take advantage of the many possibilities of bringing together the criminal justice system with health and social services, or did not know how to. Mr Clunis' symptomatology rendered him more and more irrational and violent. He killed a complete stranger in a very public, almost casual attack, wholly unprovoked by his victim. He gave no difficulty in the subsequent arrest.

It is not unique to Britain that these terrible incidents occur; the aggressors have usually been well-known to psychiatric services, but are not often in full current receipt of them. The lapses occur in spite of sound guidelines offered by government and professional bodies alike, and of legislation. For patients in England and Wales, the MHA 1983, under section 117, stipulates that the District Health Authority for the area to which a compulsorily detained person will go on discharge and the local social services authority, in conjunction with voluntary agencies, most provide after-care services until the patient no longer needs them. The Codes of Practice to the Act (Department of Health and Welsh Office, 1990, 1993) set out further guidance. More detailed advice for the after-care of those offender patients under Court-imposed Home Office restrictions on discharge is contained in separate booklets for supervising psychiatrists, social workers and hospital managers produced by the Home Office and Department of Health and Social Security (1988).

After an earlier tragedy, the killing of a social worker by one of her former clients, (Department of Health and Social Security 1988), the Royal College of Psychiatrists (1991b) issued a statement on good practice in the care, discharge and community management of all recognised psychiatric patients. The NHS and Community Care Act 1990 similarly requires multidisciplinary planning and review of care for every patient. The Department of Health circular, issued jointly with the Department of Social Services, expands on this Care Programme Approach (HC(90)23/LASSL(90)11). If community care and treatment are to be effective, the health and social services systems must be very responsive indeed. If they are, it is very doubtful whether legislation to place more constraints on the patients in the community would offer significant advantages (see also pages 582–3 above).

Following the Clunis tragedy (Ritchie *et al.*, 1994) in England, the Secretary of State for Health announced yet a further requirement – that mental health service providers establish and maintain supervision registers that identify those people with a severe mental illness who may be a significant risk to themselves or others, whether by violence or neglect. The NHS Management Executive has issued guidelines (HSG(94)5) on inclusion and practice, emphasising that the prime purpose is to prevent the patient falling through the network of services. The patient should be aware of placement on the register (unless this knowledge would be detrimental to his health). The 'basic' data suggested in the guidance are very extensive, and appropriate confidentiality potentially at risk. The nature of the registers provides no immediate solution for patients like Mr Clunis, who do not or cannot remain conveniently within one set of administrative boundaries. As with any other explicit government code or guidance, however, failure to comply could leave clinicians vulnerable in any civil law suit.

Treatment

General issues

In forensic psychiatry in the UK the provision of treatment and related services is at least as important as any other activity. As in all other branches of psychiatry, treatment is principally directed at the underlying disorder, whatever the presenting behaviour. Insofar as there are areas in treatment of patients that are special, although not exclusive, to forensic psychiatry, they are to do with the assessment and management of risk of violence or other dangerous behaviour.

Record keeping has to be exceptionally scrupulous. Not only should every interaction with a patient, telephone call, piece of advice given, prescription, piece of correspondence and every report be accurately and clearly recorded and filed in chronological order, but every source should be clearly noted, and, as far as possible, the information should be verified. During the 1980s a series of pieces of legislation in the UK gave rise to ever-increasing possibilities for the patient to access his own records (e.g. Data Protection Act 1984, The Access to Medical Reports Act 1988), culminating in the Access to Health Records Act 1990, which extended access to all manually held records made on or after 1 November 1991. Some discretion is allowed for the withholding of information that might be harmful to the patient, and information from a third party. This may be particularly important in forensic psychiatry, where adequate assessment of risk requires that professional staff encourage potential victims, e.g. family members, to be entirely candid about what they have experienced and what they fear. Nevertheless, good practice dictates encouraging the patient to take reasonable access to his records, and in particular to those reports that become semi-public documents, for example reports to the courts. Experience of doing this has generally been good (e.g. Parrott *et al.*, 1988). It is usually unwise, however, to let patients keep copies of reports, as they rarely have the means of safeguarding their own confidentiality. This caution applies also to written information as recommended under supervision register guidelines in England and Wales. This should be kept to the minimum, probably a note that in the event of concern, it would be of extreme importance to contact a psychiatrist or key worker whose names and contact numbers are prominent.

Another key issue in record keeping relates to the extent of confidentiality between people working with the patient. Clinical teamwork is essential in forensic psychiatric practice, and this may make sharing of information appropriate even though the sharing may go beyond traditional professional boundaries. It may be important, for example, to include non-professional people, such as hostel staff, who have a need to know about risk of violence, firesetting, sexual deviancy or self-harm. This area of work poses a particular challenge, too, for psychotherapists. Many would regard it as ethically impossible to share with anyone else anything that is disclosed in the course of psychotherapy. This is generally a perfectly defensible position, but those who wish to adhere to it rigidly should probably not be working with serious offender patients. In the USA, the duty to reveal threats of harm to others, not only to other professionals but also to the potential victims, has been enshrined in law following *Tarasoff*. In all jurisdictions it is good practice to establish as far as possible and at an early stage what limits to confidentiality there may be, and to make sure that the patient understands these. Nevertheless, the offender patient must enjoy as much protection of confidentiality as is possible. A serious threat in certain cases may be posed by the media. Staff must be advised to have contingency plans for safeguarding privileged information, or, in the case of film crews on hospital premises, for preventing absolutely transmission of any material from which patients can be identified. Journalists often archive material, and patients are often seduced by a few cigarettes or the promise of a moment's seeming glory to give revealing interviews, which they subsequently regret when they are trying to resettle in the community and a documentary is networked or repeated.

Risk assessment

The most important reason for the recording and sharing of information as just described is the assessment and management of the risk of violent or other dangerous behaviour. Prevention is the ideal, but not always possible.

Specific strategies for managing dangerous behaviour will vary according to setting. The ability of psychiatrists to predict dangerous behaviour even among people with a mental disorder has been subject to repeated challenge, not least by psychiatrists themselves. Acknowledgement of ability in this area also implies responsibility, and perhaps liability if harm is committed by a patient. While due modesty remains appropriate, Lidz & colleagues (1993) have shown that not only can clinicians provide better than chance predictions of violent behaviour within a mentally disordered population, but predictions using clinical data are better than those relying solely on actuarial data (including previous violence). In their series, however, this applied only to male patients. Clinicians consistently and considerably underpredicted violence among women. Here it is important to get the most popular statement about violence prediction in perspective. Previous violence is often specified as the best predictor of future violence, but anyone who relies solely on this as a guideline will make some terrible mistakes. The problem arises because a number of studies, even among people with a mental disorder, have shown a statistical association between past and previous violence (or past and previous offending), and in some cases this has been the most statistically significant association among those measured. The results may certainly mean that when there is a clear history of past violence, particularly repeated violence, then the risk of future violence may be three or more times greater. Attributable risk is, however, very small; for example, Harry & Steadman (1988) showed that in a sample of discharged psychiatric patients, including people with personality disorder, only 5% of post-discharge offending could be accounted for by previous offending history. As newer generations of researchers turn to the measurement in samples with a mental disorder or more illness-specific factors of their predecessors, qualities of the illness in fact emerge as much better predictors of violence (e.g. Werner *et al.*, 1984; Palmstierna *et al.*, 1989).

Monahan (1984) led the way to more rational approaches to the assessment of dangerousness, arguing that a position that it could not be done at all is as untenable as the notion that all-or-nothing predictions could be good for all time. He and his team (Steadman *et al.*, 1994) have suggested that the next generation of risk research must bear seven characteristics. Some could with advantage be applied to risk assessment in practice:

1. Dangerousness must be disaggregated into its component parts – the variables used to predict violence ('risk factors'), the amount and type of violence being predicted ('harm'), and the likelihood that harm will occur ('risk').
2. A rich array of theoretically chosen risk factors in multiple domains must be chosen.
3. Harm must be scaled in terms of seriousness and assessed with multiple measures.
4. Risk must be treated as a probability estimate that changes over time and context. (Points 5 and 6 are primarily research recommendations).
7. Managing risk as well as assessing risk must be a goal.

The cue domains for risk factors they suggest are *dispositional factors* – demographic (age, gender, race, social class) and personality (personality style, anger, impulsiveness, psycho-pathy); *historical factors* – including social and family, psychiatric treatment and criminal; *contextual factors* – including perceived stress, social support and means for violence; and *clinical factors* – including diagnosis, symptoms, functioning and substance abuse, to which might be added treatment arrangements and capacity for complying. The MacArthur team remains modest about the approach, as the resulting system is still under evaluation, but the model is well based theoretically.

UK clinicians may be reassured that the NHS Management Executive (1993) takes a pragmatic view of risk assessment, noting that 'by its very nature, health care is a risk activity'. This summary extends to service provision as well as individual patient care. Again, the emphasis is on rational assessment with associated management of risk. The recommended sequence is of accurate observation, followed by competent analysis of the consequent information, resulting in elimination of those risks that can be eliminated and limitation of those that cannot. Those risks that are taken must be the result of a positive decision and the outcome monitored and fed back into the system for further improvement of practice.

Specific strategies for managing dangerous behaviour will vary according to setting. It may be worth emphasising too that, although an absence of security or constraint or medication can increase risk in some circumstance, so can their excessive or exclusive use. In the in-patient setting, Weaver *et al.* (1978*a,b*), for example, showed that disruptive behaviour on a locked ward decreased once staff had encouraged and enabled patients to take more responsibilities and lessened some of the restrictions by attending to:

1. the low level of activity on the ward by organising work and occupational therapy;
2. the dependence of patients on staff by offering opportunities for responsible decision making;
3. the avoidance of social isolation by increasing social activities between patients and staff.

Seclusion and restraint

There are few professional clinical staff working with seriously violent in-patients who can envisage being able to manage safely in the foreseeable future without the possibility of occasionally using restraints or seclusion, although most would prefer to, and one or two do advocate the attempt.

There is a serious difficulty in offering guidance on the use of seclusion, the locking of a patient alone in a room against his will, and that is that there is very little research on its effect. For England and Wales the Code of Practice (Department of Health and Welsh Office, 1993) and, for the wider UK, the Royal College of Psychiatrists (1990*b*) have nevertheless produced guidelines that contain a great deal of common sense. Seclusion should be taken as a special event in the patient's life, which requires special documentation and special monitoring. There is some evidence that if seclusion is prolonged, previously non-psychotic people may develop psychotic symptoms, and indeed the so-called prison psychoses (Nitsche & Williams, 1913) may well have been simply responses to the sensory deprivation of solitary confinement. Grassian (1983) has documented the onset of similar, apparently environmentally dependent disorders in a latter day American prison. By contrast, there is some evidence that there may be some advantage in seclusion for people with an established psychosis (e.g. Reitman & Cleveland, 1964), although, insofar as this is true, the advantage might lie in the reduction in sensory input rather than seclusion itself. No one has examined the relative impact of the components of seclusion, nor of the reliability or validity of indicators that seclusion, once started, may safely be discontinued. The danger that seclusion will be construed as a punitive measure, even if not so intended, is certainly present. Mattson & Sacks (1978) have suggested that seclusion should not be regarded as a treatment in itself, but as a means of providing an environment in which some other treatment, almost invariably medication, can be given the chance to take effect in safety. Nurses can have respite, shift emphasis in care, regain a lost therapeutic alliance and/or tackle other contributory ward problems. As with restraint, the Lion & Soloff (1984) axiom is all important:

> The staff restraining the patient today will be seeking a therapeutic alliance tomorrow.

Lion *et al.* (1981) had previously pointed out that over half of the assaults on staff in one state hospital in the USA had occurred while the patients were being restrained. A number of techniques have developed for disengaging violent patients and immobilising them. If these techniques are to be practised safely for staff and patients alike, they should be learned through practical demonstration and regular retraining. Staff should be clear about their roles, and, in any planned restraint, one member of staff should adopt a leadership role and continue to talk and negotiate with the patient throughout. Apart from the important goals of avoiding injury or pain, every effort must be made to minimise the humiliation for the patient.

Medication

There is no one substance that stands out as clearly superior to any other for violence that is associated with mental disorder. A discussion of the relative merits of different preparations is included in Taylor *et al.* (1993c). It is important to recognise that, while violence is not uncommonly driven by psychotic symptoms and thus medication specific for such symptoms important, coincident high arousal is often another key problem. In these circumstances, medication that reduces arousal while targeting psychotic symptoms is ideal, but in an acute emergency even the more sedative neuroleptics may be required in doses disproportionate to their antipsychotic effects. Both short-term and longer-term risks for the patient follow. In the short-term the chances of cardiac dysrhythmias may be at their highest on administration of sudden substantial boluses of neuroleptic. In the longer-term patients may remain on very much higher doses of neuroleptics than are necessary because it took a large amount to gain control in a very dangerous situation, and no one has the courage to begin the withdrawal process in case the violence re-emerges. In an acute crisis, therefore, it may be in the patient's best interests to combine a neuroleptic with something more sedative, such as a barbiturate or a benzodiazepine, on the strict understanding that this will be discontinued as soon as the crisis has passed. Whatever the choice, close nursing care will be necessary for a patient receiving high doses of medication. The patient should not be left unobserved or infrequently attended, even if quiet. Where nursing staff are skilled in the management of violence, knowledgeable about a selection of medications regularly used in crisis, the particular patients under their care at any one time, and have been a part of devising emergency management plans, it can be most beneficial to the patients for the doctor to prescribe flexibly. This means that, within clearly defined limits, the nursing staff may choose the precise dose of a medication or medications to be given in the event of crisis. Personal experience with colleagues on one specialist unit confirmed that nurses would choose the oral route for administration in nearly 80% of cases, the lowest dose range in 20% of cases and the highest dose range in only one-half of cases in spite of the established capacity of this group of patients for serious violence (McLaren *et al.*, 1990). The Royal College of Psychiatrists has produced an important, practical consensus statement on the use of high-dose antipsychotic medication (Thompson, 1994).

Beyond the immediately dangerous clinical situation, where the problem is more one of lack of prompt response to the specific treatment than an acutely violent emergency, rather than escalating the dose of neuroleptic straight away it may be worth considering the addition of ECT to hasten the therapeutic response in people with schizophrenia, whether or not there are accompanying affective symptoms (Taylor, 1990). It should perhaps be emphasised, though, that there are no grounds for considering ECT as a specific treatment for violence.

In spite of the difficulties in monitoring, and of gaining the patient's consent and commitment to the investigations as much as to the treatment, clozapine should not be ruled out for people with treatment-resistant schizophrenia who are also violent. There have been successes in this group as in any other treatment-resistant groups (Maier, 1992). The great unknowns lie in the risk of very serious 'rebound' violence accompanying rebound psychosis in those patients for whom the medication has to be stopped abruptly and in the longer-term capacity for compliance in a group of people for whom freedom from symptoms at all times is essential for safety. For other classes of neuroleptic, depot preparations exist. These not only allow the clinician to be certain that a patient has received medication, but also a patient who misses a treatment will be at least partly protected for a few days, allowing the clinical team a little time to locate him, and take appropriate action.

Medical services in the criminal justice system

All psychiatrists will sometimes work in non-medical settings, or in close conjunction with colleagues who have a different specialist training, or different ethical codes of practice. For psychiatrists working with mentally disordered offenders, these will include lawyers, police officers, prison staff, probation officers and voluntary workers. It is essential that each group understands the strengths, limitations and aims of the others. There are a number of ethical codes that apply to psychiatrists (e.g. the Declaration of Geneva, the International Code of Medical Ethics, the Declaration of Hawaii). They have in common the theme that the patient is at the heart of consideration, but the more recent reflect greater sensitivity to the complexities of the interaction between the doctor, the patient and wider society. The Principles of Medical Ethics of the American Medical Association with Annotations Applicable to Psychiatry (American Psychiatric Association, 1989a) fully acknowledges additional duties to society, other health professionals and self, and details how these interests might be balanced; it explicitly includes continuing education among ethical duties.

Medical contact with the police

The police often constitute the first point of contact between psychiatrist and patient (e.g. Szmukler et al., 1981; Rogers & Faulkner, 1987; Teplin, 1985), but it is not uncommon for psychiatrists to find themselves working in conjunction with the police through a third party, for example in the event of a case conference called by social services about children on an at risk register. In addition the psychiatrist may take the initiative in seeking police help or advice, for individual cases, or for guidance on crime prevention strategies for the hospital or service. The police may seek psychiatric help for the management of people who are manifestly unwell, but also in relation to the interviewing of a witness or suspect of crime. In England and Wales, the interviewing of people in police custody is covered by the Police and Criminal Evidence Act 1984 (PACE). This requires that anyone thought to be mentally ill or mentally handicapped has an 'appropriate' adult with him during any interview. In the case of incoherence a doctor must be summoned. False confession as a major reason for miscarriage of justice is of concern on both sides of the Atlantic (Gudjonsson, 1992; Wrightsman & Kassin, 1993); courts in England are tightening controls over confession evidence, but concern has been expressed that the opposite is happening in the USA (Williamson, 1993).

Psychiatry and other medical services in prisons

In places where people are held pending trial on criminal charges – police cells, cells in the courts, town jails, remand prisons – or in prison when they are serving a custodial sentence, medical conditions, including mental disorders, pose common and important problems. In England and Wales there is a dedicated health care service for prisoners, under Home Office control. Over the years the service has been the focus of much criticism and advice (e.g. Smith, 1984; Gunn, 1985; House of Commons, 1986), a number of internal reports, and reviews jointly with other bodies (e.g. Department of Health, Home Office 1993; the Royal Colleges of Physicians, General Practitioners and Psychiatrists 1992). Real progress remains slow. Some European countries have developed more satisfactorily responsive systems (e.g. Koenraadt, 1993), but the problem of ensuring adequate health facilities in penal institutions is not unique to Britain. Steadman *et al* (1989) described efforts in the USA to improve health services for jail detainees, including litigation to establish their rights to 'reasonable access' to appropriately qualified medical advice and treatment; lack of funds are not a legally acceptable excuse for its absence. Steadman and colleagues, and most other commentators including the American Psychiatric Association (1989*b*) emphasise that jail is, and should remain, primarily a correctional facility. The risks of pretending that jails can be transformed into places of satisfactory and ethical treatment are acknowledged (Roth, 1980). Nevertheless, Steadman and colleagues recommend nine services as essential, and attempt to define minimum standards for most of them. They are:

1. intake screening;
2. psychological evaluations;
3. assessment and provision of reports for the courts;
4. use of psychotropic medication;
5. substance abuse counselling;
6. psychological therapy;
7. 'infirmary' care (emphasising that a prison does not provide true hospital in-patient care);
8. arrangements for external hospitalisation;
9. individual case management.

The extent to which services are required for the assessment and treatment of mental disorder is indicated by a 1992 survey questionnaire to staff in 1391 local jails in the USA (Torrey *et al.*, 1992), effectively covering about two-thirds of the jail population. Among the findings, it was noted that 29% of jails held seriously mentally ill people without any criminal charges against them, often because there were no other facilities for them. More than one out of every 14 inmates was suffering from a serious mental illness (schizophrenia, manic-depressive illness or related condition). This would mean that in the USA there would be over 30 000 seriously mentally ill people in jail in any one day. The rates are very broadly in line with the findings in relation to pre-trial prisoners in two different parts of England (Taylor & Gunn, 1984; Coid, 1988), a type of prison population that would have much in common with the US jail intake. A Scottish survey, by contrast, found a high rate of health problems, including asthma, but very little mental illness (Davidson et al., 1995), which may reflect a greater availability to psychiatric beds and services in a smaller country with a smaller population. With greater resources much, it seems, may be done for the mentally disordered offender.

In a 5% sample of sentenced prisoners in England, the rate of psychotic illness was only a little higher (1.9%) than that in the general community, but still accounted for between 700 and 1000 people in the prison population, many with immediate assessment and treatment needs (Gunn et al., 1991). Given the sampling strategy in this study, and the combined use of interview and records data in reaching a diagnosis and estimating treatment needs, it was possible also to make reasonably accurate statements about the extent of other psycho-pathology. Nearly 40% of these sentenced prisoners, making an approximate total of up to 15 000 people, had at least one psychiatric diagnosis, personality disorder and substance abuse accounting for much of the additional need.

People with personality disorders or abusing alcohol or other drugs are still very badly served by the health services in most countries. As a result, prisons have been forced to set up specialist services. In the UK, Grendon prison was opened in 1962, as the first such unit in the country to run almost entirely on therapeutic community lines. Prisoners choose to apply for selection, and, once accepted, their continued presence in the prison depends on their continuing commitment to treatment, to an extent on the views of the other prisoners and absolutely on non-violence. The men in Grendon in the 1970s demonstrably responded to the regime in terms of mental state, attitudes and behaviour while there (Gunn et al., 1978). After 10 years the reoffending rates were no better and no worse than those for men from an ordinary prison, but other indices of adjustment and the context of the reoffending were lacking (Robertson & Gunn, 1987). A further study (Genders & Player, 1994) has shown that it has proved possible to maintain and develop the regime in the prison. Studies of smaller prison units in other countries, operating for similarly serious male offenders on similar principles, have tended to show the same sort of results, with the period of residency coinciding with a significant change for the men, but the longer-term untested or looking more uncertain (de Montmollin et al., 1986; Cooke, 1989). It is one of the puzzles of psychiatry that clinicians should accept as obvious for the other major mental disease that dominates forensic psychiatric practice – schizophrenia – that specific treatment must continue indefinitely beyond any residence in hospital, but expect the impact of a period in a therapeutic community to last beyond departure without benefit of continued work.

Psychiatry, the Courts and the probation service

The extent of psychiatric disorder among offenders, perhaps particularly among those in custodial populations, has been one of the principal factors (other than prison overcrowding) that has generated new systems for diversion from the criminal justice system. For some cases diversion occurs once the whole process of charge, trial, conviction and even sentencing has taken place, and examples of use of mental health legislation to facilitate this have been discussed. A currently popular application, however, is very early diversion. In England the Crown Prosecution Service (CPS) is the body responsible for prosecution on the majority of criminal charges. Two major schemes for diversion are administered by the probation service, following experience in the USA. One, the Bail Information Scheme, depends on provision to the CPS of *verified* information about a consenting defendant. This might include information about treatment for mental disorder. No opinions are expressed, but the information may allow the CPS to take a course of action previously not envisaged, or make the evidence available to the court to do so. The other scheme is Public Interest Case Assessment (PICA). In deciding whether to proceed with a prosecution, the CPS must balance two principal factors – the quality of the evidence against the individual in question and the 'public interest'. Here the probation service additionally provides evidence for the CPS to assist it in determining 'whether the public interest requires a prosecution'. The CPS considers likely costs set beside likely penalty, or the likelihood of 'irreparable harm' for the very young, old or ill.

The USA-based Vera Institute of Justice co-operated with probation services in England and Wales to evaluate the impact of pilot bail schemes (Stone, 1988) and the PICA/discontinuance project (Stone, 1989) and demonstrated a clear impact. On this background a number of projects for diversion with specific psychiatric input have grown up. The models vary, from engaging the presence or on-call availability of a psychiatrist at a larger court, to having a standing panel for rapid assessment and guidance on cases. Blumenthal & Wessely (1992) provided an overview of such schemes in England, and Torrey *et al.* (1992) in the USA.

When proceedings continue, the offender is convicted and yet mental disorder is an important factor, it is surprising that, in those jurisdictions where it is an option, there has been a decline in the use of the probation order with a condition of psychiatric treatment. This is another key opportunity for psychiatry to work with the probation service, indeed for a psychiatrist to work in formal contract between the probation officer and the patient–client. The subject of the order must make valid consent in court to such an arrangement, but failure to comply can leave him vulnerable to re-sentencing when he is returned to the court.

Forensic psychiatry and voluntary bodies

Whether for victims and survivors of crime, or for the offenders, voluntary bodies and pressure groups have a large part to play in the support, management and treatment of the clientele of forensic psychiatry. Mawby & Gill (1987) provide a useful introduction to the development and range of such services for victims in the UK and in the USA. Taylor *et al.* (1993a) note some of the agencies and models in the UK for offenders and their families. The largest is the National Association for the Care and Resettlement of Offenders (NACRO), which engages in many activities from community project planning, through individual offender work to research and pressure group activities. Others include the Howard League for Penal Reform, the Prison Reform Trust, Women in Prison and the National Council for the Welfare of Prisoners Abroad, tending to the more specific activities indicated in their names.

Assessment for legal purposes

Writing report for courts or other statutory bodies

The skills that the courts and the non-health service bodies are perhaps most likely to seek from forensic psychiatrist are the abilities to recognise accurately links between the mental state of any given individual and his antisocial actions, together with his responsibility for them; to predict dangerousness and to develop, demonstrate and carry out a plan for the safe and effective management of risk. Most reports for courts or statutory bodies will require presentation of data relevant to these matters. If such a report is to be made, the process must be explained to the patient. For someone referred specifically for a psychiatric report for a court, statutory agency or outside body (such as an employing or housing authority), matters are relatively straightforward in that a full explanation of the risks and benefits can be given to the patient before he consents to any assessment. Not uncommonly, however, reports are required for a patient already in treatment, and here the situation is more complicated. Risks for the treating clinician when shifting to the role of report writer include the possibility that information that could and should remain confidential to the therapeutic relationship spills over into the report. Information that is not directly relevant to the pertinent legal consideration should generally be withheld, as far as possible only verified information used, and speculation kept to a minimum. Reference to people other than the patient may have to be included, but detail is rarely necessary and, unless specific permission from the relative or contact has been obtained, the precise identity of the individual should remain protected. In general, other agencies are sympathetic to issues of privacy. Magistrates and judges, for example, if requested so to do, will almost invariably avoid full disclosure of the report in open court; it is wise, however, to act at all times on the assumption that once a report has been made available outside psychiatric professional channels, the psychiatrist ceases to have any certain control over the destiny of the information contained in it.

Writing reports for the criminal courts

The psychiatrist may be required to give evidence at any of the phases of the hearing – the pre-trial stage, the trial stage or the sentencing stage.

At the pre-trial stage the issue is that of competence to stand trial, and therefore the mental state and its impact *at the time of the hearing*. In England and Wales, and some other common law jurisdictions too, this is generally dealt with pragmatically, largely outside the court room. For minor charges it is unlikely to be construed as being in the public interest to pursue the case against an incompetent patient. In other cases, every effort may be made to delay the hearing and maximise the chance of the alleged offender being well enough to be tried. For a very few serious cases, where recovery has not taken place, nor seems likely within a reasonable period of time, then the case may be sent to a Crown Court for a hearing on fitness to plead under the Criminal Procedure (Insanity and Unfitness to Plead) Act 1991 [CP (I and UP) Act 1991]. The fitness case is heard before a jury, but in the event of a finding of fitness a new jury would have to be sworn in for the trial. In the event of a finding of unfitness, a trial of the facts may proceed. If the facts are proved, then the defendant is given a psychiatric disposal, which may be tailored to community placement or hospitalisation according to needs and risks. In the UK fitness hearings are unusual (30–40 cases per year in England and Wales).

In common law countries, in order for a conviction to be recorded on most crimes, two elements in the crime must be proven. There must be adequate evidence that an unlawful act or omission has been committed by the person under examination and that the act or omission caused the offending consequence – the *actus reus* – and there must be evidence that the person had the state of mind necessary to commit the crime – the *mens rea*. The exceptions to this rule are the crimes of strict liability, such as careless driving. *Mens rea* may include intentionality, recklessness, malice, competence and responsibility. Excuses, therefore, may include mistake, accident, provocation, duress and insanity. Most cultures hold that extreme youth is a bar to full responsibility; China considers extreme old age in the same light. All excuses are matters for the court to decide, but psychiatrists may be called to give evidence on mental state that would assist the Court in a decision about mental responsibility. In England and Wales, for almost all cases, mitigation and flexibility in disposal is dealt with in the sentencing phase of the hearing. A murder conviction in the UK, however, still carries a mandatory penalty of life imprisonment, so it remains as important to hear the *mens rea* evidence as *actus reus* evidence during the trial phase of the hearing. Under the CP (I and UP) Act 1991, the insanity defence may apply as well to murder as to any other crime, but is very rarely used. In England and Wales there are some special mental disorder defences that are only applicable to homicide. One is under the Infanticide Act 1939, which allows that if a woman kills her child with 12 months of its birth, in circumstances that would otherwise amount to murder, but that *at the time of the killing* 'the balance of her mind was disturbed by reason of her not having fully recovered from the effects of giving birth . . . or lactation . . .' then she may be convicted of infanticide, an offence punishable as if she had been found guilty of manslaughter. Thus, in contrast to the insanity defence, which if successful results in a not guilty verdict, the woman is found guilty of an offence, but a lesser offence which permits flexibility in sentencing or disposal. The other, more widely applicable psychiatric defence lies in a plea of diminished responsibility, under the Homicide Act 1957. This allows that 'Where a person is a party to the killing of another, he shall not be convicted of murder if he was suffering from such an abnormality of mind . . . as substantially impaired his mental responsibility for his acts in doing or being a party to the killing'. In *Byrne*, in 1960, the term abnormality of mind was clarified: '. . . a state of mind so different from that of the ordinary human being that the reasonable man would term it abnormal . . .' Space does not permit an extended discussion of the relevance of drug and alcohol use to these defences, suffice it to say that it is relatively small, since self-induced intoxication would be no defence, and issues only really arise when the accused may have unknowingly taken a substance, or the substance use may have been so heavy and prolonged that some consequent relevant disease has supervened. Again, it is for the Court (in these cases the jury) to formulate an opinion about the extent to which mental disorder may have impaired responsibility. The psychiatrist simply provides pertinent evidence and should try to avoid going further. For a fuller discussion of this, and the interesting but rare cases of automatism and sleep-related defences, see Gunn *et al.* (1993*b*). The same volume also offers a comparative survey of medico-legal systems (Harding, 1993), which includes illustrations of the similarities and differences in the legal processing and management of cases in four different jurisdictions. Perhaps the most striking difference between common law countries is the application of the insanity defence in the USA. Its use is very little different in practice from that in the UK, on which it is based, but it is more widely applied.

In the great majority of British cases, most mentally disordered offenders who have been shown to have committed the *actus reus* are found guilty of the offence and the psychiatric report has its impact, if any, at the sentencing phase of the hearing. The Court may allow evidence of psychiatric disorder *at the time of the offence* in mitigation, and impose a lesser sentence. Perhaps more importantly, this may lead to a recommendation for some form of medical disposal, particularly if it seems likely that the mental state caused or influenced the offending. A medical disposal may also be appropriate if the mental state is disordered by the time of sentencing, even if this was not obvious at the time of the offence. In relation to more serious offending a real dilemma can be posed if the person had an abnormal and pertinent mental state at the time of the offence, but has recovered by the time of sentencing (Dell, 1984). The nature of most of the disorders linked with offending, however, is that they tend to be chronic or recurrent, and it may be important to emphasise this.

Any recommendation from a psychiatrist at this stage should be in the patient's interests, but take account of the wider societal implications. It must be practical, and, where appropriate, backed with the agreement of other interested parties. It is not acceptable, for example, to recommend a probation order, with or without a condition of treatment, unless the probation service, and usually a specific officer, has agreed to implement such an order. An exception to this rule of background agreement may be where it is important that a hospital bed or service be made available, but the reporting doctor has not been able to locate one. In England and Wales in such circumstances, a court may summon the relevant health authority to give an account of their service provision (section 39 MHA 1983). The doctor should be thoroughly familiar with the provision that he is recommending, for two reasons. The more important is that the chances of a successful outcome depend principally on the goodness of fit between the prospective patient and the facility proposed, and the doctor cannot assess this adequately without knowing the facility as well as the patient; the other is that many magistrates and judges will not be familiar with the range of psychiatric and social provisions. The chances that a court will accept a particular recommendation are enhanced by a full case being presented in the report; if this is not done more details may be requested. If the psychiatrist has no practical recommendation to make, he has to be candid about that. This may mean that some punitive measure, perhaps imprisonment, is the only option left open to the court. It is never, however, ethical for a psychiatrist to recommend punishment, and there may be some pitfalls along this road to which the less experienced are particularly vulnerable. Where an individual has been convicted of a serious offence, if a psychiatrist argues that that individual has, and had at the time of the offence, an untreatable mental disorder, according to sentencing guidelines for England and Wales (Thomas, 1979), this may be tantamount to inviting a sentence of life imprisonment. Although some treatment may prove possible if an individual receives a sentence of imprisonment, it is misleading, even unethical to lead a judge into thinking that this will necessarily be the case, or that it would be the same as treatment in hospital. Further, some specialist regimes are only open to people serving a sentence of above a certain length, so a suggestion that the offender be offered such an opportunity could, effectively, be a recommendation for a longer sentence.

Reports for civil matters

Psychiatric reports may also be required for arbitration panels or special bodies (such as the Criminal Injuries Compensation Board, in England) and for civil courts. The issues include compensation, care or custody of children and, rarely, a challenge to a will. The principles behind assessment for such purposes are very similar to those for criminal hearings. People may have been referred by lawyers explicitly for an assessment for legal proceedings, but if they have a serious mental disorder will need treatment. It may not be appropriate for the assessing doctor to provide that, but he should ensure at the least that the patient is made aware of the need for treatment, that it would be possible, and how to go about getting it. In many cases, it would even be important to make the necessary links or referral for the person.

Concluding remarks

Psychiatrists have a duty to assist the courts as far as possible when asked, and to be mindful of public and individual safety. These tasks may change relationships with patients in ways that are important and must be communicated to the patient. Even, however, when the primary purpose of seeing a patient is the provision of a report, the psychiatrist is not absolved from a duty of care to that individual.

Acknowledgements

Grateful thanks are due to Professor John Gunn for his generous comments and to Nengi Charles and Devinder Sandhu for great patience in preparing the manuscript.

Appendix: cases cited

Bolam	Bolam v. Friern Hospital Management Committee [1975] WLR 582
Byrne	R v. Byrne [1960] 2 QB 396; [1960] 3 All ER 1; 44 Cr App Rep 246.
Canons Park Mental Health Review Tribunal	R v. Canons Park Mental Health Review Tribunal, Ex Parte A [1993]

Re F.	*Re F* [1990] 2 AC 1; [1990] 2 All ER 545
Sidaway	*Sidaway v. Board of Governors of Bethlem Royal and Maudsley Hospital* [1985] 1 All ER 643; [1985] AC 871 (HL)
Tarasoff	*Tarasoff v. Regents of University of California* 1178 Cal Rptr 129 539 P (2d) 553 (1974)
	Tarasoff v. Regents of University of California 551 P (2d) 333 1312 Cal Rptr 14 (1976)

Abbreviations in legal cases cited

AC	Appeal Cases
All ER	All England Law Reports
Cal Rptr	California Reporter
Cr App Rep	Criminal Appeal Reports
HL	House of Lords
P	Probate, Divorce and Admiralty
QB	Queen's Bench Cases
R	Rex or Regina (i.e. British Crown)
WLR	Weekly Law Reports

PART IV

PRINCIPLES OF TREATMENT

24

Biological treatments in psychiatry

L. S. PILOWSKY and R. W. KERWIN

Introduction

Historically, drugs have been used to alleviate mental suffering since Hippocratic medicine began. In this century, physical treatments have become ever more critical to the rational management of psychiatric disorders. Though psychotropic treatment was initially applied in an empirical and arbitrary fashion, psychopharmacology is now a field governed by coherent methodology, based on available scientific evidence.

Biological treatments should naturally be considered part of a whole therapeutic strategy, which also includes psychological and social techniques. This chapter will focus on clinical therapeutics of psychotropic agents, rather than their basic psychopharmacology (see Leonard, 1992). The topics to be covered will be: drug evaluation, pharmacokinetics, general issues in psychotropic drug prescribing, psychotropic drug classification, and the action and use of drugs in each major class. In the final section, electroconvulsive therapy (ECT) will be discussed under the general topic of affective disorders.

Drug evaluation

Prior to the twentieth century, evaluation of a potentially useful treatment was haphazard and inefficient. Some studies anticipated the present methodology, for example, comparison of different treatments for scurvy in the late eighteenth century (Pocock, 1991), though most investigators had no appreciation of the scientific method. Greater appreciation of the importance of critical appraisal of treatments occurred throughout the nineteenth and early twentieth centuries.

The first clinical trial now widely acknowledged to have had a properly randomised control group was for streptomycin in the treatment of pulmonary tuberculoses (Medical Research Council, 1948). Bradford-Hill, of the Medical Research Council, pioneered and developed clinical trial methodology in the UK from the 1950s. He characterised the controlled trial as 'an experiment carefully and ethically designed to answer a precisely framed question' (Hill, 1955). The clinical trial therefore concerns itself with the objective and efficient prospective comparison of concurrently randomly allocated treatments (Johnson, 1989). Uncontrolled trials are inherently less neutral, and have been shown to be more likely to lead to a positive recommendation of the new treatment under investigation.

Modern clinical trials for new drugs have two parallel goals: establishment of a novel treatment's safety and efficacy, and identification of an effect superior both to the non-specific consequences of receiving any therapy (the placebo effect), and other drug treatments for the same condition. To achieve these aims objectively, investigations must follow particular rules in order to eliminate bias in favour of one or other treatment. In the development of a drug within the pharmaceutical industry, there are generally four main phases of experimentation, once neurochemical studies *in vitro*, behavioural tests in animals and animal toxicology data have suggested a new compound could be both safe in, and useful for humans (Pocock, 1991). The current evaluation phases are as follows; phase I trials: clinical pharmacology and toxicology; phase II trials: initial clinical investigation for a treatment effect; phase III trials: full-scale evaluation of treatment; phase IV trials: post-marketing surveillance. The compound must also be synthesised and produced easily. For reviews of the detailed methodology of clinical trials, the reader is referred to Pocock (1991), Yevich (1991), and Johnson (1989). The general points are outlined below.

Phase I trials are generally conducted in healthy young males. These trials last about three to six months, and are intended to test both the safety and dose levels of the experimental agent (Yevich, 1991). A single acute dose is initially administered, and subsequently in repeated doses up to three or four times a day. Just under three-quarters of new drugs pass phase I trials (Yevich, 1991), with failures eliciting unacceptable side-effects, or demonstrating suboptimal pharmacokinetic profiles.

Phase II trials are aimed both at defining dose ranges, and assessing the drug's effectiveness at treating target symptoms. Investigators have some idea of useful dose levels from toxicology and phase I data, but the level usually requires titration up or down to maximise the benefit:risk ratio. Techniques such as positron emission tomography and single photon emission tomography are being increasingly employed to assess directly the occupancy of different doses of psychotropic drugs that target distinct neurotransmitter receptor systems in the living human brain (Smith *et al.*, 1988; Farde *et al.*, 1989; Pilowsky *et al.*, 1992). Phase II studies are usually conducted in an open, non-blinded fashion. Sufficient numbers of patients are required so that individual variability due to factors such as age, gender and illness duration average out over all treatment groups. Two types of control may be used, 'positive' (an approved drug already used in the treatment of the condition) and 'negative' (a placebo drug). Where multiple controls are used, more complicated trial design is often employed, with single blind, or double blind, randomised protocols. About a third of drugs pass phase II testing, failing if efficacy is not demonstrated.

Phase III clinical trials involve large numbers of patients (hundred or thousands), and may last one to several years. In these studies, drug effectiveness is verified, long-term complications and adverse reactions identified, and interactions with other drugs and illnesses monitored. Particular subgroups of patients are studied at this stage, the elderly, or children, and those with renal or hepatic impairment. A quarter of drugs will survive phases I to III. Upon completion of these studies, all the data is submitted by the sponsoring company to the drug-licensing body for approval and registration. Once the drug is approved, phase IV, or post-marketing surveillance begins. An ever larger database on the drug is gathered and rare adverse reactions, not picked up in phase III trials, may be monitored. If these are serious, and outweigh the benefits of treatment, the drug may not survive phase IV. A recent example of this is the withdrawal of the substituted benzamide antipsychotic, remoxipride, from the UK market following the occurrence of aplastic anaemia (Kerwin, 1994).

Pharmacokinetics

Pharmacokinetics describes the way in which a drug is handled by the body, and distributed to its site of action. To exert an effect a drug must reach the site of action at a critical concentration, which is maintained over a critical period of time. This, and the efficacy:toxicity profile is determined by pharmacokinetic factors (Greenblatt, 1993; Preskor, 1993). There are essentially four pharmacokinetic phases in drug delivery to the brain, outlined below.

Absorption

The bioavailability of a drug is the fraction of the administered dose reaching the systemic circulation. For psychotropic drugs given orally this is generally high ($\approx 90\%$ of administered dose is absorbed). Intravenous administration produces rapid drug entry to the circulation, circumventing first-pass metabolism (see below). This is useful in emergency situations, where therapeutic levels of drug must be obtained quickly. The obvious disadvantage lies in the danger of producing toxic and irreversible drug levels inadvertently. Slow intravenous bolus administration, titrating against behavioural outcome, is advisable, using the minimum achievable dose. If there are antagonists of the drug in question (for example flumazenil for benzodiazepines), these should be readily available. Intramuscular injections are also commonly used in psychiatry, both during emergencies and as long-acting depot formulations. Blood flow through muscle tissue can increase tenfold during emotional excitement, leading to rapid uptake of drug during agitated episodes, so lower drug doses should be used (Lader, 1983; Thompson, 1994).

Some drugs, for example diazepam, are poorly absorbed intramuscularly. Depot formulations dissolve into the fatty tissue of the muscle and are subsequently absorbed very slowly. Given orally, psychotropics may be absorbed throughout the length of the entire gastrointestinal tract. Most absorption generally occurs over the stomach and jejunum. Psychotropics generally are lipophilic at physiological pH levels, and so passively cross the jejunal mucosa. Absorption is slowed by a full stomach, which delays gastric emptying into the small intestine. Emptying is also delayed by anticholinergic effects of psychoactive drugs. Some drugs are formulated in slow-release preparations, so the tablet dissolves slowly, or active agent is leached out of an inert matrix.

Distribution

The lipophilicity of psychotropics increases their volume of distribution, particularly to adipose tissue. Increased volume of distribution is associated with rapid disappearance of the drug from plasma, and therefore a shorter duration of action (Greenblatt, 1993). Patients who have more fatty tissue will have a greater volume of distribution than those with lean body mass. As weight gain is a common side-effect for certain psychotropic drugs, the pharmacokinetics of the drug, and so the dosage required, will change with body weight. Older patients have a greater volume of distribution, as the proportion of lean tissue mass decreases with age. Distribution to the brain is also determined by drug binding to plasma proteins, mostly albumin or glycoproteins (Lader, 1983), which affects their capacity to cross the blood–brain barrier. The greater the degree of binding (which is competitive and reversible) the smaller the amount of free drug available for interaction with its cellular target. Psychotropic drugs are highly protein bound (80–95%), and small fluctuations in the degree of binding due to alterations in circulating plasma protein levels can make large differences to drug action, as happens in liver or renal disease. The dosage must be adjusted accordingly in these conditions. Nevertheless, the high degree of lipid solubility of psychotropics favours easy passage through the blood–brain barrier. Lithium, as a small cation, also diffuses readily into the brain.

Metabolism

Conversion or biotransformation of an administered drug into active and inactive metabolites is an essential component for its eventual clearance from the body. After oral absorption, drugs pass through the liver, which may metabolise most of the dose (so-called first-pass metabolism). For most medications used in clinical psychiatry, clearance is limited only by hepatic blood flow (high clearance drugs), and not by the capacitance of liver enzyme/metabolic systems (low clearance drugs). First-pass metabolism is therefore high. In the case of antipsychotic drugs some patients may need depot medication to negate this factor. The clearance rate and volume of distribution combine to determine a drug's elimination half life ($t_{1/2}$), the time required for plasma concentration to decline by 50%. Lader (1983) has summarised the implications of plasma half-life for routine drug prescribing (see Table 24.1).

Most psychotropic drugs (with the exception of lipid-insoluble agents such as lithium) must be metabolised in the liver, to become hydrophilic prior to renal excretion. Two main varieties of liver cytochrome enzymes are responsible for over 90% of the biotransformation of drugs in psychiatric clinical practise (Greenblatt, 1993). Cytochrome P450 IID6 exists in genetically determined polymorphic forms with the consequence that individuals may be slow or fast metabolisers of drugs, mainly affecting the risk of side effects (e.g. slow and fast acetylators of isoniazid). Slow metabolisers are likely to develop higher plasma concentrations of many classes of psychotropic drugs.

The version P450 IIIA4 does not demonstrate polymorphisms, but is susceptible to induction or inhibition by other compounds. Some drugs induce their own metabolism (for example, barbiturates, phenytoin, glutethimide, chlorpromazine, imipramine). Agents such

Table 24.1. *Implications of the plasma half-life to prescribing (Lader, 1983)*

---

*Dosage intervals can be up to $\frac{2}{3}$ the $t_{1/2}$ without large fluctuations in drug concentration
*It takes 4 to 5 half-lives to reach steady-state concentrations in the body. These levels will be attained slowly in drugs with long half-lives
*Doubling the dose does not double plasma concentrations because the rate of metabolism also increases

---

as orphenadrine, caffeine, ethanol, cigarettes and cortisol and sex hormones may also induce metabolism, up to 50% in some cases. It should be noted that many metabolites of psychotropics themselves have biological activity, for example diazepam and its metabolites, amitryptiline and nortryptiline, imipramine and desipramine, and fluoxetine and norfluoxetine.

Excretion

Only water-soluble, ionised compounds dissolved in free plasma can be excreted by the renal system. This may be affected by the urine pH. For example, amphetamine, a weak base, is excreted rapidly in acidic urine but erratically and slowly in an alkaline environment (Lader, 1983). Most psychotropic drugs are excreted through the kidney, but some may be excreted in bile.

General issues in psychiatric drug prescribing

Knowledge of the pharmacokinetic behaviour of psychotropic drugs helps determine prescribing patterns, taking account of the need to achieve and maintain steady-drug concentrations (i.e. maintenance of a stable drug concentration despite intermittent dosing), with convenience and acceptability of dosing intervals to patients and minimising the risk:benefit ratio by avoiding very high peaks or low troughs of drug concentration. These issues will be discussed, as well as the precautions necessary in pregnancy, or in breastfeeding women, and the elderly (see also Crammer *et al.*, 1982; Silverstone & Turner, 1982).

Therapeutic drug monitoring

Many pharmacokinetic factors alter the level of free drug in plasma, the ultimate determinant of drug action. Most psychotropic drugs vary greatly in plasma concentration between individuals. Haloperidol, for example, shows a one to ten-fold difference in steady-state concentrations between individual patients on the same dose (Forsman, 1976).

The usefulness of plasma drug assays is questionable in terms of predicting efficacy, because the relationship between steady-state levels and therapeutic effect appears highly variable (Greenblatt, 1993). Also, plasma assays measure total drug concentrations, whereas the free, unbound portion is of greater relevance. The consensus appears to be that therapeutic drug monitoring of psychotropic drugs is useful only for determining compliance and reducing toxicity, particularly in drugs with a small therapeutic window, the most obvious example being lithium. Antipsychotics such as haloperidol demonstrate a U-shaped curve in responding patients, with the appearance of extrapyramidal side-effects at high plasma levels, and no further improvement in psychiatric symptoms (Baldessarini *et al.*, 1988; Santos *et al.*, 1989). Preskorn (1993) lists features of drugs for which therapeutic monitoring could help in rational prescribing decisions. These include: drugs with many different actions at differing concentrations; those with a small therapeutic index; a large interindividual variability in metabolism; drugs in which early detection of toxicity is necessary but difficult clinically; those with a long delay in onset of therapeutic action; and well-defined concentration–response relationships between beneficial effects, nuisance effects, and toxic drug effects.

Prescribing in practise

The existence of the placebo effect highlights the importance of setting the right psychological conditions for drug prescribing, even for active drugs. The physician must be familiar with a few drugs in each class of psychotropics, preferably with usefully distinct side-effect profiles. The drugs should usually be tried and tested, or, in the case of new drugs, show strong clinical evidence for an advantage over older therapies. After a thorough history and examination, a treatment plan will be formulated, which may include a defined list of short- and long-term target symptoms. Intervals for reassessment must be clarified early, before therapy is regarded as having failed. These should be based on a working knowledge of the prescribed drug's pharmacokinetics and suspected pharmacodynamics (see above).

Practical prescribing takes account of the patient's needs and daily activities. Dosing times and intervals may be adjusted accordingly wherever possible. The minimum dose possible should be given, starting with a small test dose and titrating upwards with regular assessment intervals. Patients and their carers require all the potential benefits, side-effects and drug interactions explained, as well as the presumed mechanism of action and rationale for a particular treatment. Some examples of interactions include the reduction of chlorpromazine absorption by antacids and the inhibition of sympathomimetic amine metabolism by monoamine oxidase inhibitors.

If this is not done, patients and carers will find less appropriate sources of information that could obstruct therapy (Nesbit, 1994). Without clear, instructive guidelines, compliance is poor. One survey of the medicine cabinets of 500 households in the north of England found 43 000 unused tablets and capsules (Silverstone & Turner, 1982). Even for in-patients, compliance cannot be assumed. Studies screening in-patients' urine found approximately one-fifth (19%) were not taking their drugs, even though these were given out by nursing staff (Hare & Willcox, 1967; Ballinger *et al.*, 1974). Psychiatric patients with remitting or chronic disorders often stop medication when improvement begins. It is critical, therefore, that all the people closely involved with the patient are aware of the need to continue medication, or consult their physician, even when the patient has improved.

Treatment failure

Before the drug is discarded as inadequate, sufficient time for treatment must be allowed. These times vary between drugs and will be specifically discussed for each psychotropic. Non-compliance or poor compliance should be considered first (certainly before increasing drug dosage), and another formulation tried (syrups rather than tablets, for example). Interactions affecting pharmacokinetics should be excluded (see above). Psychosocial stressors may outweigh therapeutic effects of drugs, which are generally palliative rather than curative. Assuming the most optimal drug dose has been tried for a reasonable length of time, several options are open. After a complete review of the course of the illness and the success or otherwise of previous treatment, the drug could be changed to a chemically distinct drug in the same class, an additional drug added, or an alternative treatment attempted. Sometimes a period off all medication is indicated, before trying new drugs, to ensure that drug side-effects (e.g. anticholinergic psychosis) are not accounting for treatment resistance. Particular alternatives within drug classes will be covered below.

It is a generally accepted principle of good prescribing that the minimum number of different psychotropics necessary be given (Muijen & Silverstone, 1987). This is particularly true where more than one drug of the same class is prescribed. Combination prescribing is none the less common, varying between 45 to 97% in three hospitals surveyed in London (Muijen & Silverstone, 1987). This practice has become increasingly justifiable for certain conditions where synergistic, or adjunctive effects are sought (for example, an oral and a depot antipsychotic in schizophrenia, or lithium and an antipsychotic in affective disorder), but clearly increases the risk of toxicity, side-effects, and non-compliance. Where drugs are given together, the clinician should be aware of the potential drug interactions and side-effects. Nelson (1993) has summarised this area.

Prescribing in pregnancy and to breastfeeding mothers

Mental illness during pregnancy may itself present a serious threat to maternal and fetal well-being. The risks must be carefully weighed against the effects of treatment on fetal development. Most psychotropic drugs do not show teratogenicity (above background levels of 1–2%) (Crammer et al., 1982), thus where there is significant danger of severe mental breakdown, prescribing should continue (with close fetal monitoring, where indicated). Conversely, where there is no apparent risk of serious relapse, drugs are to be avoided. There has been controversy with respect to the effects of lithium and carbamazepine given during the first trimester of pregnancy. Lithium has been associated, in some studies, with cardiovascular anomalies (Loudon, 1987). A recent prospective follow-up study of 148 women using lithium in the first trimester, found no difference in congenital anomalies compared to a control group, suggesting that lithium was not a major human teratogen (Jacobson et al., 1992). The researchers recommended that women with major affective disorder be allowed to continue the drug, providing ultrasound and fetal echocardiography were performed throughout pregnancy.

One prospective study of carbamazepine given in pregnancy found a pattern of malformation in the newborn including minor craniofacial defects, fingernail hypoplasia

Table 24.2. *Safety of psychotropic drugs in pregnancy and the puerperium (Loudon, 1987)*

Benzodiazepines	No excess of palatal deformities
	May see withdrawal symptoms after birth
	Bolus doses > 30 mg during delivery, or sustained prenatal treatment may lead to 'floppy infant syndrome'
Antipsychotics	No long-term effects on child as a result of use after the first trimester (prochlorperazine teratogenic if used in the 6th to 10th week of pregnancy)
Tricyclic antidepressants	As for antipsychotics
Lithium and carbamazepine	An association with birth defects (see text)
Breastfeeding and psychotropic drugs	
Diazepam	Contraindicated; crosses into breast milk, high levels of metabolites in newborn
Antipsychotics	
Tricyclic antidepressants	Clinically unimportant amounts transfer into breast milk
Monoamine oxidase inhibitors	
Lithium	Contraindicated; crosses into breast milk; may get toxicity in newborn

(Avoid all wherever possible.)

and developmental delay (Jones *et al.*, 1989). The drug is therefore to be avoided in early pregnancy. Loudon (1987) has reviewed the area of psychotropic drug prescribing in pregnancy and breastfeeding. The general recommendations are shown in Table 24.2

Psychotropic drug prescribing and age

Certain pharmacokinetic factors alter with increasing age. A relative loss of lean tissue mass results in an increased volume of distribution for some drugs. Liver function is less influenced by age than by other variables (especially drug interactions and disease). A decline in renal function may be important for some drugs. In general, relatively lower doses of drugs are required, avoiding polypharmacy. In young children, renal and hepatic capacity is greater. With higher lean tissue mass, they have a smaller volume of distribution, thus the half-life of delivered drugs is shorter, and higher doses are necessary proportional to body weight.

Psychotropic drug classification

There are many different ways of classifying psychotropic drugs. As the focus is on clinical therapeutics, the drugs will be described according to their clinical use, though these categories may encompass pharmacologically distinct medications (see Table 24.3). The chapter will review each therapeutic category.

Table 24.3. *Classification of Drug Treatment in Psychiatry*

Drug group	Other names	Main clinical use
Antipsychotics	Neuroleptics, major tranquilizers, antischizophrenics	Mania/schizophrenia, psychotic agitation
Antiparkinsonians	Anticholinergics	Drug-induced parkinsonism and tardive dyskinesia
Antianxiety drugs	Sedatives, hypnotics, ataractics, minor tranquilizers, anxiolytics	Anxiety, insomnia, aggressive behaivour
Antidepressants		Depression, phobic illnesses, neuroses
Mood stabilisers		Prophylaxis of bipolar disorders, resistant depression, psychoses
Psychostimulants		Narcolepsy, hyperkinetic disorders

After Tyrer, P., *Essentials of Postgraduate Psychiatry*, 2nd edition.

Antipsychotic drugs

In 1950, it was noted that promethazine, a phenothiazine compound with antihistaminic properties, also acted as a sedative. Other phenothiazines were synthesised with this application in mind. One of these, chlorpromazine, was a uniquely powerful sedative in animals, apparently inducing in warm-blooded animals conditions similar to those of cold-blooded or hibernating animals, a so-called artificial 'hibernation'. The French scientist Laborit, and others, were proposing that shock treatment (used in a wide range of mental conditions at the time) worked by acting on diencephalic structures in the brain responsible for arousal. It was felt that a drug that induced such powerful effects in animals may be similarly therapeutic. Chlorpromazine was first given to 38 psychotically agitated patients in 1950, with dramatic benefits (Deniker, 1970). The report of Delay & Deniker (1952), that chlorpromazine was particularly effective against psychotic symptoms previously resistant to shock or sleep therapy, ushered in the modern age of psychopharmacology.

The new drugs were dubbed neuroleptics (referring to these drugs' capacity to produce extrapyramidal side-effects (Deniker, 1970)). This and the term antipsychotic are used interchangeably, though they have slightly different meanings. Other compounds were to follow; the butyrophenones (the archetype, haloperidol, was synthesised from pethidine-like compounds by Janssen in 1957) (Janssen, 1970), the thioxanthenes (synthesised by Lundbeck in 1957–1958) (Ravn, 1970), and many more. Table 24.4 shows a classification of antipsychotics by molecular structure. Many of the original antipsychotics did not undergo the level of rigorous phase I to IV trials that new drugs must comply with, but were fully accepted as specifically useful in psychosis after controlled studies in the early 1960s. Indeed

Table 24.4. *Classification of antipsychotic drugs: examples from each class*

Phenothiazines	chlorpromazine
(aliphatic side chains)	levopromazine
	triflupromazine
(piperidine side chain)	thioridazine
	mesoridazine
	pericyazine
(piperazine side chains)	prochlorperazine
	trifluoperazine
	fluphenazine
	perphenazine
Thioxanthenes	thiothixene
	flupenthixol
	clopenthixol
	chlorprothixene
Azepines (dibenzodiazepines)	loxapine
	clozapine
Butyrophenones	haloperidol
	droperidol
	benperidol
	trifluoperidol
	spiroperidol
Diphenylbutylpiperidines	pimozide
	fluspirilene
Substituted benzamide	sulpiride
	remoxipride
Benzixasoles	risperidone
Indoles	oxypertine
	molindone
Rauwolfia alkaloids	reserpine

Deniker (1970) commented that when chlorpromazine was first studied in patients, more was known of its effects on human, than on animal behaviour and physiology.

Pharmacokinetics

The prototypical neuroleptic chlorpromazine has an extremely complex metabolic pathway, generating at least 75 detected metabolites (many more are hypothesised), some of which have psychotropic effects (Usdin, 1978). Other antipsychotics, for example butyrophenones, thiothanxenes, and dibenzoazepines, have simpler pathways, involving one or two main steps, to render molecules hydrophilic by oxidative metabolism. Chlorpromazine is almost completely excreted in the urine in the form of glucuronide. There is no consistent relationship between type of metabolic pathway, and response to chlorpromazine.

Antipsychotics are lipophilic compounds, and pass easily through the jejunum. They are >90% protein-bound in plasma, with large volumes of distribution. Phenothiazines have a high first-pass metabolism (over 75% for chlorpromazine and fluphenazine), and thus a low oral bioavailability, providing some justification for giving lower doses by the intramuscular depot route. The plasma half-lives tend to be short, ranging from 10 to 20 hours, with a longer clinical duration of action than the half-life would indicate.

As discussed above, the relationship between plasma antipsychotic drug concentration and clinical response is weak, and a U-shaped concentration:response curve has been demonstrated for haloperidol (Smith *et al.*, 1984; Santos *et al.*, 1989). No therapeutic advantage was conferred in one study by having patients treated at low, medium, or high haloperidol plasma levels (Volavka *et al.*, 1992). There is close correspondence between plasma haloperidol levels and the degree of striatal D2 receptor blockade measured *in vivo* (Smith *et al.*, 1988), though the relationship between striatal D2 receptor occupancy by these drugs, and symptomatic improvement is unclear (Wolkin *et al.*, 1989; Pilowsky *et al.*, (1993).

Pharmacodynamics

Antipsychotic drugs are thought to exert their therapeutic effect through blockade of post-synaptic dopamine receptors. It is this action that had led to the suggestion that dopaminergic overactivity could be a neurochemical substrate for schizophrenia (Crow, 1980). There is a direct, linear correlation between clinical potency (in terms of average daily dose) and affinity for dopamine receptors in striatal tissue (Creese *et al.*, 1976; Seeman *et al.*, 1976). This relationship has not been described for other receptor types, including alpha adrenergic, histaminergic, or serotonergic (Peroutka & Snyder, 1980). More convincingly, the Northwick Park group compared two isomers of the thioxanthene drug, flupenthixol (Johnstone *et al.*, 1978). The α-isomer was 1000 times more potent than the β-isomer at blocking post-synaptic dopamine receptors, but otherwise had an identical pharmacological profile. Therapeutic antipsychotic activity was restricted to the α-isomer, while the β-isomer resembled placebo. This study remains the strongest indirect evidence that antipsychotic action is exerted through an effect on central dopamine receptors. Further research established that the correlation between clinical potency and receptor blockade was true for non-adenylate cyclase-linked dopamine receptors (D2 receptors) and not for adenylate cyclase-linked D1 receptors (Kerwin, 1992). Recently, molecular genetic researchers have discovered and cloned dopamine receptor subtypes; D1-like (D5) and D2-like (D3 and D4) (Sokoloff *et al.*, 1990; Van Tol *et al.*, 1991). The physiological relevance of these receptors is unclear, but the finding that the D2-like receptors are localised to limbic, rather than striatal regions, suggests they could be important selective targets for antipsychotic drugs (Sokoloff *et al.*, 1990; Kerwin, 1994).

Positron emission tomography (PET) and single photon emission tomography (SPET) nuclear medicine techniques allow the detection and localisation of injected radiolabelled ligands in the living human brain. The pharmacodynamic effects of antipsychotic drugs may now be directly evaluated in patients. Farde *et al.* (1989) showed a 65–85% occupancy of striatal D2 receptors by 12 chemically distinct antipsychotic drugs. The relationship between this and clinical response was tested in a prospective, double-blind PET study of increasing doses of the sulpiride-like drug, raclopride. A direct correlation was found between the

Table 24.5. *Unwanted pharmacologic side-effects of antipsychotic drugs*

Autonomic nervous system	Cycloplegia, dry mouth, difficulty urinating, constipation	Muscarinic cholinergic blockade
	Orthostatic hypotension, impotence, failure to ejaculate	Alpha-adrenergic blockade
Central nervous system	Parkinson's syndrome, akathisia, acute dystonias, tardive dyskinesia	Dopamine receptor blockade ?Supersensitive dopamine receptors
	Toxic confusional state	Muscarinic cholinergic blockade
	Sedation	Alpha adrenergic blockade
Endocrine system	Amenorrhea–galactorrhea Impotence, infertility	Dopamine, receptor blockade, hypothalamic–pituitary axis
Skin (especially phenothiazines)	Erythematous reaction, excezma/urticaria, photosensitive rashes, grey/blue/purple tinge	?Autoimmune
Eye (especially chlorpromazine, thioridazine)	Conjuctival pigmentation, corneolenticular pigmentation, retinal pigmentation (doses over 800 mg/day thioridazine over 300 mg/day chlorpromazine)	?Autoimmune
Body weight	Increased, especially low potency drugs	?Central effect on hypothalamic appetite control, possible 5-HT antagonism

degree of striatal D2 receptor blockade by raclopride and symptomatic improvement (Nordstrom *et al.*, 1993). Though these data apparently provide strong evidence for a simple therapeutic effect of antipsychotics at D2 receptors, the situation is more complex.

The onset of the antipsychotic effect is often delayed at least two to three weeks after central D2 receptor occupancy is clearly established (Horneykiewicz, 1982). Typical antipsychotic-treated schizophrenic patients who fail to respond show equal, or higher, levels of striatal D2 receptor blockade compared with responders (Wolkin *et al.*, 1989; Pilowsky *et al.*, 1993). Furthermore, the atypical drug clozapine is markedly effective in a proportion of these unresponsive patients, and shows a paradoxically diminished level of striatal D2 receptor occupancy, with good clinical improvement (Pilowsky *et al.*, 1992).

There is no doubt that the dopamine system is a critical target for antipsychotic drug action. A widely held view is that selective action at mesolimbic and mesocortical dopamine projections is required for the beneficial effects of these drugs, and that blockade of nigrostriatal systems is responsible for parkinsonian side-effects (Bradley, 1986). The growing recognition of 'atypical' antipsychotic drugs, that have therapeutic effects without extrapyramidal side-effects, has excited interest in regional differences in D2 occupancy by various drugs, distinct effects on D2-like receptors, and other neurotransmitter receptor systems as selective targets for antipsychotic drug action, most notably serotonergic systems. This area has been meticulously reviewed (Deutsch *et al.*, 1991; Gerlach, 1991; Reynolds, 1992; Kerwin, 1994).

Table 24.6. *Antipsychotic drug-induced movement disorders*

	Onset	Main features	Management
Acute Dystonic reaction	Early (hours to days)	Fixed muscle postures with spasm; trismus, opisthotonos, torticollis. Rarely, oculogyric crises (mouth open, eyes staring upwards, head back). More common in young males	Dramatic response to i.m. or i.v. anti-parkinsonian, e.g. benztropine, procyclidine. Treat immediately
Parkinsonian symptoms	Medium term (weeks)	Tremor, mask-like facies, rigidity, festinating gait. Akathisic restlessness	Routine anti-parkinsonian treatment not recommended. Prescribe when symptoms appear, or if on high dosage of antipsychotic drugs. Switch to low potency drugs, e.g.: thioridazine
Tardive dyskinesia	Long-term (months to years)	Orofacial dyskinesia, lip smacking, tongue rotating. Choreoathetoid movements of head, neck and trunk. Increased risk with age, brain damage, female sex, chronic use of anti-parkinsonian drugs	No satisfactory treatment. Decrease in antipsychotic may temporarily worsen. Minority improve spontaneously

Side-effects

Antipsychotic drugs affect other neurotransmitters as well as dopamine, leading to a range of autonomic, cardiovascular and central nervous side-effects (see Table 24.5). These side-effects are generally dose-dependent and predictable, based on the individual pharmacodynamic profile of the medication involved. In general, high-potency D2 blockers (for example, haloperidol, pimozide) show a greater degree of extrapyramidal side-effects, and fewer autonomic side-effects. Low potency antipsychotics (e.g. thioridazine, chlorpromazine, fluphenazine, trifluoperazine) have the opposite profile. The drug-induced movement disorders and their general management are shown in Table 24.6.

Antipsychotic treatment may also be associated with idiosyncratic, unpredictable side-effects, which are qualitatively abnormal and unrelated to the normal pharmacology of the drug, for example cholestatic jaundice (associated with eosinophilia, declining in frequency), skin rashes, and agranulocytosis. A further rare idiosyncratic reaction to antipsychotic therapy is the neuroleptic malignant syndrome (NMS). The onset is usually after 2 to 28 days, and is characterised by muscular rigidity, akinesia, pyrexia, clouding of consciousness, and autonomic changes including hypertension, sweating and pallor. There is neutrophilia and raised creatinine phosphokinase and potassium levels. It is a medical emergency.

Immediate cessation of antipsychotic treatment, and transfer to an intensive care environment is usually indicated. Edwards (1986) has reviewed the area in detail.

Clozapine

Up to a third of schizophrenic patients do not respond, or respond poorly, to typical antipsychotic medication. Until recently, the outlook was uniformly pessimistic. In 1988 a definitive study found clear efficacy of clozapine over chlorpromazine in treating at least a third of this 'treatment resistant' group (Kane *et al.*, 1988). The *in vitro* and *in vivo* behaviour of clozapine has triggered a major resurgence of interest in the neuropharmacology of schizophrenia, and thus merits a brief discussion in its own right.

Clozapine, a dibenzazepine, was originally synthesised as an antidepressant in the early 1960s (Hippius, 1989), but its effect on animals appeared similar to that of chlorpromazine. Clinical trials confirmed that it was an excellent antipsychotic drug (Deutsch *et al.*, 1991), and the received wisdom that extrapryramidal side-effects were a necessary corollary for a useful neuroleptic, began to be challenged (Hippius, 1989). However, reports of deaths from agranulocytosis in Finnish patients receiving clozapine, led to its withdrawal from the market in the early 1970s. Interest remained because several double-blind clinical trials had suggested clozapine was superior to haloperidol in treatment-resistant schizophrenic patients (Deutsch *et al.*, 1991). When the Clozaril Multicentre Collaborative Trial (Kane *et al.*, 1988) confirmed clozapine's high antipsychotic potency even in the most resistant patient group, it was reintroduced, with restrictions, in the UK and USA in 1990. Because of the risk of agranulocytosis, clozapine is licensed for use only in psychotic patients who have proven lack of responsiveness to typical antipsychotic therapy (failing to respond to adequate trials of at least two chemically distinct classes of typical antipsychotic drugs). Patients on the drug must show clinical improvement and be able to comply with routine blood tests. Blood sample results are monitored by a centralised service, which immediately notifies local medical and pharmacy services if a decrease in white cells is identified. Clozapine prescription is stopped until the white cell count normalises. The prescription is also withheld if the patients fails to comply with blood testing.

Compared to classical antipsychotics, clozapine produces a short-lasting elevation in plasma prolactin, and elevates both striatal HVA (homovanillic acid) and dopamine content (Coward *et al.*, 1989). ^{3}H-spiperone is poorly displaced from binding sites by the drug (Kohler *et al.*, 1981). Studies in experimental animals also suggest that the drug has relatively modest D2 receptor potency, being non-cataleptogenic in animals, and weakly opposing apomorphine-induced stereotypies (Kohler *et al.*, 1981; Andersen *et al.*, 1986). Extrapyramidal side-effects are rare in patients treated with clozapine. Elucidating clozapine's neuropharmacology is critical to the search for a safe compound with a similar mode of action. However, its pharmacological profile is broad; with affinity for a large number of receptors (including dopamine D1/D2, D4, 5-HT$_2$, 5-HT$_3$, histamine, alpha-1 receptors, and anticholinergic activity) (Reynolds, 1992; Moore *et al.*, 1993).

PET and SPET studies of clozapine-treated patients have shown a low level of striatal D2 receptor occupancy by the drug (Brucke *et al.*, 1992; Farde *et al.*, 1992), associated with few extrapyramidal side-effects. Pilowsky *et al.* (1992) showed that patients poorly responsive to typical antipsychotic drugs, who subsequently improved on clozapine, had markedly lower levels of striatal D2 receptor blockade. Thus clozapine does not appear to work primarily through a direct action, at least on striatal D2 receptors. The search for its pharmacological target(s) continues.

There are now atypical antipsychotic drugs, distinct from clozapine, in development, or available for routine clinical use. These drugs represent an important step forward in obtaining therapeutic effect with minimal extrapyramidal side-effects, and some are beginning to be regarded as first-line treatments for schizophrenia (Kerwin, 1994).

Clinical use of antipsychotics

Antipsychotic drugs are primarily used to treat schizophrenia and schizophreniform disorders, affective psychosis (especially mania and hypomania) and acute agitation. The specificity and efficacy of neuroleptics has been established beyond doubt (Hirsch, 1986). The main effects on psychosis are as follows: specific effects on psychotic symptoms; sedative effects on psychotic agitation; prevention of further symptom development and relapse in treated patients. There are generally three phases of drug treatment: early (acute); middle (stabilising) and late (maintenance or long-term therapy). Specific treatment strategies for schizophrenia are discussed in detail elsewhere, but will be covered briefly here, focusing only on drug treatment.

Choice of drug

Antipsychotic drugs do not differ appreciably among themselves in terms of efficacy (the exception being clozapine in the treatment-resistant group) (Kane et al., 1988). A survey of 134 double-blind studies, comparing 21 different neuroleptics against chlorpromazine, found no advantage of any one drug over chlorpromazine (Davis & Garver, 1978). Furthermore, there is no clear advantage of different drugs in treating particular psychotic symptoms. The choice of drug at all stages of treatment is based either on the particular side-effect profile for the individual patient (for example, a more sedating antipsychotic in the agitated patient), on the pharmaceutical formulation (drugs that may be given either as injections, orally, or by depot) and on the pharmacokinetics (for example, pimozide may be given once a day).

The treatment of acute psychosis has dual aims: control of agitated or aggressive behaviour (with a time-scale of minutes to hours), and alleviation of psychotic symptoms (which has an irreducible time-scale of several days to weeks). Drugs of choice at this stage are those with flexibility of administration, that may safely be given intramuscularly, intravenously, or orally (for example, haloperidol). Attempts to achieve steady-state antipsychotic concentrations by rapid intravenous loading ('rapid neuroleptisation') are no longer considered useful. Behavioural control for aggressive behaviour should be achieved by a pure sedative (benzodiazepine, unless medically contraindicated), alone, or in combination with an antipsychotic, lowering the required dose of each (Drugs and Therapeutics Bulletin, 1991) (see Table 24.7).

Once the patient is stabilised, maintenance therapy with an oral, or depot formulation can

Table 24.7. *Pharmacological management of behavioural emergencies*

1. Use benzodiazepine alone (lorazepam/diazepam) or in combination with a high potency neuroleptic (haloperidol/droperidol)
2. Give dose benzodiazepine (lorazepam i.m. or i.v. 1–3 mg/diazepam *only* i.v. up to 20 mg) and/or (if benzodiazepine contraindicated)
3. Give haloperidol/droperidol i.m. or i.v. up to 20 mg
   Advantage of i.v. route: greater flexibility, more control over dose levels, rapid onset (seconds to minutes)
   Advantage of i.m. route: no problem with access, slower onset (5 to 30 minutes)
4. When giving i.v. medication, deliver at 1 mg per minute for up to 5 mg, then wait 5 to 15 minutes to assess effect on target behaviours (e.g. degree of struggle against physical restraint).
5. Do not use i.v. sedation outside a hospital setting without rescusitation backup available.
6. If sedation not obtained by the above, may need further medication or other strategies (behavioural, ECT); therefore urgent consultation with senior specialist colleagues will be necessary before proceeding.
7. In patients well known to treating team, with good tolerance to antipsychotic medication, in whom long-term treatment must be initiated, zuclopenthixol acetate (a medium-term injectable antipsychotic) may be used. This is not a first-line treatment for a behavioural emergency.

commence. The drug choice will be one that is simple to take and that particularly minimises extrapyramidal side-effects. These side-effects are subjectively distressing, stigmatising, discourage compliance, and may be mistaken for psychopathology (e.g. akathisia).

One conventional neuroleptic that can be given as a single oral daily dose is pimozide, though the dose ceiling is now limited by suspected cardiotoxic effects. Concerning atypical neuroleptics, a recent double-blind placebo-controlled comparison of fixed-dose haloperidol and risperidone (at doses up to 16 mg in 2 mg increments) in 388 patients, showed risperidone (at a dose of 6 mg/day) was more effective than both haloperidol and placebo, and had the same level of extrapyramidal side-effects as placebo (Marder & Meibach, 1994). Though superiority over haloperidol was claimed, the dose of haloperidol was fixed at 20 mg, which clinical studies would suggest is higher than its optimal level (Van Putten *et al.*, 1990).

Depot formulations provide a therapeutic tissue concentration of at least a week's duration in a single subcutaneous or intramuscular injection. A survey of six double-blind studies found that depot antipsychotic administration reduced relapse by an average of 15% compared to oral treatment (probably an underestimate, given that the severity of relapse is also attenuated by depot) (Glazer & Kane, 1992). In a thorough review of the area, Glazer & Kane (1992) have recommended depot to establish compliance in patients refractory to oral agents. The depot approach was not associated with a higher incidence of unwanted side-effects, indeed lower doses are achievable as the first-pass effect is avoided, and constant steady-state tissue levels maintained. There are several depot formulations available (fluphenazine, flupenthixol, clopenthixol, haloperidol, pipothiazine), but no consistent advantage has been noted for one above another, and the choice again comes down to side-effect profiles and preferred dosing intervals. Dosage varies greatly, and flexibility of management has been advised, tailored to clinical response. Maintenance treatment will need to continue indefinitely, at the lowest possible dose, as cessation of treatment and drug holidays have been associated with increased relapse rates (Hirsch, 1986).

Dosage

Antipsychotic dose levels are a trade-off between clinical improvement and the appearance of side-effects. A review of the available placebo-controlled studies of chlorpromazine demonstrated efficacy above placebo in all studies where the dose of chlorpromazine was equal to or above 500 mg for at least six weeks (Davis & Garver, 1978). Treatment failure cannot be considered to have occurred before this time period, or below this dose range. A study of survival rates to relapse on very low (5 mg) or conventional (25 mg) doses of depot fluphenazine found significantly higher rates (64%) on the conventional than the low (31%) dose (Marder et al., 1987).

Recently, high-dose antipsychotic regimes have come under scrutiny, despite the wide margin of safety of these drugs (Goldney et al., 1988). The UK Royal College of Psychiatrists advisory panel recognised that megadose therapy (2000 mg chlorpromazine equivalents) was indicated rarely in some individuals, for short periods during acute relapse. The decision to go above British National Formulary recommended dose limits should ideally be made by the consultant-led multidisciplinary team after due consideration. The scientific evidence to support antipsychotic megadoses was acknowledged to be, at the very least, limited (Thompson, 1994).

Anti-anxiety drugs

Sedative–hypnotic drugs are among the most frequently prescribed drugs worldwide. Though the term sedative implies a depressant effect on arousal, causing drowsiness, newer drugs are more specifically anxiolytic. The older drugs (see Table 24.8) were highly sedative, and have now largely been abandoned except for particular indications.

The use of sedatives/hypnotics has occurred throughout history, alcohol being the most ubiquitous example. Various alkaloids, chloral hydrate, paraldehyde, and bromides were extensively used over the last century, but were ousted in the early twentieth century by barbiturates, themselves to be replaced, in the 1960s by the benzodiazepines. The benzodiazepines, and other modern anxiolytics, will be the focus of this section (see Table 24.9).

Benzodiazepines

The chemical structure of the benzodiazepine molecule was first synthesised in the 1930s as part of a study of theoretical chemistry by Sternbach. Named Ro-5-0690, its significance remained unknown, and it remained literally on the shelf until 1957, when, during a routine laboratory clear-up, it was rediscovered, and the pharmacological profile evaluated in animals. It was found to be an extremely effective hypnotic/sedative and muscle relaxant (Cohen, 1970). Clinical testing followed in the late 1950s and the benzodiazepine

Table 24.8. *Anti-anxiety drugs (now superseded)*

Barbiturates	phenobarbitone amylobarbitone quinalbarbitone	Narrow therapeutic range, safety low. Dangerous in overdose and in withdrawal (risk fatal seizures/respiratory depression). Not as effective as benzodiazepines. Phenobarbitone still used in epilepsy
Propanediols	meprobomate	Powerful muscle relaxants. Not superior to benzodiazepines. Produce oversedation
Chloral derivatives	chloral hydrate	Not superior to benzodiazepines. Paraldehyde similar but seldom used (in diluted form in children)

Table 24.9. *Modern anxiolytic drugs*

Benzodiazepines	diazepam
	chlordiazepoxide
Piperazinylpyramadine	buspirone
Cyclopyrrolone	zopiclone
MAOIs	phenelzine
SSRIs	fluoxetine
	fluvoxamine
	paroxetine
Antipsychotic (low dose)	flupenthixol
Antidepressant (low dose)	dothiepin
	amitriptyline
Beta-blockers	propanolol
Antihistamines	promathazine

compound was clearly a therapeutic sedative in patients. The first benzodiazepine introduced into the US was chlordiazepoxide (Librium), which was marketed and immediately widely accepted by the medical profession. The pace of research quickened and soon more potent, shorter-acting compounds were introduced. Table 24.10 shows a classification of benzodiazepines.

Pharmacokinetics

Benzodiazepines are rapidly and completely absorbed through the gut. Protein binding is over 95% and, as they are very lipophilic drugs, passage into the brain is rapid. The metabolic pathways of long-acting benzodiazepines is complex, as N-desmethylation results in an active metabolite, desmethyldiazepam, that is slowly metabolised ($t_{1/2}$ approximately 72 hours or more). Both chlordizepozide and diazepam ($t_{1/2}$ 36 hours) are converted to this metabolite, which may then surpass the original drug in concentration. Desmethyldiazepam is subsequently oxidised to oxazepam, conjugated with glucuronate, and excreted. Drugs without the desmethyl, or other long-lived metabolites (oxazepam, temazepam, lorazepam), have half-lives less than 24 hours.

Table 24.10. *The classification of benzodiazepines and their clinical usage*

Group	Benzodiazepines in group
Short-acting parent drugs and active metabolites (< 15 h)	triazolam
	temazepam
	lormetazepam
	lorazepam
	oxazepam
Short-acting parent drug, long acting metabolites	chlordiazepoxide
	clorazepate
	ketazolam
	prazepam
	medazepam
Long-acting parent drug and long-acting metabolites	diazepam
	clobazam
	nitrazepam
	flurazepam
	flunitrazepam
	clonazepam

From Tyrer (1986), previous edition.

Pharmacology

A precise mechanism explaining the sedative–hypnotic action of benzodiazepines has not been clarified (Trevor & Way, 1988). Initial studies implicated serotonergic systems in their mode of action. With the availability of [³H] diazepam, a central benzodiazepine receptor has been identified and intensively studied (Williams, 1991). Though the complex pharmacology is still uncertain, the strongest evidence suggests that benzodiazepines target GABAergic systems, though they are not simple direct post-synaptic GABA-receptor agonists or presynaptic re-uptake blockers (Lader, 1983). Electrophysiology shows that benzodiazepines potentiate GABAergic transmission throughout the brain and spinal cord. Benzodiazepine receptors have now been identified, and are functionally coupled to GABA-responsive chloride channels, though an endogenous benzodiazepine has not been discovered.

Physiologically, benzodiazepines depress activity in reticular and limbic systems, sparing the cerebral cortex. Arousal is lowered by effects of diffuse activating systems of the brain. GABAergic enhancement is thought to induce muscle relaxation, and general inhibition leads to the anticonvulsant properties of these drugs (Lader, 1983). Sedation occurs at the lowest effective doses of benzodiazepines and it is not clear whether this is distinct from the anxiolytic properties of the drugs.

Clinical uses of benzodiazepines

The benzodiazepines are used to alleviate aggression, anxiety, induce sleep and anaesthesia, in the treatment of epilepsy, as muscle relaxants, and to treat alcohol withdrawal. Despite

623

energetic marketing of different benzodiazepine drugs, there are no clinically significant advantages of one drug over another, and, like antipsychotics, the choice of drug depends largely on the side-effect profile. Longer-acting benzodiazepines are more useful where a slow tailing off of effect is desirable, for example in the treatment of alcohol withdrawal (where a stepped dose-reduction regime is given), or in status epilepticus. Shorter-acting drugs are more suitable for the treatment of short-lived conditions, including insomnia, or behavioural emergencies (see above); for brief anaesthesia, or preoperative relaxation. Prescribing should be limited to one to three weeks (maximum) for short-lived conditions.

The use of benzodiazepines for long-term treatment of neurotic disorders including generalised anxiety, panic, phobic and obsessive-compulsive disorders is controversial, and behaviour therapy is considered the essential, if not primary treatment modality. Combinations of these treatments are now being tried on targeted populations with different neurotic disorders, and it appears that while both drugs and behavioural treatment produce significant gains, those from behaviour therapy are sustained once treatment is withdrawn (O'Sullivan et al., 1991; Marks et al., 1993; Merriam, 1994). The exact place of benzodiazepines for treatment of chronic neurotic disorders is still under evaluation. Other drugs, including D2 antagonists, and serotonin reuptake inhibitors (SSRIs) are also employed to treat anxiety in chronic neurotic conditions, but particularly where there is comorbidity, most often with depressive symptoms (see below). These drugs are similarly being assessed to determine their most useful place in this area, as little is still known about their comparative safety, specificity and efficacy. Rasmunssen et al. (1993), have reviewed the area in depth.

Unwanted side-effects

At high doses, benzodiazepine treatment is associated with drowsiness and sedation, and a detached feeling. Ataxia, dizziness, and disorientation may occur, particularly in the elderly. Alcohol potentiates their effects, and should not be taken with the drugs. Paradoxical aggressive feelings are said to occur on benzodiazepines, but one large survey of all published controlled studies of benzodiazepines found an incidence of 1%, the same as placebo (Dietch & Jennings, 1988). Dosage adjustment may be necessary if this is a problem. Less specific rare side-effects include nausea, weight gain, skin rashes and agranulocytosis. The benzodiazepines are not dangerous in overdose, requiring respiratory support until the effects have worn off. They are contraindicated in patients with chronic obstructive airways disease or respiratory failure.

Psychological and physical dependence does occur at high or normal doses, and a withdrawal syndrome is clearly seen after continuous treatment for as short a time as three weeks, if medication is stopped abruptly. The onset may be delayed until the active metabolites are completely excreted. Withdrawal symptoms are unpleasant, and manifold. They include, for example, rebound insomnia, anxiety, agitation, restlessness, perceptual and sensory hypersensitivity, sweating, amnesia and weight gain (Tyrer et al., 1981). For this reason, all benzodiazepine prescriptions should be carefully monitored, used for short periods only where absolutely necessary, and withdrawal performed slowly.

Buspirone

Buspirone is the prototypical non-benzodiazepine anxiolytic, which is apparently effectively 'anxioselective', relieving anxiety with minimal sedative or muscle-relaxant effects. It is a partial agonist at serotonergic $5-HT_{1a}$ receptors, rather than the GABA-BZ receptor complex, thus it is perhaps more active at cortical regions. Its introduction has reawakened interest in serotonergic hypotheses of anxiety, as preclinical data has shown that enhancing serotonergic activity by giving 5-HT agonists is anxiogenic (Iversen, 1984). The drug is metabolised hepatically to an active metabolite with anxiolytic effects which is then excreted (Trevor & Way, 1988). Several second-generation buspirone-like anxiolytics have now been developed, including, for example, gepirone and ipsapirone (Williams, 1991).

Zopiclone

Zopiclone is the most recent hypnotic to come on the market. It appears to act through the GABA-BZ receptor complex, but at a different site from the benzodiazepines. In animals, it has similar properties to the benzodiazepines, but is primarily sedative in man (Hallstrom, 1994). The drug is rapidly absorbed orally. It has an elimination half-life of three to six hours, and a duration of action of six to eight hours. An active metabolite has similar kinetics. The clinical indication for zopclone is mainly that of short term treatment of insomnia, in which it produces sleep without impairing REM (dream sleep), and, in contrast to benzodiazepines, slow wave (deep sleep) is extended. The unwanted side-effects and contraindications are the same as for the benzodiazepines, and so its prescription must also be carefully monitored, with slow withdrawal.

Antidepressants

Neurochemical theories for affective disorders

The notion that catecholamines may be involved in the aetiology of depressive disorders was consequent upon the realisation that amine depletion with drugs like reserpine was associated with depressive reactions.

It was subsequently realised that early antidepressants enhanced monoaminergic neurotransmission in a variety of ways. Thus monoamine oxidase inhibitors, the first antidepressants to be introduced (Kerwin, 1990), prevented the enzymatic breakdown of catecholamines and indoleamines, leading to increased levels presynaptically (Baldessarini *et al.*, 1988), whereas tricyclic antidepressants prevent the reuptake-dependent inactivation of these neurotransmitters. Since that time, there has been a huge amount of research searching for the underlying deficit in aminergic systems. (For a full discussion, see the review by Willner, 1990*b*). The basis of the monoaminergic hypothesis can be summarised as follows (see Reveley & Campbell, 1986).

1. Drugs that deplete monamines are depressants.
2. Most antidepressants enhance monaminergic transmission at some point in the synaptic signalling process.

3. Reduction in amines and their metabolites in CSF in depressed patients.
4. Variable post-mortem data, the most consistent being elevation in cortical 5-HT$_2$ binding.

The acute effects of antidepressants on amine systems cannot account for the irreducible delay in the onset of symptom relief. Therefore, most workers agree that the effect of antidepressant is mediated by changes in receptor numbers and sensitivity arising as secondary phenomena. The literature on this is very confusing as both pre- and post-synaptic receptors of a variety of types are differentially affected. The topic has been reviewed by Lader & Harrington (1990). In summary, the most consistent changes are upregulation of beta receptors (Bannerjee *et al.*, 1977), down-regulation of alpha receptors (Brown *et al.*, 1980) and reduced activity of mesolimbic dopamine systems (Chiodo & Antelman, 1980).

Clinical pharmacology of individual groups of antidepressants

Tricyclic antidepressants

Tricyclics were synthesised from chlorpromazine by converting a two-dimensional three-ring structure to a three-dimensional ring structure, leading to an unexpected revision of their properties. The first tricyclic, imipramine, is an iminodibenzyl derivative similar to chlorpromazine.

The best-known action of tricyclics is to block the reuptake of catechol and indoleamines, thereby increasing the amounts and duration of neurotransmitter in the synaptic cleft during impulse transmission. Although non-selective, tertiary amines (imipramine, clomipramine and amitryptyline) have a higher ratio of serotonin to noradrenaline reuptake blockade, secondary amines (desiprimine, nortryptyline) have a higher ratio for noradrenaline uptake blockade. The homeostatic consequences of this in the longer term include β-receptor downregulation, α_2 desensitization and α_1 sensitisation (see Willner, 1990*b*). Which of these represents the mode of action is an open question. The association of endogenous imipramine-binding sites at 5-HT reuptake sites strongly implicates the 5-HT system (Langer *et al.*, 1980; this will be discussed more fully under SSRIs). However, in view of the complexity of the pharmacology and multiplicity of compensatory effects, it is sensible to think of traditional tricyclics as having multiple therapeutically useful intervention sites (Sugrue, 1983).

Clinical uses

Early tricyclics, imipramine and amitryptaline, were the subject of multiple clinical trials throughout the 1950s, 1960s and 1970s. They demonstrated the usefulness of tricyclics in patients with vegetative or biological symptoms and that apart from differences in their sedative profiles, there was overall little to choose between any of the first generation tricyclics (Morris & Beck, 1974). More recent tricyclics, which include maprotiline, trazodone, amoxapine and buproprion, have been found to be equi-effective as traditional tricyclics, but their niche in clinical practice is not objectively determined (Prien & Levine, 1984).

The efficacy of tricyclics has never been in doubt. About 80% of patients with biological symptoms will respond (Lader, 1982). Administration reduces relapse rates from 50% to 10% (Rogers *et al.*, 1981). Neurophysiological effects of tricyclics related to response include profound effects on sleep, the EEG and the neuroendocrine axis. Stage 4 sleep is decreased and REM sleep prolonged (Gaillard, 1979). Unlike the other clinical parameters the sleep effect is acute and patients can be reassured that their sleep disturbance will resolve in days. Acute antidepressants decrease α rhythms on the EEG but increase other EEG waveform components, both slow and fast (Lader & Bhanji, 1980). Tricyclics are epileptogenic at higher doses.

The individual properties of tricyclics as either sedating (e.g. trimipramine, amitriptyline) or not (e.g. clomipramine) are well known and made use of in different clinical contexts. Other individual properties include the anxiolytic effects of dothiepin and the good tolerability of lofepramine (Mindham, 1982).

Pharmacokinetics

Tricyclics are rapidly absorbed through the gastrointestinal mucosa with peak plasma levels occurring three to four hours later. There is up to 70% first-pass metabolism. Being lipid soluble they have a high volume of distribution and also undergo rapid hepatic metabolism. The rate of elimination varies widely from a half life of 6–20 hours for imipramine to 70 hours for protriptyline. Steady-state concentrations are usually achieved within seven days of continuous treatment, although there may be a 20-fold variability in genetically influenced hepatic metabolism (Alexanderson *et al.*, 1969). The drug is highly plasma bound (90–95%), leading to interaction with other tightly bound drugs such as oral anticoagulants and non-steroidal analgesics.

Most information about plasma levels and clinical response is available for imipramine. A therapeutic window of 50–200 µg/ml is apparent, with a linear relationship to clinical responsivity being apparent within that range (Burrows *et al.*, 1974). The relationship of clinical responsivity to plasma level is relatively understudied and more variable for other tricyclic drugs.

Side-effects

Side-effects are related to peripheral anticholinergic and alpha adrenergic effects of the drugs. CNS effects include sedation, cognitive impairment and fine tremor. Miscellaneous effects include dermatogical, haematological, and cardiac electrophysiological effects. These are all enumerated in Table 24.11. The main problems include anticholinergic effects such as dry mouth, failure to accommodate, urinary retention and cardiovascular effects such as blood pressure lability and arrhythmias. Central nervous system effects include sedation and precipitation of mania.

Overdose

The most serious problem with tricyclics is their toxicity in overdose. At the peak of their use in the early 1980s there were 400 deaths/year in the UK (Lader, 1982). The adverse effects

627

Table 24.11. *Unwanted effects of tricyclic antidepressants*

Autonomic	Dry mouth
	Blurred vision (failure to accommodate)
	Sweating
	Urinary retention
	Precipitation of glaucoma
	Paralytic ileus
	Ejaculatory failure
CNS	Sedation
	Tremor
	Seizures
	Cognitive impairment
	Mania
CVS	Tachycardia
	Hypotension (postural)
	Atrioventricular block
Dermatological	Drug sensitivity
Haematological	Neutropenia: rare
	Agranulocytosis: rare
Miscellaneous	Weight gain

that appear may include coma, myoclonus, anticholinergic crisis, tachycardias and arrhythmias. There is no direct evidence that tricyclics are teratogenic but their use is best avoided in pregnancy.

It follows then that the major contraindications to tricyclic treatment include glaucoma, prostatism, cardiovascular disorders and blood dyscrasias.

Monamine oxidase inhibitors

MOA-Is have a long history, being amongst the first drugs to be used in psychiatry (Dally, 1958). First reports stressed their efficacy in ECT-resistant and atypical depressive states (West & Dally, 1959). Indiscriminate use and popularity of the tricylics plus the results of the Medical Research Council trial (1965) led to the conclusion that they may be no better than placebo in more serious depressive states. These facts, along with the discovery of alarming and potential fatal interactions with tyramine-containing foods (Wright, 1978), led to a sharp decline in their popularity. However, they are now re-emerging. It is now realised that the MRC trial was biased to select a group of patients who would respond better to tricyclics than MAO-Is. The tyramine reactions may have been numerically over-reported (Pare, 1985) and a spate of clinical trials in atypical depressions, phobic and mixed depressive/neurotic disorders has helped to re-establish a niche for them (Nutt & Glue, 1989). In addition, newer MAO-Is are available, which may be enzyme-specific and whose effects are reversible.

Chemical structures

MAO-Is are hydrazine derivates similar to iproniazid or non-hydrazine derivatives. These include isocarboxazid, nialamide, phenelzine and others, including tranylcypromine, an amphetamine derivative.

Pharmacology and mode of action

Traditional MAO-Is are non-competitive and non-selective inhibitors of both monoamine oxidase A, which catalyses noradrenaline and serotonin, and monoamine oxidase B, which catalyses dopamine. This brings about an increased amount of monoamines presynaptically available for release (Spector *et al.*, 1963). Newer drugs (see later) may be both selective for MOA-A or B and be reversible, thereby pre-empting the interaction with tyramine. MAO-A inhibitors are most relevant to the treatment of depression and these have been acronymised as RIMAs – reversible inhibitors of monoamine A. Longer-term adaptive changes also occur with MAO-Is, including downregulation of α_2 and β receptors and upregulation of imiprimine binding sites (Murphy *et al.*, 1984). As with tricyclics, it remains impossible to correlate response of specific psychopathology with biochemical changes evoked by MAO-Is. Therefore, their clinical use remains empirical and independent of the underlying biochemistry of the drugs.

Clinical uses of MAO-Is

Primary treatment for depression   The earliest clinical trials reported efficacy of 25–75% in a wide variety of depressive illnesses (Dally, 1958; Pare & Sandler, 1959). 'Obstinate' depression and atypical depressive states were most improved. It is worth mentioning here the classic MRC trial of 1965, which studied 250 patients randomly assigned to open-label treatment of ECT, imipramine, phenelzine or placebo. ECT and imipramine were far superior and phenelzine conferred no advantage over placebo. Although very influential, retrospective experience tells us that this trial was an inadequate assessment of MAO-Is as patients with atypical or mixed neurotic conditions were excluded. Phenelzine was found to be useful in 'neurotic depression' 'depressive anxiety' and phobic depression (Robinson *et al.*, 1973; Tyrer, 1973).Hydrazine derivatives are metabolised via acetylation and this reaction can occur at different rates in individual patients, therefore acetylation phenotype is important in determining response to these drugs (Paykel *et al.*, 1982). There is a general consensus now that MAO-Is are useful in atypical and mixed neurotic states (Bass & Kerwin, 1989). Liebowitz & Klein (1979) stressed that patients with reverse biological features (overeating, daytime somnolence and high libido) may have a particularly good response to MAO-Is.

Resistant depression   Resistant depression can be thought of in two different frameworks: intractable illness despite adequate tricyclic/ECT or other pharmacotherapies; or elderly or medically frail patients who are unable to tolerate full doses of antidepressants. Intractable illness usually necessitates combination therapy. Combination with tricyclics is safe with close monitoring. The drugs should be given at opposite ends of the day to avoid coincident plasma peaks (MAO-Is in the morning, tricyclics at night). High-potency combinations, e.g. tranylcypromine and clomipramine, should be avoided. The best combination is phenelzine and amitryptyline (Beaumont, 1973). There is some dissent in the literature due to the inherent variability of these types of illness but rigorous trials do show superiority over monotherapy (Sethnna, 1974). Interestingly, tricyclics can block the tyramine reaction due to tricyclic blockade of tyramine uptake. However, it is most important *not* to abandon dietary precautions (Pare *et al.*, 1982).

There has been some occasional value in combining MAO-Is with lithium, tryptophan or second-generation antidepressants. MAO-Is should *never* be combined with selective serotonin reuptake inhibitors.

MAO-Is may be of value when phobic symptoms predominate (Sheehan *et al.*, 1980). Social phobia may be particularly responsive to MAO-Is (Liebowitz *et al.*, 1988). The role of MAO-Is compared to other drugs and behavioural treatments has not been established.

The use of MAO-Is in personality disorder is controversial. Traditional wisdom was that a stable premorbid personality was a prerequisite for a good outcome with MAO-Is (Tyrer *et al.*, 1983). However, some studies (Nies & Robinson, 1982) state that attention-seeking, acts of deliberate self-harm and histrionic features predict a favourable outcome and Cowdry & Gardener (1988) have shown a mood stabilising effect superior to carbamazepine in borderline personality disorder.

Pharmacokinetic and side-effects

The pharmacokinetics of older MAO-Is are relatively poorly understood. They have rapid gastrointestinal absorption with plasma peaks at 2–3 hours. They have a very short plasma half-life of 1–2 hours. However, during redistribution they bind irreversibly to the enzyme, greatly prolonging their pharmacodynamic action. Hydrazines are metabolised by acetylation (see earlier for clinical comment). Eighty per cent blockade of MAO-A is seen after two weeks. Restoration of normal monoamine oxidase activity currently takes about one to two weeks. (An important practice to note is that two weeks should elapse before changing patients from an MAO-I to a high potency tricyclic or SSRI).

MAO-Is produce anticholinergic effects such as dry mouth and blurred vision. This is less than with tricyclics. Glaucoma and prostatism are contraindications. Hypertensive crises with tyramine-containing foods are the main problem and rigorous adherence to a tryamine-free diet is mandatory.

New monoamine oxidase inhibitors

Recent attempts have been made to develop MAO-Is that are reversible, thereby preventing the tyramine reaction, or selective to MAO-A or B, improving the clinical benefit/side-effect ration. MAO-B inhibitors (which prevent dopamine catabolism) are reserved for neurological conditions such as parkinsonism and have no role in psychiatric conditions. MAO-A inhibitors may well be useful antidepressants (Sunderland *et al.*, 1985). Studies with the new reversible MAO-IA inhibitor moclobemide have proved useful in otherwise MAO-I resistant patients with usefulness even in endogenous subtypes (Priest, 1989).

Selective serotonin reuptake inhibitors (SSRIs)

Over the past ten years a new class of antidepressants has emerged. These were developed from early studies that indicated that tricyclic antidepressant binding was particularly associated with serotonergic neurons; this subsequently engendered a specific serotonin hypothesis for depression and stimulated the search for more specific serotonin reuptake inhibitors. Those now clinically available include citalopram, fluoxetine, fluvoxamine, paroxetine and sertraline.

Chemical class

SSRIs have a range of structures, which are quite distinct from the tricyclic class of compounds. The SSRIs have emerged hand in hand with a specific serotonin hypothesis of depression. This is based on the following observations (Coppen & Doogan, 1988):

1. Low concentration of 5-H1AA in depressed patients, which normalise on clinical recovery.
2. Reduced serotonin uptake into platelets from depressed patients.
3. Blunted prolactin response to serotonergic agonists.
4. Increased 5-HT_2 binding sites in post-mortem suicide victims.

There is a significant problem of multiple non-replication of these types of study in the literature. However, SSRIs are an interesting and effective class of compounds that do have impressive neurochemical selectivity and whatever the fundamental aetiology of depression, they almost certainly work with a net effect to facilitate serotonergic transmission (Chaput *et al.*, 1988).

Pharmacology and mode of action

All the SSRIs are potent reversible inhibitors of high-affinity reuptake of serotonin (5-HT). At higher concentrations the drugs also inhibit noradrenaline and dopamine uptake. Ratios for this effect vary considerably but the ratio for paroxetine, for example, is 320:1 serotonin to noradrenaline and 1800:1 serotonin to dopamine compared to 0.9:1 and 43:1 respectively for amitryptyline. Paroxetine is the most potent 5-HT uptake blocker whereas citalopram is the most selective. Sertraline has an unusual profile in that it blocks dopamine uptake more potently than noradrenaline. The reverse holds for all the other SSRIs (Johnson, 1991). As a result of serotonin reuptake blockade, all the drugs reduce serotonergic turnover, as judged by reduced levels of 5-hydroxyindole acetic acid (5-HIAA – the major metabolite of 5-HT) (e.g. Brunello, *et al.*, 1986).

The vast majority of studies show little or no effect on the turnover of other monoamines. Like tricyclics, chronic SSRI intake produces transynaptic regulatory changes in monoaminergic receptors, but these are very limited. Fluoxetine and paroxetine have virtually no such effects, whereas sertraline and fluvoxamine produce a modest downregulation of β-receptors. Alpha and dopamine receptors are unaffected with chronic treatment. As might be expected, all SSRIs produce local down-regulation of 5-HT receptors, principally 5-HT$_{1A}$ and 5-HT$_2$ receptors (see Deakin, 1988 for discussion of these effects).

Large numbers of studies have been published showing that SSRIs are as effective as tricyclics in the treatment of major depression (see review by Boyer & Feighner, 1991) with insomnia, gastrointestinal disturbance and anxiety being the major side-effects. Certainly, in terms of mood elevation, SSRIs are comparable, but they lack effects on insomnia and sleep disturbances. In addition, SSRIs have a shorter latency – as early as one week. SSRIs are useful in all age groups but are particularly useful in elderly patient or patients with somatic concern who may not tolerate the side-effects of older antidepressants. There are fewer reports of SSRIs' usefulness in maintenance treatment and most information is available for fluoxetine (e.g. Montgomery et al., 1988). SSRIs are certainly effective over placebo in preventing relapse and what studies there are suggest they are likely to be as good as imipramine. Evidence is also available that suggests that SSRIs are frequently helpful in patients who are resistant to other treatment (Tyrer et al., 1987). Some clinical trials also suggest a role for SSRIs in obsessive-compulsive disorder and mixed anxiety/depression syndromes (Montgomery, 1989).

Considerable focus has centred on a possible role for SSRIs in eating disorders because of the role of serotonin in satiety control and as a neurotransmitter controlling the hypothalamic set point for weight (Breisch et al., 1976), and weight and appetite loss. A large trial to study the effects of fluoxetine in 382 patients with bulimic symptoms was found to be superior to placebo in reducing the frequency of binge eating and vomiting cycles. In addition, depression, abnormal eating attitudes and carbohydrate craving (Enas et al., 1989) were also improved. Fluoxetine has subsequently been licensed for control of bulimic symptoms.

Antimanic agents

Lithium

The antimanic effects of the simple salt lithium carbonate have been recognised since 1949, when Cade showed marked improvement in eight out of ten manic patients but not in patients with dementia praecox. The biochemical and physiological effects of lithium are legion. Early studies on brain-specific effects concentrated on the ability of lithium to stimulate choline uptake and acetylcholine synthesis (Jope et al., 1980). Lithium alters adrenylate cyclase activity (Ebstein & Belmaker, 1979) and a wide range of ATP-dependent neurotransmitter processes including uptake and release (Glen, 1979). Most recent interest has focused on lithium's effect on the inositol phosphate-dependent second messenger pathways leading to accumulation in inositol; 1,4,5-phosphate second messenger in brain tissue (Hokin, 1993). None of these effects have been unequivocally correlated to the therapeutic actions of lithium. The clinical users of lithium can be summarised as follows:

Table 24.12. *Side-effects of lithium*

Thirst	
Polyuria	Dose-dependent and reversible
Tremor	
Hypothyroidism	
Hyperthyroidism	
Anorexia	
Nausea	
Diarrhoea	
Weight gain	
Acne	
Renal parenchymal damage	
Renal damage	
Confusion	
Disorientation	Encephalopathy due to
Ataxia	lithium toxicity
Seizure	

(i)   Acute mania – note lithium is non-sedating
(ii)   Prophylaxis of bipolar affective disorder
(iii) Prophylaxis of recurrent unipolar depression
(iv) Acute episodes of depression resistant to other forms of treatment
(v)   Schizoaffective disorder
(vi) Control of aggressive behaviour.

All studies of lithium in unipolar depression show good efficacy but it does not appear superior to tricylics acutely or in controlling relapse. For this reason it is, therefore, reserved as second line or combination therapy.

In schizoaffective disorder, Prien *et al.* (1972) and Brockington *et al.* (1978) have concluded that lithium is no better than chlorpromazine except in 'mild' cases where lithium should be considered as first-line or adjunctive treatment, allowing those milder cases to be free from extrapyramidal side-effects. The side-effects of lithium are shown in Table 24.12. Many of these effects occur close to the therapeutic plasma concentration and therefore plasma monitoring of lithium is standard practice. Standard practice is to obtain lithium levels every two to three days during the loading phase, every two weeks until the desired plasma level is obtained, and thereafter every six weeks. A therapeutic range of 1.0–1.5 during the acute illness is usually recommended and 0.6–1.00 for the prophylactic phase treatment.

Lithium has a relatively slow elimination of 20 hours and so can be given once daily. The distal renal tubule efficiently concentrates lithium and so the drug is contraindicated in patients with renal tubular pathology and dehydrating conditions; diuretics, especially thiazides, are also contraindications to lithium treatment. The standard selection criterion for starting lithium is two episodes over 12 months. However, the overall severity of each episode should guide treatment. Patients must have normal renal, endocrine and neurological functions.

Electroconvulsive therapy

The observation that convulsions can influence mood has been known since the eighteenth century and Landholdt's classical view of the reciprocal relationship between epilepsy and schizophrenia is well-known (Landholdt, 1953). This, however, was not supported by research (Slater, 1969). ECT remains a valuable treatment for severe affective disorder and some treatment-resistant psychoses.

Most workers agree that convulsions increase the turnover of dopamine, noradrenaline and 5-HT: Grahame-Smith et al. (1978) showed that the behavioural response to stimulation of 5-HT and dopamine receptors was enhanced following ECT. Pandey et al. (1979) additionally demonstrated increased sensitivity of β-adrenergic receptors. In human studies, Cooper et al. (1968) demonstrated an increase in serotonin metabolites in CSF from patients recently treated with ECT.

Evidence for efficacy of ECT

Like many classical therapeutic interventions in medicine, such as warfarin and digoxin, the usefulness of ECT in psychiatry grew up before the culture of the scientific clinical trial was developed. However, the MRC (1965) trial of antidepressants compared ECT with imipramine, phenelzine and placebo. ECT was superior to imipramine in efficacy but its effect was waning at four weeks to equal that of imipramine. Methodologically sound trials of ECT versus anaesthetic only, include Cronholm & Ottoson (1960); Robin & Harris (1962) and Wilson et al. (1963); in all cases ECT had a significantly better outcome than placebo or tricyclic. Other studies are discussed in Chapter 11.

Indications for ECT

Many studies throughout the latter half of the century have confirmed the efficacy of ECT in major depression where biological features and delusions predominate (e.g. Roth, 1959; Kiloh & Garside, 1963); on the other hand, neurotic patients respond unpredictably and, at best, achieve only very short-term improvement (Slater & Roth, 1969). The MRC antidepressant trial of 1965 compared ECT with imipramine, phenelzine and placebo in a large group of endogenously depressed patients and found comparable improvement rates for ECT and imipramine. In view of inherent doubts about ECT, many clinical trials have assessed which patient subgroups may respond to ECT. The most influential study (Carney et al., 1965) showed that features of endogenous depression such as early morning wakening, somatic and paranoid delusions, retardation and absence of neurotic traits predicted ECT response. These features also predict good outcome with tricyclics (Kiloh et al., 1962) and may simply reflect a treatment-responsive syndrome. Studies comparing categorical diagnoses (Mintel & Mandel, 1979) suggest psychotic depressives and depressed bipolars do best. No biological markers for depression (e.g. dexamethasone suppression) directly predict response.

There are no controlled clinical trials of ECT in mania. Retrospective studies of

ECT-treated manics show good response and fewer relapses (Black *et al.*, 1987*b*). The most severely disturbed manics seem to do well after one or two applications (McCabe & Norris, 1977). Small *et al.* (1988) showed that manics responded more rapidly to ECT than to drug therapy.

ECT was, particularly in the USA, widely used as second- or third-line treatment for schizophrenia. There is no evidence that the core symptoms of schizophrenia respond to ECT. Salzman (1980), reviewing the literature, found no scientific evidence for efficacy. The only recent British trial, by Taylor & Fleminger (1980), found improvement in the short-term but this was not sustained beyond 16 weeks. ECT may still have a place in catatonic schizophrenia (now very rare) and schizoaffective disorder (Van Valkenburg & Clayton, 1985).

Side-effects and contraindications

There are no absolute contraindications to ECT except the presence of raised intracranial pressure. Relative contraindications include cardiovascular and other cerebral disorder and the use of ECT is weighed up against the dangers of the psychiatric illness and the safety of the drug treatment in these cases. All ECT is, of course, modified and so the convulsion is not a risk, the main risk being that of a very short duration anaesthetic. Side-effects include headache, nausea, dizziness, and short-term retrograde amnesia. Short-term dysphasia will occur if the shock is given to the non-dominant hemisphere. Occasional post-ictal confusional states may occur. Age itself is not a contraindication to ECT.

Unilateral or bilateral?

A huge literature exists on this (see Kiloh, 1980). Unilateral ECT produces less confusion and memory disturbance. It is, however, less reliable, less effective in severe illness, may require more application and more skill and technical sophistication. For these reasons many clinicians prefer bilateral treatment.

25

Psychotherapy

STIRLING MOOREY AND RUTH WILLIAMS

A. BEHAVIOURAL AND COGNITIVE THERAPIES

Introduction

Behavioural and cognitive therapies are a group of psychological treatments that have in common a focus on the modification of symptoms and overt behaviour. In contrast to psychodynamic approaches, which see symptoms as markers of more significant underlying unconscious pathology, behavioural and cognitive therapies tend to take presenting problems at face value. These problems have been learned and can therefore be unlearned through active techniques that manipulate behaviour, thoughts and beliefs. Behavioural and cognitive therapies also share a commitment to empiricism – theories must be backed by scientific evidence, and techniques must be shown to be effective through well-designed single case-studies or randomised controlled trials. The applicability of these techniques is wide. Cognitive and behavioural techniques are of major importance in the treatment of anxiety disorders, depression, eating disorders and sexual dysfunctions. Beyond this core group of disorders, the methods can be applied to enhance coping and change unwanted behaviours in conditions as diverse as cancer, chronic pain, schizophrenia and to challenging behaviours in people with learning difficulties.

Early behaviour therapies were based on either classical (Pavlovian) conditioning or operant (Skinnerian) conditioning, but increasingly theoretical advances in social psychology, cognitive psychology and empirical research in abnormal psychology have contributed to the range of therapeutic strategies available.

Development of behavioural and cognitive psychotherapies

Although Watson, the founder of behaviourism, reported the case of an experimentally induced phobia in an 11-month-old child (Watson & Rayner, 1920), and one of his followers (Jones, 1924) applied methods of deconditioning anxiety to children with phobias, behaviour therapy did not become a formal treatment until the pioneering work of Joseph Wolpe in the 1950s. *Systematic desensitisation* is a technique in which phobic patients are taught deep muscle relaxation, and then imagine feared stimuli in an increasing hierarchy of anxiety (Wolpe, 1958). Wolpe's method was based on the premise that one physiological state (relaxation) was incompatible with another (anxiety), a concept termed reciprocal inhibition. Subsequently, many behavioural interventions have been thought to depend on the process of *habituation*. This process, which is still incompletely understood, is one in which repeated exposure to a stimulus leads to a decrement in orienting responses and arousal. In systematic desensitisation, the principle of keeping increments in anxiety to a minimum meant that the method often needed vary small graded steps and was therefore slow and time-consuming. An alternative more rapid technique, called *flooding* or *implosion* (Stampfl & Levis, 1967), involved exposure to the feared stimulus at maximal intensity until the anxiety habituated. This approach is more rapid and effective, but can cause great distress to the patient. A more humane alternative is a graded exposure programme, where the patient constructs a hierarchy of feared situations and confronts them a step at a time. *Graded exposure in vivo* has become the basic technique of much behaviour therapy. It was initially found to be effective in simple phobias (Watson & Marks, 1971), then applied to agoraphobia (Mathews *et al.*, 1981) and obsessive compulsive disorder (Marks *et al.*, 1975).

Deconditioning strategies arose from classical conditioning theory. Another strand of behaviour therapy has been the application of operant conditioning principles in what some have termed 'behaviour modification'. This approach emphasises the single case-study, since each patient's problem behaviour is determined by a unique set of environmental factors that trigger it and reinforce it. A detailed *behavioural analysis* (Kanfer & Saslow, 1965) is required before a therapy programme is constructed. Behaviour modification has been used in treating problem behaviour in children (e.g. elective mutism: Sanok & Stiefell, 1979), people with learning difficulties (Yule & Carr, 1980), and in the rehabilitation of schizophrenics (Ayllon & Azrin, 1968).

When applied in institutional settings, these methods can take the form of a *token economy* (Ayllon & Azrin, 1968; Paul & Lentz, 1977) where absence of unwanted behaviours and the enactment of desirable behaviours are rewarded with tokens, which can then be exchanged for more tangible rewards such as food, cigarettes, etc. For ethical and other reasons, e.g. problems in generalisation from the controlled into the natural environment, token economies are much less common now than in the 1960s and 1970s, but many operant principles can still be employed in behaviour therapy, where subtle environmental rewards for symptoms may go unnoticed if a careful behavioural analysis is not carried out.

Probably the most striking change in behavioural psychotherapy over the last 20 years has been the increasing interest in mental events. Once eschewed as out of the range of the behaviourists' field of inquiry, and by some even labelled epiphenomena, thoughts, images and beliefs are now at the forefront of therapists' consciousness. Albert Ellis and A.T. Beck were pioneers of these *cognitive therapies*. Ellis' rational emotive therapy (Ellis, 1962) and Beck's cognitive therapy (Beck, 1976) see emotional disorder and behavioural problems as secondary to irrational beliefs or faulty information processing. Beck's systematic approach to identifying the cognitive disorder associated with diagnoses such as depression (Beck *et al.*, 1979) and anxiety (Beck *et al.*, 1985), as well as his efforts to test the efficacy of his therapy, have led to a widening acceptance of the cognitive model among behaviourists. Beck and Ellis were psychoanalysts. From a more traditional psychology background, Donald Meichenbaum (Meichenbaum, 1977) developed *cognitive behaviour modification*. Meichenbaum's work with self-verbalisations of children with attention deficit disorder (Meichenbaum & Goodman, 1971), schizophrenics (Meichenbaum & Cameron, 1973) and self-instructional methods in general has been highly influential. There is now a spectrum from straightforward behavioural techniques at one end to cognitive therapy at the other. Different patients require different mixes, but most therapists will use both cognitive and behavioural techniques in their practice. This integration of the two approaches has led to the use of the term *cognitive behaviour therapy*.

Principles of assessment

Behavioural and cognitive therapies may sometimes appear to be technique-bound, using almost a cookbook approach. This is a misunderstanding derived in part from the fact that research studies of behavioural and cognitive therapies use operational definitions of exactly what techniques should be used, and often employ manuals describing how the therapy should be conducted. Clinical practice needs to be more flexible, and for this type of therapy to be effective it needs to be grounded in a good formulation of the individual patient's problems. The basis of this is a *cognitive behavioural analysis*.

Both behavioural and cognitive therapies are essentially problem-solving therapies. The starting point is the presenting problem as defined by the patient. A detailed description of the problem is taken, trying to define behaviourally exactly what happens, when it happens and in what circumstances. Particular attention is given to the cues or triggers for the problem, what actually happens, and the consequences such as any rewarding effects of the behaviour. The current attempts at coping and their success are also examined. It is important to assess the frequency of the problems, initially from the patient's description and then from self-monitoring or observation.

In building up a picture of the problem behaviour or emotional difficulty, attention is paid to four systems: behavioural, cognitive, affective and physiological. For instance, if someone has anger problems the therapist will want to know what thoughts or images go through the patient's mind when the anger is triggered, what the anger feels like and how strong it is, what physical changes occur, such as raised heart rate or muscular tension, and finally what the person does as a result of the anger.

This cross-sectional assessment needs to be put into the context of the person's life as a whole. Still in the here and now, the therapist tries to understand how the problem affects the person's social, personal and work functioning. What factors might be maintaining the problem such as avoidance (important in phobias and obsessions) or reinforcement (in problem behaviours such as violence, sexual deviations etc.)? Looking at the history, the therapist asks about the duration of the problems, previous episodes and other psychological problems. The history can give indications of predisposing factors, triggers for episodes and past strengths and coping abilities.

Wherever possible, cognitive and behavioural therapists use objective measures such as direct observation of the problem, the use of behavioural tests (e.g. at what distance can a spider phobic tolerate a spider in the room?), self-monitoring, and standardised question-naires (e.g. the Beck Depression Inventory).

Finally, the issue of motivation is a difficult one. It is not easy to measure or assess objectively. For most therapy the patient must be prepared to carry out the behavioural assignments or to try using the cognitive techniques and must give an undertaking to do this both in the session and in the form of homework tasks.

Principles of treatment

Exposure therapy

Exposure therapy is a simple but highly effective technique used particularly in the treatment of phobias and obsessive-compulsive disorders. As with many cognitive and behavioural techniques, active participation of the client is necessary for the therapy to be effective. The first step in therapy therefore involves the explanation of the rationale of exposure. Patients are taught about the nature and function of anxiety and told that symptoms, although unpleasant, are not dangerous. They are told that with exposure the anxiety symptoms will gradually diminish with time. The patient and therapist then construct a hierarchy of feared situations, and the patient is encouraged to systematically confront these feared situations in a graded way. The hierarchy is constructed so that there is a gradual increase in the feared characteristics of the stimuli at each stage. For example, a patient with a spider might find size, movement and hairiness as the salient features that induce fear. Exposure could start with looking at pictures of spider, then television programmes. The next step might be to hold a toy spider. Exposure to live spiders could then begin with small spiders seen at a distance and brought progressively closer. Once the patient can tolerate holding a small spider in the hand the process is repeated with bigger, livelier and more hairy specimens. Part of the skill of therapy is working out a list of feared stimuli that allows as rapid a progress as possible without the patient becoming overwhelmed with anxiety.

Initial sessions may require therapist-aided exposure, but most patients can then go on to carry out homework assignments on their own. Exposure is more effective if it is in real life rather than imagination (Emmelkamp & Wessels, 1975), prolonged rather than brief (Stern & Marks, 1973) and practised regularly with self-exposure tasks (McDonald et al., 1978). Spouses may be employed as co-therapists to help patients with exposure assignments (Mathews et al., 1981). Modelling has also been employed as an aid to exposure (Bandura, 1971): if a patient is too frightened to approach a feared stimulus, the therapist can model a coping response, e.g. by approaching and handling a spider. More recent work has shown that many patients can carry out self-exposure effectively with only minimal intervention from the therapist (Marks, 1987),

In obsessive-compulsive disorder, exposure is combined with *response prevention*. Obsess-ional fears are neutralised by rituals, such as checking, handwashing, etc. For example, a patient with contamination fears became anxious when exposed to household dust because he feared that it might contain lead and other toxic materials and if his hands became contaminated he might inadvertently poison someone. He avoided situations where he feared he might be contaminated, but also carried out prolonged handwashing rituals to neutralise the obsession when he was contaminated. Therapy consisted of a combination of graded and prolonged exposure to feared stimuli with the additional component of preventing any neutralising rituals. The patient and therapist jointly constructed a hierarchy of graded steps involving increasing fears of contamination (e.g. from dusting the hospital office accompanied by the therapist to cleaning the toilet at home). Beforehand the patient agreed to refrain from carrying out attempts to clean his hands. In treating obsessions, attention needs to be given to covert rituals (saying things or repeating phrases, etc.) and to generalisation from safe situations where the therapist sanctions exposure to more dangerous situations outside the control of the therapist.

Operant conditioning

Operant conditioning techniques are based on the principle that behaviour that is followed by pleasant consequences is likely to increase in frequency, while behaviour that is followed by unpleasant consequences will be less likely to be repeated (the so called *Law of Effect*; Thorndike, 1898). Through a careful behavioural analysis, the links between the circumstances in which a particular behaviour occurs and the consequences of the behaviour are established. To change a behaviour, operant techniques can address either the setting conditions or the reinforcing consequences. Changing *stimulus control* involves changing the cues for a particular behaviour. For example, if someone with insomnia spends much of the night awake in bed thinking or reading, bed becomes associated with behaviours other than sleeping. Part of therapy is to institute the rule 'beds are for sleeping' and ensure that when the sufferer has been awake for more than 10 minutes he gets out of bed, returning when he feels sleepy again.

The behavioural analysis will show how unwanted behaviour is being reinforced or how desirable behaviour is not receiving reinforcement. What is aversive or rewarding will vary between individuals and cannot be assumed. In the past, behaviour modification has relied too much on tangible rewards like food or cigarettes, where in fact human behaviour is reinforced by more subtle factors like social contact and praise. Undesirable behaviour can be reduced by punishment, or by withholding reinforcement until the behaviour is extinguished, or discontinues. *Aversive techniques* can be effective but often elicit aversive emotional reactions that complicate the process of relearning. They are also contentious ethically. In practice they are confined to cases where the behaviour to be punished is life-threatening or has dire social consequences, e.g. substance misuse and some sexual deviations. More commonly, undesirable behaviour is reduced by replacing it with a more socially acceptable behaviour, which is reinforced, e.g. orgasmic reconditioning in sexual problems. Wherever possible, therapists look for ways to reinforce prosocial behaviour by pairing it with a reward. The closer the time relationship between the behaviour and the reward the better. Of course, the target behaviour is not always present at the beginning of therapy. Initially it may be necessary to reward an approximation to the desired goal and then to shape the response by rewarding successively closer approximations.

Operant conditioning techniques lend themselves well to single case study designs. A behaviour that is to be increased is measured at baseline and a change observed with the intervention. When the intervention is stopped the behaviour is seen to decrease in frequency. A direct causal relationship can be established, but the strength of this method is also its weakness, because in many situations the clinician wants the behavioural change to persist when therapy has stopped. There are various ways in which generalisation of behavioural change can be encouraged. One method is to degrade the relationship between stimulus and response by giving only intermittent *reinforcement*. Theorists have argued that by giving the patient more responsibility for regulating and rewarding his or her own behaviour improvements can be maintained after therapy (Kanfer & Karoly, 1972).

Skills training

Another important component of any cognitive-behavioural work is skills training. This approach is not based on a single model of learning, and in fact often uses operant techniques to help reinforce and maintain gains in skills. The skills training approach usually involves a cognitive-behavioural analysis of the skills deficits, followed by teaching the skill and a period of practice with feedback within the session as well as practice outside the session. This method has been applied to a variety of skills. Problem-solving was originally introduced by D'Zurilla & Goldfried (1971). There is evidence that some patients who experience repeated life crises and resort to parasuicide have problem-solving deficits (Hawton & Catalan, 1987). Problem-solving training has been used with crisis intervention and suicidal patients (Hawton & Catalan, 1987). Difficulties in interpersonal skills are found in people with chronic mental illness, marital problems and in the parents of children with behavioural problems. *Social skills training* has been used in depression (Bellack *et al.*, 1983), social phobia (Trower *et al.*, 1978), and schizophrenia (Falloon, 1988). A skills training approach is also used in *assertiveness training*, and *anxiety management training*.

Relaxation and *biofeedback* can also be conceptualised as skills. They are often taught in behaviour therapy as coping skills. Ost (1987) has developed a form of *applied relaxation* in which the patient is taught a simple relaxation technique and learns how to apply it in everyday settings. Bernstein & Borkovec (1973) describe another useful method. The training involves practising to detect and control the muscular sensations involved in tension and relaxation. The patient is taught to go through cycles of inducing tension and then relaxing the tension away, progressing to deeper levels of relaxation as all the muscles of the body are covered. Training then proceeds to practising relaxation with self-instruction so that the individual may begin to apply control of tension when it is induced by environmental stimuli. Generalisation may be improved by the use of cue stickers in the environment to prompt the use of the developing skill.

Cognitive therapy

Cognitive techniques are frequently used in combination with the treatment methods described above. However, cognitive therapy as a treatment in its own right has been shown to be effective in depression, generalised anxiety, panic and hypochondriasis.

The next section describes cognitive therapy in some detail and indicates how it uses behavioural techniques from within a *cognitive* model as well as purely cognitive interventions.

General characteristics

Cognitive therapy, like other behavioural and cognitive-behavioural approaches, is a time-limited, structured therapy aimed at helping individuals cope with emotional problems and achieve symptom relief as well as deal with associated life problems. The therapy takes place in weekly 50 minute sessions (12–20 sessions in total) spaced over 3–6 months. It is a directive, educational approach based upon the cognitive model of emotional disorder and not a string of techniques thrown arbitrarily together. Its successful application rests upon a sound therapeutic relationship being established in which patient and therapist work together to achieve joint therapeutic goals. Beck coined the term 'collaborative empiricism' to describe the special nature of the relationship in cognitive therapy where patient and therapist test out the hypotheses of the cognitive model as applied to the patient's problems. The therapy teaches a sceptical approach to cognitive events, encourages achieving distance from thoughts as a prelude to learning to modify them and thereby gain control over powerful negative feelings.

Beck's cognitive model (Beck, 1976)

Whereas formerly negative thinking had been seen as a symptom of an emotion such as depression, a consequence of an emotional disorder/brain state, Beck introduced the notion that thinking had a causative status, that depressive symptoms develop as a result of the activation of maladaptive information processing structures that affect the way information is subjected to selective attention; memories are selectively recalled, particular meaning is attached to events and events responded to. Beck hypothesised that these structures are laid down in childhood and embody immature, global and absolute features of cognition in relation to childhood experiences. Once formed they can remain inactive or latent for many years only to be reactivated by an event that resembles the information content of the earlier events. The result of the structure's activation is that current information becomes processed in a biased way, resulting in thought content that is dominated by negative thinking about the self, the world and the future (the cognitive triad). It is this conjunction of negative cognitions or beliefs that Beck hypothesised to be responsible for the development of the full range of symptoms: motivational, affective, physiological, behavioural and cognitive. A vicious circle develops between symptoms and thoughts such that more symptoms result in more negative thinking and more negative thoughts result in more intense symptoms, leading to a potential spiralling downward into more severe states.

Therapy overview

The initial phase of therapy concentrates on listening to the patient's account of their problems and forming a conceptualisation in terms of the cognitive model of the patient's problems. At the same time, the patient is introduced to the ideas and structure of the therapy including the use of homework assignments. Behavioural techniques are used to test out negative thoughts with a view to initial symptom management. As symptoms improve, thought monitoring is introduced and then challenging of negative thoughts to deal with distorted perceptions and inferences. The final stages of therapy deal with the identification and challenging of dysfunctional assumptions and preparation for future problems as a means of relapse prevention.

Behavioural techniques

Behavioural technology is utilised in cognitive therapy in many ways: in the manner in which problems are identified and defined in concrete and measurable terms; in the use of concrete goal-setting; in the use of monitoring tasks throughout therapy. Behavioural techniques are used as a major therapeutic tool to manage symptoms whenever mood is intense at the beginning of therapy or at later stages in therapy. The aim in cognitive terms is to decrease the frequency of negative thinking and thus to improve symptoms. Techniques called upon will depend on the particular problems the patient presents but frequently involve increasing the patient's level of activity and engagement in pleasant and rewarding tasks and interactions to increase his or her experience of positive feelings of pleasure, achievement and relaxation and to reduce negative ruminations. At all times these interventions are used in sessions to furnish evidence for the cognitive model, to point out where predictions are erroneous, where positive experiences are dismissed or minimised, where self-expectations are unrealistic and how these negative interpretations contribute to emotional responses and behavioural and environmental consequences.

Cognitive techniques

Cognitive techniques are used by the therapist from the first session in applying the cognitive model to the patient's problems and pointing out less damaging alternatives, particularly those arising from the patient's own specific experiences.

Formal cognitive techniques are introduced to the patient when symptom intensity is decreasing and specific episodes of negative thinking can be identified. Probably the principal technique in use is a diary to monitor upsetting experiences and associated negative thoughts on a daily basis. The patient is likely to need considerable help in sessions to identify the specific thoughts in question and in the use of a structured monitoring sheet. Excellent self-help reading material is available to aid the process of explanation (e.g. Fennell, 1989). Techniques such as *mental action replay* are used to bring an incident vividly back to mind in session with a view to identifying negative automatic thoughts. Other techniques include role-play of interpersonal scenarios or exposure to specific cues or bodily sensations that are subject to misinterpretation.

After learning to identify thoughts, the patient is introduced to ways of challenging them, that is, subjecting them to scrutiny to assess their accuracy and usefulness. It is important that the therapist does not take on a too hectoring or bullying stance in this work. Beck emphasises the use of *Socratic questioning* in challenging thoughts, that is using questions that lead the patient in coming to his/her own conclusions. Persuading or arguing with the patient is likely to be counterproductive. In many cases the patient's thoughts may well be true, in which case the therapist needs to help the patient find the underlying meaning that makes the thought so arousing of emotion. For example, a negative thought such as 'she didn't look at me' may be true. It is only when the meaning of the consequences of this being true is explored that the distortion becomes apparent – the patient may say 'she didn't look at me, because she doesn't love me any more'.

There are five principal ways of challenging thoughts:

1. What is the evidence to support and contradict this idea? The patient is taught to weigh the thought against the balance of relevant evidence, thus bringing into focus the evidence against, which tends to be overlooked as a result of selective memory bias. Often the evidence may be insufficient and a behavioural experiment may be devised to gather relevant evidence, often involving important behavioural changes, e.g. expressing feelings or revealing weakness to test out other people's reactions.
2. Is there an alternative way of looking at this and what is the evidence with respect to the alternative? The patient is taught to open up the range of their perspective and to frame the event/thought in a different way. Looking at the event through someone else's eyes may aid this process.
3. What is the effect of thinking this way? The patient can remind him/herself of the dysfunctionality of the negative interpretation and how it may lead to self-defeating consequences, including confirmation of the negative thought.
4. What cognitive error am I making? The patient can spot their overgeneralisations, black-and-white thinking, etc. as an aid to answering the negative thought.
5. Supposing the thought is true, what does it mean about you, the world, the future? The patient can then challenge both the validity of the underlying thought and the reasoning by which he/she reaches it.

As a result of these challenges the patient can produce answers to his or her original thought that may effect their emotions. Often patients will need several sessions to work on and finally deal with key disturbing thoughts that have troubled them for some time.

After several weeks spent in monitoring negative automatic thoughts and the events that cue them, the therapist will have a clearer idea about the patient's underlying dysfunctional assumptions, i.e. the basic beliefs about the subjective meaning of events that are associated with emotional disorders. It is important that these are derived collaboratively with the patient rather than delivered as an interpretation, as the patient must acknowledge them to take the work to this more abstract level and indeed they can be so idiosyncratic that the patient's active co-operation in identifying them is essential.

Challenging dysfunctional assumptions can involve the same questioning as in dealing with automatic thoughts. However, their more abstract nature makes them less susceptible to challenges with reference to the evidence. More use is made of pointing to their dysfunctionality, to the consequences of holding such beliefs with regard to negative emotional states, goal attainment and other people's welfare. Finally, challenging involves further behavioural change and experiment in acting contrary to these beliefs and testing out the consequences. One of the implications of this work, later in therapy, is that it involves placing the patient up against his/her vulnerability and acts to strengthen their ability to deal with negative events.

The final stages in therapy include the recapitulation of what has been learned in therapy and the formulation of a plan to deal with future problems.

Applications of cognitive and behavioural therapy

Phobias

There is now a substantial body of clinical and research evidence for the effectiveness of behaviour therapy in phobias. Exposure is most effective with simple phobias such as animal phobias, and there is now evidence that one long exposure session may be sufficient for many patients (Ost, 1989; Ost et al., 1991). About two-thirds of agoraphobics are successfully treated with exposure alone (Mathews et al., 1981), and these gains are maintained at two year follow-up (Munby & Johnston, 1980). Social phobia has also been effectively treated with exposure. (Butler et al., 1984). These effects are not due to non-specific factors (Gelder et al., 1973). Despite these successes a percentage of patients do not improve, and this had led to an interest in combining cognitive techniques with exposure. There is some evidence that adding anxiety management or cognitive procedures enhances the effects of exposure in social phobia (Butler et al., 1984; Butler, 1989; Mattick & Peters, 1988). The cognitive emphasis is on identifying the idiosyncratic meaning of the phobic stimulus. In agoraphobia this is often related to fears of losing control or passing out, and it has been suggested that by devising specific behavioural experiments in combination with cognitive techniques much briefer exposure times might be possible. One study (van den Hout et al., 1994) found specific effects of cognitive therapy and exposure in panic and agoraphobia: cognitive therapy reduces panic frequency, but does not overcome avoidance, whereas exposure reduces agoraphobic avoidance but not panic.

Obsessive-compulsive disorder

Until the advent of behaviour therapy the prognosis for obsessive-compulsive disorder was very poor. Exposure with response prevention has produced a median success rate of 75% improvement in patients who are able to complete treatment. This is superior to the results from drug trials. Foa & Goldstein (1978) showed that a combination of exposure and response prevention seems to be most effective. Marks (1987) recommends home-based exposure as the most efficient form of treatment. In severe cases this may need to be preceded by a brief hospital admission. In hospital, 24-hour response prevention has been shown to produce a success rate of 85% (Foa & Goldstein, 1978). In most therapist-aided exposure the therapist uses modelling, but this does not seem to substantially improve results (Emmelkamp, 1982). Involving the family in treatment may enhance the effects of exposure (Emmelkamp, 1982). Despite the successes of behaviour therapy, 50% of patients with OCD are not helped because of treatment refusal, dropout or failure (Salkovskis, 1989). The role of cognitive techniques in the treatment of OCD remains controversial. An early study did not show any benefits of adding self-instructional training to exposure (Emmelkamp *et al.*, 1980), but others have demonstrated that cognitive therapy was as effective as exposure (Emmelkamp *et al.*, 1988; van Oppen *et al.*, 1995). With patients who experience obsessional ruminations but do not ritualise, exposure has been less effective.

Generalised anxiety, panic disorder and hypochondriasis

The application of exposure therapy to generalised anxiety and panic is limited because there are not always clear-cut phobic situations or signs of avoidance. Cognitive therapy has a great deal to offer these patients. Beck's model of anxiety stresses the way in which the anxious patient develops a view of the self as vulnerable, the world as dangerous and threatening and the future as unpredictable. As with depression, therapy involves teaching the patient the cognitive model of anxiety, then helping to identify and challenge negative automatic thoughts. Butler *et al.* (1991) compared cognitive therapy and behaviour therapy and found a superiority for cognitive therapy, particularly at six month follow-up.

The cognitive model of panic (Clark, 1986) stresses the specific interpretations the patient makes about the physical symptoms associated with panic. According to this model, catastrophic misattributions are made about symptoms such as palpitations, dizziness, faintness, breathlessness, etc., which are really due to autonomic manifestations of anxiety, but are seen as signs of impending death, madness or loss of control. A vicious circle develops in which the automatic thoughts produce more anxiety and therefore more symptoms. Therapy consists of helping the patient to test his or her attributions through logical discussion and setting up behavioural experiments. Beck *et al.* (1992) showed cognitive therapy to be more effective than supportive psychotherapy. Clark *et al.* (1994) compared cognitive therapy, imipramine, applied relaxation and a waiting-list control. The active treatments were all more effective than the waiting-list, and cognitive therapy was the most effective treatment post-treatment and at follow-up. Cognitive therapy has also been shown to reduce the relapse rate in panic patients who initially respond to alprazolam (Spiegal *et al.*, 1994).

The cognitive approach to hypochondriasis is similar to panic. The model suggests that patients misinterpret bodily symptoms as signs of physical illness, but do not believe they are about to die immediately. Reassurance-seeking and avoidance act to maintain the hypo-chondriacal beliefs. Cognitive therapy helps patients set up an alternative explanation for their symptoms, while behaviour therapy stresses a ban on reassurance-seeking and overcoming avoidance. Both treatments have been shown to be effective (Salkovskis & Warwick, 1986; Warwick & Marks, 1988).

Depression

Beck's cognitive therapy (CT) has been the psychological therapy subjected to the most extensive evaluation, possibly because of the clarity with which it has been described, the author's phenomenal energy in teaching worldwide and its theoretical face-validity and attractiveness. It is now widely accepted as effective in comparison with tricyclic antidepress-ant medication (the most frequent comparison) in non-psychotic, unipolar, out-patient patients, in many settings and in various parts of the world (see Dobson, 1989 for a meta-analysis of 28 studies and Hollon *et al.*, 1991, 1993 for two cautious reviews). Studies comparing CT with other psychological treatments, though few in number using clinical referrals, have also generally produced results favourable to CT. The largest study,which also produced the poorest result for cognitive therapy, is worthy of specific comment. Elkin *et al.* (1989) mounted a large, multi-centre sample of 250 patients randomly allocated between CT, Interpersonal Psychotherapy (IPT, see below), tricyclic pharmacotherapy and placebo. This study produced few significant differences between the groups taking the sample as a whole and a significant advantage of pharmacotherapy and for IPT on some measures for more severely depressed subjects. CT did no better than placebo with more severely depressed subjects. Hollon *et al.* pointed out that between-centre differences would suggest differences in the adequacy with which CT was being carried out in this study and they question the adequacy of training and supervision of therapists. Such an observation raises the issue of CT being a practically complicated even if theoretically simple approach. Further investigation of both the effects of training on competency and of the effects of variations in competency on outcome would seem indicated, also the impact of simplified and more programmed versions of CT.

One of the most interesting theoretical aspects of CT is its claim to change underlying cognitive vulnerability to depression through the modification of dysfunctional assumptions. Several follow-up studies have indicated that such optimism may be justified (e.g. Blackburn *et al.*, 1986; Evans *et al.*, 1992). However, studies have not had sufficient statistical power to yield significant differences between groups and the difficulties, practical and theoretical, in designing a lengthy follow-up study are considerable.

Other cognitive behavioural therapies for depression emphasise the behavioural component more strongly than Beck. Lewinsohn and colleagues developed a cognitive-behavioural therapy based on operant principles targeting interpersonal behaviour. They developed a highly structured 12-session programme involving increasing pleasant interpersonal interactions and decreasing aversive interactions through a multi-component treatment including a variety of social learning tactics: planning activities, monitoring, relaxation training, cognitive skills, assertiveness training, etc. Lewinsohn *et al.* (1987) have developed a group-based educational course (the Coping with Depression Course) on the same lines and have adapted this to the treatment of adolescents and the elderly and to the prevention of depression in depression-prone individuals. Lewinsohn's behavioural approach has been compared with a waiting-list control and found effective (Hoberman *et al.*, 1988).

Becker *et al.* (1987) developed a programme composed of four components: social skills training, social perception training, practice, self-evaluation and self-reinforcement. Training is applied across different interpersonal settings. Three behavioural skills are emphasised: negative assertion (standing up for yourself), positive assertion (expressing positive feelings, giving compliments etc.) and conversational skills.

Eating disorders

Early work with patients with eating disorders concentrated on increasing weight in anorexics using an operant conditioning approach in in-patient settings. Later research showed that a structured regime of this sort had no advantage over good in-patient nursing. More recent work has focused on bulimia from a cognitive behavioural perspective. Fairburn & Cooper (1989) have suggested that bulimics have maladaptive beliefs about shape and weight, particularly a tendency to judge self-worth in terms of shape and weight. This promotes dieting. Strict dietary control and perfectionistic attitudes mean that any lapse from the diet is seen as catastrophic and leads to a temporary abandonment of all control over eating. Therapy consists of monitoring binges and food intake, adopting a more normal dietary pattern and challenging maladaptive beliefs. Fairburn et al. (1991) compared cognitive behaviour therapy (CBT), behaviour therapy and interpersonal therapy. All treatments produced improvements, but cognitive therapy was more effective than the other treatments in modifying disturbed attitudes to shape and weight and reducing extreme dieting. CBT has been found to be more effective than imipramine (Mitchell et al., 1990).

Anorexia nervosa has not been as fully investigated. Cooper & Fairburn (1984) described a series of cases of anorexia nervosa treated with CBT. Controlled trials have found cognitive and behavioural treatments of anorexia to be effective (Channon et al., 1989) with an improvement in up to two-thirds of cases (Treasure et al., 1995).

Chronic mental illness

Behavioural techniques have had a place in the rehabilitation of patients with long-term mental illness for many years. Pioneering work was done by Ayllon & Azrin (1968) using token economies. The restrictive nature of these methods does not fit well with modern principles of normalisation, which encourage patients to take an active part in their care, and in fact the token economy may not add anything to what a motivated and enthusiastic set of staff might achieve (Hall et al., 1977). Nevertheless, operant conditioning principles are still valuable in rehabilitation settings and an approach that emphasises problem definition, identifying goals and using social reinforcement is widespread in the rehabilitation field. Many programmes combine a skills approach with social reinforcement. A set of skills that need to be developed are identified with the patient, and a graded approach to attaining the skills developed

Recent developments in work with schizophrenia have used cognitive behavioural family interventions to teach problem solving skills (Falloon, 1988), reduce high expressed emotion (Leff et al., 1982) and to teach patients and families to recognise early signs of relapse (Birchwood et al., 1989). These interventions have had real effects on relapse rates.

Another exciting development is the application of cognitive behavioural principles in coping with psychotic symptoms (Tarrier et al., 1990) and even challenging delusional ideas (Kingdon & Turkington, 1994; Fowler et al., 1995).

Learning difficulties

Operant conditioning techniques have been widely used with adults and children with learning difficulties (Yule & Carr, 1980). Recent work has increased the sophistication of the learning theory by looking at the social and cognitive aspects of challenging behaviour. Self-injurious behaviour can be seen as an attempt to communicate, and therefore teaching the person an effective way of communicating their needs to their carers can reduce the challenging behaviour (Durand, 1990).

Neurotic problems are now also receiving attention. Allen (1989) has described *behavioural relaxation training* specifically developed for people with learning difficulties. Anger management training has also been applied with this client group (Black *et al.*, 1988), and Williams & Moorey (1989) have described case reports of cognitive behavioural work with three clients with anger and anxiety problems. Lindsay *et al.* (1993) reported two case-studies of cognitive therapy for depression in this client group.

Conclusions

There is not space in this chapter to describe all the applications of cognitive and behavioural methods. We have not been able to cover the use of these techniques with children (Meyers & Craighead, 1984), substance misuers (e.g. Marlett & Gordon, 1985; Moorey, 1989), sexual deviation (Laws, 1989) and in behavioural medicine (e.g. Hodes & Moorey, 1993; Moorey & Greer, 1989). Cognitive behavioural techniques (summarised here as exposure therapy, operant conditioning, skills training and cognitive therapy) have a wide application across the whole spectrum of psychiatric work and beyond. Their emphasis on clearly defined, teachable procedures and the measurement of change means that it has been possible to demonstrate their effectiveness. In a health service with limited resources these cost-effective treatment cannot be ignored, and all psychiatrists should have a working knowledge of them.

Psychotherapy

CHRISTOPHER DARE

B. ANALYTICALLY INFORMED

Introduction

In previous editions of this book, there have been detailed accounts as to the conduct of psychoanalytic psychotherapy, the indications for the treatment and the research basis for its use. The range of psychological treatments in mental health practice is constantly increasing and for all patients the type and intensity of psychological treatment required must be considered in setting up a rational plan of management. Parry (1992) has surveyed the current scientific status of the provision of psychotherapy within the health services. The cost of psychoanalytic psychotherapy has been considered to be problematic for its use within publically funded services (see Fahy & Wessely, 1993), although the true cost effectiveness of the treatment remains unclear (see APA Commission on Psychotherapy, 1982, Chapter 16; McGovern *et al.*, 1990; Krupnick & Pincus, 1992).

It has been the ambition of many psychiatrists, including some psychoanalytic psychotherapists, to bring their subject into line with other treatments in psychiatry. This ambition seems to remain as far as ever from fulfilment and one way of exploring the topic of the chapter is by enquiring as to why this might be so. The chapter describes some of the curious features of the subject matter, and outlines aspects of the nature of the practice of psychoanalytic psychotherapy, especially brief applications.

The nature of psychoanalytic psychotherapy

Psychoanalytic treatments have peculiar aspects which can only be understood by considering their historical evolution and the nature of the ideas informing the therapies. By the middle of the twentieth century it appeared to many that psychoanalysis had run its course. Eysenk (1952*b*, 1966) had analysed the accumulated available data and shown that psychotherapy was no more effective than the control treatments. Popper (1959) as a philosopher had enunciated a clear notion of the qualities that defined scientific research, from which it was obvious that psychoanalysis did not constitute a scientifically constructed body of knowledge. Medawar (1967), a pre-eminent biologist, had endorsed this view. Psychoanalysis was declared a non-science (and therefore nonsense) and the therapy derived from it was useless. From time to time serious commentators have felt it necessary to repeat the message, that psychoanalysis was inconsequential. And yet, at the end of the twentieth century, psychoanalysis is not only not dead, but the psychotherapy associated with it is a fast-growing body of practice. Training courses in the therapy are arduous, expensive and receive, in the main, no form of subsidy or official support and yet an enlarging group of private institutions in the UK appear to flourish and have no problem recruiting candidates for training. Graduates from the courses mostly appear to acquire a full timetable of patients in therapy. In recent years, in Britain, university degrees are being developed in the theory of psychoanalysis and postgraduate degrees and diplomas in the therapeutic practice have been established.

In Europe also, psychoanalysis is not dead. Truckle (1992) has looked at the phenomenon of the evolution of psychoanalysis in France. She shows that in the first 20 years, following the Second World War, psychoanalysis was shunned by psychiatrists, philosophers and politicians. After 1968, the situation was transformed: from there being a score or so French practitioners calling themselves psychoanalysts, there were, by the end of the 1980s many thousands claiming the title (albeit dubiously). Psychoanalytic thinking grew to be accorded a special place in literary, philosophical, social and political thinking. In Germany, Spain, Italy and Switzerland, the subject flourishes. In the Netherlands, the state had supported an enormous programme ensuring the wide availability of psychoanalytic psychotherapy. There, the enthusiasm of the patients for the treatment led to alarm in the state and private health insurance agencies paying for the treatments; state action followed to constrain the demand. In the United States, the picture is unclear. North American psychoanalysts bemoan the withering of the flow of patients available for intensive psychoanalytic treatment and a fall-off in applications for training. The starting position for this apparent decline is from a vast and prestigious organisation, membership of psychoanalytic institutions being much more numerous *per capita* than in Europe. Despite the current pessimism amongst psychoanalysts, the influence of psychoanalytic thinking has been much more widespread, in the USA in comparison with elsewhere, in the mental health fields of psychiatry, psychology and social work and in the academic faculties of philosophy, history and social sciences. At present, in the USA, although ostensibly in decline, psychoanalytic psychotherapy is widely available (along with a myriad of other psychotherapies).

Considerations as to how psychoanalytic psychotherapy can be viewed

The psychiatrist in the contemporary world can survey the phenomenon of psychoanalysis and its hold in the areas mentioned: What attitude can be taken? What is the place of psychoanalytic thinking in psychiatry and what is the clinical relevance of psychoanalytic psychotherapy?

There are a number of possible approaches for the contemporary psychiatrist:

1. The traditional dismissal can be maintained ('We shoot psychoanalysts on sight' as the author was hospitably informed in a US Department of Clinical Psychology).
2. The subject can be taken to be coherent enough to be swallowed whole and retailed as the conceptual and serviceable answer to the whole of the theory and practice in mental health.
3. The subject can be taken seriously, accepted as a conceptual system, like any other, and as a proclaimed treatment, as are so many. Both the theory and the therapy can be considered as a suitable subject for empirical testing; those aspects that pass the tests to be incorporated into the general body of knowledge and clinical activity.
4. The theory, so-called psychoanalytic psychology, can be studied without taking it to be an empirical, scientifically evolved subject. The question can be asked, what is psychoanalysis actually about? Why is it constructed as it is? What are its variants? Why do they exist? What determines their differences and their influence?
5. The theory can be declared irrelevant, and the question asked, does the psychotherapy work? With what patients? And what, if any, are the effective ingredients? What does it do if it does work?
6. Another approach is possible. The phenomenon of psychoanalysis as a whole can be observed as existing and as a subject of study, like the history of a people, or a language. Truckle (1992) has investigated the case of psychoanalysis in France using this approach. She takes no sides in any discussions as to whether psychoanalysis is 'true' or whether it works. She approaches it as a social phenomenon that languished in France and then became enormously influential publicly and intellectually. She plots the process, linking it to the events of the student and worker protests of 1968.

The point of view of this chapter excludes the possibilities (1) and (2) and is sympathetic to two approaches (4) to (6). The approach listed as (3) is taken to be mistaken.

Science and psychoanalysis

Psychoanalysis was believed by Freud, its inceptor, to be a genuine science of the mind and this view has been accepted by many subsequent adherents. However, Freud's method was modelled on that of Darwin, the enquiring observer, identifying new phenomena in nature to be shaped into an extensive innovative theoretical view (Jones, 1953a; Sulloway, 1979; Gray, 1988). Freud had been able to identify new tracts in the nervous system of the lamphrey (quoted in Sulloway 1979, page 15), to observe the pharmacological properties of cocaine (1884 but published in English, Freud, 1974) and to untangle the clinical and neuropathological picture of the aphasias using the available scientific techniques. He and his followers believed that psychoanalysis and psychoanalytic treatment evolved by means of identical and therefore scientific methods. It has been argued (e.g. by Isaacs, 1939) that the process of making an interpretation itself constitutes a genuine empirical, scientific process. Isaacs suggested that the psychoanalytic psychotherapist makes an hypothesis about the current psychological status of the patient and forms this into an interpretation. Wisdom (1967), a philosopher and psychoanalyst, has elaborated a thoughtful critique of this idea. The patient's response to the communication of the interpretation is noted, and the psychotherapist then modifies the overall understanding of the patient, in turn revising subsequent interpretations, communicates them and the cycle is repeated. Spence (1982, 1986) has described this logic as suffering from the 'fallacy of the confirming instance'(1986). However superficially plausible such a view is and whatever the aspirations and claims of psychoanalysis, it is not a subject that can be taken to be a science as are the experimental subjects of neuropharmacology or metallurgy. The methodology of the subject has diverged from the particular refining process that has characterised the detailed empirical evaluation and evolution of twentieth-century experimental psychology and psychiatry. The latter have apparently accepted a model stemming from the physical sciences. Adherents of this strategy often find psychoanalysis incomprehensible and negligible, but also, somehow, disturbing, sinister and potentially dangerous: a force, possibly, for evil with no conceivable beneficial value.

Psychoanalysis is a subject that started using a biological, scientific approach, making observations, constructing a theory, making further observations, modifying the theory, re-examining the data, and in turn, modifying the theory. It is interesting to ask the question as to why it ceased to go in the direction of descriptive biology, how it failed to incorporate other forms of experimental investigation. It is true to say that Freud and his earliest followers came to believe that they had discovered a truth that was unpalatable to most people. In particular they believed that the theory of motivation by unconscious mental contents, most derived from intense and diverse sexual drives, was largely unacceptable. This unacceptability was intrinsic, because conscious recognition of these drives has been designed out of the human mind in order to create a civilised, cultured society in which people became decorous and refined in their expression of sexual needs. The teleological, quasi-Lamarckian views implicit in this description of man's social evolution represented, perhaps, a failure on the part of the earliest psychoanalysts to fully absorb a Darwinian understanding. The result of the belief in an inevitable resistance to the acknowledgement of psychoanalysis, intensified a tendency to inspect any alterations or revisions of psychoanalytic theory as revealing a wish to discard the fundamental and unpalatable aspects.

However, this critique is incomplete because it would imply that psychoanalysis was totally rigid and unchanging and this is far from the case. It is certainly true to say that from the perspective of a psychoanalyst, reviews of psychoanalysis by non-analysts often set up an archaic version of the subject matter as an Aunt Sally to be demolished. Psychoanalysis does change, new data are incorporated, theories are radically modified and technique evolves (Figure 25.3, later in the chapter, maps some of the current diversity). It is also obvious that psychoanalysis has widened the knowledge base upon which it is built as can be seen from the incorporation of information from direct clinical and formal empirical studies of children (Spitz, 1957; Bowlby, 1969; Mahler et al., 1975; Brazelton, 1982; Stern, 1985; Emde & Sameroff, 1989; Brazelton & Cramer, 1991). Clinical, psychoanalytic studies of family interaction (Stierlin, 1975; Boszormenyi, Nagy & Spark, 1982) and of stranger groups (Bion,

1961; Foulkes, 1975) have also been conducted and are potentially sources of data for psychoanalytic theorising. The methodology remains crucially clinical in its orientation and the subject matter is of personal, subjective experience. These factors have a profound effect upon the structure of psychoanalytic thinking which, in turn, stamps its mark upon the practice of psychoanalytic psychotherapy.

It remains true to say that there is a mutual suspicion: Empirically orientated and academic psychiatrists and psychologists tend to believe that psychoanalytic psychotherapy is empty theorising conducted at the expense of denying real treatment to patients. Psychoanalytic psychotherapists often talk as though they believe that empirical studies are mere number-crunching activities that eliminate the essential differences, affects and intense subjectivity that characterises that which is human about human experience.

This chapter cannot hope to bridge this gap of suspicion. It presents two themes, a major and a minor one. The first is that of the nature of the psychoanalytic approach to psychotherapy, its application and its effectiveness. The second theme is addressed only insofar as it is needed to understand the main theme: it is to do with the nature of psychoanalytic descriptions of the human condition.

A history of psychoanalysis

In a later section, the evolution of contemporary psychoanalytic models will describe the development of object relations theory. The history of the early origins of psychoanalytic ideas is summarised in Figure 25.1.

Sigmund Freud's intellectual forebears are multiple, but in the diagram a few sources are highlighted. In the first instance, on the left, are denoted what Ellenberger (1970) has called the 'dynamic psychiatries' within which the phenomenon of hypnotism had given rise to the notion of aspects of the mind outside of consciousness that could motivate feelings and behaviour. The philosopher Wittgenstein thought that Freud was influenced by a general nineteenth century preoccupation with dynamics (1966) but the most direct influence from this source for Freud was transmitted by the famous Parisian neurologist Pierre Charcot. The diagram (Figure 25.1) shows the importance of Helmholtzian physiology, with its emphasis on experiment and reaction against 'naturphilosophie'. Hemlholtz also formed a group around himself, to promulgate his approach to his own subject, and this seems to have been in the mind of Jones (1953a) when he proposed the formation of the 'Secret Ring' or inner circle, around Freud. Figure 25.1 also represents the origins of Freud's thinking in the neurology and neuropathology of his day from his training in Brücke's laboratory (Sulloway, 1979; Gay, 1988). The concept of a dynamic, hierarchically structured functioning of the brain, the contribution of Hughlings Jackson, is also represented. Freud's model of a conscious part of the mind, on the surface, with a deeper layered unconscious, resembles the Jacksonian notion of the relationship between cortical and medullary activity with progression and regression between the layers.

In the 'inner circle' in the figure, there are three groups of oval outlines. These portray the first export of psychoanalysis outside Vienna, which are included because they also represent the formation of distinctive schools of psychoanalytic theorising which, unlike the 'early

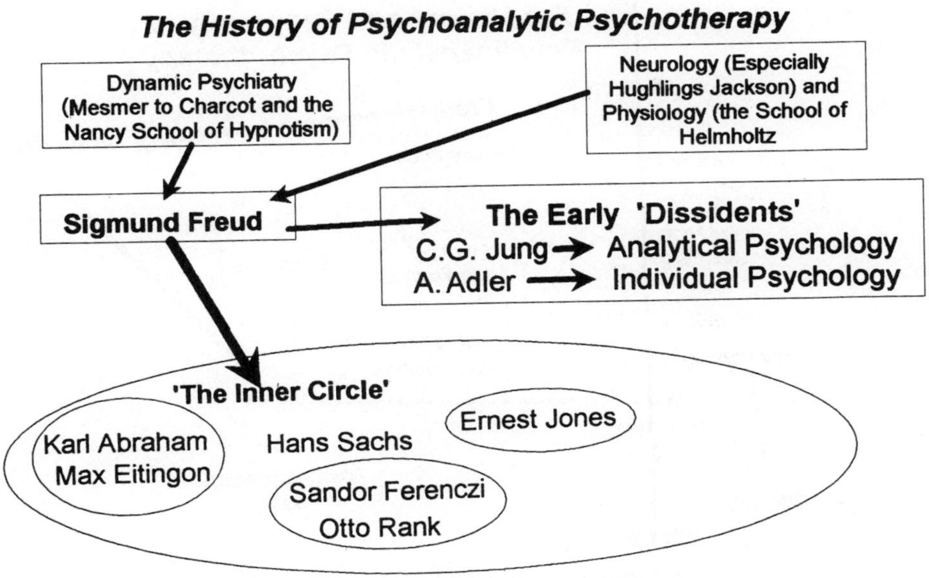

The History of Psychoanalytic Psychotherapy

Figure 25.1 The history of psychoanalytic psychotherapy. The history is assumed to derive from the work of Freud and his co-workers. The origins of Freud's approach are located in the figure as from 'dynamic psychiatry' and neurology. The history is marked by a pattern of defining deviation from a certain viewpoint as apostasy or betrayal. The 'inner circle' was created in response to fear of dissent.

dissidents' remained within the Freudian corpus. The initial spread of psychoanalysis was to Britain and central Europe. This is shown in Figure 25.2 which also places Freud's psychoanalytic daughter, Anna, alongside the inner circle. She, like Melanie Klein (1948) and Michael Balint (e.g. 1957, 1959, 1968) migrated to Britain, importing a vigorous and creative source of controversy within the British Psycho-Analytic society. Of course many psychiatrists came from the Usa to train in Vienna and, with the rise of Nazism, a large number of psychoanalysts migrated from middle Europe to the USA as well as to Britain. In America, Anna Freud had a larger influence than in Britain, to which she had come, and it was in the United States that psychoanalytic psychotherapy came to have its greatest grip, for a while, on the practice of psychiatry in general. In Figure 25.2, Franz Alexander (e.g. Alexander & French, 1946), Sandor Ferenczi (Ferenczi, 1912, 1924; Ferenczi & Rank, 1925), Otto Rank (e.g. 1924; Ferenczi & Rank, 1925) and Michael Balint (1959) are highlighted as representing those early psychoanalysts who experimented with the shortening and intensification of the course of psychoanalytic therapy. Their relationship with contemporary varieties of briefer psychodynamic psychotherapy will be mentioned in a later section.

The further evolution of psychoanalytic conceptualisation broadened the scope of psychoanalytic psychology and psychotherapeutic practice and needs to be described, briefly. Figure 25.3 identifies some major themes. Again, the starting point of the diagram are the early co-workers of Freud and a number of lines of development are stressed. A 'Viennese' line consisted of close colleagues of Anna Freud (e.g. 1936, 1965) included Heinz

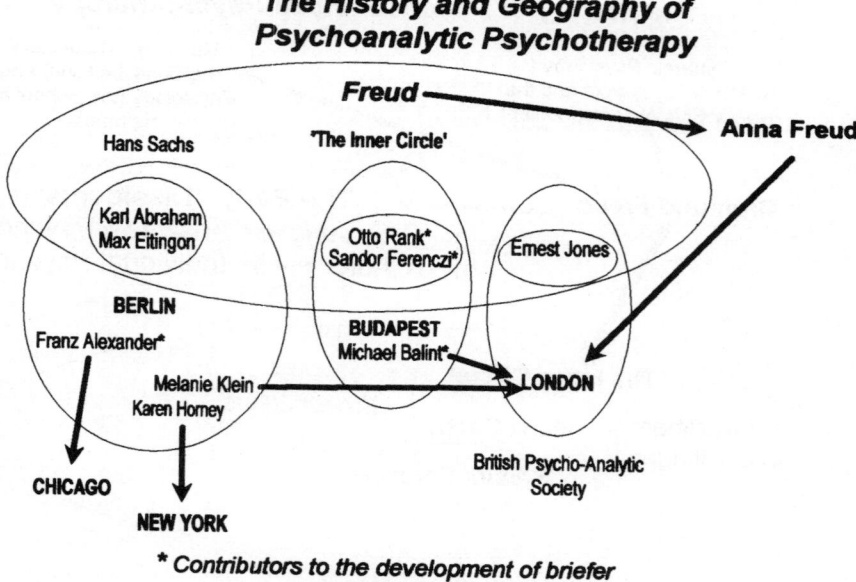

The History and Geography of Psychoanalytic Psychotherapy

* Contributors to the development of briefer
therapies

Figure 25.2 The history and geography of psychoanalytic psychotherapy. Freud's daughter, Anna, is given importance alongside the 'inner circle'. The figure shows the spread, first to middle Europe and then to Britain and the United States. The need to find briefer, less intensive forms of therapy than formal psychoanalysis is also shown by an asterix against some names.

Hartmann (e.g. 1939, 1964). This was especially influential in the East Coast Universities of America and became defined within the USA as a school of Ego Psychology. An emphasis was placed upon those aspects of the mind that were responsive to the demands of reality as opposed to the areas of the mind most responsive to the demands of the instinctual drives (the 'id'). Erik Erikson (1950, 1959) was an important member of this group and evolved a theory of development that took account of socio-cultural variables (Erikson, 1950, 1959). This type of thinking was associated with an inter-personal approach to psychiatry as embodied in the work of Harry Stacks Sullivan (e.g. 1953) and Karen Horney (e.g. 1939), a migrant from Berlin. These interpersonal approaches to psychoanalysis are important in the origins of the theory and practice of psychodynamic marital and family therapy. Otto Kernberg (e.g. 1975, 1980), a New York based psychoanalyst of Argentinian origins, has been a potent force to integrate object relations thinking with ego psychology. He was influenced by another New York psychoanalyst, Margaret Mahler (e.g. 1968; Mahler *et al.*, 1975), who, like René Spitz (1957, 1965), combined psychoanalytic understanding with direct observation of child behaviour. The work of both Mahler and Spitz led in the direction of a focus on the sense of self and of identity, which contributed, on the one hand, to object relations theory and, on the other, to a new development in psychoanalysis, self psychology (e.g. Kohut, 1971). Direct observation of infants and children has had a profound effect upon present day psychoanalytic thinking. This is shown in Figure 25.3 as a square box

The Development of Psychoanalysis

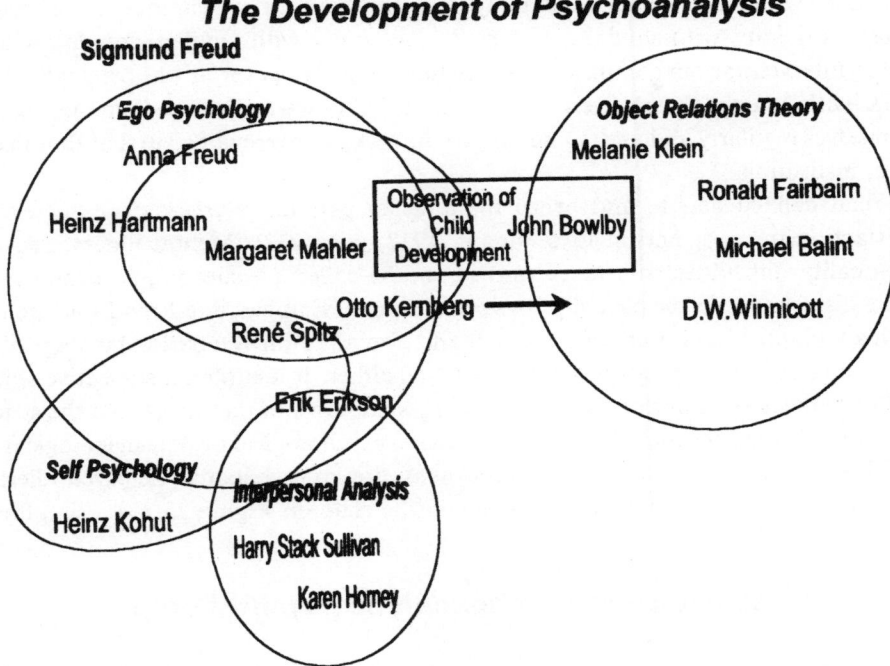

Sigmund Freud

Ego Psychology
Anna Freud
Heinz Hartmann
Margaret Mahler
René Spitz

Observation of Child Development   John Bowlby

Otto Kernberg →

Object Relations Theory
Melanie Klein
Ronald Fairbairn
Michael Balint
D.W.Winnicott

Erik Erikson

Self Psychology
Heinz Kohut

Interpersonal Analysis
Harry Stack Sullivan
Karen Horney

Figure 25.3 The development of psychoanalysis. Four main 'schools' of psychoanalysis are shown: ego psychology, object relations theory, self psychology and interpersonal psychoanalysis. Links are suggested by the overlapping ellipses. Observational studies of child development are shown as being outside of psychoanalysis, but as contributing to the development of psychoanalysis of all schools. Interpersonal psychoanalysis, also known as post-Freudian psychoanalysis, is not considered as being truly psychoanalytic by the other schools.

linking ego psychology and object relations theory. The gap between the two is to allow for the vast field of child observation studies, which are in no way reliant upon psychoanalytic conceptualisation but which are increasingly being taken into the psychodynamic model. John Bowlby is an important person in this area, utilising ethological and other biological models of child behaviour to formulate an attachment theory version of psychodynamic thinking (Bowlby, 1969, 1973, 1980). Bowlby, as a psychoanalyst trained originally by Kleinian teachers, is placed within the British object relations school, but also has a role outside of psychoanalytic thinking as the originator of the attachment theory model of psychology.

The conduct of psychoanalytic psychotherapy

Against this background, describing in a general way the nature and diversity of the theory and historical personages of psychoanalysis, can be placed the clinical practice associated with the subject. Psychoanalytic psychotherapeutic techniques have been applied to psychotherapy with children, with psychotic adults, with families, couples, with groups and to interventions in complex social organisations. However, it was originally devised to work with young or relatively young adults who were disturbed enough to commit themselves regularly and over some time to the task, but were not so ill that they need reside in an institution.

Freud defined health, and hence the aims of psychoanalysis, as the achievement of satisfaction in work and in love (Freud, 1912, page 232). Mental illness, neurotic and personality difficulties, substance misuse and so-called psychosomatic problems can all cause disturbance in the capacity to work and love. Emphasising Freud's adage identifies both a theoretical end point of treatment and also a person at a particular stage of life, not too young nor too old, not too ill but not well either. It identifies a subjective state, being dissatisfied with life, but not overwhelmed by symptoms to the extent that the stridency of the patient's need compels the offer of a specific psychological or pharmacological relief. A decision-making tree leading to the implementation of psychoanalytic psychotherapy with this type of patient is described elsewhere in the chapter. Figure 25.7 is a simplified plan.

The structure of psychoanalytic psychotherapy

A person selected or self-selected for psychoanalytic psychotherapy will have a tendency towards specific expectations and attitudes towards personal difficulties. In Figure 25.4, which schematises the practice, these pre-existing expectations, hopes and wishes bringing the patient to treatment are described by the initial transferences (the top left hand side of the diagram). These expectations have an effect upon the patient's first responses to the manner, style and person of the psychotherapist. In addition, patients in psychoanalytic psychotherapy must find a way to talk about themselves other than to ask for direct help for their specific symptoms; this, in interaction with the initial expectations, contributes to the development of the initial working alliance (Figure 25.4).

In persevering with the treatment, patients will learn to avoid having a defined agenda and to rely upon discovering in themselves a stream of thoughts, memories, fantasies and dreams in which the patient and the therapist will discover patterns of wishes and needs that are evolved in a construction, the meaning of their symptoms. This gradually leads to an established therapeutic alliance – a co-operative, active willing participation which, as portrayed in Figure 25.4, exists alongside of and interacts with the transference, that is the unconsciously derived tendency to perceive and to experience the therapist as resembling a significant figure from the patient's past.

Because of the need to work with transferences in the context of coexisting conscious wishes to undergo and co-operate in the treatment, the therapist presents the patient with an unusual relationship. In most socialising in which a person reveals intimate details of his or her innermost, private life, there is some mutuality in the exchange. On the other hand, if there is no intimate exchange, the relationship will tend to be formal and to have a clear business. It is strange to go to see someone on a formal, professional basis, and to talk in an unstructured, inconsequential but intense, personal, and intimate manner. It is peculiar

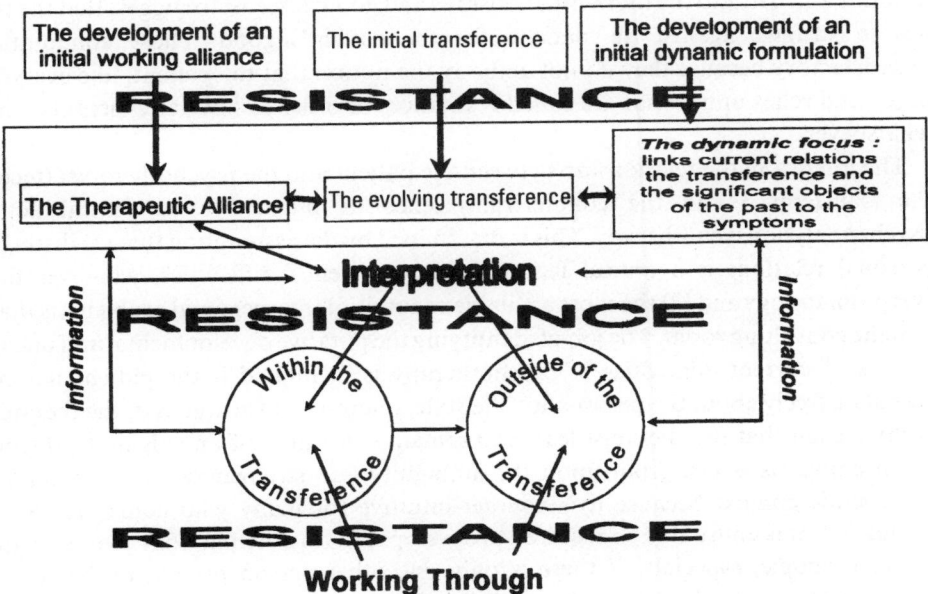

Figure 25.4 The structure of psychoanalytic psychotherapy. The diagram shows than an established therapeutic alliance, an evolving transference and a dynamic focus develop from an initial working alliance, transference and assessment but always in the face of **resistance**. Interpretation addresses transference material, including factors to do with the therapeutic alliance, as well as extra-transferential material. No interpretation is a single event, for a working through of all avenues of change is necessary.

when the interlocutor does not answer many sensible questions that the patient puts and reveals little of him- or herself. The making of direct remarks about the characteristics of the other is uncommon in most social circumstances. Patients and doctors, for example, often talk to each other about the patient's illness, symptoms or treatment almost as though 'gossiping' about a third person. The opening remark of many conversations is: 'How are you?' but only the briefest reply is customary, and a prolonged account in response would seem self centred or merited only by unusual circumstances.

A further, important and special activity of the psychoanalytic psychotherapist has already been mentioned; it is the focus upon the process, the patterning of the relationship evolving between the patient and the therapist (that is to say upon the evolving transference) in preference to the overt subject brought up by the patient. The patient has certain predictable rights and expectations of the therapist as a professional undertaking a specific task. This aspect is necessary to form the basis of the therapeutic alliance, which varies over time and is influenced by the patient's unfolding psychopathology. The psychotherapist has to work to facilitate the development of this therapeutic alliance, especially by exploring and interpreting aspects that hinder the work of healing, that is to say be exploring resistance. In Figure 25.4, resistance is shown as operating at all stages of treatment. The word itself has come to have some unfortunate connotations as it tends to imply the patient as being negative and bad and the therapist as positive and good; it seems to suggest that the therapist has to struggle against the patient, for the patient's good. Those connotations are unsatisfactory because they do not embody the notion that the patient, like everyone else, needs and relies upon what are called resistances in order to have any mental equilibrium whatsoever.

The interest in the relationship between the patient and the psychotherapist (technically, the transference and the countertransference) is pursued as a central activity of psychoanalytic psychotherapy. This is determined by the assumption that (1) disturbance of personal relations is a crucial feature of any patient's difficulties, whatever the other symptomatology and (2) the most available example of interpersonal problems is that which is in the consulting room. The job of identifying the putative developmental and unconscious origins of current difficulties in psychotherapy is facilitated if the patient has room to speculate freely about the personality, life style, interests and attitudes of the therapist. This is the reason that the therapist learns to remain something of an enigma to the patient.

An emphasis is being put upon the ambiguity and strangeness of the psychoanalytic therapeutic context because it is counter-intuitive for many who come into a 'helping' profession. It is unusual to be required to develop skills in noticing what goes on in the space between people, especially if there is only one other person present in the room (as in individual therapy). As these 'odd' qualities of the psychoanalytic style of conversation are not accidental but essential components of the technique, they have to be learned by the would-be therapist. To allow for transference work in an 'uncluttered' way, the trainee also has to acquire the habit of setting up regular, predictable and precisely timed treatment sessions. Without a baseline of reliability and predictability, issues of personal vulnerability and sensitivities to separation on the patient's part may not be revealed. The more general aspects of therapeutic relationships, the offer of a genuine interest in, respect for and concern about the patient, is as necessary in psychoanalytic psychotherapy as in other forms of treatment. However, a psychoanalytic psychotherapist will not regularly or directly show support and approval as this otherwise limits the sorts of transferences that will be evoked to the rather positive and superficial aspects. Psychoanalytic psychotherapists expect to work with the negative and oppositional aspects of the person and a too-ready recourse to friendliness and helpfulness will militate against such feelings, in many patients. This means that some patients will find psychoanalytic psychotherapy uncomfortable and difficult to tolerate. Careful interpretation of the patient's discomfort and of their requests for more warmth can usually reduce the danger of the patient exiting from what otherwise might be worked through to a useful outcome.

All aspects described so far derive from the special subject matter of psychoanalytic psychotherapy. This is the process of finding the meaning of the subjective experience of the patient, the establishment of a revised, more coherent and realistic history of the individual; an understanding of the important patterns of relationships in which the patient tends to become involved. This work is conducted in such a manner as to enable patients to find themselves, as much as possible, in control of their own destiny. Many of the 'medical models' of psychiatry are helpful in allowing patients to believe that they are not responsible for everything that happens to them. This liberates psychiatric patients from the detrimental consequences of being blamed and rejected for their strange of obnoxious behaviour. The negative effect of such a model is that it tends to diminish patients' ability to be in charge of their own lives. The usual manner of relating to medical practitioners, that patients have learned, is to describe and focus upon their complaints and problems as they see them. Previous encounters in medical consultations have led the patient to believe that having told the doctor the problem, a prescription, a treatment plan or reassurance as to the need for neither, will be given. Hence, early in psychoanalytic physiotherapy, the patients' tendency to be preoccupied with and to talk about their symptoms. The absence of the customary, medical-type response, may affront the patient, but in persevering with the psychoanalytic psychotherapy, the patient attempts to adapt to the novel treatment situation and seeks an alternative subject matter.

The natural turn of people's preoccupations and the preferential attention and interest of the psychanalytic psychotherapist leads the patient, soon, to talk a great deal about his or her parents. Rather rapidly, patients in psychoanalytic psychotherapy come to see themselves as the victim of childhood experiences. In later stages of treatment, this perception will be modified as patients explore not so much how others are responsible for their difficulties but rather what they themselves do, what their part is in creating their own predicaments. Learning to forgive others as well as themselves is the content of the ending phase of many psychotherapeutic treatments. It also entails an alteration in the therapeutic alliance, for, initially, the therapist has to be relatively unconditional in accepting the patient's version of the story of their parents' failures. Later, the psychotherapist may have to be more confrontational, challenging the patients' views of themselves as victims and pressing them to contemplate their own contributions.

The characteristic activity of the psychoanalytic psychotherapist is that of interpretation. It is shown in Figure 24.5 as being directed towards transference and non-transference elements of the patient's discourse. It is also shown as being directed towards the maintenance of the therapeutic alliance. Interpretation is a communication to the patient about what the therapist believes is going on between the patient and therapist, at the moment. It is likely to make connections between the current situation and hypothesised groups of mental processes within the patient, some of which make links with symptomatic behaviours, some to patterns of relationships in the current life of the patient and some to the mental structures that have been built up as an outcome of infantile and childhood personal relationship experience. There is an interchange between the initial dynamic formulation, as show in the diagram, based upon the referring information and the material of the assessment interview(s), the nature of the therapeutic alliance, as it becomes established, and the transference. The multiple sources of information establish what is shown in the diagram as the dynamic focus, which provides the basis for the content of interpretation and for the sort of emotional relationship that the therapist attempts to make with the patient.

Different schools of psychoanalytic thinking vary as to the extent to which the structures of what is being called the dynamic focus are thought to derive from actual experience. All psychoanalysts acknowledge the impact of external reality. Some follow the lead of such analysts as Bowlby (1969, 1973, 1980) in believing that the adult personality has been dominated by the real experiences within significant family-of-origin attachments. The internal world, by this view, is an accurate 'map' of actual happenings in the life of the person. Such an 'environmentalist' view is in some ways opposed by those that see the internal world of the person as largely structured by the relics of experiences largely distorted by the workings of the patient's mind. Such influences include powerful, innate urges, for example those of sexuality, aggression and destructive envy. In addition, mechanisms of mental functioning thought to characterise the immature person, defense mechanisms such as projection and spitting, for example, are also thought to give primitive colouring and gross distortion of reality, altering the patient's remembrances and fantasies concerning his or her early existence. Whatever their school of allegiance, all psychoanalytic psycho-therapists are interested in evidence in their patients of maladaptive ways of thinking that interfere with obtaining a reasonably integrated, sustainable and balanced view of themselves and the world in which they live. The jargon of the psychoanalytic discourse creates a vocabulary designed to evoke the way the mind can operate on reality, using such mechanisms as primitive envy, sadistic cruelty, intense defences, e.g. projection (the fantasy of disposing unwanted parts of the self by seeing them as existing only in others), spitting (the refusal to accept the admixture of good and bad qualities in the self or others), pathological narcissism (the need to deny that the world does not revolve around the self), concrete thinking (the failure to have developed a language of emotion and of symbolic thinking), sexualisation (the impact of childhood sensuality on adult desires).

Clearly, it is in the making of interpretations that psychoanalytic psychotherapists address those aspects of analytic thinking referred to earlier in the chapter as psychoanalytic psychology. Any statement describing an aspect of someone beyond the simplest behav-ioural observation, is likely to reveal theoretical ideas about human nature. It has been suggested that any observation, put into language, reveals a conceptualisation about that which is observed. This is most especially obvious in the field of complex descriptions of workings of the mind.

It is not possible for a psychotherapist to make an interpretation without calling on some theoretical view as to the workings of the mind. For this reason psychoanalytic psycho-therapists should be as sophisticated as possible in their understanding of the implicit and explicit models of the mind employed in the formulation of interpretations. There are a wide range of such models, evolved in different schools of psychoanalysis, often employing specialist vocabularies but usually drawing upon much of the terminologies common to other schools. For example, Anna Freud (1936) described the specific defence mechanism, projection, mentioned above, whereby an unacceptable aspect of the self that might be inflicted on another person, is experienced as existing in another person and inflicted on the self. Thus a person full of obvious anger and resentment against authority, but nonetheless denying it, might describe an episode suggesting that the boss was being hostile to the employee. He might also believe, without foundation, that the therapist is angry with him, the patient, in fact the therapist was feeling quite calm and it is the patient that is angry. The situation is complicated by the fact that the patient may be driven to discover ways to get under the skin of the therapist so that the therapist does indeed feel some anger. This process of 'unloading' painful and difficult affects is not reserved to anger and hostility. Shame, guilt or sexual arousal may all be sources of distress or discomfort to the patient and may be attributed to others, including the therapist.

Anna Freud (1936) distinguished the process of projection from a related but slightly different mechanism, externalisation. In this the person disposes of an unwanted aspect of the self by believing it to be a quality existing in others but does not experience that quality as returned and redirected to the self.

> A patient may, for instance, express delight in his own autoerotism, and be convinced that everyone, except himself, and including the psychotherapist, is ashamed of masturbation. Detailed discussion suggests that the patient carries out his masturbation only after taking extreme precautions against discovery, hinting at his own high level of shame, a shame denied in himself as it might limit his own pleasure but re-located as existing exclusively in others. The hypothesised mechanism is that the patient, in order to enjoy his masturbation free from inhibition or self reproach, comes to believe that it is only other people who suffer such feelings.

Psychoanalysts other than followers of Anna Freud use the word projection to include both of the above-described mechanisms. The process whereby the other person actually experiences feelings that derive from the patient who is attempting to gain relief from the possession of these feelings, is called projective identification, and idea developed by Klein (1948) and her followers, but now widely used in all schools of psychoanalysis (Kernberg, 1975).

The elucidation of the precise meaning and clinical usefulness of the wide range of defence mechanisms is an important part of psychoanalytic clinical scholarship. The contemporary of Anna Freud, Otto Fenichel (1945), took great care to distinguish between introjection, a process of forming a clear recognition of the specific qualities and characteristics of another person, and identification in which the person uses knowledge of another person acquired by introjection and attempts to shape aspects of the self on the model of the other.

> An example of introjection without identification was provided by a patient, a professional actor, who had an extraordinary facility for learning his allocated part. He described a capacity whereby he had only to read through a script two to three times for the acquisition of his own lines, entry prompts and so forth. In therapy sessions, this extremely rapid assimilation of what the psychotherapist said was quite evident. However, the therapist also felt that, although the patient seemed to hear, to understand and to be able to repeat the interpretations, it was all done too quickly, too glibly, there was no evidence of the patient trying to take notice of what he had taken in from the therapist. The material of the psychotherapy, as of a play, was remembered and could be recalled if required, but it had no apparent psychological impact. In this patient, the process of introjection seemly cut off from identification rather exactly. When the psychotherapist talked of the fate of the interpretations to the patient and likened it to the patient's style of learning scripts, the patient acknowledged that he believed that there was some lack of conviction in his acting. He had a successful career but he himself realised that there was justice in the occasional critical reviews that implied an emotional shallowness. Indeed he had taken care not to accept parts that would reveal this defect in his craft. Further work with the patient concentrated on the extent to which in his childhood, brought up by his mother on her own, he had had to protect himself from her complex and frequently contradictory demands on him. It seemed that he had had to learn not to identify with her needs of him, i.e. avoid making them part of himself, because they were so often bewilderingly incompatible both with his own needs and with other of her requirements.

Identification, then, is a process whereby the person recognises and assimilates characteristics and constructs aspects of the personality from these qualities. An introjected image has to be available for the process of identification subsequently to take place. Melanie Klein

(1948) in her elaboration of the concept of projective identification integrated the ideas of identification and projection. In projective identification, the person experiences the other as containing aspects of the self and is, hence, unable to make a clear distinction between that which constitutes and motivates the other from the self. In intimate relationships, projective identification is used to describe the extent to which each person in the relationship believes in the identity of purpose and interest of the partner. The mechanism of projective identification can be associated with confusion, poor interpersonal boundaries and inadequate reality testing but it is also that which enables us to make empathic contact with others.

When studying any one scheme of psychoanalytic thinking the reader has to understand the specific meanings attached to the technical jargon that is used, and must not assume consistent usage between different schools. The language of psychoanalytic psychotherapy focuses upon three areas: (1) mechanisms of mental functioning and the dynamic functioning of the mind; (2) the development of personal psychological differences and (3) the psychological development of the person, especially during the years of infancy and early childhood. These areas, it must be emphasised, are all described from the point of view of subjective experience although as shown in Figure 25.3, direct observation of infant and child behaviour is being incorporated into many schools of psychoanalytic thought.

The attempt to address individual differences, to make sense of personal development and to help the patient understand how his or her mind works is what the psychoanalytic psychotherapist offers as the essence of the treatment. Freud believed that such personalised knowledge, that is 'insight' had a potentially curative value although he was often pessimistic about the actual power of psychoanalysis to change people. It is probably true to say that few psychoanalytic psychotherapists nowadays have strong conviction that self knowledge alone produces powerful therapeutic benefit, but nonetheless the activity of psychoanalytic psychotherapy is governed by the generation and sharing of an understanding of the working of the patient's mind. Indeed it is likely that most mental health practitioners have an open or covert belief that self-knowledge must be helpful or even, in some sense, morally right. This conviction may account for the popularity of psychoanalytic psychotherapy among many intellectually aspirant people, including psychiatrists. The pursuit of such self-knowledge can be a strong motivation, on its own, for people to enter into psychoanalytic psychotherapy, and may account, in part, for the continued existence of the treatment in the absence of empirical proof of it having specific efficacy.

Psychoanalytic psychotherapy, object relations and the process of change in treatment

The current clinical practices of psychoanalytic psychotherapists rely heavily upon the notion of transference, and the theoretical reasons for this have to be grasped in order to understand this preoccupation. It is strongly connected to beliefs about the curative process. Having given up the notion that insight on its own is a curative ingredient in the treatment, psychoanalytic psychotherapists have not abandoned a faith in the efficacy of their activity. Indeed the persistence and commitment of their patients to the long-lasting and often disconcerting, uncomfortable treatment fuels the belief that many practitioners have that if only the patient can be seen often enough and for long enough then benefit will accrue. Psychoanalytic psychotherapists now suggest different conceptualisation of the means whereby patients might change in the treatment. The emphasis follows from observations made many years ago by the psychoanalyst Strachey (1934). He suggested that what was changed in treatment was the relationship between the patient and internal versions of significant figures in the formative years. This theory has been of enormous influence in psychoanalysis. It will be elaborated here, to provide an outline of contemporary thinking. As a result of changes in the general theory of psychoanalytic motivation, psychoanalysts have come to downgrade the importance of biologically derived motivational systems, that is sexuality, and to emphasise the effect of patterns of personal relationships. For example, in early writings on sexuality (Freud, 1905; Abraham, 1924), children under the age of 4 to 5 years were thought to be governed by drives for gratification of an essentially self-centred nature. Freud and his early colleagues had suggested that the frustration of the toddler's natural curiosity about and pleasure in sphincter activity and excretion, produced effects on the developing mind of the child so that secret, unconscious derivatives of anal sensuality could be identified in the structure of, for example, the obsessional personality. Freud and these early psychoanalysts believed that it was not the child's frustration by the parent that was forming his or her personality, but the frustration of the pleasures of anal sensuality. It was believed that it was only by the time that the child became aware of having conflicting needs for exclusive love from the two opposite sexed parents, that the relationship with other people, as people, began to impinge on the evolving structure of the patient's mind. This was at the time of the notorious Oedipus phase. This phase was dominated, Freud believed, by the child coming to realise an intense and essentially possessive, sexualised love for the parent of the opposite sex[1]. The possessive longing for exclusive rights to the one parent was believed to spur the development of fear for the consequences of the jealous opposition of the same-sexed parent. Later, the child would become aware of a wish to be loved by both parents, which would further complicate the feelings of the child within the family and have, Freud believed, life-long results in predisposing all people to minor or major neurotic features. Eventually, Freud thought that a major agency of the mind came about as a result of the Oedipus experience. In order to cope with the implicit unresolvability of the jealousies and rivalries of the three-person Oedipal situation, the child attempted to withdraw to some extent, the retreat being potentiated by the demands to function in the society of school, commenced at about that time. Freud suggested that at the time of the child giving up expectation of gratification of sexual longing for the opposite-sex parent (out of fear of the consequent hostility of the same-sex parent) a crucial mental structure evolved. This structure, which he named the superego, took over from the external parent in setting ideals and prohibitions governing the child's behaviour. The child began to comply with standards and rules not because of the presence of law enforcer, a parent, but because the superego functioned as an internal enforcer. The notion that a part of the person was structured on the basis of external persons had profound implications for the subsequent development of the psychoanalytic theory of the person and for the conduct of therapy.

---

[1] The idea of a child having an incestuous love for his mother was described before Freud. For example, the novelist Stendahl (see Ellenberger, 1970, p. 505) has described his attachment to his mother in this way.

As time went on, psychoanalysts realised that it had been a mistake to have disregarded the intense attachment to and involvement in the relationship with the mother that is observable in even the youngest babies. Ultimately a new model of the mind came out of the further elaboration of the concept of the superego. The personality came to be postulated as being structured both by the need to make relationships and by the consequences of those relationships. Initially, this idea was introduced, against great opposition, by Melanie Klein in her formulation of the superego as being perceptible in the youngest infants (Klein, 1948). It is true to say that the opposition was made easy by her contention that she could re-create the thoughts and fantasies of even the smallest children from their play and that she could discern patterns of thoughts that were also directly present in the minds of adults. Through controversy about the nature of the fantasy life of infants, psychoanalysts failed, for some time, to realise their mistake in denying the relationship that existed between the infant and the earliest caretakers. A fundamental shift in psychoanalytic thinking occurred as this attitude was worked through in the clinical discussions of child and adult psychoanalytic material. The concept of a mind shaped by drives was replaced by that of psychological structuring under the impact of object relationships. Seminal for this was Freud's notion, as described above, of the superego. This is seen as an inner representation of the child's image of the parental ambitions, rules, prohibitions, ideals and aspirations. The superego, as the description given shows, was conceived of as bearing the mark of many aspects of the parents. It is not seen simply as an internalised and literal memory trace of the actual people but a complex mixture of how the parents really were and what the child had made of them at the varying stages of family life. The child's superego was also thought of by Freud (1923) as containing aspects of the parents' own wishes, expectations, fears and hopes, that is of their own superego. Aided by (and sometimes, for some psychoanalysts, despite) empirical studies by developmental psychologists sympathetic to psychoanalysis, all psychoanalysts have come to accept that infants are motivated not by purely autoerotic sexual drives but by an intense focus upon and interaction with the primary caretakers. Many psychoanalysts have responded to this change in theory, elaborating theories of the mind and of psychological development determined by the impact of the emotionally significant caretakers of the child. These developments have been portrayed in Figures 25.2 and 25.3 earlier in this chapter. There is a continuing tension within psychoanalysis with regard to the preoccupation with inner autochthonous forces as opposed to the power of the external experience. This is reflected by a suspicion of any reliance upon empirical studies, from whatever source, other than upon the data of the consulting room. All English-speaking psychoanalysts would, however, advocate a view that those aspects of human psychology that are most relevant to the conduct of psychotherapy are dominated by the vicissitudes of the relationships between the person and his or her primary objects throughout the life-cycle. (This is not necessarily true of the Lacanians of the francophone world).

The account of the development of psychoanalytic theory has been for the purpose of introducing contemporary views of the potential sources of change in psychoanalytic psychotherapy. Relationships in the actual world (insofar as they are under the influence of the person, the patient), are thought of as deriving from the motivational structures, the object relations. Relationships with familiar attachment objects of childhood are internalised and are necessarily connected to memories of the self, at the same time. An internal object, therefore, is strictly speaking an internalised other in interaction with the self. As internal objects are formed, in the course of development, certain configurations of relationships are associated with positive affects and others with negative affects. Naturally, those object relations linked to negative patterns are likely to lead to the avoidance of situations that threaten to repeat the unpleasantness of the past. However, the internal object relationships may lead to attempts at what can be termed 'curative' repetition.

> For example, in marital relationships, it is often obvious that each of the partners is, in important ways, trying to address parent/child relationships in the spouse relationship. A man can be seen to be trying to persuade his wife that the proper way to behave is an expression of his childhood experiences with his mother, whilst his wife tries to get him to do something like a mother or father. Sometimes the repetition is in pursuit of mastering perceived problems in the primary relationship. For instance, a woman who has experienced her father, though much loved, as very critical may find herself committed to a partner who is also very critical. Some physical or characterological aspect of the man may remind the wife of her father and lead her to expect the positive and gratifying qualities of her childhood. Her spouse's potential for love may have an intense meaning for his wife. She hopes that she can 'cure' his tendency to criticism, can win him over, by her love (for example by her sexuality), to offer her his unconditional approval. It is as though she marries him to gain an approximation to her childhood times with her father but hopes that in the new edition of her relationship with a crucial man the ending will be different. The pain of his criticism, that persists as a continuing hurt in her memory, can be overcome in the present. Of course this may be thought of as a high-risk strategy because the repetition may be too much like the first experience. On the other hand if her hopes are fulfilled she will not simply have a happy marriage in the present but the hurt of the past may be alleviated.

Putative mental structures, such as these, have to be worked upon repetitively in psychoanalytic psychotherapy and this is why the notion of working through is given prominence in Figure 25.4.

Psychoanalysis and brief psychotherapy

Figures 25.2 and 25.5 indicate members of the early group of psychoanalytic practitioners who developed an interest in shortening the duration of psychoanalytic treatment. This has to be put into the context of the practice, in that era, in which treatment lasted about 12 to 18 months. The sense that psychoanalysis lasted too long was also expressed succinctly in one of Freud's last papers ('Analysis terminable and interminable', 1937) in which he mused pessimistically on the forces opposing change in people. Sandor Ferenczi (Ferenczi & Rank, 1925), one of Freud's closest colleagues, experimented with what he called 'active' techniques. These altered the usual injunctions against giving advice, as recommended at that time. Two groups of indications for activity were considered by Frenczi, in phobic and obsessional patients. In the former, Ferenczi suggested pressuring the patient to enter the phobic situation, to encounter dogs, to go out alone, to travel by train, or whatever was the feared situation. He argued that by imposing such an injunction upon the patient, the relevant psychodynamic material became more readily available. The relationship of this treatment suggestion with de-conditioning, using a behavioural paradigm, is

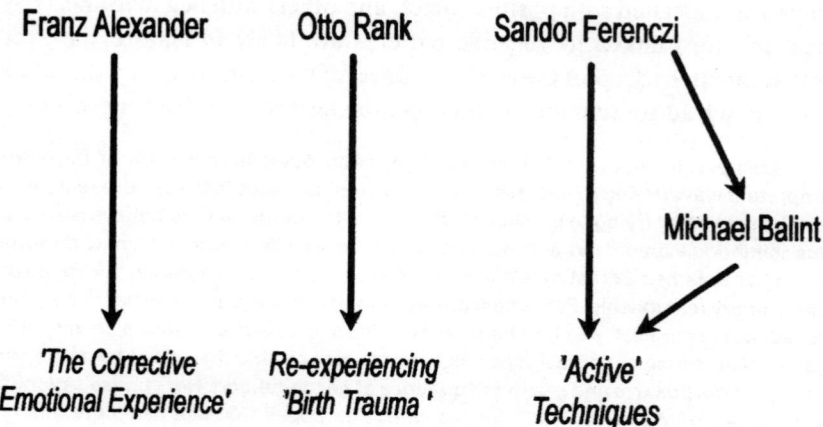

The Evolution of Briefer Psychotherapies

Figure 25.5 The evolution of briefer psychotherapies. The figure summarises early attempts to identify therapeutic ingredients in psychoanalytic psychotherapy that could be utilised to create briefer treatments. Together with the concept of insight, which in part is a strongly cognitive concept, the corrective emotional experience, re-experiencing intense affect (like that of alleged 'birth trauma') and 'active techniques', the figure covers many current lines of thought and practice.

obvious. In working with obsessional patients, whose compulsive behaviour and style of thinking militated against becoming independent of the therapist, Ferenczi advocated the necessity of the psychoanalyst nominating a time for ending at a stage when the patient might believe that the termination date was too soon. In the contemporary world, whilst formal psychoanalytic treatments have lengthened to between 4 and 8 years, economic need has compelled the establishment of short-term treatments, which are, indeed, the rule in most health service or otherwise state-supported treatment centres. There is ample evidence of the effectiveness of short-term treatments and very little evidence of the particular or additional advantage of longer-term, open-ended treatments. This, however, derives from an artifact: it is methodologically much more difficult to set up satisfactory controlled studies of long-term open-ended treatments. The exigencies of the time scale of PhD requirements has resulted in vast numbers of studies, within departments of psychology, of brief psychological treatments, including time-limited psychodynamic psychotherapies. By reason of economic and research constraints Ferenczi's advocacy of occasional enforcement of time limits on psychoanalytic treatments has become the rule in psychoanalytic psychotherapy, outside of private practice.

Another aspect of Ferenczi's technical additions to the practice of psychoanalytic psychotherapy is also relevant to current practice and controversy. He came to believe that many patients in psychoanalysis needed evidence of warmth and commitment from the psychoanalyst, which was in contrast to the metaphor of the psychoanalyst as mirror that Freud himself had advocated (Freud, 1911–1915). Freud was always aware of the danger of a professionally originating warmth slipping into a unprofessional misconduct, especially where the psychoanalyst was a man and the patient a younger women. Freud's technical suggestions for the practice of psychotherapy seemed to propose a cold, uninvolved, rigidly neutral and unbending attitude. In that context, Ferenczi's experiments caused concern without suggestions of impropriety: What would happen if the demonstration of warmth and affection became the rule? However, in the last two decades, following the work of Truax and his colleagues (Truax *et al.*, 1966), outcome studies of psychological treatment have repeatedly demonstrated that evidence of empathy and warmth are crucial ingredients of effect psychological interventions. Although the neutrality and ambiguity on the part of the psychoanalyst remain sensible admonitions for the practice of psychotherapy, in general, it is also true that patients need to know of the therapist's interest and involvement. The need to empathise with patients in psychological treatment is generally agreed; less obvious is how empathy can be demonstrated to all patients. Paranoid patients, for example, are unlikely to experience a psychotherapist's empathy, but this is also true for people who use narcicisstic defences. It is with regard to the latter group of patients that the psychoanalyst Heinz Kohut (1971, 1977) developed both specific theories ('self psychology') and treatment techniques.

Otto Rank (e.g. 1924), a non-medical co-worker of Freud worked with Ferenczi on the development of active treatments, but also evolved a theory of birth trauma. He suggested that all anxiety was modelled upon its first manifestation, in the pain and anguish of the birth experience. Rank (1924) suggested that identifying, as soon as possible, the roots of adult anxieties in the birth experience, would shorten treatment. The idea of birth trauma has been rejected by psychoanalysis, but there is cogency in (and experimental evidence for) the notion that it is necessary to create an emotional intensity to sustain the impact of brief therapy. Contemporary advocates of short-term psychoanalytic psychotherapy (as well as those proposing other types of brief psychotherapy) have shown the usefulness of both maintaining a single focus for treatment and of establishing a high level of emotional impact during its course.

A further important attempt at shortening psychoanalytic psychotherapy was inaugurated by Franz Alexander (a Berliner who moved to Chicago) (see Alexander & French, 1946) when he suggested that the psychotherapist should seek to engage the patient in an enactment that avoided past pain in relationships and offered a new relationship, that is that provided a 'corrective emotional experience'. The suggestion was that the therapist identified the nature of the patient's relationship with parents in childhood, assessed the deficits in that experience that contributed to the adult problems and then sought, in psychotherapy, to avoid repeating the pattern of the problematic relationship. In crude form such an enactment, though achievable in life, is probably impossible in a professional relationship. Modern psychotherapeutic technique has an aspiration to address the tendency that patients have to enter into patterns of interaction that represent repitition or avoidance of past relationship patterns. As with the ideas mentioned so far, the innovations intended to shorten therapy all have limitations, but appear repeatedly in contemporary efforts to achieve the same ends.

Varieties of Brief Psychodynamic Psychotherapies

Short-Term Psychotherapy: A Self Psychological Approach - H.S.Baker, 1991

Brief SASB-Directed Reconstructive Learning Therapy - L.S.Benjamin, 1991

Intensive Short-Term Dynamic Psychotherapy - H. Davanloo, 1980

Short-Term Dynamic Therapy of Stress Response Syndromes - M.J. Horowitz, 1991

Short-Term Supportive-Expressive Psychoanalytic Psychotherapy - L. Luborsky, 1984

Focal Psychoanalytic Psychotherapy - D. Malan, 1963, 1976a, 1976b.

Time Limited Psychotherapy - J. Mann, 1973.

Dynamic Supportive Psychotherapy - H. Pinsker et al., 1991

Brief Adaptive Psychotherapy - J. Pollack & A. Horner, 1985

Short-Term Anxiety Provoking-Psychotherapy - Sifneos, 1979

The Vanderbilt Approach - H.H. Strupp & J.L. Binder, 1984

Cognitive Analytic Therapy - A. Ryle, 1990

(Derived, in part, from. P. Crits-Christoph & J.P. Barber, 1991)

Figure 25.6 Varieties of brief psychodynamic psychotherapies.

Brief psychodynamic psychotherapies today

Crits-Christoph & Barber (1991) have summarised the situation: 'The multitude of brief psychodynamic psychotherapies puts a burden on practitioners and researchers about how to distinguish between them, which form to choose, and for which purpose' (p. 323). These authors emphasised that the conduct of brief therapy, patient selection and therapist training are closely linked. The therapist must, they point out, be able and prepared to make an assessment within a few sessions and keep to the focus. Barber and Crits-Christoph review the wide range of conditions for which brief psychoanalytic psychotherapy has been claimed to be efficacious. They also show that some exponents of the treatment suggest a narrow applicability whilst others make broader propositions. If patients are to be assigned to such therapies on the basis of controlled trials, then there is bound to be certain arbitrariness. Research in the area, although extensive, is determined by many rather chancy factors. For example, the methodology of psychotherapy has been bedeviled by problems of consensually acceptable outcome measures. This has led some, such as the present author, to work in a field where outcome measurement is relatively simple (in this instance, restricting eating disorder). The relative ease or difficulty in acquiring research funds or identifying sufficiently homogeneous patient groups is likewise a strong influence in the choice of patients chosen for research. Thus there may be quite marked skewing of the available research base for the application of these therapies.Of course, health service funding agencies have had an ulterior interest in short-term psychotherapy. A US insurance company is credited with the first investigation into the efficacy of brief forms of treatment (Avnet, 1962, 1965).

Figure 25.6, which is partly derived from the chapter headings of Crits-Christoph & Barber (1991), lists twelve variants on the theme. As mentioned already, the list is disparate as to the extent to which these therapies have been subjected to formal empirical evaluation, both as to their separateness (i.e. by process research) or their efficacy (outcome research).

The earliest author in the list to develop brief psychoanalytic psychotherapy, was Strupp, who drew upon the traditions of classical psychoanalysis but was also influenced by the neo-Freudian tradition (interpersonal psychoanalysis) (Figure 25.3). Strupp's work is incorporated in the Vanderbilt Psychotherapy Research Team's efforts which have addressed both the process and outcome of their form of brief psychotherapy – Time-Limited Dynamic Psychotherapy (TLDP). In keeping with traditional long-term psychoanalytic treatments (and against the usual suggestions for non-intensive treatments at the time he first began his researches) Strupp advocated a focus on the management of hostility in the therapeutic relationship both as manifested directly by the patient and as revealed in the subjective responses of the therapist to the patient (i.e. in the countertransference v Sandler et al., 1992, pp. 81–98). Strupp says:

> 'Our research has called forceful attention to the overriding importance of the dyadic *interactions* [original emphasis] between patient and therapist over the course of therapy, with special emphasis on the early phases. Thus, our approach forms part of a movement toward a greater integration of classical and interpersonal psychoanalytic theory and technique – in short, nothing less than a reconceptualization of transference and countertransference phenomena in interactional terms'[2].
>
> Binder & Strupp, 1991, p. 138)

Strupp has used a conceptualisation of the crucial themes of the material of psychoanalytic psychotherapy that he terms the Cyclical Maladaptive Pattern (CMP). This cycle is a sequence of self-generated acts, in a context of specific expectations of others, their actual response and the nature of the treatment of the self that is meted out in that context. This idea that brief therapy requires a consistent focus of interpretations is a common theme in the adaptation of techniques of long-term psychoanalytic psychotherapy to brief work. In the model of TLDP the therapist is advised to bring the CMP in relation to the nature of the patient–therapist interaction. The empirical support for the efficacy of TLDP is summarised by Binder & Strupp (1991) and includes detailed process investigation as well as control trial studies.

Almost at the same time as Strupp's first experiments, Mann (1973), was advocating the use of a brief, ten-session therapy, for selected patients. He focuses upon the identification of the main painful affect from which the patient suffers, the main childhood event that is linked by the patient to such pain. This is seen as a focus or central issue. The brevity of the therapy and the re-creation of separation pain enforced by the termination of treatment is used to explore the patient's traumas around separation (and/or loss).

Malan (1963, 1976a.b), like Strupp and Mann, has used a conceptual system close to orthodox psychoanalysis. He was influenced by the Hungarian psychoanalyst, Balint (Balint et al., 1972), who had envisioned a focal psychotherapy that also addressed the relationship between an intensely recalled childhood experience and the current psychological pain. Balint had propounded ideas for the theoretical possibility of brief, psychoanalytic therapy by means of the detailed exposition of a particular case. Malan, through the use of a

---

[2] This conceptualisation of transference and countertransference in dyadic, interpersonal terms is especially relevant to the present author's attempts to demonstrate links between psychoanalytic psychotherapy and marital and family therapy theory and practice (see Dare, 1986, 1988, etc).

Balint-type training/treatment workshop, systematically explored the clinical scope and effectiveness of brief psychoanalytic psychotherapy (Malan, 1963, 1976a. b). He, like Mann, advocated and presented ample clinical examples in support of his belief, that the brief treatment was effective when it emphasised the psychological relevance of the phenomena of separation and loss. He recommended dealing with these through consistent interpretation of the transference. He did not use a control trial technique to demonstrate efficacy but produced a large number of examples of the range of successes available with the treatments. Their duration was from four to 40 sessions.

Sifneos (e.g. 1972, 1979) likewise was working in the 1960s to modify classical psychoanalytic technique. His therapy is designated by a acronym STAPP – Short-Term Anxiety Provoking Therapy. Sifneos and his co-workers have evolved techniques to assess motivational elements within patients that are believed to predict suitability for short-term treatment. The technique of the therapy relies on focusing upon intense feelings aroused by discussion of interpersonal conflicts. The assumption of maladaptive styles of relating that have to be challenged has similarities to aspects of Cognitive Therapy as portrayed by Beck and his colleagues (e.g. Beck et al., 1979, 1990) but is psychoanalytic in style with its preoccupation with defences and triangular interpersonal conflicts (Oedipal problems). The style is confrontative and arousing and the number of sessions is not pre-set, being of the same order as that proposed by Malan. Although there are several well-conducted follow-up studies of a series of patients treated by STAPP, there appear to have been no controlled studies.

The next acronymously identified example of brief psychoanalytic psychotherapy is that associated with the work of Habib Davanloo (1978, 1980), – Intensive Short-Term Dynamic Psychotherapy (ISTDP). Davanloo, as with the other workers so far mentioned, specifies origins both in Freud's technical papers (1911–1915) and by latter-day innovators. Unlike the other psychoanalysts so far mentioned, he also cited the influence of the work of Lindemann (1944), whose clinical work with the survivors of a disastrous fire in a dancehall is a landmark both in the development of crisis theory approaches to psychological treatments and also in the psychology of grieving. Davanloo (1978, 1980) used a technique that is very confrontational, emphasising the accurate identification of the affects of the patient and challenging the observed psychological processes, especially those that are resisting change of attitude and self perception. He pointed out that the best way to select patients for his form of brief psychotherapy was by making the assessment interview a 'mini therapy'. If the patient can manage the confrontation and challenge of the assessment interview then he or she can probably use the treatment. If they become confused and overwhelmed by anxiety in the assessment state, then the therapy is contraindicated. The psychotherapy is itself seen as establishing a crisis for the patient, within which change is hopefully optimalised. Constant interpretation of the transference of the patient to the therapist is accentuated alongside of the other confrontations within the therapy. This is especially true when feelings about the psychotherapist are seen as heightening the resistance of the patient to progress in treatment and in the termination phase – another regular theme of brief therapies using psychodynamic thinking. Davanloo (1980) himself has reported three series of follow-up studies with patients seen for about 20 sessions. A group at the Beth Israel Medical Centre in New York have used a comparison of ISTDP with both Brief

Adaptive Psychotherapy (BAP) and a waiting-list control, to study the treatment's efficacy, systematically. The two treatments have been shown to be equally effective both with regard to target complaints and social adjustment, in comparison with the waiting-list control (Winston, 1985; Winston et al., 1991).

The next group of workers (Luborsy, Pinsker, and Pollack) represent a new, evolving approach to the subject, whereby the research needs are given strong precedence over the proving of a particular viewpoint. The tendency within psychoanalytic psychotherapy research has been for the researchers to have an axe to grind – to wish to prove that their life's work in psychoanalysis has not been in vain.

Luborsky (1984; Luborsky et al., 1988) trained at the Menninger Clinic, wherat was conducted one of the few serious attempts at the evaluation of formal psychoanalysis and long-term psychanalytic psychotherapy (Wallerstein, 1986). He has been concerned to explore two conceptually separate aspects of psychoanalytic psychotherapy, the element of the practice that facilitates emotional expression and the supportive aspects. The whole concept of 'support' in clinical work is itself a hoary topic, difficult to ignore but hard to quantify. Alongside these distinctions, Luborsky (Luborsky, 1984; Luborsky & Mark, 1991) has also had his own attempt at defining the nature of the focus. He uses yet another acronym, the CCRT, the Core Conflictual Relationship Theme, which has a clear categorical relationship to the other usages mentioned so far:

'The CCRT is a general relationship pattern that recurrently becomes activated although with variations, throughout therapy and perhaps throughout life'.
(Luborsky & Mark, 1991, p. 119)

Luborsky is unusual amongst psychoanalytic psychotherapists in that he accepts that a treatment manual, prescribing in detail the nature of the therapy in such a way that others can utilise it, is essential in the scientific establishment of the treatment. He has published the manual (Luborsky, 1984) and there are unpublished specific instances of the treatment for different diagnostic groups (including severe depression and drug dependency). These have been used to study the efficacy of psychodynamic psychotherapy in the specific disorders.

Horowitz (1988) is also an advocate of the incorporation of normal standards and techniques of psychological treatment evaluation into the field of psychodynamic psycho-therapy. His starting point was in working with patients attempting to overcome the effects of stressful events (the first work he conducted in this area was before the elaboration of the concept of Post Traumatic Stress Disorder in the DSM classifications) (Horowitz, 1986). He uses the notion of the personal schema (originally developed from the neurological concept of the body schema, as a psychologically useful idea, by Bartlett, 1932) as an organising principle for his model of psychodynamic therapy and therapeutic change. This concept has been used by other psychoanalysts (e.g. Sandler's concept of the representational word; Sandler et al., 1963), forming a useful link between psychoanalytic and cognitive behaviour therapy. As with the whole spectrum of contemporary applications of psychoanalysis to brief therapy, transference interpretations and the work on the ending of therapy are all considered to be important by Horowitz. He has a useful categorisation of 'levels of interpretation' (see Table 25.5 in Horowitz, 1991). He considers there to be a range from working with current stressful situations to dealing with 'unconscious scenarios and impulsive agendas' (Horowitz, 1991, p.193). Horowtiz has been especially associated with the development of measures of assessment and outcome in psychotherapy, using them to evaluate outcome in a series of 52 cases of pathological grief reaction (Horowtiz *et al.*, 1984).

Horowitz's technique of brief dynamic psychotherapy has also been used in a study of the treatment of depression (Thompson *et al.*, 1987), comparing the therapy with a cognitive and a behavioural treatment conditions. The fact that the psychodynamic psychotherapy was as effective as the other therapies is particularly interesting because the patients were elderly.

For long, psychodynamic therapists have proposed a distinction between supportive and analytic forms of psychotherapy. In principle, the distinction is clear; supportive therapies offer support, envisioned as some form of psychological equivalent of a crutch, helping the patient survive a psychosocial crisis or an illness: analytic therapies facilitate the patient's expression of psychological state, the therapy analyses and speaks to the patient about a psychological construction or interpretation to the imputed meaning of what the patient has communicated. This distinction is difficult to maintain in a simple form, either in practice (or theory). Even the most banal, would-be supportive, remark is likely to contain an element of the therapist's views as to the nature of the patient's state and functioning, i.e. it has an interpretative component. On the other hand, an analytic approach cannot be maintained unless the patient feels sufficiently supported (psychological 'holding' or containment is the common phrase). The distinction has become coloured by value judgements being made in which support has been seen as a commonplace non-specific activity requiring little professional skill. Analytic work has been seen as a 'purer' more professional art. It is certainly true to say that the acquisition of skills in psychodynamic psychotherapy requires serious study and detailed supervision (as well as the experience of personal therapy). However, supportive therapy with disturbed, psychologically damaged people with severe relationship difficulties, makes considerable demands upon the professional. Tact, sympathy, firmness, psychological insight and knowledge of the specific disorder require great skill and to be able, in addition, to be useful is difficult. In one of our own studies (Russell *et al.*, 1987; Dare *et al.*, 1990; Dare & Szmukler, 1991; Szmukler & Dare, 1991) in the psychotherapy of anorexia nervosa, we have found that an individual, supportive therapy used as a control treatment was superior in one group of patients (those with late onset anorexia nervosa) to the specific form of psychotherapy (family therapy).

Currently there is interest in the measurement of the supportive and expressive components of brief psychoanalytic psychotherapy. There is a long-standing and distinguished theoretical basis for the conceptualisation of a psychoanalytic psychotherapy that is also deliberately supportive. In Figure 25.3, on the evolution of psychoanalysis, a place was given to an ego-psychological school of psychoanalysis. This can be linked specifically to Anna Freud (e.g. 1936, 1965) and a fellow Viennese, Hartmann (1939, 1964). The ego psychological school was particularly interested in adaptational and problem-solving aspects of mental functioning and in the manner whereby unconscious processes interfered with these processes. By this paradigm, supportive psychotherapy is directed towards 'enhancing the ego'. This is not simply a matter of being concerned about raising the patient's self-esteem but it is also concerned with their capacity to keep track on reality and to adapt appropriately to that reality. A psychoanalytic approach assumes that there are always unconscious mental systems tending to impose the needs and wishes of an inner psychological reality upon the external reality.

There is no doubt that an ego-psychological approach to a supportive form of psychodynamic psychotherapy will converge with cognitive behavioural therapy. This is evident in the approaches both of Beck (Beck *et al.*, 1979), the originator of cognitive therapy, and of contemporary versions such as the dialectical cognitive therapy of Linehan, 1993 (which takes psychological conflicts as a central phenomenon of personality difficulties).

The Beth Israel Medical Center group in New York shows the influence of Hartmann. The group (Winston *et al.*, 1986; Pinsker *et al.*, 1991) have described a conceptualisation of a Dynamic Supportive Psychotherapy (DSP) which they have developed alongside of Brief Adaptive Therapy (BAT, see above). They have devised a method of specifying and measuring the admixture of supportive and other therapeutic ingredients, and have investigated the treatment's efficacy in comparison with ISTDP and BAP (Pinsker *et al.*, 1991). The supportive therapists used more directive and information giving statements, they offered more self-disclosure, used clarifications and interpretations, but did not confront or use transference analysis. The preliminary results of these studies are particularly interesting in that they suggest that at the end of treatment the more confrontational as opposed to the more supportive therapies are associated with identifiable differences in the patients' defensive styles, although all three treatments were symptomatically effective.

In the list of brief psychodynamic therapies provided in Figure 25.6, reference is made to the work of Benjamin (1986). This is a technique based on a system of measurement of the dynamics of interpersonal relationships. The therapy thus specifies a methodology for the measurement of process and of outcome (Structural Analysis of Social Behaviour, SASB). As such it represents one type of solution to the problem of assaying psychotherapy. Most psychotherapies have evolved as essentially clinical activities being guided by clinical skills, intuitions and inspirations. The complexity of the theoretical conceptualisations and the multiplicity of interventive technique has intensified the difficulties of scientific evaluation of the treatments. Benjamin's solution to these problems is to make a close integration of the research technology and the treatment. This is an approach that resembles that of Shapiro (see Philips, 1986) who uses a non-psychodynamic interpersonal and problem-solving therapy based upon a technique for measuring target problems (the Personal Questionnaire, PQ).

Benjamin's work is only mentioned here as an example of an attempt to measure psychodynamics. Her form of therapy (Benjamin,1986, 1991) is of interest also, in that it shows the influence both of psychodynamic thinking but also of cognitive therapies. Her approach specifies, clearly, the role of learning new patterns and in this it resembles Klerman's (1984) interpersonal psychotherapy, which has links with the theories and practice of Sullivan (1953).

Lastly, in this summary of brief, psychodynamic therapies, will be mentioned Ryle's Cognitive Analytic Therapy. This too integrates cognitive techniques and psychodynamic thinking. The technique is highly structured, the therapist and the patient working together to develop a plan or mental map of the main problems, how relationships in the present are affected and what connections can be made with experiences in the course of growing up. This map bears some resemblance to the focus or core relationship patterns that are the subject matter of most brief dynamic therapies. The defining feature of CAT is that the patient and therapist concretely create a plan showing the structure of the problems, which then becomes the basis for planned, sequential work. The patient has a copy of the plan, which is worked upon in and between sessions. The therapy is brief, with 12 weekly sessions being followed by fortnightly meetings for two months with a final follow-up one month later. The patient–therapist relationship and transference is not a focus and the model of change is largely cognitive. CAT is being formally studied in the treatment of anorexic and bulimic patients at the Maudsley Hospital Eating Disorder Unit.

The decision to use psychoanalytic psychotherapy

In the preceding sections on methods of brief psychodynamic psychotherapy, the evaluation of the treatments in differing conditions was mentioned. Thus examples of the evidence for the therapies in the elderly depressed (Thompson et al., 1987), in cocaine habituation (Woody et al., 1983), in a variety of personality disorders, and so on, has been mentioned. Many of the available studies use some form of assessment of suitability for psychoanalytic psychotherapy as a criterion for admission to a formal study. In others, as in Woody et al's (1983) investigation of psychotherapy for cocaine habituation, there were no such admission criterion. Likewise, in our own studies (e.g. Dare, 1994), comparing psychoanalytic psychotherapy of eating disorder with other psychotherapies, we have selected the patients by diagnosis not by suitability for one or other form of treatment. In research, testing the applicability of psychodynamic therapy for a psychiatric population, the strategy of selecting for diagnosis, not for suitability, is sensible and easier to interpret. However, when it comes to making the decision, in practice, specific motivation is a major factor. The Penn Project group have carried out extensive studies of factors predicting a good outcome from individual psychodynamic psychotherapy. This work has been summarised and linked to many other studies by Luborsky et al. (1988). They show that psychological mindedness, combined with medium degrees of distress (depressive or anxiety, for example) are associated with better outcome than low motivation and either low or very high levels of distress.

Figure 25.7 shows a decision-making diagram. The starting point is a patient with a wide range of psychological problems associated with a psychiatric illness, a physical illness or a relationship difficulty. The presence of psychotic symptoms, at presentation, is a contraindication to exploratory psychotherapy. Figure 25.7 suggests that there are circumstances in which psychoanalytic psychotherapy can be helpful in manic-depressive illness. Some patients with a history of manic-depressive disorder want to explore the subjective connectedness and psychological concomitants of their breakdown. Psychodynamic psychotherapy has been used by clinicians within the Maudsley Psychotherapy Unit. It has been used, for example when the patient is stabilised upon lithium, and has been claimed to reduce the subsequent admission rate.

For selecting non-psychotic patients for psychoanalytic psychotherapy, the specific symptomatology is less important than the context within which it occurs. The more specific the complaint of the patient and the more that the patient is asking for relief from that

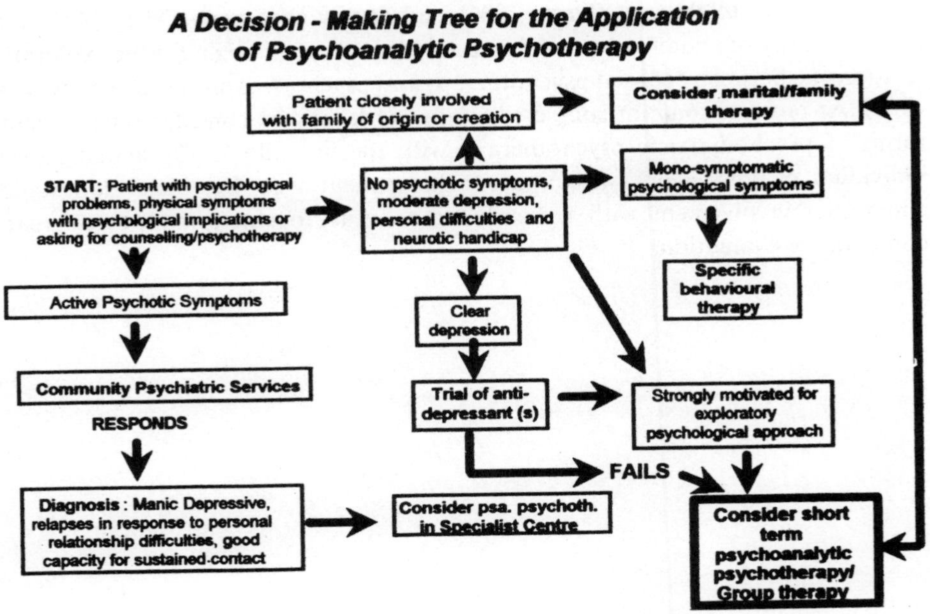

A Decision - Making Tree for the Application of Psychoanalytic Psychotherapy

Figure 25.7 A decision-making tree for the application of psychoanalytic psychotherapy. The figure assumes a context of a mental health care setting. Level of disturbance, nature of particular symptomatology and motivation for an exploratory psychological treatment are all important. Separate lines for group or individual psychoanalytic psychotherapy are not suggested because so little data contribute to the making of such a differentiation. The provision of marital and family forms of therapy are assumed to be available in parallel to individual psychotherapy, an assumption that is not always justified by reality.

particular complaint, the more specific remedies of a pharmacological or behavioural psychological kind are the treatment of first choice. Psychodynamic psychotherapy is indicated: (1) the more the patient has relatively diffuse but disabling and pervasive complaints; (2) the more their colouring is of existential discontent; (3) the more that there is a request for self-understanding. Motivation for self-understanding is complicated. It can be a contraindication to exploratory psychotherapy if the dominant aspect is the wish to place blame for the patient's condition exclusively upon others. Sometimes a patient referred for psychotherapy turns out to be filled with a sense of grudge, for which unburdening upon a psychotherapists is seen as 'the answer'. If the unburdening and blame of others is the sole motivation, it is not part of a wish to change and to overcome the pain of the past and in this sense is not an indication for psychoanalytic psychotherapy.

Figure 25.7 shows an additional complication. In an earlier section, attention was drawn to the role of life-cycle location in defining the aims of exploratory psychotherapy. This consideration is also embodied in the figure, which suggests that where a patient is closely involved in a family of origin or creation then a strategy of conjoint therapy might be equivalent to an individual psychotherapy. The author has been concerned to demonstrate clear conceptual links between the practice of individual psychoanalytic psychotherapy and couple or marital therapy (Dare, 1986) and family therapies (Dare, 1981, 1988). The psychotherapy of anorexia nervosa has been taken as a paradigm for the exploration of the relationship between conjoint psychotherapy and psychodynamic psychotherapy (see Dare, 1991). At present, conjoint couple or family work may be considered equivalent to brief forms of psychodynamic psychotherapy with the individual. The actual indication for individual or joint work with a particular patient who has close, longstanding and committed involvement with a family or a sexual partner, requires a great deal of comparative evaluation.

References

Abas, M. A., Sahakian, B. J. & Levy, R. (1990) Neuropsychological deficits and CT scan changes in elderly depressives. *Psychol. Med.*, 2

Abel, K. M., O'Keane, V. & Murray, R. M. (1996) Enhancement of the prolactin response to D-Fenfluramine in drug naive schizophrenic patients. *Br. J. Psychiat.* (in press).

Aber, J. L., Allen, J. P., Carlson, V. & Cicchetti, D. (1989) The effects of maltreatment on development during early childhood. In *Child Maltreatment: Theory and Research on the Causes and Consequences of Child Abuse and Neglect* (ed. D. Cicchetti & V. Carlson). Cambridge University Press, Cambridge, pp. 579–619.

Abercrombie, N., Hill, S. & Turner, B. (1988) *Dictionary of Sociology*, 2nd edn. Penguin Books, London.

Abraham, K. (1924) A short study of the development of the libido, viewed in the light of mental disorder. In *Selected Papers on Psycho-analysis*. Hogarth Press, London, 1953, pp. 418–501.

Abrams, R. & Taylor, M. A. (1983) The genetics of schizophrenia: a reassessment using modern criteria. *Am. J. Psychiat.*, **140**, 171–5.

Abramson, L. Y., Seligman, M. E. P. & Teasdale, J. D. (1978) Learned helplessness in humans: critique and reformulation. *J. Abnorm. Psychol.*, **87**, 49–74.

Achenbach, T. M. & Edelbrock, C. S. (1978) The classification of child psychopathology: a review and analysis of empirical efforts. *Psychol. Bull.*, **85**, 1275–301.

Acker, C. (1986) Neurophsychological deficits in alcoholics; the relative contributions of gender and drinking history. *Br. J. Addiction.*, **81**, 395–403.

Ackernecht, E. H. (1982) The history of psychosomatic medicine. *Psychol. Med.*, **12**, 17–24.

Adamovich, B. B., Henderson, J. A. & Auerback, S. (1984) *Cognitive Rehabilitation of Closed Head Injury Patients*. College Hill Press, San Deigo.

Adams S. (1961) The PTCO project. In *The Sociology of Punishment and Correction* (ed. N. Johnston, L. Savitz & M. E. Wolfgang). Wiley, New York, pp. 213–24.

Adams, S. (1991) Prescribing of psychotropic drugs to children and adolescents. *Br. Med. J.*, **302**, 217.

Adcock, M. & White, R. (eds.) (1985) *Good Enough Parenting*. British Agency for Adoption and Fostering, London.

Adelstein, A. & White, G. (1976) Alcoholism and Mortality. *Population Genetics*, **6**, 7–13, HMSO.

Adityanjee & Murray, R. M. (1991) The role of genetic predisposition in alcoholism. In *International Handbook of Addiction Behaviour* (ed. I. B. Glass). Routledge, London, pp. 41–7.

Advisory Council on the Misuse of Drugs (1982) *Treatment and Rehabilitation Report*. Department of Health and Social Security, London.

Advisory Council on the Misuse of Drugs (1984) *Prevention*. London Home Office, London.

REFERENCES

Advisory Council on the Misuse of Drugs (1988) *AIDs and Drug Misuse Part I*. London, Department of Health, London.

Advisory Council on the Misuse of Drugs (1989) *AIDs and Drug Misuse Part II*. London Department of Health, London.

Advisory Council on the Misuse of Drugs (1993) *AIDs and Drug Misuse Update*. London Department of Health, London.

Advisory Council on the Misuse of Drugs (1994) *Drug misuse and the Criminal Justice System. Part II. Policing drug misusers and the community*. London, HMSO.

Agras, W. S. (1993) Short term psychological treatments for binge eating. In *Binge Eating, Nature Assessment and Treatment* (ed. C. G. Fairburn & G. T. Wilson). Guildford Press, New York, pp. 270–86.

Agras, W. W., Rossiter, E. M., Arnow, B. *et al.* (1992) Pharmacological and cognitive–behavioural treatment for bulimia nervosa: a controlled comparison. *Am. J. Psychiat.*, **149**, 82–7.

Akbarian, S., Burney, W. E., Potkin, S. G. *et al.* (1993) Altered distribution of nicotinamide adenine phosphate-diaphorase cells in frontal lobe of schizophrenics implies disturbance of cortical development. *Arch. Gen. Psychiat.*, **50**, 169–77.

Akiskal, H. S. (1983) Dysthymic disorder: psychopathology of proposed chronic depressive subtypes. *Am. J. Psychiat.*, **140**, 11–20.

Akiskal, H. S. & McKinney, W. T. (1975) Overview of recent research in depression: Integration of ten conceptual models into a comprehensive clinical frame. *Arch. Gen., Psychiat.*, **32**, 285–305.

Albee, G. (1969) Emerging concepts of mental illness and models of treatment: the psychological point of view. *Am. J. Psychiat.*, **125**, 870.

Albert, M. (1981) *Clinical Aspects of Dysphasis*. Springer-Varlay, Vienna.

Alderson, M. R. (1985) National trends in self-poisoning in women. *Lancet*, **i**, 974–5.

Alessi, N. E., McManus, M., Grapentine, W. L. & Brickman, A. (1984) The characterisation of depressive disorders in serious juvenile offenders. *J. Affect. Disorders*, **6**, 9–17.

Alexander, F. & French, T. M. (1946) *Psychoanalytic Therapy*. Ronald Press, New York.

Alexanderson, D., Price-Evans, D. & Sjoquist, F. (1969) Steady state plasma levels and nortriptyline in twins. Influence of genetic factors and drug therapy. *Br. Med. J.*, **4**, 764–8.

Allderidge, P. (1974) Criminal insanity: Bethlem to Broadmoor. *Proc. Roy. Soc. Med.*, **67**, 897–904.

Allderidge, P. (1979) Hospitals, madhouses and asylums: cycles in the care of the insane. *Br. J. Psychiat.*, **134**, 321–34.

Allebeck, P. & Allgulander, C. (1990) Suicide among young men: psychiatric illness, deviant behaviour and substance abuse. *Acta Psychiat. Scand.*, **81**, 565–70.

Allebeck, P., Varla, A., Kristjansson, E. & Wistedt, B. (1987) Risk factors for suicide among patients with schizophrenia. *Acta Psychiat. Scand.*, **76**, 414–19.

Allebeck, P. & Wistedt, B. (1986) Mortality in schizophrenia. A ten-year follow-up based on the Stockholm county in-patient register. *Arch. Gen. Psychiat.*, **43**, 650–3.

Allen, E. A. (1989) Behavioural treatment of anxiety and related disorders in adults with a mental handicap: a review. *Mental Handicap Res.*, **2**, 47–60.

Allgulander, C. (1994) Suicide and mortality patterns in anxiety neurosis and depressive neurosis. *Arch. Gen. Psychiat.*, **51**, 702–12.

Alloway, R. & Bebbington, P. (1987) The buffer theory of social support – a review of the evidence. *Psychol. Med.*, **17**, 91–108.

Allport, G. W. (1937) Personality: A psychological interpretation. Holt, New York.

Almond, J. W. (1995) Will bovine spongiform encephalopathy transmit to humans? *Br. Med. J.*, **311**, 1415–16.

Altemus, M., Swedo, S., Leonard, H. *et al.* (1994) Changes in cerebrospinal fluid neurochemistry during treatment of obsessive-compulsive disorder with clomipramine. *Arch. Gen. Psychiat.*, **51**, 794–803.

Altschule, M. D. (1976) Evolution of the concept of schizophrenia. In *The Biology of the Schizophrenic Process* (ed. S. Wolf & B. B. Berle). Plenum Press, New York and London, pp. 1–16.

Alzheimer, A. (1895) Die Arteriosklerotische atrophie des gehirns. *Allq. Z. Psychiat.*, **51**, 809–11.

Alzheimer, A. (1907) Uber eine eigenartige Erkrankung des Hirnide Allemeine Zeitschift fur psychiatric und psychisch. *Gerichtliche Medicin*, **64**, 146–8.

Aman, M. G. (1987) Overview of pharmacotherapy. Current status and future direction. *J. Ment. Defic. Res.*, **31**, 121–30.

Aman, M. G. (1991) *Assessing Psychopathology and Behaviour Problems in Persons with Mental Retardation. A Review of Available Instruments.* DHSS, Rockville, MD.

Aman, M. G., Singh, N. N., Stewart, A. W. & Field, C. J. (1985) The Aberrant Behaviour Checklist: a behaviour rating scale for the assessment of treatment effects. *Am. J. Ment. Defic.*, **89**, 485–91.

Ambrosini, P. J., Bianchi, M. D., Rabinovich, H. & Elia, J. (1993) Antidepressant treatments in children and adolescents: I. Affective disorders. *J. Am. Acad Child Adol Psychiat.*, **32**, 1–6.

American Association on Mental Retardation (1993) *Mental Retardation. Definition, Classification and Systems of Support*, 9th Edn. AAMR, Washington, DC.

American Psychiatric Association (1980) *Diagnostic and Statistical Manual of Mental Disorders*, Third edn. American Psychiatric Association, Washington, DC.

American Psychiatric Association (1987) *Diagnostic and Statistical Manual of Mental Disorders*, Third edn – Revised. American Psychiatric Association, Washington, DC.

American Psychiatric Association (1989*a*) *The Principles of Mental Ethics of the American Medical Association with Annotations Applicable to Psychiatry.* American Psychiatric Association, Washington, DC.

American Psychiatric Association (1989*b*) Position statement on psychiatric services in jails and prisons. *Am. J. Psychiat.*, **146**, 1244.

American Psychiatric Association (1992) Practice guidelines for eating disorders. *Am. J. Psychiat.*, **150**, 208–28.

American Psychiatric Association (1993) DSM-IV draft criteria (3/1/93), Washington, DC.

American Psychiatric Association (1994) *Diagnostic and Statistical Manual of Mental Disorders*, fourth edn. American Psychiatric Association, Washington, DC.

APA Commission on Psychotherapies (1982) *Psychotherapy Research: Methodological and Efficacy Issues.* American Psychiatric Association, New York.

Ames, D. (1991) Epidemiological studies of depression among the elderly in residential and nursing homes. *Internat. J. Geriat. Psychiat.*, **6**, 347–54.

Amsterdam, J. D., Maislin, G. & Potter, L. (1994) Fluoxetine efficacy in treatment of resistant depression. *Prog. Neuro. Psychopharmacol. Biol. Psychiat.*, **18**, 243–61.

Ancoli-Israel, S., Kripke, D. F. & Mason, W. (1987) Characteristics of obstructive and central sleep apnoea in the elderly: an interim report. *Biol. Psychiat.*, **22**, 741–50.

Anderson, D. H., Nielsen, E. B., Grovald, F. C., *et al.* (1986) Some atypical neuroleptics inhibit ^{3}H-SCH-23390 binding *in vivo. Eur. J. Pharmacol.*, **120**, 143–4.

Anderson, C., Hogarty, G. & Reiss D. (1980) Family treatment of adult schizophrenic patients: a psycho-educational approach. *Schiz. Bull.*, **6**, 490–505.

Anderson, J. R. (1980) *Cognitive Psychology and its Implications.* Freeman, San Francisco.

Anderson, J., Martin, J., Mullen, P. *et al.* (1993) Prevalence of childhood sexual abuse experiences in a community sample of women. *J. Am. Acad. Child Adol. Psychiat.*, **32**, 911–19.

Anderson, P. (1988) Excess mortality associated with alcohol consumption. *Br. Med. J.*, **297**, 824–6.

Anderson, P. (1990) *Management of Drinking Problems.* World Health Organization, Geneva.

Anderson, P. (1996) Screening and Brief Intervention. In *Oxford Textbook of Medicine* (ed. D. J. Weatherall, J. G. G. Ledingham & D. A. Warrell). Oxford University Press, Oxford.

Anderson, P. & Lehto, G. (1994) Prevention policies. *Br. Med. Bull.*, **50**, 171–85.

Andreasen, N. C. (1979) Thought, language and communication disorders. *Arch. Gen. Psych.*, **36**, 1315–30.

Andreasen, N. C. (1986) Scale for the assessment of thought, language and communication. *Schiz. Bull.*, **12**, 473–82.

Andreasen, N. C. (1987) Creativity and mental illness: prevalence rates in writers and their first-degree relatives. *Am. J. Psychiat.*, **144**, 1288–92.

Andreasen, N. C. & Carpenter, W. T. (1993) Diagnosis and Classification of Schizophrenia. *Schiz. Bull.*, **19**, 199–214.

Andreasen, N. C., Swayze, V., Flaum, M. *et al.* (1990) Ventricular abnormalities in affective disorder: clinical and demographic correlates. *Am. J. Psychiat.*, **147**, 893–900.

Andreason, S., Allebeck, P., Engstrom, A. *et al.* (1987) Cannabis and Schizophrenia – a longitudinal study of Swedish conscripts. *Lancet.* **ii**, 1483–5.

Andrews, E., Bellard, J. & Ryan-Williams, G. (1986) Monosymptomatic hypochondriacal psychosis manifesting as delusions of infestation: case studies of treatment with haloperidol. *J. Clin. Psychiat.*, **47**, 188–90.

Andrews, G. (1991) Anxiety, personality and anxiety disorders. *Int. Rev. J. Psychiat.*, **3**, 293–302.

Andrews, G., Stewart, G., Allen, R. *et al.* (1990) The genetics of six neurotic disorders: a twin study. *J. Affect. Disorders*, **19**, 23–9.

Angst, J. (1986) The course of affective disorders. *Psychopathology*, **19**, (suppl 2), 47–52.

Angst, J., Baastrup, P., Grof, P. *et al.* (1973) The course of monopolar depression and bipolar psychoses. *Psychiatria Neurologia Neurochirurgia*, **76**, 489–500.

Angst, J. & Dobler-Mikola, A. (1985) The Zurich Study. VI. A continuum for depression to anxiety disorders: *Eur. Arch. Psychiat. Neurol. Soc.*, **235**, 179–86.

Angst, J. & Vollrath, M. (1991) The natural history of anxiety disorders. *Acta Psychiat. Scand.*, **84**, 446–52.

Annegers, J. F., Hauser, W. A. & Elveback, L. R. (1979) Remission of seizures and relapse in patients with epilepsy. *Epilepsia*, **20**, 729–37.

Annis, H. M., Davis, G. S., Graham, H. (1988) A controlled trial of relapse prevention procedures based on self-efficacy theory. Unpublished manuscript, ARF, Toronto.

Anon, J. S. (1976) P-LI-SS-IT (Permission-Limited Information-Specific Suggestions-Intensive Therapy) Behavioural treatment of sexual problems. In *Brief Therapy*, Harper and Row, Hagerstown, M.D. pp. 43–132.

Anthony, E. J. (1957) An experimental approach to the psychopathology of childhood: encopresis. *Br. J. Med. Psychol.*, **30**, 146–75.

Anthony, J. C., Folstein, M., Romanowski, A. J. *et al.* (1985) Comparison of the lay Diagnostic Interview Schedule and a standardised psychiatric diagnosis. *Arch. Gen. Psychiat.*, **42**, 667–75.

Anthony, W., Cohen, M., Farkas, M. *et al.* (1988) The chronically mentally ill and case management – more than a response to a dysfunctional system. *Commun. Ment. Health J.*, **24**, 21–8.

Appelbaum, P. & Roth, L. H. (1984) Involuntary treatment in medicine and psychiatry. *Am. J. Psychiat.*, **141**, 202–5.

Appels, A. (1990) Mental precursors of myocardial infarction. *Br. J. Psychiat.*, **156**, 465–71.

Appleby, L. (1991) Suicide during pregnancy and in the first postnatal year. *Br. Med. J.*, **302**, 137–40.

Appleby, L., Amos, T., Doyle, U. *et al.* (1996) General practitioners and young suicides. A preventive role for primary care. *Br. J. Psychiat.*, **168**, 330–3.

Appleby, L. & Desai, P. (1985) Documenting the relationship between homelessness and psychiatric hospitalisation. *Hosp. Commun. Psychiat.*, **36**, 732–5.

Appleby, L., Fox, H., Shaw, M. & Kumar, R. (1989) The psychiatrist in the obstetric unit. Establishing a liaison service. *Br. J. Psychiat.*, **154**, 510–15.

Appleby, L., Gregoire, A., Platz, C. *et al.* (1994) Screening women for high risk of postnatal depression. *J. Psychosom. Res.*, **38**, 539–45.

Appleby, L. & Warner, R. (1993) Parasuicide: features of repetition and the implications for intervention. *Psychol. Med.*, **23**, 13–16.

Aracharya, S. & Ekdawi, M. (1982) Day hospital rehabilitation, a six year study. *Soc. Psychiat.*, **17**, 1–5.

Arie, T. (1970) The first year of the Goodmayes psychiatric service for old people. *Lancet*, **ii**, 1179–82.

Arie, T. (1977) Thoughts on rationing and responsibility. *Age and Ageing*, **6** (suppl). 104–7.

Arie, T., Jolley, D. (1982) Making services work: organisation and style of psychogeriatric services. In *The Psychiatry of Late Life* (ed. R. Levy & F. Post). Blackwell, Oxford, pp. 222–51.

Arndt, I. O., Dorozynsky, L., Woody, G. E. *et al.* (1992) Desipramine treatment of cocaine dependence in methadone maintained patients. *Arch. Gen. Psychiat.*, **49**, 888–93.

Arthur, A. (1964) Theories and explanations of delusions: A review. *Am. J. Psychiat.*, **121**, 105–15.

Asberg, M. (1976) Treatment of depression with tricyclic drugs: pharmacokinetic and pharmacodynamic aspects. *Pharmacopsychiat. Neuropsychopharmacol.*, **9**, 18–26.

Asberg, M., Traskman, L. & Thoren, T. (1976) 5HIAA in cerebrospinal fluid: a biochemical suicide predictor? *Arch. Gen. Psychiat.*, **33**, 1193–7.

Ashton, J. R. (1980) Psychosocial outcome of induced abortion. *Br. J. Obset. Gynecol.* **87**, 1115–22.

Astrom, M. Adolffson, R. & Asplund, K. (1993) A 3 year longitudinal study. *Stroke*, **24**, 976–82.

Asubel, D. (1961) Personality disorder in disease. *Am. Psychol.*, **16**, 69–74.

Atkinson, R. M. (1991) Alcohol and drug abuse in the elderly. In *Psychiatry in the Elderly* (ed. R. Jacoby & C. Oppenheimer). Oxford Medical Publishers, Oxford, pp. 819–852.

Audit Commission (1986) *Making a Reality of Community Care*. HMSO, London.

Avnet, H. H. (1962) *Psychiatric Insurance: Financing short-term ambulatory treatment*. The New York Group Health Insurance Company, New York.

Avnet, H. H. (1965) How effective is short-term therapy? Appraisal of mental health after short-term ambulatory psychiatric treatments. In *Short-term Psychotherapy* (ed. L. R. Wolberg). Grune & Stratton, New York.

Ayllon, T. & Azrin, N. H. (1968) *The Token Economy*. Appleton-Century-Crofts, New York

Azrin, N. H. (1976) Improvements in the community reinforcement approach to alcoholism. *Behav. Res. Ther.*, **14**, 339–48.

Azrin, N. H., Sneed, T. J. & Fox, R. M. (1974) Dry-bed training: rapid elimination of childhood enuresis. *Behav. Res. Ther.*, **12**, 147–56.

Baastrup, P. C., Poulson, J. C., Schou, M. (1970) Prophylactic lithium: double-blind discontinuation in manic-depressive and recurrent depressive disorders. *Lancet* **ii**, 326–30.

Babor, T. F., Ritson, E. B., & Hodgson, R. J. (1986) Alcohol related problems in the primary health care setting; a review of early intervention strategies. *B. J. Addiction* **81**, 23–46.

Bachman, J. G., O'Malley, P. M. & Johnson, L. D. (1984) Drug use among young adults the impact of role status and social environment. *J. Personal. Soc. Psychol.*, **47**, 629–45.

Bachrach, L. (1984) *The Homeless Mentally Ill and Mental Health Services; an Analytical Review of the Literature*. US Dept. of Health and Human Services, Washington.

Bachrach, L. (1986) Deinstitutionalisation: what do the numbers mean? *Hosp. Commun. Psychiat.*, **37**, 118–21.

Bachrach, L. (1992) What do we know about homelessness among mentally ill persons? *Hosp. Commun. Psychiat.* **43**, 453–64.

Bagley, C. (1973) Occupational class and symptoms of depression. *Soc. Sci. Med.*, **7**, 327–39.

Bahar, E. (1989) Development and Mental Health. A psychiatric Epidemiological study in Developing Country: An Enquiry in Palembang, Indonesia. Phd thesis. The Australian National University.

Bahar E., Henderson, A. S. & MacKinson, A. J. (1992) An epidemiological study of mental health and socioeconomic conditions in Sumatra, Indonesia. *Acta Psychiat. Scand.*, **85**, 257–63.

Bailey, A., Bolton, P., Butler, L. *et al.* (1993) Prevalence of the fragile X anomaly amongst autistic twins and singletons. *J. of Child Psychol. Psychiat.*, **34**, 673–88.

Bailey, A., Le Couteur, A., Gottesman, I. I. *et al.* (1995) Autism as a strongly genetic disorder: evidence from a British twin study. *Psychol. Med.*, **25**, 63–77.

Bailey, S. (1993) Health in young persons' establishments: treating the damaged and preventing harm. *Crim. Behav. Ment. Health*, **3**, 349–67.

Baillarger, J. (1853) Note on the type of insanity with attacks characterised by two regular periods, one of depression and one of excitation. *Bulletin of Acadamie Nationale de Medecine*, **19**, 340.

Baker, A. W. & Duncan, S. P. (1985) Child sexual abuse: a study of prevalence in Great Britain. *Child Abuse and Neglect*, **9**, 457–67.

REFERENCES

Baker, H. & Wills, U. (1979) School phobic children at work. *Br. J. Psychiat.*, **135**, 561–4.

Baker, P., Piven, J., Schwart, S. & Patil, S. (1994) Duplication of chromosome 15q11–13 in two individuals with autistic disorder. *J. Autism Devel. Disorders*, **24**, 529–35.

Baker, H. A. (1991) Shorter-term psychotherapy: A self psychological approach. In *Handbook of Short-term Dynamic Psychotherapy* (ed. P. Crits-Christoph & J. P. Barker). Basic Books, New York, pp. 287–322.

Baker, R. & Hall, J. N. (1988) REHAB: a new assessment instrument for chronic psychiatric patients. *Schiz. Bull.*, **14**, 95–113.

Baldessarini, R. J., Cohen, B. M. & Teicher, M. H. (1988) Significance of neuroleptic dose and plasma level in the pharmacological treatment of psychoses. *Arch. Gen. Psychiat.*, **45**, 79–91.

Baldwin J. & Oliver, J. E. (1975) Epidemiology and family characteristics of severely abused children. *Br. J. Prev. Soc. Med.*, **29**, 205–21.

Baldwin, R. (1988) Delusional and non-delusional depression in late life: evidence for distinct sub-types. *Br. J. Psychiat.*, **152**, 39–44.

Baldwin, R. C. (1990) Age of onset of depression in the elderly. *Br. J. Psychiat.*, **156**, 445–6.

Baldwin, R. C. (1991) Depressive illness In *Psychiatry in the Elderly* (ed. R. Jacoby & C. Oppenheimer). Oxford Medical Publications, Oxford, pp. 676–710.

Baldwin, R. C. (1993) Late life depression and structural brain changes: A review of recent magnetic resonance imaging research. *Internat. J. Geriat. Psychiat.*, **8**, 115–124.

Baldwin R. C. & Byrne, E. J. (1989) Psychiatric aspects of Parkinson's disease. *Br. Med. J.*, **299**, 3–4.

Baldwin R. & Jolley, D. J. (1986) The prognosis of depression in old age. *Br. J. Psychiat.*, **149**, 574–583.

Bales, R. F. (1946) Cultural differences in rates of alcoholism. *Quart. J. Stud. Alcolhol*, **6**, 480–99.

Balint, M. (1957) *The Doctor, his Patient and the Illness*. Pitman Medical, London.

Balint, M. (1959) *Thrills and Regression*. Hogarth, London.

Balint, M. (1968) *The Basic Fault*. Tavistock Publications, London.

Balint, M., Ornstein, P. H. & Balint, E. (1972) *Focal Psychotherapy: An Example of Applied Psychoanalysis*. Tavistock, London.

Balkom, A., van Oppen, P., Vermeulen, A. *et al.* (1994) A meta-analysis on the treatment of obsessive-compulsive disorder: a comparison of antidepressants behaviour therapy and cognitive treatment. *Clin. Psychol. Rev.*, **14**, 359–81.

Ball, C. J. (1991) The vascular origins of the Charles Bonnet syndrome: four cases and a review of the pathogenic mechanisms. *Internat. J. Geriat. Psychiat.*, **6**, 673–9.

Ball, D. M. & Murray, R. M. (1994) Genetics of alcohol misuse. *Br. Med. Bull.*, **50**, 18–35.

Ball, J. C. & Ross, A. (1991) *The Effectiveness of Methadone Maintenance Treatment: Patients, Programs, Services, and Outcome*. Springer-Verlag, New York.

Ball, W. A. & Whybrow, P. C. (1993) Biology of depression and mania. *Curr. Opin. Psychiat.*, **6**, 27–34.

Ballinger, B. R., Simpson, E. & Stewart, M. J. (1974) An evaluation of a drug administration system in a psychiatric teaching hospital. *Br. J. Psychiat.*, **125**, 202–7.

Bancroft, J. (1974) *Deviant Sexual Behaviour: Modification and Assessment*. Clarendon Press, Oxford.

Bancroft, J. (1989) *Human Sexuality and its Problems*. Churchill Livingstone, Edinburgh.

Bancroft, J. & Coles, L. (1976) Three years' experience in a sexual problems clinic. *Br. Med. J.*, **1**, 1575–7.

Bancroft J. & Wu, F. C. W. (1983) Changes in erectile responsiveness during androgen therapy. *Arch. Sexual Behaviour.* **12**, 59–66.

Bancroft, J. H. J. & Marzack, P. (1977) The repetitiveness of self-poisoning and injury. *Br. J. Psychiat.*, **131**, 394–9.

Bancroft, J. H. J., Reynolds, F., Simkin, S. & Smith, J. (1975) Self-poisoning and self-injury in the Oxford area. *Br. J. Prevent. Soc. Med.*, **29**, 170–7.

Bandura, A. (1971) *Principles of Behaviour Modification*. Holt, Rhinehart & Winston, New York.

Bandura, A. (1977a) Social Learning Theory. Prentice Hall, Englewood Cliffs.

Bandura, A. (1977b) Self-efficacy: toward a unifying theory of behavioural change. *Psychol. Rev.*, **84**, 191–215.

Banks, M. & Jackson, P. (1982) Unemployment and risk of minor psychiatric disorder in young people: cross sectional and longitudinal evidence. *Psychol. Med.*, **12**, 786–98.

Bannerjee, S. P., Kung, L. S., Riggi, S. J. & Chanda, S. K. (1977) Development of β-adrenergic subsensitivity by antidepressants. *Nature*, **268**, 455–6.

Barham, P. (1993) *Schizophrenia and Human Value*. Free Association Books, London.

Barkley, R. (1990) *Attention Deficit Hyperactivity*. Guildford Press, New York.

Barkley, R. A., Fischer, M., Edelbrock, C. S. & Smallish, L. (1990) The adolescent outcome of hyperactive children diagnosed by research criteria. I. An 8-year prospective follow-up study. *J. Am. Acad. Child Adol. Psychiat.*, **29**, 546–57.

Barlow, D., Vermilyea, J., Blanchard, E. *et al.* (1985) The phenomenon of panic. *J. Abnorm. Psychol.*, **94**, 320–8.

Baron-Cohen, S. (1989) The autistic child's theory of mind: a case of specific developmental delay. *J. Child Psychol. Psychiat.*, **30**, 285–97.

Baron-Cohen, S., Tager-Flusberg, H. & Cohen, D. (1993) *Understanding Other Minds: Perspectives from Autism*. Oxford University Press, Oxford.

Barr, L. C. (1988) The surgical complications of drug abuse. *Surgery*, **60**, 1420–4.

Barraclough, B. (1981) Suicide and epilepsy. In *Epilepsy and Psychiatry* (ed. E. H. Reynolds & M. R. Trimble). Churchill Livingstone, Edinburgh, pp. 72–6.

Barraclough, B., Bunch, J., Nelson, B. & Sainsbury, P. (1974) A hundred cases of suicide: clinical aspects. *Br. J. Psychiat.*, **122**, 95–6.

Barrowclough, C., Tarrier, N., Watts, S. *et al.* (1987) Assessing the functional value of relatives' knowledge about schizophrenia: a preliminary report. *Br. J. Psychiat.*, **151**, 1–8.

Barsky, A. (1979) Patients who amplify bodily sensations. *Ann. Internal Med.*, **91**, 63–70.

Barsky, A., Wool, C., Barnett, M. & Cleary, P. (1994) Histories of childhood trauma in adult hypochondriacal patients. *Am. J. Psychiat.*, **151**, 397–401.

Barsky, A., Wyshak, G. & Klerman, G. (1992) Psychiatric comorbidity in DSM-IIIR hypochondriasis. *Arch. Gen. Psychiat.*, **49**, 101–8.

Barta, P. E., Pearlsson, G. D., Powers, R. E. *et al.* (1990) Auditory hallucinations and smaller superior temporal gyrus volume in schizophrenia. *Am. J. Psychiat.*, **147**, 1457–62.

Barlett, F. C. (1932) *Remembering: A Study in Experimental and Social Psychology*. Cambridge University Press, London.

Bass, C. & Benjamin, S. (1993) The management of chronic somatisation. *Br. J. Psychiat.*, **162**, 472–80.

Bass, C. & Gardner, W. N. (1985) Respiratory and psychiatric abnormalities in chronic symptomatic hyperventilation. *Br. Med. J.*, **290**, 1387–90.

Bass, C. & Gardner, W. (1989) Hyperventilation in clinical practice. *Br. J. Hosp. Med.*, **41**, 73–81.

Bass, C. & Kerwin, R. W. (1989) Rediscovering monoamine oxidase inhibitors. *Br. Med. J.*, **298**, 345–6.

Bassett, T., Braisby, D., Edwards, S. & Newbiggin, K. (1991) Involving service users in community mental health services. In *Community Mental Health Centres/Teams* (ed. R. Echlin). Good Practices in Mental Health.

Bassuk, E. (1984) The homelessness problem. *Scientific American*, **251**, 40–6.

Baumeister, A. A. (1989) Causes of severe maladaptive behaviour in persons with severe mental retardation: a review of hypotheses. Presentation given to the National Institute of Health, Bethesda, MD.

Bauer, M. S. & Whybrow, P. C. (1986) The effect of changing thyroid function of cyclic affective illness in a human subject. *Am. J. Psychiat.*, **143**, 633–6.

Baxter, L., Phelps, M., Mazziotta, J. *et al.* (1985) Cerebral metabolic rates for glucose in mood disorders. *Arch. Gen. Psychiat.*, **42**, 411–47.

Baxter, L., Schwartz, J., Bergman, K. *et al.* (1992) Caudate glucose metabolic rate changes with both drug and behaviour therapy for obsessive-compulsive disorder. *Arch. Gen. Psychiat.*, **49**, 681–9.

Baxter, L. R. Jr., Schwartz, J. M., Phelps, M. E. *et al* (1989) Reduction of prefrontal cortex glucose metabolism common to three types of depression. *Arch. Gen. Psychiat.*, **46**., 243–50.

Bear, D. M. & Fedio, P. (1977) Qualitative analysis of interictal behaviour in temporal lobe epilepsy. *Arch. Neurol.*, **34**, 454–67.

Beardslee, W. R., Son, L. & Vaillant, G. E. (1986) Exposure to parental alcoholism during childhood and outcome in adulthood: a prospective longitudinal study. *Br. J. Psychiat.*, **149**, 584–91.

Beary, M. D., Lacey, J. H. & Merry, J. (1986) Alcoholism and eating disorders in women of fertile age. *Br. J. Addiction.* **81**, 685–9.

Beaumont G. (1973) Drug interactions with clomiprimine (Anafranil). *J. Internat. Med. Res.*, **1**, 480–4.

Beaumont, G. (1989) The toxicity of antidepressants. *Br. J. Psychiat.*, **154**, 457–8.

Bebbington, P. (1985) Three cognitive theories of depression. *Psych. Med.*, **15**, 739–69.

Bebbington, P. E. (1988) The social epidemiology of clinical depression. In *Handbook of Studies in Social Psychiatry* (ed. A. S. Henderson & G. Burrows). Elsevier, Amsterdam, pp. 87–102.

Bebbington, P. E. (1990) Population surveys of psychiatric disorder and the need for treatment. *Soc. Psychiat. Psychiat. Epidemiol.*, **25**, 33–40.

Bebbington, P. E. (1991) The epidemiology of affective disorders. In *Social Psychiatry: Theory, Methodology and Practice* (ed. P. E. Bebbington). Transaction, New Brunswick, NJ, pp. 265–304

Bebbington, P. E. (1993) Transcultural aspects of affective disorder. *Internat. Rev. Psychiat.*, **5**, 145–56.

Bebbington, P. E., Bowen, J. & Ramana, R. (1995) Life events and psychosis. In *Stressful Life Events* (ed. T. W. Miller). International Universities Press, pp. 89–118.

Bebbington, P. E., Brugha, T., MacCarthy, B. *et al.* (1988) The Camberwell Collaborative Depression Study. I. Depressed probands: Adversity and the form of depression. *Br. J. Psychiat.*, **152**, 754–65.

Bebbington, P. E. & Hill, P. D. (1985) *A Manual of Practical Psychiatry*. Blackwell Scientific, Oxford.

Bebbington, P. E., Hurry, J. & Tennant, C. (1981*a*) Psychiatric disorders in selected immigrant groups in Camberwell, *Soc. Psychiat.*, **16**, 43–51.

Bebbington, P. E., Hurry, J. & Tennant, C. (1986) Adversity and working class vulnerability to minor affective disorder. *J. Affect. Disord.*, **11**, 115–20.

Bebbington, P. E., Hurry, J., Tennant C. *et al.* (1981*b*) Epidemiology of mental disorders in Camberwell. *Psychological Medicine*, **11**, 561–80.

Bebbington, P., Katz, R., McGuffin, P. *et al.* (1989) The risk of minor depression before the age 65: Results from a community survey. *Psychol. Med.*, **19**, 393–400.

Bebbington, P. E. & Kuipers, L. (1994) The predictive utility of Expressed Emotion in schizophrenia: an aggregate analysis. *Psychol. Med.*, **24**, 707–18.

Bebbington, P. E., Marsden, L. & Brewin, C. R. (1996) Measuring the need for psychiatric treatment in the general population: the community version of the Needs for Care Assessment. *Psychol. Med.*, **26**, 229–36.

Bebbington, P. E., Tennant, C. & Hurry, J. (1991) Adversity in groups with an increased risk of minor affective disorder. *Br. J. Psychiat.*, **158**, 40–5.

Bebbington, P. E., Wilkins, S., Jones, P. *et al.* (1993) Life events and psychosis: Initial results from the Camberwell Collaborative Psychosis Study. *Br. J. Psychiat.*, **162**, 72–9.

Bech, P. (1981) Rating scales for affective disorders: their validity and consistency. *Acta Psychiat. Scand.*, Supplement **295**, 1–99.

Bech, P. (1992) Symptoms and assessment of depression. In *Handbook of Affective Disorders* (ed. E. S. Paykell). Churchill Livingstone, London, pp. 3–12.

Bech, P., Allerup, P., Gram, L. F. *et al.* (1981) The Hamilton Depression Scale. Evaluation of objectivity using logistic models. *Acta Psychiat. Scand.*, **63**, 290–9.

Bech, P., Bolwig, T. G., Kramp, P. *et al* (1979) The Bech-Rafaelson Mania Scale and the Hamilton Depression Rating Scale. *Acta Psychiat. Scand.*, **59**, 420–30.

Bech, P., Gram, L. F., Dein, E. *et al.* (1975) Quantitative rating of depressive states. *Acta Psychiat. Scand.*, **51**, 161–70.

Beck, A. T. (1976) *Cognitive Therapy and the Emotional Disorders*. International Universities Press, New York.

Beck, A. (1979) *Cognitive Therapy of Depression*. Guilford Press, New York.

Beck, A. T., Emery, G. & Greenberg, R. L. (1985) *Anxiety Disorders and Phobias: a Cognitive Perspective*. Basic Books, New York.

Beck, A. T., Epstein, N., Brown, G. *et al.* (1988*b*) An inventory for measuring clinical anxiety: psychometric properties. *J. Consult Clin. Psychol.*, **56**, 893–7.

Beck, A. T., Freeman, A. & Associates (1990) *Cognitive Therapy and Personality Disorders*. Guildford Press, New York.

Beck, A. T., Rush, A. J., Shaw, B. F. & Emery G. (1979) *Cognitive Therapy of Depression*. Guildford Press, New York.

Beck, A. T., Sokol, L., Clark, D. A. *et al.* (1992) Focused cognitive therapy of panic disorder: a cross over design and one year follow-up. *Am. J. Psychiat.*, **147**, 778–83.

Beck, A. T., Steer, R. A. & Garbin, M. G. (1988*a*) Psychometric properties of the Beck Depression Inventory: twenty-five years of evaluation. *Clin. Psychol. Rev.*, **8**, 77–100.

Beck, A. T., Steer, R. A., Kovacs, M. & Garrison, B. (1985) Hopelessness and eventual suicide: a 10-year prospective study of patients hospitalised with suicidal ideation. *Am. J. Psychiat.*, **142**, 559–63.

Beck, A. T., Ward, C. H., Mendelson, M. *et al.* (1961). An inventory for measuring depression. *Arch. Gen. Psychiat.*, **4**, 561–71.

Beck, A. T., Ward, C. H. Mendelson, M. (1962) Reliability of psychiatric diagnoses II. A study of consistency of clinical judgement ratings. *Am. J. Psychiat.*, **119**, 351–7.

Becker, H. (1963) *Outsider Studies in the Sociology of Deviance*. The Free Press, New York.

Becker, R. E., Heimberg, R. G. & Bellack, A. S. (1987) *Social Skills Training Treatment for Depression*. Pergamon Books Inc., UK.

Becker, J. V., Skinner, L. J., Abel, G. G. & Cichon, J. (1986) Level of post assault functioning in rape and incest victims. *Arch. Sexual Behaviour*, **15**, 37–49.

Beerforth, M., Conlon E., Field, V. *et al.* (eds) (1990) *Whose Service is it Anyway? Users' Views of Co-ordinating Community Care*. Research and Development for Psychiatry (RDP), London.

Begleiter, H., Porjes, B., Bihari, B. & Kissin, B. (1984) Event related potentials in boys at risk from alcoholism. *Science*, **225**, 1493–6.

Beigel, A., Murphy, D. & Bunney, W. E. (1971) The manic-state rating scale. *Arch. Gen. Psychiat.*, **25**, 256–62.

Bell, R. (1985) *Holy Anorexia*. Chicago University Press, Chicago.

Bellack, A. S., Hersen, M. & Himmelhock, J. M. (1983) A comparison of social skills training, pharmacotherapy and psychotherapy for depression. *Behav. Res. Therapy.*, **21**, 101–7.

Bellak, L. (1958) *Schizophrenia: a Review of the Syndrome*. Logos Press, New York.

Benbow, S. M. (1987) Liaison referrals to a department of psychiatry for the elderly. *Internat. J. Geriat. Psychiat.*, **2**, 235–40.

Benbow, S. M. (1988) Family therapy in the elderly. In *Current Approaches to Affective Disorders in the Elderly*. Duphar, Southampton, pp. 44–6.

Benbow, S. M. (1989) The role of electroconvulsive therapy in the treatment of depressive illness in old age. *Br. J. Psychiat.*, **155**, 147–52.

Benbow, S. M. (1991) ECT in late life. *Internat. J. Geriat. Psychiat.*, **6**, 401–6.

Bench, C. J., Friston, L. K. J., Brown, R. G. *et al.* (1993) Regional cerebral blood flow in depression measured by positron emission tomography. The relationship with clinical dimensions. *Psychol. Med.*, **23**, 579–90.

Benjamin, L. S. (1986) *Interpersonal Diagnosis and Treatment: The SASB Approach*. Guildford Press, New York.

Benjamin, L. S. (1987) Use of the SASB dimensional model to develop treatment plans for personality disorder: Narcissism. *J. Personality Disorders*, **1**, 43̂70.

Benjamin, L. S. (1991) Brief SASB-directed reconstructive learning therapy. In *Handbook of short-term dynamic psychotherapy* (ed. P. Crits-Christoph & J. P. Barber). Basic Books, New York, pp. 248–86.

Benjamin, R. S., Costello, E. J. & Warren, M. (1990) Anxiety disorders in a paediatric sample. *J. Anxiety Disord.*, **4**, 293–316.

REFERENCES

Benjamin, S., Decalmer, P. & Haran, D. (1982) Community screening for mental illness: a validity study of the General Health Questionnaire. *Br. J. Psychiat.*, **140**, 174–80

Bennett, D. (1978) Social forms of psychiatric treatment. In *Schizophrenia: Towards a New Synthesis* (ed. J. Wing). Academic Press, London and Ontario. pp. 211–32.

Benson, D. F. (1973) Psychiatric Aspects of Aphasia. *Br. J. Psychiat.*, **123**, 555–66.

Benson, D. F., Gardner, H. & Meadows, J. C. (1976) Reduplicative paramnesia. *Neurology*, **23**, 147–151.

Beresin, E. V. (1988) Delirium in the elderly. *J. Geriat. Psychiat. Neurol.*, **1**, 127–43.

Berg, I. (1982) When truants and school refusers grow up. *Br. J. Psychiat.*, **141**, 208–10.

Berg, J. M. & Gosse, G. C. (1990) Specific mental retardation disorders and problem behaviours. *Internat. Rev. Psychiat.*, **2**, 53–60.

Bergem, A. L. M., Dahl, A. A., Guldberg, C. & Hansen, H. (1990) Langfeldt's schizophreniform psychoses fifty years later. *Br. J. Psychiat.*, **157**, 351–4.

Berger, M., Yule, W. & Rutter, M. (1975) Attainment and adjustment in two geographical areas. II. The prevalence of specific reading retardation. *Br. J. Psychiat.*, **126**, 510–19.

Berglund, M. (1984) Suicide in alcoholism. A prospective study of 88 suicides: I. The multidimensional diagnosis at first admission. *Arch. Gen. Psychiat.*, **41**, 888–91.

Berglund, M. & Nilsson, K. (1987) Mortality in severe depression. A prospective study including 103 suicides. *Acta Psychiat. Scand.*, **76**, 372–80.

Bergmann, K. (1971) The neurosis in old age. In Recent developments in psychogeriatrics (ed. D. W. K. Kay & A. Walk). *British Journal of Psychiatry*, special publication No: 6, pp. 39–50.

Bernadt, M. W. & Murray, R. (1986) Psychiatric disorder, drinking and alcoholism: what are the links? *Br. J. Psychiat.*, **148**, 393–400.

Bernadt, M. W., Mumford, J., Taylor, C. *et al.* (1982) Comparison of questionnaire and laboratory tests in the detection of excessive drinking and alcoholism. *Lancet*, **1**, 325–8.

Berney, T. (1992) Autistic disorders. *Current Opinion in Psychiatry.*, **5**, 683–6.

Berney, T., Kolvin, I., Bhat, S. R. *et al* (1981) School phobia: a therapeutic trial with clomipramine and short-term outcome. *Br. J. Psychiat.*, **138**, 110–18.

Bernstein, D. A. & Borkovec, T. D. (1973) *Progressive Relaxation Training: a manual for the helping professions*. Chapman, Illinois.

Berrettini, W. H., Cappellari, C. B., Nurnberger, J. I. & Gershon, E. S. (1987) Beta-adrenergic receptor on lymphoblasts. A study of manic-depressive illness. *Neuropsychobiology*, **17**, 15–18

Berrettini, W. H., Ferraro, T. N., Goldin, L. R. *et al* (1994) Chromosome 18 DNA markers and manic-depressive illness: Evidence for a susceptibility gene. *Proc. Natl. Acad. Sci.*, **91**, 5918–21.

Berridge, V. & Edwards, G. (1987) *Opium and the People. Opiate Use in Nineteenth-Century England.* Yale University Press, New Haven and London.

Berrios, G. E. (1981) Stupor: a conceptual history. *Psychol. Med.*, **11**, 677–88.

Berrios, G. (1992) History of the affective disorders. In *Handbook of Affective Disorders* (ed. E. G. Paykel). Churchill Livingstone, Edinburgh, pp. 43–56.

Berrios, G. E. (1993) European views on personality disorders: a conceptual history. *Compreh. Psychiat.*, **34**, 14–30.

Berrios, G. G. & Brook, P. (1984) Visual hallucinations and sensory delusions in the elderly. *Br. J. Psychiat.*, **144**, 662–64.

Bertagnoli, M. W. & Borchart, C. M. (1990) A review of ECT for children and adolescents. *J. Am. Acad. Child Adol. Psychiat.*, **29**, 302–7.

Bertelsen, A., Harvald, B. & Hauge, M. (1977) A Danish twin study of manic-depressive disorders. *Brit. J. Psychiat.*, **130**, 330–51.

Berthier, M. L. (1994) Corticocallosal anomalies in Asperger syndrome. *Am. J. Roentgenol.*, **162**, 236–7.

Betts, T. A. (1993) Neuropsychiatry In *A Textbook of Epilepsy* (ed. J. Laidlaw, A. Richens & D. Chadwick). Churchill Livingstone, London, pp. 397–457.

Beaumont, P. J. V., Russell, J. D. & Touyz, S. W. (1995) Psychological concerns in the maintenance of dieting disorders. In *Handbook of Eating Disorders* (ed. G. Szmukler, C. Dare & L. Treasure). Willey, London, pp. 221–42.

Beutler, L. E., Thornby, J. I. & Karacan, I (1978) Psychological variables in the diagnosis of insomnia. In *Sleep Disorders: Diagnosis and Treatment* (ed. R. L. Williams & I. Karacan). Wiley, New York, pp. 61–100.

Bhanji, S. & Mattingly D. (1988) *Medical Aspects of Anorexia Nervosa*. Wright, London.

Bicknell, J. (1983) The psychopathology of handicap. *Br. J. Med. Psychol.*, **56**, 167–78.

Biegon, A. & Israeli, M. (1988) Regionally selective increases in B-adrenergic receptor density in the brains of suicide victims. *Brain Res.*, **442**, 199–203.

Bienenfeld, D., Wheeler, B. G. (1989) Psychiatric services to nursing homes: A liaison model. *Hosp. Commun. Psychiat.*, **40**, 793–4.

Biernacki, P. (1986) *Pathways away from Heroin Addiction: Recovery Without Treatment*. Temple University, Philadelphia.

Bifulco, A., Brown, G. W. & Alder, Z. (1991) Early sexual abuse and clinical depression in adult life. *Br. J. Psychiat.*, **159**, 115–22.

Binder, J. L. & Strupp, H. H. (1991) The Vanderbilt approach to time-limited dynamic psychotherapy. In *Handbook of Short-term Dynamic Psychotherapies* (ed. P. Crits-Christoph & J. P. Barber). Basic Books, New York, pp. 137–65.

Binswanger, L. (trans by Mendel W. M. & Lyons, J) (1959) The case of Ellen West. I *Existence a New Dimension in Psychiatry and Psychiatry* (ed. R. May, E. Angel & Ellenberger), pp. 237–364.

Bion, W. R. (1961) *Experience in Groups and other Papers*. Tavistock, London.

Birchwood, M., Smith, J., MacMillan F. *et al.* (1989) Predicting relapse in schizophrenia: the development and implementation of an early signs monitoring system using patients and families as observers, a preliminary investigation. *Psychological Medicine*, **19**, 649–656.

Bird, H. R., Canino, G., Rubio-Stipec, M. *et al.* (1988) Estimates of the prevalence of childhood maladjustment in a community survey in Puerto Rico. *Arch. Gen. Psychiat.*, **45**, 1120–6.

Birtchnel, J. (1972) Early parent death and psychiatric diagnosis. *Soc. Psychiat.*, **7**, 202–10.

Bishop, D. V. M. (1989) Autism, Asperger's syndrome and Semantic Pragmatic Disorder: Where are the boundaries? *Br. J. Disord. Commun.*, 24, 107–21.

Bishop, D. V. M. & Adams, C. (1989) Conversational characteristics of children with semantic-pragmatic disorders. II. What features lead to a judgement of inappropriacy? *Br. J. Disord. Commun.*, **24**, 241–63.

Bishop, K., Briggs, P. & Schmidt, U (1994) Identification and immediate management of the oral changes associated with eating disorders. *Brit. J. Hosp. Med.*, **52**, 326–42.

Black, D. & Kaplan, T. (1988) Father kills mother: issues and problems encountered by a child psychiatric team. *Br. J. Psychiat.*, **153**, 624–30.

Black, D., Noyes, R., Goldstein, R. & Blum, N. (1992) A family history study of obsessive-compulsive disorder. *Arch. Gen. Psychiat.*, **49**, 362–8.

Black, D., Wesner, R., Bowers, W. & Gabel, J. A. (1993) A comparison cf fluvoxamine, cognitive therapy, and placebo in the treatment of panic disorder. *Arch. Gen. Psychiat.*, **50**, 44–50.

Black, D., Winokur, G. & Nasrallah, A. (1987*a*) Suicide in subtypes of major affective disorder. *Arch. Gen. Psychiat.*, **44**, 878–80.

Black, D. W., Winour, G. & Nasrallah, A. (1987*b*) Treatment of mania: a naturalistic study of electroconvulsive therapy versus lithium in 438 patients. *J. Clin. Psychiat.*, **48**, 132–9.

Black, F. W. (1976) Cognitive deficits in patients with unilateral war-related frontal lobe lesions. *J. Clin. Psychol.*, **32**, 366–72.

Black, L., Cullen, C., Dickens, P. & Turnbull, J. (1988) Anger control. *Br. J.Hosp. Med.*, **39**, 325–9.

Blackburn, I. M., Eunson, K. M. & Bishop, S. (1986) A two year naturalistic follow-up of depressed patients treated with cognitive therapy and pharmacotherapy, each alone and in combination. *Br. J. Psychiat.*, **139**, 181–9.

Blackburn, I. M., Bishop, S., Glen, A. I. M. *et al.* (1981) The efficacy of cognitive therapy in depression:

a treatment trial using cognitive therapy and pharmacotherapy, each alone and in combination. *Br. J. Psychiat.*, **139**, 181–9.

Blackburn, I. M., Loudon, J. B. & Ashworth, C. M. (1977) A new scale for measuring mania. *Psychol. Med.*, **7**, 453–8.

Blackburn, R. (1982) *The Special Hospitals Assessment of Personality and Socialisation.* Unpublished MS, Ashworth Hospital, Liverpool.

Blackburn, R. (1987) Two scales for the assessment of personality disorder in antisocial populations. *Personality and Individual Differences*, **8**, 81–93.

Blackburn, R. (1988) On moral judgements and personality disorders: The myth of the psychopathic personality revisited. *Br. J. Psychiat.*, **153**, 505–12.

Blackburn, R. (1992) Criminal behaviour, personality disorder, and mental illness: the origins of confusion. *Crim. Behav. Men. Health*, **2**, 66–77.

Blackburn, R. (1993) *The Psychology of Criminal Conduct.* Wiley, Chichester.

Blackwood, D. H., St Clair, D. M. & Muir, W. J. (1991) Auditory P300 and eye tracking dysfunction in schizophrenic pedigrees. *Arch. Gen. Psychiat.*, **48**, 899–909.

Blakemore, C. (1990) *The Mind Machine.* BBC, London.

Bland, R. C., Newman, S. C. & Orme, H. (1988) Epidemiology of psychiatric disorders in Edmonton. *Acta Psychiat. Scand.*, **77**, (Suppl. 338).

Blane, D., Davey Smith, G., Bartley, M. (1990) Social differences in years of potential life lost: site trends and principal causes. *Br. Med. J.*, **301**, 429–32.

Blanz, B., Schmidt, M. H. & Esser, G. (1991) Familial adversities and child psychiatric disorders. *J. Child Psychol. Psychiat.*, **32**, 939–50.

Blaxter, M. (1990) *Health and Lifestyles.* Routledge, London.

Blazer, D., George, L. K., Landerman, R. *et al.* (1985) Psychiatric disorders: a rural/urban companion. *Arch. Gen. Psychiat.*, **45**, 1078–84.

Blazer, D., Hughes, D. C. & George, L. K. (1987) The epidemiology of depression in an elderly community population. *The Gerontologist*, **27**, 281–7.

Blazer, D., Swartz, M., Woodbury, M. *et al* (1988) Depressive symptoms and depressive diagnoses in a community population. *Arch. Gen. Psychiat.*, **45**, 1078–84.

Bleeker, J. A. C. (1994) Dementia services: a continental European view. In *Dementia* (ed. A. Burns & r. Levy). Chapman & Hall Medical, London, pp. 581–99.

Blessed, G., Tomlinson, B. & Roth, M. (1968) The association between quantative measures of dementing and senile change in cerebral grey matter of elderly subjects. *Br. J. Psychiat.*, **114**, 797–811.

Bleuler, E. (1911) *Dementia Praecox or the Group of Schizophrenias* (translated by J. J. Zinkin, 1950). International Universities Press, New York.

Bleuler, E. (1950) *Dementia Praecox or the Group of Schizophrenias* (translated by I. L. Abell). Grune and Stratton, New York.

Bleuler, M. (1974) The long-term outcome of the schizophrenic psychoses. *Psychol. Med.*, **4**, 244–54.

Blum, K., Noble, E. P., Sheridan, P. J. *et al.* (1990) Allelic association of human dopamine D2 receptor gene in alcoholism. *J. Amer. Med. Assoc.*, **263**, 2055–60.

Blume, S. B. (1986) Women and alcohol; a review. *J. Amer. Med. Assoc.*, **256**, 1467–70.

Blumenthal, S. & Wessely, S. (1992) National survey of current arrangements for diversion from custody in England and Wales. *Br. Med. J.*, **305**, 1322–5.

Blumstein, A. & Cohen, J. (1987) Characterising criminal careers. *Science* **237**, 985–91.

Blumstein, A., Cohen, J., Roth, J. & Fisher, C. (1986) *Criminal Careers and Career Criminals.* National Academy Press, Washington DC.

Blundell E. & Hill, A. J. (1993) Binge eating: psychobiological mechanism. In *Binge Eating: Nature, Assessment and Treatment* (ed. C. G. Fairburn & G. T. Wilson). pp. 206–24.

Boardman, J. (1987) *The Mental Health Advice Centre in Lewisham. Service Usage: Trends from 1978–1984.* Research Report No. 3. The National Unit for Psychiatric Research and Development, Lewisham.

Bohman, M. (1978) Some genetic aspects of alcoholism and criminality. *Arch. Gen. Psychiat.*, **35**, 269–76.

Bohman, M., Sigvardsson, S. & Cloninger, C. R. (1981) Maternal inheritance of alcohol abuse. Cross fostering analysis of adopted women. *Arch. Gen. Psychiat.*, **38**, 965–9.

Boller, F. & Grafman, J. (1983) Acalulia: Historical development and current significance. *Brain and Cognition.*, **2**, 205–23.

Bolton, D., Collins, S. & Steinberg, D. (1983) The treatment of obsessive-compulsive disorder in adolescence. *Br. J. Psychiat.*, **142**, 456–64.

Boon, F. (1991) Encopresis and sexual assault. *J. Am. Acad. Child Adol. Psychiat.*, **30**, 509–10.

Boone, K. B., Miller, M. L., Lesser, I. M. *et al.* (1992) Neuropsychological correlates of white-matter lesions in healthy elderly subjects. *Arch. Neurol.*, **49**, 549–54.

Bond, M. R. (1978) Psychological and psychiatric aspects of pain. *Anaesthesia*, **33**, 355–62.

Bonhoeffer, K. (1909) Exogenous psychoses (translated 1974). In *Themes and Variations in European Psychiatry* (ed. S. R. Hirsch & M. Shepherd). J. Wright, Bristol, pp. 47–64.

Boreham, J. (1983) A follow-up study of 54 persistent school refusers. *Assoc Child Psychol. Psychiat. News*, **15**, 8–14.

Boss, M. (1949) *Meaning and Content of Sexual Perversions.* Grune and Stratton, New York.

Boszormenyi-Nagy, I. & Spark, G. (1982) *Invisible Loyalties: Reciprocity in Intergenerational Family Therapy.* Harper Row, New York.

Bourne, S. (1968) The psychological effects of stillbirths on women and their doctors. *J. R. Coll. Gen. Pract.*, **16**, 103–12.

Bowen, D., Smith, C., White, P. & Davidson, A. (1976) Neurotransmitter transmitted enzymes as indices of hypoxia in senile dementia and other abiotrophies. *Brain*, **99**, 159–96.

Bower, W. H. & Altschule, M. D. (1956) The use of progesterone in the treatment of postpartum psychosis. *N. Engl. J. Med.*, **254**, 157–60.

Bowlby, J. (1951) *Maternal Care and Mental Health.* World Health Organization.

Bowlby, J. 1969) *Attachment and loss Vol I: Attachment.* Hogarth Press, London.

Bowlby, J. (1973) *Attachment and Loss Vol II: Separation: anxiety and anger.* Hogarth Press, London.

Bowlby, H. (1980) *Attachment and Loss Vol. III: Loss, sadness and depression.* Hogarth Press, London.

Bowling, A. (1991) *Measuring Health. A Review of Quality of Life Measurement Scales.* Open University Press, Buckingham.

Boyer, W. F. & Feighner, J. P. (1991) The efficacy of selective serotonin reuptake inhibitors in depression. In *Selective Serotonin Reuptake Inhibitor.* (ed. J. P. Fergmer & W. F. Boyer). Wiley, Chichester and New York, pp. 89–108.

Boyle, M. (1990) *Schizophrenia: A Scientific Delusion?* Routledge, London and New York.

Bozarth, M. (1991) Drug Addiction as a psychobiological process. In *Addictions Controversies*, (ed. D. M. Warburton), Harwood Academic Publishers, Chur, Switzerland, pp. 112–34.

Brabbins, C. J. (1992) Charles Bonnet syndrome. *Internat. J. Geriat. Psychiat.*, **7**, 455–7.

Bradbury, T. N. & Miller, G. A. (1985) Season of birth in schizophrenia: A review of evidence, methodology, and etiology. *Psychol. Bull.*, **98**, 569–94.

Bradley, A. M. (1988) Keep coming back: the case for a valuation of Alcoholics Anonymous. *Alcohol Health and Research World*, **12**, 192–9.

Bradley, B. & Mathews, A. (1983) Negative self schemata in clinical depression. *Br. J. Clin. Psychol.*, **22**, 173–81.

Bradley, P. B. (1986) Pharmacology of antipyschotic drugs, In *The Psychopharmacology and Treatment of Schizophrenia* (ed. P. Bradley & S. Hirsch). Oxford Med. Pubs., Oxford, pp. 27–70.

Brain, W. R. (1965) *Speech Disorders: Aphasia, Apraxia & Agnosia* (2nd edn). Butterworth, London.

Brain Committee (1965) *2nd Report on the Departmental Committee on Morphine and Heroin Addiction.* HMSO, London.

Bramble, D. (1992) A survey of lithium use in the elderly. *Internat. J. Geriat. Psychiat.*, **7**, 819–36.

Brandenburg, N. A., Friedman, R. M. & Silver, S. E. (1990) The epidemiology of childhood psychiatric disorders: prevalence findings from recent studies. *J. Am. Acad. Child Adol. Psychiat.*, **29**, 76–83.

REFERENCES

Brandon, D. (1991) *Innovation Without Change: Consumer Power in Psychiatric Services*. Macmillan, London.

Brandon, A. & Brandon, D. (1987) *Consumers as Colleagues*. MIND Publications, London.

Brandt, L. B. & Mackenzie, T. B. (1987) Obsessive-compulsive disorder–exacerbation during pregnancy. *Int. J. Psychiat. Med.*, **17**, 361–5.

Braun, P., Kochansky, G., Shapiro, R. *et al.* (1981) Overview: deinstitutionalisation of psychiatric patients, a critical review of outcome studies. *Am. J. Psychiat.*, **138**, 736–74.

Brazelton, T. B. (1982) *Infants and Mothers*. Delacorte Press, New York.

Brazelton, T. B. & Cramer, B. G. (1991) *The Earliest Relationship: Parents, Infants and the Drama of Early Attachment*. Karanc Books, London.

Breakey, W. R., Goodell, H., Lorenz, P. L. & McHugh, P. (1974) Hallucinogenic drugs as precipitants of schizophrenia. *Psychol. Med.*, **4**, 255–61.

Breeze, E. (1985) *Differences in Drinking Patterns Between Selected Regions*. HMSO, London.

Breier, A., Charney, D. & Heninger, G. (1985) The diagnostic validity of anxiety disorders and their relationship in depressive illness. *Am. J. Psychiat.*, **142**, 782–7.

Breisch, S. T., Zanlan, F. P. & Hobel, B. G. (1976) Hyperphagia and obesity following serotonin depletion by intraventricular p-chlorophenylanine. *Science*, **192**, 382–5.

Brent, D. (1987) Correlates of medical lethality of suicide attempts in children and adolescents. *J. Am. Acad. Child Adol. Psychiat.*, **26**, 87–91.

Brent, D., Perper, J. & Allman, C. (1987) Alcohol, firearms and suicide among youth: temporal trends in Allegheny County, Pennsylvania, 1960–1983. *J. Am. Med. Assoc.*, **257**, 3369–72.

Breslau, N. (1987) Inquiring about the bizarre: false positives in Diagnostic Interview Schedule for Children (DISC) ascertainment of obsessions, compulsions and psychotic symptoms. *J. Am. Acad. Child Adol. Psychiat.*, **26**, 639–44.

Breslau, N. & Davis, G. (1987) Posttraumatic stress disorder: the etiologic specificity of wartime stressors. *Am. J. Psychiat.*, **144**, 578–83.

Brettle, R., Strang, J. & Farrell, M. (1990) Clinical features of HIV infection and AIDS in drug takers. In *AIDS and Drug Misuse* (ed. J. Strand & G. Stimson). Routledge, London, pp. 38–53.

Brewer, C. (1977) Incidence of post-abortion psychosis: a prospective study. *Br. Med. J.*, **1**, 476–7.

Brewin, C., Wing, J., Mangen, S *et al.* (1987) Principles and practice of measuring needs in the long-term mentally ill: the MRC Needs of Care Assessment. *Psychol. Med.*, **17**, 871–981.

Bridges, K. W. & Goldberg, D. P. (1985) Somatic presentation of DSM-III psychiatric disorder in primary care. *J. Psychosom. Res.*, **29**, 563–9.

Bridges, K., Goldberg, D., Evans, B. & Sharpe, T. (1991) Determinants of somatisation in primary care. *Psychol. Med.*, **21**, 473–84.

Bridgewater, R., Leigh, S., James, O. F. W. & Potter, J. F. (1987) Alcohol consumption and dependence in elderly patients in an urban community. *Br. Med. J.*, **295**, 884–5.

Bridgman, P. W. (1927) *The Logic of Modern Physics*. Macmillan, New York.

Brierley, C. E., Szabaldi, E., Rix, K. J. *et al.* (1988) The Manchester nurse rating scales for the daily simultaneous assessment of depressive and manic ward behaviours. *J. Affect. Disorders*, **15**, 45–54.

Brindley, G. S. (1983) Cavernosal alpha-blockade: a new treatment for investigating and treating erectile impotence. *Br. J. Psychiat.*, **143**, 332–7.

Bristow, M. F. & Clare, A. W. (1992) Prevalence and characteristics of at risk drinkers among elderly acute medical in-patients. *Br. J. Addiction*, **87**, 291–4.

British Medical Journal (1938) Charge of procuring abortion: Mr. Bourne acquitted. **2**, 199–205.

Broadhead, E., Blazer, D., George, L. & Tse, C. (1990) Depression, disability days and days lost from work in a prospective epidemiological survey. *J. Am. Med. Assoc.*, **264**, 2524–8.

Broadhead, J. & Jacoby, R. J. (1990) Mania in old age: a first prospective study. *Internat. J. Geriat. Psychiat.*, **5**, 215–22.

Brockington, I., Kandell, R., Keller, J *et al.* (1978) Trials of lithium, chlorpromazine and amitriptyline in schizoaffective patients. *Br. J. Psychiat.*, **133**, 162–8.

Brockington, I. F., Kelly, A., Hall, P. & Deakin, W. (1988) Premenstrual relapse of puerperal psychosis. *J. Affect. Disord.*, **14**, 287–92.

Brockington, I. F., Kendell, R. E., Kellett, J. M. *et al.* (1978) Trials of lithium, chlorpromazine and amitriptyline in schizoaffective patients. *Br. J. Psychiat.*, **133**, 162–8.

Brockington, I. F., Kendell, R. E. & Leff, J. P. (1978) Definitions of schizophrenia: concordance and prediction of outcome. *Psychol. Med.*, **8**, 387–98.

Brockington, I. F., Kendell, R. E. & Wainwright, S. (1980*b*) Depressed patients with schizophrenic or paranoid symptoms. *Psychol. Med.*, **10**, 665–75.

Brockington, I. F. & Kumar, R. (1982) Drug addiction and psychotropic drug treatment during pregnancy and lactation. In *Motherhood and Mental Illness* (ed. I. F. Brockington & R. Kumar). Academic Press, London, pp. 239–55.

Brockington, I. F. & Leff, J. (1979) Schizoaffective psychosis: definitions and incidence. *Psychol. Med.*, **9**, 91–99.

Brockington, I. F., Perris, C., Kendell, R. E. *et al* (1982) The course of outcome of cycloid psychosis. *Psychol. Med.*, **12**, 97–105.

Brockington, I. F., Wainwright, S. & Kendell, R. E. (1980*a*) Manic patients with schizophrenic or paranoid symptoms, *Psychol. Med.*, **10**, 73–83.

Brockington, I. F., Winokur, G. & Dean, C. (1982). Puerperal Psychosis. In *Motherhood and Mental Illness* (ed. I. F. Brockington & R. Kumar). Academic Press, London, pp. 37–69.

Brodaty, H. & Andrews, G. (1983) Brief psychotherapy in family practice. *Br. J. Psychiat.*, **143**, 11–19.

Brody, H., Meikle, S. & Gerritse, R. (1971) Therapeutic abortion: a prospective study I. *Am. J. Obstet. Gynecol.*, **109**, 347–53.

Bromet, E. J., Dunn, L. O., Connell, M. O. *et al* (1986) Long-term reliability of diagnosing lifetime major depression in a community sample. *Arch. Gen. Psychiat.*, **43**, 435–40.

Brook, J. S., Whiteman, M., Gordon, A. S. *et al.* (1986) Onset of adolescent drinking: A longitudinal study of intrapersonal and interpersonal antecedents. *Adv. Alcohol Sub. Abuse*, **5**, 91–110.

Brooke, D., Edwards, G. & Andrews, T. (1993) Doctors and substance misuse: type of doctors, types of problems. *Addiction*, **88**, 655–63.

Brooker, C., Tarrier, N., Barrowclough, C. & Goldberg, D. (1992) Skills for Community Psychiatric Nurses working with the seriously mentally ill: Report of a pilot trial of psycho-social intervention. In *Community Psychiatric Nursing: a Research Perspective* (ed. C. Brooker & E. White). Chapman, London.

Brooks, D. N., Campsie, L., Symington C. *et al.* (1986) The five year outcome of severe blunt head injury. *J. Neurol. Neurosurg. Psychiat.*, **49**, 764–70.

Brooner, R. K., Bigelow, G., Stain, E. & Schmidt, C. W. (1990) Intravenous drug abusers with antisocial personality disorders: increased HIV risk behaviour. *Drug and Alcohol Dependence*, **26**, 39–44.

Brown, A. & Cooper, A. F. (1987) The impact of a liaison psychiatry service on patterns of referral in a general hospital. *Br. J. Psychiat.*, **150**, 83–7.

Brown, G. W. (1974) Meaning, measurement and stress of life events. In *Stressful Life Events: Their Nature and Effects* (ed. B. S. Dohrenwend & B. P. Dohrenwend). John Wiley, New York, pp. 217–43.

Brown, G. W., Andrews, B., Bifulco, A. *et al.* (1986) Social support, self-esteem and depression. *Psychol. Med.*, **16**, 813–32.

Brown, G., Andrews, B., Harris, T. *et al.* (1986) Social support, self-esteem and depression. *Psychol. Med.*, **16**, 813–31.

Brown, G. W., Bifulco, A. & Harris, T. (1987) Life events, vulnerability and onset of depression: some refinements. *Br. J. Psychiat.*, **150**, 30–42.

Brown, G. W. & Birley, J. L. T. (1968) Crises and life changes and the onset of schizophrenia. *J. Health Soc. Behav.*, **9**, 203–14.

Brown, G. W., Birley, J. L. T. & Wing, J. K. (1972) Influence of family life on the source of schizophrenic disorders: a replication. *Br. J. Psychiat.*, **121**, 241–58.

Brown, G. W., Bone, M., Dalison, B. M. & Wing, J. K. (1966) *Schizophrenia and Social Care*, Maudsley Monograph no 17. Oxford University Press, Oxford.

Brown, G. W., Carstairs, G. M. & Topping, G. C. (1958) The post hospital adjustment of chronic mental patients. *Lancet*, **ii**, 685–9.

REFERENCES

Brown, G. W., Davidson, S., Harris, T. *et al* (1977) Psychiatric disorder in North Uist and London. *Soc. Sci. Med.*, **11**, 367–77.

Brown, G. W., Davidson, S., Harris, T. O. (1978). *Social Origins of Depression*. Tavistock, London.

Brown, G. W. & Harris, T. O. (1978) *Social Origins of Depression*. Tavistock, London.

Brown, G. & Harris, T. (1993) Aetiology of anxiety and depressive disorders in an inner-city population. I. Early adversity. *Psychol. Med.*, **23**, 143–54.

Brown, G. W., Harris, T. O., & Copeland, J. R. (1977) Depression and loss. *Br. J. Psychiat.*, **130**, 1–18.

Brown, G., Harris, T. & Eames, M. (1993) Aetiology and anxiety and depressive disorders in an inner-city population. II. Comorbidity and adversity. *Psychol. Med.*, **23**, 155–65.

Brown, G., Harris, T. & Hepworth C. (1995) Loss, humiliation and entrapment among women developing depression: a patient and non-patient comparison. *Psychol. Med.*, **25**, 7–21.

Brown, G. W., Lemyre, L. & Bifulco, A. (1992) Social factors and recovery from anxiety and depressive disorders: a test of specificity. *Br. J. Psychiat.*, **161**, 44–54.

Brown, G. W. & Rutter, M. L. (1966) The measurement of family activities and relationships. *Human Relations*, **19**, 241–63.

Brown, J. (1977) *Mind, Brain and Consciousness*. Academic Press, London.

Brown, J., Doxey, J. C. & Handley, S. (1980) Effects of alpha-adrenoceptor agonists and antagonists and of antidepressant drugs on pre and post synaptic alpha adreno receptors. *Eur. J. Pharmacol.*, **67**, 33–40.

Brown, R. A. (1980) Conventional education and controlled drinking education courses with convicted drunken drivers. *Behav. Ther.*, **11**, 632–42.

Brown, R. G. & Marsden, C. D. (1988) Subcortical dementia: The neuropsychological evidence. *Neuro. Sci.*, **25**, 363–87.

Brown, R., Strathdee, G., Christie-Brown, J. & Robinson, P. (1988) A comparison of referrals to primary care and hospital out-patient clinics. *Br. J. Psychiatrist.*, **153**, 168–73.

Bruch, H. (1978) *The Golden Cage: The Enigma of Anorexia Nervosa*, Open Books, England.

Brucke, T., Roth, J., Podrecka, I. *et al* (1992) Striatal dopamine D_2 blockade by typical and atypical neuroleptics. *Lancet*, **339**, 497.

Brugha, T. S., (1988) Social support. *Curr. Opin. Psychiat.*, **1**, 206–11.

Brugha, T. S. (1989) Social psychiatry. In *The Instruments of Psychiatric Research* (ed. C. Thompson). John Wiley & Sons, Chichester, pp. 253–70.

Brugha, T., Bebbington, P. E., MacCarthy, B. *et al.* (1987) Social networks, social support and types of depressive illness. *Acta Psychiat. Scand.*, **76**, 664–73.

Brugha, T., Bebbington, P., Tennant, C. *et al.* (1985) The List of Threatening Experiences: a subset of 12 life event categories with considerable long-term contextual threat. *Psychol. Medic.*, **15**, 189–94.

Brugha, T. S. & Conroy, R. (1985) Categories of depression: reported life events in a controlled design. *Br. J. Psychiat.*, **147**, 641–6.

Brugha, T. S., Wing, J. K. & Smith, B. L. (1989) Physical ill-health of the long-term mentally ill in the community. Is there an unmet need? *Br. J. Psychiat.*, **155**, 777–82.

Brumberg, J. J. (1988) *Fasting Girls: The Emergence of Anorexia Nervosa as a Modern Disease*. Harvard University Press, Cambridge, Mass.

Brunello, M., Riva, M. Voltera, A. *et al* (1986) Biochemical changes in rat brain after acute and chronic administration of fluvoxamine, a selective 5-HT uptake blocker. Comparison with desmethylimiprine. *Adv. Pharmacother.*, **2**, 186–9.

Brunswick, A. F., Messeri, P., Aidala A. A. (1990) Hanging drug use patterns and treatment behaviour: A longitudinal study of urban black youth. In *Drug and Alcohol Abuse Prevention* (ed. R. R. Watson). Humana Press, New Jersey.

Bruton, C. J. *et al* (1990) Schizophrenia and the brain. *Psychol. Med.*, **20**, 285–304.

Bruun, R. D. & Budman, C. L. (1992) The natural history of Tourette syndrome. In *Tourette Syndrome: Genetics, Neurobiology and Treatment, Advances in Neurology* (ed. T. N. Chase., A. J. Friedhoff & D. J. Cohen). Raven Press, New York, pp. 1–6.

Bryan, K. L. (1989) *The Right Hemisphere Language Battery*. Whurr Publishers, Southampton.

Buchanan, A., Reed, A., Wessely, S. *et al.* (1993) Acting on Delusions II: The phenomenological correlates of acting on delusions. *Br. J. Psychiat.*, **163**, 77–83.

Buchsbaum, M., Cappelletti, J., Ball, R. *et al.* (1984*a*) Positron emission tomographic image measurement in schizophrenia and affective disorders. *Ann Neurol.*, Suppl. **15**, 157–165.

Buchsbaum, M., DeLisi, L., Holcomb, H. *et al.* (1984*b*) Anterposterior gradients in cerebral glucose use in schizophrenia and affective disorders. *Arch. Gen. Psychiat.*, **41**, 1159–66.

Buchsbaum, M., Wu, J., DeLisi, L. *et al.* (1986) Frontal cortex and basal ganglia metabolic rates assessed by positron emission tomography with [^{18}F]2-dexyglucose in affective illness. *J. Affect. Disorders*, **10**, 137–152.

Buckland, R. P., O'Donovan, M. C. & McGuffin, P. (1992) Changes in dopamine D_1, D_2 and D_3 receptors mRNA levels in rat brain following antipsychotic treatment. *Psychopharmacol.*, **106**, 479–83.

Buglass, D. & Horton, J. (1974) The repetition of parasuicide: a comparison of three cohorts. *Br. J. Psychiat.*, **125.**, 168–74.

Buist, A., Norman, T. R. & Dennerstein, L. (1990) Breast feeding and the use of psychotropic medication: a review. *J. Affect. Disord.*, **19**, 197–206.

Bundey, S., Hardy, C., Vickers, S., Kilpatrick, M. W. & Corbett, J. A. (1994) Duplication of the 15q11-13 region in a patient with autism, epilepsy and ataxia. *Devel. Med. Child Neurol.*, **36**, 736–42.

Burack, J. A. & Volkmar, F. R. (1992) Development of low- and high-functioning autistic children. *J. Child Psychol. & Psychiat.*, **33**, 607–16.

Burgess, A. W., Hadman, C. R. & McCormack, A. (1987) Abused to abuser – antecedents of socially deviant behaviours. *Am. J. Psychiat.*, **144**, 1431–6.

Burns, A., Carrick, J., Ames, D. *et al* (1989) the cerebral cortical appearance in late paraphrenia. *Internat. J. Geriat. Psychiat.*, **4**, 31–34.

Burns, A., Howard, R. & Pettit, W. (1995) *Alzheimer's Disease: A Medical Companion*. Blackwell Scientific Publications, Oxford.

Burns, A., Jacoby, R. & Levy, R. (1990) Psychiatric phenomena in Alzheimer's Disease. *Br. J. Psychiat.*, **157**, 72–94.

Burns, A., Jacoby, R. & Levy, R. (1991) Neurological signs in Alzheimer's Disease. *Age and Ageing*, **20**, 45–51.

Burns, A. & Levy, R. (1992) Clinical diversity in late onset Alzheimer's Disease. Maudsley Monograph No. 34. Oxford University Press, Oxford, pp. 7–25.

Burns, A. & Pearlson, G. D. (1994) *Computed Tomography in Alzheimer's Disease*. In *Dementia* (ed. A. Burns & R. Levy). Chapman and Hall, London.

Burns, B. H. & Howell, J. B. L. (1969) Disproportionately severe breathlessness in chronic bronchitis. *Quart. J. Med.*, **38**, 277–94.

Burns, B. H. & Nichols, M. A. (1972) Factors related to the localisation of symptoms to the chest in depression. *Br. J. Psychiat.*, **121**, 405–9.

Burke, K. C., Burke, J. D., Regier, D. A. & Rae, D. S. (1990) Age of onset of selected mental disorders in five community populations. *Arch. Gen. Psychiat.*, **47**, 511–18.

Burgos, O. K. (1972) *The Seventh Mental Measurements Yearbook*. Gryphon Press, New Jersey.

Burrows, G., Scoggins, B. A., Turecek, L. R. & Davies, B. (1974) Plasma nortriptyline and clinical response. *Clin. Pharmacol. Therapeut.*, **16**, 639–44.

Busatto, G., Pilowsky, L. S., Costa, D. *et al.* (1995) $GABA_A$ receptor changes in schizophrenia assessed using ^{123}I-Iomazenil single photon emission tomography (SPET) – a preliminary report. *Schiz. Res.*, **15**, 78–9.

Bushnell, J. A., Wells, E., Hornblow, A. R. *et al.* (1990) Prevalence of three bulimia syndromes in the general population. *Psychol. Med.*, **20**, 671–80.

Bushnell, J. A., Wells J. E. R. McKenzie, J. M. *et al* (1994) Bulimia comorbidity in the general population and in the clinic. *Psychol. Med.*, **24**, 605–13.

Butler, G. (1989) Issues in the application of cognitive and behavioural strategies to the treatment of social phobia. *Clin. Psychol. Rev.*, **9**, 91–106.

Butler, G., Cullington, A., Munby, M. *et al.* (1984) Exposure and anxiety management in the treatment of social phobia. *J. Consult. Clin. Psychol.*, **52**, 642–50.

Butler, G., Fennell, M., Robson, P. & Gelder, M. (1991) Comparison of behaviour therapy and cognitive behaviour therapy in the treatment of generalised anxiety disorder. *J. Consult. Clin. Psychol.*, **59**, 167–75.

Butler, R. N. (1968) Towards a psychiatry of the life cycle: implications of sociopsychologic studies of the ageing process for the psychotherapeutic situation. In *Ageing in Modern Society* (ed. A. Simon & L. J. Epstein). Psychiatric research reports of the American Psy. Association, Washington, pp. 233–48.

Bynum, W. (1983) Psychiatry in its historical context. In *Handbook of Psychiatry 1. General Psychopathology* (ed. M. Shepherd & O. L. Zangwill). Cambridge University Press, Cambridge, pp. 11–38.

Byrne, E. J. (1987) Reversible dementia. *Internat. J. Geriat. Psychiat.*, **2**, 73–81.

Byrne, E. J., Lennox, G. G., Godwin-Austen, R. B. *et al.* (1991) Dementia associated with cortical Lewy bodies. *Dementia*, **2**, 283–4.

Byrne, E. J., Lennox, G. & Lowe, J. (1989) Diffuse Lewy Body Disease. *J. Neurol. Neurosurg. Psychiat.*, **52**, 709–17.

Cade, J. F. (1949) Lithium salts in the treatment of psychotic excitement. *Med. J. Australia*, **2**, 349–53.

Cadoret, R. J. & Gath, A. (1978) Inheritance of alcoholism in adoptees. *Br. J. Psychiat.*, **132**, 252–8.

Cahalan, D. (1992) *An Ounce of Prevention*. Jossey-Bass, San Francisco.

Caine, E. D. (1981) Pseudodementia. *Arch. Gen. Psychiat.*, **38**, 1359–64.

Caine, E. D., McBride, M. C., Chiverton, P. *et al.* (1988) Tourette syndrome in Monroe County school children. *Neurology*, **38**, 472–5.

Caine, E. D., Lyness, J. M., King, D. A. & Connors, L. (1994) Clinical and aetiological heterogeneity of mood disorders in elderly patients. In *Diagnosis and treatment of depression in late life. Results of the NIH concensus development conference* (ed. L. S. Schneider, C. F. Reynolds, B. D. Lobowitz & A. J. Friedhoff). American Psychiatric Press, Washington DC, pp. 25–53.

Calloway, S. P. & Dolan, R. J. (1989) Endocrine changes and clinical profiles in depression. In *Life Events and Ilness* (ed. G. W. Brown & T. Harris). Guildford Press, London.

Calloway, S. P., Dolan, R. J., Fonagy, P. *et al* (1984a) Endocrine changes and clinical profiles in depression: I. The dexamethasone suppression test. *Psychol. Med.*, **14**, 749–58.

Calloway, S. P., Dolan, R. J., Fonagy, P. *et al* (1984b) Endocrine changes and clinical profiles in depression: II. The thyrotropin-releasing hormone test. *Psychol. Med.*, **14**, 759–66.

Calnan, M. (1988) Lay Evaluation of Medicine and Medical Practice: Report of the Pilot Study. *Internat. J. Health Services*, **18**, 311–23.

Cameron, N. (1944) Experimental analysis of schizophrenic thinking in language and thought in schizophrenia. In *Language and Thought in Schizophrenia* (ed. J. Kasanin). University of California Press, pp. 50–64.

Campbell, S. B. & Ewing, L. J. (1990) Follow-up of hard-to-manage preschoolers: adjustment at age 9 and predictors of continuing symptoms. *J. Child Psychol. Psychiat.*, **31**, 871–89.

Canadian Medical Association Journal Special Supplement (1991) Preventing alcohol problems; the challenge for medical education, **143**.

Cannon, M., Jones, P. B., Kargin, M. *et al* (1995) Predictors of adult psychosis in children who present to a child psychiatry clinic. *Schizo. Res.*, **15**, 191.

Cannon, T. D., Mednik, S. A., Parnas, J. *et al.* (1993) Developmental brain abnormalities in the offspring of schizophrenic mothers. *Arch. Gen. Psychiat.*, **50**, 551–64.

Cannon, W. B. (1927) The James–Lange theory of emotion: a critical examination and an alternative theory. *Am. J. Psychol.*, **39**, 106–24.

Cantor, C. H., Hill, M. A. & McLachlan, E. K. (1989) Suicide and related behaviour from river bridges. A clinical perspective. *Br. J. Psychiat.*, **155**, 829–35.

Cantor-Graae, E., McNeil, T. F., Sjostrom, K. *et al.* (1994) Obstetric complications and their relationship to other aetiological risk factors in schizophrenia. *J. Nerv. Ment. Diseases*, **182**, 645–50.

Cantwell, D. P., Sturzenburger, S., Burroughs, J. *et al.* (1977) Anorexia nervosa: an affective disorder? *Arch. Gen. Psychiat.*, **34**, 1087–90.

Capelhorn, J. R., Bell, J., Kleinbaum, D. G. & Gebski, V. J. (1993) Methadone dose and heroin use during maintenance treatment. *Addiction*, **88**, 119–24.

Capgras, J. & Reboul-Lachand, J. (1923) Illusion des sosies dansan défine systematisé chronique. *Bulletin de la Société Clinique de Médecine Mentale*, **2**, 6–16.

Carlson, G. A. (1990) Child and adolescent mania – diagnostic considerations. *J. Child Psychol. Psychiat.*, **31**, 331–41.

Carlsson, A. & Lindquist, M. (1963) Effect of chlorpromazine or haloperidol on formation of 3-methoxytrymanine and normetanephrine in mouse brain. *Acta Pharmacol.*, **20**, 140–4.

Carmines, E. G. & Zeller, R. A. (1979) *Reliability and Validity Assessment*. Sage, Beverly Hills.

Carney, M. W. P., Roth, M. & Garside, R. F. (1965) The diagnosis of depressive syndromes and the prediction of ECT response. *Br. J. Psychiat.*, **14**, 659–74.

Caron, C. & Rutter, M. (1991) Comorbidity in child psychopathology: concepts, issues and research strategies. *J. Child Psychol. Psychiat.*, **32**, 1063–80.

Carpenter, S., Yassa, R. & Ochs, R. (1982) A pathologic basis for Kleine–Levin syndrome. *Arch. Neurol.*, **39**, 25–8.

Carpenter, W. T., Bartko, J. J., Carpenter, C. L. & Strauss, J. S. (1976) Another view of schizophrenia subtypes. A report from the International Pilot Study of Schizophrenia. *Arch. Gen. Psychiat.*, **33**, 508–16.

Carpenter, W. T., Douglas, W. H. & Wagman, A. M. I. (1988) Deficit and non-deficit forms of schizophrenia. *Am. J. Psychiat.*, **145**, 247–53.

Carroll, B. J., Feinberg, M., Smouse, P. E. *et al.* (1981) The Carroll Rating Scale for depression. Development, reliability and validation. *B. J. Psychiat.*, **138**, 194–200.

Carse, J., Panton, N. & Watt, A. (1958) A district mental health service. The Worthing Experiment. *Lancet*, **i**, 39–41.

Carter, C. M., Urbanowitz, M., Hemsley, R. *et al.* (1993) Effects of a few-food diet in attention deficit disorder. *Arch. Dis. Child.*, **69**, 564–8.

Casey, P. R. & Tyrer, P. J. (1986) Personality, functioning and symptomatology. *J. Psychiat. Res.*, **20**, 363–74.

Castle, D. J. & Murray, R. M. (1991) The neurodevelopmental basis of sex differences in schizophrenia. *Psychol. Med.*, **21**, 565–75.

Castle, D., Scott, K., Wessely, S. & Murray, R. M. (1993b) Does social deprivation during gestation and early life predispose to later schizophrenia? *Soc. Psychiat. Psychiat. Epidemiol.*, **28**, 1–4.

Castle, D. J., Sham, P. C., Wessely, S. & Murray, R. M. (1994) The subtyping of schizophrenia in men and women: a latent class analysis. *Psychol. Med.*, **24**, 41–51.

Castle, D. J., Wessely, S. & Murray, R. M. (1993a) Sex and schizophrenia: effects of diagnostic stringency, and associations with premorbid variables. *Br. J. Psychiat.*, **162**, 658–64.

Catalan, J., Gath, D. Anastasiades, P. (1991) Evaluation of a brief psychological treatment for emotional disorders in primary care. *Psychol. Med.*, **21**, 1013–18.

Catalan, J., Gath, G., Edmonds, G. *et al.* (1984) The effects of non-prescribing of anxiolytics in general practice. I Controlled evaluation of psychiatric and social outcome. II Factors associated with outcome. *Br. J. Psychiat.*, **144**, 593–610.

Catalan, J., Marzack, P., Hawton, K. E. *et al* (1980) Comparison of doctors and nurses in the assessment of deliberate self-poisoning patients. *Psycholog. Med.*, **10**, 483–91.

Catalano, R. C., Morrison, D. M., Wells, E. A. *et al.* (1992) Ethnic differences in family factors related to early drug initiation. *J. Studies in Alcohol.*, **53**, 208–17.

Cattell, R. B. (1957) *Personality and Motivation: Structure & Measurement*. World Books, Yonkers-on-Hudson.

Centers for Disease Control (1988) Health status of Vietnam veterans. *J. Am. Med. Assoc.*, **259**, 2701–19.

Central Statistical Office (1992) *Annual Abstract of Statistics*. Government Statistical Service, London.

Chadwick, O., Anderson, R., Bland, J. & Ramsey, J. (1989) Neuropsychological Consequences of Volatile Substance Abuse: a population based study of secondary school pupils. *Br. Med. J.*, **298**, 1679–84.

Challis, D. (1986) *Case Management in Community Care*. Gower, Aldershot.

Champion, L. (1990) The relationship between social vulnerability and the occurrence of severely threatening life events. *Psychol. Med.*, **20**, 157–61.

Chandola, C. A., Robling, M. R., Peters, T. J., Melville-Thomas, G. & McGuffin, P. (1992) Pre- and perinatal factors and the risk of subsequent referral for hyperactivity. *J. Child Psychol. Psychiat.*, **33**, 1077–90.

Channon, S., de Silva, P., Hemsley, D. & Perkins R. (1989) A controlled trial of cognitive-behavioural and behavioural treatment of anorexia nervosa. *Behav. Res. Ther.*, **27**, 529–35.

Chapman, P. L. H. & Huygens, I. (1988) An evaluation of three treatment programmes for alcoholism: experimental study with six and 18-month follow-ups. *Br. J. Addict.*, **83**, 67–81.

Chaput, Y., Blier, P. & de Montigny, C. (1988) Acute and long-term effects of antidepressant serotonin (5-HT) reuptake blockers on the efficacy of 5-HT transmission: Electrophysiological studies on the rat central nervous system. *J. Pharmacol. Exp. Therap.*, **246**, 359–70.

Charney, D., Goodman, W., Price, L. *et al* (1988) Serotonin function in obsessive-compulsive disorder: a comparison of the effects of tryptophan and m-CPP in patients and healthy subjects. *Arch. Gen. Psychiat.*, **45**, 177–85.

Charney, D. S. & Nelson, J. C. (1981) Delusional and nondelusional unipolar depression. Further evidence for distinct subtypes. *Am. J. Psychiat.*, **138**, 328–33.

Charney, D., Wood, S., Krystal, J. *et al.* (1992) Noradrenergic neuronal dysregulation in panic disorder: the effects of intravenous yohimbine and clonidine in panic disorder patients. *Acta psychiat. Sand.*, **86**, 273–82.

Checkley, S. A. (1992) Neuroendocrine mechanisms and the precipitation of depression by life events. *Br. J. Psychiat.*, **160**, 7–17.

Chesterman, L. P., Taylor, P. J., Cox, T. *et al.* (1994) Multiple measures of cerebral state in dangerous, mentally disordered in-patients. *Crim. Behav. Ment. Health*, **4**, 228–39.

Chick, J. (1989) Delirium tremens: try to spot it early. *Br. Med. J.*, **298**, 3–4.

Chick, J., Lloyd, G. & Gombie, E. (1985) Counselling problem drinkers in medical wards; a controlled study. *Br. Med. J.*, **290**, 965–7.

Chick, J. D. & Ritson, E. B. (1989) Alcoholism – Advice versus extended treatment. *Br. J. Addiction*, **84**, 817–19.

Chick, J. D., Ritson, B., Connaughton, J. *et al.* (1988) Advice versus extended treatment for alcoholism: A controlled study. *Br. J. Addiction*, **83**, 159–70.

Childress, A. R., Ehrman, R., McLellan, A. T. & O'Brien, C. P. (1988) 'Conditioned craving and arousal in cocaine addiction'. Problems of drug dependence, NIDA Monograph Series, DHSS pub no. (ADM) 88–1564, pp. 74–80.

Childress, A. R., McLellan, A. T., & O'Brien, C. P. (1986) Abstinent opiate abusers exhibited conditioned craving, conditioned withdrawal and reductions in both through extinction. *Br. J. Addiction*, **81**, 655–60.

Chiodo, L. A. & Antelman, S. M. (1980) Repeated tricyclics induce a progressive dopamine autoreceptor subsensitivity independent of daily drug treatment. *Nature*, **287**, 451–54.

Chodoff, P. (1982) Hysteria and women. *Am. J. Psychiat.*, **139**, 545–51.

Chowdhury, N., Hicks, R. C. & Kreitman, N. (1973) Evaluation of an aftercare service for parasuicide patients. *Soc. Psychiat.*, **8**, 67–81.

Christie Brown, J. R. W. (1990) Transsexualism. In *Principles and Practice of Forensic Psychiatry* (ed. R. Bluglass & P. Bowden). Churchill Livingstone, Edinburgh, pp. 705–10.

Christodoulou, G. N. (1977) The syndrome of Capgras. *Br. J. Psychiat.*, **130**, 556–64.

Chua, S. & Murray, R. M. (1995) The neurodevelopmental theory of schizophrenia: evidence concerning structure and neuropsychology. *Acta Neuropsychiat.*, **7**(3), 568–70.

Clare, A. (1985) Freud's cases: the clinical basis of psychoanalysis. In *The Anatomy of Madness. Essays in the History of Psychiatry. People and Ideas* (ed. W. F. Bynum, R. Porter & M. Shepherd). Tavistock, London, pp. 271–288.

Clare, A. W. (1976) *Psychiatry in Dissent. Controversial Issues in Thought and Practice.* Tavistock Press, London.

Clare, A. W. & Tyrrell, J. (1994) Psychiatric aspects of abortion. *Ir. J. Psychol. Med.,* **11,** 92–8.

Clare, I. C. H. & Gudjonsson, G. H. (1992) *Devising and Piloting and Experimental Version of the Notice to Detained Persons.* The Royal Commission on Criminal Justice Research Study No. 7. HMSO, London.

Claridge, G. (1972) The schizophrenias as nervous types. *Br. J. Psychiat.,* **121,** 1–17.

Clark, A. N. G., Mankikar, G. D. & Gray, I (1975) Diogenes syndrome. A clinical study of gross neglect in old age. *Lancet,* **1,** 366–73.

Clark, D. M. (1986) A cognitive approach to panic. *Behav. Res. Ther.,* **24,** 461–70.

Clark, D. M., Salkovskis, P. M. Hackmann, A. *et al.* (1994) A comparison of cognitive therapy, applied relaxation and imipramine in the treatment of panic disorder. *Br. J. Psychiat.,* **164,** 759–69.

Clark, R. & Goate, A. (1993) Molecular genetics of Alzheimer's disease. *Arch. Neurol.,* **50,** 1164–70.

Clayden, G. & Agnarsson, U. (1991) *Constipation in Childhood.* Oxford University Press, Oxford.

Cleckley, H. (1976) *The Mask of Sanity,* 5th edn. C. V. Mosby, St Louis.

Clifford, C. A., Fulker, D. W., Murray, R. M. (1984) Genetic and environmental influences on drinking patterns in normal twins. In *Alcohol Related Problems* (ed. N. Krasner, J. S. Madden & R. J. Walker). John Wiley & Sons, Chichester.

Clifford, C., Murray, R. & Fulker, D. (1984) Genetic and environmental influences on obsessional traits and symptoms. *Psychol. Med.,* **14,** 791–800.

Cloninger, C. R. (1987) Neurogenetic adaptive mechanisms in alcoholism. *Science,* **236,** 410–16.

Cloninger, C. R., Bohman, M. & Sigvardsson, S. (1981) Inheritance of alcohol abuse: cross fostering analysis of adopted men. *Arch. Gen. Psychiat.,* **38,** 861–8.

Cloninger, C. R., Marton, R. L., Guze, S. B. & Clayton, P. J. (1985) Diagnosis and prognosis in schizophrenia. *Arch. Gen. Psychiat.,* **42,** 15–25.

Cloninger, C., Reich, T. & Guze, S. (1975) The multifactorial model of disease transmission III: Familial relationship between sociopathy and hysteria (Briquet's Syndrome). *Br. J. Psychiat.,* **127,** 23–32.

Closser, M. H. & Blow, F. C. (1993) Special Populations: Women, ethnic minorities and the elderly. In *Recent Advances in Addictive Disorders, Psychiatric Clinics in North America* (ed. N. S. Miller), **16,** 199–209. W. B. Saunders, Philadelphia.

Clum, G., Clum G. & Surls, R. A. (1993) A meta-analysis for treatments for panic disorder. *J. Consult. Clin. Psychol.,* **61,** 317–29.

Clunis Report – J. H. Ritchie, D. Dick & R. Lingham (1994) *The Report of the Enquiry into the Care and Treatment of Christopher Clunis.* HMSO, London.

Cochrane, R. & Bal, S. (1990) Drinking habits of Sikh, Hindu, Muslim and white men in the west Midlands: a community survey. *Br. J. Addiction.,* **85,** 759–69.

Coekin, M. & Gairdner, D. (1960) Faecal incontinence in children: the physical factor. *Br. Med. J.,* **ii,** 1175–80.

Cogill, S., Caplan, H. L., Alexandra, H. *et al.* (1986) Impact of maternal postnatal depression on cognitive development of young children. *Br. Med. J.,* **292,** 1165–7.

Cohen, C. (1991) Integrated community services. In *Comprehensive Review of Geriatric Psychiatry* (ed. J. Sadavoy, L. Lazarus & L. Jarvik). American Psychiatric Press, Washington pp. 613–34.

Cohen, I. (1970) The benzodiazepines. In *Discoveries in Biological Psychiatry* (ed. F. J. Ayd & B. Blackwell). J. B. Lippincott, Philadelphia, pp. 130–42.

Cohen, L. J., Test, M. A. & Brown, R. L. (1990) Suicide and schizophrenia: data from a prospective community treatment study. *Am. J. Psychiat.,* **147,** 602–7.

Cohen, L. S., Friedman, J. M., Jefferson, J. W. *et al* (1994) A re-evaluation of risk of in utero exposure to lithium. *J.A.M.A.,* **271,** 146–50.

Cohen, P., Cohen, J., Kasen, S. *et al* (1993) An epidemiological study of disorders in late childhood and adolescence. I. Age- and gender-specific prevalence. *J. Child Psychol. Psychiat.*, **34**, 851–77.

Cohen-Cole, S. A. & Stoudemire, A. (1987) Major depression and physical illness. Special considerations in diagnosis and biological treatment. *Psych. Clin. N. Am.*, **10**, 1–17.

Cohn, A. H. & Daro, D. (1987) Is treatment too late: what ten years of evaluative research tells us. *Child Abuse and Neglect*, **11**, 433–42.

Coid, B., Lewis, S. W. & Revely, A. M. (1993) A twin study of psychosis and criminality. *Br. J. Psychiat.*, **162**, 87–92.

Coid, J. (1983) The epidemiology of abnormal homicide and murder followed by suicide. *Psychol. Med.*, **13**, 855–60.

Coid, J. (1988) Mentally abnormal prisoners on remand. I. Rejected or accepted by the NHS? II. Comparison of services provided by Oxford and Wessex regions. *Br. Med. J.*, **296**, 1979–82, 1783–4.

Coid, J. (1992) DSM-III diagnosis in criminal psychopaths a way forward. *Crim. Behav. Ment. Health*, **2**, 78–94.

Coid, J. W. (1993) A survey of bed occupancy in medium security, 21st November, 1993. Unpublished discussion paper for the Department of Health. Available from the author, Hackney Hospital, London, UK.

Colby, K. M. (1960) *An Introduction to Psychoanalytic Research*. Basic Books, New York.

Cole, A. J., Fillett, J. P. & Fairbairn A. (1992) A case of senile self-neglect in a married couple: 'Diogenes a Deux'. *Internat. J. Geriat. Psychiat.*, **7**, 839–41.

Coleman, S. E. (1933) Misidentification and non recognition. *J. Ment. Sci.*, **79**, 42–51.

Coles, R. J., Van Abendorff, R. & Herzberg, J. L. (1991) The impact of the new community mental health team on an inner city psychogeriatric service. *Internat. J. Geriat. Psychiat.*, **6**, 31–39.

Collighan, G., MacDonal, A., Hertzberg, J. *et al* (1993) An evaluation of the multidisciplinary approach to psychiatric diagnosis in the elderly. *Br. Med. J.*, **306**, 821–4.

Collings, S. & King, M. (1994) Ten-year follow-up of 50 patients with bulimia nervosa. *Br. J. Psychiat.*, **164**, 80–7.

Collins, J. J. & Bailey, S. L. (1990) Traumatic stress disorder and violent behaviour. *J. Traum. Stress*, **3**, 203–20.

Collis, I. & Lloyd, G. (1992) Psychiatric aspects of liver disease. *Br. J. Psychiat.*, **161**, 12–22.

Comfort, A. (1972) What is a Doctor? *Lancet*, **1**, 971–4.

Comings, D. E. (1990) *Tourette Syndrome and Human Behaviour*. Duarte Press, Duarte, CA.

Condou, S. (1989) *L'aide a domicile en Europe a l'harizon 1992, Union National*. ADMR, Paris.

Connell, P. H. (1958) *Amphetamine Psychosis*. Maudsley Monograph number 5. Oxford University Press, London.

Conners, C. K. (1973) Rating scales for use in drug studies with children. *Psychopharmacology Bulletin (Special Issue: Pharmacotherapy of Children)*, 24–84.

Connolly, J. (1976) Life events before myocardial infarction. *J. Human Stress*, **2**, 3–17.

Constantinidis, J. (1978) Is Alzheimer's Disease a major form of senile dementia? In *Alzheimer's Disease – senile dementia and related disorders* (ed. R. Katzman, R. Terry & K. Bick). Raven Press, New York, pp. 15–26.

Cook, C. C. H. (1988a) The Minnesota Model in the management of drug and alcohol dependency: miracle, method or myth? Part I The philosophy and the programme *Br. J. Addiction.*, **83**, 625–34.

Cook, C. C. H. (1988b) The Minnesota Model in the management of drug and alcohol dependency: miracle, method or myth? Part II Evidence and conclusions. *Br. J. Addiction.*, **83**, 735–48.

Cook, C. C. H. & Gurling, H. M. D. (1994) The D2 dopamine receptor gene and alcoholism: a genetic effect in the liability for alcoholism. *J. Roy. Soc. Med.*, **87**, 400–3.

Cook, D. A. G., Fox, C. A., Weaver, C. M. & Rooth, F. G. (1991) The Berkeley group: ten years' experience of a group for non-violent sex offenders. *Br. J. Psychiat.*, **151**, 238–43.

Cooke, D. J. (1989) Containing violent prisoners: an analysis of the Barlinnie Special Unit. *Br. J. Criminol.*, **29**, 129–43.

Cooke, R. A., Chambers, J. B., Singh, R. *et al*. (1994) The QT interval in anorexia nervosa. *Br. Heart J.*, **72**, 69–73.

Cooke, R. E. (1984) Atlanto-axial instability in individuals with Down's syndrome. *Adapted Physical Activity Quarterly*, **1**, 194–6.

Cookson, J. C. (1985) The neuroendocrinology of mania. *J. Affect. Disord.*, **8**, 233–41.

Cooley, C. H. (1909) *Social Organisation: a Study of the Larger Mind.* C. Scribner's & Sons, New York.

Cooper, A. J. (1974) A blind evaluation of a penile ring: a sex aid for impotent males. *Br. J. Psychiat.*, **124**, 402–6.

Cooper, A. J. (1987) Preliminary experience with a vacuum constriction device (VCD) as a treatment for impotence. *J. Psychosom. Res.*, **31**, 413–18.

Cooper, A. J., Moir, A. J. B. & Guldberg, H. C. (1968) Effect of electroconvulsive shock on the cerebral metabolism of dopamine and 5-hydroxytryptamine. *J. Pharm. Pharmacol.*, **20**, 729–30.

Cooper, B. (1987) Psychiatric disorders among elderly patients admitted to hospital medical wards. *J. Roy. Soc. Med.*, **80**, 13–16.

Cooper, B. (1991) Late-life mental disorder and primary health care: a review of research. In *Primary Health Care and Psychiatric Epidemiology* (ed. B. Cooper & M. R. Eastwood). Routledge, London, pp. 213–33.

Cooper B. (1992) Sociology in the context of social psychiatry. *Br. J. Psychiat.*, **161**, 594–8.

Cooper, B. & Eastwood, R. (eds) (1992) *Primary Health Care and Psychiatric Epidemiology.* Routledge, London.

Cooper, J. E. (1970) The Leyton Obsessional Inventory. *Psychol. Med.*, **1**, 48–64.

Cooper, J. E., Kendell, R. E., Gurland, B. J. *et al.* (1972) Psychiatric Diagnosis in New York and London. Maudsley Monograph No. 20. Oxford University Press, London.

Cooper, J. E. & Sartorius, N. (1977) Cultural and temporal variations in schizophrenia. *Br. J. Psychiat.*, **130**, 50–5.

Cooper, P. J. (1993) *Bulimia Nervosa.* Robinson Press.

Cooper, P. J., Campbell, E. A., Day, A. *et al* (1988) Non-psychotic psychiatric disorder after childbirth: a prospective study of prevalence, incidence, course and nature. *Br. J. Psychiat.*, **152**, 799–806.

Cooper, P. J. & Fairburn, C. G. (1984) Cognitive-behaviour therapy for anorexia nervosa: some preliminary findings. *J. Psychosom. Res.*, **28**, 493–9.

Cooper, P. J. & Fairburn, C. G. (1986) The depressive symptoms of bulimia nervosa. *Br. J. Psychiat.*, **148**, 268–74.

Cooper, P. J. & Goodyer, I. (1993) A community sample of depression in adolescent girls. I. Estimates of symptom and syndrome prevalence. *Br. J. Psychiat.*, **163**, 369–74.

Cooper, Z. & Fairburn, C. G. (1987) The Eating Disorder Examination. A semi-structured interview for the assessment of the specific psychopathology of eating disorders. *Internat. J. Eat. Disorders*, **6**, 1–8.

Copas, J. B., Freeman-Browne, D. L. & Robin, A. A. (1971) Danger periods for suicide in patients under treatment. *Psychol. Med.*, **1**, 400–4.

Copeland, J. R. M., Davidson, I. A., Dewey, M. E. *et al.* (1992) Alzheimer's disease, other dementias, depression and pseudodementia: prevalence incidence and three-year outcome in Liverpool. *Br. J. Psychiat.*, **151**, 230–9.

Copeland, J. R. M., Dewey, M. E., Wood, N. *et al.* (1987) Range of mental illness among the elderly in the community: Prevalence in Liverpool using the GMS-AGECAT package. *Br. J. Psychiat.*, **150**, 815–23.

Copeland, J. & Hall, W. (1992) A comparison of predictors of treatment drop out of women seeking drug and alcohol treatment in a specialist women and two traditional mixed sex treatment services. *Br. J. Addiction*, **87**, 883–90.

Coppen, A. (1967) The biochemistry of affective disorders. *Br. J. Psychiat.*, **113**, 1237–64.

Coppen, A. & Ghose, K. (1978) Peripheral alpha-adrenoreceptor and central dopamine receptor activity in depressive patients. *Psychopharmacology* (Berlin) **59**, 171–7.

Coppen, A. & Metcalfe, M. (1965) Effect of a depressive illness on MPI scores. *Br. J. Psychiat.*, **111**, 236–9.

Coppen, A., Montgomery, S. A., Rao, V. *et al.* (1978) Continuation therapy with amitriptyline in depression. *Br. J. Psychiat.*, **133**, 206–10.

Coppen, A. J. & Doogan, D. P. (1988) Serotonin and its place in the pathogenesis of depression. *J. Clin. Psychiat.*, **49**, 4–11.

Corbett, J. (1981) Epilepsy and mental retardation. In *Epilepsy and Psychiatry* (ed. E. H. Reynolds & M. R. Trimble). Churchill Livingstone, Edinburgh, pp. 138–46.

Corbett, J. A., Harris, R. & Robinson, R. G. (1975) Epidemiological issues. In *Mental Retardation and Developmental Disabilities*, Vol. VII. (ed. J. Wortis). Brunner Mazel, New York. pp. 79–111.

Corbett, J. A., Trimble, M. R. & Nichol, T. C. (1985) Behavioural and cognitive impairments in epileptic children. *J. Am. Acad. Child Psychiat.*, **24**, 17–23.

Coryell, W. (1981) Obsessive compulsive disorder and primary unipolar depression. *J. Nerv. Ment. Disease*, **169**, 220–4.

Coryell, W., Endicott, J. & Keller, M. (1987) The importance of psychotic features to major depression: course and outcome during a 2-year follow-up. *Acta Psychiat. Scand.*, **75**, 78–85.

Coryell, W., Keller, M., Endicott, J. *et al.* (1989) Bipolar II illness: course and outcome over a five-year period. *Psychol. Med.*, **19**, 129–41.

Coryell, W., Keller, M., Lavori, P. & Endicott, J. (1990) Affective syndromes, psychotic features and prognosis. I. Depression. *Arch. Gen. Psychiat.*, **47**, 651–7.

Coryell, W., Noyes, R. & Clancy, J. (1983) Panic disorder and primary unipolar depression: background and outcome. *J. Affect. Disorder.*, **5**, 311–17.

Coryell, W., Noyes, R. & House, J. D. (1986) Mortality among out-patients with anxiety disorders. *Am. J. Psychiat.*, **143**, 508–10.

Coser, R. L. (1976) Suicide and the relational system: a case study in a mental hospital. *J. Health Soc. Behav.*, **17**, 318–27.

Costello, E. J. (1989) Developments in child psychiatric epidemiology. *J. Am. Acad. Child Adol. Psychiat.*, **28**, 836–41.

Cotard, J. (1882) Du delire des negations. In *Themes and Variations in European Psychiatry*, 1974 (ed. M. Shepherd & S. Hirsch). John Wright & Sons, Bristol.

Cotterill, J. A. (1981) Dermatological non-disease: A common and potentially fatal disturbance of cutaneous body image. *Br. J. Dermatol.*, **104**, 611–19.

Cotton, N. S. (1979) The familial incidence of alcoholism. *J. Studies in Alcohol*, **40**, 89–116.

Coward, D. M., Imperato, A., Urwyler, S. *et al.* (1989) Biochemical and behavioural properties of clozapine. *Psychopharmacology*, **99**, S6–S12.

Cowdry, W. L. & Gardener, D. L. (1988) Pharmacotherapy of Borderline Personality Disorder. *Arch. Gen. Psychiat.*, **45**, 111–19.

Cowe, L., Lloyd, D. J. & Dawling, S. (1982) Neonatal convulsions caused by withdrawal from maternal clomipramine. *Br. Med. J.*, **284**, 1837–8.

Cowen, P. J. (1993) Serotonin receptor subtypes in depression: Evidence from studies in neuroendocrine regulation. *Clino–Neuropharmacol.*, **16**, 6–18.

Cowen, P. J. & Charig, E. M. (1987) Neuroendocrine responses to intravenous tryptophan in major depression. *Arch. Gen. Psychiat.*, **44**, 958–66.

Cowley, D. S. & Roy-Byrne, P. P. (1989) Panic disorder during pregnancy. *J. Psychosom. Obstet. Gynecol.*, **10**, 193–210.

Cox, A. D. (1991) Is Asperger's syndrome a useful diagnosis? *Arch. Dis. Child.*, **66**, 259–62.

Cox, A. D. (1993) Social factors in child psychiatric disorder. In *Principles of Social Psychiatry* (ed. D. Bhugra & J. Leff). Blackwell Scientific, Oxford, pp. 203–33.

Cox, B. D., Blaxter, M., Buckle, A. L. J. *et al.* (1987) *The Health and Lifestyle Survey*. Health Promotion Research Trust, Cambridge.

Cox, J. L., Murray, D. & Chapman, G. (1993) A controlled study of the onset, duration and prevalence of postnatal depression. *Br. J. Psychiat*, **163**, 27–31.

Craft, M., Bicknell, J. & Hollins, S. (eds.) (1987) *Mental Handicap. A Multi-disciplinary Approach*. Ballière Tindall.

Craig, T. K. J., Boardman, A. P., Mills, K. *et al.* (1993) The South London somatisation study. I: Longitudinal course and the influence of early life experiences. *Br. J. Psychiat.*, **163**, 579–88.

Craddock, M. & Owen, M. J. (1996) Candidate gene association studies in psychiatric genetics: a SERTain future? *Molec. Psychiat.* (in press).

Crammer, J. L. (1984) The special characteristics of suicide in hospital in-patients. *Br. J. Psychiat.*, **145**, 460–76.

Crammer, J., Barraclough, B. & Heine, B. (1982) *The Use of Drugs in Psychiatry*, 2nd edn. Royal College of Psychiatrists, Gaskell, London.

Crawford, A. (1986) Adults at risk: a comparison of heavy drinkers in three areas of Britain. *Drug and Alcohol Dependence*, **18**, 301–9.

Creed, F. (1981) Life events and appendicectomy. *Lancet*, **1**, 1381–5.

Creed, F. (1985) Life events and physical illness. *J. Psychosom, Res.*, **29**, 113–23.

Creed, F. (1992) The future of liaison psychiatry in the UK. *Internat. Rev. Psychiat.*, **4**, 99–107.

Creed, F. & Guthrie E. (1987) Psychological factors in the irritable bowel syndrome. *Gut*, **28**, 1307–18.

Creed, F. & Marks B. (1989) Liaison psychiatry in general practice: a comparison of the liaison-attachment schema and the shifted out-patient clinic models. *J. Roy. Coll. Gen. Pract.*, **39**, 514–17.

Creer, C. (1978) Social work with patients and their families. In *Schizophrenia: Towards a New Synthesis* (ed. J. Wing). Academic Press, London and Orlando, pp. 233–51.

Creese, I., Burt, D. R. & Snyder, S. H. (1976) Dopamine receptor binding predicts clinical and pharmacological potencies of antischizophrenic drugs. *Science*, **192**, 481–3.

Cregler, M. & Mark, H. (1986) Medical complications of cocaine use. *N. Engl. J. Med.*, **315**, 1495–500.

Creighton, F. J., Black, D. L. & Hyde, C. E. (1991) 'Ecstasy' psychosis and flashbacks. *Br. J. Psychiat.*, **159**, 713–15.

Crisp, A. (1980) *Anorexia Nervosa: Let Me Be.* Academic Press, London.

Crisp, A. H., Callender, J. S., Halek, C. & Hsu, L. K. G. (1992) Long term mortality in anorexia nervosa: a twenty year follow-up of the St Georges's and Aberdeen cohorts. *Br. J. Psychiat.*, **161**, 104–7.

Crisp, A. H., Norton, K., Gowers, S. *et al.* (1991) A controlled study of the effect of therapies aimed at adolescent and family psychopathology in anorexia nervosa. *Br. J. Psychiat.*, **159**, 325–33.

Critchley, M. (1953) *The Parietal Lobes.* Hafner, New York.

Critchley, M. (1962) Periodic hypersomnia and megagraphia in adolescent males. *Brain*, **85**, 627–56.

Critchley, M. (1964) The neurology of psychotic speech. *Br. J. Psychiat.*, **110**, 353–64.

Critchley, E. & Cantor, H. (1984) Charcot's hysteria renaissant. *Br. Med. J.*, **289**, 1785–1788.

Crits-Christoph, P. & Barber, J. P. (eds.) (1991) *Handbook of Short-term Dynamic Psychotherapies.* Basic Books, New York.

Croft-Jeffreys, C. & Wilkinson, G. (1989) The cost of neurosis in UK general practice, 1985. *Psychol. Med.*, **19.**, 549–58.

Cronbach, L. J., Gleser, G. C., Nander, H. *et al.* (1972) *The Dependability of Behavioural Measurements: Theory of Generalisability for Scores and Profiles.* John Wiley & Sons, New York.

Cronholm, B. & Ottoson, J. O. (1960) Experimental studies of the therapeutic action of electroconvulsive therapy in endogenous depression: The role of the electrical stimulation and of the seizures studied by variation of stimulus intensity and modification of seizure discharge. *Acta Psychiat. Scand.*, whole Suppl. 145.

Cross-National Collaborative Panic Study: Second Phase Investigators. (1992) Drug treatment of panic disorder: comparative efficacy of alprazolam, imipramine and placebo. *Br. J. Psychiat.*, **160**, 191–202.

Crossley, D., Myers, M. P. & Wilkinson, G. (1992) Assessment of psychological care in general practice. *Br. Med. J.*, **305**, 1333–6.

Crow, T. J. (1980) Molecular pathology of schizophrenia. *Br. Med. J.*, **280**, 66–8.

Crow, T. J. (1986) The continuum of psychosis and its implication of the structure of the gene. *Br. J. Psychiat.*, **149**, 419–29.

Crow, T. J. (1987) Recurrent and chronic psychoses. *Br. Med. Bull.*, **43**, 469–79.

Crow, T. J. (1990) Nature of the genetic contribution to psychotic illness – a continuum viewpoint. *Acta Psychiatr. Scand.*, **81**, 401–8.

Crow, T. J., Johnstone, E. C. & Owen, F. (1979) Research on schizophrenia. In *Recent Advances in Clinical Psychiatry*, vol. 3 (ed. K. Granville-Grossman). Churchill Livingstone, Edinburgh, pp. 1–36.

Crowe, M. & Jones, M. (1992) Sex therapy: the successes, the failures, the future. *Br. J. Hosp. Med.*, **48**, 474–82.

Crowe, M. J. & Qureshi, M. J. H. (1991) Pharmacologically induced penile erection (PIPE) as a maintenance treatment for erectile impotence: a report of 41 cases. *Sexual and Marital Therapy*, **6**, 273–9.

Crowe, M. & Ridley, J. (1986) The negotiated timetable: a new approach to marital conflicts involving male demands and female reluctance for sex. *Sexual and Marital Therapy*, **1**, 157–73.

Crowe, M. & Ridley, J. (1990) *Therapy with Couples: a behavioural-systems approach to marital and sexual problems*. Blackwell Scientific, Oxford.

Crowe, R., Noyes, R., Paul, D. & Slymen, D. (1983) A family history study of panic disorders. *Arch. Gen. Psychiat.*, **40**, 1065–9.

Crystal, H. A., Wofson, L. & Ewing, S. (1988) Visual hallucinations as the first symptom of Alzheimer's disease. *Am. J. Psychiat.*, **145**, 1318.

Cummings, E. M. & Davies, P. T. (1994) Maternal depression and child development. *J. Child Psychol. Psychiat.*, **35**, 73–112.

Cummings, J. L. & Benson, D. F. (1988) Psychological dysfunction accompanying subcortical dementia. *Ann. Rev. Med.*, **39**, 53–61.

Cummings, J. L. & Benson, D. F. (eds.) (1992) *Dementia: a Clinical Approach*, 2nd edn. Butterworth-Heinemann, Boston.

Cummings, J. & Duchen, L. W. (1981) Kluver–Bucy syndrome in Pick disease. *Neurology*, **31**, 1415–22.

Cummings, J., Hebben, N. A., Obler, L. & Leonard, P. (1980) Nonaphasic misnaming and other neurobehavioural features of an unusual toxic encephalopathy. *Cortex*, **16**, 315–23.

Cummings, J. & Victoroff, J. (1991) Non cognitive neuropsychiatric syndromes in Alzheimer's disease. *Neuropsychiat. Neuropsychol. Behav. Neurol.*, **3**, 140–58.

Curfs, L. M., Verhulst, F. C. & Fryns, J. P. (1991) Behavioural and emotional problems in youngsters with Prader-Willi syndrome. *Genetic Counselling*, **2**, 33–41.

Curran, P. S. (1988) Psychiatric aspects of terrorist violence: Northern Ireland 1969 to 1987. *Br. J. Psychiat.*, **153**, 470–5.

Currie, S., Heathfield, K. W. G., Henson, R. A. & Scott, D. M. (1971) Clinical course and.prognosis of temporal lobe epilepsy. *Brain*, **94**, 173–90.

Cutting, J. (1978*a*) A reappraisal of alcoholic psychoses. *Psychol. Med.*, **8**, 285–95.

Cutting, J. (1978*b*) Study of anosognosia. *J. Neurol. Neurosurg. Psychiat.*, **41**, 548–55.

Cutting, J. (1980) Physical illness and psychosis. *Br. J. Psychiat.*, **136**, 109–19.

Cutting, J. (1983) Acute organic reactions. In *Handbook of Psychiatry*, Vol. 2, (ed. M. Lader). Cambridge University Press, Cambridge, pp. 119–127.

Cutting, H. (1985) *The Psychology of Schizophrenia*. Churchill Livingston, London.

Cutting, J. (1986) Atypical psychosis. In *Essentials of Postgraduate Psychiatry*, 2nd edn. (ed. P. Hill, R. M. Murray & A. Thorley). Grune & Stratton Inc, London, pp. 425–43.

Cutting, J. C., Clare, A. W. & Mann, A. H. (1978) Cycloid psychosis: an investigation of the diagnostic concept. *Psychol. Med.*, **8**, 637–48.

Dahlgren, L. & Willander, A. (1989) Are special treatment facilities for female alcoholics needed? A controlled 2-year follow-up study from a specialised female unit versus a mixed male/female treatment facility. *Alcoholism: Clin. Exper. Res.*, **13**, 499–504.

Dally, P. J. (1958) Indications for use of iproniazid in psychiatric practice. *Br. Med. J.*, **i**, 1338–9.

Dalton, K. (1980) *Depression after Childbirth*. Oxford University Press, Oxford.

Damasio H. & Damasio, A. R. (1980) The anatomical basis of conduction aphasia. *Brain.*, **103**, 337–50.

Dare, C. (1981) Psychoanalysis and family therapy. In *Development in Family Therapy* (ed. S. Walrond-Skinner). Routledge & Kegan Paul, London, pp. 281–97.

Dare, C. (1986) Psychoanalytic marital therapy. In *Clinical Handbook of Marital Therapy* (ed. N. S. Jacobson & A. S. Gurman). New York, Guildford, pp. 13–28.

Dare, C. (1988) Psychoanalytic family therapy. In *Family Therapy in Britain* (ed. E. Street & W. Dryden). Open University Press, Milton Keynes, pp. 23–50.

Dare, C. (1991) The place of psychotherapy in the management of anorexia nervosa. In *Psychotherapy in Psychiatric Practice* (ed. J. Holmer). Churchill Livingstone, Edinburgh, pp. 395–418.

Dare, C. (1994) Psychoanalytic psychotherapy of eating disorder. In *Treatment of Psychiatric Disorders: The DSM IV Edition* (ed. G. O. Gabbard). American Psychiatric Press Inc, Washington DC.

Dare, C. & Crowther, C. (1995) Psychodynamic models of eating disorders. In *Handbook of Eating Disorders: Theory, Treatment & Research* (ed. G. Szmuckler, C. Dare & J. Treasure). John Wiley & Sons, Chichester, pp. 124–140.

Dare, C., Eisler, I., Russell, G. F. M. & Szmukler, G. (1990) Family therapy for anorexia nervosa: Implications from the results of a controlled trial of family and individual therapy. *J. Marital and Family Therapy*, **16**, 39–57.

Dare, C. & Szmukler, G. (1991) The family therapy of early onset, short history anorexia nervosa. *Family Approaches to Eating Disorders* (ed. D. B. Woodside & L. Shekter-Wolfson). American Psychiatric Press, Inc, Washington DC. pp. 1–22.

Darke, S., Hall, W., Ross, M. & Wodak, A. (1994*a*) Benzodiazepine use and HIV risk-taking behaviour among injecting drug users. *Addiction*.

Darke, S., Hall, W. & Swift, W. (1994*b*) Prevalence, symptoms and correlates of anti-social personality disorder among methadone maintenance clients. *Drug and Alcohol Dependence*, **34**(3), 253–7.

Darke, S., Wodak, A., Hall, W. *et al.* (1992) Prevalence and predictors of psychopathology among opioid users. *Br. J. Addiction*, **87**, 771–6.

Davanloo, H. (ed.) (1978) *Basic Principles in Short-term Dynamic Psychotherapy*. Spectrum, New York.

Davanloo, H. (ed.) (1980) *Short-term Dynamic Psychotherapy*. Jason Aronson, New York.

David, A. S. & Appleby, L. (1992) Diagnostic criteria in schizophrenia: accentuate the positive. *Schiz. Bull.*, **18**, 551–7.

David, A. S. & Cutting, J. C. (1990) Affect, affective disorder and schizophrenia: a neuropsychological investigation of right hemisphere function. *Br. J. Psychiat.*, **156**, 491–5.

David, A. S. & Cutting, J. C. (eds.) (1994) *The Neuropsychology of Schizophrenia*. Lawrence Erlbaum Assocs, East Sussex.

Davidson, E. A. & Summerskill, W. H. J. (1956) Psychiatric aspects of liver disease. *Postgrad. Med. J.*, **32**, 487–94.

Davidson, J. (1992) Drug therapy of post-traumatic stress disorder. *Br. J. Psychiat.*, **160**, 309–14.

Davidson, J. & Foa, E. (1991) Diagnostic issues in post traumatic stress disorder: considerations for DSM-IV. *J. Abn. Psychol.*, **160**, 346–55.

Davidson, J., Hughes, D., George, L. & Blazer, D. (1993) The epidemiology of social phobia: findings from the Duke Epidemiological Catchment Area Study. *Psychol. Med.*, **23**, 709–18.

Davidson, J., Hughes, D., Blazer, D. & George, L. (1991) Post-traumatic stress disorder in the community: a epidemiological study. *Psychol. Med.*, **21**, 713–21.

Davidson, M., Humphreys, M., Johnstone, E. C. & Cunningham Owens, D. G. (1995) Prevalence of psychiatric morbidity among remand prisoners in Scotland. *Br. J. Psychiat.*, **167**, 545–8.

Davidson, R., Bunting, B. & Raistrick, D. (1989) The homogeneity of the alcohol dependence syndrome: a factorial analysis of the SADD questionnaire. *Br. J. Addiction*, **84**, 907–15.

Davies, J. M., Fann, W. E., El-Yousef, M. K. *et al.* (1973) Clinical problems in treating the aged with psychotropic drugs. *Ad. Behav. Biol.*, **6**, 11–125.

Davis, J. M. & Garver, D. L. (1978) Neuroleptics, clinical use in psychiatry. In *Handbook of*

Psychopharmacology (ed. L. L. Iversen, S. D. Iversen & S. H. Snyder). Plenum Press, London, pp. 129–60.

Davis, J. M. & Janowsky, D. S. (1974) Recent advances in the treatment of depression. *Br. J. Hosp. Med.*, February, 219–28.

Davis, R., Olmstead, M. P. & Rockert, W. (1990) Brief group psychoeducation for bulimia nervosa: Assessing the clinical significance of change. *J. Consult. Clini. Psychol.*, **58**, 882–5.

Davison, K. & Bagley, C. R. (1969) Schizophrenia-like psychoses associated with organic disorders of the central nervous system. In *Current Problems in Neuropsychiatry* (ed. R. Herrington). Headley Brothers, Ashford, Kent.

Davison, K. (1976) Drug-induced psychoses and their relationship to schizophrenia. In *Schizophrenia Today* (ed. D. Kemali, G. Bartholini & D. Richter). Pergamon Press, Oxford.

Davison, K. (1981) Toxic psychosis. *Br. J. Hosp. Med.*, **26**, 530–7.

Dawe, S., Griffiths, P., Gossop, M. & Strang, J. (1991) Should opiate addicts be involved in controlling their own detoxification? A comparison of self-regulated versus fixed negotiable schedules. *Br. J. Addiction*, **86**, 977–82.

Dawe, S., Powell, J., Richards, D. *et al.* (1993) Does post withdrawal cue exposure improve outcome in opiate addiction – A controlled trial. *Addiction*, **88**, 1233–45.

Dawson, D. A., Harford, T. C. & Grant, B. F. (1992) Family history as a prediction of alcohol dependence. *Alcohol: Clin. Exper. Res.*, **16**, 572–5.

Dawson, E., Parfitt, E., Roberts, Q. *et al.* (1995) linkage studies of bipolar disorder in the region of the Darier's disease gene on chromosome 12q23–24.1. *Am. J. Med. Genet.*, **60**, 94–102.

Day, K. (1983) A hospital-based psychiatric unit for mentally handicapped adults. *Mental Handicap*, **11**, 137–140.

Day, K. (1985) Psychiatric disorder in the middle-aged and elderly mentally handicapped. *Br. J. Psychiat.*, **147**, 660–7.

Day, R., Neilsen, J. A., Koren, A. *et al.* (1987) Stressful life events preceding the acute onset of schizophrenia: a cross-national study from the World Health Organization. *Culture, Medicine and Psychiatry*, **11**, 123–206.

Deakin, J. F. W. (1988) 5HT$_2$ receptors, depression and anxiety. *Pharmacol. Biochem. Behav.*, **29**, 819–82.

Dean, M. (1992) Bedlam Lives On. *Lancet*, **340**, 1398–99.

Dean, C. & Gadd, E. (1990) Home treatment for acute psychiatric illness. *Br. Med. J.*, **301**, 1021–4.

Dean, C., Williams, J. R. & Brockington, I. F. (1989) Is puerperal psychosis the same as bipolar manic depressive disorders? A family study. *Psychol. Med.*, **19**, 637–47.

Deb, S. & Hunter, D. (1991*a*) Psychopathology of people with mental handicap and epilepsy. II: Psychiatric illness. *Br. J. Psychiat.*, **159**, 826–30.

Deb, S. & Hunter, D. (1991*b*) Psychopathology of people with mental handicap and epilepsy. III: Personality disorder. *Br. J. Psychiat.*, **159**, 830–4.

de Figueiredo, J. M., & Boerstler, H. (1992) Ageing and co-morbidity among low-income psychiatric out-patients. *Internat. J. Psychiat.*, **7**, 875–8.

Defries, J. C., Fulker, D. W. & LaBuda, M. C. (1987) Evidence for a genetic aetiology in reading disability of twins. *Nature*, **329**, 537–9.

de Girolamo, G. & Reich, J. H. (1993) *Personality Disorders*. WHO, Geneva.

De Jong, R. N. (1977) CNS manifestations of diabetes mellitus. *Postgrad. Med J.*, **61**, 101–7.

De Jong, C. A. J., Van Den Brink, W., Harteveld, F. M. *et al.* (1993) Personality disorders in alcoholics and drug addicts. *Compreh. Psychiat.*, **34**, 87–94.

De la Pena, A. (1978) Towards a physiologic conceptualism of insomnia. In *Sleep Disorders: Diagnosis and Treatment* (ed. R. L. Williams & I. Karecan). Wiley, New York, pp. 101–43.

Delay, J. & Deniker, P (1952) Le traitement des psychoses par un methode neurolytique derivee de l'hibernotherapie (le 4560 RP utilise-seul en cure prolongee et continue). In *Le Congres de Psychiatrie et de Neurologie de langue francaise* (ed. P. Cossa). Maisson, Luxembourg, pp. 497–502.

De Leon, G., Skodol, A. & Rosenthal, M. (1973) The Phoenix Therapeutic Community for Drug Addicts. *Arch. Gen. Psychiat.*, **28**, 131–5.

Dell, S. (1984) *Murder into Manslaughter*. Maudsley Monograph No. 17. Oxford University Press, Oxford.

Demaret, A. (1991) De la grossesse nerveuse a l'anorexie mentale *Acta Psychiat. Belg.*, **91**, 11–22.

Dement, W. C., Carskadon, M. & Ley, R. (1973) The prevalence of narcolepsy. *Sleep Res.*, **2**, 147.

Dement, W. C., Zarcone, V., Varner, V. *et al.* (1972) The prevalence of narcolepsy. *Sleep Res.*, **1**, 148.

Demitrack, M., Dale, J., Straus, S. *et al.* (1991) Evidence for impaired activation of the hypothalamic-pituitary adrenal axis in patients with chronic fatigue syndrome. *J. Clin. Endocrinol. Metab.*, **73**, 1224–34.

De Montmollin, M. J., Zimmerman, E., Bernheim, J. & Harding, T. W. (1986) Sociotherapeutic treatment of delinquents in prison. *Internat. J. Offender Ther. Comp. Criminol.*, **30**, 25–34.

De Morsier, G. (1938) Les hallucinations, etude oto-neuro-ophtalmologique. *Revue Otoneurophtalmologique*, **16**, 244–352.

Deneau, G., Yanagita, T. & Seevers, M. H. (1969) Self-administration of psychoactive substances by the monkey: a measure of psychological dependence. *Psychopharmacologica*, **16**, 30–48.

Deniker, P. (1970) Introduction of neuroleptic chemotherapy into psychiatry. In *Discoveries in Biological Psychiatry* (ed. F. J. Ayd & B. Blackwell). J. B. Lippincott, Philadelphia (pubs), pp. 155–65.

Dening, T. (1992) Community psychiatry of old age. A UK perspective. *Internat. J. Geriat. Psychiat.*, **7**, 757–66.

Dennehy, J., Appleby, L., Thomas, C. S. & Faragher, B. (1996) A case control study of suicide by discharged psychiatric patients. *British Medical Journal.* (in press).

Dent, H. & Stephenson, G. (1979) An experimental study of the effectiveness of different techniques of questioning child witnesses. *Br.J. Soc. Clin. Psychol.*, **18**, 41–51.

De Paermentier, F., Cheetham, S. C., Crompton, M. R. (1990) Brain B-adrenoceptor binding sites in antidepressant-free depressed suicide victims. *Brain Res.*, **525**, 71–7.

Department of Health (1989) *Caring for People: Community Care in the next Decade and Beyond*. HMSO, London.

Department of Health (1991*a*) *Drug Misuse and Dependence. Guidelines on Clinical Management*. HMSO, London.

Department of Health (1991*b*) *Health of the Nation*. HMSO, London.

Department of Health (1991*c*) *The Clinical Guidelines for the Management of Drug Dependence*. HMSO, London.

Department of Health (1991*d*) *Working Together under the Children Act 1989*. HMSO, London.

Department of Heath (1992) *The Health of the Nation. A Strategy for Health in England*. HMSO, London.

Department of Health (1993*a*) *The Health of the Nation*. HMSO, London.

Department of Health (1993*b*) *Mental Illness Key Area Handbook*. Appendix 3.2, HMSO, London, p. 43.

Department of Health (1994) *On the State of the Public Health 1993*. HMSO, London.

Department of Health (1995) *A Handbook on Child and Adolescent Mental Health*. Department of Health, London.

Department of Health, Home Office (1992) (Reed Report) *Review of Health and Social Services for Mentally Disordered Offenders and Others Requiring Similar Services Final Summary Report*. HMSO, London, Cm2088.

Department of Health, Home Office (1993) *Review of Health and Social Services by Mentally Disordered Offenders and Others Requiring Similar Services Vol. 2. Service Needs*. HMSO, London.

Department of Health and Social Security (1974) *Revised Report of the Working Party on Security in NHS Psychiatric Hospitals* (The Glancy Report). HMSO, London.

Department of Health and Social Security (1975) *Better Services for the Mentally Ill*, Cmnd 6233. HMSO, London.

Department of Health and Social Security (1978) *Collaboration in Community Care.* Central Health Services Council, HMSO, London.

Department of Health and Social Security (1981) *Care in Action.* HMSO, London.

Department of Health and Social Security (1985) *Reform of Social Security.* HMSO, London.

Department of Health and Social Security (1988) *Report on the Committee of Inquiry into the Care and After-care of Miss Sharon Campbell.* HMSO, London. Cmnd 440.

Department of Health and Welsh Office (1990) *Code of Practice,* HMSO, London.

Department of Health and Welsh Office (1993) *Code of Practice. Mental Health Act 1983.* HMSO, London.

Depue, R. A., Monroe, S. M. & Shackman, S. L. (1979) The psychobiology of human disease: Implications for conceptualising the depressive disorders. In *The Psychobiology of the Depressive Disorders: Implications for the Effects of Stress* (ed. R. A. Depue). Academic Press, New York, pp. 3–20.

Der, G. & Bebbington, P. (1987) Depression in inner London. A register study. *Soc. Psychiat.,* **22,** 73–84.

Der, G., Gupta, S. & Murray, R. M. (1990) Is schizophrenia disappearing? Evidence from England and Wales 1952–1986. *Lancet,* **335,** 513–16.

des Jarlais, D. (1992) The first and second decades of AIDS among injecting drug users. *Br. J. Addiction,* **87,** 347–53.

Deutsch, A. Y., Moghaddam, B., Innis, R. B. *et al.* (1991) Mechanisms of action of atypical antipsychotic drugs: Implications for novel therapeutic strategies for schizophrenia. *Schiz. Res.,* **4,** 121–56.

Devlen, J., Maguire, P., Phillips, P. & Crowther, D. (1987) Psychological problems associated with diagnosis and treatment of lymphoma. II: Prospective study. *Br. Med. J.,* **295,** 955–7.

De Vries, L. S., Dubowitz, L. M. S., Dubowitz, V. *et al.* (1985) Predictive value of cranial ultrasound in the newborn baby: a reappraisal. *Lancet,* **i,** 137–40.

De Vries, L. B. A., Halley, D. J. J., Oostra, B. A. & Niermeijer, M. F. (1994) The fragile-X syndrome: a growing gene causing familial intellectual disability. *J. Intell. Disab. Res.,* **38,** 1–8.

De Wilde, E. J., Kienhorst, I. C. W. M., Diekstra, R. F. W. & Wolters, W. H. G. (1992) The relationship between adolescent suicidal behaviour and life events in childhood and adolescence. *Am. J. Psychiat.,* **149,** 45–51.

Dick, P., Cameron, L., Cohen, D. & Barlow N. (1985) Day and full-time psychiatric treatment: a controlled comparison. *Br. J. Psychiat.,* **147,** 246–50.

Dietch, J. T. & Jennings, R. K. (1988) Aggressive dyscontrol in patients treated with benzodiazepines. *J. Clin. Psychiatr.,* **49,** 184–8.

Dikmen, S., Matthews, C. G. & Harley, J. P. (1977) Effect of early versus late onset of major motor epilepsy on cognitive intellectual performance. *Epilepsia,* **18,** 31–6.

Dilling, H., Weyerer, S. & Fichter, M. (1989) The upper Bavarian studies. *Acta Psychiat. Scand.,* **79** (Suppl. 348), 113–240.

Dinan, T. H. (1993) A rational approach to the non-responding depressed patient. *Int. Clin. Psychopharmacol.,* **8,** 221–3.

Dinan, T. G. (1994) Glucocorticoids and the genesis of depressive illness. A psychobiological model. *Br. J. Psychiat.,* **164,** 365–71.

DiNicola, V. F. (1990) Anorexia multiform: self starvation in historical and cultural context II: Anorexia nervosa as a culture reactive syndrome. *Transcult. Psychiat. Res. Rev.,* **27,** 245–86.

Ditta, S. D., George, C. F., Singh, S. M. (1992) HLA-D-region genomic DNA restriction fragments in DRW15 (DR2) familial narcolepsy. *Sleep,* **15,** 48–57.

Dobson, K. S.. (1989) A meta-analysis of the efficacy of cognitive therapy for depression. *J. Consult. Clin. Psychol.,* **57,** 414–19.

Dobson, A. & Culhane, M. (1991) Social work and the elderly mentally ill. In *Psychiatry in the Elderly* (ed. R. Jacoby & C. Oppenheimer). Oxford University Press, Oxford, pp. 513–34.

Dodge, K. A., Bates, J. E. & Pettit, G. S. (1990) Mechanisms in the cycle of violence. *Science,* **250,**

1678–83.

Dodrill, C. B. & Temkin, N. R. (1989) Motor speed is a contaminating factor in evaluating the 'cognitive' effects of phenytoin. *Epilepsia*, **30**, 453–7.

Dohrenwend, B. P., Stueve, A., Skodol, A. E. & Link, B. (1993) *Life events vulnerability and schizophrenia episodes: A case-control study*. Paper presented at WPA Section of Epidemiology and Community Psychiatry Symposium, Groningen, Netherlands. Sept 1–3.

Dohrenwend, R. S., Cook, D. & Dohrenwend, B. P. (1981) Measurement of social functioning in community populations. In *What is a Case?* (ed. J. K. Wing, P. Bebbington & L. Robins). Grant McIntyre, London, pp. 183–201.

Dolan, B. & Coid, J. (1993) *Psychopathic and Antisocial Personality Disorders. Treatment and Research Issues*. Gaskell (Royal College of Psychiatrists), London.

Dolan, R. J., Bench, C. J., Brown, R. G. *et al.* (1992) Regional cerebral blood flow abnormalities in depressed patients with cognitive impairment. *J. Neurol. Neurosurg. Psychiat.*, **55**, 768–73.

Dolan, R. J., Calloway, S. P. & Mann, A. H. (1985a) Cerebral ventricular size in depressed subjects. *Psych. Med.*, **15**, 873–8.

Dolan, R. J., Calloway, S. P., Fonagy, P. *et al.* (1985b) Life events, depression and hypothalamic–pituitary–adrenal axis function. *Br. J. Psychiat.*, **147**, 429–33.

Doll, R. & Peto, R. (1981) The causes of cancer. *J. Nat. Cancer Inst.*, **66**, 1191–308.

Donnai, D., Charles, N. & Harris, R. (1981) Attitude of patients after 'genetic' termination of pregnancy. *Br. Med. J.*, **282**, 621–2.

d'Orban, P. T. (1993) Female offenders. In *Forensic Psychiatry: Clinical, Legal and Ethical Issues* (ed. J. Gunn & P. J. Taylor). Butterworth–Heinemann, Oxford, pp. 599–623.

Dorus, W. (1988) Lithium carbonate treatment of depressed and non-depressed alcoholics in double-blind placebo controlled study. Presented at the annual meeting of the Research Society on Alcoholism, June 3 1988.

Douglas, A., Matson, I. C. & Hunter, S. (1989) Sex therapy for women incestuously abused as children. *Sex. Marital Ther.*, **4**, 143–60.

Douglas, V. I. (1988) Cognitive deficits in children with attention deficit disorder with hyperactivity. In *Attention Deficit Disorder – Criteria, Cognition, Intervention* (ed. L. Bloomingdale & J. Sergeant). Pergamon, New York, pp. 65–81.

Downey, G., Feldman, S., Khuri, J. & Friedman, S. (1994) Maltreatment and childhood depression. In *Handbook of Depression in Children and Adolescents* (ed. W. M. Reynolds & H. F. Johnston). Plenum Press, New York, pp. 481–509.

Drake, R. E. & Cotton, P. G. (1986) Depression, hopelessness and suicide in chronic schizophrenia. *Br. J. Psychiat.*, **148**, 554–9.

Drake, R. E., Gates, C., Cotton, P. G. & Whitaker, A. (1984) Suicide among schizophrenics. Who is at risk? *J. Nerv. Ment. Dis.*, **172**, 613–17.

Drejer, K., Theilgaard, A., Teesdale, T. W. *et al.* (1985) A prospective study of young men at high risk for alcoholism. A neuropsychological assessment. *Alcoholism, Clin. Exp. Res.*, **9**, 498–502.

Drugs and Therapeutics Bulletin (1991) Management of behavioural emergencies, **29**, 62–4.

Drummond, D. C. (1990) The relationship between alcohol dependence and alcohol related problems in clinical population. *Br. J. Addiction* **85**, 357–66.

Drummond, D. C., Cooper, T. & Glautier, S. (1990) Conditioned learning in alcohol dependence: implications for one exposure treatment. *Br. J. Addiction.* **85**, 125–44.

Dubin, W. R. (1989) The role of fantasies, counter-transference and psychological defenses in patient violence. *Hosp. Comm. Psychiat.*, **40**, 1280–3.

Dubos, R. (1968) *Man, medicine and environment*. Pall Mall Press, London.

Du Bow, F. L. & Becker, T. M. (1976) Patterns in victim advocacy. In *Criminal Justice and the Victim* (ed. N. McDonald). Sage, Beverly Hills.

Duncan-Jones, P., Fergusson, D. M., Ormel, J. & Horwood, L. J. (1990) A model of stability and change in minor psychiatric symptoms: results from three longitudinal studies. *Psychol. Med.*, Monograph Suppl. 18.

Dunner, D. L., Fleiss, J. L. & Fieve, R. R. (1976) The course of development of mania in patients with recurrent depression. *Am. J. Psychiat.*, **133**, 905–8.

Dunner, D. L., Murphy D., Stallen, F. & Fieve, R. R. (1979) Episode frequency prior to lithium treatment in bipolar manic-depressive patients. *Compreh. Psychiat.*, **20**, 511–15.

Durand, V. M. (1990) *Severe Behaviour Problems: A Functional Communication Training Approach.* Guilford Press, New York.

Durand, V. M. & Crimmins, D. (1988) Identifying the variables maintaining self injurious behaviour. *J. Autism Devel. Disord.*, **17**, 17–28.

Durham, R., Murphy, T., Allan, T. *et al.* (1994) Cognitive therapy, analytic therapy and anxiety management training for generalised anxiety disorder. *Br. J. Psychiat.*, **165**, 315–23.

Durkheim, E. (1951) *Suicide* (Trans. J. A. Spalding & G. Simpson). Free Press, New York.

Dworkin, R. J., Friedman, L. C., Telschow, R. L. *et al* (1990) The longitudinal use of the Global Assessment Scale in multiple-rater situations. *Commun. Ment. Health J.*, **26**, 335–44.

Dyck, R. J., Bland, R. C. M., Newman, S. C. & Om, H. (1988) Suicide attempts and psychiatric disorders in Edmonton. *Acta Psychiat. Scand.*, **77**, (Suppl. 338) pp. 64–71.

Dytrych, Z., Matejcek, Z., Schuller, V. *et al.* (1975) Children born to women denied abortion. *Fam. Plann. Perspect.*, **7**, 165–71.

D'Zurilla, T. J. & Goldfried, M. R. (1971) Problem solving and behaviour modification. *J. Abnorm. Psychol.*, **78**, 107–26.

Eagles, J. M. & Whalley, L. J. (1985) Ageing and affective disorders: the age at first onset of affective disorders in Scotland; 1969–1978. *Br. J. Psychiat.*, **147**, 180–7.

Eames, P. (1992) Hysteria following brain injury. *J. Neurol. Neurosurg. Psychiat.*, **55**, 1046–53.

Earls, F. (1994) Oppositional defiant and conduct disorders. In *Child and Adolescent Psychiatry: Modern Approaches* (ed. M. Rutter, E. Taylor & L. Hersov). Blackwell Scientific, Oxford, pp. 308–29.

Eaton, W. W. (1980) *The Sociology of Mental Disorders.* Praeger, New York.

Eaton, W. W. & Kessler, L. G. (1985) *Epidemiologic Field Methods in Psychiatry: The NIMH Epidemiologic Catchment Area Program.* Academic Press, Orlando, Fla.

Eaton, W. & Keyl, P. (1990) Risk factors for the onset of Diagnostic Interview Schedule/DSM-III agoraphobia in a prospective, population based study. *Arch. Gen. Psychiat.*, **47**, 819–24.

Eaton, W., Kramer, M., Anthony, J. et al. (1989) The incidence of specific DIS/DSM-III mental disorders: data from the NIMH Epidemiologic Catchment Area Program. *Acta Psychiat. Scand.*, **79**, 163–78.

Eaton, L. F. & Menolascino, F. J. (1982) Psychiatric disorders in the mentally retarded: types, problems and challenges. *Am. J. Psychiat.*, **139**, 1297–303.

Eaton, W. W. & Ritter, C. (1988) Distinguishing anxiety and depression with field survey data. *Psychol. Med.*, **18**, 155–66.

Ebrahim, S., Dallosso, H., Morgan, K. *et al.* (1988) Causes of ill health among a random sample of old and very old people: possibilities for prevention. *J. Roy. Coll. Physic. Lond.*, **22**, 105–7.

Ebstein, R. P. & Belmaker, R. H. (1979) Lithium and brain adenylate cyclase. In *Lithium; Controversies and Unsolved Issues.* (ed. T. Cooper, S. Gershon, N. Kline & M. Schou). Excerpta Medica, London, pp. 703–29.

Edeh, J. & Toone, B. (1987) Relationship between interictal psychotheology and the type of epilepsy. Results of a survey in general practice. *Br. J. Psychiat.*, **151**, 95–101.

Edwards, J. G. (1986) The untoward effects of antipsychotic drugs; pathogenesis and management, In *The Psychopharmacology and Treatment of Schizophrenia* (ed. P. Bradley & S. Hirsch). Oxford Med. Pubs., Oxford, pp. 403–43.

Edwards, G. (1984) Drinking in longitudinal perspective; career and natural history. *Br. J. Addiction*, **79**, 175–83.

Edwards, G. (1987) *The Treatment of Drinking Problems.* Blackwell, Oxford.

Edwards, G. (1989) Addictions as challenge to general psychiatry. *Internat. Rev. Psychiat.*, **1**, 5–8.

Edwards, G., Anderson, P., Babor, T. F. *et al.* (1994) *Alcohol policy and the public good.* Oxford Medical Publications, Oxford University Press.

Edwards, G., Arif, A. & Hodgson, R. (1981) Nomenclature and classification of drug related problems: a WHO memorandum. *Bull. WHO*, 225–242.

Edwards, G. & Gross, M. M. (1976) Alcohol dependence: provisional description of a clinical syndrome. *Br. Med. J.*, **1**, 1058–61.

Edwards, G., Gross, M. M., Keller, M. *et al.* (1977a) *Alcohol Related Disabilities.* WHO Offset Publication No. 32, WHO, Geneva.

Edwards, G. & Lader, M. (1992) *The Nature of Dependence.* Oxford University Press, Oxford.

Edwards, G. E., Orford, J., Egert, S. *et al.* (1977b) Alcoholism. a controlled trial of treatment and advice. *J. Stud. Alcohol*, **38**, 1004–31.

Edwards, G., Strang, J. & Jaffe, J. (eds) (1993) *Drugs, Alcohol and Tobacco: Making the Science and Policy Connections.* Oxford University Press, Oxford.

Einfeld, S. L. (1990) Guidelines for the use of psychotropic medication in individuals with developmental disabilities. *Austr. N.Z. J. Devel. Disabil.*, **16**, 71–3.

Einfeld, S. L. & Tonge, B. J. (1991) Psychometric and clinical assessment of psychopathology in developmentally disabled children. *Austr. N.Z. J. Devel. Disabil.*, **17**, 147–67.

Ellenberger, H. F. (1970) *The Discovery of the Unconscious: The History of Dynamic Psychiatry.* Allen Lane, the Penguin Press, London.

Elias, R. (1993) *The Political Manipulation of Crime Victims.* Sage, Newbury Park, CA.

Elkin, I., Shea, T., Watkins, J. T. *et al* (1989) NIMH treatment of depression collaborative research program. I. General effectiveness of treatments. *Arch. Gen. Psychiat.*, **46**, 971–82.

Elliott, D. S., Huizinga, D. & Menard, S. (1989) *Multiple Problem Youth.* Springer-Verlag, New York.

Elliott, S. A. (1989) Psychological strategies in the prevention and treatment of postpartum depression. *Baillières Clin. Obstet. Gynaecol.*, **3**, 879–903.

Ellis, A. (1962) *Reason and Emotion in Psychotherapy.* Lyle Stuart, New York.

Ellis, H. D. & de Pauw, K. W. (1994) The cognitive neuropsychiatric origins of the Capgras delusion. In *The Neuropsychology of Schizophrenia* (ed. A. S. David & J. C. Cutting). Lawrence Erlbaum Assocs, Hove, East Sussex. pp. 317–36.

Ellis, P. M., Mellsop, G. W., Beeston, R. & Cooke, R. R. (1991) Platelet tritiated imipramine binding in patients suffering from mania. *J. Affect. Disorders.*, **22**, 105–10.

Elvy, G. A., Wells, J. E. & Baird, K. A. (1988) Attempted referral as intervention for problem drinking in the general hospital. *Br. J. Addiction*, **83**, 83–9.

Emde, R. & Sameroff, A. (1989) *Relationship Disturbances.* Basic Books, New York.

Emmelkamp, P. M. G. (1982) *Phobic and Obsessive-compulsive Disorders: Theory Research and Practice.* Plenum, New York.

Emmelkamp, P., Mersch, P., Vissia, E. & Van der Helm, M. (1985) Social phobia: a comparative evaluation of cognitive and behavioural interventions. *Behav. Res. Ther.*, **23**, 265–9.

Emmelkamp, P. M. G., Van der Helm, M., Van Zanten, B. & Plochg, I. (1980) Treatment of obsessive compulsive patients: the contribution of self-instructional training to the effectiveness of exposure. *Behav. Res. Ther.*, **18**, 61–6.

Emmelkamp, P. M. G., Visser, S. & Hoekstra, R. J. (1988) Cognitive therapy versus exposure *in vivo* in the treatment of obsessive-compulsives. *Cogn. Ther. Res.*, **12**, 103–14.

Emmelkamp, P. M. G. & Wessels, H. (1975) Flooding in imagination versus flooding *in vivo* for agoraphobics. *Behav. Res. Ther.*, **13**, 7–15.

Emerson, E., Barret, S., Bell, C. *et al.* (1987) *Developing Services for People with Severe Learning Difficulties and Challenging Behaviours.* Institute of Social and Applied Psychology, University of Kent.

Emerson, T. R., Milne, J. R. & Gardner, A. J. (1981) Cardiogenic dementia – a myth? *Lancet*, **ii**, 743–4.

Emrick, C. D. (1989) Alcoholics Anonymous: Membership characteristics and effectiveness as treatment. In *Recent Developments in Alcoholism: Emerging Issues in Treatment.* Vol. 7, (ed. M. Galanter). Plenum Press, New York, pp. 37–53.

Enas, G. G., Pope, H. G. & Vevine, L. R. (1989) Fluoxetine in bulimia nervosa: A double blind study. In *New Research Program and Abstracts*. American Psychiatric Association, 142nd Annual Meeting (abstract). APA Press, New York, p. 204.

Endicott, J. & Spitzer, R. L. (1978) A diagnostic interview: the Schedule for Affective Disorders and Schizophrenia. *Arch. Gen. Psychiat.*, **35**, 837–44.

Endicott, J., Spitzer, R. L., Fleiss, J. L. *et al.* (1976) The global assessment scale. *Arch. Gen. Psychiat.*, **33**, 766–71.

Engel, G. L. (1967) A psychological setting of somatic disease: The 'giving-up, given up' complex. *Proc. Roy. Soc. Med.*, **60**, 553–5.

Engel, G. L. (1977) The need for a new medical model: a challenge for biomedicine. *Science*, **196**, 129–36.

English, H. (1929) Three cases of the 'conditioned fear response'. *J. Abnorm. Soc. Psychol.*, **34**, 221–5.

Enoch, M. D. & Trethowan, W. H. (1979) *Uncommon Psychiatric Syndromes* (2nd edn). John Wright & Sons, Bristol.

Epling, W. F. & Pierce, W. D. (1984) Activity based anorexia in rats as a function of opportunity to run on an activity wheel. *Nutr. Behav.*, **2**, 37–49.

Epstein, L. J. (1976) Symposium on age differentiation in depressive illness. Depression in the elderly. *J. Gerontol.*, **31**, 278–82.

Epstein, L. J., Mills, C. & Simon, A. (1970) Antisocial behaviour of the elderly. *Compreh. Psychiat.*, **11**, 36–42.

Epstein, S. (1979) The stability of behaviour: 1. On predicting most of the people much of the time. *J. Personal. Soc. Psychol.*, **37**, 1097–125.

Erb, J. L., Gwirtsman, H. E., Fuster, J. M. & Richeimer, S. H. (1987) Bulimia Associated with Frontal Lobe Lesions. *Int. J. Eat. Dis.*, **8**(1), 117–21.

Erikson, E. H. (1950) *Childhood and society*. Norton, New York.

Erikson, E. H. (1959) Identity and the life cycle. *Psychological Issues Monograph*, International Universities Press, New York.

Erikson, K. (1964) Notes on the sociology of deviance. In *The Other Side* (ed. H. Becker). The Free Press, New York.

Escobar, J., Golding, J., Hough, R. *et al.* (1987) Somatization in the community: relationship to disability and use of services. *Am. J. Pub. Health*, **77**, 837–40.

Epsie, C., Montgomery, J. & Gillies, J. (1988) The development of a psychosocial behaviour scale for the assessment of mentally handicapped people. *J. Intell. Disabil. Res.*, **32**, 395–403:

Esquirol, J. E. D., (1833) *Observations of the Illusions of the Insane*. Renshaw and Rush, London.

Essau, C. A. & Wittchen, H.-U. (1993) An overview of the Composite International Diagnostic Interview (CIDI). *Internat. J. Meth. Psychiat. Res.*, **3**, 79–85.

Esser, G., Schmidt, M. H. & Woerner, W. (1990) Epidemiology and course of psychiatric disorders in school-age children. Results of a longitudinal study. *J. Child Psychol. Psychiat.*, **31**, 243–63.

Essex, B., Doig, R., Renshaw, J. (1990) Pilot study of records of shared care for people with mental illnesses. *Br. Med. J.*, **300**, 1442–6.

Evans, M. D., Hollon, S. D., de Rubeis, R. J. *et al.* (1992) Differential relapse after cognitive therapy and pharmacotherapy. *Arch. Gen. Psychiat.*, **49**, 802–8.

Evans, M. E., Copeland, J. R. M. & Dewy, M. E. (1991) Depression in the elderly in the community: effect of physical illness and selected social factors. *Internat. J. Geriat. Psychiat.*, **6**, 787–95.

Everall, I. P., Luthert, P. J. & Lautos, P. L. (1991) Neuronal loss in the frontal cortex of HIV infection. *Lancet*, **337**, 119–21.

Everitt, B. S., Gourlay, A. J. & Kendell, R. E. (1971) An attempt at validation of traditional psychiatric syndromes by cluster analysis. *Br. J. Psychiat.*, **199**, 319–412.

Ewing, J. A. (1984) Detecting alcoholism: The CAGE questionnaire. *J. Am. Med. Assoc.*, **252**, 1905–7.

Eysenk, H. J. (1952a) *The Scientific Study of Personality*. Routledge & Kegan Paul, London.

Eysenk, H. J. (1952b) The effects of psychotherapy: An evaluation. *J. Consult. Psychol*, **16**, 319–24.

Eysenk, H. J. (1966) *The effects of psychotherapy.* International Science Press, New York.

Eysenk, J. H. (1975) *The Future of Psychiatry.* Methuen, London.

Eysenk, H. J. & Eysenk, S. B. G. (1964) *Manual of Eysenk Personality Inventory.* University of London Press, London.

Eysenk H. J. & Eysenk, S. B. G. (1975) *Manual of the Eysenk Personality Inventory.* Hodder & Stoughton, London.

Faedda, G. L., Tondo, L., Baldessarini, R. J. (1993) Outcome of rapid vs gradual discontinuation of lithium in treatment of bipolar disorders. *Arch. Gen. Psychiat.*, **50**, 448–55.

Fahy, T. A. (1991) Obsessive-compulsive symptoms in eating disorders. *Behav. Res. Ther.*, **29**, 113–16.

Fahy, T. A. & O'Donoghue, G. (1991) Eating disorders in pregnancy (editorial). *Psychol. Med.*, **21**, 577–80.

Fahy, T. A. & Morrison, J. J. (1993) The clinical significance of eating disorders in obstetrics (editorial). *Br. J. Obstet. Gynaecol.*, **100**, 708–10.

Fahy, T. A., Osacar, A. & Marks, I. (1993) History of eating disorders in female patients with obsessive compulsive disorder. *Internat. J. Eat. Disorders*, **14**, 439–45.

Fahy, T. & Wessely, S. (1993) Should purchasers pay for psychotherapy? *Br. Med. J.*, **307**, 576–8.

Fairburn, C. G. (1981) A cognitive behavioural approach to the management of bulimia. *Psychol. Med.*, **11**, 707–11.

Fairburn, C. G. (1985) Cognitive behavioural treatment for bulimia nervosa. In *Handbook of Psychotherapy for Anorexia Nervosa and Bulimia* (ed. D. M. Garner & P. E. Garfinkel). Guildford Press, New York, pp. 160–92.

Fairburn, C. G. & Cooper, P. J. (1989) Eating Disorders. In *Cognitive Behaviour Therapy for Psychiatric Problems* (ed. K. Hawton, P. M. Salkovskis, J. Kirk & D. M. Clark) Oxford Medical Publications, Oxford, pp. 277–314.

Fairburn, C. & Cooper, Z. (1993) The eating disorder examination. In *Binge Eating: Nature, Assessment and Treatment* (ed. C. G. Fairburn & T. G. Wilson). Guildford Press, London, pp. 317–60.

Fairburn, C. G., Jones, R., Peveler, R. C. *et al.* (1991) Three psychological treatments for bulimia nervosa: a comparative trial. *Arch. Gen. Psychiat.*, **48**, 463–9.

Fairburn, C. G., Jones, R., Peveler, R. C. *et al.* (1993) Psychotherapy and bulimia nervosa. Longer-term effects of interpersonal psychotherapy, behaviour therapy and cognitive behaviour therapy. *Arch. Gen. Psychiat.*, **50**, 416–28.

Fairbairn, C. G., Wu, F. C. W., McCulloch, D. K. *et al.* (1982) The clinical features of diabetic impotence: a preliminary study. *Br. J. Psychiat.*, **140**, 447–52.

Fairweather, D. S. (1991) Delirium. In *Psychiatry in the Elderly* (ed. R. Jacoby & C. Oppenheimer). Oxford Medical Publications, Oxford, pp. 647–75.

Falkowski, B. (1991) Group Psychotherapy. In *The International Handbook of Addiction Behaviour* (ed. I. B. Glass). Routledge, London.

Falloon, I. R. H. (ed.) (1988) *Handbook of Behavioural Family Therapy.* Unwin Hyman, London.

Falloon, I. R. H., Boyd, J. L., McGill, C. W. *et al.* (1982) Family management in the prevention of exacerbations of schizophrenia. A controlled study. *N. Engl. J. Med.*, **306**, 1437–40.

Falloon, I. & Pederson, J. (1985) Family management in the prevention of morbidity of schizophrenia. The adjustment of the family unit. *Br. J. Psychiat.*, **147**, 156–63.

Falret, J. P. (1854) *Clinical Lectures on Mental Medicine, General Symptomatology.* Baillière, Paris.

Famularo, R., Kinscherff, R. & Fenton, T. (1992) Psychiatric diagnoses of maltreated children: preliminary findings. *J. Am. Acad. Child Adol. Psychiat.*, **31**, 863–7.

Farber, E. A. & Egeland, B. (1987) Invulnerability among abused and neglected children. In *The Invulnerable Child* (ed. E. J. Anthony & B. Cohler). Guildford Press, New York, pp. 253–88.

Farde, L., Nordstrom, A. L., Weisel, F-A. *et al.* (1992) Positron emission tomographic analysis of central D1 and D2 receptor occupancy in patients treated with classical neuroleptics and clozapine. *Arch. Gen. Psychiat.*, **49**, 538–44.

Farde, L., Weisel, F-A., Nordstrom, A-L. & Sedvall, G. (1989) D1 and D2 dopamine receptor occupancy during treatment with conventional and atypical neuroleptics. *Psychopharmacol.*, **99**, S28–S31.

Farde, L., Wiesel, F. A., Stone-Elander, S. *et al.* (1990) D2 dopamine receptors in neuroleptic-naive schizophrenic patients. *Arch. Gen. Psychiat.*, **47**, 213–19.

Faris, R. B. L. & Dunham, H. W. (1939) *Mental Disorders in Urban Areas. An Ecological Study of Schizophrenia and Other Psychoses.* University of Chicago Press, Chicago.

Farmer, A. E. & Griffiths, H. (1992) Labelling and illness in primary care: comparing factors influencing General Practitioner's and Psychiatrist's decisions regarding patient referral to mental illness services. *Psychol. Med.*, **22**, 717–23.

Farmer, A., Jones, I., Hillier, J. *et al.* (1995) Neurasthenia revisited: ICD-10 and DSM-IIIR psychiatric syndromes in chronic fatigue patients and comparison subjects. *Br. J. Psychiatry*, **167**, 503–6.

Farmer, A. E., Katz, R., McGuffin, P. & Bebbington, P. (1987) A comparison between the Present State Examination and the Composite International Diagnostic Interview. *Arch. Gen. Psychiat.*, **44**, 1064–68.

Farmer, A. E. & McGuffin, P. (1989) The classification of the depressions: contemporary confusion revisited. *Br. J. Psychiat.*, **155**, 437–43.

Farmer, A. E., McGuffin, P. & Gottesman, I. I. (1987) Twin concordance for DSM-III schizophrenia. *Arch. Gen. Psychiat.*, **44**, 634–41.

Farmer, R., Tanah, T., O'Donnell, I. & Catalan, J. (1992) Railway suicide; the psychological effects on drivers. *Psychol. Med.*, **22**, 407–14.

Farmer, A. E., Wessley, S., Castle, D. & McGuffin, P. (1992) Methodological issues in using a polydiagnostic approach to define psychotic illness. *Br. J. Psychiat.*, **161**, 824–30.

Farravelli, C., Webb, T., Ambonetti, A. *et al.* (1985) Prevalence of traumatic early life events in 31 agoraphobic patients with panic attacks. *Am. J. Psychiat.*, **142**, 1493–4.

Farrell, B. A. (1979) Mental illness: a conceptual analysis. *Psychol. Med.*, **9**, 21–35.

Farrell, M. (1992) Physical complications of Drug Abuse. In *The International Handbook of Addiction Behaviour* (ed. I. B. Glass). Routledge, London, pp. 120–5.

Farrell, M. (1994) Opiate withdrawal. *Addiction*, **89**, 1471–6.

Farrell, M., Chrome I. B. & Strang, J. (1996) Assessing substance use and misuse. In *Oxford Textbook of Medicine* (ed. D. J. Weatherall, J. G. G. Ledingham & D. A. Warrell). Oxford University Press, Oxford.

Farrell, M. & Strang, J. (1992) Working where the risks are. In *Healthy drug users and HIV prevention. The Working Paper.* (ed. B. Evans, S. Sandberg & W. Stuart). Health Education Authority, London, pp. 154–86.

Farrell, M., Ward, J., Mattick R. *et al.* (1994) Methadone maintenance treatment in opiate dependence: a review. *Br. Med. J.*, **309**, 997–1001.

Farrington, D. P. (1978) The family backgrounds of aggressive youths. In *Aggression and Antisocial Behaviour in Childhood and Adolescence* (ed. L. Hersov, M. Berger & D. Straffer). Pergamon, Oxford, pp. 73–93.

Farrington, D. P. (1979) Environmental stress, delinquent behaviour, and convictions. In *Stress and Anxiety*, Vol 6 (ed. I. G. Sarason & C. D. Spielberger). Hemisphere, Washington DC, pp. 93–107.

Farrington, D. P. (1981) The prevalence of convictions. *Br. J. Criminol.*, **21**, 173–5.

Farrington, D. P. (1986) Stepping stones to adult criminal careers. In *Development of Antisocial and Prosocial Behaviour* (ed. D. Olweus, J. Block & M. R. Yarrow). Academic Press, New York, pp. 359–84.

Farrington, D. P. (1988*a*) Advancing knowledge about delinquency and crime: the need for a coordinated programme of longitudinal research. *Behav. Sci. Law*, **6**, 307–31.

Farrington, D. P. (1988*b*) Studying changes within individuals: the causes of offending. In *Studies of Psychological Risk* (ed. M. Rutter). Cambridge University Press, Cambridge, pp. 158–83.

Farrington, D. P. (1991) Childhood aggression and adult violence: early precursors and later-life outcomes. In *The Development and Treatment of Childhood Aggression* (ed. D. J. Pepler & K. H. Rubin). Erlbaum, Hillsdale, NJ, pp. 5–29.

Farrington, D. P. (1993) The Psychosocial Milieu of the Offender. In *Forensic Psychiatry: Clinical, Legal and Ethical Issues* (ed. J. Gunn & P. J. Taylor). Butterworth–Heinemann, Oxford, pp. 252–85.

Farrington, D. P. & Hawkins, J. D. (1991) Predicting participation, early onset and later persistence in officially recorded offending. *Crim. Behav. Ment. Health*, **1**, 1–33.

Farrington, D. P., Snyder, H. & Finnegan, T. (1988) Specialisation in juvenile court careers. *Criminology*, **26**, 461–88.

Farrington, D. P. & West, D. J. (1993) Criminal, penal and life histories of chronic offenders: risk and protective factors and early identification. *Crim. Behav. Ment. Health*, **3**, 492–523.

Fawcett, J., Scheftner, W. A., Fogg, L. *et al* (1990) Time-related predictors of suicide in major affective disorder. *Am. J. Psychiat.*, **147**, 1189–94.

Fawcett, J., Scheftner, W., Clark, D. *et al.* (1987) Clinical predictors of suicide in patients with major affective disorders: a controlled prospective study. *Am. J. Psychiat.*, **144**, 35–40.

Federal Bureau of Investigation (1988) *Age-Specific Arrest Rates and Race-Specific Arrest Rates for Selected Offenses 1965–1986*. US Department of Justice, Washington, DC.

Fedoroff, J. P., Starkstein, S. E., Forrster, A. W. *et al.* (1992) Depression in patients with acute traumatic brain injury. *Am. J. Psychiat.*, **149**, 918–23.

Feighner, J. P., Robins, E., Guze, S. B. *et al* (1972) Diagnostic criteria for use in psychiatric research. *Arch. Gen. Psychiat.*, **26**, 57–67.

Feinberg, G. (1984) White haired offenders: an emergent social problem. In *Elderly Criminals* (ed. W. Wilbanks & P. K. H. Kim). University Press of America, Lanham, MD, pp. 83–108.

Feinberg, M., Carroll, B. J., Smouse, P. E. *et al* (1981) The Carroll Rating Scale for Depression 3. Comparison with other rating instruments. *Br. J. Psychiat.*, **138**, 105–9.

Feinmann, C., Harris, M. & Cawley, R.(1984) Psychogenic facial pain: Presentation and treatment. *Br. Med. J.*, **288**, 436–8.

Feinstein, A. & Dolan, R. (1991) Predictors of post-traumatic stress disorder following physical trauma: an examination of the stressor criterion. *Psychol. Med.*, **21**, 85–91.

Fenichel, O. (1945) *The Psychoanalytic Theory of Neurosis*. W. W. Norton, New York.

Fennell, M. J. V. (1989) Depression. In *Cognitive Behaviour Therapy for Psychiatric Problems*. Oxford Medical Publications, Oxford, pp. 169–234.

Fenton, G. W. (1986) Epilepsy and hysteria. *Br. J. Psychiat.*, **149**, 28–37.

Fenton, G. W. (1975) Clinical disorders of Sleep. *Br. J. Hos. Med.*, **14**, 120–45.

Fenton, G. W. (1980) Epilepsy and automatism. *J. Irish. Med. Ass.*, **73** (Suppl. 10).

Fenton, G. W. (1981) Psychiatric disorders of epilepsy. In *Epilepsy and Psychiatry* (ed. E. H. Reynolds & M. R. Trimble). Churchill Livingstone, Edinburgh, pp. 12–26.

Fenton, G. W. & Standage, K. (1993) The EEG in Psychiatry. *Psychiat. Bull.*, **17**, 601–3.

Fenton, F., Tessier, L., Struening, E. *et al.* (1982) *Home and Hospital Psychiatric Treatment*. Croom Helm, London.

Ferenczi, S. (1912) *Sex in psychoanalysis*. Basic Books, New York, 1950.

Ferenczi, S. (1924) *Thalassa: A theory of geniality*. Psychoanalytic Quarterly, Albany, 1938.

Ferenczi, S. & Rank, O. (1925) *The Development of Psychoanalysis*. The Nervous and Mental Diseases Publishing Co, New York.

Ferguson, B. & Tyrer, P. (1989*a*) Rating instruments in psychiatric research. In *Research Methods in Psychiatry* (ed. C. Freeman & P. Tyrer). Gaskell, London.

Ferguson, B. & Tyrer, P. (1989*b*) Personality disorders. In *The Instruments of Psychiatric Research* (ed. C. Thompson), pp. 239–51. John Wiley & Sons, Chichester.

Fergusson, D. M., Horwood, L. J. & Shannon, F. T. (1986) Factors related to the attainment of nocturnal bladder control: an 8-year longitudinal study. *Paediatrics*, **78**, 884–90.

Fichter, M. M., Quadflieg, N. & Rief, W. (1992) The German longitudinal bulimia nervosa study. I. In *The Course of Eating Disorders* (ed. W. Herzog, H. C. Deter & W. Vandereycken). Springer Verlag, Berlin, pp. 133–49.

Fichter, M. M., Quadflieg, N. & Rief, W. (1994) Course of multi-impulsive bulimia. *Psychol. Med.*, **24**, 591–604.

Fillmore, K. M. & Midanik, (1984) Chronicity of drinking problems among men. A longitudinal study. *J. Stud. Alcohol*, **45**, 288–36.

Finch, E. J. L., Groves, I. P., Feinmann, C. & Farmer, R. (1995) A low threshold methadone treatment programme – the first two months. *Addict. Res.*, **3**(1), 63–71.

Finch, E. J. L. & Katona, C. L. E. (1989) Lithium augmentation in the treatment of refractory depression in old age. *Internat. J. Geriat. Psychiat.*, **4**, 41–6.

Fink, P. (1992a) Surgery and medical treatment in persistent somatizing patients. *J. Psychosom. Res.*, **36**, 439–47.

Fink, P. (1992b) The use of hospitalisations by persistent somatizing patients. *Psychol. Med.*, **22**, 173–80.

Finlay-Jones, R. (1989) Anxiety. In *Life Events and Illness* (ed. G. Brown & T. Harris). Hyman, London, pp. 95–112.

Finlay-Jones, R. & Brown, G. (1981) Types of stressful life event and the onset of anxiety-depressive disorder. *Psychol. Med.*, **11**, 803–15.

Finlay-Jones, R. A. & Murphy, E. (1979) Severity of psychiatric disorder and the 30-item General Health Questionnaire. *Br. J. Psychiat.*, **134**, 609–16.

Fitzgerald, M. (1993) *Ethnic Minorities and the Criminal Justice System*. The Royal Commission on Criminal Justice. Research Study No. 20. HMSO, London.

Fitzpatrick, R., Fletcher, A., Gore, S. *et al* (1992) Quality of life measures in health care. I: Applications and issues in assessment. *Br. Med. J.*, **305**, 1074–7.

Fischer, P. & Breakey, W. (1986) Homelessness and mental health: an overview. *Internat. J. Ment. Health*, **14**, 6–41.

Fish, F. (1967) *Clinical Psychopathology*. Wrights, Bristol.

Fish, B. (1977) Neurobiological antecedents of schizophrenia in children. *Arch. Gen. Psychiat.*, **34**, 1297–313.

Flament, M. F., Koby, E., Rapoport, J. L. *et al.* (1990) Childhood obsessive-compulsive disorder: a prospective follow-up study. *J. Child Psychol. Psychiat.*, **31**, 363–80.

Flament, M. F., Rapoport, J. L., Berg, C. J. *et al* (1985) Clomipramine treatment of childhood compulsive disorder: a double-blind controlled study. *Arch. Gen. Psychiat.*, **42**, 977–83.

Flament, M. F., Whitaker, A., Rapoport, J. *et al.* (1988) Obsessive compulsive disorder in adolescence: An epidemiological study, *J. Am. Acad. Child Adol. Psychiat.*, **27**, 764–71.

Fleminger, S. & Burns, A. (1993) The delusional misidentification syndromes in patients with and without evidence of organic cerebral disorder: a structured review of case reports. *Biol. Psychiat.*, **33**, 22–32.

Flint, A. J. (1992) The optimum duration of antidepressant treatment in the elderly. *Internat. J. Geriat. Psychiat.*, **7**, 617–19.

Flood, R. A. & Seager, C. P. (1968) A retrospective examination of psychiatric case records of patients who subsequently committed suicide. *Br. J. Psychiat.*, **114**, 443–50.

Flor, H., Birbaumer, N., Schulte, W. & Ross, R. (1985) Assessment of stress-related psychophysiological responses in chronic back pain patients. *J. Consult. Clin. Psychol.*, **53**, 354–64.

Flor-Henry, P. (1969) Psychosis and temporal lobe epilepsy. *Epilepsia*, **10**, 363–95,

Flor-Henry, P. (1976) Epilepsy and psychopathology. In *Recent Advances in Clinical Psychiatry*, vol. 2. (ed. K. Granville-Grossman). Churchill Livingstone, Edinburgh, pp. 262–95.

Fluoxetine, Bulimia Nervosa Collaborative Study Group (1992) Fluoxetine in the treatment of bulimia nervosa: a multicentre placebo-controlled double-blind trial. *Arch. Gen. Psychiat.*, **49**, 139–47.

Foa, E. G. & Goldstein, A. (1978) Continuous exposure and strict response prevention in the treatment of obsessive-compulsive neurosis. *Behav. Ther.*, **9**, 821–9.

Focault, M. (1971) *Madness and Civilisation*. Tavistock, London.

Foerster, A., Lewis, S., Owen, M. & Murray, R. M. (1991a) Premorbid personality in psychosis: effects of sex and diagnosis. *Br. J. Psychiat.*, **158**, 171–6.

Foerster, A., Lewis, S., Owen, M. & Murray, R. M. (1991b) Low birth weight and a family history of schizophrenia predict poor premorbid functioning in psychosis. *Schiz. Res.*, **5**, 3–20.

Fogel, B. S., Fretwell, M. (1985) Re-classification of depression in the medically ill elderly. *J. Am. Geriat. Society*, **33**, 446–8.

Folstein, M. F., Romanowski, A. J., Nestadt, G. *et al.* (1985) Brief report on the clinical reappraisal of the Diagnostic Interview Schedule carried out at the Johns Hopkins site of the Epidemiological Catchment Area Program of the NIMH. *Psychol. Med.*, **15**, 809–14.

Folstein, M. F., Bassett, S. S., Romanoski, A. J. *et al.* (1991) The epidemiology of delirium in the community: The Eastern Baltimore Mental Health Survey. *Internat. Psychogeriat.*, **3**, 169–79.

Ford, R. A. (1989) The psychopathology of echophenomena. *Psychol. Med.*, **19**, 627–35.

Forsman, A. (1976) Individual variability in response to haloperidol. *Proc. Roy. Soc. Med.*, **69**, (suppl. 1) 9–12.

Forssman, H. & Thuwe, I. (1966) One hundred and twenty children born after application for therapeutic abortion refused. Their mental health, social adjustment and educational level up to the age of 21. *Acta Psychiatr. Scand.*, **42**, 71–88.

Forstl, H., Almeida, O. P., Owen, A. M. *et al.* (1991) Psychiatric, neurological and medical aspects of misidentification syndromes: a review of 260 cases. *Psychol. Med.*, **21**, 905–10.

Forstl, H., Burns, A., Levy, R. *et al.* (1992) Neurologic signs in Alzheimer's disease. *Arch. Neurol.*, **49**, 1038–42.

Foster, J. R., Silver, M. & Boksay, I. J. E. (1990) Lithium use in the elderly: Diagnostic and research considerations. *Internat. J. Geriat. Psychiat.*, **5**, 1–8.

Foulkes, S. H. (1975) *Group-Analytic Psychotherapy*. Karnac Books, London, 1986.

Fowler, D., Garety, P. & Kuipers, E. (1995) *Cognitive Behaviour Therapy for Psychosis: Theory and Practice*. Wiley, Chichester.

Fowler, R. C., Rich, C. L. & Young, D. (1986) San Diego suicide study, II. Substance abuse in young cases. *Arch. Gen. Psychiat.*, **43**, 962–5.

Foy, D. W., Nunn, B. L. & Rychtarik, R. G. (1984) Broad spectrum treatment for chronic alcoholics. Effects of training in controlled drinking skills. *J. Consult. Clin. Psychol.*, **52**, 218–30.

Frances, A. (1980) The DSM-III personality disorders: a commentary. *Am. J. Psychiat.*, **137**, 1050–4.

Franceschi, M., Comola, M., Piattoni, F. *et al.* (1990) Prevalence of dementia in adult patients with trisomy 21. *Am. J. Med. Genet.* (Suppl.) **7**, 306–8.

Francis, J., Martin, D. & Kapoor, W. N. (1990) A prospective study of delirium in hospitalised elderly. *J. Am. Med. Assoc.*, **263**, 1097–101.

Frangou, S., Alarcon, G., Sharma, T. *et al.* (1994) P300 latency: a trait marker for familial schizophrenia. *Schiz. Res.*, **15**, 176.

Frank, E., Anderson, C. & Rubinstein, D. (1978) Frequency of sexual dysfunction in 'normal' couples. *N. Engl. J. Med.*, **299**, 111–15.

Frank, E., Anderson, B. P., West, D. G. & Lando, J. (1988) Depressive symptoms and adolescent rape victims. In *Advances in Adolescent Mental Health, a Research-Practice Annual: Depression and Suicide* (ed. A. R. Stiffman & R. A. Feldman). JAI Press, Greenwich.

Frank, E., Kupfer, D. J., Perel, J. M. *et al* (1990) Three-year outcomes for maintenance therapies in recurrent depression. *Arch. Gen. Psychiat.*, **47**, 1093–9.

Frankel, B. L., Coursey, R. D., Buchbinder, R. & Snyder, F. (1976) Recorded and reported sleep in chronic primary insomnia. *Arch. Gen. Psychiat.*, **33**, 615–23.

Frankish, P. (1989) Meeting the emotional needs of handicapped people: a psycho-dynamic approach. *J. Ment. Defic. Res.*, **33**, 407–14.

Franko, D. L. & Walton, B. E. (1993) Pregnancy and eating disorders: a review and clinical implications. *Int. J. Eat. Disord.*, **13**, 41–7.

Franssen, E. (1993) In *Ageing and Dementia Neurologic Signs in Ageing and Dementia* (ed. A. Burns). Edward Arnold, London, pp. 144–74.

Fraser, R. M. & Glass, I. B. (1980) Unilateral and bilateral ECT in elderly patients: A comparative study. *Acta Psychiat. Scand.*, **62**, 13–31.

Fraser, W. & Minns, R. (1992) Mental Handicap. In *Textbook of Paediatrics* (ed. A. Campbell & B. McIntosh). Churchill Livingstone, Edinburgh, pp. 854–74.

Fraser, W. I. & Rao, J. M. (1991) Recent studies of mentally handicapped young people's behaviour. *J. Child Psychol. Psychiat.*, **32**, 79–108.

Frederick, C. J. (1985) Children traumatised by catastrophic situations. In *Post-Traumatic Stress Disorder in Children* (ed. S. Eth & R. S. Pynoos). American Psychiatric Press, Washington DC, pp. 73–99.

Freeman, C. (1995) Cognitive Therapy. In *Handbook of Eating Disorders Theory Treatment & Research* (ed. G. Szmukler, C. Dare & J. L. Treasure). Wiley, Chichester.

Freeman, C. P. L., Barry, F., Dunkeld-Turnbull, J. & Henderson, A. (1988) Controlled trial of psychotherapy for bulimia nervosa. *Br. Med. J.*, **296**, 521–5.

Freeman, C. P. L., Davies, F., Morris, J. *et al.* (1991) A double-blind controlled trial of fluoxetine versus placebo. Unpublished.

Freeman, C. P. L., Weeks, D. & Kendell, R. E. (1980) ECT: patients who complain. *Br. J. Psychiat.*, **137**, 17–25.

Frenken, J. (1976) *Afkeer van Seksualiteit*. Van Loghum Slaterus, Daventer.

Freud, A. (1936) *The Ego and the Mechanisms of Defence*. Hogarth Press, London.

Freud, A. (1965) *Normality and Pathology in Childhood: Assessments of Development*. Hogarth Press, London.

Freud, S. (1895) On the grounds for detaching a particular syndrome from neurasthenia under the description 'anxiety neurosis'. *The Standard Edition of the Complete Psychological Works of Sigmund Freud*, Volume III (ed. J. Strachey). Hogarth Press, London, pp. 87–115.

Freud, S. (1905) Three essays on the theory of sexuality. *The Standard Edition of the Complete Psychological Works of Sigmund Freud*. Volume XII. Hogarth Press, London (1958), pp. 227–38.

Freud, S. (1912) Types of onset of neurosis. *The Standard Edition of the Complete Psychological Works of Sigmund Freud*. Volume XII, Hogarth Press, London, (1958), pp. 227–38.

Freud, S. (1911–1915) Papers on technique. *The Standard Edition of the Complete Psychological Works of Sigmund Freud*. Volume XII. Hogarth Press, London (1958) pp. 35–183.

Freud, S. (1917) *Mourning and Melancholia*. Standard Edition Vol. 14 (1957). Hogarth Press, London.

Freud, S. (1923) The ego and the id. *The Standard Edition of the Complete Psychological Works of Sigmund Freud*. Volume XIX. Hogarth Press, London (1958) pp. 3–66.

Freud, S. (1937) Analysis, terminable and interminable *The Standard Edition of the Complete Psychological Works of Sigmund Freud*. Volume XXIII. Hogarth Press, London (1958).

Freud, S. (1974) *Cocaine Papers* (ed. R. Byke). Stonehill Publishers, New York.

Freund, K. (1980) Therapeutic sex drive reduction. *Acta Psychiat. Scand.*, **62**, Suppl. 287.

Frezza, M., DiPadova, C., Pozzato, G. *et al* (1990) High blood alcohol levels. The rate of decreased alcohol dehydrogenase activity and first pass metabolism. *N. Engl. J. Med.*, **322**, 95–7.

Frick, P. J., Lahey, B. B., Hartdagen, S. & Hynd, G. W. (1989) Conduct problems in boys: relations to maternal personality, marital satisfaction and socioeconomic status. *J. Clin. Child Psychol.*, **18**, 114–20.

Friedman, M. & Rosenman, R. H. (1959) Association of specific overt behaviour pattern with blood and cardiovascular findings. *J. Amer. Med. Ass.*, **169**, 1085–96.

Friedman, M., Thoresen, C. E., Gill, J. J. *et al.* (1986) Alteration of Type A behaviour and its effect on cardiac recurrences in post-myocardial infarct patients: summary results of the Recurrent Coronary Prevention Project. *Am. Heart J.*, **112**, 653–65.

Friedman, T. & Gath, D. (1989) The psychiatric consequences of spontaneous abortion. *Br. J. Psychiat.*, **155**, 810–3.

Frijda, N. H. (1986) *The Emotions*. Cambridge University Press, Cambridge.

Frischer, M. (1992) Estimating the prevalence of injecting drug use in Glasgow. *Br. J. Addiction*, **87**, 235–43.

Frith, C. (1992) *The Cognitive Neuropsychology of Schizophrenia*. Lawrence Erlbaum, Hove.

Fritz, G. S., Stoll, K. & Wagner, N. (1981) A comparison of males and females who were sexually molested as children. *J. Sex. Marital Ther.*, **7.**, 54–9.

Fromm, E., Oberlander, M. I. & Gruenewald, D. (1970) Perceptual and cognitive process in different states of consciousness: the waking state and hypnosis. *J. Proj. Tech. Assess.*, **34**, 375–87.

Fry, J. & Sandler, G. (1988) Domiciliary consultations: some fact and questions. *Br. Med. J.*, **297**, 337–8.

Fryers, T. (1992) Epidemiological research related to mental retardation. *Curr. Opin. in Psychiat.*, **5**, 650–5.

Fuchs, T. & Lauter, H. (1992) Charles Bonnet syndrome and musical hallucinations in the elderly. In *Delusions and Hallucinations in Old Age* (ed. C. Katona & R. Levy). Gaskell, London, pp. 187–98.

Fuhrer, R., Antonucci, T. C., Gagnon, M. *et al* (1992) Depressive symptomatology and cognitive functioning: an epidemiological survey in an elderly community sample of France. *Psychol. Med.*, **22**, 159–72.

Fukuda, K., Straus, S. E., Hickie H. *et al*. (1994) The chronic fatigue syndrome: a comprehensive approach to its definition and study. *Ann. Intern. Med.*, **121**, 953–9.

Fuller, R. K. L., Branchey, D. R., Brightwell *et al* (1986) Disulfiram treatment and alcoholism. A veterans administration cooperative study. *J. Am. Med. Assoc.*, **256**, 1449–55.

Futen, L. J., Morely, J. E., Gross, P. L. *et al* (1989) Depression. *J. Am. Geriat. Soc.*, **37**, 459–72.

Fydrich, T., Dowdall, D. L. & Chambless, D. L. (1992) Reliability and validity of the Beck Anxiety Inventory. *J. Anx. Disorders*, **6**, 55–61.

Fyer, A., Mannuzza, S., Chapman, T. *et al*. (1993) A direct interview family study of social phobia. *Arch. Gen. Psychiat.*, **50**, 286–93.

Gadow, K. (1992) Paediatric psychopharmacotherapy: a review of recent research. *J. Child Psychol. Psychiat.*, **33**, 153–95.

Gagnon, J. H. (1975) Sex research and social change. *Arch. Sex. Behav.*, **4**, 111–41.

Gaillard. (1979) Brain catecholaminergic activity in relation to sleep. In *Sleep Research* (ed. R. G. Priest, A. Fletcher & J. Ward). MTP Press Ltd., Lancaster, pp. 35–41.

Galaburda, A. M., Sherman, G., Rosen, G. *et al* (1985) Developmental dyslexia: four consecutive patients with cortical anomalies. *Ann. Neurol.*, **18**, 222–33.

Galante, R. & Foa, D. (1986) An epidemiological study of psychic trauma and treatment effectiveness for children after a natural disaster. *J. Am. Acad. Child Adol. Psychiat.*, **25**, 357–63.

Gale, S. W., Mesnikoff, A., Fine, J. *et al*. (1980) Study of suicide in state mental hospitals in New York City, *Psychiat. Quart.*, **52**, 201–13.

Garbarino, J. (1989) Troubled youth, troubled families: the dynamics of adolescent maltreatment. In *Child Maltreatment: Theory and Research on the Causes of Consequences of Child Abuse and Neglect* (ed. D. Cicchetti & V. Carlson). Cambridge University Press, Cambridge, pp. 685–706.

Garety, P. (1985) Delusions: problems in definition and measurement. *Br. J. Med. Psychol.*, **58**, 25–34.

Garety, P. A., Kuipers, L., Fowler, D. *et al*. (1994) Cognitive behavioural therapy for drug resistant psychosis. *Br. J. Med. Psychol.*, **67**, 259–73.

Garety, P. & Morris, I. (1984) A new unit for long-stay psychiatric patients: organisation, attitudes and quality of care. *Psychol. Med.*, **14**, 183–92.

Garfinkel, P. E. & Garner, D. M. (1982) *Anorexia Nervosa: A Multidimensional Perspective*. Brunner/Mazel, New York.

Garner, D. M., Fairburn, C. G. & Davis, R. (1987) Cognitive behavioural treatment of bulimia nervosa. *Behav. Modif.*, **11**, 398–431.

Garner, D. M. & Garfinkel, P. E. (1979) The eating attitudes test: An index of the symptoms of anorexia nervosa. *Psychol. Med.*, **9**, 273–9.

Garner, D. M., Garfinkel, P. E. & Irvine, M. J. (1986) Integration and sequencing of treatment approaches for eating disorders. *Psychother. Psychosom.*, **46**, 67–75.

Garner, D. M., Garfinkel, P. E., Schwartz, D. & Thompson, M. (1980) Cultural expectations of thinness in women. *Psychol. Rep.*, **47**, 483–91.

Garner, D. M., Olmsted, M. P., Bohr, Y. *et al*. (1982) The eating Attitudes Test: psychometric features and clinical correlates. *Psychol. Med.*, **12**, 871–8.

Garner, D. M., Olmsted, M. P. & Polivy, J. (1983) Development and validation of a multidimensional eating disorder inventory for anorexia nervosa and bulimia nervosa. *Int., J. Eat. Dis.*, **2**, 15–34.

Garrido, V. & Redondo, S. (1993) Institutionalisation of young offenders. *Crim. Behav. Ment. Health*, **3**, 336–48.

Garrison, W. & Earls, F. (1985) Change and continuity in behaviour problems from the pre-school period through school entry: an analysis of mothers' reports. In *Recent Research in Developmental Psychopathology* (ed. J. E. Stevenson). Pergamon, Oxford, pp. 51–65.

Garro, A. J. & Lieber, C. S. (1990) Alcohol and cancer. *Ann. Rev. Pharmacol. Toxicol.*, **30**, 219–49.

Gartner, A. F., Marcus, R. N., Halmi, K. A. *et al.* (1989) DSM-IIIR personality disorder in patients with eating disorders. *Am. J. Psychiat.*, **146**, 1585–91.

Gater, R., Ameida, E. S., Barreintos, G. *et al.* (1991) The pathways to psychiatric care: a cross-cultural study. *Psychol. Med.*, **21**, 761–74.

Gath, A. & Gumley, D. (1986) Behaviour problems in retarded children with special reference to Down's syndrome. *Br. J. Psychiat..*, **149**, 156–61.

Gawin, F. H., Kleber, H. D. & Byck, R. (1987) Desipramine facilitation of initial cocaine abstinence. *Arch. Gen. Psychiat.*, **46**, 117–21.

Gay, P. (1988) *Freud: A Life for our Times*. J. M. Dent, London

Gebhard, P., Gagnon, J., Pomeroy, N. & Christenson, C. (1965) *Sex Offenders*. Harper and Row, New York.

Gedye, A. (1990) Dietary increase in serotonin reduces self injurious behaviour in a Down's syndrome adult. *J. Ment. Defic. Res.*, **34**, 195–203.

Gelder, M. G., Bancroft, J. H. J., Gath, D. H. *et al* (1973) Specific and non-specific factors in behaviour therapy. *Br. J. Psychiat.*, **123**, 445–62.

George, D. T., Ladenheim, J. A. & Nutt, D. J. (1987) Effect of pregnancy on panic attacks. *Am. J. Psychiat.*, **144**, 1078–9.

Gelineau, J. B. E. (1880) De la narcolepside. *Gaz Hop Paris*, **55**, 626–8.

Geller, J. L. (1990) Clinical guidelines for the use of involuntary out-patient treatment. *Hosp. Comm. Psychiat.*, **41**, 749–55.

Geller, B., Cooper, T. B., Graham, D. L. *et al.* (1992) Pharmacokinetically designed double-blind placebo-controlled study of nortriptyline in 6- to 12-year-olds with major depressive disorder. *J. Am. Acad. Child Adol. Psychiat.*, **31**, 34–44.

Genders, E. & Player, E. (1994) *Grendon: A Study of a Therapeutic Prison*. Clarendon Press, Oxford.

General Accounting Office (1977) *Returning the Mentally Disordered to the Community: the Government Needs to do More*. Government Printing Office, Washington DC.

Gerard, K. (1990) Determining the contribution of residential care to the quality of life of children with severe learning difficulties. *Child Care Health and Development*, **16**, 177–88.

Gerlach, J. (1991) New antipsychotics: classification, efficacy and adverse effects. *Schiz. Bull.*, **17**, 289–309.

Gershon, E. S. (1989) Recent developments in genetics of manic-depressive illness. *J. Clin. Psychiat.*, **50**, 4–7.

Gershon, E. S., Bunney, W. F. & Leckman, J. F. (1976) The inheritance of affective disorders: a review of data and hypotheses. *Behav. Genet.*, **6**, 227–61.

Gershon, E., Hamovit, J. H., Guroff, J. J. & Nurnberger, J. I. (1987) Birth cohort changes in manic and depressive disorders in relatives of bipolar and schizoaffective patients. *Arch. Gen. Psychiat.*, **44**, 314–9.

Gerstein, D. R. & Harwood, H. J. (1900) (eds.) *Treatment Drug Problems. Vol 1: A Study of Evolution Effectiveness, and Financing of Public and Private Drug Treatment Systems*. National Academy Press, Washington.

Ghubash, R., Hamdi, E. & Bebbington, P. E. (1992) The Dubai Community Psychiatric Survey: Prevalence and socio-demographic correlates. *Soc. Psychiat. Psychiat. Epidemiol.*, **27**, 53–61.

Ghubash, R., Hamdi, E. & Bebbington, P. E. (1994) The Dubai Community Psychiatric Survey: III: Acculturation and the prevalence of psychiatric disorder. *Psychol. Med.*, **24**, 121–31.

Gibb, W. R. G. (1989) Dementia and Parkinsons Disease. *Br. J. Psychiat.*, **154**, 596–614.

Gibbens, T. C. N., Soothill, K. L. & Pope, P. (1977) *Medical Remands in the Criminal Courts*, Maudsley Monograph No 25. Oxford University Press, Oxford.

Gibbons, J. S., Butler, J., Urwin, P. & Gibbons, J. L. (1978) Evaluation of a social work service for self-poisoning patients. *Br. J. Psychiat.*, **133**, 111–18.

Giel, R. & Horn, G. ten (1982) Patterns of mental health care in a Dutch register area. *Soc. Psychiat.*, **17**, 117–23.

Giles, D. E., Biggs, M. M., Rush, A. J. & Roffwarg, H. P. (1988) Risk factors in families of unipolar depression, I: Psychiatric illness and reduced REM latency. *J. Affect. Disorders.*, **14**, 51–9.

Gillberg, C. L. (1992) Autism and autistic-like conditions: subclasses among disorders of empathy. *J. Child Psychol. Psychiat.*, **33**, 813–42.

Gillberg, C., Carlstrom, G. & Rasmussen, P. (1983) Hyperkinetic disorders in children with perceptual, motor and attentional deficits. *J. Child Psychol. Psychiat.*, **24**, 233–46.

Gillberg, C., Rastam, M. & Gillberg, C. (1994) Anorexia nervosa outcome: Six-year controlled longitudinal study of 51 cases including a population cohort. *J. Am. Acad. Child, Adolesc. Psychiat.*, **33**, 729–39.

Gillberg, I. C. & Gillberg, C. (1989) Asperger syndrome: some epidemiological considerations. *J. Child Psychol. Psychiat.*, **30**, 631–8.

Gillis, L. & Egert, S. (1973) *The Psychiatric Out-patient: Clinical and Organisational Aspects.* Faber & Faber, London.

Gjerris, A., Bech, P., Bolwig, T. G. *et al.* (1983) The Hamilton Anxiety Scale. Evaluation of homogeneity and inter-observer reliability in patients with depressive disorders. *J. Affect. Disorders*, **5**, 163–70.

Glanz, A., Byrne, C., Jackson, P. (1989) The role of community pharmacies in the prevention of AIDS among injecting drug misusers: findings of a survey in England and Wales. *Br. Med. J.*, **299**, 1076–9.

Glaser, D. (1993) Emotional Abuse. In *Ballière's Clinical Paediatrics. International Practice & Research, Child Abuse.* Vol 1. No 1, pp. 251–65.

Glass, I. B. (1994) *The International Handbook of Addiction Behaviour.* Routledge, London.

Glass, I. B. (1989*a*) Alcoholic hallucinosis; a psychiatric enigma I. The development of the idea. *Br. J. Addiction.*, **84**, 29–41.

Glass, I. B. (1989*b*) Alcoholic hallucinosis: II a psychiatric enigma and follow-up studies. *Br. J. Addiction*, **84**, 151–64.

Glass, I. B. & Jackson, P. (1988) Maudsley Hosptial survey: prevalence of alcohol problems and other psychiatric disorders in a hospital population. *Br. J. Addiction.*, **83**, 1105–11.

Glass, I. B. & Marshall, J. (1991) Alcohol and mental illness, cause or effect? In *International Handbook of Addiction Behaviour.* Routledge, London, pp. 152–63.

Glass-Crome, I. B. (1992) Training: a vital ingredient for alcohol treatment services. *Curr. Opin. Psychiat.*, **5**, 436–40.

Glass-Crome, I. B. (1994) Gender related issues in alcohol problems research – a special need group? In *Biological Aspects of Alcoholism* (ed. B. Tabakoff & P. Holtman). WHO, Geneva.

Glassman, A. H., Kantor, S. J. & Shostak, M. (1975) Depression, delusions and drug response. *Am. J. Psychiat.*, **132**, 716–19.

Glatt, M. M., Rosin, A. & Jauha, P. (1978) Alcoholism and the elderly. *Age & Ageing.*, **7**, (suppl) 64–6.

Glazer, W. M., Kane, J. M. (1992) Depot neuroleptic therapy: an underutilised treatment option. *J. Clin. Psychiat.*, **53**, 426–33.

Glen, A. I. M. (1979) The effects of lithium on cell membranes. In *Lithium Controversies and Unresolved Issues.* (ed. T. Cooper, S. Gershon, N. Kline & M. Schou). Excerpta Medica, pp. 768–88.

Gloag, D. (1984) Unmet need in chronic disability. *Br. med. J.*, **289**, 211–12.

Gloning, K. (1977) Handedness and aphasia. *Neuropsychologia*, **15**, 355–8.

Glover, G. R., Flannigan, C., Feeney, S. *et al.* (1994) Admissions of British Caribbeans to mental hospitals: Is it a cohort effect? *Soc. Psychiat. Psychiat. Epidemiol.*, **29**, 282–4.

Glover, V., Liddle, P., Taylor, A. *et al* (1994) Mild hypomania (the Highs) can be a feature of the first postpartum week. Association with later depression. *Br. J. Psychiat.*, **164**, 517–21.

Glueck, S. & Gleuck, E. T. (1968) *Delinquents and Non-Delinquents in Perspective*. Harvard University Press, Cambridge, Mass.

Goethe, K. F., Mitchell, J. E. Marshal, D. W. *et al*. (1989) Neuropsychological and neurological functions of human immunodeficiency virus seropositive asymptomatic individuals. *Arch. Neurol.*, **46**, 129–31.

Godber, C., Rosenvinge, H., Wilkinson, D. & Smithies, J. (1987) Depression in old age: prognosis after ECT. *Intern. J. Geriat. Psychiat.*, **2**, 19–24.

Godfrey, C. & Maynard, A. (1992) A health strategy for alcohol; setting targets and choosing policies. YARTIC occasional paper. Centre for Health Economics, York.

Goh, S. E., Salmons, P. H. & Whittington, R. M. (1989) Hospital suicides: are there preventable factors? Profile of the psychiatric hospital suicide. *Br. J. Psychiat.,* **154**, 247–9.

Goldacre, M., Seagroatt, V. & Hawton, K. (1993) Suicide after discharge from psychiatric in-patient care. *Lancet*, **342**, 283–6.

Goldberg, B. (1993) Violence, death and associated factors on a mentally handicapped ward. Letter, *J. Intellect. Disabil. Res.*, **37**, 111–12.

Goldberg, D. P. (1972) *Detecting Psychiatric Illness by Questionnaire*. Maudsley Monograph 22. Oxford University Press, Oxford.

Goldberg, D. (1986) Implementation of mental health policies in the North West of England. In *The Provision of Mental Health Services in Britain: the Way Ahead* (ed. G. Wilkinson & H. Freeman). Royal College of Psychiatrist, Gaskell, London.

Goldberg, D. P. & Blackwell, B. (1970) Psychiatric Illness in General Practice: a detailed study using a new method of case identification. *Br. Med. J.*, **ii**, 439–43.

Goldberg, D. & Bridges, K. (1988) Somatic presentation of psychiatric illness in primary care settings. *J. Psychosom. Res.*, **32**, 137–44.

Goldberg, D. P., Bridges, K., Duncan-Jones, P. & Grayson, D. (1987) Dimensions of neurosis seen in primary care settings. *Psychol. Med.*, **17**, 461–70.

Goldberg, D. P., Cooper, B., Eastwood, M. R. *et al.* (1970) A standardised psychiatric interview for use in community settings. *Br. J. Prevent. Soc. Med.*, **24**, 18–23.

Goldberg, D., Gask, L. & O'Dowd, T. (1989) The treatment of somatisation: teaching techniques of re-attribution. *J. Psychosom. Res.*, **33**, 689–95.

Goldberg, D. & Huxley, P. (1980) *Mental Illness in the Community*. Tavistock, London.

Goldberg, D. & Huxley, P. (1992) *Common Mental Disorders. A Bio-Social Model*. Routledge, London.

Goldberg, D., Kay, C. & Thompson, L. (1976) Psychiatric morbidity in general practice and the community. *Psychol. Med.*, **6**, 565–9.

Goldberg, D. P., Steele, J. J., Smith, C. & Spivey, L. (1980) Training family doctors to recognise psychiatric illness with increased accuracy. *Lancet*, **ii**, 521–3.

Goldberg, D. & Williams, P. (1988) *A users guide to the General Health Questionnaire*. NEFR-Nelson, Berkshire.

Goldberg, S. M. & Morrison, S. L. (1963) Schizophrenia and social class. Br. J. Psychiat., **109**, 785–802.

Goldberg, S. C. Halmi, K. A., Eckert, R. C. *et al.* (1979) Cyproheptidine in anorexia nervosa. *Br. J. Psychiat.*, **134**, 67–7).

Goldie, N. & Freden, L. (1991) A crisis of closure and openness: the present state of Swedish mental health system in the light of a policy of sectorisation. *Soc. Sci. Med.*, **32**, 499–506.

Golding, J., Smith, R. & Kashner, M. (1991) Does somatization disorder exist in men? *Arch. Gen. Psychiat.*, **48**, 231–5.

Goldman, H. (1981) Defining and counting the chronically mentally ill. *Hosp. Commun. Psychiat.*, **32**, 21–7.

Goldman, H., Adams, N. & Taube, C. (1983*a*) Deinsitutionalisation; the data demythologised. *Hosp. Commun. Psychiat.*, **34**, 129–34.

Goldman, H., Morrissey, J. & Bachrach, L. (1983*b*) Deinstitutionalisation in international perspective: variations on a theme. *Internat. J. Ment. Health*, **11**, 153–65.

Goldman, H. H., Skodol, A. E. & Lave, T. R. (1992) Revising axis V for DSM-IV: a review of measures of social functioning. *Am. J. Psychiat.*, 149, 1148–56.

Goldney, R. D., Spence, N. D. & Bowes, J. A. (1988) The safe use of high dose neuroleptics in a psychiatric intensive care unit. *Aust. N.Z. J. Psychiat.*, 20, 370–5.

Goldstine, K. (1944) Methodological approach to the study of schizophrenic thought disorder. In *Language and Thought in Schizophrenia* (ed. J. Kasanin). University of California Press, pp. 17–40.

Goldstein, M., Anderson, L. T., Reuben, R. & Dancis, J. (1985) Self-mutilation in Lesch-Nyhan disease is caused by dopaminergic denervation. *Lancet*, i, 388–9.

Goldstein, R., Weissman, M., Adams, P. *et al.* (1994) Psychiatric disorders in relatives of probands with panic disorder and/or major depression. *Arch. Gen. Psychiat.*, 51, 383–94.

Goldthorpe, J. & Hope, K. (1974) *The Social Grading of Occupations: A New Approach and Scale.* Oxford University Press, London.

Gonzalez, J. P., Brogden, R. N. (1988) Naltrexone. A review of its pharmacodynamic and pharmacokinetics properties and therapeutic efficacy in the management of opioid dependence. *Drugs*, 35, 192–213.

Goodchild, M. E. & Duncan-Jones, P. (1985) Chronicity and the General Health Questionnaire. *Br. J. Psychiat.*, 146, 55–61.

Goodman, R. & Graham, P. (1996) Psychiatric problems in children with hemiplegia. *Br. Med. J.*, 312, 1065–9.

Goodman, R. & Stevenson, J. (1989) A twin study of hyperactivity, I & II. *J. Child Psychol. Psychiat.*, 30, 671–710.

Goodwin, D. W., Schulsinger, F., Hermansen, L. *et al.* (1973) Alcohol problems in adoptees raised apart from alcoholic biological parents. *Arch. Gen. Psychiat.*, 28, 238–43.

Goodwin, F. K. & Jamison, K. R. (eds.) (1990) *Manic-Depressive Ilness.* OUP, New York.

Goodwin, G. (1994) Recurrence of mania after lithium withdrawal. Implications for the use of lithium in the treatment of bipolar affective disorder: *Br. J. Psychiat.*, 164, 149–52.

Goodwin, J. (1988) Post-traumatic symptoms in abused children. *J. Traum. Stress*, 4, 475–88.

Goodyer, I. Kolvin, I. & Gatzanis, S. (1987) The impact of recent undesirable life events on psychiatric disorder in childhood and adolescence. *Br. J. Psychiat.*, 151, 179–84.

Goodyer, I. M., Cooper, P. J., Vize, C. M. & Ashby, L. (1993) Depression in 11–16 year-old girls: the role of past parental psychopathology and exposure to recent life events. *J. Child Psychol. Psychiat.*, 34, 1103–15.

Gorman, D. M. (1994) Alcohol misuse and the predisposing environment. *Br. Med. Bull.*, 50, 36–49.

Gordon, E., Krajuhin C., Kelly, P. *et al.* (1986) A neuropsychological study of somatization disorder. *Comp. Psychiat.*, 27, 295–301.

Gorman, J., Papp, L., Coplan, J. *et al* (1994) Anxiogenic effects of CO_2 and hyperventilation in patients with panic disorder. *Am. J. Psychiat.*, 151, 547–53.

Gossop, M., Darke, S., Griffiths, P. *et al.*, (1995) The severity of dependence scale (SDS): psychometric properties of the SDS in English and Australian samples of heroin, cocaine and amphetamine users. 90:5, pp. 607–614

Gossop, M., Johns, A. & Green, L. (1986) Opiate withdrawal: inpatient versus outpatient programmes and preferred versus random assignment to treatment. *Br. Med. J.*, 293, 103–4.

Gossop, M., Green L., Phillips, G., Bradley, B. (1989) Lapse, relapse and survival among opiate addicts after treatment: A prospective follow-up study. *Br. J. Psychiat.*, 154, 348–53.

Gossop, M., Strang, J., Griffiths, P., Powis, B. (1994) Cocaine: changes in initiation route of administration and degree of dependence. *Br. J. Psychiat.*, 164, 660–5.

Gostavson, R., Wahlstrom, J., Johannisson, J. & Holmqvist, D. (1991) Chromosomal aberrations in the mildly mentally retarded. *J. Ment. Defic. Res.*, 35, 240–6.

Gottesman, I. I. (1991) *Schizophrenia Genesis: The Origins of Madness.* W. H. Freeman and Company, New York.

Gottesman, I. I., Shields, J. & Hanson, D. R. (1982) Schizophrenia: the epigenetic puzzle. Cambridge University Press, Cambridge.

Gould, M. S. & Shaffer, C. (1986) The impact of suicide in television movies: evidence of imitation. *N. Engl. J. Med.*, **315**, 690–4.

Gowers, S., Norton, K., Yeldum, D. *et al.* (1988) The St George's prospective treatment study of anorexia nervosa: a discussion of the methodological problems. *Int. J. Eat. Disord.*., **8**, 445–54.

Grahame, P. (1984) Schizophrenia in old age. *Br. J. Psychiat.*, **145**, 493–5.

Graham, P. (1993) Lecture on hyperactivity: Maudsley Bequest Series, January 26th 1993.

Grahame-Smith, D. G., Green, A. R. & Costain, D. W. (1978) Mechanism of the antidepressant action of electroconvulsive therapy. *Lancet*, **i**, 254–7.

Grassian, S. (1983) Psychopathological effects of solitary confinement. *Am. J. Psychiat.*, **140**, 1450–4.

Gray, J. (1982) The neuropsychology of anxiety: an enquiry into the functions of the septohippocampal system. Oxford University Press, Oxford.

Gray, J. A., Feldon, J. Rawlins, J. N. *et al.* (1991) The neuropsychology of schizophrenia. *Behav. Brain Sci.*, **14**, 1–20.

Greenberg, D. (1983) Age and crime. In *Encyclopedia of Crime and Justice* (ed. S. H. Kandish). Macmillan, New York, pp. 30–5.

Greenberg, M. T. & Kusche, C. A. (1993) *Promoting Social and Emotional Development in Deaf Children: the PATHS Project.* University of Washington, Seattle.

Greenblatt, D. J. (1993) Basic pharmacokinetic principles and their application to psychotropic drugs. *J. Clin. Psychiat.*, **54** (suppl), 8–14.

Greenswag, L. R. (1987) Adults with Prader-Willi syndrome: a survey of 232 cases. *Devel. Med. Child Neurol.*, **29**, 145–52.

Greer, H. S., Lal, S., Lewis, S. C. *et al.* (1976) Psychosocial consequences of therapeutic abortion. Kings Termination Study III. *Br. J. Psychiat.*, **128**, 74–9.

Greer, S., & Bagley, C. (1971) Effects of psychiatric intervention in attempted suicide: a controlled study. *Br. Med. J.*, **i**, 310–12.

Greer, S., Moorey, S., Baruch, J. D. R. *et al* (1992) Adjuvant psychological therapy for patients with cancer: a prospective randomised trial. *Br. Med. J.*, **304**, 675–80.

Greer, S. & Morris, T. (1975) Psychological attributes of women who develop breast cancer: A controlled study. *J. Psychosom. Res.*, **19**, 147–53.

Griffith, J. D., Cavanagh, J., Held, J. & Oates, J. A. (1972) Dextroamphetamine: evaluation of psychomimetic properties in man. *Arch. Gen. Psychiat.*, **26**, 97–100.

Griffiths, P., Gossop, M., Powis, B. & Strang, J. (1993) Reaching hidden populations of drug users by privileged access interviewers: methodological and practical issues. *Addiction*, **88**, 1617–26.

Griffiths, P., Powis, B., Gossop, M. & Strang, J. (1994) Transitions in patterns of heroin administration: a study of heroin chasers and heroin injectors. *Addiction*, **89**, 301–9.

Griffiths, R. (1988) *Community Care: an Agenda for Action.* HMSO, London, p. V.

Grinker, R., Werble, B. & Drye, R. (1968) *The Borderline Syndrome.* Basic Books, New York.

Gronwall, D. & Wrightson, P. (1975) Cumulative effect of concussion. *Lancet*, **ii**, 995–7.

Gross, M. M., Rosenblatt, S. M., Chartoff, S. *et al.* (1971) Evaluation of acute alcoholic psychosis and related states. *Quart. J. Stud. Alcohol*, **32**, 611–19.

Grossman, L. S., Harrow, M., Goldberg, J. F. & Fichtner, C. G. (1991) Outcome of schizoaffective disorder at two long-term follow-ups: comparisons with outcome of schizophrenia and affective disorders. *Am. J. Psychiat.*, **148**, 1359–65.

Group for the Advancement of Psychiatry (GAP) (1994) *Forced into Treatment. The Role of Coercion in Clinical Practice.* American Psychiatric Association Press, Washington DC.

Grove, W., Andreasen, N. C., Clayton, P. J. *et al.* (1987) Primary and secondary affective disorders: Baseline characteristics of unipolar patients. *J. Affect. Disord.*, **13**, 249–57.

Grubin, D. & Prentky, R. (1993) Sexual psychopathy laws. *Crim. Behav. Ment. Health*, **3**, 381–92.

Grundy, E. (1992) Sociodemographic change and the elderly population of England and Wales. *Internat. J. Geriat. Psychiat.*, **7**, 75–82.

Gudjonsson, G. H. (1987) A parallel form of the Gudjonsson Suggestibility Scale. *Br. J. Clin. Psychol.*, **26**, 215–21.

Gudjonsson, G. H. (1992) *The Psychology of Interrogations, Confessions and Testimony*. Wiley, Chichester.

Gudjonsson, G. H., Clare, J., Rutter, S. & Pearse, J. (1993) *Persons at Risk During Interviews in Police Custody: The Identification of Vulnerabilities*. The Royal Commission on Criminal Justice Research Study No. 12. HMSO, London.

Gudjonsson, G. H. & Clark, N. K. (1986) Suggestibility in police interrogation: a social psychological model. *Soc. Behav.*, **1**, 83–104.

Gudjonsson, G. H. & Gunn, J. (1982) The competence and reliability of a witness in the criminal court: a case report. *Br. J. Psychiat.*, **141**, 624–7.

Guilleminault, C. & Dement, W. C. (1988) Sleep apnoea syndromes and related sleep disorders. In *Sleep Disorders: Diagnosis and Treatment* (ed. R. L. Williams, I. Karacan & C. A. Moore). Wiley, New York, pp. 47–761.

Gull, W. W. (1874) Anorexia nervosa (apepsia hysterica, anorexia hysterica) *Trans. Clin. Soc. Lond.*, 7, 22–8.

Gunn, J. (1977) *Epileptics in Prison*. Academic Press, London.

Gunn, J. (1985) Psychiatry and the prison medical service. In *Secure Provision* (ed. L. Gostin). Tavistock, London, pp. 126–52.

Gunn, J. (1986) Education and Forensic Psychiatry. *Can. J. Psychiat.*, **31**, 273–9.

Gunn, J. (1996) Stress disorders and medico legal issues. *International Review of Psychiatry* Vol 2. (ed. J. Davidson & A. C. McFarlane). American Psychiatric Press, Inc., Washington, DC (in press).

Gunn, J., Blackburn, R., Hill, J. *et al.* (1993a) Personality disorders in *Forensic Psychiatry: Clinical, Legal & Ethical Issues* (ed. J. Gunn & P. J. Taylor). Butterworth–Heinemann, Oxford, pp. 373–406.

Gunn, J., Briscoe, O., Carson, D. *et al.* (1993b) The law, adult mental disorder and the psychiatrist in England and Wales. In *Forensic Psychiatry: Clinical, Legal & Ethical Issues* (ed. J. Gunn & P. J. Taylor). Butterworth–Heinemann, Oxford, pp. 21–115.

Gunn, J. & Fenton, G. (1971) Epilepsy, automatism and crime. *Lancet*, **i**, 173–6.

Gunn, J., Grounds, A., Mullen, P. & Taylor, P. J. (1993c) Secure institutions: their characteristics and problems. In *Forensic Psychiatry. Clinical, Legal & Ethical Issues* (ed. J. Gunn & P. J. Taylor). Butterworth–Heinemann, Oxford, pp. 794–825.

Gunn, J., Maden, A. & Swinton, M. (1991) *Mentally Disordered Prisoners*. Home Office, London.

Gunn, J. & Robertson, G. (1976) Psychopathic personality: a conceptual problem. *Psychol. Med.*, **6**, 631–4.

Gunn, J., Robertson, G., Dell, S. & Way, C. (1978) *Psychiatric Aspects of Imprisonment*. Academic Press, London.

Gunn, J. & Taylor, P. J. (1993a) *Introduction to Forensic Psychiatry: Clinical, Legal & Ethical Issues* (ed. J. Gunn & P. J. Taylor). Butterworth–Heinemann, Oxford, pp. 1–20.

Gunn, J. & Taylor, P. J. (1993b) Ethics in forensic psychiatry. In *Forensic Psychiatry: Clinical, Legal & Ethical Issues* (ed. J. Gunn & P. J.Taylor). Butterworth–Heinemann, Oxford, pp. 857–84.

Gupta, S. & Murray, R. M. (1991) The changing incidence of psychiatry. Schizophrenia: fact or artefact? *Directions in Psychiatry*, **11**, 1–7.

Gur, R. E, Skolnick, B. E., Gur, R. C. *et al.* (1983) Brain function in psychiatric disorders: I. Regional cerebral blood flow in medicated schizophrenics. *Arch. Gen. Psychiat.*, **40**, 1250–4.

Gur, R. E., Skolnick, B., Gur, R. C. *et al.* (1984) Brain function in psychiatric disorders: II. Regional cerebral blood flow in medicated unipolar depressives. *Arch. Gen. Psychiat.*, **41**, 695–9.

Gurling, H. M. D., Murray, R. M. (1984) Alcoholism and genetics: old and new evidence. In *Alcohol Related Problems* (ed. N. Krasner, J. S. Madden & R. J. Walker). John Wiley & Sons, Chichester, pp. 127–36.

Gurling, H. M. D., Murray, R. M., Clifford, C. A. (1981) Investigations into the genetics of alcohol dependence and into its effect on brain function. In *Twin Research* 3 Part C (ed. L. Gedda, P. Parisi & W. E. Nance). Alan R. Liss, New York, pp. 77–87.

Gustafson, L. (1987) Frontal lobe degeneration of the non-Alzheimer type. II Clinical picture and differential diagnosis. *Arch. Gerontol. Geriat.*, **6**, 209–23.

Gustafson, L., Risberg, J., Silfverskiold, P. (1981) Cerebral blood flow in dementia and depression. *Lancet*, **1**, 275.

Guthrie, E., Creed, F., Dawson, D. & Tomenson, B. (1993) A randomised controlled trial of psychotherapy in patients with refractory irritable bowel syndrome. *Br. J.Psychiat.*, **163**, 315–21.

Guze, S. (1975) The validity and significance of hysteria (Briquet's Syndrome). *Am. J. Psychiat.*, **132**, 138–41.

Guze, S. B., Cloninger, C. R., Martin, R. & Clayton, P. J. (1986) Alcoholism as a medical disorder. *Compreh Psychiat.*, **27**, 501–10.

Guze, S. B. & Robins, E. (1970) Suicide and primary affective disorder. *Br. J. Psychiatry*, **117**, 437–8.

Hachinski, V. C., Iliff, L. D., Zilka, E. *et al.* (1975) Cerebral blood flow in dementia. *Arch. Neurol.*, **32**, 632–7.

Häfner, H. & Böker, W. (1973) *Crimes of Violence by Mentally Abnormal Offenders* (trans. H. Marshall 1982) Cambridge University Press, Cambridge.

Hagberg, B., Hagberg, G., Lewerth, A. & Lindberg, U. (1981) Mild mental retardation in Swedish school children. *Acta Paediat. Scand.*, **70**, 441–4.

Hagnell, O. (1986) The 25-year follow-up of the Lundby study: incidence and risk of alcoholism, depression and disorders of the senium. In *Mental Disorders in the Community: Findings from Psychiatric Epidemiology* (ed. J. Barret & R. M. Rose). Guilford Press, New York.

Haggerty, J. J. Jr., Simon, J. S., Evans, D. L. & Nemeroff, C. B. (1987) Relationship of serum TSH concentration and antithyroid antibodies to diagnosis and DST response in psychiatric inpatients. *Am. J. Psychiat.*, **144**, 1492–3.

Hagnell, O., Grasbeck, A., Öjesjö, L. & Otterbeck, L. (1993) Mental tiredness in the Lundby study: Incidence and course over 25 years. *Acta Psychiat. Scand.*, **88**, 316–21.

Hagnell, O., Öjesjö, L., Otterbeck, L & Rosman, B. (1994) Prevalence of mental disorders, personality traits and mental complaints in the Lundby Study. *Scand. J. Soc. Med.*, Suppl 50.

Haines, A. P., Imeson, J. D. & Meade, T. W. (1987) Phobic anxiety and ischaemic heart disease. *Br. Med. J.*, **295**, 297–9.

Hall, A. & Crisp, A. H. (1987) Brief psychotherapy in the treatment of anorexia nervosa – outcome at one year. *Br. J. Psychiat.*, **151**, 185–91.

Hall, D., Hill, P. & Elliman, D. (1994) *The Child Surveillance Handbook*, Second Edn. Radcliffe Medical Press, Oxford.

Hall, J. N., Baker, R. D. & Hutchinson, K. (1977) A controlled evaluation of token economy procedures with chronic schizophrenic patients. *Behav. Res. Ther.*, **15**, 261–83.

Hall, M. & Chng, P. (1982) Antenatal care in practice. In *Effectiveness and Satisfaction in Antenatal Care* (ed. M. Enkin & I. Chalmers). Heinemann, London, pp. 60–8.

Hall, R. C. W., Gardner, E. R., Stickney, S. K. *et al.* (1980) Physical illness manifesting as psychiatric disease. *Arch. Gen. Psychiat.*, **37**, 989–95.

Hall, R. C. W., Hoffman, R. S., Beresford, T. P. *et al.* (1989) Physical illnesses encountered in patients with eating disorders. *Psychosomatics.*, **30**, 174–91.

Hallas, C., Fraser, W. & MacGillivray, R. (1982) *Care and Training of the Mentally Handicapped.* Wrights, Bristol.

Hallstrom, C. (1994) Drugs in focus: 12. Zopiclone. *Prescribers Journal*, **34**, 115–19.

Halmi, K. A. (1985) Rating scales in the eating disorders. *Psychopharmacol. Bull.*, **21**, 1001–3.

Halmi, K. A., Eckert, G. D., Ela du T. & Cohen, J. (1986) Anorexia Nervosa: treatment efficacy of cyproheptides and amitryptine. *Arch. Gen. Psychiat.*, **43**, 177–81.

Halmi, K. A., Eckert, E., Marchi, P. A. *et al.* (1991) Comorbidity of psychiatric diagnoses in anorexia nervosa. *Arch. Gen. Psychiat.*, **48**, 712–18.

Hamer, D. H., Hu, S., Magnuson, V. L. *et al.* (1993) A linkage between DNA markers on the X chromosome and male sexual orientation. *Science*, **261**, 321–7.

Hamilton, M. (1985) *Fish's Clinical Psychopathology*, 2nd edn. Wright, Bristol.

Hamilton, M. (1959) The assessment of anxiety states by rating. *Br. J. Med. Psychol.*, **32**, 50–5.

Hamilton, M. (1960) A rating scale for depression. *J. Neurol. Neurosurg. Psychiat.*, **23**, 56–62.

Hamilton, M. (1967) Development of a rating scale for primary depressive illness. *Br. J. Soc. Clin. Psychol.*, **6**, 278–96.

Hamilton, J. A. & Sichel, D. A. (1992) Prophylactic measures. In *Postpartum Psychiatric Illness* (ed. J. A. Hamilton & P. N. Harberger). University of Pennsylvania Press, Philadelphia, pp. 219–34.

Hamilton, L. H., Brooks Gunn, J. & Warren, M. P. (1985) Sociolcultural influences on eating disorders in professional female ballet dancers. *Int. J. Eat. Dis.*, **4**, 465–77.

Hammersley, R., Forsyth, A. & Lavelle, T. (1990) The criminality of new drug users. *Br. J. Addiction.*, **85**, 1583–94.

Hammond, J. E. & Toseland, P. A. (1970) Placental transfer of chlorpromazine. *Arch. Dis. Child*, **45**, 139–40.

Hannah, P., Cody, D., Glover, V. *et al.* (1993) The tyramine test is not a marker for postnatal depression: early postpartum euphoria may be. *J. Psychosom. Obstet. Gynaecol.*, **14**, 295–304.

Hansen, V. (1987) Psychiatric service within primary care. Mode of organisation and influence on admission rates to a mental hospital. *Acta Psychiat. Scand.*, **76**, 121–8.

Hansson, L. (1989) Utilisation of psychiatric in-patient care. *Acta Psychiatr. Scand.*, **79**, 571–78.

Happé, F. (1994) Current psychological theories of autism: the 'Theory of Mind' account and rival theories. *J. Child Psychol. Psychiat.*, **35**, 215–29.

Harding, C. M., Brooks, G. W., Ashikaga, T. *et al.* (1987) The Vermont Longitudinal Study II. *Am. J. Psychiat.*, **144**, 727–35.

Harding, T. W. (1993) A comparative survey of medical legal systems. *Forensic Psychiatry: Clinical, Legal & Ethical Issues* (ed. J. Gunn & P. J. Taylor). Butterworth–Heinemann, Oxford, pp. 118–66.

Harding, T. W., de Arango, M. V., Baltazar, J. *et al.* (1980) Mental disorders in primary health care: a study of their frequency and diagnosis in four developing countries. *Psychol. Med.*, **10**, 231–41.

Hardy, J. (1989) Slow virus dementias: Prion gene holds the key. *Trends Neurosci.*, **12**, 168–9.

Hardy, J. & Allsop. I. (1991) Amyloid predisposition as the central event in the aetiology of Alzheimers disease. *Trends Pharmacol.*, **12**, 383–8.

Hare, E. H. (1973) A short note on pseudo-hallucinations. *Br. J. Psychiat.*, **122**, 469–76.

Hare, E. H. (1983) Was insanity on the increase? *Br. J. Psychiat.*, **142**, 439–55.

Hare, E. H., Price, J. S. & Slater, E. (1972) Parental social class in psychiatric patients. *Br. J. Psychiat.*, **121**, 515–24.

Hare, E. H. & Willcox, D. R. C. (1967) Do psychiatric in-patients take their pills? *Br. J. Psychiat.*, **113**, 1435–39.

Hare, R. D. (1991) *The Hare Psychopathy Checklist – Revised.* Multi-health Systems, Toronto.

Hare, R. D., Harpur, T. J., Hakstian, A. R. *et al.* (1990) The revised psychopathy checklist: reliability and factor structure. *Psychol. Assess. J. Consult. Clin. Psychol.*, **2**, 338–41.

Hare, R. D. & Hart, S. D. (1993) Psychopathy, mental disorder, and crime. In *Mental Disorder and Crime* (ed. S. Hodgins). Sage, Newbury Park, CA, pp. 104–15.

Hare, R. D., Hart, S. D. & Harpur, T. J. (1991) Psychopathy and the DSM-IV criteria for antisocial personality disorder. *J. Abnorm. Psychol.*, **100**, 391–8.

Harper, N. (1988) Planned short-stay admission to a geriatric unit: one aspect of respite care. *Age and Ageing*, **17**, 199–204.

Harré, R. (1986) *The Social Construction of Emotion.* Blackwell, London.

Harrington, R. (1992) The natural history and treatment of child and adolescent affective disorders. *J. Child Psychol. Psychiat.*, **33**, 1287–302.

Harrington, R., Fudge, H., Rutter, M. *et al.* (1990) Adult outcomes of child and adolescent depression. I. Psychiatric status. *Arch. Gen. Psychiat.*, **47**, 465–73.

Harrington, R. C., Fudge, H., Rutter, M. *et al.* (1993) Child and adult depression: a test of continuities with data from a family study. *Br. J. Psychiat.*, **162**, 627–33.

Harris, B. (1994) Biological and hormonal aspects of postpartum depressed mood. Working towards strategies for prophylaxis and treatment. *Br. J. Psychiat.*, **164**, 288–92.

Harris, B., Fung, H., Johns, S. *et al.* (1989) Transient post-partum thyroid dysfunction and postnatal depression. *J. Affect. Disord.*, **17**, 243–49.

Harris, B., Lovett, L., Newcombe, R. G. *et al.* (1994) Maternity blues and major endocrine changes: Cardiff puerperal mood and hormone study. *Br. Med. J.*, **308**, 949–53.

Harris, B., Othman, S., Davis, J. A. *et al* (1992) Association between postpartum thyroid dysfunction and thyroid antibodies and depression. *Br. Med. J.*, **305**, 152–6.

Harris, T., Brown, G. W. & Bifulco, A. (1986) Loss of parent in childhood and adult psychiatric disorder: The Walthamstow Study 1. The role of lack of adequate parental care. *Psychol. Med.*, **16**, 641–60.

Harrison, G. (1994) New or old antidepressants? *Br. Med. J.*., **309**, 1280–1.

Harrison, P., McLaughlin, D. & Kerwin, R. (1991) Decreased hippocampal expression of a glutamate receptor gene in schizophrenia. *Lancet*, **337**, 450–2.

Harrison, G., Owens, D., Holton, A. *et al.* (1988) A prospective study of severe mental disorder in Afro-Caribbean patients. *Psychol. Med.*, **18**, 643–57.

Harrow, M. & Prosen, M. (1979) Schizophrenia thought disorders; bizarre associations and intermingling. *Am. J. Psychiat.*, **136**, 293–6.

Harry, B. & Steadman, H. J. (1988) Arrest rates of patients treated at a community mental health centre. *Hosp. Comm. Psychiat.*, **39**, 862–6.

Hartlage, L. C., Green, J. M. & Offutt, L. (1972) Dependency in epileptic children. *Epilepsia*, **13**, 27–30.

Hartmann, H. (1939) *Ego Psychology and the Problem of Adaptation.* International Universities Press, New York.

Hartmann, H. (1964) *Essays in Ego Psychology.* Hogarth Press, London.

Hartnoll, R., Lewis, R., Daviaud, E. & Mitcheson, M. (1985) *Drug Problems: Assessing Local Needs.* Institute of the Study of Drug Dependence (London, Drug Indicators Project).

Hartnoll, R., Mitcheson, M., Battersby, M. *et al.* (1983) Evaluation of heroin maintenance in controlled trial. *Arch. Gen. Psychiat.*, **37**, 877–84.

Hartshorne, H. & May, M. A. (1928) *Studies in the Nature of Character. Vol. 1. Studies in Deceit.* Macmillan, New York.

Harvey, I., Persaud, R., Ron, M. A. *et al.* (1994) Volumetric MRI measures in bipolars compared with schizophrenics and healthy controls. *Psychol. Med.*, **24**, 689–99.

Harvey, I., Ron, M., du Boulay, G. (1993) Reduction of cortical volume in schizophrenia on magnetic resonance imaging. *Psychol. Med.*, **23**, 591–604.

Hasegawa, K. & Imai, Y. (1994) Psychogeriatric services of demented elderly in Japan. In *Dementia* (ed. A. Burns & R. Levy). Chapman & Hall Medical, London, pp. 601–10.

Hasin, D. S. & Skodol, A. E. (1989) Standardised diagnostic interviews for psychiatric research. In *The Instruments of Psychiatric Research* (ed. C. Thompson). John Wiley & Sons, Chichester, pp. 19–57.

Hatfield, A. B., Spanish, L. & Zipple, A. M. (1987) Expressed emotion: a family perspective. *Schiz. Bull.*, **13**, 221–6.

Haw, C. & Lanceley, C. (1987) Patients at a psychiatric walk-in clinic. Who, how, why and when. *Bull. Roy. Coll Psychiat.*, **11** 329–32.

Hawkins, J. D., Catalanu, R. F. Miller, J. T. (1992) Risk and protective factors for alcohol and other drug problems in adolescence and early adulthood. Implications for substance abuse prevention. *Psychol. Bull.*, **112**, 64–105.

Hawton, K. (1982) Attempted suicide in children and adolescents. *J. Child Psychol. Psychiat.*, **23**, 497–503.

Hawton, K. (1985) *Sex Therapy: A Practical Guide.* Oxford Medical Publications, Oxford.

Hawton, K. (1987) Assessment of suicide risk. *Br. J. Psychiat.*, **150**, 145–53.

Hawton, K., Bancroft, J. H. J., Catalan, J. *et al* (1981) Domiciliary and out-patient treatment of self-poisoning patients by medical and non-medical staff. *Psychol. Med.*, **11**, 169–77.

Hawton, K. & Catalan, J. (1987) *Attempted Suicide: A Practical Guide to its Nature and Management.* Oxford University Press, Oxford.

Hawton, K., Catalan, J., Martin, P. & Fagg, J. (1986) Long-term outcome of sex therapy. *Behav. Res. Ther.*, **24**, 377–85.

Hawton, K., Cole, D., O'Grady, J. & Osborn, M. (1982) Motivational aspects of deliberate self-poisoning in adolescents. *Br. J. Psychiat.*, **141**, 286–91.

Hawton, K., Crowel, J., Simkin, S. & Bancrofrt, J. (1978) Attempted suicide and suicide among Oxford University students. *Br. J. Psychiat.*, **132**, 506–9.

Hawton, K. & Fagg, J. (1988) Suicide and other causes of death following attempted suicide. *Br. J. Psychiat.*, **152**, 259–66.

Hawton, K. & Fagg, J. (1992a) Trends in deliberate self-poisoning and self-injury in Oxford, 1976–1990. *Br. Med. J.*, **304**, 1409–11.

Hawton, K. & Fagg, J. (1992b) Deliberate self-poisoning and self-injury in adolescents: a study of characteristics and trends in Oxford 1976–1989. *Br. J. Psychiat.*, **161**, 816–23.

Hawton, K., Fagg, J., Platt, S. & Hawkins, M. (1993) Factors associated with suicide after parasuicide in young people. *Br. Med. J.*, **306**, 1641–4.

Hawton, K., McKeown, S., Day, A. *et al.* (1987) Evaluation of out-patient counselling compared with general practitioner care following overdoses. *Psychol. Med.*, **17**, 751–61.

Hawton, K., Simkin, S., Fagg, J. & Hawkins, M. (1995) Suicide in Oxford University students, 1976–1990. *Br. Med. J.*, **166**, 44–50.

Hay, E. M., Huddy, A., Black, D. *et al.* (1994) A prospective study of psychiatric disorder and cognitive function in systemic lupus erythematosus. *Ann Rheum. Dis.*, **53**, 298–303.

Hayashi, T., Watnabe, T., Kiton, H. & Sekine, T., (1992) Multivariate analyses of CT findings in typical schizophrenia and atypical psychosis. *Jap. J. Psychiat. Neurol.*, **46**, 699–709.

Hayden, T. L. (1980) Classification of elective mutism. *J. Am. Acad. of Child Psychiat.*, **19**, 118–33.

Hayslip, C. C., Fein, H. G., O'Donnell, V. M. *et al.* (1988) The value of serum antimicrosomal antibody testing in screening for symptomatic post partum thyroid dysfunction. *Am. J. Obstet. Gynecol.*, **159**, 203–9.

Hazell, P., O'Connell D., Heathcote, D. *et al.* (1995) Efficacy of tricyclic drugs in treating child and adolescent depression: a meta-analysis. *Br. Med. J.*, **310**, 897–901.

Heath Departments of Great Britain (1989) *General Practice in the National Health Service: the 1990 contract*. Appendix A. 19–30. Health Departments of Great Britain.

Health Education Authority (1992a) *Tomorrows Young Adults*. London.

Health Education Authority (1992b) *Todays Young Adults*. London.

Heather, N. & Robertson, I. (1985) *Problem drinking: the new approach*. Penguin, Harmondsworth.

Heathfield, K., Croft, P. & Swash, M. (1973) Syndrome of transient global amnesia. *Brain*, **96**, 729–36.

Heaton-Ward, A. (1977) Psychosis in mental handicap. *Br. J. Psychiat.*, **130**, 525–33.

Hecaen, F. (1981) Apraxia. In *Handbook of Clinical Neuropsychology* (ed. S. B. Filskov & T. J. Boll). Wiley, New York, pp. 257–86.

Hecker, E. (1871) Die Hebephrenic. *Virchows Archiv. fur Pathologische Anatomie*, **52**, 392–449.

Hedlund, J. L. & Viewig, B. W. (1979) The Hamilton Rating Scale for depression: a comprehensive review. *J. Operat. Psychiat*, **10**, 149–65.

Hedstrom, P. & Ringen, S. (1987) Age and income in contemporary society: a research note. *J. Soc. Policy*, **16** (2), 227–39.

Hellerstein, D., Frosch, W. & Koeningsberg, H. W. (1987) The clinical significance of command hallucinations. *Am. J. Psychiat.*, **144**, 219–21.

Helzer, J. E. (1987) Epidemiology of alcoholism. *J. Consult. Clin. Psychol.*, **55**, 284–92.

Helzer, J. E. & Pryzbek, T. (1988) The co-occurrence of alcoholism with other psychiatric disorders in the general population and its impact on treatment. *J. Studies on Alcohol*, **49**, 219–24.

Helzer, J. E., Robins, L. N., McEvoy, L. T. *et al.* (1985) A comparison of clinical and diagnostic interview schedule diagnoses. *Arch. Gen. Psychiat.*, **42**, 657–66.

Helzer, J., Robins, L. & McEvoy, L (1987) Post-traumatic stress disorder in the general population. Findings from the Epidemiological Catchment Area Survey. *N. Engl. J. Med.*, **317**, 1630–4.

Helzer, J. E., Robins, L. N. & Taylor, J. R. (1985) The extent of long-term moderate drinking among alcoholics discharged from medical and psychiatric facilities. *N. Engl. J. Med.*, **312**, 1678–2.

Hempel, C. G. (1961) *Introduction to Problems of Taxonomy in Field Studies in the Mental Disorders* (ed. J. Zubin). Grune & Stratton, New York, pp. 3–22.

Henderson, A. F., Gregoire, A. J. P., Kumar, R. C. & Studd, J. W. W. (1991) Treatment of severe postnatal depression with oestradiol skin patches. *Lancet*, **338**, 816–17.

Henderson, D. K. (1939) *Psychopathic States*. London.

Henderson, M. & Freeman, C. L. (1987) A self-rating scale for bulimia: The BITE. *Br. J. Psychiat.*, **150**, 168–78.

Henderson, S., Byrne, D. G. & Duncan-Jones, P. (1981) *Neurosis and the Social Environment*. Academic Press, Sydney.

Henderson, S., Duncan Jones, P., Byrne, D. G. *et al* (1979) Psychiatric disorder in Canberra. *Acta Psychiat. Scand.*, **60**, 355–74.

Henn, F. A. (1996) The psychobiology of depression: data for animal models. In *New Research in Psychiatry* (ed. H. Hafner of E. M. Wolpert). Hogrede & Huber, Seattle, pp. 1–10.

Hennekens, C. H. & Buring, J. E. (1987) *Epidemiology in Medicine*. Little, Brown and Company, Boston.

Henry, J. (1992) Ecstasy and the dance of death. *Br. Med. J.*, 305–306.

Henry, J. A., Alexander, C. A. & Sener, E. S. (1995) Relative mortality from overdose of antidepressants. *Br. Med. J.*, **310**, 221–4.

Her Majesty's Stationary Office. (1989) *Working for Patients*. HMSO, London.

Herman, C. P. & Mack, D. (1975) Restrained and unrestrained eating. *J. Personality.*, **43**, 77–109.

Herrmann, M., Bartels, C. & Wallesch, C. N. (1993) Depression in acute and chronic aphasia: Symptoms, patho-anatomical-clinical correlations and functional implications. *J. Neurol. Neurosurg. Psychiat.*, **56**, 672–8.

Hersov, L. A. (1960a) Persistent non-attendance at school. *J. Child Psychol. Psychiat.*, **1**, 130–6.

Hersov, L. A. (1960b) Refusal to go to school. *J. Child Psychol. Psychiat.*, **1**, 137–45.

Hersov, L. A. (1985) School refusal. In *Child and Adolescent Psychiatry: Modern Approaches*, Second edn (ed. M. Rutter & L. Hersov). Blackwell, Oxford, pp. 382–99.

Herzog, D. B., Keller, M. B., Lavorie, P. W. *et al*. (1992) The prevalence of personality disorders in 210 women with eating disorders. *J. Clin. Psychiat.*, **53**, 147–52.

Heston, L. L. & Denney, D. (1968) Interactions between early life experience and biological factors in schizophrenia. In *The Transmission of Schizophrenia* (ed. D. Rosenthal & S. Kety). Pergamon Press, Oxford, pp. 363–76.

Heston, L. L. & Shields, J. (1968) Homosexuality in twins. *Arch. Gen. Psychiat.*, **18**, 149–60.

Hewett, L. J., Nixon, S. J., Glenn, S. W. & Parsons, O. A. (1991) Verbal fluency deficits in female alcoholics. *Psychology*, **47**, 716–19.

Hibbert, G. & Chan, M. (1989) Respiratory control: its contribution to the treatment of panic attacks: a controlled study. *Br. J. Psychiat*, **154**, 232–6.

Hibbert, G. & Pilsbury D. (1989) Hyperventilation: is it a cause of panic attacks? *Br. J. Psychiat*, **155**, 805–9.

Hill, A. B. (1955) *Introduction to medical statistics* (5th edn), *Lancet*. London.

Hill, D. (1953) Psychiatric disorders of epilepsy. *Med. Press*, **229**, 473–5.

Hill, O. W. (1968) Psychogenic vomiting. *Gut.*, **9**, 348–52.

Hill, P. (1986) Child psychiatry. In *Essentials of Postgraduate Psychiatry*, second edn (ed. P. Hill, R. Murray & A. Thorley). Grune & Stratton, London, pp. 81–137.

Hill, P. (1989) *Adolescent Psychiatry*. Churchill Livingstone, Edinburgh.

Hill, P. (1990) Behavioural psychotherapy with children. *Internat. Rev. Psychiat.*, **1**, 257–66.

Hill, P. (1994a) Adjustment disorders. In *Child and Adolescent Psychiatry: Modern Approaches*, third edn (ed. M. Rutter, E. Taylor & L. Hersov). Blackwell Scientific, Oxford, pp. 375–91.

Hill, P. (1994b) Sleep disorders in depression and anxiety: issues in childhood and adolescence. *J. Psychosom. Res.*, **38**, Suppl. 1, 61–7.

Hill, P. (1994c) Contribution from the Child & Adolescent Section. In *Purchasing Psychiatric Care*. Royal College of Psychiatrists, London.

Hill, R. M., Desmond, M. M. & Kay, J. L. (1966) Extrapyramidal dysfunction in an infant of a schizophrenic mother. *J. Pediatr.*, **97** 589–95.

Hiller, W., Zaudig, M. & Mobour, W. (1991) Development of diagnostic checklists for use in routine clinical care. *Arch. Gen. Psychiat.*, **47**, 782–4.

Hinde, R. A. (1979) *Towards Understanding Relationships*. Academic Press, London.

Hindler, C. G., Crisp, A. H., McGuigan, S. & Joughlin, N. (1994) Anorexia nervosa; change over time in age of onset, presentation and duration of illness. *Psychol. Med.*, **24**, 719–30.

Hinkle, L. E. & Wolff, H. G. (1957) The nature of man's adaptation to his total environment and the relation of this to illness. *Arch. Int. Med.*, **99**, 442–60.

Hinton, J. & Withers, E. (1971) The usefulness of clinical tests of the sensorium *Br. J. Psychiat.*, **119**, 9–18.

Hippius, H. (1989) The history of clozapine. *Psychopharmacology*, **99**, S3–S5.

Hirsch, S. (1986) Clinical treatment of schizophrenia. In *The Psychopharmacology and Treatment of Schizophrenia* (ed. P. Bradley & S. Hirsch). Oxford Med. Pubs., Oxford, pp. 286–339.

Hirsch, S. (1988) *Psychiatric Bed and Resources: Factors Influencing Bed Use and Service Planning.* Gaskell, The Royal College of Psychiatrists, London.

Hirsch, S. R. & Leff, J. P. (1975) *Abnormalities in the Parents of Schizophrenics.* Maudsley Monograph No. 22. Oxford University Press, Oxford.

Hirschfeld, R. M. A., Klerman, G. A., Clayton, P. J. *et al.* (1983) Assessing personality: effects of the depressive state on trait measurement. *Am. J. Psychiat.*, **140**, 695–9.

Hirschfeld, D. R., Rosenbaum, J. F., Biederman, J. *et al.* (1992) Stable behavioural inhibition and its association with anxiety disorder. *J. Am. Acad. Child Adol. Psychiat.*, **31**, 103–11.

Hoberman, H. H., Lewinsohn, P. M. & Tilson, M. (1988) Group treatment of depression: individual predictions of outcome. *J. Consult. Clin. Psychol.*, **56**, 393–8.

Hobson, R. P. (1993) *Autism and the Development of Mind.* Laurence Erlbaum Association, Hillsdale, NJ.

Hodes, M., Eisler, I. & Dare, C. (1991) Family therapy for anorexia nervosa in adolescence: a review. *J. Royal Soc. Med.*, **84**, 359–62.

Hodes, M. & Moorey, S. (1993) *Psychological Treatment in Disease and Illness.* Gaskell, London.

Hodge, J. E. (1992) Addiction to violence: a new model of psychopathy. *Crim. Behav. Ment. Health*, **2**, 212–23.

Hodgins, S. (1992) Mental disorder, intellectual deficiencies and crime. *Arch. Gen. Psychiat.*, **49**, 476–83.

Hodgson, R. (1993) Psychological treatments, the research and policy connections. In *Drugs, Alcohol and Tobacco: Making the Science and Policy Connections* (ed. G. Edwards, J. Strang & J. Jaffe). Oxford University Press, Oxford, pp. 199–210.

Hodgson, R. J. & Rachman, S. (1977) Obsessional compulsive complaints. *Behav. Res. Ther.*, **15**, 389–95.

Hoek, H. W. (1993) Review of the epidemiological studies of eating disorders. *Int Rev. Psychiat.*, **5**, 61–74.

Hoek, H. W. (1991) The incidence and prevalence of anorexia nervosa and bulimia nervosa in primary care. *Psychol. Med.*, **21**, 455–60.

Hoenig, J. R., Kenna, J. C. (1979) EEG abnormalities and transsexualism. *Br. J. Psychiat.*, **134**, 293–300.

Hofman, A., Rocca, W., Brayne, C. *et al* (1991) The prevalence dementia in Europe. *Intern. J. Epidemiol.*, **20**, 736–48.

Hogarty, G. E., Goldberg, S. C., Schooler, N. R. & Ulrich, R. F. (1974) Drugs and sociotherapy in the aftercare of schizophrenic patients. *Arch. Gen. Psychiat.*, **31**, 603–8.

Hokin, L. E. (1993) Lithium increasing accumulation of second messenger 1,4,5-triphosphate in brain cortex slices in species ranging from mouse to monkey. *Adv. Enz. Regul.*, **33**, 299–312.

Holden, J. M., Sagovsky, R. & Cox, J. L. (1989) Counselling in a general practice setting: Controlled study of health visitors' intervention in treatment of post-natal depression. *Br. J. Psychiat*, **298**, 223–6.

Holden, N. (1987) Late paraphrenia or the paraphrenias. *Br. J. Psychiat.*, **150**, 635–9.

Holder, H., Longabaugh, R., Miller, W. R. & Rubonis, A. V. (1991) The cost effectiveness of treatment for alcohol problems: a first approximation. *J. Studies on Alcohol.*, **52**, 517–40.

Hollander, E., Schiffman, E., Cohen B. *et al.* (1990) Signs of central nervous system dysfunction in obsessive-compulsive disorder. *Arch. Gen. Psychiat.*, **47**, 27–32.

Hollander, E., Decaria, C., Nitescu, A. *et al.* (1992) Serotonergic function in obsessive-compulsive disorder: behavioural and neuroendocrine responses to oral-M-chlorophenylpiperazine and fenfluramine in patients and healthy volunteers. *Arch. Gen. Psychiat.*, **49**, 21–28.

Hollingshead, A. B. & Redlich, F. C. (1958) *Social Class and Mental Illness: A Community Study.* Wiley, New York.

Hollister, L. (1986) Health aspects of cannabis. *Pharmacol. Rev.*, **38**, 1–20.

Hollon, S. D., Shelton, R. C. & Davis, D. D. (1993) Cognitive therapy for depression: conceptual issues and clinical efficacy. *J. Consult. Clin. Psychol.*, **61**, 270–5.

Hollon, S. D., Shelton, R. C. & Loosen, P. T. (1991) Cognitive therapy and pharmacotherapy for depression. *J. Consult. Clin. Psychol.*, **59**, 88–99.

Holloway, F. (1988) Day care and community support. In *Community Care in Practice* (ed. A. Lavender & F. Holloway). Wiley, Chichester.

Holloway, F. (1990) Caring for people: a critical review of British Government policy for the community care of the mentally ill. *Psychiat. Bull.*, **14**, 641–5.

Holmes, F. (1936) An experimental investigation of a method of overcoming children's fears. *Child Devel.*, **7**, 6–30.

Holmes, S. J. & Robins, L. N. (1987) The influence of childhood disciplinary experience on the development of alcoholism and depression. *J. Child Psychol. Psychiat.*, **28**, 399–415.

Holmes, T. H. & Rahe, R. H. (1967). The Social Readjustment Rating Scale. *J. Psychosom. Res.*, **11**, 213–18.

Holsboer, F., Gerken, A., Stalla, G. K. & Muller, O. A. (1987) Blunted aldosterone and ACTH release after human CRH administration in depressed patients. *Am. J. Psychiat.*, **144**, 229–31.

Holsboer, F., von Bardeleben, U., Gerken, A. *et al.* (1984) Blunted corticotrophin and normal cortisol response to human corticotrophin-releasing factor in (h-CRF) in depression. *N. Engl. J. Med.*, **311**, 1127.

Holzman, P. S. (1988) A single dominant gene can account for eye tracking dysfunctions and schizophrenia in offspring of discordant twins. *Arch. Gen. Psychiat.*, **45**, 641–7.

Home Office (1988) *Criminal Statistics, England and Wales 1987.* HMSO: London Cmnd. 498.

Home Office (1989) *Criminal Statistics England and Wales 1988.* HMSO: London, Cmnd. 847.

Home Office (1994) *Statistics on the Misuse of Drugs in the United Kingdom.* HMSO, London.

Home Office, Department of Health and Social Security (1974) *Interim Report of the Committee on Mentally Abnormal Offenders.* London, HMSO Cmnd. 5698.

Home Office, Department of Health and Social Security (1975) *Report of the Committee on Mentally Abnormal Offenders* (The Butler Report). London, HMSO Cmnd. 6244.

Hook, K. (1963) Refused abortion: a follow-up study of 249 women whose applications were refused by the National Board of Health in Sweden. *Acta Psychiatr. Neurol. Scand, Suppl. 39,* **168**, 1–156.

Hooper, S. T. & Willis, W. G. (1989) *Learning Disability Subtyping.* Springer-Verlag, New York.

Hope, T. & Patel, V. (1993) Assessment of behavioural phenomena in dementia In: *Ageing and Dementia: a methodological approach* (ed. A. Burns). Edward Arnold, London, pp. 221–36.

Hopkins A. (1981) *Epilepsy: The Facts.* Oxford University Press, Oxford.

Horder, E. (1990) *Medical Care in Three Psychiatric Hostels.* Hampstead and Bloomsbury District Health Authority, Hampstead and South Barnet GP Forum and the Hampstead Department of Community Medicine.

Horder, J. (1988) Working with general practitioners. *Br. J. Psychiat.*, **153**, 513–20.

Horn, G. ten., Giel, R., Gulbinat, W. & Henderson, J. (eds) (1986) *Psychiatric Case Registers in Public Health. A Worldwide Inventory, 1960–1985).* Elsevier, Amsterdam.

Horn, W. F., Oalongo, N. S., Pascoe, J. M. *et al.* (1991) Additive effects of psychostimulants, parent training, and self-control therapy with ADHD children. *J. Am. Acad. Child Adol Psychiat.*, **30**, 233–40.

Hornstra, R. A. (1962) The psychiatric hospital and the community. Paper read at the Annual Workshop in Community Health, Candler, N. Carolina.

Horney, K. (1939) *New Ways in Psychoanalysis*. W. W. Norton, New York.

Horneykiewicz, O. (1982) Brain catecholamines in schizophrenia – a good case for schizophrenia. *Nature*, **299**, 484–6.

Horowitz, J. M. (1978) *Image Formation and Cognition* (2nd edn). Appleton, Century, Crofts, New York.

Horowitz, M. J. (1986) *Stress Response Syndromes*, 2nd edn. Jason Aronson, Northvale, NJ.

Horowitz, M. J. (1988) *Introduction to Psychodynamics: A New Synthesis*. Basic Books, New York.

Horowitz, M. J. (1991) Short-term dynamic therapy of stress response syndromes. In *Handbook of short-term Dynamicp psychotherapies* (ed. P. Crits-Christoph & J. P. Barber). Basic Books, New York, pp. 166–98.

Horowitz, M. J., Marmar, C., Weiss, D. *et al.* (1984) Brief psychotherapy of bereavement reactions. *Arch. Gen. Psychiat.*, **41**, 438–48.

Horvath, T., Friedman, J. & Meares, R. (1980) Attention in hysteria: a study of Janet's hypothesis by means of habituation and arousal methods. *Am. J. Psychiat.*, **137**, 217–21.

Hoult, J. & Reynolds, I. (1984) Schizophrenia: a comparative trial of community oriented and hospital oriented psychiatric care. *Acta Psychiat. Scand.*, **69**, 359–72.

House, A. (1987) Mood disorder after stroke: a review of the evidence. *Internat. J. Geriat. Psychiat.*, **2**, 211–21.

House of Commons (1985) *Second Report from the Social Services Committee, Session 1984–85, Community Care*. HMSO, London.

House of Commons (1986) *Third Report from the Social Services Committee, Session 1985–6 Prison Medical Service*. HMSO, London.

House of Commons (1990) The National Health Service and Community Care Act. HMSO, London.

Howard, R. Forstl, H., Naguib, M. *et al.* (1991) First rank symptoms in late paraphrenia: Cortical structural correlates. *Br. J. Psychiat.*, **160**, 108–9.

Howard, R., Castle, D., Wessely, S. & Murray, R. M. (1993) A comparative study of 470 cases of early onset and late onset schizophrenia. *Br. J. Psychiat.*, **163**, 352–7.

Hoyer, G. & Lund, E. (1993) Suicide among women related to number of children in marriage. *Arch. Gen. Psychiat.*, **50**, 134–7.

Hrubec, Z. & Omenn, G. S. (1981) Evidence of genetic predisposition to alcoholic cirrhosis and psychosis. *Alcohol. Clin. Exper.*, **5**, 207–15.

Hser, Y., Anglin, D. & Powers, K. (1993) A 24-year follow-up of Californian narcotic addicts. *Arch. Gen. Psychiat.*, **50**, 577–84.

Hsu, L. K. G. & Sobkiewicz, T. A. (1991) Body image disturbance: Time to abandon the concept of eating disorders. *Internat. J. Eat. Disorders.*, **10**, 15–30.

Huber, G., Gross, G., Schuttler, R. & Linz, M. (1980) Longitudinal studies of schizophrenic patients. *Schiz. Bull.*, **6**, 592–605.

Hunter, D. & Wistow, G. (1987) Mapping the organisational context. 1 Central departments, boundaries and responsibilities. In *Community Care in Britain: Variations on a Theme* (ed. D. Hunter & G. Wistow). King Edward's Hospital Fund for London, London.

Hupkens, C. L., Knibbe, R. A. & Drop, M. J. (1993) Alcohol consumption in the European Community: uniformity and diversity in drinking patterns. *Addiction*, **88**, 1391–404.

Hurry, J. & Sturt, E. (1981) Social performance in a population sample: relation to psychiatric symptoms. In *What is a Case?* (ed. J. K. Wing, P. Bebbington & L. Robins). Grant McIntyre, London, pp. 202–13.

Hurry, J., Tennant, C. & Bebbington, P. E. (1980) Selective factors leading to psychiatric referral. *Acta Psychiat. Supplementum*, **285**, 315–23.

Huss, M. (1849–51) *Alcoholismus chronicus eller Chronsik alkoholsjukdom* (Alcoholismus chronicus or

Chronic alcohol disease), 2 vols. Stockholm–German edn: Chronische Alkoholkrankheit oder Alcoholismus chronicus. Stockholm and Leipzig, 1852.

Huxley, P. J., Goldberg, D. P., Maguire, P. & Kincy, V. (1979) The prediction of the course of minor psychiatric disorders. *Br. J. Psychiat.*, **135**, 535–43.

Hwu, H-G., Yeh, E-K. & Change, L-Y. (1989) Prevalence of psychiatric disorders in Taiwan defined by the chinese Diagnostic Interview Schedule. *Acta Psychiat. Scand.*, **79**, 136–47.

Hymas, N., Lees, A., Bolton, D. *et al.* (1991) The neurology of obsessional slowness. *Brain*, **114**, 2203–33.

Hymas, N., Naguib, M., Levy, R. (1989) Late paraphrenia – a follow-up study. *Internat. J. Geriat. Psychiat.*, **4**, 23–9.

Ihlen, B. M., Amundsen, A. & Tronnes, L. (1993) Reduced alcohol use in pregnancy and changed attitudes in the population. *Addiction*, **88**, 389–94.

Iles, S. (1989) The loss of early pregnancy. *Baillières Clin. Obstet. Gynaecol.*, **3**, 769–90.

Iles, S. & Gath, D. (1993) Psychiatric outcome of termination of pregnancy for foetal abnormality. *Psychol. Med.*, **23**, 407–13.

Iliffe, S., Haine, A., Booroof, A. *et al.* (1991) Alcohol consumption by elderly people: a general practice survey. *Age and Ageing*, **20**, 120–3.

Illich, I. (1974) Medical nemesis. *Lancet*, **1**, 918–22.

Impastato, D. J., Gabriel, A. R. & Lardaro, H. H. (1964) Electric and insulin shock therapy during pregnancy. *Dis. Nerv. System*, **15**, 542–6.

Ineichen, B., Harrison, G. & Morgan, H. (1984) Psychiatric hospital admission in Bristol. 1. Geographical and ethnic factors. *Br. J. Psychiat.*, **145**, 50–504.

Ingram. I. M. (1961) Obsessional illness in mental hospital patients. *J. Ment. Sci.*, **107**, 381–402.

Insel, T. (1992) Towards a neuroanatomy of obsessive compulsive disorder. *Arch. Gen. Psychiat.*,**49**, 739–44.

Intagliata, J. (1982) Improving the quality of care for the chronic mentally disabled: the role of case management. *Schiz. Bull.*, **982**, 655–74.

Insel, T. R. & Akiskal, H. S. (1986) Obsessive-compulsive disorder with psychotic features: a phenomenological analysis. *Am. J. Psychiat.*, **143**, 1527–33.

Institute of Medicine (1990) *Broadening the Base of Treatment for Alcohol Problems*. National Academy Press, Washington DC.

Ireland, M., English, C., Cross, I. *et al.* (1991) A *de nova* translocation (3;17)(q26.3;q23.1) in a child with Cornelia de Lang syndrome. *J. Med. Genet.*, **28**, 639–40.

Issac, G. (1992) Misdiagnosed bipolar disorder in adolescents in a special educational school and treatment program. *J. Clin. Psychiat.*, **53**, 133–6.

Isaacs, S. (1939) Criteria for interpretation. *Internat. J. Psycho-anal.*, **20**.

Isacsson, G., Holmgren, P., Wasserman, D. & Bergman, U. (1994) Use of antidepressants among people committing suicide in Sweden. *Br. Med. J.*, **308**, 506–8.

Iversen, S. D. (1984) 5-HT and anxiety. *Neuropharmacol.*, **23**, 1553–60.

Iwata, B., Dorsey, N., Slifer, K. *et al.* (1982) Towards a functional analysis of self injury. *Analy. Intervent. Develop. Disabil.*, **2**, 3–20.

Jablensky, A., Sartorius, N., Ernberg, G. *et al.* (1992) Schizophrenia: manifestations, incidence and course in different cultures. A World Health Organization Ten-Country Study. *Psychol. Med.* Monograph supplement 20.

Jacobson, E. (1938) *Progressive Relaxation*. University of Chicago Press, Chicago.

Jacobson, R. (1986) Female alcoholics: a controlled CT brain scan and clinical study. *Br. J. Addiction*, **81**, 661–9.

Jacobson, S. J., Jones, K., Johnson, K. *et al.* (1992) Prospective multicentre study of pregnancy outcome after lithium exposure during the first trimester. *Lancet*, **339**, 530–3.

Jacobvitz, D., Sroufe, L. A., Stewart, M. & Leffert, N. (1990) Treatment of attentional and hyperactivity problems in children with sympathomimetic drugs: a comprehensive review. *J. Am. Acad. Child Adol. Psychiat.*, **29**, 677–88.

Jacoby, R. J. (1981) Depression in the elderly. *Br. J. Hosp. Med.*, **25**, 40–7.

Jacoby, R. J. (1991) Manic illness In *Psychiatry in the Elderly* (ed. R. Jacoby & C. Oppenheimer). Oxford Medical Publications, Oxford, pp. 720–6.

Jacoby, R. J. & Levy, R. (1980) Computed tomography in the elderly: 3. Affective disorder. *Br. J. Psychiat.*, **136**, 270–5.

Jacoby, R. J., Levy, R. & Bird, J. M. (1981) Computed tomography and the outcome of affective disorder: A follow-up study of elderly patients. *Br. J. Psychiat.*, **139**, 288–92.

Jaffe, J. (1990) Drug addiction and drug abuse. In *Textbook of Pharmacology and Therapeutics.* (ed. Goodman and Gillman). Macmillan, New York, pp. 522–72.

Jaffe, J. & Martin, W. (1990) Opioid analgesics and antagonists. In *Textbook of Pharmacology and Therapeutics* (ed. Goodman and Gillman). Macmillan, New York, pp. 485–521.

Jagger, C. & Lindesay, J. (1993) The epidemiology of senile dementia In *Ageing and Dementia* (ed. A. Burns). Edward Arnold, London, pp. 41–57.

James, I. & Savage, I. (1984) Beneficial effects of nadolol on anxiety-induced disturbances of performance in musicians: a comparison with diazepam and placebo. *Am. Heart J.*, **4**, 1150–55.

James, W. (1890) *The Principles of Psychology*. Holt, New York.

Janson, C. G. (1984) *Project Metropolitan: A Presentation and Progress Report*. University of Stockholm Department of Sociology, Stockholm.

Janssen, P. A. J. (1970) The butyrophenone story. In *Discoveries in Biological Psychiatry*, (ed. F. S. Ayd & B. Blackwell). J. B. Lippincott, Philadelphia, pp. 165–80.

Jarman, B. (1983) Identification of underprivileged areas. *Br. Med. J.*, **286**, 1705–9.

Jarman, B. (1984) Underprivileged areas: validation and distribution of scores. *Br. Med. J.*, **289**, 1587–92.

Jarvik, L. S., Mintz, J., Steur, J. & Gerner, J. (1982) Treating geriatric depression:. a 26 week interim analysis *J. Am. Geriat. Soc.*, **30**, 713–17.

Jarvik, L. F. & Russell, D. (1979) Anxiety, ageing and the third emergency reaction. *J. Gerontol.*, **34**, 197–200.

Jarvis, T. J. (1992) Implications of gender for alcohol treatment research: a quantitative and qualitative review. *Br. J. Addiction,.*, **87**, 1249–62.

Jaspers, K. (1963) *General Psychopathology* (translated from 7th edn by J. Hoenig & M. W. Hamilton). Manchester University Press, Manchester.

Jehu, D. (1988) *Beyond Sexual Abuse. Therapy with Women who Where Childhood Victims*. John Wiley, Chichester.

Jehu, D. (1991) Post-traumatic stress reactions among adults molested as children. *Sexual and Marital Therapy*, **6**, 227–43.

Jellinek, E. M. (1952) Phases of alcohol addiction. *Quart. J. Stud. Alcohol*, **13**, 673–84.

Jellinek, E. M. (1960) *The Disease Concept of Alcoholism*. Hillhouse Press, New Haven.

Jenkins, A., Teasdale, G., Hadley, M. D. M. *et al.* (1986) Brain lesions detected by magnetic resonance imaging in mild and severe head injuries. *Lancet*, **ii**, 445–6.

Jenkins, H. (1990) Family therapy – developments in thinking and practice. *J. Child Psychol Psychiat.*, **31**, 1015–26.

Jenkins, R. (1985) Sex differences in minor psychiatric morbidity. *Psychol. Med.* **15**, (Suppl. 7)

Jenkins, R. & Meltzer, H. (1994) The National Psychiatric Morbidity Survey of Great Britain – an Overview. *Soc. Psychiat. Psychiatr. Epidemiol.*, **6**, 349–56.

Jenkins, R., Smeeton, N. & Shepherd, M. (188). Classification of mental disorder in primary care. *Psychological Medicine Monograph* Supplement 12.

Jenner, F. A., Monteiro, A. C. D., Zagalo-Cardoso, J. A. & Cunha-Olivera, J. A. (1993) *Schizophrenia: A Disease or Some Ways of Being Human?* Sheffield Academic Press, Sheffield.

Jennett, B. & Bond, M. (1975) Assessment of outcome after severe brain damage. *Lancet*, **i**, 480–4.

Jennett, B. & MacMillan, R. (1981) Epidemiology of head injury. *Br. Med. J.*, **i**, 101–4.

Jennett, B. & Plum, F. (1972) Persistent vegetative state after brain damage. *Lancet*, **i**, 734–7.

Jennings, C., Barraclough, B. M. & Moss, J. R. (1978) Have the Samaritans lowered the suicide rate? A controlled study. *Psychol. Med.*, **8**, 412–22.

Jessor, R. (1976) Predicting time and onset of marijuana use: a developmental study of high school youth. *J. Consult. Clin. Psychol.*, **44**, 125–34.

Jessor, R. & Donovan, J. (1991) *Beyond Adolescence. Problem behaviour and Young Adult Development*. Cambridge University Press, Cambridge.

Jessor, R. & Jessor S. L. (1977) *Problem Behaviour and Psychosocial Development: a Longitudinal Study of Youth*. Academic Press, New York.

Jessor R, Donovan, J. E. Costa F. M. (1991) *Beyond Adolescence: Problem Behaviour and Young Adolescent Development*. Cambridge University Press, Cambridge.

Jick, S. S., Dean, A. D. & Jick, H. (1995) Antidepressants and suicide. *Br. Med. J.*, **310**, 215–18.

Jitapunkul, S., Pillay, I. & Ebrahim, S. (1992) Delirium in newly admitted elderly patients. A prospective study. *Quart. J. Med.*, **300**, 307–14.

Johnson, A. M. (1991) The comparative pharmacological properties of selective serotonin reuptake inhibitors in animals. In *Selective Serotonin Reuptake Inhibitors* (ed. J. P. Feighner & W. F. Boyer). John Wiley, Chichester/New York, pp. 37–70.

Johnson, A. M., Wadsworth, J., Wellings, K. *et al.* (1992) Sexual lifestyles and HIV risk. *Nature*, **360**, 410–12.

Johnson, A., Wadworth, J. Wellings, K. & Field, J. (1994) *Sexual Attitudes and Lifestyles*. Blackwell Scientific Publications, Oxford.

Johnson, D. A. W. (1981) Depression: treatment compliance in general practice. *Acta Psychiat. Scand.*, **63**, (Suppl 290), 447–53.

Johnson, J. (1993) Catatonia: the tension insanity. *Br. J. Psychiat.*, **162**, 733–8.

Johnson, J. C., Gottlieb, G. L., Sullivan, E. *et al.* (1990) Using DSM-III criteria to diagnose delirium in elderly general medical patients. *J. Gerontol.*, **45**, M113–119.

Johnson, J., Weissman, M. M. & Klerman, G. L. (1992). Service utilization and social morbidity associated with depressive symptoms in the community. *J. Am. Med. Assoc.*, **267**, 1478–83.

Johnson, P., Conrad, C. & Thompson, D. (eds) (1989) *Working Versus Pensioners: International Justice in an Ageing World*. Manchester University Press, Manchester.

Johnson, S. & Thornicroft G. (1993). The sectorisation of psychiatric services in England and Wales. *Soc. Psychiat Psychiat Epidemiol.*, **28**, 45–7.

Johnson, T. (1989) Methodology of clinical trials in psychiatry In *Research Methods in Psychiatry* (ed. C. Freeman & P. Tyrer). Gaskell (pubs), Royal College of Psychiatrists, London, pp. 12–46.

Johnston, B. B., Naylor, G. J., Dick, E. G. *et al.* (1980) Prediction of clinical course of bipolar manic depressive illness treated with lithium. *Psychol. Med.*, **10**, 326–34.

Johnston, D. W. (1993) The current status of the coronary prone behaviour pattern. *J. Roy. Soc. Med.*, **86**, 406–9.

Johnstone, A. & Goldberg, D. (1976) Psychiatric screening in general practice.: A controlled trial. *Lancet*, **i**, 605–8.

Johnstone, E. C. (1994) Brain imaging, psychopathology and neurology. In *Search for the Causes of Schizophrenia* Vol III (ed. H. Hafner & W. F. Gattaz). Springer-Verlag, Berlin, pp. 129–40.

Johnstone, E. C., Crow, T. J., Frith, C. D. *et al.* (1976) Cerebral ventricular size and cognitive impairment in chronic schizophrenia. *Lancet*, **ii**, 924–26.

Johnstone, E. C., Crow, T. J., Frith, C. D. *et al* (1978) Mechanism of the antipsychotic effect in the treatment of acute schizophrenia. *Lancet*, **1**, 848–51.

Johnstone, E. C., Crow, T. J., Frith, C. D. *et al.* (1978) Mechanisms of the antipsychotic effect in the treatment of acute schizophrenia. *Lancet*, **i**, 848–51.

Johnstone, E. C., Crow, T. J., Frith, C. D. & Owens, D. G. C. (1988) The Northwick Park 'functional' psychosis study: diagnosis and treatment response. *Lancet*, **ii**, 119–25.

Johnstone, E. C., Frith, C. D., Crow, T. J. *et al.* (1992) The Northwick Park 'functional' psychosis study: diagnosis and outcome. *Psychol. Med.*, **22**, 331–46.

Johnstone, E., Cunningham-Owens, D., Frith, C. *et al.* (1980) Neurotic illness and its response to anxiolytic and antidepressant medication. *Psychol. Med.* **10**, 321–8.

Johnstone, E. C., Owens, D. G. C., Crow, T. J. *et al.* (1989) Temporal lobe structure as determined by nuclear magnetic resonance in schizophrenia and bipolar affective disorder. *J. Neurol. Neurosurg. Psychiat.*, **52**, 736–41.

Johnstone, E., Owens, D., Gold, A. *et al.* (1984) Schizophrenic patients discharged from hospital – a follow-up study. *Br. J. Psychiat.*, **145**, 586–90.

Joint Committee on Higher Psychiatric Training (1995) *Handbook*, 7th edn, Occasional Paper OP27. Royal College of Psychiatrists, London.

Jolley, D. J. (1993) Psychiatric services for the elderly doctors should be in the front line. *Br. Med. J.*, **306**, 1411.

Jolley, D. J. & Arie, T. (1978) Organisation of psychogeriatric services. *Br. J. Psychiat.*, **132**, 1–11.

Jolley, D. J. & Arie, T. (1992) Developments in psychogeriatric services. In *Recent Advances in Psychogeriatrics* 2 (ed. T. Arie). Churchill Livingstone, Edinburgh, pp. 117–35.

Jolley, D. J. & Hodgson, S. (1985) Alcoholism and the elderly: a tale of women and our times. In *Recent Advances in Geriatric Medicine* 3 (ed. B. Isaacs). Churchill Livingstone, Edinburgh, pp. 113–22.

Jones, M. C. (1924) The elimination of children's fears. *J. Exper. Psychol.*, **7**, 383–90.

Jones, D. H. (1992) *Interviewing the Sexually Abused Child* (4th edn). Gaskell, London.

Jones, E. (1953a) *The life and work of Sigmund Freud, Vol 1*. Hogarth Press, London.

Jones, M. (1953b) *The Therapeutic Community*, Tavistock Press, London.

Jones, E. A., Gammal, S. H. & Martin, P. (1989) Hepatic encephalopathy – new light on an old problem. *Quart. J. Med.*, **69**, 851–67.

Jones, K. L., Lacro, R. V., Johnson, K. A. & Adams, J. (1989) Pattern of malformations in the children of women treated with carbamazepine during pregnancy. *N. Engl. J. Med.*, **320**. 1661–6.

Jones, K. L. & Smith, D. W. (1973) Recognition of foetal alcohol syndrome in early infancy. *Lancet*, **2**, 999–1001.

Jones, P. B., Rodgers, B., Murray, R. M. & Marmot, M. (1994a) Child developmental risk factors for adult schizophrenia in the British 1946 birth cohort. *Lancet*, **344**, 1398–402.

Jones, P. B., Harvey, I., Lewis, S. W. *et al.* (1994b) Cerebral ventricle dimensions as risk factors for schizophrenia and affective psychosis. an epidemiological approach to analysis. *Psychol. Med.*, **24**, 995–1011.

Jonsson, B. & Bebbington, P. (1993) Economic studies of the treatment of depressive illness. In *Perspectives in Psychiatry. Vol 4: Health Economics and Depression* (ed. S. Montgomery & F. Rouillon). Wiley, Chichester. pp. 35–48.

Jonsson, B. & Bebbington, P. E. (1994) What price depression? The cost of depression and the cost of pharmacological treatment. *Br. J. Psychiat.*, **164**, 665–73.

Jope, R. S., Jenden, D. J., Ehrlich, B. E. *et al.* (1980) Erythrocyte choline concentrations are elevated in manic patients. *Proc. Nat. Acad. Sci. USA*, **77**, 6144–6.

Jorgenson, P. & Jensen, J. (1994) What predicts the persistence of delusional beliefs? *Psychopathology*, **27**, 73–8.

Jorm, A. (1985) Subtypes of Alzheimer's Dementia: A conceptual analysis and critical review. *Psychol. Med.*, **15**, 543–53.

Jorm, A. (1990) *The Epidemiology of Alzheimer's Disease and Related Disorders*. Chapman and Hall, London.

Joseph, P., Bridgwater, J. A., Ramsden, S. S. & El Kabir, D. J. (1990) A psychiatric clinic for the single homeless in a primary care setting in inner London. *Psychiat. Bull.*, **14**, 270–1.

Jouandet, M. & Gazzaniga, M. S. (1979) The frontal lobes. In *Handbook of Behavioural Neurobiology*, Vol 2 (ed. M. S. Gazzaniga). Plenum, New York. pp. 225–59.

Jouriles, E. N., Murphy, C. M. & O'Leary, K. O. (1989) Interspousal aggression, marital discord, and child problems. *J. Consult. Clin. Psychol.*, **57**, 453–5.

Joyce, E. M. (1991) Cerebral blood flow and metabolism in affective disorders. *Internat. J. Geriat. Psychiat.*, **6**, 423–30.

Joyce, P. R. (1994) Predictors for treatment, response and treatment selection. *Curr. Opin. Psychiat.*, **7**, 26–9.

Joyce, P. R., Donal, R. A., Livesey, J. H. & Abbott, R. M. (1987) The prolactin response to metoclopramide is increased in depression and in euthymic rapid cycling bipolar patients. *Biol. Psychiat.*, **22**, 508–12.

Joyce, P. R., Oakley-Browne, M. A., Wells, J. E. *et al.* (1990) Birth cohort trends in major depression: increasing rates and earlier onset in New Zealand. *J. Affect. Disorders.*, **18**, 83–9.

Judd, F. K., Stone, J., Webber, J. E. *et al.* (1989) Depression following spinal cord injury. *Br. J. Psychiat.*, **54**, 668–71.

Kadden, R. M., Cooney, N. L., Getter, H. & Li, H. M. D. (1990) Matching alcoholics to coping skills or interactional therapies: post treatment results. *J. Consult. Clin. Psychol.*, **57**, 698–704.

Kaeser, A. C. & Cooper, B. (1971) The psychiatric out-patient, the general practitioner and the out-patient clinic; an operational study: a review. *Psychol. Med.*, **1**, 312–25.

Kagan, J., Reznick, J. S. & Snidman, N. (1988) Biological bases of childhood shyness. *Science*, **240**, 167–71.

Kahlbaum, K. L. (1973, orig. 1874) *Catatonia* (trans. G. Mora). Johns Hopkins, University Press, Baltimore.

Kahn, R. L. & Antonucci, T. C. (1980) Convoys over the life course: attachment, roles and social support. In *Life Span Development and Behaviour*, Vol. 3 (ed. P. B. Baltes & O. G. Brim). Academic Press, New York.

Kahne, M. J. (1968) Suicides in mental hospitals: a study of the effects of personnel and patient turnover. *J. Health Soc. Behav.*, **9**, 255–66.

Kaij, L. (1960) *Alcoholism in Twins*. Amquist & Wiksell, Stockholm.

Kaij, L., Malmquist, A. & Nilsson, A. (1969) Psychiatric aspects of spontaneous abortion–II: the importance of bereavement attachment and neurosis in early life. *J. Psychosom. Res.*, **13**, 53–9.

Kales, A., Soldatos, C. R., Bixteir, E. O. *et al.* (1982) Narcolepsy–cataplexy. *Arch. Neurol.*, **39**, 169–75.

Kalman, T. P. (1983) An overview of patient satisfaction with psychiatric treatment. *Hosp. Commun. Psychiat.*, **34**, 48–54.

Kandel, D. B. & Davies, M. (1986) Adult sequelae of adolescent depressive symptoms. *Arch. Gen. Psychiat.*, **43**, 255–62.

Kandel, D., Davies, M., Karus, D. & Yamaguchi, K. (1986) The consequences in young adulthood of adolescent drug involvement. *Arch. Gen. Psychiat*, **43**, 746–54.

Kane, J., Honigfeld, G., Singer, J. & Meltzer, H. Clozaril Collaborative Study Group (1988) Clozapine for the treatment-resistant schizophrenic. *Arch. Gen. Psychiat.*, **45**, 789–97.

Kanfer, F. H. & Karoly, P. (1972) Self control: a behaviouristic excursion into the lion's den. *Behav. Ther.*, **3**, 398–416.

Kanfer, F. & Saslow, G. (1965) Behavioural analysis: an alternative to diagnostic classification. *Arch. Gen. Psychiat.*, **12**, 529–38.

Kaplan, H. S. (1974) *The New Sex Therapy. Active Treatment of Sexual Dysfunction.* Brunner/Mazel, New York.

Kaponen, H. J. & Riekkinen, P. J. (1993) A prospective study of delirium in elderly patients admitted to a psychiatric hospital. *Psychol. Med.*, **23**, 103–9.

Kaponen, H., Stenback, U., Mattila, E. *et al.* (1989) Delirium in elderly persons admitted to a psychiatric hospital: Clinical cause during the acute stage and one-year follow-up. *Acta Psychiat. Scand.*, **79**, 579–85.

Karacan, I. & Howell, J. W. (1988) Narcolepsy. In *Sleep Disorders Diagnosis and Treatment* (ed. R. L. Williams., I Karacan & C. A. Moore). J Wiley & Sons, New York, pp. 87–105.

Karacan, I., Thornby, J. I. & Williams, R. L. (1983) Sleep disturbance: a community survey. In *Sleep/Wake Disorders: Natural History, Epidemiology, and Long-term Evolution* (ed. C. Guilleminault & E. Lugaresi). Raven Press, New York, pp. 37–60.

Karacan, I., Williams, R. L., Little, R. C. & Salis, P. J. (1973) Insomniacs. In *Sleep: Physiology, Biochemistry, Psychology, Pharmacology, Clinical Implications* (ed. W. Koella & P. Levin). Karger, Basel, pp. 120–132.

Kasanin, J. (1933/1994) The acute schizoaffective psychoses. *Am. J. Psychiat.*, **151**, 144–54.

Kashani, J. H., Niels, C. B., Hoeper, E. W. *et al.* (1987) Psychiatric disorders in a community sample of adolescents. *Am. J. Psychiat.*, **144**, 584–9.

Kashani, J. H. & Orvaschel, H. (1988) Anxiety disorders in mid-adolescence: a community sample. *Am. J. Psychiat.*, **145**, 960–4.

Kasovits, Y. G., Tsakiris, F., Marks, I. M. *et al.* (1986) Past history of anorexia nervosa in women with obsessive compulsive disorder. *Internat. J. Eat. Disorder*, **5**, 1069–75.

Katon, W., Kleinman, A. & Rosen, G. (1982) Depression and somatisation: A review. Part I. *Am. J. Med.*, **72**, 127–35.

Katon, W., Lin, E., Von Korff, M. *et al.* (1991) Somatization: a spectrum of severity. *Am. J. Psychiat.*, **148**, 34–40.

Katon, W., von Korff, M., Lin, E. *et al.* (1990) Distressed high utilisers of medical care: DSM-IIIR diagnoses and treatment needs. *Gen. Hosp. Psychiat.*, **12**, 355–63.

Katona, C. L. E. (1994) The management of depression in old age. In *Depression in Old Age*. John Wiley, Chichester, pp. 93–121.

Katschnig, H. (1986) Measuring life stress. In *Life Events and Psychiatric Disorders: Controversial Issues* (ed. H. Katschnig). Cambridge University Press, Cambridge, pp. 74–106.

Katz, M., Cole, J. O. & Lowery, H. A. (1969) Studies of the diagnostic process: the influence of symptom perception, past experience and ethnic background on diagnostic decision. *Am. J. Psychiat.*, **125**, 937–7.

Katz, R. & McGuffin, P. (1987) Neuroticism in familial depression. *Psychol. Med.*, **17**, 155–61.

Kavanagh, D. J. (1992) Recent developments in expressed emotion and schizophrenia. *Br. J. Psychiat.*, **160**, 601–20.

Kay, D. W. K., Beamish, P. & Roth, M. (1964) Old age mental disorders in Newcastle upon Tyne. Part I: A study of prevalence. *Br. J. Geriat. Psychiat.*, **110**, 146–58.

Kay, D. W. K., Henderson, A. S., Scott, R. *et al.* (1985) Dementia and depression among the elderly living in the Hobart community: the effect of the diagnostic criteria on the prevalence rates. *Psychol. Med.*, **15**, 771–88.

Kay, G., Sargeant, M., McGuffin, P. *et al.* (1993) The lymphoblast beta-adrenergic receptor in bipolar depressed patients: characterisation and down regulation. *J. Affect. Disorders*, **27**, 163–72.

Kazdin, A. E. (1990) Childhood depression. *J. Child Psychol. Psychiat.*, **31**, 121–60.

Kazdin, A. E., Esveldt-Dawson, K., French, N. H. & Unis, A. S. (1987) Effects of parent management training and problem-solving skills training combined in the treatment of antisocial child behaviour. *J. Am. Acad. Child Adol Psychiat.*, **26**, 416–24.

Kazdin, A. E., Matson, J. L. & Senatore, V. (1983) Assessment of depression in mentally retarded adults. *Am. J. Psychiat.*, **140**, 1040–3.

Kearns, N. P., Cruickshank, C. A., McGuigan, K. J. *et al.* (1982) A comparison of depression rating scales. *Br. J. Psychiat.*, **141**, 45–9.

Keck, P. E., McElroy, S. L., Strakowski, S. M. & West, S. A. (1994) Pharmacologic treatment of schizoaffective disorder. *Psychopharmacol.*, **114**, 529–38.

Kellam, S. G., Rebok, G. W., Ialongo, N. & Mayer, L. S. (1994) The course and malleability of aggressive behaviour from early first grade into middle school: results of developmental epidemiologically-based trial. *J. Child Psychol Psychiat.*, **35**, 259–81.

Keller, O. J. & Vedder, C. B. (1968) The crimes that old people commit. *The Gerontologist*, **8**, 43–50.

Kelly, R. (1975) The post traumatic syndrome. *Forensic Sci.*, **6**, 17–24.

Kelly, W. F., Checkley, S. A. & Bender, D. A. (1989) Cushing's syndrome, tryptophan and depression. *Br. J. Psychiat.*, **142**, 16–19.

Kennedy, P. (1971) Efficacy of a regional poison treatment centre. *Br. Med. J.*, **iv**, 255–7.

Kennedy, W. A. (1965) School phobia: rapid treatment of fifty cases. *J. Abnorm. Psychol.*, **70**, 285–9.

Kendell, R. E. (1968) *The Classification of Depressive Illness*. OUP, Oxford, Maudsley Monograph No. 18.

Kendell, R. E. (1973) Psychiatric diagnoses: a study of how they are made. *Br. J. Psychiat.*, **122**, 437–45.

Kendell, R. E. (1975) *The Role of Diagnosis in Psychiatry*. Blackwell Scientific Publications, Oxford.

Kendell, R. E. (1976) The classification of depressions: A review of contemporary confusion. *Br. J. Psychiat.*, **129**, 15–28.

Kendell, R. E. (1979) Alcoholism: a medical or political problem: *Br. Med. J.*, **i**, 367–71.

Kendell, R. (1983) Hysteria. *Med. Internat.*, **34**, 1614–17.

Kendell, R. E. (1984) The beneficial consequences of the United Kingdom's declining per capita consumption of alcohol in 1979–1982. *Alcohol and Alcoholism*, **19**, 271–276.

Kendell, R. E. (1989) Clinical Validity. *Psychol. Med.*, **19**, 45–55.

Kendell, R. E. (1991*a*) Chronic fatigue, viruses, and depression. *Lancet*, **337**, 160–2.

Kendell, R. E. (1991*b*) Suicide in pregnancy and the puerperium. *Br. Med. J.*, **302**, 126–7.

Kendell, R. E. (1993) Paranoid and other psychoses. In *Companion to Psychiatric Studies*. Churchill Livingstone, Edinburgh, pp. 459–71.

Kendell, R. E., Chalmers, J. C. & Platz, C. (1987) Epidemiology of puerperal psychosis. *Br. J. Psychiat.*, **150**, 662–73.

Kendell, R. E., de Roumani, M. & Ritson, E. B. (1983) Influence of an increase in excise duty on alcohol consumption and its adverse effects. *Br. Med. J.*, **ii**, 809–11.

Kendell, R., Di Scipio, W. (1968) Eysenck Personality Inventory scores of patients with depressive illness. *Br. J. Psychiat.*, **114**, 767–70.

Kendell, R. & Di Scipio, W. (1970) Obsessional symptoms and obsessional personality traits in depressive illness. *Psychol. Med.*, **1**, 65–72.

Kendell, R. E. & Gourlay, J. (1970) The clinical distinction between the affective psychoses and schizophrenia. *Br. J. Psychiat.*, **117**, 261–6.

Kendell, R. E., Malcolm, D. E. & Adams, W. (1993) The problem of detecting changes in the incidence of schizophrenia. *Br. J. Psychiat.*, **162**, 212–18.

Kendell, R. E., Pichot, P. & von Cranach, M. (1974) Diagnostic criteria of English, French and German psychiatrists. *Psychol. Med.*, **4**, 187–95.

Kendell, R. E., Rennie, D., Clarke, J. A. & Dean, C. (1981) The social and obstetric correlates of psychiatric admission in the puerperium. *Psychol. Med.*, **11**, 341–350.

Kendell, R. E., Wainwright, S., Hailey, A. & Shannon, B. (1976) The influence of childbirth on psychiatric morbidity. *Psychol. Med.*, **6**, 297–302.

Kendler, K. S. (1980) The nosological validity of paranoia. *Arch. Gen. Psychiat.*, **37**, 699–706.

Kendler, K. S. (1985) A twin study of individuals with both schizophrenia and alcoholism. *Br. J. Psychiat.*, **147**, 48–53.

Kendler, K. S. (1991) Mood-incongruent psychotic affective illness. *Arch. Gen. Psychiat.*, **48**, 362–9.

Kendler, K. S. & Diehl, S. R. (1993) The genetics of schizophrenia: a current, genetic-epidemiologic perspective. *Schiz. Bull.*, **19**, 261–85.

Kendler, K. S., Glazer, W. M. & Morgenstern, H. (1983) Dimensions of delusional experience. *Am. J. Psychiat.*, **140**, 466–9.

Kendler, K. S. & Gruenberg, M. A. (1984) An independent analysis of the Copenhagen sample of the Danish Adoption Study of schizophrenia. *Arch. Gen. Psychiat.*, **41**, 555–64.

Kendler, K. S., Heath, A. C., Neale, M. C. *et al.* (1992) A population-based twin study of alcoholism in women. *JAMA.*, **268**, 1877–82.

Kendler, K. S., Kessler, R. C., Heath, A. C. *et al.* (1991) Coping: a genetic epidemiological investigation. *Psychol. Med.*, **21**, 337–46.

Kendler, K. S., McGuire, M., Gruenberg, A. M. *et al.* (1993*a*) The Roscommon family study I. Methods, diagnosis of probands and risk of schizophrenia in relatives. *Arch. Gen. Psychiat.*, **50**, 527–40.

Kendler, K. S., McGuire, M., Gruenberg, A. M. *et al.* (1993*b*) The Roscommon family study. II. The risk of nonschizophrenic noneffective psychoses in relatives. *Arch. Gen. Psychiat.*, **50**, 645–52.

Kendler, K. S., McLean, C., Neale, M. *et al.* (1991) The genetic epidemiology of bulimia nervosa. *Am. J. Psychiat.*, **148**, 1627–37.

Kendler, K., Neale, J., Kessler, R. *et al.* (1992) Generalised anxiety disorder in women: a population based twin study. *Arch. Gen. Psychiat.*, **49**, 267–72.

Kendler, K., Neale, M., Kessler, R. *et al.* (1993*c*) Panic disorder in women: a population-based twin study. *Psychol. Med.*, **23**, 397–406.

Kendler, K., Neale, M., Kessler, R. *et al.* (1993*d*) Major depression and phobias: the genetic and environmental sources of co-morbidity. *Psychol. Med.*, **23**, 361–71.

Kendler, K. S. & Robinette, C. D. (1983) Schizophrenia in the National Academy of Science-National Research Council Twin Registry. *Am. J. Psychiat.*, **140**, 1551–63.

Kendler, K.S., Silberg, J. L., Neale, M. C. *et al* (1991) The family history method: whose psychiatric history is measured? *Am. J. Psychiat.*, **148**, 1501–4.

Kendrick, T., Sibbald, B., Addington-Hall, J. *et al.* (1993) distribution of mental health professionals working on site in English and Welsh general practices. *Br. Med. J.*, **307**, 544–6.

Kendrick, A., Sibbald, B., Burns, T. & Freeling, P. (1991) Role of general practitioners in care of long term mentally ill patients. *Br. Med. J.*, **302**, 508–11.

Kenyon, F. (1964) Hypochondriasis: a clinical study. *Br. J. Psychiat.*, **110**, 478–88.

Kernberg, O. (1975) *Borderline Conditions and Pathological Narcissism.* Jason Aronson, New York.

Kernberg, O. (1980) *Internal World and External Reality.* Jason Aronson, New York.

Kerr, M. P. (1994) Antidepressant prescribing: a comparison between general practitioners and psychiatrists. *Br. J. Gen. Pract.*, June, 275–6.

Kerwin, R. W. (1990) Monoamine oxidase inhibitors. 30 years of progress? *Internat. Rev. Psychiat.*, **2**, 179–85.

Kerwin, R. W. (1992) A history of frontal and temporal lobe aspects of the neuropharacology of schizophrenia. *J. Psychopharmacol* **6**(2), 186–96.

Kerwin, R. W. (1994) The new atypical antipsychotics. *Br. J. Psychiat.*, **164**, 141–8.

Kerwin, R. W., Patel S. & Meldrum, B. (1990) Receptor autoradiographic characterisation of glutamate receptors in human and schizophrenic hippocampus. *Neuroscience*, **39**, 25–32.

Kessel, N. & Grossman, G. (1965) Suicide in alcoholics. *Br. Med. J.*, **ii**, 1671–2.

Kessler, R. C., Brown, R. L. & Broman, C. L. (1981) Sex differences on psychiatric help-seeking: evidence from four large surveys. *J. Health Soc. Behav.*, **22**, 49–64.

Kessler, R. C., McGonagle, K. A., Zhao, S. *et al.* (1994) Lifetime and 12 month prevalence of DSM-IIIR psychiatric disorders in the United States. *Arch. Gen. Psychiat.*, **51**, 8–19.

Ketter, T. A., Pazzaglia, P. J. & Post, R. M. (1992) Synergy of carbamazepine and valproic acid in affective illness. Case report and review of the literature. *J. Clin. Psychopharmacol.*, **12**, 276–81.

Kety, S. S. (1974) From rationalisation to reason. *Am. J. Psychiat.*, **131**, 957–63.

Kety, S. S., Rosenthal, L., Wender, P. H. *et al.* (1975) Mental illness in the biological and adoptive families of adopted individuals who have become schizophrenic. In *Genetic Research is Psychiatry* (ed. R. R. Fieve, D. Rosenthal & H. Brill). Johns Hopkins University Press, Baltimore, pp. 147–65.

Kety, S. S. *et al.* (1976) Mental illness in the biological and adoptive families of individuals who have become schizophrenic. *Behav. Genet.*, **6**, 219–25.

Kety, S. S., Wender, P. H., Jacobsen, B. *et al.* (1994) Mental illness in the biological relatives of schizophrenic adoptees. Replication of the Copenhagen study in the rest of Denmark. *Arch. Gen. Psychiat.*, **51**, 442–55.

Keys, A., Brozak, J., Henshall, A. *et al.* (1950) *The Biology of Human Starvation*, vol 11. University of Minnesota Press, Minneapolis, pp. 850–7.

Khantzian, E. J. (1985) The self medication hypothesis of addictive disorders: focus on heroin and cocaine dependence. *Am. J. Psychiat.*, **142**, 1259–64.

Khantzian, E. J. & Treece, C. (1985) DSM-III psychiatric diagnosis of narcotic addicts. Recent findings. *Arch. Gen. Psychiat.*, **42**, 1067–71.

Kiesler, C. (1982) Mental hospitals and alternative care. *Am. Psychol.*, **4**, 354–60.

Kiloh, L. G. (1980) ECT, its place and value in present day psychiatry. In *Advances in Human Psychopharmacology* (ed. G. Burrows & J. S. Werry). Aijar Press, Greenwich.

Kiloh, L. G., Andrews, G. & Neilson, M. (1988) The long-term outcome of depressive illness. *Br. J. Psychiat.*, **153**, 752–7.

Kiloh, L. G., Ball, R. B. & Garside, R. F. (1962) Prognostic factors in the treatment of depressive states with imipramine. *Br. Med. J.*, **i**, 1225–7.

Kiloh, L. G. & Garside, R. F. (1963) The independence of neurotic depression and endogenous depression. *Br. J. Psychiat.*, **109**, 451–63.

King, E. & Barraclough, B. (1990) Violent death and mental illness. A study of a single catchment area over 8 years. *Br. J. Psychiat.*, **156**, 714–20.

King, M. B. (1991) The natural history of eating pathology in attenders to primary medical care. *Int. J. Eat. Disorders*, **10**, 379–87.

King, M. B. (1993) *AIDS, HIV and Mental Health*. Cambridge University Press, Cambridge.

Kingdon, D. (1989) Mental health services: results of a survey of English district plans. *Psychiat. Bull.*, **13**, 77–8.

Kingdon, D. G. & Turkington D. (1994) *Cognitive Behaviour Therapy of Schizophrenia*. Lawrence Erlbaum, Hove.

Kingdon, D., Turkington, D. & John, C. (1994) Cognitive behaviour therapy of schizophrenia. The amenability of delusions and hallucinations to reasoning [editorial]. *Br. J. Psychiat.*, **164**, 581–7.

Kingsley, S. & Towell, D. (1989) Designing local processes for service development (paper 4) In *Managing Psychiatric Services in Transition*. King's Fund Centre, London.

Kinsey, A. C., Pomeroy, W. B. & Martin, C. E. (1948) *Sexual Behaviour in the Human Male*. Saunders, Philadelphia.

Kinsey, A. C., Pomeroy, W. B., Martin, C. E. & Gebhard, P. H. (1953) *Sexual Behaviour in the Human Female*. Saunders, Philadelphia.

Kleber, H. D., Weissman, M. M., Rounsaville, B. J. *et al.* (1983) Imipramine as treatment for depression in addicts. *Arch. Gen. Psychiat.*, **40**, 649–53.

Klee, H., Faugier, J., Hayes, C. *et al.* (1990) AIDs related risk behaviour, polydrug use and temazepam. *Br. J. Addiction.*, **85**, 1125–32.

Klein, D. (1964) Delineation of two drug responsive anxiety syndromes. *Psychopharmacologia.*, **5**, 397–408.

Klein, D. (1993) False suffocation alarms, spontaneous panics, and related conditions: an integrative hypothesis. *Arch. Gen. Psychiat.*, **50**, 306–17.

Klein, D. (1994) Pregnancy and panic disorder. *J. Clin. Psychiat.*, **55**, 293–4.

Klein, D. N., Depue, R. A. & Slater, J. F. (1985) Cyclothymia in the adolescent offspring of parents with bipolar affective disorder. *J. Abnorm. Psychol.*, **94**, 115–27.

Klein, D. F., Mannuzza, S., Chapman, T. & Fyer, A. J. (1992*a*) Child panic revisited. *J. Am. Acad. Child Adol. Psychiat.*, **31**, 112–16.

Klein, M. (1934) *A Contribution to the Psychogenesis 1921–1945* (1948). Hogarth Press, London, 282–310.

Klein, M. (1948) *Contributions to Psycho-analysis*. Hogarth, London.

Klein, M. (1946) Notes on some schizoid mechanisms. *The Writings of Melanie Klein: Volume III: Envy and gratitude and other works*. Hogarth Press, London, 1975, pp. 1–24.

Klein, M. (1955) On identification. *The Writings of Melanie Klein: volume III: Envy and gratitude and other works*. Hogarth Press, London, 1975, pp. 141–25

Klein, R. (1991) The politics of change. *Br. Med. J.*, **320**, 1102–3.

Klein, R. G. (1994) Anxiety disorders. In *Child and Adolescent Psychiatry: Modern Approaches*, third edn. (ed. M. Rutter, E. Taylor & L. Hersov). Blackwell Scientific, Oxford. 351–74.

Klein, R. G., Koplewicz, H. S. & Kanner, A. (1992*b*) Imipramine treatment of children with separation anxiety disorder. *J. Am. Acad. Child Adol., Psychiat.*, **31**, 21–8.

Kleinman, A. (1986) *Social Origins of Stress and Disease: Depression, Neurasthenia and Pain in Modern China*. Yale University Press, New Haven.

Kleist, K. (1930) (Translated 1987) Alogical thought disorder. In *The Clinical Roots of the Schizophrenic Concept* (ed. J. Cutting & M. Shepherd). Cambridge University Press, Cambridge, pp. 75–79.

Klerman, G. L. (1984) *Interpersonal Psychotherapy of Depressions*. Basic Books, New York.

742

Klerman, G. L. (1988) Drugs and psychotherapy. In *Handbook of Psychotherapy and Behaviour change* (ed. S. B. Garfield & A. B. Bergen). John Wiley, New York, pp. 773–814.

Klerman, G. L. Lavori, P. W., Rice, J. *et al.* (1985) Birth-cohort trends in rates of major depressive disorder among relatives of patients with affective disorder. *Arch. Gen. Psychiat.*, **421**, 689–93.

Klerman, G. L., De Mascio, A., Weissman, M. M. *et al.* (1974) Treatment of depression by drugs and psychotherapy. *Am. J. Psychiat.*, **131**, 186–91.

Klerman, G. L. & Weissman, M. M. (1989) Increasing rates of depression. *J. Am. Med. Assoc.*, **261**, 2229–35.

Kligman, D. & Goldberg, D. A. (1975) Temporal lobe epilepsy and aggression. *J. Nerv. Ment. Disease.*, **160**, 324–41.

Klimes, I., Mayou, R. A., Pearce, M. J. *et al.* (1990) Psychological treatment for atypical non-cardiac chest pain: a controlled evaluation. *Psychol. Med.*, **20**, 605–11.

Kline, P. (1993) *The Handbook of Psychological Testing*. Routledge, London.

Knesper, D. J. (1978) Psychiatric manpower for state mental hospitals. a continuing dilemma. *Arch. Gen. Psychiat.*, **35**, 19–24.

Knop, J., Teasdale, T., Goodwin, D. W. *et al.* (1988) Genetic aspects of alcoholism. Proceedings of the satellite symposium on alcohol and genetics. In *Genetic Aspects of Alcoholism: Proceedings of the Satellite Symposium on Alcohol and Genetics* 137th edn. (ed. K. Kiianmaa, B. Tabakoff & T. Saito). The Finnish Foundation for Alcohol Studies, 117–26.

Koch, J. A. (1891) *Die Psychopathischen Minderwertigkeiten*. Ravensburg: Maier.

Koehler, K. (1979) First rank of schizophrenia: Questions concerning clinical boundaries. *Br. J. Psychiat.*, **134**, 236–48.

Koenigsberg, H., Pollak C., Fine, J. & Kakuma, T. (1994) Cardiac and respiratory activity in panic disorder: effects of sleep and sleep lactate infusions. *Am. J. Psychiat.*, **151**, 1148–52.

Koenraadt, F. (1993) Forensic mental hospitals according to Dutch standards. *Crim. Behav. Ment. Health.*, **3**, 322–34.

Kohler, C., Haglund, L., Ogren, S. O. *et al.* (1981) Regional blockade by neuroleptic drugs of *in vivo* ^{2}H spiperone binding in the rat brain. Relation to blockade of apomorphine induced hyperactivity and stereotypes. *J. Neur. Trans.*, **52**, 163–73.

Kohn, M. L. (1973) Social class and schizophrenia: a critical review and reformulation. *Schiz. Bull.*, **7**, 60–79.

Kohut, H. (1971) *The Analysis of the Self: a Systematic Approach to the Psychoanalytic Treatment of Narcissistic Personality Disorders*. International Universities Press, New York.

Kohut, H. (1977) *The Restoration of the Self*. International Universities Press, New York.

Kolb, L. (1987) A neuropsychological hypothesis explaining posttraumatic stress disorder. *Am. J. Psychiat.*, **144**, 989–95.

Koller, H., Richardsons, S. A., Katz, M. & McClaren, J. (1983) Behavioural disturbance since childhood among a 5-year birth cohort of all mentally retarded young adults in a city. *Am. J. Ment. Defic.*, **87**, 386–95.

Kolvin, I., Barrett, M. L., Bhate, S. R. *et al.* (1991) The Newcastle Child Depression Project: diagnosis and classification of depression. *Br. J. Psychiat.*, **159** (suppl. 11), 9–21.

Kolvin, I. & Fundudis, T. (1981) Effective mute children: psychological development and background factors. *J. Child Psychol. Psychiat.*, **22**, 219–32.

Kolvin, I., Garside, R. F., Nicol, A. R., Macmillan, A., Wostenholme, F. & Leitch, I. M. (1981) *Help Starts Here*. Tavistock, London.

Kosten, T. R., Morgan, C. M., Falcione, J. *et al.* (1992) Pharmacotherapy for cocaine abusing methadone maintained patients using amantadine or desipramine. *Arch. Gen. Psychiat.*, **49**, 893–4.

Kovacs, M. (1985) The natural history and course of depressive disorders in childhood. *Psychiat. Annals.*, **15**, 387–9.

Kovacs, M., Feinberg, T. L., Crouse-Novak, M. *et al.* (1984*a*) Depressive disorders in childhood. I. A longitudinal prospective study of characteristics and recovery. *Arch. Gen. Psychiat.*, **41**, 229–37.

Kovacs, M., Feinberg, T. L., Crouse-Novak, M. *et al.* (1984*b*) Depressive disorders in childhood. A longitudinal study of the risk for a subsequent major depression. *Arch. Gen. Psychiat.*, **41**, 643–9.

Kovaks, M., Gatsonis, C., Paulauskas, S. L. & Richards, C. (1989) Depressive disorders in children IV. A longitudinal study of comorbidity with a risk for anxiety disorders. *Arch. Gen. Psychiatry*, **46**, 776–82.

Kozak, M. & Foa, E. (1994) Obsessive, over-valued ideas, and delusions in obsessive-compulsive disorder. *Behav. Res. Ther.*, **32**, 342–53.

Kraepelin, E. (1896*a*) Der psycholgische Versuch in der Psychiatrie. *Psycholog. Arbeit*, **1**.

Kraepelin, E. (1896*b*) *Psychiatrie*. 5th edition. Barth, Leipzig.

Kraepelin, E. (1913) Psychiatrie, Vol 3, Part 2. Translated as *Dementia Praecox and Paraphrenia*. Livingstone, Edinburgh.

Kraepelin, E. (1919) *Dementia Praecox and Paraphrenia* (translated R. M. Barclay), E & S Livingstone, Edinburgh.

Kraepelin, E. (1921) *Manic-Depressive Insanity and Paranoia* (translated R. M. Barclay). E & S Livingstone, Edinburgh.

Kramer, M. (1961) Some problems for international research suggested by observations as differences in first admission rates to the mental hospitals of England and Wales and of the United States. In *Proceedings of the Third World Congress of Psychiatry*, **3**, 153–60.

Kratochwill, T. R. (1981) *Selective Mutism*. Lawrence Erlbaum, New York.

Krauthammer, C. & Klerman, G. L. (1978) Secondary mania. *Arch. Gen. Psychiat.*, **35**, 1333–9.

Krch, F. D. (1991) Epidemiologie des troubles des conduites alimentaires en tchecoslovaquie. *Neuropsychiatrie de L'Enfance*, **39**, 311–22.

Kreitman, N. (1976) The coal gas story. *Br. J. Prevent. Soc. Med.*, **30**, 86–93.

Kreitman, N. (1977) *Parasuicide*. Wiley, London.

Kreitman, N. (1988) Suicide, age and marital status. *Psychol. Med.*, **18**, 121–8.

Kreitman, N., Sainsbury, P., Morrisey, J. *et al.* (1961) The reliability of psychiatric assessment: an analysis. *J. Ment. Sci.*, **107**, 887–908.

Kretschmer, E. (1918) *Die Sensitive Beziehungswan*. Springer, Berlin.

Kristenson, H., Ohlin, H., Hulten-Nosslin, M. *et al.* (1983) Identification and intervention of heavy drinking in middle-aged men: results and follow-up of 24–60 months of long-term study with randomised controls. *Alcohol Alcoholism: Clin. Exp. Res.*, **7**, 203–9.

Kroenke, K. & Mangelsdorff, D. (1989) Common symptoms in ambulatory care: incidence, evaluation, therapy and outcome. *Am. J. Med.*, **86**, 262–6.

Kroenke, K. & Price, R. (1993) Symptoms in the community: prevalence, classification and psychiatric comorbidity. *Arch. Int. Med.*, **153**, 2474–80.

Kroenke, K., Wood, D., Mangelsdorff, D. *et al.* (1988) Chronic fatigue in primary care: prevalence, patient characteristics and outcome. *J. Am. Med Assoc.*, **260**, 929–34.

Kroll, J., Carey, K., Hagedorn, D. *et al.* (1986) A survey of homeless adults in urban shelters. *Hosp. Comm. Psychiat.*, **37**, 283–6.

Krug, D. A., Arick, J. R. & Almond, P. J. (1988) *Autism Behaviour Checklist. Autism Screening Instrument for Educational Planning*. ASIEP Education Company, Portland, OR.

Krupnick, J. L. & Pincus, H. A. (1992) The cost-effectiveness of psychotherapy: A plan for research. *Am. J. Psychiat.*, **149**, 1295–305.

Kua, E. H. (1993) The depressed elderly Chinese living in the community. A five-year follow-up study. *Internat. J. Geriat. Psychiat.*, **8**, 427–30.

Kuipers, L. & Bebbington, P. E. (1988) Expressed emotion research in schizophrenia: theoretical and clinical implications. *Psychol. Med.*, **18**, 893–910.

Kuipers, L. & Bebbington, P. E. (1990) *Working in Partnership: Clinicians and Carers in the Management of Longstanding Mental Illness*. Heinemann Medical. Oxford.

Kuipers, L. & Bebbington, P. (1991) *Working in Partnership: Clinicians and Carers in the Management of Long-term Mental Illness*. Heinemann, Oxford.

Kuipers, L., Leff, J. P. & Lam, D. (1992) *Family Work for Schizophrenia: A Practical Guide*. Gaskell, London.

Kumar, R. (1982) Neurotic disorders in childbearing women. In *Motherhood and Mental Illness* (ed. I. F. Brockington & R. Kumar). Academic Press, London, pp. 71–118.

Kumar, R. (1992) Mentally ill mothers and their babies: what are the benefits and risks of joint hospital admission? In *Dilemmas in the Management of Psychiatric Patients* (ed. K. Hawton & P. J. Cowen). Oxford University Press, Oxford.

Kumar, R. (1994) Postnatal mental illness: a transcultural perspective. *Soc. Psychiat. Psychiat. Epidemiol.*, **29**, 250–64.

Kumar, R. & Hipwell, A. (1994) Implications for the infant of maternal puerperal psychiatric disorders. In *Child and Adolescent Psychiatry* 3rd edn. (ed. M. Rutter, L. Hersov & E. Taylor) Blackwell, Oxford, pp. 759–75.

Kumar R. & Robson, K. M. (1978) Previous induced abortion and ante-natal depression in primiparae: preliminary report of a survey of mental health in pregnancy. *Psychol. Med.*, **8**, 711–15.

Kumar, R. & Robson, K. M. (1984) A prospective study of emotional disorders in child-bearing women. *Br. J. Psychiat.*, **144**, 35–47.

Kupfer, D. J., Frank, E., Perel, J. M. *et al.* (1992) 5-year outcome for maintenance therapies in recurrent depression. *Arch. Gen. Psychiat.*, **49**, 769–73.

Kupfer, D. J., Spiker, D. G., Rossi, A. *et al* (1983) Recent diagnostic and treatment advances in REM sleep and depression. In *Treatment of Depression: Old Controversies and New Approaches* (ed. P. Clayton & J. Barrett). Raven Press, New York, pp. 31–52.

Kushlick, A. & Blunden, R. (1974) The epidemiology of mental subnormality. In *Mental Deficiency The Changing Outlook*. (ed. A. Clarke & A. B. D. Clarke). Methuen, London.

Lacey, J. H. (1983) Bulimia nervosa, binge eating and psychogenic vomiting: a controlled treatment study and long-term outcome. *Br. Med. J.*, **286**, 1609–13.

Lacey, J. H. & Moureli, E. (1986) Bulimic alcoholics: some features of a clinical subgroup. *Br. J. Addiction*, **81**, 389–93.

Lacey, J. H. & Smith, G. (1987) Bulimia nervosa: the impact of pregnancy on mother and her baby. *Br. J. Psychiat.*, **150**, 777–81.

Laczko, F. (1990) New poverty and the old poor: pensioner's income in the European Community. *Ageing and Society*, **10**, 261–77.

Ladd, G. W. (1990) Having friends, keeping friends, making friends, and being liked by peers in the classroom: predictors of children's early school adjustment? *Child Devel.*, **61**, 1081–100.

Lader, M. (1982) Some newer antidepressants. *Hosp. Update*, **8**, 896–902.

Lader, M. (1983) *Introduction to Psychopharmacology*. Scope Publications (Upjohn), Michigan.

Lader, M. (1989) Benzodiazepine dependence. *Int. Rev. Psychiat.*, **1**, 149–56.

Lader, M. & Bhanji, S. (1980) Physiological and psychological effects of antidepressants in man. In *Psychotropic Agents Part 1. Antipsychotics and Antidepressants* (ed. F. Hoffmeister & G. Stille). Springer, Berlin, pp. 573–82.

Lader, M. & Harrington, R. (1990) *Biological Treatment in Psychiatry*. Oxford Medical Publications, Oxford.

Lader, M. & Sartorius, N. (1968) Anxiety in patients with hysterical conversion symptoms. *J. Neurol. Neursurg. Psychiat.*, **31**, 490–5.

Laegreid, L., Olegard, R., Walstrom, J. & Conrade, N. (1989) Teratogenic effects of benzodiazepine use during pregnancy. *J. Pediatr.*, **144**, 126–31.

Laessle, R. G., Zoettl, H. & Pirke, K. (1987) Meta-analysis of treatment studies for bulimia. *Internat. J. Eat. Disorders*, **11**, 97–110.

Laidlaw, J. D. D. & Khin-Maung-Zaw. (1993) *A Textbook of Epilepsy*. Churchill Livingstone, London.

Laidlaw, J., Richens, A. & Chadwick, D. (1993) *A Textbook of Epilepsy*. Churchill Livingstone, London.

Lam, D. (1991) Psychosocial family intervention in schizophrenia: a review of empirical studies. *Psychol. Med.*, **21**, 423–41.

Lamb, H. (1984) Deinstitutionalisation and the homeless mentally ill. *Hosp. Community Psychiat.*, **35**, 899–907.

Lancet Editorial (1985) Snoring and sleepiness. *Lancet*, **ii**, 925–6.

Lancet Editorial (1990) Caring for disabled people's health in Britain. *Lancet*, **335**, 577–8.

Landoldt, H. (1953) Some clinical electroencephalographic correlations in epileptic psychoses (Twilight States). *Electroencephalograph. Clin. Neurophysiol.*, **5**, 121.

Langer, S. Z., Galzin, A. M., Lee, C. R. *et al.* (1980) Antidepressant binding sites in brain and platelets. In *Antidepressants and Receptor Function*. CIBA Foundation Symposium Series, **123**, 3–29.

Langevin, R. & Stancer, H. (1979) Evidence that depression rating scales primarily measure a social undesirability response set. *Acta Psychiat. Scand.*, **59**, 70–79.

Langfeldt, G. (1939) *The Schizophreniform States*. Oxford University Press, Oxford.

Langley, G. E. & Bayatti, N. (1984) Suicides in Exe Vale Hospital 1972–1981. *Br. J. Psychiat.*, **145**, 463–7.

Langsley, D., Flomenhaft, K. & Machotka, P. (1969) Follow-up evaluation of family crisis therapy. *Am. J. Orthopsychiat.*, **39**, 753–9.

Lanktree, C., Biere, J. & Zaidi, L. (1991) Incidence and impact of sexual abuse in child out-patient sample: the role of direct enquiry. *Child Abuse & Neglect*, **15**, 447–53.

Lantos, P. & Cairns, N. (1994) The neuropathology of Alzheimer's disease. In *Dementia* (ed. A. Burns & R. Levy). Chapman & Hall Medical, London, pp. 185–208.

Larkin, B. A., Copeland, J. R. M., Dewey, M. E. *et al.* (1992) The natural history of neurotic disorder in an elderly urban population. Findings from the Liverpool study of continuing health in the community. *Br. J. Psychiat.*, **160**, 681–6.

Larsen, P. J., Hoien, T., Lundberg, I. & Odegaard, H. (1990) MRI evaluation of the size and symmetry of the planum temporale in adolescents with developmental dyslexia. *Brain & Language*, **39**, 289–300.

Lascelles, R. G. (1966) Atypical facial pain and depression. *Br. J. Psychiat.*, **112**, 651–9.

Lasègue, C. (1873) De l'anorexie hysterique. *Archieves Générales de Médecine*, **i**, 385–403.

Last, C. G., Hersen, M., Kazdin, A. *et al.* (1991) Anxiety disorders in children and their families. *Arch. Gen. Psychiat.*, **48**, 928–34.

Last, C. G., Strauss, C. C. & Francis, G. (1987) Comorbidity among childhood anxiety disorders. *J. Nerv. Ment. Disease*, **175**, 726–30.

Lavori, P. W., Klerman, G. L., Keller, M. B. *et al.* (1987) Age-period-cohort analysis of secular trends in onset of major depression: Findings in siblings of patients with major affective disorder. *J. Psychiat. Res.*, **21**, 23–35.

Law Commission (1991) Mentally Incapacitated Adults and Decision Making: an Overview. Consultation Paper No. 119. HMSO, London.

Lawrence, K. M., De Paermentier, F., Cheetham, S. C. *et al* (1990) Brain 5-HT uptake sites and labelled with (^{3}H) parozetine in antidepressant-free depressed suicides. *Brain Research*, **526**, 17–22.

Laws, A. (Ed.) (1989) *Relapse Prevention with Sex Offenders*. The Guilford Press, New York.

Lazarus, A. A. (1968) Learning theory and the treatment of depression. *Behav. Res. Ther.*, **6**, 83–9.

Lazare, A. (1973) Hidden conceptual models in clinical psychiatry. *N. Eng. J. Med.*, **288**, 345–51.

Lazarus, R. D. & Folkman, S. (1984) *Stress Appraisal and Coping*. Springer, New York.

Lazare, A. & Klerman, G. (1968) Hysteria and depression: The frequency and significance of hysterical personality features in hospitalised depressed women. *Am. J. Psychiat.*, **124**, Suppl., 48–56.

LeBlanc, M. & Fechette, M. (1989) *Male Criminal Acitivity from Childhood Through Youth*. Springer-Verlag, New York.

Lebuffe, F., Granter, S. & Wise, T. (1979) The Virginia Commitment Law: clinical characteristics of patients hospitalised involuntarily by court order. *Bull. Am. Acad. Psychiat.*, **7**, 411–21.

Leckman, J. F. & Cohen, D. J. (1994) Tic disorders. In *Child and Adolescent Psychiatry: Modern Approaches*, third edn (ed. M. Rutter, E. Taylor & L. Hersov). Blackwell Scientific, Oxford, pp. 455–66.

Leckman, J. F., Hardin, M. T., Riddle, M. A. *et al.* (1991) Clonidine treatment of Gilles de la Tourette's syndrome. *Arch. Gen. Psychiat.*, **48**, 324–8.

Leckman, J. F., Walker, D. E. & Cohen, D. J. (1993) Premonitory urges in Tourette's syndrome. *Am. J. Psychiat.*, **150**, 98–102.

Leckman, J., Weissman, M., Merikangas, K. *et al.* (1983) Panic disorder and major depression; increased risk of depression, alcoholism, panic and phobic disorders in families of depressed probands with panic disorder. *Arch. Gen. Psychiat.*, **40**, 1055–60.

Le Couteur, A., Rutter, M., Lord, C. *et al.* (1989) Autism Diagnostic Interview. A standardised investigator based instrument. *J. Autism Devel. Disorder*, **19**, 363–87.

Lee, S., Chiu, H. F. K. & Chen, C.-N (1989) Anorexia nervosa in Hong Kong – Why not more in Chinese? *Br. J. Psychiat.*, **154**, 683–8.

Lee, A. S. & Murray, R. M. (1988) The long-term outcome of Maudsley depressives. *Br. J. Psychiat.*, **153**, 741–51.

Leff, J. (1978) Psychiatrists versus patients concepts of unpleasant emotions. *Br. J. Psychiat.*, **133**, 306–13.

Leff, J. P. (1981) *Psychiatry Around the Globe: A Transcultural View.* Dekker, New York.

Leff, J. P., Hirsch, S. R., Rohde, P. *et al.* (1973) Life events and maintenance therapy in schizophrenic relapse. *Br. J. Psychiat.*, **123**, 659–60.

Leff, J., Kuipers, L., Berkowtiz, R. *et al.* (1982) A controlled trial of intervention in the families of schizophrenic patients. *Br. J. Psychiat.*, **141**, 121–34.

Leff, J., Sartorius, N., Jablensky, A. *et al.* (1992) The International Pilot Study of Schizophrenia: five-year follow-up findings. *Psychol. Med.*, **22**, 131–45.

Leff, J. P. & Vaughn, C. (1985) *Expressed Emotions in Families.* The Guilford Press, New York.

Le Grange, D., Eisler, I., Dare, C. & Russell, G. F. M. (1992) Evaluation of family treatments in adolescent anorexia nervosa: a pilot study. *Int. J. Eat. Disorders.*, **12**, 347–57.

Lehman, A. (1982) The well-being of chronic mental patients – assessing their quality of life. *Arch. Gen. Psychiat.*, **40**, 369–74.

Lehnert, H., Schrezenmeir, J. & Beyer, J. (1990) Zentralnervose appetit regulation: Mechanismen und Bedeutung fur die Entstehung der Adipositas. *Zeitschrift fur Ernahrungswissen*, **29**, 2–12.

Lehtinen, V., Lindholm T., Veijola, J. & Vaisaene, E. (1990) The prevalence of PSE-CATEGO disorders in a Finnish adult population cohort. *Soc Psychiat. Psychiat. Epidemiol.*, **25**, 187–92.

Leighton, A. H. (1959) *My Name is Legion: The Stirling County Study of Psychiatric Disorder and Sociocultural Environment.* Basic Books, New York.

Leighton, D. C., Harding, J. S., Macklin, D. B. *et al.* (1963) *The Character of Danger (Stirling County Council Study Vol. 3).* Basic Books, New York.

Lelbach, W. K. (1975) Cirrhosis in the alcoholic and its relation to the volume of alcohol abuse. *Annals of the New York Academy of Sciences*, **252**, 85–105.

Lelliott, P., Marks, I., McNamee, G. & Tobena, A. (1989) Onset of panic disorder with agoraphobia: toward an integrated model. *Arch. Gen. Psychiat.*, **46**, 1000–4.

Lemert, E. M. (1951) *Social Pathology.* McGraw–Hill, New York.

Lenane, M., Swedo, S., Leonard, H. *et al.* (1990) Psychiatric disorders in first degree relatives of children and adolescents with obsessive-compulsive disorder. *J. Am. Acad. Child Adol. Psychiat.*, **29**, 407–12.

Lennon, S. & Jolley, D. J. (1991) An urban service in South Manchester In: *Psychiatry in the Elderly* (ed. R. Levy & C. Oppenheimer). Oxford University Press, Oxford, pp. 322–38.

Leonard, B. E. (1992) *Fundamentals of Psychopharmacology.* John Wiley & Sons, New York.

Leonard, H. L., Lenane, M. C., Swedo, S. E. *et al.* (1992) Tics and Tourette's disorder: a 2 to 7 year follow-up of 54 obsessive-compulsive children. *Am. J. Psychiat.*, **149**, 1244–51.

Leonhard, K. (1959) *Anteilung der Endogen Psychosen.* Akademie Verlag, Berlin.

Leonhard, K. (1979) *The Classification of Eudogenous Psychoses* (5th edn), (trans. R. Berman, ed. E. Robins). Wiley & Sons, New York.

Leppert, P. C. & Pahlka, B. S. (1984) Grieving characteristics after spontaneous abortion: a management approach. *Obstet. Gynecol.*, **64**, 119–122.

Lesage, A. & Tansella, M. (1989) Mobility of schizophrenic patients, non-psychotic patients and the general population in a case register area. *Soc. Psychiat. Psychiat. Epidemiol.*, **24**, 271–4.

Leslie, A. M. (1987) Pretence and representation: the origins of 'theory of mind'. *Psychol. Rev.*, **94**, 412–26.

Lesser, R. & Milroy, L. (1993) *Linguistics in Aphasia*. Longman, London, pp. 186–225.

Lester, D. (1989) Changing rates of suicide by car exhaust in men and women in the United States after care exhaust was detoxified. *Crisis*, **10**, 164–8.

Lettieri, D. J., Sayers, M. & Pearson, H. W. (1985) (eds) *Theories on Drug Abuse: Selected Contemporary Perspectives* (NIDA Research Monograph 30). Rockville, Md: National Institute of Drug Abuse.

Leuchter, A. F. & Jacobsen, A. A. (1991) Quantitative measurement of brain electrical activity in delirium. *Internat. Psychogeriat.*, **3**, 231–47.

Leudar, I. & Fraser, W. (1987) Behaviour disturbance and its assessment. In *Assessment in Mental Handicap* (ed. J. Hogg & N. V. Raynes). Croom Helm, 107–28.

Leudar, I., Fraser, W. & Jeeves, M. A. (1987) Theoretical problems and practical solutions to behaviour disorders in retarded people. *Health Bull.*, **45**, 347–55.

Levine, D. N. & Finklestein, S. (1982) Delayed psychosis after right temporo-parietal stroke or trauma. *Neurology*, **32**, 267–73.

Levine, P. M., Silberfarb, P. M. & Lipowski, Z. J. (1978) Mental disorders in cancer patients. *Cancer*, **42**, 1385–91.

Levkoff, S., Clearly, P., Pitzin, B. & Evans, D. S. (1991) Epidemiology of delirium: an overview of research issues and findings. *Internat. Psychogeriat.*, **3**, 149–67.

Lewin, W. (1968) Rehabilitation after head injury. *Br. Med. J.*, **i**, 465–70.

Lewin, B., Robertson, I. H., Cay, E. L. *et al* (1992) Effects of self-help post-myocardial infarction rehabilitation on psychological adjustment and use of health services. *Lancet*, **339**, 1036–40.

Lewinsohn, P. M., Antonuccio, D. O. Breckenridge, J. & Teri, L. (1987) *The Coping with Depression Course: A Psychoeducational Intervention for Unipolar Depression*. Castalia Press, Eugene, Or.

Lewis, A. (1955) Health as a social concept. *Br. J. Sociol.*, **4**, 109–24.

Lewis, A. (1963) Medicine and the Affections of the Mind. *Brit. Med. J.*, **2**, 1549–57.

Lewis, A. (1967) *Obsessional Illness. Injuries in Psychiatry*. Routledge and Kegan Paul, London.

Lewis, A. (1974) Psychopathic Personality: a most elusive category *Psychol. Med.*, **4**, 133–40.

Lewis, A. (1975) The survival of hysteria. *Psychol. Med.*, **5**, 9–12.

Lewis, D. O. (1992) From abuse to violence: psychophysiological consequences of maltreatment. *J. Am. Acad. Child Adol. Psychiat.*, **31**, 383–91.

Lewis, E. (1976) The management of stillbirth: coping with an unreality. *Lancet*, **ii**, 619–20.

Lewis, E. & Page, A. (1978) Failure to mourn in stillbirth: an overlooked catastrophe. *Br. J. Med. Psychol.*, **51**, 237–41.

Lewis, G. (1991) Observer bias in the assessment of anxiety and depression. *Soc. Psychiat. Psychiat. Epidemiol.*, **26**, 265–72.

Lewis, G. (1992) Dimensions of neurosis. *Psychol. Med.*, **22**, 1011–18.

Lewis, G. (1994) Assessing psychiatric disorder with a human interviewer or a computer. *J. Epidemiol. Commun. Health*, **48**, 207–10.

Lewis, G. & Appleby, L. (1988) Personality disorder: the patients psychiatrists dislike. *Br. J. Psychiat.*, **153**, 44–9.

Lewis, G. & Booth, M. (1992) Regional differences in mental health in Great Britain. *J. Epidemiol. Commun. Health*, **46**, 608–11.

Lewis, G. & Booth M. (1994) Are cities bad for your mental health? *Psychol. Med.*, **24**, 913–16.

Lewis, G., David, A., Andreasson, S. & Allebeck, P. (1992) Schizophrenia and city life. *Lancet*, **340**, 137–40.

Lewis, G., Pelosi, A. J., Araya, R. *et al.* (1992) Measuring psychiatric disorder in the community: a standardised assessment for use by lay interviewers. *Psychol. Med.*, **22**, 465–86.

Lewis, G. & Wessely, S. (1990) Comparison of the General Health Questionnaire and the Hospital

Anxiety and Depression Scale. *Br. J. Psychiat.*, **157**, 860–4.

Lewis, G. & Wessley, S. (1992) The epidemiology of chronic fatigue: more questions than answers. *J. Epidem. Comm. Health*, **46**, 92–7.

Lewis, G. & Williams, P. (1989) Clinical judgement and the standardised interview in psychiatry. *Psychol. Med.*, **19**, 971–9.

Lewis, M. (1986) Principles of intensive individual psychoanalytic psychotherapy for childhood anxiety disorders. In *Anxiety Disorders of Childhood* (ed. R. Gittelman). Guilford Press, New York, pp. 233–55.

Lewis, S. W. (1990) Computerised tomography in schizophrenia 15 years on. *Br. J. Psychiat.*, **157** (suppl. 9), 16–24.

Lewis, S. W. & Murray, R. M. (1987) Obstetric complications, neurodevelopmental deviance, and risk of schizophrenia. *J. Psychiat. Res.*, **21**, 413–21.

Lewis, S. W., Owen, M. J. & Murray, W. M. (1989) Obstetric complications and schizophrenia; methodology and mechanisms. In *Schizophrenia: A Scientific Focus* (ed. S. C. Schulz & C. A. Tamminga). Oxford University Press, New York, pp. 56–68.

Leyberg, J. T. (1959) A district psychiatric service. The Bolton Pattern. *Lancet*, **i**, 282–284.

Lezak, M. D. (1983) *Neuropsychological Assessment*. Oxford University Press, New York.

Liberman, R. P. & Raskin, D. E. (1971) Depression: a behavioural formulation. *Arch. Gen. Psychiat.*, **24**, 515–23.

Liddle, P. F. (1987) Symptoms of chronic schizophrenia. *Br. J. Psychiat.*, **151**, 145–51.

Liddle, P. F., Friston, K. J., Frith, C. D. *et al.* (1992) Patterns of cerebral blood flow in schizophrenia. *Brit. J. Psychiatry*, **160**, 179–86.

Lidz, C. W., Mulvey, E. P. & Gardner, W. (1993) The accuracy of predictions of violence to others. *J. Am. Med. Assoc.*, **269**, 1007–11.

Liebowitz, M., Gorman, J., Fyer, A. *et al.* (1984) Lactate provocation of panic attacks ii: Biochemical and physiological findings. *Arch. Gen. Psychiat.*, **42**, 709–19.

Liebowitz, M., Gorman, J., Fyer, A. & Klein, D. (1985) Social phobia: a review of a neglected anxiety disorder. *Arch. Gen. Psychiat.*, **42**, 729–36.

Liebowitz, M. R., Gorman, J. M. & Fryer, A. J. (1988) Pharmacotherapy of social phobia: an interim report of a placebo controlled comparison of phenelzine and atenolol. *J. Clin. Psychiat.*, **49**, 252–7.

Liebowitz, M. R. & Klein, D. F. (1979) Hysteroid dysphoria. *Psychiat. Clin. N. Am.*, **2**, 555–75.

Lim. L. C., Lee, T. E. & Boey, M. L. (1991) Psychiatric manifestations of systemic lupus erythematosis in Singapore. a cross-cultural comparison. *Br. J. Psychiat.*, **159**, 520–3.

Lim. M. H. (1983) A psychiatric emergency clinic: a study of attendances over six months. *Br. J. Psychiat.*, **143**, 480–66.

Lin, T. (1953) A study of the incidence of mental disorder in Chinese and other cultures. *Psychiatry*, **16**, 313–36.

Lin, T., Chu, H., Rin, H. *et al.* (1989) Effects of social change on mental disorders in Taiwan: observations based on a 15-year follow-up survey of general populations in three communities. *Acta Psychiat. Scand.*, Suppl. **348**, 11–34.

Lindemann, E. (1944) Symptomatology and management of acute grief. *Am. J. Psychiat.*, **101**, 141–8.

Lindesay, J. (1991*a*) Suicide in the elderly. *Int. J. Geriat. Psychiat.*, **6**, 355–61.

Lindesay, J. (1991*b*) Anxiety disorders in the elderly. In: *Psychiatry in the Elderly* (ed. R. Jacoby & C. Oppenheimer). Oxford Medical Publications, Oxford, pp. 735–57.

Lindesay, J. & Banerjee, S. (1993) Phobic disorders in the elderly: a comparison of three diagnostic systems. *Internat. J. Gen. Psychiat.*, **8**, 387–93.

Lindesay, J., Briggs, K. & Murphy, E. (1989) The Guy's/Age Concern survey prevalence rates of cognitive impairment, depression and anxiety in an urban elderly community. *Br. J. Psychiat.*, **155**, 317–29.

Lindesay, J., MacDonald, A. & Starke, I. (1990) *Delirium in the Elderly*. Oxford Medical Publications, Oxford, pp. 80–97.

Lindholm, H. (1983) Sectorised psychiatry. *Acta Psychiat. Scand.*, **67**, Supplement 304.

Lindqvist, P. & Allebeck, P. (1990) Schizophrenia and crime. a longitudinal follow-up of 644 schizophrenics in Stockholm. *Br. J. Psychiat.*, **157**, 345–50.

Lindsay, W. R. (1991) Psychological therapies in mental handicap. In *Hallas: The Care of the Mentally Handicapped* (ed. W. Fraser, A. Green & R. MacGillivray). Butterworth, London. pp. 225–44.

Lindsay, W. R., Howells, L. & Pitcaithly, D. (1993) Cognitive therapy for depression with individuals with intellectual disabilities. *Br. J. Med. Psychol.*, **66**, 135–41.

Linehan, M. (1993) *Cognitive-Behavioural Treatment of Borderline Personality Disorder*. Guilford Press, New York.

Linehan, M. M., Armstrong, H. E., Suarez, A. *et al.* (1991) Cognitive behavioural treatment of chronically parasuicidal borderline patients. *Arch. Gen. Psychiat.*, **48**, 1060–4.

Link, B. G., Andrews, H. & Cullen, F. T. (1992) The violent and illegal behaviour of mental patients reconsidered. *Am. Sociol. Rev.*, **57**, 275–92.

Link, B. G., Cullen, F. T., Frank, J. *et al.* (1987) *Amer. J. Sociol.*, **92**, 1461–500.

Link, B. G. & Stueve, A. (1994) Psychotic symptoms and the violent/illegal behaviour of mental patients. *Mental Disorder. Developments in Risk Assessment* (ed. J. Monahan & H. J. Steadman). The University of Chicago Press, Chicago, pp. 137–59.

Linn, M. W., Caffey, E. M., Klett, J. *et al.* (1975) Drug treatment and psychotropic drugs in the aftercare of schizophrenia. *Archiv. Gen. Psychiat.*, **36**, 1055–66.

Linksy, A. S., Celby, J. P. Jr. & Straus, M. A. (1987) Social stress normative constraints and alcohol problems in American states. *Soc. Sci. Med.*, **24**, 875–83.

Lion, J. R., Snyder, W. & Merrill, G. L. (1981) Under-reporting of assaults on staff in a state hospital. *Hosp. Comm. Psychiat.*, **33**, 97–8.

Lion, J. R. & Soloff, P. H. (1984) Implementation of seclusion and restraint. In *The Psychiatric Uses of Seclusion and Restraint* (ed. K. Tardiff). American Psychiatric Press, Washington, DC. pp. 19–34.

Lipowski, I. J. (1989) Delirium in the elderly patients. *New Engl. J. Med.*, **320**, 578–82.

Lipowski, Z. J. (1990) *Delirium (Acute Confusional States)*. Oxford University Press, New York.

Lipowski, Z. J. (1992) Delirium and impaired consciousness. In *Oxford Textbook of Geriatric Medicine* (ed. J. G. Evans & T. F. Williams). Oxford Medical Publications, Oxford, pp. 490–6.

Lipowski, Z. J. (1974) Consultation-liaison psychiatry: an overview. *Am. J. Psychiat.*, **131**, 623–30.

Lipowski, Z. J. (1978) Organic brain syndromes: A reformulation. *Compr. Psychiat.*, **19**, 309–22.

Lipowski, Z. J. (1979) Consultation-liaison psychiatry: Past failures and new opportunities. *Gen. Hosp. Psychiat.*, **1**, 3–10.

Liptzin, B. & Levkoff, S. E. (1992) An empirical study of delirium subtypes. *Br. J. Psychiat.*, **161**, 843–5.

Lishman, W. A. (1968) Brain damage in relation to psychiatric disability after head injury. *Br. J. Psychiat.*, **114**, 373–410.

Lishman, W. A. (1973) The psychiatric sequelae of head injury: a review. *Psychol. Med.*, **3**, 304–18.

Lishman, A. (1987) *Organic Psychiatry* 2nd Edition, Blackwell Scientific Publications, Oxford.

Lishman, W. A. (1990) Alcohol and the brain. *Br. J. Psychiat.*, **156**, 635–44.

Liston, E. H. (1982) Delirium in the aged. *Psychiat. Clin. N. Am.*, **5**, 49–66.

Littlejohns, P. (1986) Domiciliary consultations – who benefits? *J. Roy. Coll. GPs*, **36**, 313–15.

Littlewood, R. & Lipsedge, M. (1982) *Aliens and Alienists: Ethnic Minorities and Psychiatry* 2nd edn. Penguin, Harmondsworth.

Livingston, G. (1994) Epidemiology of dementia. In *Dementia* (ed. A. Burns & R. Levy). Chapman and Hall, London.

Livingston, G., Hawkins, A., Graham, N. *et al.* (1990) The Gospel Oak Study: prevalence rates of dementia, depression and activity limitation among elderly residents in Inner London. *Psychol. Med.*, **20**, 137–46.

Livingston, G. & King, M. (1993) Alcohol abuse in an inner city elderly population. The Gospel Oak Study. *Int. J. Geriat. Psychiat.*, **8**, 511–14.

Livingston, M. G. (1986) Assessment of need for co-ordinated approach in families with victims of head injury. *Br. Med. J.*, **293**, 742–4.

Lloyd, G. (1990) Alcoholic doctors can recover. *Br. Med. J.*, **100**, 728–30.

Lloyd, G. G. (1991) *Textbook of General Hospital Psychiatry*. Churchill Livingstone, Edinburgh.

Lloyd, G.G. (1992) Functional gastrointestinal disorders: psychological factors in aetiology and management. In *Recent Advances in Gastroenterology* (ed. R. E. Pounder). Churchill Livingstone, Edinburgh, pp. 63–71.

Lloyd, G. G. & Cawley, R. H. (1983) Distress of illness? A study of psychological symptoms after myocardial infarction. *Br. J. Psychiat.*, **142**, 120–5.

Locker, D. & Dunt, D. (1978) Theoretical and methodological issues in sociological studies of consumer satisfaction with medical care. *Soc. Sci. Med.*, **12**, 283–92.

Loeber, R. (1900) Development and risk factors of juvenile antisocial behaviour and delinquency. *Clin. Psychol. Rev.*, **10**, 1–41.

Loening-Baucke, V. A., & Cruikshank, B. M. (1986) Abnormal defecation dynamics in chronically constipated children with encopresis. *J. Pediatr.*, **108**, 562–6.

Lohr, J. B. & Wisniewski, A. A. (1987) *Movement Disorders: A Neuropsychiatric Approach*. Guilford Press, New York.

Loizou, L. A., Kendall, B. E. & Marshall, J. (1981) Subcortical arteriosclerotic encephalopathy. *J. Neuro. Neurosurg. Psychiat.*, **44**, 294–304.

Longabough, R. B., McCrady, E., Fink, E. *et al.* (1983) Cost effectiveness of alcoholism treatment in partial vs in-patient settings: six month outcomes. *J. Studies on Alcohol*, **44**, 1049–71.

Loranger, A. W., Hirschself, F., Sartorius, N. & Regier, D. A. (1991) The WHO/ADAMHA international pilot study of personality disorders background and purpose. *J. Personal. Disorders*, **5**(3), 296–306.

Loranger, A. W., Lenzenweger, M. F., Gartner, A. F. *et al.* (1991) Trait-state artefacts and the diagnosis of personality disorders. *Arch. Gen. Psychiat.*, **48**, 720–8.

Lord, C. & Rutter, M. (1994) Autism and pervasive developmental disorders. In *Child and Adolescent Psychiatry: Modern Approaches* third edn (ed. M. Rutter, E. Taylor & L Hersov). Blackwell Scientific, Oxford, pp. 569–93.

Loranger, A. W., Susman, V. L., Oldham, J. M. & Russikoff, L. M. (1987) The personality disorder examination: a preliminary report. *J. Personal. Disorders.*, **1**, 1–13.

Lösel, F. (1993) The effectiveness of treatment in institutional and community settings. *Crim. Behav. Ment. Health*, **3**, 416–38.

Lott, I. T. (1982) Down's syndrome, ageing and Alzheimer disease: clinical review. *Ann. N. Y. Acad. Sci.*, **396**, 15–27.

Loudon, J. B. (1987) Prescribing in pregnancy – Psychotropic drugs. *Brit. Med. J.*, **294**, 167–9.

Lovell, D. (1994) Anorexia nervosa and bulimia nervosa: an investigation of vulnerability factor. PhD Thesis, University of Keele.

Luborsky, L. (1984) *Principles of psychoanalytic psychotherapy: a manual for supportive–expressive treatment*. Basic Books, New York.

Luborsky, L., Crits-Christoph, P., Mintz, J. & Auerbach A. (1988) *Who will benefit from psychotherapy: Predicting therapeutic outcomes*. Basic Books, New York.

Luborsky, L. & Mark, D. (1991) Short-term supportive expressive psychoanalytic psychotherapy. In *Handbook of short-term dynamic psychotherapy* (ed. P. Crits-Christoph & J. Barber). Basic Books, New York, 110–36.

Lucas, A. R., Beard, C. M., O'Fallon, W. M. & Kurland, L. T. (1991) 50-year trends in the incidence of anorexia nervosa in Rochester. Minn: a population based study. *Amer. J. Psychiat.*, **148**, 917–22.

Luce, G. G. & Segal, J. (1969) *Insomnia: A Guide for Troubled Sleepers*. Doubleday and Co, New York.

Lum, L. C. (1981) Hyperventilation and anxiety state. *J. Roy. Soc. Med.*, **74**, 1–4.

Lusznat, R. M., Murphy, D. P. & Nann, C. M. (1988) Carbamazepine vs lithium in the treatment and prophylaxis of mania. *Br. J. Psychiat.*, **153**, 198–204.

Luxon, L., Lees, A. J. & Greenwood, R. J. (1979) Neurosyphilis today. *Lancet*, **i**, 90–3.

Lynch, P., Bakal, D., Whitelaw, W. & Fung, T. (1991) Chest muscle activity and panic activity: a preliminary investigation. *Psychosomatic Med.*, **53**, 80–9.

Macalpine, I. & Hunter, R. (1974) The pathography of the past. *Times Literary Supplement*, 15 March, 256–57.

MacCarthy, B., Lesage, A., Brewin, C. *et al.* (1989) Needs for care among the relatives of long term users of day care. *Psychological Medicine*, **19**, 725–36.

MacCrimmon, D., Cleghorn, J. M., Asarnow, R. F. *et al.* (1980) Children at risk in schizophrenia. *Arch. Gen. Psychiat.*, **37**, 671–74.

MacDonald, A. (1991a) How can we measure mental health? In *Indicators for Mental Health in the Population* (eds. R. Jenkins & S. Griffiths). HMSO, London.

MacDonald, A. (1991b) Running a team. In *Working Out: Setting Up and Running Community Psychogeriatric Teams* (ed. J. Lindesay). RDP, London.

MacDonald, A. (1992a) 'Suicide prevention' by GPs? *Br. J. Psychiat.*, **161**, 574.

MacDonald, A. (1992b) Old age depression and organic brain change. In *Recent Advances in Psychogeriatrics* 2 (ed. T. Aries). Churchill Livingstone, Edinburgh, pp. 45–58.

MacDonald, A. J. D., Simpson, A. & Jenkins, D. (1989) Delirium in the elderly: a review and a suggestion for a research programme. *Int. J. Geriat. Psychiat.*, **4**, 311–19.

MacGregor, R., Pullar, A. & Cundall, D. (1994) Silent at school – elective mutism and abuse. *Arch. Dis. Childhood*, **70**, 540–1.

Mack, J. L. & Levine, R. N. (1981) The basis of visual constructional disability in patients with unilateral cerebral lesions. *Cortex*, **17**, 515–31.

MacKinnon, A., Henderson, A. & Andrews, G. (1990) Genetic and environmental determinants of the liability of trait neuroticism and the symptoms of anxiety and depression. *Psychol. Med.*, **20**, 581–90.

MacKinnon, A., Henderson, A. & Andrews, G. (1993) Parental 'affectionless control' as an antecedent to adult depression: a risk factor refined. *Psychol. Med.*, **23**, 135–41.

Macklin, R. (1973) The medical model in psychoanalysis and psychotherapy. *Compr. Psychiat.*, **14**, 49–69.

MacMahon, B. & Pugh, T. F. (1970) *Epidemiology: Principles and Methods*. Little, Brown, Boston.

MacMillan, D. (1967) Problems of a geriatric mental health service. *Br. J. Psychiat.*, **113**, 175–81.

MacMillan, D. & Shaw, P. (1966) Senile breakdown in standards of personal and environmental cleanliness. *Br. Med. J.*, ii, 1032–37.

MacMillan, H. L., MacMillan, J. H., Offord, D. R. *et al.* (1994a) Primary prevention of child physical abuse and neglect: a critical review. Part I. *J. Child Psychol. Psychiat.*, **35**, 835–56.

MacMillan, H. L., MacMillan, J. H., Offord, D. R.*et al.* (1994b) Primary prevention of child sexual abuse: a critical review. Part II. *J. Child Psychol. Psychiat.*, **35**, 857–76.

MacSween, R. M. N. (1982) Alcohol and cancer. *Br. Med. Bull.*, **38**, 31–3.

Maden, A., Curle, C., Meux, C. *et al.* (1993) The treatment and security needs of special hospital patients. *Crim. Behav. Ment. Health.*, **3**, 290–306.

Maden, A., Swinton, M., Gunn, J. (1991) Drug dependence in prison. *Br. Med. J.*, **301**, 286.

Maguire, M., Morgan, R. & Rainer, R. (1994) *The Oxford Handbook of Criminology*. Clarendon Press, Oxford.

Maher, B. (1970) *Introduction to Research in Psychopathology*. McGraw-Hill, New York.

Maher, B. A. (1972) The language of schizophrenia: a review and interpretation. *Br. J. Psychiat.*, **120**, 3–17.

Mahler, H. (1973) Health – a demystification of medical technology. *Lancet*, **1**, 829–34.

Mahler, M. S. (1968) *On human symbiosis and the vicissitudes of individuation*. International Universities Press, New York.

Mahler, M. S., Pine, F. & Bergman, A. (1975) *The Psychological Birth of the Human Infant*. Basic Books, New York.

Mai, F. (1993) Psychiatric aspects of heart transplantation. *Br. J. Psychiat.*, **163**, 285–92.

Maier, G. J. (1990) Psychopathic disorders: beyond counter-transference. *Curr. Opin. Psychiat.*, **3**, 766–9.

Maier, G. J. (1992) The impact of clozapine on 25 forensic patients. *Bull. Am. Acad. Psychiat. Law.*, **20**, 197–307.

Maier, W., Buller, R., Philipp, M. *et al.* (1988*c*) The Hamilton Anxiety Scale: reliability, validity and sensitivity to change in anxiety and depressive disorders. *J. Affect. Disorders.*, **14**, 61–8.

Maier, W., Heuser, I., Philipp, M. *et al.* (1988*b*) Improving depression severity assessment II. Content, concurrent and external validity of three observer depression scales. *J. Psychiat. Res.*, **22**, 13–19.

Maier, W., Lichtermann, D., Minges, J. *et al.* (1993) Continuity and discontinuity of affective disorders and schizophrenia. Results of a controlled family study. *Arch. Gen. Psychiat.*, **50**, 871–83.

Maier, W. & Philipp, M. (1985) Comparative analysis of observer depression scales. *Acta Psychiat. Scand.*, **72**, 239–45.

Maier, W., Philipp, M., Heuser, I. *et al.* (1988*a*) Improving depression severity assessment I. Reliability, internal validity and sensitivity to change of three observer depression scales. *J. Psychiat. Res.*, **22**, 3–12.

Maj, M., Starace, F. & Pirozzi, R. (1991) A family study of DSM-III-R schizoaffective disorder, depressive type, compared with schizophrenia and psychotic and nonpsychotic major depression. *Am. J. Psychiat.*, **148**, 612–16.

Malan, D. H. (1963) *A Study of Brief Psychotherapy*. Tavistock Publications, London.

Malan, D. H. (1976*a*) *The frontier of brief psychotherapy*. Plenum, New York.

Malan, D. H. (1976*b*) *Towards the validation of dynamic psychotherapy: A replication*. Plenum, New York.

Malebranche, N. (1980, orig. 1674) *The Search After Truth* trans. T. M. Lennon, Ohio State University Press, Columbus.

Malouf, R., Jaquette, G., Dobkin, J. & Brust, J. C. (1990) Neurological disease in human immunodeficiency virus-infected drug abusers. *Arch. Neurol.*, **47**, 1002–7.

Malt, U. (1988) The long-term psychiatric consequences of accidental injury: a longitudinal follow-up of 107 adults. *Br. J. Psychiat.*, **153**, 810–18.

Malzberg, B. (1937) Mortality among patients with involutional melancholia. *Am. J. Psychiat.*, **93**, 1231–8.

Manchanda, R., Hirsch, S. R. & Barnes, T. R. E. (1989) A review of rating scales for measuring symptom changes in schizophrenia research. In *The Instruments of Psychiatric Research* (ed. C. Thompson). John Wiley & Sons, Chichester, pp. 59–86.

Manchip, S. (1994) That stupid club. *Br. Med. J.*, **308**, 1447.

Mander A. & Loudon, J. (1988) Rapid recurrence of mania following abrupt discontinuation of lithium. *Lancet*, **ii**, 15–17.

Mann, A. H. (1977) Psychiatric morbidity and hostility in hypertension. *Psychol. Med.*, **7**, 653–9.

Mann, A. H., Jenkins, R. & Belsey, E. (1981*a*) The twelve-month outcome of patients with neurotic illness in general practice. *Psychol. Med.*, **11**, 535–50.

Mann, A. H., Jenkins, R. & Cutting, J. C. (1981*b*) The development and use of a standardised assessment of abnormal personality. *Psychol. Med.*, **11**, 839–47.

Mann, J. (1973) *Time limited psychotherapy*. Harvard University Press, Cambridge, MA.

Mann, J. J., Stanley, M., McBridge, P. A. & McEwen, B. S. (1986) Increased serotin and beta-adrenergic receptor binding in the frontal cortices of suicide victims. *Arch. Gen. Psychiat.*, **43**, 954–9.

Mann, R. E. & Smart, R. G. (1990) Alcohol problems, prevention and epidemiology: looking for the next questions. *Br. J. Addiction*, **85**, 1385–7.

Mannoni, O. (1973) The antipsychiatric movement(s). *Int. Soc. Sci. J.*, **XXV**(4) 489–503.

Mannuzza, S., Klein, R. G. Bessler, A. *et al.* (1993) Adult outcome of hyperactive boys: educational achievement, occupational rank and psychiatric status. *Arch. Gen. Psychiat.*, **50**, 565–76.

Manschreck, T. C., Maher, B. A., Ruclos, M. E. *et al.* (1982) Disturbed voluntary motor activity in schizophrenic disorder. *Psychol. Med.*, **12**, 73–84.

Marcé L. V. (1860) On a form of hypochondriacal delirium occurring consecutive to dyspepsia and characterised by refusal of food. *J. Psychol. Med. Ment. Pathol.*, **13**, 204–6.

Marder, S. R., Van Putten, T. V., Mintz, J. *et al.* (1987) Low and conventional maintenance dose therapy with fluphenazine decanoate. *Arch. Gen. Psychiat*, **151**, 825–35.

Marder, S. R. & Meibach, R. C. (1994) Risperidone in the treatment of schizophrenia. *Am. J. Psychiat.*, **151**, 825–35.

Margetts, E. L. (1950) The early history of the word 'psychosomatic'. *Canad. Med. Ass. J.*, **63**, 402–4,

Margraf, J. Barlow, D., Clark, D. & Telch, M. (1993) Psychological treatment of panic: work in progress on outcome, active ingredients and follow-up. *Behav. Res. Ther.*, **31**, 1–8.

Margraf, J., Taylor, C., Ehlers, A. *et al.* (1987) Panic attacks in the natural environment. *J. Nerv. Ment. Disease.*, **175**, 558–65.

Mari, J. J. & Williams, P. (1985) A comparison of the validity of two psychiatric screening questionnaires (GHQ-12 and SRQ-20) in Brazil, using Relative Operating Characteristic (ROC) analysis. *Psychol. Med.*, **15**, 651–9.

Markowitz, P. I. (1990) Fluoxetine treatment of self-injurious behaviour in mentally retarded patients. *J. Clin. Psychopharmacol.*, **10**, 299–300.

Marks, I. (1985) Controlled trial of psychiatric nurse therapists in primary care. *Br. Med. J.*, **290**, 1181–4.

Marks, I, M. (1987) *Fears, phobias and rituals: Panic, Anxiety and their Disorders.* Oxford University Press, New York.

Marks, I., Connolly, J. & Muijen, M. (1988) The Maudsley Daily Living Programme. *Bull. Roy. Coll. Psychiat.*, **12**, 22–4.

Marks, I. & Gelder, M. (1966) Different ages of onset in varieties of phobias. *Am. J. Psychiat.*, **123**, 2218–21.

Marks, I., Gray, S., Cohen, D. *et al.* (1983) Imipramine and brief therapist-aided exposure in agoraphobics having self-exposure homework. *Arch. Gen. Psychiat.*, **40**, 153–62.

Marks, I., Greist, J., Basoglu, M. *et al.* (1992) Comment on the second phase of the cross-national collaborative panic study. *Br. J. Psychiat.*, **160**, 202–5.

Marks, I. M., Hodgson, R. & Rachman, S. (1975) Treatment of chronic OCD 2 years after *in vivo* exposure. *Br. J. Psychiat.*, **127**, 349–64.

Marks, I. M., Lelliott, P., Basoglu, M. *et al.* (1988) Clomipramine, self-exposure and therapist-aided exposure for obsessive-compulsive rituals. *Br. J. Psychiat.*, **152**, 522–34.

Marks, I. & O'Sullivan, G. (1989) Anti-anxiety drugs and psychological treatment effects in agoraphobia/panic and obsessive-compulsive disorders. In *Psychopharmacology of Anxiety* (ed. P. Tyrer). Oxford University Press, Oxford, pp. 196–242.

Marks, I. M., Stern, R. S., Mawdon, D. *et al.* (1980) Clomipramine and exposure for obsessive-compulsive rituals: I. *Br. J. Psychiat.*, **136**, 1–25.

Marks, I. M., Swinson, R. P., Basoglu, M. *et al.* (1993) Alprazolam and exposure therapy alone and combined in panic disorder with agoraphobia: a controlled study with London and Toronto. *Brit. J. Psychiat.*, **162**, 776–87.

Marks, J. N., Goldberg, D. P. & Hillier, V. F. (1979) Determinants of the general practitioner's ability to detect psychiatric illness. *Psychol. Med.*, **9**, 337–54.

Marks, M. N., Wieck, A., Checkley, S. A. & Kumar, R. (1992) Contribution of psychological and social factors to psychotic and non-psychotic relapse after childbirth in women with previous histories of affective disorder. *J. Affect. Disord.*, **29**, 253–64.

Marlett, G. A. & Gordon, J. R. (1985) *Relapse Prevention: Maintenance Strategies in the Treatment of Addictive Behaviours.* Guilford Press, New York.

Marmot, M. G. (1981) Alcohol and mortality: a U-shaped curve. *Lancet*, **1**, 580–3.

Marmot, M. G. & Bruner, E. (1991) Alcohol and cardiovascular disease: the status of the U-shaped curve. *Br. Med. J.*, **303**, 565–8.

Marsden, C. D. (1986) Hysteria: A neurologist's view. *Psychol. Med.*, **16**, 277–88.

Marsden, C. D. & Harrison, M. J. G. (1972) Outcome of investigation of patients with presenile dementia. *Br. Med. J.*, **ii**, 249–52.

Marsden, C. D. & Jenner, P. (1980) The pathophysiology of extrapyramidal side-effects of neuroleptic drugs. *Psychol. Med.*, **10**, 55–72.

Marshall, E. J., Syed, G. M. S., Fenwick, P. B. C., Lishman, W. A. (1993) A pilot study of schizophrenia-like psychosis in epilepsy using single photon emission computerised tomography. *Br. J. Psychiat.*, **163**, 32–6.

Martikainen E. K., Urponen, H., Partinen, M. *et al.* (1992) Daytime sleepiness: a risk factor in community life. *Acta Neurol. Scand.*, **86**, 337–41.

Martin, R. L., Cloninger, C. R., Guze, S. B. & Clayton, P. J. (1985) Mortality in a follow-up of 500 psychiatric out-patients. *Arch. Gen. Psychiat.*, **42**, 47–54.

Martin, R. L., Cloninger, R., Guze, S. B. & Clayton, P. J. (1985) Mortality in a follow-up of 500 psychiatric out-patients II. Cause-specific mortality. *Arch. Gen. Psychiat.*, **42**, 58–66.

Masters, W. H. & Johnson, V. E. (1966) *Human Sexual Response.* Little, Brown and Co., Boston.

Masters, W. H. & Johnson, V. E. (1970) *Human Sexual Inadequacy.* Little, Brown and Co., Boston.

Masserman, J. & Carmichael, H. T. (1936) Diagnosis and prognosis in psychiatry. *J. Ment. Sci.*, **84**, 893–946.

Mathers, D. C., Ghodse, A. H., Caan, W. & Scott, S. A. (1991) Cannabis use in a large sample of acute psychiatric admissions. *Br. J. Addiction*, **86**, 779–84.

Mathews, A. M., Gelder, M. G. & Johnstone, D. W. (1981) *Agoraphobia: Nature and Treatment.* Tavistock, London.

Matson, J. L., Gardner, W. I., Coe, D. A. & Sovner, R. (1991) A scale for evaluating emotional disorders in severely and profoundly mentally retarded persons. *Br. J. Psychiat.*, **159**, 404–9.

Matsuki, K., Grumet, F. C. Lin, X. *et al.* (1992) DQ (rather than DR) gene marks susceptibility to narcolepsy. *Lancet*, **399**, 1052.

Mattick, R. P. & Peters, L. (1988) Treatment of severe social phobia: effects of guided exposure with and without cognitive restructuring. *J. Consult. Clin. Psychol.*, **56**, 251–60.

Mattson, M. R. & Sacks, M. H. (1978) Seclusion: uses and complications. *Am. J. Psychiat.*, **135**, 1210–3.

Maughan, B. & Yule W. (1994) Reading and other learning disabilities. In *Child and Adolescent Psychiatry: Modern Approaches*, third edn (ed. M. Rutter, E. Taylor & L Hersov). Blackwell Scientific, Oxford, pp. 647–65.

Mavissakalian, M. & Perel, J. (1985) Imipramine in the treatment of agoraphobia: dose-response relationship. *Am. J. Psychiat.*, **142**, 1032–6.

Mavreas, V. & Bebbington, P. E. (1988) Greeks, British Greek Cypriots and Londoners: a comparison of psychiatric morbidity. *Psychol. Med.*, **18**, 433–42.

Mawby, R. I. & Gill, M. L. (1987) *Crime Victims: Needs, Services and The Voluntary Sector.* Tavistock, London.

Mawson, D. (1985) Delusions of poisoning. *Medicine, Science and the Law*, **25**, 279–87.

Mayhew, P., Maung, N. A. & Mirrlees-Black, C. (1993) *The 1992 British Crime Survey.* Home Office Research Study 132. HMSO: London.

Mayou, R. (1989) Atypical chest pain. *J. Psychosom. Res.*, **33**, 393–406.

Mayou, R. (1995) Medico-legal aspects of road traffic accidents. *J. Psychosom. Res.*, **39**, 789–98.

Mayou, R., Bryant, B. & Duthie, R. (1993) Psychiatric consequences of road traffic accidents. *Br. Med. J.*, **307**, 647–51.

Mayou, R. & Hawton, K. (1986) Psychiatric disorder in the general hospital. *Br. J. Psychiat.*, **149**, 172–90.

McAllister, T. W. (1981) Cognitive functioning in the affective disorders. *Compr. Psychiat.*, **22**, 572–86.

McArdle, P., O'Brien, G. O. & Kolvin, I. (1995) Hyperactivity: prevalence and relationship with conduct disorder. *J. Child Psychol. Psychiat.*, **36**, 279–303.

McBride, W. G. (1972) Limb deformities associated with iminodibenzyl hydrochloride. *Med. J. Aust.*, **1**, 492.

McCabe, M. S. & Norris, B. (1977) ECT versus chlorpromazine in mania. *Biol. Psychiat.*, **12**, 245–46.

McCance, C., Olley, P. C. & Edward, V. (1973) Long-term psychiatric follow-up. In *Experience with Abortion* (ed. G. Horobin). Cambridge University Press, London, pp. 245–300.

McClelland, H. A. (1981) Psychiatric disorders. In *Textbooks of Adverse Drug Reactions* (ed. D. M. Davies). Oxford University Press, Oxford, pp. 479–502.

McClelland, R. J. (1985) A neurophysiological investigation of minor head injury. In *Clinical and Experimental Neuropsychophysiology* (ed. D. Papakostopoulos, S. Butler & I. Martin). Croom Helm, London, pp. 615–34.

McClure, G. M. G. (1987) Suicide in England and Wales 1975–1984. *Br. J. Psychiat.*, **150**, 309–14.

McCord, J. (1977) A comparative study of two generations of native Americans. In *Theory in Criminology* (ed. R. F. Meier). Sage, Beverly Hills, CA. pp. 83–92.

McCord, J. (1978) A thirty-year follow-up of treatment effects. *Am. Psychologist*, **33**, 284–9.

McCord, J. (1988) Parental behaviour in the cucle of aggression. *Psychiatry* **51**, 14–23.

McCormack, H. M., Horne, D. J. de L. & Sheather, S. (1988). Clinical applications of visual analogue scales: a critical review. *Psychol. Med.*, **18**, 1007–19.

McCrady, B. S. & Miller, W. R. (Eds) (1993) *Research on Alcoholics Anonymous*. Rutgers, New Jersey.

McCrone, P. & Phelan M. (1995) Diagnosis and length of psychiatric in-patient stay. *Psychol. Med.*, **24**, 1025–30.

McDonald, C. (1969) Clinical heterogeneity in senile dementia. *Br. J. Psychiat.*, **115**, 267–71.

McDonald, R., Sartory, G., Grey, S. J. *et al.* (1978) Effects of self-exposure instructions on agoraphobic patients. *Behav. Res. Ther.*, **17**, 83–5.

McDonnell, R. & Maynard, A. (1985) Estimation of life years lost from alcohol-related premature death. *Alcohol and Alcoholism*, **20**, 435–43.

McFall, M. E., McKay, P. W. & Donovan, D. M. (1991) Combat-related PTSD and psychosocial adjustment problems among substance abusing veterans. *J. Nerv. Ment. Disease.*, **179**, 33–8.

McFarlane, A. (1988*a*) Relationship between psychiatric impairment and a natural disaster: the role of distress. *Psychol. Med.*, **18**, 129–39.

McFarlane, A. (1988*b*) The aetiology of post-traumatic stress disorders following a natural disaster. *Br. J. Psychiat.*, **152**, 116–121.

McGee, J. J., Menolascino, F., Hobbs, D. & Menonsch, P. E. (1987) *Gentle Teaching: A Non-aversive Approach to Helping Persons with Mental Retardation*. Human Sciences, New York.

McGee, R., Feehan, M., Williams, S. *et al.* (1990) DSM-III disorders in a large sample of adolescents. *J. Am. Acad. Child Adol. Psychiat.*, **29**, 611–19.

McGee, R., Makinson, T., Williams, S. *et al.* (1984) A longitudinal study of enuresis from five to nine years. *Aust. Paed. J.*, **20**, 30–42.

McGhie, A. & Chapman, J. (1961) Disorders of attention and perception in early schizophrenia. *Br. J. Psychiat.*, **34**, 103–16.

McGillis, D. & Smith, P. (1983) *Compensating Victims of Crime: An Analysis of American Programs*. National Institute of Justice, Washington DC.

McGlashan T. H. (1984) The Chestnut Lodge follow-up study, II. Long-term outcome of schizophrenia in the affective disorders. *Arch. Gen. Psychiat.*, **41**, 586–601.

McGovern, D. & Cope, R. V. (1987) First psychiatric admission rates of first and second generation Afro-Caribbeans. *Soc. Psychiat.*, **22**, 139–49.

McGovern, M. P., Lyons, J. S. & Pomp, H. C. (1990) Capitation payment systems and public mental health care: implications for psychotherapy with the seriously mentally ill. *Am. J. Orthopsychiat.*, **60**, 298–304.

McGrath, J. & Murray, R. M. (1995) Risk factors for schizophrenia from conception to birth. In *Schizophrenia* (ed. S. Hirsch & D. Weinberger). Blackwell Scientific, Oxford. pp. 187–205.

McGregor, S., Ettori, B. Roscomber, R. *et al.* (1991) *The Central Funding Initiative*. London Institute for the Study of Drug Dependence.

McGuffin, P., Farmer, A., Gottesman, I. I. *et al.* (1984) Twin concordance of operationally defined schizophrenia: confirmation of familiality and heritability. *Arch. Gen. Psychiat.*, **41**, 541–5.

McGuffin, P., Farmer, A. E. & Harvey, I. (1991) A polydiagnostic application of operational criteria in studies of psychotic illness: development and reliability of the OPCRIT system. *Arch. Gen. Psychiat.*, **48**, 764–70.

McGuffin, P. & Katz, R. (1986) Nature, nurture and affective disorders. In *The Biology of Depression* (ed. J. W. K. Deakin). Gaskell Press, London, pp. 26–51.

McGuffin, P., Katz, R., Aldrich, J. & Bebbington, P. E. (1988a) The Camberwell Collaborative Depression Study. II. The investigation of family members. *Br. J. Psychiat.*, **152**, 766–74.

McGuffin, P., Katz, R. & Bebbington, P. E. (1988b) The Camberwell Collaborative Depression Study, III. Depression and adversity in the relatives of depressed probands. *Br. J. Psychiat.*, **152**, 775–82.

McGuffin, P., Katz, R. & Rutherford, J. (1991) Nature, nurture and depression: a twin study. *Psychol. Med.*, **21**, 329–35.

McGuffin, P., Murray, R. M. & Reveley, A. M. (1987) Genetic influences on the functional psychoses. *Br. Med. Bull.*, **43**, 531–56.

McGuffin, P., Owen, M. J., O'Donovan, M. (1994) *Seminars in Psychiatric Genetics*. Gaskell Press, London.

McGuire, A. & Drummond, M. (1993) Economic evaluation in health care: an introduction for psychiatrists. *Soc. Psychiat. Psychiat. Epidemiol.*, **28**, 211–17.

McGuire, A., Duncan, J. S. & Trimble, M. R. (1992) Effects of vigabatrine on cognitive function and mood when used as add-on therapy in patients with intractable epilepsy. *Epilepsia*, **33**, 128–34.

McGuire, P., Bench, C., Frith, C. *et al.* (1994) Functional anatomy of obsessive-compulsive phenomena. *Br. J. Psychiat.*, **164**, 459–64.

McGuire, P. & Fahy, T. (1991) Chronic paranoid psychosis following use of MDMA ('Ecstasy'). *Brit. Med. J.*, **302**, 697.

McGuire, P., Jones, P., Harvey, I. (1994) Cannabis and acute psychosis. *Schiz. Res.*, **13**, 161–8.

McGuire, P. K., Shah, G. M. S. & Murray, R. M. (1993) Increased blood flow in Broca's area during auditory hallucinations in schizophrenia. *Lancet*, **342**, 703–6.

McGuire, P. Silbersweig, D., Wright, I. *et al.* (1996) Abnormal monitoring of inner speech: the physiological basis of auditory hallucinations. *Lancet* (in press).

McIntosh, I. D. (1982) Alcohol related disabilities in general hospital patients: a critical assessment of the evidence. *Int. J. Addict.*, **17**, 609–39.

McIver, S. (1991) *Obtaining the Views of Users of Mental Health Services*. King's Fund Centre, London.

McKeith, I., Perry, R., Fairbairn, A. *et al* (1992) Operational criteria for senile dementia of Lewy Body Type. *Psych. Med.*, **22**, 911–22.

McKenna, P. J. (1984) Disorders with overvalued ideas. *Br. J. Psychiat.*, **145**, 579–83.

McKenry, P. C., Tishler, C. L. & Kelley C. (1982) Adolescent suicide: a comparison of attempters and nonattempters in an emergency room population. *Clin. Pediatr.*, **21**, 266–70.

McKenzie, J. M. & Joyce, P. R. (1992) Hospitalisation for anorexia nervosa. *Int. J. Eat. Disorders.*, **11**, 235–41.

McKeon, P. & Murray, R. (1987) Familial aspects of obsessive-compulsive neurosis. *Br. J. Psychiat.*, **151**, 528–34.

McKinley, W. W., Brooks, D. N., Bond, M. R. (1983) Postconcussional symptoms, financial compensation and outcome of severe blunt head injury. *J. Neurol. Nerosurg. Psychiat.*, **46**, 1084–91.

McLaren, S., Browne, F. W. A. & Taylor, P.J. (1990) A study of psychotropic medication given 'as required' in a regional secure unit. *Br. J. Psychiat.*, **156**, 732–5.

McLean, E. & Liebowitz, J. (1989) Towards a working definition of the long-term mentally ill. *Psychiat. Bull.*, **13**, 251–2.

McLellan, A. T., Luborsky, L., Erdlen, F. R. *et al.* (1980) Addiction severity index: A diagnostic/evaluation profile of substance abuse patients. In *Substance Abuse and Psychiatric Illness* (ed. E. Goltheil, A. T. McLelland & K. A. Druley). Pergamon Press, New York, pp. 151–9.

McNeil, T. F. & Kaij, L. (1978) Obstetric factors in the development of schizophrenia: complications in the births of pre-schizophrenics and in reproductions by schizophrenic parents. In *The Nature of Schizophrenia: New Approaches to Research and Treatment* (ed. L. C. Wynne, R. L. Cromwell & S. Matthysse). John Wiley & Sons, New York, pp. 401–29.

Meadow, R. (1989a) Epidemiology. In *ABC of Child Abuse* (ed. R. Meadow). British Medical Association, London, pp. 1–4.

Meadow, R. (1989*b*) Munchausen syndrome by proxy. In *ABC of Child Abuse* (ed. R. Meadow). British Medical Association, London, pp. 37–9.

Meadows, G., Turner, T., Campbell, L. *et al.* (1991) Assessing schizophrenia in adults with mental retardation: a comparative study. *Br. J. Psychiat.*, **158**, 103–5.

Mechanic D. (1962) The concept of illness behaviour. *J. Chron. Dis.*, **15**, 189–94.

Mechanic D. (1986) The concept of illness behaviour: culture, situation and personal predisposition. *Psychol. Med.*, **16**, 1–7.

Mechanic, D. (1987) Correcting misconceptions in mental health policy: Strategies for improved care of the seriously mentally ill. *The Millbank Quarterly*, **65**, 203–30.

Medawar, P. B. (1967) *The Art of the Soluble*. Methuen, London.

Medical Research Council (1948) Streptomycin treatment of pulmonary tuberculosis. *Br. Med. J.*, **i**, 925–9.

Medical Research Council (1965) Clinical trial of the treatment of depressive illness. *Br. Med. J.*, **i**, 881–6.

Medical Research Council Drug Trial Sub Committee (1981) Continuation therapy with lithium and amitriptyline in unipolar depressive illness: a controlled clinical trial. *Psychol. Med.*, **11**, 409–16.

Mednick, S. A. & Christiansen, K. O. (1977) *Biosocial Bases of Criminal Behaviour*. Gardner Press, New York.

Mednick, S. A., Machon, R. A., Huttenen, M. O. *et al.* (1988) Adult schizophrenia following prenatal exposure to an influenza epidemic. *Arch. Gen. Psychiat.*, **45**, 189–92.

Mednick, S. A., Parnas, J. & Schulsinger, F. (1987) The Copenhagen High-Risk Project, 1962–86. *Schiz. Bull.*, **13**, 485–95.

Meichenbaum, D. (1977) *Cognitive Behaviour Modification: An Integrative Approach*. Plenum Press, New York.

Meichenbaum, D. & Cameron, R. (1973) Training schizophrenics to talk to themselves: a means of developing attentional controls. *Behav. Ther.*, **4**, 515–34.

Meichebaum, D. & Goodman, J. (1971) Training impulsive children to talk to themselves: a means of developing self-control. *J. Abnorm. Psychol.*, **77**, 115–26.

Mello, N. K. & Mendelson, J. H. (1971) Drinking patterns during work contingent and non contingent alcohol acquisition. In *Recent Advances in Studies of Alcoholism* (ed. N. K. Mello & J. H. Mendelson), pp. 647–86. Publication No/HSM/71–9045 US Government Printing Office, Washington DC.

Mellor, C. S. (1970) First rank symptoms of schizophrenia. *Br. J. Psychiat.*, **17**, 15.

Mellsop, G., Varghese, F., Joshua, A. S. & Hicks, A. (1982) Reliability of axis II of DSM-III. *Am. J. Psych.*, **139**, 1360–1.

Meltzer, E. S. & Kumar, R. (1985) Puerperal mental illness, clinical features and classification: a study of 142 mother and baby admissions. *Br. J. Psychiat.*, **147**, 647–54.

Meltzer, H. Y. (1994) Mechanisms of action of atypical drugs. In *Biology of Schizophrenia and Affective Disorder* (ed. S. J. Watson & H. Akie). Raven Press, New York.

Meltzer, H., Gill, B. & Petticrew, M. (1995) *OPCS Surveys of Psychiatric Morbidity in Great Britain*. Report No. 1. The prevalence of psychiatric morbidity among adults aged 16–64 living in private households in Great Britain, HMSO, London.

Mendels, J., Weinstein, N. & Cochrane, C. (1972) The relationship between depression and anxiety. *Arch. Gen. Psychiat.*, **27**, 649–53.

Mendez, M. F., Lanska, D. J., Manon-Espaillat, R. *et al* (1989) Causative factors for suicide by overdose in epileptics. *Arch. Neurol.*, **46**, 1065–8.

Mendlewicz, J. & Rainer, J. D. (1977) Adoptive study supporting genetic transmission in manic-depressive illness. *Nature*, **268**, 327–29.

Menninger, K. (1963) *The Vital Balance: the Life Process in Mental Health and Illness*. Viking Press, New York.

Merikangas, K. & Angst, J. (1994) A longitudinal study of neurasthenia. *Psychol. Med..*, **24**, 1013–24.

Merriam, A. E. (1994) Biological treatment of neuroses. *Curr. Opin. Psychiat.*, **7**, 154–9.

Merson, S., Tyrer, P., Onyett, S. *et al.* (1992) Early intervention in psychiatric emergencies: a controlled clinical trial. *Lancet*, **339**, 1311–14.

Mesulam, M. M. (1981) A cortical network for directial attention and unilateral neglect. *Ann. Neurol.*, **10**, 309–25.

Mesulam, M. M., Waxman, S. G., Geschwind, N. & Sabin, T. D. (1976) Acute confusional states with right middle cerebral artery infarctions. *J. Neurol. Neurosurg. Psychiat*, **39**, 80–9.

Metzger, D., Woody, G. E., De Philippis, D. *et al.* (1991) Risk factors for needle-sharing among methadone-treated patients. *Am. J. Psychiat.*, **148**(5) 636–40.

Metzner, J. J. (1992) A survey of university – prison collaboration and computerised tracking systems in prisons. *Hosp. Comm. Psychiat.*, **43**, 713–16.

Meyer, R. (1986) How to understand the relationship between psychopathology and addictive disorders: Another example of the chicken and the egg. In: *Psychopathology and Addictive Disorders* (ed. R. Meyer). The Guilford Press, New York, 3–16.

Meyer-Bahlburg, H. F. C. (1977) Sex hormones and male homosexuality in comparative perspective. *Arch. Sex. Behav.*, **6**. 297–302.

Meyers, A. W. & Craighead, W. E. (1984) *Cognitive Behaviour Therapy with Children*. Plenum Press, New York.

Micale, M. (1990) Hysteria and its historiography; the future perspective. *History of Psychiatry.*, **1**, 33–124.

Micale, M. (1993) On the 'disappearance' of hysteria. A study in the clinical deconstruction of a diagnosis. *Isis.*, **84**, 496–526.

Michael, A., Joseph, A. & Pallen, A. (1994) Delusions of pregnancy. *Br. J. Psychiat.*, **164**, 244–6.

Miers, D. (1978) *Responses to Victimisation*. Professional Books, Abingdon.

Miller, B., Lesser, I. & Boone, K. (1991) Brain lesions in cognitive function in late life psychosis. *Br. J. Psychiat.*, **158**, 76–82.

Miller, F. J., Kolvin, I. & Fells, H. (1985) Becoming deprived: a cross-generation study based upon the Newcastle upon Tyne 1000 family survey. In *Longitudinal Studies in Child Psychology and Psychiatry* (ed. A. R. Nicol). Wiley, Chichester, pp. 233–40.

Miller, H. C. (1961) Accident neurosis. *Br. Med. J.*, **i**, 919–25.

Miller, K. & Klauber, G. T. (1990) Desmopressin acetate in children with severe primary nocturnal enuresis. *Clin. Ther.*, **12**, 357–66.

Miller, R. D. (1992) Involuntary civil commitment to out-patient treatment: an update. *Hosp. Comm. Psychiat.*, **43**, 79–80.

Miller, W. (1983) Motivational interviewing with problem drinkers. *Behav. Psychother.*, **11**, 147–72.

Miller, W. R. & Hester, R. K. (1986) The effectiveness of alcoholism treatment: What research reveals. In *Treating Addictive Behaviours* (ed. W. R. Miller & N. Heather). Premium Press, New York, pp. 121–84.

Miller, W. R. & Rollnick, S. (1991) *Motivational Interviewing: Preparing People to Change Addictive Behaviour*. Guilford Press.

Milton, O. & Wahler, R. G. (1969) Perspectives and trends. In *Behaviour Disorders* (ed. O. Milton & R. G. Wahler). Lippincott, New York.

Milstein, V. (1988) EEG topography in patients with aggressive violent behaviour. In *Biological Contributions to Crime Causation* (ed. T. E. Moffitt & S. A. Mednick). Dordrecht, Martinus Nijhoff, pp. 40–52.

Ministry of Health (1961) *Special Hospitals: Report of a Working Party* (The Emery Report). HMSO, London.

MIND Publications (1983) *Common Concerns*. London.

Mindham, R. H. S. (1970) Psychiatric symptoms in parkinsonism. *J. Neurol. Neurosurg. Psychiat.*, **33**, 188–91.

Mindham, R. H. (1982) Tricylic antidepressants. In *Drugs in Psychiatric Practice* (ed. P. Tyrer). Butterworth, London, pp. 219–48.

Mindham, R. H. S., Howland, C. & Shepherd, M. (1973) An evaluation of continuation therapy with tricyclic antidepressants in depressive illness. *Psychol. Med.*, **3**, 5–17.

Minkowski, E. (1970) *Lived Time* (translated by N. Metzell). Northwestern University Press, Evanston.

Mintel, R. E. & Mandel, M. R. (1979) The treatment of psychotic major depressive disorder with drugs and electroconvulsive therapy. *J. Nerv. Ment. Dis.*, **167**, 726–33.

Mirin, S. M., Weiss, R. D. & Michael, J. (1988) Psychopathology in substance abusers: diagnosis and treatment. *Am. J. Drug Alcohol Abuse*, **14**, 139–47.

Mischel, W. (1968) *Personality and Assessment.* Wiley, New York.

Mischel, W. & Peake, P. K. (1982) Some facets of consistency: replies to Epstein, Funder and Bem. *Psychol. Rev.*, **90**, 394–402.

Misri, S. & Sivertz, K (1991) Tricyclic drugs in pregnancy and lactation: a preliminary report. *Int. J. Psychiat. Med.*, **21**, 157–71.

Mitchell, A. (1985) Psychiatrists in primary health care settings. *Br. J. Psychiat*, **147**, 371–9.

Mitchell, J. E., Pyle, R. L. Eckert, E. D. *et al.* (1990) A comparison study of antidepressants and structured intensive group psychotherapy in the treatment of bulimia nervosa. *Arch. Gen. Psychiat.*, **47**, 149–57.

Mitcheson, M. (1994) Drug clinics in the 1970s. In *The British System* (ed. J. Strang & M. Gossop). Oxford University Press, Oxford, pp. 178–91.

Moberg, D. O. (1953) Old Age and crime. *J. Crim. Law, Criminol. Police Sci.*, **43**, 764–76.

Modestin, J. (1985) Antidepressive therapy in depressed clinical suicides. *Acta Psychiat. Scand.*, **71**, 111–16.

Moffatt, M. E. K., Kato, C. & Pless, I. B. (1987) Improvements in self-concept after treatment of nocturnal enuresis: randomised control trial. *J. Pediatr.*, **110**, 647–52.

Moffit, T. E. & Silva, P. A. (1988*a*) Neuropsychological deficit and self-reported delinquency in an unselected birth cohort. *J. Am. Acad. Child Adol. Psychiat.*, **27**, 233–40.

Moffit, T. E. & Silva, P. A. (1988*b*) Self-reported delinquency: results from an instrument for New Zealand. *Austr. N.Z. J. Criminol.*, **21**, 227–40.

Mollica, R. (1983) From asylum to community. *New Engl. J. Med.*, **308**, 367–73.

Monahan, J. (1984) The prediction of violent behaviour: toward a second generation of theory and policy. *Am. J. Psychiat.*, **141**, 10–15.

Monahan, J. (1988) Risk assessment of violence among the mentally disordered: generating useful knowledge. *Int. J. Law and Psychiatry*, **11**, 249–57.

Monahan, J. (1992) Mental disorder and violent behaviour. *Am. Psychol.*, **47**, 511–21.

Monahan, J. & Steadman H. (1983) Crime and mental disorder: an epidemiological approach. In *Crime and Justice: An Annual Review of Research, Vol. 3* (ed. N. Morris & M. Tonry). University of Chicago Press, Chicago, pp. 145–89.

Monck, E., Graham, P., Richman, N. & Dobbs, R. (1994) Adolescent girls II: Background factors in anxiety and depressive states. *Br. J. Psychiat.*, **165**, 770–80.

Monck, E., Sharland, E., Bentovim, A. *et al.* (1995) *Child Sexual Abuse: A Descriptive and Treatment Study.* HMSO, London.

Montgomery, E. A., Fenton, G. W., McClelland, R. *et al.* (1991) The psychobiology of minor head injury. *Psychol. Med.*, **21**, 375–84.

Montgomery, S. A. (1989) Fluoxetine in the treatment of anxiety, agitation and suicidal thoughts. In *Psychiatry Today VII World Congress of Psychiatry Abstracts* (ed. C. N. Stefanis, C. R. Soldatos & A. D. Rabavilas). Elsevier, New York.

Montgomery, S. A. & Asberg, M. (1979) A new depression scale designed to be sensitive to change. *Br. J. Psychiat.*, **134**, 382–9.

Montgomery, S. A., Dufour, S., Brion, S. *et al.* (1988) The prophylactic efficacy of fluoxetine in unipolar depression. *Br. J. Psychiat.*, **153**, 69–76.

Moodley, P. & Thornicroft, G. (1988) Ethnic group and the compulsory admission of psychiatric patients. *Medicine, Science and the Law*, **28**, 324–8.

Moore, E., Kuipers, L. & Ball, R. (1992) Staff patient relationships in the case of the long-term mentally ill: a content analysis of EE interviews. *Soc. Psychiatry Psychiatric Epidemiol.*, **27**, 28–34.

Moore, N. A., Calligaro, D. O., Wong, D. T. *et al* (1993) The pharmacology of olanzapine and other new antipsychotic agents. *Curr. Opin. Invest. Drugs*, **2**, 281–93.

Moorey, S. (1989) Cognitive therapy with drug abusers. In *Cognitive Therapy in Clinical Practice: an Illustrative Casebook* (ed. J. Scott, J. M. G. Williams & A. T. Beck). Routledge, London, pp. 157–82.

Moorey, S. & Greer, S. (1989) *Psychological Therapy for Patients with Cancer: A New Approach*. Heinemann, Oxford.

Moorey, S., Greer, S., Watson, M. *et al* (1991) The factor structure and factor stability of the Hospital Anxiety and Depression Scale in patients with cancer. *Br. J. Psychiat.*, **158**, 255–9.

Morgan, H. G., Barton, J., Pottle, S. *et al.* (1976) Deliberate self-harm: a follow-up study of 279 patients. *Br. J. Psychiat.*, **128**, 361–8.

Morgan, H. G., Burns-Cox, C. J., Pocock, H. & Pottle, S. (1975) Deliberate self-harm: clinical and socio-economic characteristics of 368 patients. *Br. J. Psychiat.*, **127**, 564–74.

Morgan, H. G., Jones, E. M. & Owen, J. H.(1993) Secondary prevention of non-fatal deliberate self-harm. The green card study. *Br. J. Psychiat.*, **163**, 111–12.

Morgan, H. G. & Priest, P. (1984) Assessment of suicide risk in psychiatric in-patients. *Br. J. Psychiat.*, **145**, 467–9.

Morgan, H. G. & Priest, P. (1991) Suicide and other unexpected deaths among psychiatric in-patients. The Bristol Confidential Inquiry. *Br. J. Psychiat.*, **158**, 368–74.

Morgan, H. G., Purgold, J. & Welbourne, J. (1983) Management and outcome in anorexia nervosa: a standardised prognosis study. *Br. J. Psychiat.*, **143**, 282–7.

Morgan, K., Dallosso, H. M., Arie, T. *et al.* (1987) Mental health and psychological well-being among the old and the very old living at home. *Br. J. Psychiat.*, **150**, 801–7.

Morgan, K., Lilley, J., Aire, T. *et al.* (1993) The incidence of dementia in a representative British sample. *Br. J. Psychiat.*, **163**, 467–70.

Morley, S. & Snaith, P. (1992) Principles of psychological assessment. In *Research Methods in Psychiatry* 2nd end. (ed. C. Freeman & P. Tyrer). Gaskell, London, pp. 135–52.

Mori, E. & Yamadori, A. (1987) Acute confusional state and acute agitated delirium occurrence after infarction in the right middle cerebral artery territory. *Arch. Neurol.*, **44**, 1139–43.

Morris, J. B. & Beck, A. T. (1974) The efficacy of antidepressant drugs: a review of research. *Arch. Gen. Psychiat.*, **30**, 667–74.

Morris, P. L. P., Robinson, P. G., Andozeyewski, P. *et al.* (1993) Association of depression with 1-year post stroke mortality. *Am. J. Psychiat.*, **150**, 124–9.

Morris, R. J. & Kratochwill, T. R. (1983) *Treating Children's Fears and Phobias*. Pergamon, New York.

Morris, R. G. & Morris, L. W. (1991) Cognitive and behavioural approaches with the depressed elderly. *Int. Geriat. Psychiat.*, **6**, 407–13.

Morrisey, J. & Levine, I. (1987) Researchers discuss latest findings, examine needs of homeless mentally ill persons. *Hosp. Comm. Psychiat.*, **38**, 811–12.

Morrison, J. R.(1982) Suicide in a psychiatric practice population. *J. Clin. Psychiat.*, **43**, 348–52.

Morton, R. (1946) *Phthisiologia seu Exercitiones de Phthisis*. Smith, London.

Mosbach, P. & Leventhal, H. (1988) Peer group identification and smoking: implications for prevention. *J. Abnorm. Psychol.*, **97**, 238–45.

Moser, J. (1991) What does a national alcohol policy look like? In *International Handbook of Addiction Behaviour*. Routledge, London, pp. 313–19.

Mosher, L. (1983) Radical deinstitutionalisation: the Italian experience. *Int. J. Ment. Health*, **11**, 129–36.

Mosher, J. F. & Yanagisko, K. L. (1991) Public health, not social warfare: A public health approach to illegal drug policy. *J. Pub. Health Policy*, **12**, 278–323.

Moskovitz, J. M. (1989) The primary prevention of alcohol problems: A critical review of the research literature. *J. Studies in Alcohol*, **50**, 54–88.

Moskowitz, S. B., Chalmers, T. C. & Sacks, H. (1983) Deficiencies of clinical trials of alcohol withdrawal. *Alcoholism*, **7**, 42–6.

Moss, S. C. (1991) Age and functional abilities of people with a mental handicap. Evidence from the Wessex mental handicap responses. *J. Ment. Defic. Res.*, **35**, 430–45.

Moss, S. C., Goldberg, D., Simpson, N. *et al.* (1993) *The Psychiatric Assessment Schedule for Adults with Developmental Disorders (PAS-ADD10)*. The Hester Adrian Centre, University of Manchester.

Mott, J., Mirlees-Black, C. (1995) *Self Reported Drug Misuse in England and Wales: Findings From the 1992 British Crime Survey*. Research and Planning Unit Paper 89. Home Office, London.,

Mountjoy, C. Q. & Roth, M. (1982) Studies in the relationship between depressive disorders and anxiety states. Part I. Rating scales. *J. Affec. Dis.*, **4**, 127–47.

Mowat, R. R. (1966) *Morbid Jealousy and Murder*. Tavistock Publications, London.

Mowbray, R. M. (1972) The Hamilton Rating Scale for depression: a factor analysis. *Psychol. Med.*, **2**, 272–80.

Mowrer, O. H. (1960) *Learning Theory and Behaviour*. Wiley, New York.

Mueller, D. P., Edwards, D. W. & Yarvis, R. M. (1977) Stressful life events and psychiatric symptomatology: change or undesirability. *J. Health Soc. Behav.*, **18**, 307–17.

Mueller, E. & Silverman, N. (1989) Peer relations in maltreated children. In *Child Maltreatment: Theory and Research on the Causes and Consequences of Child Abuse and Neglect* (ed. D. Cicchetti & V. Carlson). Cambridge University Press, Cambridge, pp. 529–78.

Mueser, K. T., Yarnold, P. R., Levinson, D. F. *et al.* (1990) Prevalence of substance abuse in schizophrenia: demographic and clinical correlates. *Schiz. Bull.*, **16**, 31–56.

Mufson, L., Moreau, D., Weissman, M. M. & Klerman, G. L. (1993) *Interpersonal Psychotherapy for Depressed Adolescents*. Guilford Press, New York.

Muijen, M., Marks, I. M., Connolly, J. *et al.* (1992) The daily living programme: preliminary comparison of community versus hospital-based treatment for the seriously mentally ill facing emergency admission. *Br. J. Psychiat.*, **160**, 379–84.

Muijen, M. & Silverstone, T. (1987) A comparative hospital survey of psychotropic drug prescribing. *Br. J. Psychiat.*, **150**, 501–4.

Mullen, P. E. (1990) A phenomenology of jealousy. *Aust. N.Z. J. Psychiat.*, **24**, 17–28.

Mullen P. E. (1991) Jealousy: the pathology of passion. *Br. J. Psychiat.*, **158**, 593–601.

Mullen, P. E., Gunn, J., Mawson, D. & Noble, P. (1993*b*) Deception, self-deception, and dissociation. In *Forensic Psychiatry. Clinical, Legal & Ethical Issues* (ed. J. Gunn & P. J. Taylor). Butterworth–Heiniemann, Oxford, pp. 407–34.

Mullen, P. E., Martin, J. L., Anderson, J. C. *et al.* (1993*a*) Childhood sexual abuse and mental health in adult life. *Br. J. Psychiat.*, **163**, 721–32.

Mullen, P. E. & Pathé M. (1994) The pathological extensions of love. *Br. J. Psychiat.*, **165**, 614–23.

Mullen, P. E., Romans-Clarkson, S. E., Walton, V. A. & Herbison, G. P. (1988) Impact of sexual and physical abuse on women's mental health. *Lancet*, **i**, 841–5.

Mumford, D. B. & Whitehouse, A. M. (1988) Bulimia Nervosa among Asian schoolgirls. *Br. Med. J.*, **297** (6650), 718.

Mumford, D. B., Whitehouse, A. M. & Platts, M. (1991) Sociocultural correlates of eating disorders among Asian schoolgirls in Bradford. *Br. J. Psychiat.*, **158**, 222–8.

Munby, M. & Johnson, D. W. (1980) Agoraphobia: the long-term follow-up of behavioural treatment. *Br. J. Psychiat.*, **137**, 418–27.

Munro, A. (1980*a*) *Delusional Hypochondriasis: A Description of Monosymptomatic Hypochondriacal Psychosis (MHP)*. Clarke Institute of Psychiatry Monograph Series, Number 5, University of Toronto.

Munro, A. (1980*b*) Monosymptomatic hypochondriacal psychosis. *Br. J. Hosp. Med.*, **24**, 34–38.

Munby, M. & Johnston, G. W. (1980) Agoraphobia: the long-term follow-up of behavioural treatment. *Br. J. Psychait.*, **137**, 418–27.

Munro, A. (1988) Monosymptomatic hypochondriacal psychosis. *Br. J. Psychiat.*, **153** (Suppl. 2), 37–40.

Murphy, D. L., Garrick, N. A., Aulakh, C. C. & Cohen, R. M. (1984) New contributions from basic science to understanding the effects of monoamine oxidase inhibiting antidepressants. *J. Clin. Psychiat.*, **45**, 37–43.

Murphy, E. (1983) The prognosis of depression in old age. *Br. J. Psychiat.*, **142**, 111–19.

Murphy, E. (1988) Community care: II Possible solutions. *Br. Med. J.*, **296**, 6–8.

Murphy, E. & Brown, G. W. (1980) Life events, psychiatric disturbances and physical illness. *Br. J. Psychiat.*, **136**, 326–38.

Murphy E., Smith R., Lindesay, J. & Slattery, J. (1988) Increased mortality in late-life depression. *Br. J. Psychiat.*, **139**, 288–92.

Murphy, G. E., Armstrong, J. W., Hermele, S. L. *et al* (1979) Suicide and alcoholism. Interpersonal loss confirmed as a predictor. *Arch. Gen. Psychiat.*, **36**, 65–9.

Murphy, J., Monson, R., Oliver, D. *et al.* (1987) Affective disorders and mortality. *Arch. Gen. Psychiat.*, **44**, 473–80.

Murphy, J., Olivier, D., Sobol, A. *et al.* (1986) Diagnosis and outcome: depression and anxiety in a general population. *Psychol. Med.*, **16**, 117–26.

Murphy, J., Olivier, D., Monson, R. *et al.* (1988) Incidence of depression and anxiety: the Stirling County Study. *Am. J. Pub. Health*, **78**, 534–40.

Murphy, J. M., Sobol, A. M., Oliver, D. C. *et al.* (1989) Prodromes of depression and anxiety. The Stirling County Study. *Br. J. Psychiat..*, **155**, 490–5.

Murphy, M. (1990) Methods of forecasting mortality for population projections. In *Population Projections, Trends, Methods and Uses*. OPCS' Occasional Paper 38. OPCS, London.

Murray, L. (1992) The impact of postnatal depression on infant development. *J. Child Psychol. Psychiat.*, **33**, 543–61.

Murray, R. M. (1980) An epidemiological and clinical study of alcoholism in the medical profession. In *Aspects of Alcohol and Drug Dependence* (ed. J. S. Madden *et al.*). Pitman Medical, London.

Murray, R. (1986) Schizophrenia. In *Essentials of Postgraduate Psychiatry* (ed. P. Hill, R. Murray & A. Thorley). Grune and Stratton, London, pp. 3–36.

Murray, R. M. (1994) Neurodevelopmental schizophrenia: the rediscovery of dementia praecox. *Br. J. Psychiat.*, **165**, 6–12.

Murray, R. M., Cooper, J. E. & Smith, A. (1979) The Leyton obsessional inventory: an analysis of the responses of 73 obsessional patients. *Psychol. Med.*, **9**, 305–11.

Murray, R. M., Oon, M. C. H., Smith, A. L. *et al.* (1979) A possible association between raised urinary DMT and certain psychotic symptoms. *Arch. Gen. Psychiat.*, **36**, 644–49.

Murray, R. M. & Lewis, S. W. (1987) Is schizophrenia a neurodevelopmental disorder? *Br. Med. J.*, **295**, 681–2.

Murray, R. M., Lewis, S. & Reveley, A. M. (1985). Towards an aetiological classification of schizophrenia. *Lancet*, **i**, 1023–6.

Murray, R. M., O'Callaghan, E., Castle, D. J. & Lewis, S. W. (1992) A neurodevelopmental approach to the classification of schizophrenia. *Schiz. Bull.*, **18**, 319–32.

Murray Parkes, C., Brown, G. W. & Monck, E. M. (1962) The general practitioner and the schizophrenic patient. *Br. Med. J.*, **1**, 972–6.

Musetti, L., Perugi, G., Soriani, A. *et al.* (1989) Depression before and after 65. A re-examination. *Br. J. Psychiat.*, **155**, 330–6.

Musto, D. (1987) *The American Disease: Origins of Narcotic Control.* Oxford University Press, Oxford.

Myers, D. H. & Neal, C. D. (1978) Suicide in psychiatric patients. *Br. J. Psychiat.*, **133**, 38–44.

Myers, J. K., Wissman, M. M., Tischler, G. L. *et al.* (1984) Six month prevalence of psychiatric disorders in three communities. *Arch. Gen. Psychiat.*, **41**, 959–67.

Naeser, M. A., Alexander, M. P., Helm-Estabrooks, N. *et al.* (1982) Aphasia with predominantly subcortical lesion sites: description of three capsular/putaminal aphasia syndromes. *Arch. Neurol.*, **39**, 2–14.

Naguib, N. & Levy, R. (1987) Late paraphrenia – neuropsychological impairment and structural brain abnormalities on computer tomography. *Br. J. Geriat. Psychiat.*, **2**, 83–90.

Naik, P. & Jones, R. (1993) Response of visual hallucinations to blindfolding. *Int. J. Geriat. Psychiat.*, **8**, 357–353

Naranjo, C. S. & Sellers, E. M. (eds) (1985) *Research Advances in New Psychopharmacological Treatments for Alcoholism.* Elsevier Science Publishing, New York.

Naranjo, C. & Sellers, E (eds) (1991) *Novel Pharmacological Interventions for Alcoholism.* Verlag, New York.

Nasrallah, H. A., McCalley-Whitters, M. & Jacoby, C. G. (1982) Cerebral ventricular enlargement in young manic males: a controlled study. *J. Affective Disorders*, **4**, 15–19.

Nasser, M. (1988) Comparative study of the prevalence of abnormal eating attitudes among Arab female students from both London and Ciaro Universities. *Psychol. Med.*, **16**, 621–25.

National Institute of Mental Health (1980) *Mental Health Services in Primary Care Settings: Report of a Conference* (ed. D. L. Parron & F. Solomon). Supt. of Docs., US Government Printing Office, Washington.

National Institute of Mental Health (1987) *Towards a Model for a Comprehensive Community-Based Mental Health System.* NIMH, Washington DC.

Nayani, T. & David, A. S. (1995) The auditory hallucination: a phenomenological survey. *Psychol. Med.*, **26**, 177–89.

Nazareth, I. & King, M. B. (1933) The urethral syndrome: a controlled evaluation. *J. Psychosom. Res.*, **37**, 737–43.

Neary, D. (1990) Dementia of frontal lobe type. *J. Am. Geriat. Soc.*, **38**, 71–2.

Neary, D., Snowden, J., Northen, B. & Goulding, P. (1988) Dementia of frontal lobe type. *J. Neurol. Neurosurg. Psychiat.*, **51**, 353–61.

Nelson, J. C. (1993) Combined treatment strategies in psychiatry. *J. Clin. Psychiat.*, **54** (suppl 9), 42–9.

Nemeroff, C. B., Owens, M. J., Bissette, G. (1988) Reduced corticotrophin releasing factor binding sites in the frontal cortex of suicide victims. *Arch. Gen. Psychiat.*, **45**, 577–9.

Nemeroff, C. B., Widerlov, E., Bissette, G. *et al.* (1984) Elevated concentrations of corticotrophin-releasing factor-like immunoreactivity in depressed patients. *Science*, **226**, 1342–4.

Nesbit, F. (1994) Noncompliance with psychiatric drug prescriptions. *Am. J. Psychiat.*, **151**, 783–4.

Neuberger, M. (1943) The doctrine of the healing power of nature. Translated Boyd L. J. In *Handbook of Psychiatry 1 General Psychopathology* Chap. 1. Bynum, W. F.. Psychiatry in its historical context (ed. M. Shepherd & O. L. Zangwill). Cambridge University Press, Cambridge.

Newburn, T. (1989) *The Settlement of Claims at the Criminal Injuries Compensation Board.* Home Office Research Study No. 112. HMSO, London.

Newcomb, M. D. & Bentler, P. M. (1988) *Consequences of Adolescent Drug Use.* Sage, Berverly Hills.

Newmann, J. P., Engel, R. J. & Jensen, J. E. (1991) Age differences in depressive symptoms experiences. *J. Gerontol.*, **46**, 224–35.

Newson-Smith, J. (1983) Who cares for the adult brain damaged? *Psychiat. Bull.*, **7**, 181–3.

Newsom-Smith, J. G. B. & Hirsch, S. R. (1979*a*) Psychiatric symptoms in self-poisoning patients. *Psychol. Med.*, **9**, 493–500.

Newson-Smith, J. G. B. & Hirsch, S. R. (1979*b*) A comparison of social workers and psychiatrists in evaluating parasuicides. *Br. J. Psychiat.*, **134**, 335–42.

Neziroglu, F., Anemone, R. & Yaryura-Tobias, J. A. (1992) Onset of obsessive-compulsive disorder in pregnancy. *Am. J. Psychiat.*, **149**, 947–50.

NHS Management Executive (1993) Risk management in the NHS. BAPS, HPU, DSS Distribution Centre, Heywood, Lancs. OL10 2PZ.

Nicol, A. R., Smith, J., Kay, B. *et al.* (1988) A focussed casework approach to the treatment of child abuse: a controlled comparison. *J. Child Psychol. Psychiat.*, **29**, 703–11.

Nicol, R., Stretch, D. & Fundudis, T. (1993) *Preschool Children in Troubled Families.* John Wiley, Chichester.

Nielsen, S. (1900) The epidemiology of anorexia nervosa in Denmark from 1973 to 1987: a nationwide survey of psychiatric admissions. *Acta Psychiat. Scand.*, **81**, 507–14.

Nies, A. & Robinson, M. D. (1982) Monamine oxidase inhibitors. In *Handbook of Affective Disorders* (ed. E. S. Paykel). Churchill Livingstone, Edinburgh, pp. 246–61.

Nihira, K., Foster, R., Shelhaas, M. & Lelland, H. (1974) *AAMD Adaptive Behaviour Scale*. American Association on Mental Deficiency, Washington DC.

Nijkamp, P., Pacolet, J., Spinnewyn, H. *et al.* (1990) *Services for the Elderly in Europe. A Cross-National Comparative Study*. Catholic University Leuven, Free University Amsterdam.

Nilsson, L. V. & Persson, G. (1984) Prevalence of mental disorders in an urban sample examined at 70, 75 and 79 years of age. *Acta Øsych Scand.*, **69**, 519–27.

Nisbett, R. & Ross, L. (1980) *Human Inference: strategies and shortcomings of social judgement*. Prentice Hall, Englewood Cliffs.

Nitsche, P. & Williams, K. (1913) The history of prison psychoses. *Nervous and Mental Disease Monograph Series No. 13*. Journal of Nervous and Mental Disease Publishing Co., New York.

Noble, E. P. (1991) Genetic studies in alcoholism – CNS functioning and molecular biology. *Psychiat. Annals.*, **21**, 215–29.

Noble, E. P. (1993) The D_2 dopamine receptor gene: a review of association studies in alcoholism. *Behav. Genet.*, **23**, 119–29.

Noble, E. P., Blum, K., Ritchie, T. *et al* (1991) Allelic association of the D2 dopamine receptor gene with receptor-binding characteristics in alcoholism. *Arch. Gen. Psychiat.*, **48**, 648–54.

Nordstrum, A. L., Farde, L., Weisel, F. A. *et al.* (1993) Central D2 dopamine receptor occupancy in relation to antipsychotic drug effects: a double blind PET study of schizophrenic patients. *Biol. Psychiat.*, **33**, 227–35.

Noreik, K. & Odegaard, O. (1966) Psychosis in Norwegians with a background of higher education. *Br. J. Psychiat.*, **112**, 43–55.

Norman, R. M. G. & Malla, A. K. (1993) Stressful life events and schizophrenia I and II. *Br. J. Psychiat.*, 162, 161–74.

Norman, R. M. G. & Malla, A. K. (1993) Stressful life events and schizophrenia I: a review of the research. *Br. J. Psychiat.*, 162, 161–6.

Norman, W. T. (1963) Toward an adequate taxonomy of personality attributes: replicated factor structure in peer nomination personality ratings. *J. Abn. Soc. Psychol.*, **66**, 574–83.

Norton, K. (1992) Personality disordered individuals: the Henderson hospital model treatment. *Criminal Behaviour and Mental Health.*, **2**, 180–91.

Novaco, R. W. (1975) *Anger control: The Development and Evaluation of an Experimental Treatment*. Heath, Lexington, MA.

Noyes, R., Clancy, J., Crowe, R. *et al.* (1983) The familial prevalence of anxiety neurosis. *Arch. Gen. Psychiat.*, **35**, 1067–74.

Noyes, R., Clarkson, C., Crowe, R. *et al.* (1987) A family history study of generalised anxiety disorder. *Am. J. Psychiat.*, **144**, 1019–24.

Noyes, R., Kathol, R, Fisher, M. *et al.* (1993) The validity of DSM-IIIR hypochondriasis. *Arch. Gen. Psychiat.*, **50**, 861–970.

Nutt, D. (1990) The pharmacology of human anxiety. *Pharmacol. Therap.*, **47**, 233–66.

Nutt, D. & Glue, P. (1989) Monoamine oxidase inhibitors: Rehabilitation from recent research. *Br. J. Psychiat.*, **154**, 287–91.

Nutt, D., Glue, P., Lawson, C. & Wilson (1990) Flumazenil provocation of panic attacks. *Arch. Gen. Psychiat.*, **47**, 917–25.

Nutt, D. & Lawson, C. (1992) Panic attacks: A neurochemical overview of models and mechanisms. *Br. J. Psychiat.*, **160**, 165–78.

Oates, M. (1988) The development of an integrated community-orientated service for severe postnatal mental illness. In *Motherhood and Mental Illness 2: Causes and Consequences* (ed. R. Kumar & I. F. Brockington). Wright, London, pp. 133–58.

Oates, M. (1989) Management of major mental illness in pregnancy and the puerperium. *Baillières Clin. Obstet. Gynaecol.*, **3**, 905–20.

O'Callaghan, E., Sham, P., Takei, N. (1991) Schizophrenia after prenatal exposure to 1957 A2 influenza epidemic. *Lancet*, **337**, 1248–50.

O'Connor, D., Pollitt, P. & Hyde, J. (1989) The prevalence of dementia as measured by the CAMDEX. *Acta Psychiat. Scand.*, **79**, 190–8.

O'Connor, M., Johnson, G. H. & James, D. I. (1981) Intrauterine effects of phenothiazines. *Med. J. Aust.*, **1**, 416–17.

O'Connor, P. & Brown, G. W. (1984) Supportive relationships: fact or fantasy? *J. Soc. Personal Relationships*, **1**, 159–75.

Oddy, M., Humphrey, M. & Uttley, D. (1978) Subjective impairment and social recovery after closed head injury. *J. Neurol. Neurosurg. Psychiat.*, **41**, 611–16.

Odegaard, O. (1932) Emigration and insanity. *Acta Psychiat.*, (Suppl). **4**.

Odegaard, O. (1975) Social and ecological factors in the etiology, outcome, treatment and prevention of mental disorders In *Psychiatrie der Gegenwart., Bd. 3: Soziale und angewandte Psychiatrie.2 Auflage* (ed. K. P. Kisker, J.-E Meyer & H. Muller). pp. 151–198. Springer, Heidelberg.

Office of Population Censuses and Surveys (1991) *Drinking in England and Wales in the late 1980s.* HMSO, London.

Office of Population Censuses and Surveys (1995) *Mortality Statistics 1993.* HMSO, London.

Office of Technology Assessment (1990) *Confused Minds, Burdened Families: Finding Help for People with Alzheimer's Disease and Other Dementias.* US Government Printing Office, Washington DC.

Offord, D. R., Boyle, M. H., Szatmari, P. *et al.* (1987) Ontario Child Health Study: II. Six-month prevalence of disorder and rates of service utilisation. *Arch. Gen. Psychiat.*, **44**, 832–6.

Offord, D. R. & Cross, L. A. (1969) Behavioural antecedents of adult schizophrenia. *Arch. Gen. Psychiat.*, **21**, 267–83.

Ogborne, A. C. (1989) Some limitations of Alcoholics Anonymous. In *Recent Developments in Alcoholism; Emerging Issues in Treatment*, Vol 7, (ed. M. Galanter). Plenum Press, New York, pp. 55–65.

Ogborne, A. C. & Glaser, F. B. (1981) Characteristics of the affiliates of Alcoholics Anonymous: A review of the literature. *J. Studies on Alcohol*, **42**, 661–75.

O'Hara, M. W., Schlechte, J. A., Lewis, D. A. & Wright, E. J. (1991) Prospective study of postpartum blues biologic and psychosocial factors. *Arch. Gen. Psychiat.*, **48**, 801–6.

O'Hara, M. & Zekoski, E. M. (1988) Postpartum depression: a comprehensive review. In *Motherhood and Mental Illness 2: Causes and Consequences* (ed. R. Kumar & I. F. Brockington). Wright, London, pp. 17–63.

O'Hara, M. W., Zekoski, E. M., Phillips, L. H. & Wright, E. J. (1990) Controlled prospective study of postpartum mood disorders: comparison of childbearing and non-childbearing women. *J. Abnorm. Psychol.*, **99**, 3–15.

Okano, T. & Nomura, J. (1992) Endocrine study of the maternity blues. *Prog. Neuropsychopharmacol. Biol. Psychiat.*, **16**, 921–32.

O'Keane, V. & Dinan, T. G. (1991) Prolactin and cortisol responses to D-fenfluramine in major depression: Evidence for diminished responsibility of central serotonergic function. *Am. J. Psychiat.*, **148**, 1009–15.

Old Age Depression Interest Group (1993) How long should the elderly take antidepressants? A double blind placebo-controlled study of continuation/prophylaxis therapy with dothiepin. *Br. J. Psychiat.*, **162**, 175–182.

Oldham, P. D., Pickering, G., Fraser Roberts, J. A. & Sowry, G. S. C. (1960) The nature of essential hypertension. *Lancet*, **1**, 1085–1093.

Oliver, J. P. J. (1991) The Social Care Directive: development of a quality of life profile for use in community services for the mentally ill. *Soc. Work Soc. Sci. Rev.*, **3**, 5–45.

Ollendick, T. H., Mattis, S. G. & King, N. J. (1994) Panic in children and adolescents: a review. *J. Child Psychol. Psychiat.*, **35**, 113–34.

Olmsted, P. M., Davis, R., Rockert, W. *et al.* (1991) Efficacy of a brief group of psychoeducational intervention for bulimia nervosa. *Behav. Res. Ther.*, **29**, 71–83.

Oltmanns, T. F. & Maher, B. A. (eds) (1987) *Delusional Beliefs*. John Wiley, New York.

Olweus, D. (1979) Stability of aggressive reaction patterns in males: a review. *Psychol. Bull.*, **86**, 852–75.

Ong, Y., Martineau, F., Lloyd, C. & Robins, I. (1987) A support group for the depressed elderly. *Int. Geriat. Psychiat.*, **2**, 119–23.

Onstead, S., Skre, I., Torgersen, S. *et al.* (1991) Twin concordance for DSM-IIIR schizophrenia. *Acta Psychiat. Scand.*, **83**, 395–401.

Oppenheim, J. (1991) *'Shattered Nerves': Doctors, Patients and Depression in Victorian England.* Oxford University Press.

Oppenheimer, D. R. (1968) Microscopic lesions in the brain following head injury. *J. Neurol. Neurosurg., Psychiat.*, **31**, 299–306.

Oppenheimer, E., Tobutt, C., Taylor, C. & Andrew, T. (1994) Death and survival in a cohort of heroin addicts from London clinics: a 22-year follow-up study. *Addiction*, **89**(10) 1299–308.

Orbach, S. (1986) *The Hunger Strike. The Anorectic's Struggle as a Metaphor for Our Age.* Norton, New York.

Orbach, S. (1978) *Fat is a Feminist Issue: The Anti-Diet Guide to Permanent Weight Loss.* New York.

Oreland, L., Wiiberg, A., Asberg, M. *et al.* (1981) Platelet MAO activity and monoamine metabolites in cerebro-spinal fluid in depressed and suicidal patients and in healthy controls. *Psychiat. Res.*, **4**, 21–9.

Orley, J. & Wing, J. K. (1979) Psychiatric disorders in two African villages. *Arch. Gen. Psychiat.*, **36**, 513–20.

Ormel, J. Von Korff, M., Van Den Brink, W. *et al.* (1993) Depression, anxiety and social disability show synchrony of change in primary care patients. *Am. J. Pub. Health*, **83**, 385–90.

Ormel, J., Von Korff, M., Ustun, B. *et al.* (1994) Common mental disorders and disability across cultures: results from the WHO collaborative study on psychological problems in general health care. *J. Am. Med. Assoc.*, **272**, 1741–8.

Orr, S., Piman, R., Lasko, N. & Herz, L. (1993) Psychophysiologic assessment of posttraumatic stress disorder imagery in World War II and Korean combat veterans. *J. Abn. Psychol.*, **102**, 152–9.

Orrell, M. & Bebbington, P. E. (1995) Life events and dementia. I. Admission deterioration and social environmental change. *Psychol. Med.*, **25**, 373–85.

Osler, M., Morgall, J. M., Jensen, B. & Osler, M. (1992) Repeat abortion in Denmark. *Dan. Med. Bull.*, **39**, 89–91.

Osontokun, B. O., Ogunniyi, A. O. & Lekwauwa, U. G. (1992) Alzheimer's disease in Nigeria. *Afr. J. Med. Med. Sci.*, **21**, 71–7.

Ost, L. G. (1987) Applied relaxation: description of coping techniques and review of controlled studies. *Behav. Res. Ther.*, **25**, 397–410.

Ost, L. G. (1989) One session treatment for specific phobias. *Behav. Res. Ther.*, **27**, 1–7.

Ost, L. G., Salkovskis, P. M. & Hellstrom, K. (1991) One session therapist directed exposure vs self-exposure in the treatment of spider phobia. *Behav. Ther.*, **22**, 407–22.

O'Sullivan, G., Noshirvani, H., Marks, I. M. *et al.* (1991) Six year follow-up after exposure and clomipramine therapy for obsessive-compulsive disorder. *J. Clin. Psychiat.*, **52**, 150–5.

Oswald, I. (1962) *Sleeping and Waking*. Elsevier, Amsterdam.

Otto, U. (1972) Suicidal acts by children and adolescents. *Acta Psychiat. Scand.*, Suppl. 233, 5–123.

Ounsted, C. & Lindsay, J. (1981) Long-term outcome of temporal lobe epilepsy in childhood. In *Epilepsy and Psychiatry* (ed. E. H. Reynolds & M. R. Trimble). Churchill Livingstone, Edinburgh, pp. 185–215.

Ovenstone, I. M. K. & Kreitman, N. (1974) Two syndromes of suicide. *Br. J. Psychiat.*, **124**, 336–45.

Overall, J. E. (1974) The Brief Psychiatric Rating Scale in psychopharmacology research. In *Psychological Measure in Psychopharmacology* (ed. P. Pichot). Karger, Basel.

Overall, J. E. & Gorham, D. R. (1962) The Brief Psychiatric Rating Scale (BPRS). *Psychol. Reports*, **10**, 799–812.

Ovretweit, J. (1986) *Case Responsibility in Multi-Disciplinary Teams (BIOSS)*. Good Practices in Mental Health, London.

Owen, J. B. (1990) Weight control and appetite: nature over nurture. *Animal Breeding Abstracts*, **58**, 583–91.

Pai, S. & Kapur, R. (1982) Impact of treatment intervention on the relationship between dimensions of clinical psychopathology, social dysfunction and burden on the family of psychiatric patients. *Psychol. Med.*, **12**, 651–8.

Paffenbarger, R. S. (1964) Epidemiological aspects of para-partum mental illness. *Br. J. Prev. Soc. Med.*, **18**, 189–95.

Paffenbarger, R. S. Jr. & McCabe, L. J. Jr. (1966) The effect of obstetric and perinatal events on risk of mental illness in women of childbearing age. *Am. J. Public Health*, **56**, 400–7.

Palazzoli, M. (1974) *Self-Starvation. From Individual to Family Therapy in the Treatment of Anorexia Nervosa*. Jason Aronson, New York.

Palmstierna, T., Lasserius, R. & Wistedt, B. (1989) Evaluation of the brief rating scale in relation to aggressive behaviour by acute involuntarily admitted patients. *Acta Psychiat. Scand.*, **79**, 313–16.

Pandey, G. N., Dysken, M. W., Garva, D. L. *et al.* (1979) Beta adrenergic receptor function in affective illness. *Am. J. Psychiat.*, **36**, 675–8.

Pantellis, C., Taylor, J. & Campbell, P. (1988) The South Camden schizophrenia survey. *Psychiat. Bull.*, **12**, 98–101.

Panting, A. & Merry, P. (1972) Long-term rehabilitation of severe head injuries. *Rehabilitation*, **38**, 33–7.

Papp, L., Klein, D., Martinez J. *et al.* (1993) Diagnostic and substance specificity of carbon dioxide induced panic. *Am. J. Psychiat.*, **150**, 250–7.

Pare, C. M. B. (1985) The present status of manoamine oxidase inhibitors. *Br. J. Psychiat.*, **154**, 287–91.

Pare, C. M. B., Kline, N., Hallstrom, C. *et al.* (1982) Will amitryptaline prevent the cheese reaction of monoamine oxidase inhibitors? *Lancet*, **ii**, 182–6.

Pare, C. M. B. & Raven. H. (1970) Psychiatric sequelae of therapeutic abortion: follow-up of patients referred for termination of pregnancy. *Lancet*, **i**, 635–8.

Pare, C. M. B. & Sandler, M. (1959) A clinical and biochemical study of a trial of iproniazid in the treatment of depression. *J. Neurol. Neurosurg. Psychiat.*, **22**, 247–51.

Parke, R. D. & Collmer, C. W. (1975) Child abuse. an interdisciplinary analysis. In *Review of Child Development Research*, Vol V (ed. E. M. Hetherington). University of Chicago Press, Chicago, pp. 509–91.

Parkes, J. D. (1993) Daytime sleepiness. *Br. Med. J.*, **306**, 772–5.

Parker, G. (1979) Reported parental characteristics of agoraphobics and social phobics. *Br. J. Psychiat.*, **135**, 555–60.

Parker, G. (1987) Are the lifetime prevalence estimates in the ECA study accurate? *Psychol. Med.*, **17**, 275–82.

Parker, G. (1992) Early environment. In *Handbook of Affective Disorders*, 2nd edn. (ed. E. S. Paykel). Churchill Livingstone, Edinburgh.

Parkin, A. J. (1982) *Memory and Amnesia: an Introduction*. Blackwell, Oxford.

Parkinson, I. S., Ward, M. K., Feest, T. G. *et al.* (1979) Fracturing dialysis osteodystrophy and dialysis encephalopathy. *Lancet*, **i**, 406–9.

Parrott, J., Strathdee, G. & Brown, P. (1988) Patient access to psychiatric records: the patient's view. *J. Roy. Soc. Med.*, **81**, 520–2.

Parry, G. (1992) Improving psychotherapy services. Applications of research, audit and evaluation. *Br. J. Clin. Psychol.*, **31** 3–19.

Parsons, T. (1951*a*) *The Social System*. The Free Press, Glencoe, Illinois.

Parsons, T. (1951*b*) Illness and the role of the physician: a sociological perspective. *Am. J. Orthopsychiat.*, **21**, 452–60.

Partenen, J., Bruun, K. & Markkanen, T. (1966) *Inheritance of Drinking Behaviour*. The Finnish Foundation for Alcohol Studies, Helsinki.

Pasamanick, B., Scarpitty, F. & Dinitz, S. (1967) *Schizophrenics in the Community*. Appleton-Century-Crofts, New York.

Passini, F. & Norman, W. (1966) A universal conception of personality structure? *J. Personal. Soc. Psychol.*, **4**, 44–9.

Passouant, P., Cadilhac, J. & Baldy-Moulinier, M. (1967) Physio-patholgie des hypersomnies. *Rev. Neurol.*, **116**, 585–629.

Patmore, C. & Weaver, T. (1990) Rafts on an open sea. *Health Service Journal*, 11th October, 1510–12.

Patrick, V., Dunner, D. L. & Fieve, R. R. (1978) Life events and primary affective illness. *Acta Psychiat. Scand.*, **58**., 48–55.

Patterson, D. G. (1992) Neurobiology of Substance Abuse. *Curr. Opin. Psychiat.*, **5**, 66–8.

Patterson, G. R. (1982) *Coercive Family Process*. Castalia Press, Eugene, Oregon.

Patterson, G. R. & Stoolmiller, M. (1991) Replications of a dual failure model for boys' depressed mood. *J. Consult. Clin. Psychol.*, **59**, 491–8.

Patton, G. C., Johnson-Sabine, E., Wood, K. *et al.* (1990) Abnormal eating attitudes in London schoolgirls – a prospective epidemiological study – outcome at 12 month follow-up. *Psychol. Med.*, **20**, 383–94.

Patton, G. C. (1988) Mortality and eating disorders. *Psychol. Med.*, **18**, 947–51.

Pattison, E. M., Sobell, M. B. & Sobell, L. C. (eds) (1977) *Emerging Concepts of Alcohol Dependence*. Springer, New York.

Paul, G. L. & Lentz, R. J. (1977) *Psychosocial Treatment of the Chronic Mental Patient*. Harvard University Press, Cambridge, MA.

Paykel, E. (1975) Suicide attempts and recent life events. *Arch. Gen. Psychiat.*, **32**, 327–33.

Paykel, E. S. (1983) Methodological aspects of life events research. *J. Psychosom. Res.*, **27**, 341–52.

Paykel, E. (1990) Innovations in mental health in the primary care system. In *Mental Health Service Evaluation* (ed. I. Marks & R. Scott). Cambridge University Press, Cambridge.

Paykel, E. S. & Cooper, Z. (1992) Life events and social stress. In *Handbook of Affective Disorders* (ed. E. S. Paykel). Churchill Livingstone, London, pp. 149–70.

Paykel, E. S., Emms, E. M., Fletcher, J. & Rassaby, E. S. (1980) Life events and social support in puerperal depression. *Br. J. Psychiat.*, **136**, 339–46.

Paykel, E. S., Myers, J. K. & Dienelt, M. N. (1969) Life events and depression: a controlled study. *Arch. Gen. Psychiat.*, **21**, 753–60.

Paykel, E. S., West, P. S., Rowan, P. R. & Parker, P. R. (1982) Influence of acetylator phenotype on antidepressant effects of phenelzine. *Br. J. Psychiat.*, **141**, 243–8.

Payne, R. L. & Graham Jones, J. (1987) Measurement and methodological issues in social support. In *Stress and Health: Issues in Research Methodology* (eds. S. V. Kasl & C. L. Cooper). Wiley, Chichester, pp. 167–205.

Payne, R. W. (1973) Cognitive abnormalities. In *Handbook for Abnormal Psychology* (ed. H. J. Eysenck), 2nd edn. Pitman Medical, London.

Peachey, J. E. & Annis, H. M. (1985) New strategies for using the alcohol-sensitising drugs. In *Research Advances in New Psychopharmacological Treatments for Alcoholism* (ed. C. A. Narianjo & E. M. Sellers). Excerpta Medica, Amsterdam, pp. 199–216.

Pearlson, G. D. (1994) Structural neuro-imaging in neuropsychiatry. In *Brain Imaging in Psychiatry* (ed. S. W. Lewis & N. P. Higgins). Blackwell Scientific Publications Ltd, Oxford.

Peck, C. C., Pond, S. M. & Becker, C. E. (1981) An evaluation of the effects of lithium in the treatment of chronic alcoholism. *Alcoholism: Clin. Exp. Res.*, **5**, 252–5.

Peet, M. & Harvey, N. S. (1991) Lithium maintenance – a standard education programme for patients. *Br. J. Psychiat.*, **158**, 197–204.

Pelever, R. & Fairburn, C. (1990) Eating disorders in women who abuse alcohol. *Br. J. Addict.*, **85**, 1633–8.

Pennington, B. F., Gilger, J. W., Pauls, D. *et al* (1991) Evidence for major gene transmission of developmental dyslexia. *J. Am. Med. Assoc.*, **266**, 1527–34.

Pequignot, G., Tuyns, A. G. & Berta, J. L. (1978) Ascitic cirrhosis in relation to alcohol consumption. *Int. J. Epidemiol.*, **7**, 113–20.

Perednia, C., Van Vreckem, E. & Vandereycken, W. (1989) Parent counselling: from guidance to treatment. In *The Family Approach to Eating Disorders* (ed. W. Vandereycken, E. Kog & J. Vanderlinden). PMA Publishing, New York, pp. 249–61.

Perez, M. M. & Trimble, M. R. (1980) Epileptic psychosis: diagnostic comparison with process schizophrenia. *Br. J. Psychiat.*, **137**, 245–9.

Perez, M. M., Trimble, M. R., Murray, N. M. F. *et al.* (1985) Epileptic psychosis: an evaluation of PSE profiles. *Br. J. Psychiat.*, **146**, 155–63.

Peroutka, S. J. & Snyder, S. H. (1980) Relationship of neuroleptic drug effects at brain dopamine, serotonin, alpha-adrenergic and histaminergic receptors to clinical potency. *Am. J. Psychiat.*, **137**, 1518–22.

Perpina, C., Hemsley, D., Treasure, J. & De Silva, P. (1993) Is their selective information processing of food and body works specific to patients with eating disorders? *Int. J. Eat. Disorders.*, **14.**, 359–66.

Perrin, S. & Last, C. G. (1992) Do childhood anxiety measures measure anxiety? *J. Abnorm. Child Psychol.*, **20**, 567–78.

Perris, C. (1966) A study of bipolar (manic-depressive) and unipolar recurrent depressive psychoses. *Acta Psychiat. Scand.*, suppl. 194.

Perris, C., Beskow, J. & Jacobson, L. (1980) Some remarks on the incidence of successful suicide in psychiatric care. *Soc. Psychiat.*, **15**, 1616–6.

Persaud, R. & Marks, I. (1995) A pilot study of exposure control of chronic auditory hallucinations in schizophrenia. *Br. J. Psychiat.*, **167**, 45–50.

Perry, A., Tomlinson, B., Blessed, G. *et al.* (1978) Correlation of cholinergic abnormalities with senile plaques and mental test scores in senile dementia. *Br. Med. J.*, **II**, 1457–9.

Peters, T. J. (1996) The physical complications of alcohol misuse. In *Oxford Textbook of Medicine* (ed. D. J. Weatherall, J. G. G. Ledingham & D. A. Warrell), pp. 4276–8.

Petrie, A. (1952) *Personality and the Frontal Lobes*. Routledge and Paul, London.

Peveler, R. & Fairburn C. (1990) Eating disorders in women who abuse alcohol. *Br. J. Addict.*, **85**, 1633–8.

Philips, J. P. N. (1986) Shapiro personal questionnaire and generalised personal questionnaire techniques: a repeated measures individualised outcome measurement. In *The Psychotherapeutic Process: A Research Handbook* (ed. L. S. Greenberg & W. M. Pinsof). Guilford, New York. pp. 557–89.

Phillips, K., McElroy, S., Keck, P. E. *et al* (1993) Body dysmorphic disorder: 30 cases of imagined ugliness. *Am. J. Psychiat.*, **150**, 302–8.

Philpot, M. P. (1986) Biological factors in depression in the elderly: In *Affective Disorders in the Elderly* (ed. E. Murphy). Churchill Livingstone, Edinburgh, pp. 53–77.

Philpot, N. & Burns, A. (1989) Reversible dementias. In *Dementia Disorders* (ed. C. Katona). Chapman & Hall, London, pp. 142–59.

Piccinelli, M. & Wilkinson, G. (1994) Outcome of depression in psychiatric settings. *Br. J. Psychiat.*, **164**, 297–30.

Pichot, P., Bailly, R. & Overall, J. E. (1966) Les sterotypes diagnostiques des psychoses chez les psychiatres Francais. Comparison avec les stereotypes Americains. *Proceedings of the Fifth International Congress of the Collegium Internationale Neuropsychopharmacologicum.* Excerpta Medica International Congress Series No. 129.

Pickens, R. W., Svikis, D. S., McGue, M. *et al.* (1991) Heterogeneity in the inheritance of alcoholism: a study of male and female twins. *Arch. Gen. Psychiat.*, **48**, 19–28.

Pierce, D. (1987) Deliberate self-harm in the elderly. *Int. Geriat. Psychiat.*, **2**, 105–10.

Piletz, J. E., Serasua, M. Magsood, C. *et al.* (1991) Relationship between membrane fluidity and adrenoceptor binding in depression. *Psychiat. Res.*, **38**, 1–12.

Pilgrim, D. & Rogers, A. (1993) Mental Health Service Users' Views of Medical Practitioners. *J. Interprof. Care.*, **7**, 167–76.

Pilgrim, J. A. & Mann, A. H. (1990) Use of the standardised assessment of personality to determine the prevalence of personality disorder in psychiatric in-patients. *Psychol. Med.*, **20**, 985–92.

Pilgrim, J. A., Mellors, J. D., Boothby, H. A. *et al* (1993) Inter-rater and temporal reliability of the standardised assessment of personality and the influence of informant characteristics. *Psychol. Med.*, **23**, 779–86.

Pilowsky, I. (1978) A general classification of abnormal illness behaviour. *Br. J. Med. Psychol.*, **51**, 131–7.

Pilowsky, I. (1985) Cryptotrauma and accident neurosis. *Br. J. Psychiat.*, **147**, 310–11.

Pilowsky, I. (1988) Abnormal illness behaviour. In *Handbook of Social Psychiatry* (ed. A. S. Henderson & G. Burrows). Elsevier, Amsterdam, pp. 305–15.

Pilowsky, L. S., Costa, D. C., Ell, P. J. *et al.* (1992) Clozapine, single photon emission tomography and the D2 dopamine receptor blockade hypothesis of schizophrenia. *Lancet*, **340**, 199–202.

Pilowsky, L. S., Costa, D. C., Ell, P. J. *et al.* (1993) Antipsychotic medication, D2 dopamine receptor blockade and clinical response – a 123 IBZM SPET (single photon emission tomography) study. *Psychol. Med.*, **23**, 791–9.

Pilowsky, L. & Murray, R. M. (1991) Why don't preschizophrenic children have delusions and hallucinations? *Behavioural and Brain Sciences*, **14**, 41–2.

Pinsker, H., Rosenthal, R. & McCullough, L. (1991) Dynamic supportive psychotherapy. In *Handbook of Short-term Dynamic Psychotherapy* (ed. P. Crits-Christoph & J. P. Barker), pp. 220–47.

Piran, N. & Kaplan, A. S. (eds) (1990) *A Day Hospital Group Treatment Programme for Anorexia Nervosa and Bulimia Nervosa*. Brunner Mazel, New York.

Pitt, B. (1968) Atypical depression following childbirth. *Br. J. Psychiat.*, **136**, 339–46.

Pitt, B. (1986) Characteristics of depression in the elderly. In *Affective Disorders in the Elederly* (ed. E. Murphy). pp. 41–51.

Pitt, B. (1991) Depression in the general hospital setting. *Br. J. Geriat. Psych.*, **6**, 363–70.

Pitts, F. & McClure, J. (1967) Lactate metabolism in anxiety neurosis. *New Eng. J. Med.*, **277**, 1329–36.

Plant, M. A. (1979) *Drinking Careers: Occupations, Drinking Habits and Drinking Problems*. Tavistock, London

Plant, M. I. (1990) *Women and Alcohol: a Review of International Literature on the Use of Alcohol*. World Health Organization, Geneva.

Platt, S., Hawton, J., Kreitman, H. *et al* (1988) Recent clinical and epidemiological trends in parasuicide in Edinburgh and Oxford: a tale of two cities. *Psychol. Med.*, **18**, 405–18.

Platt, S. & Kreitman, N. (1984) Trends in parasuicide and unemployment among men in Edinburgh 1968 to 1982. *Br. Med. J.*, **289**, 1029–32.

Platt, S. & Kreitman, N. (1985) Parasuicide and unemployment among men in Edinburgh. *Psychol. Med.*, **15**, 113–23.

Pliszka, S. R. (1989) Effect of anxiety on cognition, behaviour, and stimulant response in ADHD. *J. Am. Acad. Child & Adol. Psychiat.*, **28**, 882–7.

Plomin, R. (1990) The role of inheritance in behaviour. *Science*, **248**, 183–8.

Plomin, R., McLearn, G. E., Smith, D. L. *et al.* (1996) DNA markers associated with high and low IQ: the IQ and QTL project. *Behav. Genet.* (in press).

Plomin, R., Owen, M. J. & McGuffin, P. (1994). The genetics basis of complex human behaviours. *Science*, **26**, 1733–9.

Plomin, R., Rende, R. & Rutter, M. (1991) Quantitative genetics and developmental psychopathology. In *Internalising and Externalising Expressions of Dysfunction: Rochester Symposium on Developmental Psychopathology*. Vol. II. (ed. D. Cicchetti & S. L. Toth). Lawrence Erlbaum, Hillside, NJ, pp. 155–202.

Plum, F. & Posner, J. (1980) *Diagnosis of Stupor and Coma*. F. A. Davis, Philadelphia.

Pocock, S. J. (1991) *Clinical Trials*. John Wiley and Sons, Chichester.

Podoll, K., Schwam, M. & Noth, J. (1990) Charles Bonnet-syndrome bei einem Parkinson – patienten mit biedseitigem visusverlust. *Nervenarzt.*, **61**, 52–6.

Pond, D. (1981) Epidemiology of the psychiatric disorders of epilepsy. In *Epilepsy and Psychiatry* (ed. E. H. Reynolds & M. R. Trimble). Churchill Livingstone, Edinburgh, pp. 291–5.

Pond, D. & Bidwell, B. H. (1960) A survey of epilepsy in 14 general practices. *Epilepsia*, 1, 285–99.

Pogue-Geile, M. F., Garrett, A. H., Brunke, J. J. & Hall, J. K. (1991) Neuropsychological impairments are increased in siblings of schizophrenic patients. *Schiz. Res.*, 4, 390.

Pohl, R., Yeragani, V., Balon, R. & Lycaki H. (1988) The jitteriness syndrome in panic disorder patients treated with antidepressants. *J. Clin. Psychiat.*, 49, 100–104.

Pokorny, A. D. (1966) A follow-up study of 618 suicidal patients. *Am. J. Psychiat.*, 122, 1109–16.

Pokorny, A. D. (1983) Prediction of suicide in psychiatric patients. Report of a prospective study. *Arch Gen Psychiat.*, 40, 249–57.

Polak, P. & Kirby, M. (1976) A model to replace psychiatric hospitals. *J. Nerv. Ment. Dis.*, 162, 13–22.

Polich, J. M., Armor, D. J. & Braiker, H. B. (1981) *The Course of Alcoholism.* Wiley, New York.

Polich, J., Haier, R. J., Buchsbaum, M. & Bloom, F. E. (1988) Assessment of young men at risk for alcoholism with P300 from a visual discrimination task. *J. Studies in Alcohol*, 49, 186–90.

Polivy J. & Herman, C. P. (1985) Dieting and binging: a causal analysis. *Am. Psychol.*, 40, 193–201.

Polkinghome Report (1989) *Review of the Guidance on the Research Use of Fetuses and Fetal Material.* HMSO, London.

Pollak, O. (1950) *The Criminality of Women.* University of Pennsylvania Press, New York.

Pollack, J. & Horner, A. (1985) Brief adaptations-oriented psychotherapy. In *Clinical and Research Issues in Short-term Dynamic Psychotherapy* (ed. A. Winston). American Psychiatric Press, Washington DC.

Pollit, J. (1957) Natural history of obessional states. *Br. J. Psychiat.*, 1, 194–8.

Pollitt, J. (1972) The relationship between genetic and precipitating factors in depressive illness. *Br. J. Psychiat.*, 1221, 67–70.

Pollock, V. E. (1992) Meta-analysis of subjective sensitivity to alcohol in sons of alcoholics. *Am. J. Psychiat.*, 149, 1534–8.

Pollock, V. E., Volavka, J., Goodwin, D. W. *et al.* (1983) The EEC after alcohol administration in men at risk for alcoholism. *Arch. Gen. Psych.*, 40, 857–81.

Pond, S. M., Becker, C. E. & Vandervoort, R. (1981) An evaluation of the effects of lithium in the treatment of chronic alcoholism I: clinical results. *Alcoholism Clin. Exper. Res.*, 5, 247–51.

Pop, d. J., De Rooy, H. A. M., Vader, H. L. *et al.* (1991) Postpartum thyroid dysfunction and depression in an unselected population. *N. Engl. J. Med.*, 324, 1815–16.

Pope, H. G., Jonas, J. M., Cohen, B. M. *et al.* (1982) Failure to find schizophrenia in first degree relatives of shizophrenic probands. *Am. J. Psychiat.*, 139, 826.

Pope, H. G. & Lipinsky, J. F. (1978) Diagnosis in schizophrenia and manic depressive illness. *Arch. Gen. Psychiat.*, 35, 811–28.

Popper, K. (1959) *The Logic of Scientific Discovery.* Hutchinson, London.

Porporino, F. J. & Baylis, E. (1993) Designing a progressive penology: the evolution of Canadian Federal Corrections. *Clin. Behav. Ment. Hlth.*, 3, 268–9.

Porter, R. J. (1993) Classification of epileptic seizures and epileptic syndromes. In *A Textbook of Epilepsy* (ed. J. Laidlow, A. Richens & D. Chadwick). Churchill Livingstone, London, pp. 1–22.

Porter, T. L., Levine, J. & Dinneen, M. (1993) Shifts of dependency in the resolution of *folie à deux.* *Br. J. Psychiat.*, 162, 704–6.

Posey, T. B. & Losch, M. E. (1983) Auditory hallucinations of hearing voices in 375 normal subjects. *Imagination Cognition & Personality*, 2, 99–113.

Post, F. (1965) *The Clinical Psychiatry of Late Life.* Pergamon Press, Oxford, pp. 77–105.

Post, F. (1966) *Persistent Persecutory States of the Elderly.* Pergamon, Oxford.

Post, F. (1982) Paranoid disorders. In *Handbook of Psychiatry* vol. 3. (ed. J. K. Wing & L. Wing). Cambridge University Press, Cambridge.

Post, F. (1982) Functional disorders I: Description, incidence and recognition. In *Psychiatry of Late Life* (ed. R. Levy & F. Post). Blackwell, Oxford, pp. 180–1.

Post, F. (1986) The factor of ageing in affective illness. In *Recent Developments in Affective Disorders* (ed. A. Coppen & A. Walk). Headley Bros, Ashford, pp. 105–16.

Pounder, D. J. (1985) Suicide by leaping from multistorey car parks. *Medicine, Science and the Law,* **25,** 179–88.

Powell, G. E. (1981) *Brain Function Therapy.* Gower, Aldershot.

Powell, M. (1987) Data note 8: Alcohol data in the European Community. *Br. J. Addiction,* **82,** 559–66.

Preskorn, S. H. (1993) Pharmacokinetics of psychotropic agents: why and how they are relevant to treatment. *J. Clin. Psychiat.,* **54** (suppl), 3–8.

Preston, S., Hines, L., Eggers, M. (1989) Demographic conditions responsible for populations ageing. *Demography,* **26,** 691–704.

Prettyman, R. J. & Cordle, C. (1992) Psychological aspects of miscarriage: attitudes of the primary health care team. *Br. J. Gen. Pract.,* **42,** 97–9.

Price, R. W., Sidtis, J. & Rosenblum, M. (1988) The AIDS dementia complex – some current questions. *Ann. Neurol.,* **23,** 27–33.

Prichard, J. C. (1835) *A Treatise of Insanity.* Sherwood Gilbert and Pipers, London.

Prien, R., Caffey, E. & Klett, C. (1972) A comparison of lithium carbonate and chlorpromazine in the treatment of schizoaffecting. *Arch. Gen. Psychiat.,* **27,** 182–9.

Prien, R. F., Kupfer, D. J., Mansky, P. A. *et al.* (1984) Drug therapy in the prevention of recurrences in unipolar and bipolar affective disorders. *Arch. Gen. Psychiat.,* **4,** 1096–194.

Prien, R. F. & Levine, J. (1984) Research and methodological issues to evaluate the therapeutic effectiveness of antidepressant drugs. *Psychopharmacol. Bull.,* **20,** 250–7.

Priest, R. G. (1989) (Ed) Depression and reversible monoamine oxidase inhibitors: New perspectives. *Br. J. Psychiat.,* Suppl 6.

Prior, M. (1992) Childhood temperament. *J. Child Psychol. Psychiat.,* **33,** 249–79.

Pritchard, C. (1992) Changes in elderly suicides in the USA and the developed world 1974–1987: Comparison with current homicide. *Int. Geriat. Psychiat.,* **7,** 125–34.

Procci, W. R. (1976) Schizo-affective psychosis: fact or fiction? *Arch. Gen. Psychiat.,* **33,** 1167–78.

Prochaska, J. O. & DiClemente, C. C. (1983) Stages and processes of self-change of smoking: towards a more integrative model of change. *J. Consult. Clin. Psychol.,* **51,** 390–5.

Prochaska, J. O. & DiClemente, C. C. (1985) *The Transtheoretical Approach: Crossing Traditional Boundaries of Therapy.* Dow Jones-Irwin, Homewood, IL.

Pugh, T. F., Jerath, B. K., Schmidt, W. M. & Reed, R. B. (1963) Rates of mental disease related to childbearing. *N. Engl. J. Med.,* **268,** 1224–23.

Puig-Antich J., Perel, J. M., Lupatkin, W. *et al.* (1987) Imipramine in prepubertal major depressive disorders. *Arch. Gen. Psychiat.,* **44,** 81–9.

Pujal, J., Leal, S. Fluia, X. & Conde, C. (1989) Psychiatric aspects of normal pressure hydrocephalus. A report of five cases. *Br. J. Psychiat.,* **154,** 77–80.

Pulkkinen, L. (1988) Delinquent development: theoretical and empirical considerations. In *Studies of Psychosocial Risk* (ed. M. Rutter). Cambridge University Press, Cambridge, pp. 184–99.

Pullen, I., Wilkinson, G., Wright, A. & Pereira Grey, D. (1994) *Psychiatry and General Practice Today.* Gaskell, London.

Pullen I. & Yellowlees, A. (1988) Scottish psychiatrists in primary health care settings: a silent majority. *Br. J. Psychiat.,* **153,** 633–6.

Pynoos, R., Goenjian, A., Tashjian, M. *et al.* (1993) Post-traumatic stress reactions in children after the 1988 Armenian earthquake. *Br. J. Psychiat.,* **163,** 239–47.

Pyorala, E. (1990) Trends in alcohol consumption in Spain, Portugal, France and Italy from the 1950s until the 1980s. *Br. J. Addict.,* **85,** 469–77.

Quality Assurance Project (1991) (a) Treatment outlines for borderline, narcissistic and histrionic personality disorders. (b) Treatment outlines for avoidant, dependent and passive – aggressive personality disorders. *Austral. N.Z. J. Psychiat.,* **25,** 391–403; 404–11.

Rabins, P., Perlson, G., Jayaram, G. *et al.,* (1987) Increased VBR in late onset schizophrenia. *Am. J. Psychiat.,* **144,** 1216–18.

Rachman, S. (1974) Primary obsessional slowness. *Behav. Res Ther.,* **12,** 9–18.

Rachman, S. J. & Hodgson, R. J. (1968) Experimentally induced 'sexual fetishism': replication and development. *Psychol. Rec.*, **18**, 25–7.

Rachman, S. J. & Hodgson, R. J. (1980) *Obsessions and Compulsions*. Prentice Hall, Englewood Cliffs.

Rail, D., Scholtz C. & Swash, M. (1981) Post-encephalitic parkinsonism: current experience. *J. Neurol. Neurosurg, Psychiat.*, **44**, 670–6.

Ramon, S. (1988) Community care in Britain. In *Community Care in Practice* (ed. A. Lavender & F. Holloway). F. Wiley & Sons.

Rampling, D. (1985) Ascetic ideals and anorexia nervosa. *J. Psychiat. Res.*, **19**, 89–94.

Rank, O. (1924) *The Trauma of Birth*. Harper & Row, New York, 1973.

Rao, J. M. (1990) A population based study of mild mental handicap in children: preliminary analysis of obstetric associations. *J. Ment. Defic. Res.*, **34**, 59–65.

Rapin, I. & Allen, D. (1983) Developmental language disorders: nosologic considerations. *Neuropsychology of Language, Reading and Spelling* (ed. U. Kirk). Academic Press, New York.

Rapoport, J. (1991) Recent advances in obsessive-compulsive disorder. *Neuropsychopharmacology*, **5**, 1–10.

Rapoport, J., Buchsbaum, M. S., Weingartner, H. *et al* (1980) Dextroamphetamine. Its cognitive and behavioural effects in normal and hyperactive boys and normal men. *Arch Gen. Psychiat.*, **37**, 933–43.

Raskin, V. D. (1993) Psychiatric aspects of substance use disorders in childbearing populations. *Psychiatric Clinics of North America: Recent Advances in Addictive Studies* (ed. N. S. Miller), **16** 157–65. W. B. Saunders, Philadelphia.

Rasmunssen, A. A., Eisen, J. L. & Plat, M. T. (1993) Current issues in the pharmacologic management of obsessive-compulsive disorder. *J. Clin. Psychiat.*, **54**, suppl. 6, 4–9.

Rastam, M. & Gillberg, G. (1992) Background factors of anorexia nervosa. *Eur. Child Adol. Psychiat.*, **1**, 54–65.

Rastam, M., Gillberg, C. & Garton, M. (1989) Anorexia nervosa in a Swedish urban region: a population based study. *Brit. J. Psychiat.*, **155**, 642–6.

Ratnasuriya, R. H., Eisler, I., Szmukler, G. I & Russell, G. F. M. (1991) Anorexia nervosa: outcome and prognostic factors after 20 years. *Br. J. Psychiat.*, **158**, 495–502.

Rauch, S., Jenike, M., Alpert, N. *et al* (1994) Regional cerebral blood flow measured during symptom provocation in obsessive-compulsive disorder using oxygen-15 labelled carbon dioxide and positron emission tomography. *Arch. Gen. Psychiat.*, **51**, 62–70.

Rausch, J. L., Montiero, M. G. & Schuckit, M. A. (1991) Platelet serotonin uptake in men with family histories of alcoholism. *Neuropsychopharmacology*, **4**, 83–6.

Ravn, J. F. (1970) The history of the thioxanthenes. In: *Discoveries in Biological Psychiatry* (ed. F. J. Blackwell). J. B. Lippincott, Philadelphia, pp 180–94.

Rawnsley, K. (1967) An international diagnostic exercise. *Proceedings of the Fourth World Congress of Psychiatry*, **4**, 2683–6. Excerpta Medica Foundation, Amsterdam.

Rehman, A. U., St. Clair, D. & Platz, C. (1990) Puerperal insanity in the 19th and 20th centuries. *Br. J. Psychiat.*, **156**, 861–5.

Regier, D. A., Burke, J. R., Manderscheid, R. W. & Burns, B. J. (1985) The chronically mentally ill in primary care. *Psychol. Med.*, **15**, 265–73.

Regier, D. A., Farmer, M. E., Rae, D. *et al.* (1993) One-month prevalence of mental disorder in the United States and sociodemographic characteristics: The epidemiologic catchment area study. *Acta Psychiat. Scand.*, **88**, 35–47.

Regier, D., Narrow, W. & Rae, D. (1990) The epidemiology of anxiety disorders: the epidemiological catchment area (ECA) experience *J. Psychiat. Res.*, **24** (suppl. 2), 3–14.

Reich, J. H., Yates, W. & Nduaguba, M. (1989) Prevalence of DSM-III personality disorders in the community. *Social Psychiatry*, **24**, 12–16.

Reid, A. H. (1980) Diagnosis of psychiatric disorder in the severely and profoundly retarded patient. *J. Roy. Soc. Med.*, **73**, 607–9.

Reid, A. H. (1983) Psychiatry of mental handicap: a review. *J. Roy. Soc. Med.*, **76**, 587–9.

Reid, A. H. & Ballinger, B. R. (1987) Personality Disorder in mental handicap. *Psychol. Med,* **17,** 983–9.

Reid, W. H. (1985) The anti-social personality: a review. *Hosp. Comm. Psychiat.,* **36,** 831–7.

Reiss, A. J. & Roth, J. A. (Eds.) (1993) *Understanding and Preventing Violence.* National Academy Press, Washington DC.

Reiss, S. (1988) *The Reiss Test Screen.* Diagnostic Systems Inc.

Reiss, S. (1993) Assessment of psychopathology in persons with mental retardation. In *Psychopathology and Mental Retardation* (2nd edn) (ed. J. L. Matson & R. P. Barrett). Grune & Stratton, New York. pp. 17–40.

Reiss, S., Levitan, G. W. & Szysko, J. (1982) Emotional disturbance and mental retardation: Diagnostic overshadowing. *Am. J. Ment. Defic.,* **86,** 567–4.

Reitman, B. & Cleveland, S. (1964) Changes in body image following sensory deprivation in schizophrenia and control groups. *J. Abn. Soc. Psychol.,* **68,** 168–76.

Remick, R. A. & Maurice, W. L. (1978) ECT in pregnancy. *Am. J. Psychiat,* **135,** 761–2.

Renshaw, J., Hampson, R., Thomason, C. *et al.* (1988) *Care in the Community: The First Steps.* Gower, Aldershot.

Renton, C.A., Affleck, J. W., Carstairs, G. M. & Forrest, A. D. (1963) A follow-up of schizophrenic patients in Edinburgh. *Acta Psychiat. Scand.,* **39,** 548–600.

Repp, A. & Felce, D. (1990) A micro-computer system used for evaluative and experimental research in mental handicap. *Ment. Hand. Res.,* **3,** 21–32.

Rett Syndrome Diagnostic Criteria Workshop (1988) Diagnostic criteria for Rett syndrome. *Ann. Neurol.,* **23,** 425–8.

Reveley, A., Reveley, M., Clifford, C. & Murray, R. M. (1982) Cerebral ventricular size in twins discordant for schizophrenia. *Lancet,* **i,** 540–1.

Reveley, A. M., Reveley, M. A. & Murray, R. M. (1984) Cerebral ventricular enlargement in non-genetic schizophrenia: a controlled study. *Br. J. Psychiat.,* **144,** 89–93.

Reveley, M. & Campbell, I. C. (1986) Neurochemistry. In *The Scientific Principles of Psychopathology* (ed. P. McGuffin, M. Shanks & R. J. Hodgson). Academic Press, London, Orlando and New York, pp. 57–95.

Rey, J. M. & Hutchins, P. (1993) Childhood hyperactivity. *Med. J. Aust.,* **159,** 289–91.

Reynolds, C. F., Kupfer, D. J., Hock, P. R. *et al.* (1988) Reliable discrimination of elderly depressed and demented patients by electroencephalographic sleep data. *Arch. Gen Psychiat.,* **45,** 258–64.

Reynolds, E. H. (1968) Epilepsy and schizophrenia. *Lancet,* **i,** 398–401.

Reynolds, G. P. (1992) Developments in the drug treatment of schizophrenia. *Trends Pharmacol. Sci.,* **13,** 116–21.

Reynolds, J. (1669) *A Discourse on Prodigious Abstinence.* Royal College of Psychiatrists, London.

Reynolds, J. (1869) Three cases of paralysis dependent on idea. *Br. Med. J.,* 1869, **ii** 483–5.

Reynolds, W. M. (1994) Depression in adolescents: contemporary issues and perspectives. In *Advances in Clinial Child Psychology.* Vol. 16 (ed. T. H. Ollendick & R. J. Prinz). Plenum Press, London. pp. 261–316.

Rich, C. L., Fowler, R. C., Fogarty, L. A. & Young, D. (1988) San Diego suicide study. III. Relationship between diagnoses and stressors. *Arch. Gen. Psychiat.,* **45,** 589–92.

Richman, N. (1993) Children in situations of political violence. *J. Child Psychol. Psychiat.,* **34,** 1286–302.

Richman, N., Stevenson, J. E. & Graham, P. J. (1975) Prevalence of behaviour problems in three-year-old children: an epidemiological study in a London borough. *J. Child Psychol. Psychiat.,* **16,** 277–87.

Rifkin, L., Lewis, S., Jones, P. B. *et al* (1994) Low birth weight and schizophrenia. *Br. J. Psychiat.,* **165,** 357–62.

Riley, A. J., Goodman, R. E., Kellett, J. M. & Orr, R. (1989) Double-blind trial of yohimbine hydrochloride in the treatment of erection inadequacy. *Sexual and Marital Therapy,* **4,** 17–26.

Riley, D. (1986) An audit of obstetric liaison psychiatry in 1984. *J. Reprod. Infant Psychol.,* **4,** 99–115.

Rimland, B. (1993) Editorial. *Autism Res. Rev*, **7**, 5–7.

Ritchie, J. H., Dick, D. & Lingham, R. (1994) *The Report of the Inquiry into the Treatment of Christopher Clunis*. HMSO, London.

Robens, A. B. & Kertesz, A. (1983) The localisation of lesions in aphasias. In *Aphasias* (ed. A. Kertesz). Academic Press, New York, pp. 245–68.

Roberts, G. W., Done, D. J., Bruton, C. & Crow, T. J. (1990) A 'mock-up' of schizophrenia-like psychosis. *Biol. Psychiat.*, **28**, 127–43.

Robertson, G. & Gunn, J. (1987) A ten-year follow-up of men discharged from Grendon Prison. *Br. J. Psychiat.*, **151**, 674–8.

Robertson, G. & Taylor, P. J. (1985) a. Some cognitive correlates of schizophrenic illnesses. *Psychol. Med.*, **15**, 81–98. b. Some cognitive correlates of affective disorders. *Psychol. Med.*, **15**, 297–309.

Robertson, M. M. (1989) The Gilles de la Tourette Syndrome: current status. *Br. J. Psychiat.*, **154**, 147–69.

Robertson, M. M. (1994) Gilles de la Tourette syndrome – an update. *J. Child Psychol. Psychiat.*, **35**, 597–611.

Robertson, N.C. (1979) Variations in referral patterns to the psychiatric services by general practitioners. *Psychol. Med.*, **9**, 355–64.

Robin, A. & Harris, J. A. (1962) A controlled comparison of imipramine and electroplexy. *J. Ment. Sci.*, **108**, 217–19.

Robins, E. & Guze, S. B. (1972) Classifcation of affective disorders: the primary-secondary, the endogenous-reactive, and the neurotic-psychotic concepts. In *Recent Advances in the Psychobiology of the Depressive Illnesses* (ed. T. A. Williams, M. M. Katz & J. A. Shield), US Government Printing Office, Washington DC. pp. 283–93.

Robins, H. S. & Michelson, J. B. (1988) *Illustrated Handbook of Drug Abuse Recognition and Diagnosis*. Year Book Medical Publishers, Chicago and London.

Robins, E., Murphy, G. E., Wilkinson, R. H. *et al.* (1959) Some clinical considerations in the prevention of suicide based on a study of 134 successful suicides. *Am. J. Pub. Health*, **49**, 888–99.

Robins, L. N. (1966) *Deviant Children Grown Up: A Sociological and Psychiatric Study of Sociopathic Personality*. Williams and Wilkins, Baltimore.

Robins, L. N. (1978) Sturdy predictors of adult antisocial behaviour: replications from longitudinal studies. *Psychol. Med.*, **8**, 611–22.

Robins, L. N. (1985) Epidemiology: reflections on testing the validity of psychiatric interviews. *Arch. Gen. Psychiat.*, **42**, 918–24.

Robins, L. N. (1993) Vietnam veterans' rapid recovery from heroin addiction: a fluke or normal expectation. *Addiction*, **88**, 1041–54.

Robins, L. N., Helzer, J. E., Crougha, J. *et al.* (1981) National Institute of Mental Health Diagnostic Interview Schedule; its history, characteristics and validity. *Arch. Gen. Psychiat.*, **38**, 381–9.

Robins, L. N., Helzer, J. E., Weissman, M. M. *et al.* (1984) Lifetime prevalence of specific psychiatric disorders in three sites. *Arch. Gen. Psychiat.*, **41**, 949–58.

Robins, L. N., Helzer, J. E., Orvaschel, H. *et al.* (1985) The Diagnostic Interview Schedule. In *Epidemiologic Field Methods in Psychiatry: The NIMH Epidemiologic Catchment Area Program* (ed. W. W. Eaton & L. G. Kessler). Academic Press, Orlando, Flo. pp. 143–70.

Robins, L., Helzer, J. & Przybeck, T. (1986) Substance abuse in the general population. In *Mental Disorders in the Community. Progress and Challenges* (ed. J. Barrett & R. Rose). Guilford Press, New York.

Robins, L. N. & Price, R. K. (1991) Adult disorders predicted by childhood conduct problems: results from the NIMH Epidemiologic Catchment Area project. *Psychiatry*, **54**, 116–32.

Robins, L. N. & Regier, D. A. (eds) (1991) *Psychiatric Disorder in America: The Epidemiological Catchment Area Study*. The Free Press, New York, NY.

Robins, L. N. & Sartorius, N. (1993) Editorial. *Internat. J. Meth. Psychiat. Res.*, **3**, 63–5.

Robins, L, N., Wing, J., Wittche, H. U. *et al.* (1988) The Composite International Diagnostic

Interview. An Epidemiological instrument suitable for use in conjunction with different diagnostic systems and in different cultures. *Arch. Gen. Psychiat.*, **45**, 1969–77.

Robinson, A. (1984) *Respite Care Services for Families with a Handicapped Child.* National Children's Bureau, London.

Robinson, D. S., Kayser, A., Corcell, J. *et al.* (1973) The monoamine oxidase inhibitor phenelzine, in the treatment of depressive anxiety states: a controlled clinical trial. *Arch. Gen. Psychiat.*, **29**, 407–13.

Robson, M. H., France, R. & Bland, M. (1984) Clinical psychologist in primary care. Controlled clinical and economic evaluation. *Br. Med. J.*, **288**, 1805–8.

Rocca, W. A., Hofman, A., Brayne, C. *et al* (1991) The prevalence of vascular dementia in Europe: facts and fragments from 1980–1990 studies. *Ann. Neurol.*, **30**, 817–24.

Roche Report (1978) *Frontiers of Psychiatry.* Hoffman La Roche, Nutley, N. J.

Roe, A. & Burks, B. (1945) Adult adjustment of foster-children of alocholic and psychotic parentage and the influence of the foster home. In *Memoirs of the Section of Alcohol Studies.*

Rogers, A. & Faulkner, A. (1987) *A Place of Safety.* MIND, London.

Rogers, A., Pilgrim D. & Lacey, R. (1993) *Experiencing Psychiatry: Users' Views of Services.* Macmillan, London.

Rogers, H. J., Sector, R. G. & Trounee, J. R. (1981) *A Textbook of Clinical Pharmacology.* Hodder & Stoughton, UK.

Rolleston Report (1926) *Report of the Departmental Committee on Morphine and Heroin Addiction.* HMSO, London.

Romanoski, A. J., Folstein, M. F., Nestadt, G. *et al.* (1992) The epidemiology of psychiatrist-ascertained depression and DSM-III depressive disorders: Results from the Eastern Baltimore Mental Health Survey Clinical Reappraisal. *Psychol. Med.*, **22**, 929–655.

Romans, S., Walton, V., McNoe, B. *et al.* (1993) Otago women's health survey: 30-month follow-up. I: Onset patterns of non-psychotic psychiatric disorder. *Br. J. Psychiat.*, **163**, 733–738.

Romelsjo, A. & Agren, G. (1985) Has mortality related to alcohol decreased in Sweden? *Br. Med. J.*, **291**, 167–70.

Rooth, F. G. (1971) Indecent exposure and exhibitionism. *Br. J. Hosp. Med.*, **5**, 521–33.

Rorsmann, B. (1973) Suicide in psychiatric patients: a comparative study. *Soc. Psychiat.*, **8**, 55–66.

Rose, G. (1992) *The Strategy of Preventive Medicine.* OUP, Oxford.

Rose, G. & Barker, D. J. P. (1978) What is a case? Dichotomy or continuum? *Br. Med. J.*, **2**, 873–4.

Rose, G. & Barker, D. J. P. (1986) *Epidemiology for the Unitiated* (2nd edn). British Medical Journal, London.

Rose, S. (1993) *The Making of Memory.* Beniam, London.

Rosen, A., Hadzi-Pavlovic, D. & Parker, G. (1989) The life skills profile: a measure assessing function and disability in schizophrenia. *Schiz. Bull.*, **15**, 325–37.

Rosenbaum, J. F., Biederman, J., Gersten, M. *et al.* (1988) Behavioural inhibition in children of parents with panic disorder and agoraphobia. *Arch. Gen. Psychiat.*, **45**, 463–70.

Rosenhan, D. L. (1973) On being sane in insane places. *Science*, **179**, 250–8.

Rosenman, R. H., Brand, R. J., Jenkins, C. D. *et al.* (1975) Coronary heart disease in the Western collaborative group study: Final follow-up experience of 8 and a half years. *J. Amer. Med. Assoc.*, **233**, 872–7.

Rosenthal, D., Wender, P., Kety, S. *et al.* (1971) The adopted-away offspring of schizophrenics. *Am. J. Psychiat.*, **128**, 307–11.

Rosenthal, M. S. (1991) Therapeutic Communities. In *The International Handbook of Addiction Behaviour* (ed. B. Illana Glass). Routledge, London, pp. 258–63.

Rosin, A. J. & Glatt, M. M. (1971) Alcohol excess in the elderly. *Quart. J. Stud. Alcohol.*, **32**, 53–9.

Ross, E. D. & Rush, A. J. (1981) Diagnosis and neuroanatomical correlates of depression in brain-damaged patients. *Arch. Gen. Psychiat.*, **38**, 1344–54.

Ross, H. E. & Glaser, F. B. (1989) Psychiatric screening of alcohol and drug patients: the validity of the GHQ-60. *Am. J. Drug Alcohol Abuse*, **15**(4), 429–42.

Rossman, B., Mieza, M. & Melman, A. (1990) Penile vein ligation for corporal incompetence. An evaluation of short-term and long-term results. *J. Urology*, **144**, 679–82.

Roth, L. (1980) Correctional psychiatry. In *Modern Legal Medicine, Psychiatry and Forensic Science* (ed. W. J. Curran, A. L. McGarry & C. S. Petty). Davis, Philadelphia.

Roth, M. (1955) The natural history of mental disorder in old age. *J. Ment. Sci.*, **101**, 281–301.

Roth, M. (1959) The phenomenology of depressive states. *Can. Psychiat. Assoc. J.*, **4** (Special Supplement) 32–54.

Roth, M. (1976) Schizophrenia and the theories of Thomas Szasz. *Br. J. Psychiat.*, **129**, 317–25.

Roth, M. Gurney, C., Garside, R. F. *et al.* (1972) Studies in the classification of affective disorders: the relationship between anxiety states and depressive illnesses I. *Br. J. Psychiat.*, **121**, 147–161.

Rothenberg, A. (1986) Eating disorders as a modern obsessive-compulsive syndrome. *Psychiatry*, **49**, 45–53.

Rounsaville, B. J., Anton, S. F., Carroll, K. *et al.* (1991) Psychiatric diagnoses of treatment seeking cocaine abusers. *Arch. Gen. Psychiat.*, **48**, 43–51.

Rounsaville, B. J., Dolinksy, Z. S., Babor, T. F. & Meyer, R. E. (1987) Psychopathology as a predictor of treatment outcome in alcoholics. *Arch. Gen. Psychiat.*, **44**, 505–13.

Rounsaville, B. J., Weissman, M. M., Kleber, H. D. & Wilber, C. (1982) Heterogeneity of psychiatric diagnosis in treated opiate addicts. *Arch. Gen. Psychiat.*, **39**, 161–6.

Rourke, B. (1988) The syndrome of non-verbal learning disabilities. *Clin. Neuropsychol*, **2**, 293–330.

Rovner, B. W., German, P. S., Broadhead, J. *et al.* (1990) The prevalence and mangement of dementia in nursing homes. *Int. Psychogeriat. J.*, **2**, 13–24.

Rovner, B. W., Kafonek, S., Filipp, L. *et al.* (1986) Prevalence of mental illness in a community nursing home. *Am. J. Psychiat.*, **143**, 1446–9.

Rowland, N., Maynard, A., Beveridge, A. *et al.* (1987) Doctors have no time for alcohol screening. *Br. Med. J.*, **295**, 95–6.

Roy, A. (1982*a*) Risk factors for suicide in psychiatric patients. *Arch. Gen. Psychiat*, **39**, 1089–95.

Roy, A. (1982*b*) Suicide in chronic schizophrenia. *Br. J. Psychiat.*, **141**, 613–17.

Roy, A. (1990) Suicide in twins. *Arch. Gen. Psychiat.*, **48**, 29–31.

Roy, A. Breier, A., Doran, A. R. *et al.* (1985) Life events and depression: relation to subtypes. *J. Affect. Disorders*, **9**, 143–8.

Royal College of General Practitioners (1986) *Alcohol – a Balanced View*. Royal College of General Practitioners, London.

Royal College of General Practitioners (1992) *Women and Alcohol*. HMSO, London.

Royal College of Physicians (1981) Organic mental impairment in the elderly. *J. Roy. Coll. Physic.*, **15**, 141–67.

Royal College of Physicians (1987) *The Medical Consequences of Alcohol Abuse. A Great and Growing Evil*. Tavistock, London.

Royal College of Physicians (1991) *Physical Signs of Sexual Abuse in Children*. Royal College of Physicians, London.

Royal College of Physicians & Royal College of Psychiatrists (1989) *Care of Elderly People with Mental Illness: Specialist Services and Medical Training*. RCP & RCPsych. London.

Royal College of Physicians, Royal College of General Practitioners & Royal College of Psychiatrists (1992) *Report of the Working Party of Three Medical Royal Colleges on the Education and Training of Doctors in the Health Care Service for Prisoners*. Available from the College.

Royal College of Physicians & Royal College of Psychiatrists (1995) *The Psychological Care of Medical Patients: Recognition of Need and Service Provision*. RCP & RCPsych. London.

Royal College of Psychiatrists (1986) *Alcohol – Our Favourite Drug*. Tavistock, London.

Royal College of Psychiatrists (1990*a*) *The Practical Administration of Electroconvulsive Therpy (ECT)*. Gaskell, London.

Royal College of Psychiatrists (1990*b*) The seclusion of psychiatric patients. *Psychiat. Bull.*, **14**, 754–6.

Royal College of Psychiatrists (1991*a*) Services for brain injured adults – report of a working group of the Research Committee of the Royal College of Psychiatrists 1990. *Psychiat. Bull.*, **15**, 513–18.

Royal College of Psychiatrists (1991b) *Good Medical Practice in the Aftercare of Potentially Violent and Vulnerable Patients Discharged from Inpatient Psychiatric Treatment*. Royal College of Psychiatrists, London.

Royal College of Psychiatrists (1992a) *Eating Disorders*. Royal College of Psychiatrists Council Report CR 14, London.

Royal College of Psychiatrists (1992b) Report of the General Psychiatry Section Working Party on postnatal illness. *Psychiat. Bull.*, **16**, 519–22.

Royal Commission on Criminal Justice (1993) *Report*, HMSO Cm 2263, London.

Rubin, P. C. (1994) Commentary: New drugs increase doctors' choice. *Br. Med. J.*, **309**, 1282.

Rudden, M., Sweeney, J. & Frances, A. (1990) Diagnosis and clinical course of erotomanic and other delusional patients. *Am. J. Psychiat.*, **147**, 625–8.

Rudin, D. O. (1981) The choroid plexus and system disease in mental illness. II Systemic lupus erythematosus: a combined transport dysfunction model for schizophrenia. *Biol. Psychiat.*, **16**, 373–97.

Ruggeri, M. & Dall'Agnola, R. (1993) The development and use of the Verona Expectation for Care Scale (VECS) and the Verona Service Satisfaction Scale (VSSS) for measuring expectations and satisfaction with community-based psychiatric services in patients, relatives and professionals. *Psychol. Med.*, **23**, 511–23.

Rupprecht, R., Rupprecht, C., Rupprecht, M. *et al.* (1989) Triiodothyronine, thyroxine and TSH response to dexamethasone in depressed patients and normal controls. *Biol. Psychiat.*, **25**, 22–32.

Rush, A. J. Erman, M. K., Giles, D. E. *et al.* (1986) Polysomnographic findings in recently drug-free and clinically remitted depressed patients. *Arch. Gen. Psychiat.*, **43**, 878–84.

Rush, B. (1785) *An Inquiry into the Effects of Spirituous Liquors on the Human Body*. Thomas and Andrews.

Russell, G. F. M. (1970) Anorexia nervosa: its identity as an illness and its treatment. In *Modern Trends in Psychological Medicine* (ed. J. H. Price). Butterworth, London, pp. 131–64.

Russell G. F. M. (1977) Editorial: The present status of anorexia nervosa. *Psychol. Med.*, **7**, 363–7.

Russell, G. F. M. (1979) Bulimia nervosa: an ominous variant of anorexia nervosa. *Psychol. Med.*, **9**, 429–88.

Russell, G. F. M. (1985) Premenarchal anorexia nervosa and its sequelae. *J. Psychiat. Res.*, **19**, 363–69.

Russell, G. F. M. (1995) Anorexia nervosa through time. In *Handbook of Eating Disorders. Theory Treatment and Research* (ed. G. Szmukler, C. Dare & J. L. Treasure). Wiley, Chichester.

Russell, G. F. M. & Treasure, J. (1989) The modern history of anorexia nervosa: an interpretation of why the illness has changed. In *The Psychobiology of Human Eating Disorders: Preclinical and Clinical Perspectives* (ed. L. A. Schneider, S. J. Cooper & K. A. Halmi). *Ann. N.Y. Acad. Sci.*, **575**, 13–30.

Russell, G. F. M., Szmukler, G., Dare, C. & Eisler, I. (1987) An evaluation of family therapy in anorexia nervosa and bulimia nervosa. *Arch. Gen. Psychiat.*, **44**, 1047–56.

Rust, J. & Golombok, S. (1989) *Modern Psychometrics*, Routledge, London, pp. 76–7.

Rutter, D. R. (1979) The reconstruction of schizophrenic speech. *Br. J. Psychiat.*, **134**, 356–9.

Rutter, M. (1972) Relationships between child and adult psychiatric disorders. *Acta. Psych. Scand.*, **48**, 3–21.

Rutter, M. (1981) Isle of Wight and Inner London studies. In *Prospective Longitudinal Research* (ed. S. A. Mednick & E. E. Baert). Oxford University Press, Oxford.

Rutter, M. (1989a) Isle of Wight revisited: twenty five years of child psychiatric epidemiology. *J. Am. Acad. Child & Adol. Psychiat.*, **28**, 633–53.

Rutter, M. (1989b) Pathways from childhood to adult life. *J. Child Psychol. Psychiat.*, **30**, 23–51.

Rutter, M. (1995) Clinical implications of attachment concepts: retrospect and prospect. *J. Child Psychol. Psychiat.*, **36**, 549–71.

Rutter, M., Bailey, A., Bolton, P. & Le Couteur, A. (1993) Autism: syndrome definition and possible genetic mechanisms. In *Nature, Nurture and Psychology* (ed. R. Plomin & G. E. MaClearn). APA Books, Washington DC. pp. 269–84.

Rutter, M., Bailey, A., Bolton, P. & Le Couteur, A. (1994) Autism and known medical conditions, myth and substance. *J. Child Psychol. Psychiat.*, **35**, 311–22.

Rutter, M., Cox, A., Tupling, C., Berger M. & Yule, W. (1975) Attainment and adjustment in two geographical areas: I. Prevalence of psychiatric disorder. *Br. J. Psychiat.*, **126**, 493–509.

Rutter, M., Graham, P. & Yule, W. (1970) *A Neuropsychiatric Study in Childhood*. Spastics International Medical Publications, London.

Rutter, M., Graham, P., Chadwick, O. F. D. & Yule, W. (1976) Adolescent turmoil: fact or fiction? *J. Child Psychol. Psychiat.*, **17**, 35–56.

Rutter, M., Tizard, J. & Whitmore, K. (1970) *Education, Health and Behaviour*. Longman, London.

Rutz, W., Carlsson, P., von Knorring, L. & Walinder, J. (1992b) Cost-benefit analysis on an educational program for general practitioners by the Swedish Committee for the prevention and treatment of depression. *Acta Psychiat. Scand.*, **85**, 457–64.

Rutz, W., von Knorring, L. & Walinder, J. (1989b) Frequency of suicide on Gotland after systematic postgraduate education of general practitioners. *Acta Psychiat. Scand.*, **80**, 151–4.

Rutz, W., von Knorring, L. & Walinder, J. (1992a) Long-term effects of an educational programme for general practitioners given by the Swedish Committee for Prevention and Treatment of Depression. *Acta Psychiat. Scand.*, **85**, 83–8.

Rutz, W., Walinder, J., Eberhad, G. *et al.* (1989a) An educational programme on depressive disorders for general practitioners on Gotland: background and evaluation. *Acta Psychiat. Scand.*, **79**, 19–26.

Ryan, G., Sweeney, P. J. & Solola, A. S. (1980) Prenatal care and pregnancy outcome. *Am. J. Obstet. Gynecol.*, **137**, 876–81.

Ryan. N. D. (1990) Pharmacotherapy of adolescent major depression: beyond TCAs. *Psychopharmacol. Bull.*, **26**, 75–9.

Ryan, N. D., Meyer, V., Dachille, S. *et al.* (1988) Lithium antidepressant augmentation in TCA-refractory depression in adolescents. *J. Am. Acad. Child & Adol. Psychiat.*, **27**, 371–6.

Rydelius, P. A. (1988) The development of antisocial behaviour and sudden violent death. *Acta. Psychiat. Scand.*, **77**, 398–403.

Ryle, A. (1982) *Psychotherapy: A Cognitive Integration of Theory and Practice*. Academic Press, London.

Ryle, A. (1990) *Cognitive Analytic Therapy: Active Participation in Change*. J. Wiley & Sons, Chichcester.

Ryle, G. (1949) *The Concept of Mind*. Hutchinson's University Library.

Ryle, J. A. (1936) *The Natural History of Disease*. Oxford University Press, Oxford.

Ryle. J. A. (1948) *Changing Disciplines*. Oxford University Press, London.

Sabshin, M. (1966) Theoretical models in community and social psychiatry. In *Community Psychiatry* (ed. L. Roberts, S. Halbeck & M. Loeb). University of Wisconsin Press, Madison.

Sadowski, C. & Kelley, M. L. (1993) Social problem solving in suicidal adolescents. *J. Consul. Clin. Psychol.*, **61**, 121–7.

Safer, D. J. & Kruger, J. M. (1988) A survey of medication treatment for hyperactive/inattentive students. *J. Am. Med. Assoc.*, **260**, 2256–8.

Sahakian, W. W. (1970) *Psychopathology Today* (ed. W. S. Sahakian). Peacock, Itaca, Illinois.

Sainsbury, P. (1995) *Suicide in London*. Maudsley Monograph No. 1. Chapman & Hall, London.

Sainsbury, P. & Gibson, J, (1954) Symptoms of anxiety and tension and the accompanying physiological changes in the muscular system. *J. Neurol. Neurosurg. Psychiat.*, **17**, 216–24.

Salkovskis, P. M. (1989) Obsessional Disorders. In *Cognitive Behaviour Therapy for Psychiatric Problems* (ed. K. Hawton, P. M. Salkovskis, J. Kirk & D. M. Clark). Oxford Medical Publications, Oxford.

Salkovskis, P. M., Atha, C. & Storer, D. (1990) Cognitive-behavioural problem solving in the treatment of patients who repeatedly attempt suicide: a controlled trial. *Br. J. Psychiat.*, **157**, 871–6.

Salkovskis, P., Jones, D. & Clark, D. (1986) Respiratory control in the treatment of panic attacks: replication and extension with concurrent measurement of behaviour and pCO_2. *Br. J. Psychiat.*, **148**, 526–32.

Salkovskis, P. M. & Warwick, H. M. C. (1986) Morbid preoccupations, health anxiety and reassurance: a cognitive behaviour approach to hypochondriasis. *Behav. Res. Ther.*, **24**, 597–602.

Salzman, C. (1980) The use of ECT in the treatment of schizophrenia. *Am. J. Psychiat.*, **137**, 1032–41.

Salzman, C. (1983) Electroconvulsive therapy in the elderly patient. *Psychiat. Clin. N. Am.*, **5**, 191–7.

Sanchez-Craig, M., Annis H. M., Bornet, A. R. (1984) Random assignment to abstinence and controlled drinking: Evaluation of a cognitive-behavioural treatment programme for problem drinkers. *J. Consult. Clin. Psychol.*, **52**, 390–403.

Sanchez-Craig, M., Spirak, K. & Davila, R. (1991) Superior outcome of females over males after brief treatment for the reduction of heavy drinking replication and report of therapist effects. *Br. J. Addict.*, **86**, 867–76.

Sanders, D. (1985) *The Woman Book of Love and Sex*. Sphere Books, London.

Sanders, D. (1987) *The Woman Report on Men*. Sphere Books, London.

Sandler, J., Dare, C. & Holder, A. (1992) *The Patient and the Analyst*. Karnac, London.

Sandler, J., Holder, A. & Meers, D. (1963) The ego ideal and the ideal self. *The Psychoanalytic Study of the Child*, **18**, 139–58.

Sanok, R. L. & Stiefell, S. (1979) Elective mutism: generalisation of verbal responding across people and setting. *Behav. Ther.*, **10**, 357–71.

Santos, J. L., Cabranes, J. A., Almogeura, I. *et al.* (1989) Clinical implications of determination of plasma haloperidol levels. *Acta Psychiat. Scand.*, **79**, 348–54.

Sass, L. A. (1992) *Madness and Modernism*. Basic Books, New York.

Saunders, J. B. (1981) A 20-year prospective study of cirrhosis. *Br. Med. J.*, **282**, 263–6.

Saunders, J. B. (1989) The efficiency of treatment for drinking problems. *Int. Rev. Psychiat.*, **1**, 121–38.

Saunders, J. B. & Aasland, O. G. (1987) WHO collaborative project on identification and treatment of persons with harmful alcohol consumption. *Report on Phase 1. Development of a Screening Instrument*. World Health Organization, Geneva.

Saunders, J. B. & Williams, R. (1983) The genetics of alcoholism: is there an inherited susceptibility to alcohol related problems? *Alcohol and Alcoholism*, **18**, 189–217.

Savage, W. (1988). The active management of perinatal death. In *Motherhood and Mental Illness 2: Causes and Consequences* (ed. R. Kumar & I. F. Brockington). Wright, London, pp. 247–69.

Savron, G., Grandi, S., Michelacci, L. *et al* (1989) Hypochondriacal symptoms in pregnancy. *Psychother. Psychosom.*, **52**, 106–9.

Scadding, J. G. (1967) Diagnosis: the clinician and the computer. *Lancet*, **2**, 877–82.

Scarr, S. (1992) Developmental theories for the 1990s: development and individual differences. *Child Development*, **63**, 1–19.

Schacter, S. & Singer, J. (1962) Cognitive, social and physiological determinants of emotional state. *Psychol. Rev.*, **69**, 379–97.

Scharfetter, C. (1980) *General Psychopathology. An Introduction* (translated by H. Marshall). Cambridge University Press, Cambridge.

Scharfetter, C. (1975) The historical development of the concept of schizophrenia. In *Studies of Schizophrenia* (ed. M. H. Lader). Headley Brothers, Ashford, Kent, pp. 5–9.

Scheff, T. J. (1963) Decision rules, types of error, and their consequences. *Behavioural Science*, **8**, 97–107.

Scheff, T. (1966) *Being Mentally Ill*. Aldine, Chicago.

Scheff, T. (1974) The labelling theory of mental illness. *American Sociological Review*, **39**, 444–52.

Schiffer, R. B. (1983) Psychiatric aspects of clinical neurology. *Am. J. Psychiat.*, **140**, 205–7.

Schildkraut, J. J. (1965) The catecholamine hypothesis of effective disorders: a review of supporting evidence. *Am. J. Psychiat.*, **122**, 509–22.

Schipkowensky, N. (1973) Epidemiological aspects of homicide. In *World Biennial of Psychiatry and Psychotherapy*, Vol 2 (ed. S. Arieti). Basic Books, New York, pp. 192–215.

Schmale, A. H. & Iker, H. P. (1966) The affect of hopelessness and the development of cancer. *Psychosom. Med.*, **28**, 714–21.

REFERENCES

Schmidt, H. J. (1943) The use of progesterone in the treatment of postpartum psychosis. *J. A. M. A.*, **121**, 190–2.

Schmidt, H. O. & Fonda, C. P. (1956) The reliability of psychiatric diagnosis: a new look. *J. Abnorm. Soc. Psychol.*, **52**, 262–7.

Schmidt, U., Tiller, J. & Treasure, J. (1993a) Setting the scene for eating disorders: childhood care, classification and course of illness. *Psychol. Med.*, **23**, 663–72.

Schmidt, U., Tiller, J. & Treasure, J. L. (1993b) Psychosocial factors in bulimia nervosa. *Internat. Rev. Psychiat.*, **5**, 51–60.

Schmidt, U. & Treasure, J. L. (1993a) From medieval mortification to charcots rose red ribbon and beyond: modern explanatory models of eating disorders. *Internat. Rev. Psychiat.*, **5**, 3–98.

Schmidt, U. & Treasure, J. (1933b) *Getting Better Bit(e) by Bit(e)*. Laurence Erlbaum, London.

Schneck, M. K., Reisberg, B. & Ferris, S. H. (1982) An overview of current concepts of Alzheimer's disease. *Amer. J. Psychiat.*, **139**, 165–73.

Schneider, A. L. & Schneider, P. R. (1981) Victim Assistance Programmes. In *Perspectives on Crime Victims* (ed. B. Galaway & J. Hudson). Molsby, St Louis, pp. 364–73.

Schneider, C. (1930) *Psychologie der Schizophrenen*. Thieme, Leipzig.

Schneider, K. (1950) *Psychopathic Personalities* (translated by M. Hamilton).

Schneider, K. (1959) *Clinical Psychopathology* (translated by M. Hamilton). Grune & Stratton, New York.

Schneider, K. (1974) Primary and secondary symptoms in schizophrenia. In *Themes and Variations in European Psychiatry* (ed. S. Hirsch & M. Shepherd). Wrights, Bristol, pp. 40–44.

Schopf, J., Bryois, C., Jonquiere, M. & Le, P. K. (1984) On the nosology of severe psychiatric postpartum disorders. *Eur. Arch. Psychiat. Neurol. Sci.*, **234**, 54–63.

Schou, M., Goldfield, M. D., Weinstein, M. R. & Villeneuve, A. (1973) Lithium and pregnancy I: Report from the registry of lithium babies. *Br. Med. J.*, **2**, 135–6.

Schou, M. & Weeke, A. (1988) Did manic depressive patients who committed suicide receive prophylactic or continuation treatment at the time? *Br. J. Psychiat.*, **153**, 324–7.

Schreber, D. P. (1955) *Memoirs of My Nervous Illness* (translated and edited by I. MacAlpine & R. A. Hunter). R. A. Dawson, London.

Schuckit, M. A. (1987) Studies of populations at high risk for the future development of alcoholism. In *Genetics of Alcoholism* (ed. H. W. Goedde & D. P. Agarual), Alan Liss, New York.

Schuckit, M. A. (1989) *Drug and alcohol abuse*. Plenum, New York.

Schuckit, M. A. (1994) A clinical model of genetic influences in alcohol dependence. *J. Stud. Alcohol.* **55**, 5–17.

Schuckit, M. A., Butters, N., Lyn, L & Irwin, M. (1987) Neuropsychologic deficits and risk for alcoholism. *Neuropsychopharmacology*, **1**, 45–53.

Schuckit, M. A., Duthie, L. A., Mahler, H. I. M. *et al.* (1991) Subjective feelings and changes in body sway following diazepam in sons of alcoholics and control subjects. *J. Stud. Alcohol,* **52**, 601–608.

Schuckit, M. A. & Gold, E. (1988) A simultaneous evaluation of multiple markers of ethanol/placebo challenges in sons of alcoholics and controls. *Arch. Gen. Psychiat.*, **45**, 211–16.

Schulgin, A. & Schulgin, A. (1991) *Pihkal. A Chemical Love Story*. Transform Press, Berkeley, California.

Schulsinger, F., Parnas, J., Petersen, E. T. *et al.* (1984) Cerebral ventricular size in the offspring of schizophrenic mothers. A preliminary study. *Arch. Gen. Psychiat.*, **41**, 602–6.

Schulsinger, R., Kety, S., Rosenthal, D. & Wender, P. (1979) A family study of suicide. In *Origins, Prevention and Treatment of Affective Disorders* (ed. M. Schow & E. Strongren). Academic Press, New York.

Schulte, B. (1989) Reform of Guardianship Laws in Europe – A Comparative and Interdisciplinary Approach. In *An Aging world: Dilemmas and Challenges for Law and Social Policy* (ed. K. Eekelaar & D. Pearl), pp. 591–6.

Scott, A. I. F. & Freeman, C. P. L. (1992) Edinburgh primary care depression study: treatment outcome, patient satisfaction and cost after 16 weeks. *Br. Med. J.*, **304**, 883–8.

782

Scott, D. B. (1986) Mortality related to anaesthesia in Scotland. *Health Bull.*, **44**, 43–58.

Scott, M. L., Golden, C. J., Reudrich, S. L. & Bishop, R. J. (1983) Ventricular enlargement in major depression. *Psychiat. Res.*, **8**, 91–3.

Scott, M. & Stradling, S. (1994) Post-traumatic stress disorder without the trauma. *Br. J. Clin, Psychol.*, **33**, 71–4.

Scull, A. (1984) Was insanity increasing? *Br. J. Psychiat.*, **144**, 432.

Searle, J. R. (1969) *Speech Acts: An Essay in the Philosophy of Language*. Cambridge University Press, Cambridge.

Secretaries of State for Health, Wales, Northern Ireland and Scotland (1989) *Working for Patients*. HMSO, London.

Secretaries of State for Health, Social Security, Wales and Scotland. *Caring for People, Community Care in the Next Decade and Beyond* (Cmnd 849), HMSO, London, p.21

Seeman, P., Lee, T., Chau-Wong, M. & K. (1976) Antipsychotic drug doses and neuroleptic/dopamine receptors. *Nature*, **261**, 717–19.

Seligman, M. (1970) On the generality of the laws of learning. *Psychol. Rev.*, **77**, 406–18.

Seligman, M. E. P. (1976) Reversal of performance deficits and perceptual deficits in learned helplessness and depression. *J. Abnorm. Psychol.*, **85**, 11–26.

Sellar, C., Hawton, K. & Goldacre, M. J. (1990) Self-poisoning in adolescents: hospital admission and deaths in the Oxford region 1980–1985. *Br. J. Psychiat.*, **156**, 866–70.

Selzer, B. & Sherwin, I. (1983) A comparison of clinical features in early and late onset primary degenerative dementia. *Arch. Neurol.*, **40**, 143–6.

Semans, J. H. (1956) Premature ejaculation, a new approach. *South. Med. J.*, **49**, 353–7.

Senatore, V., Matson, J. L. & Kazdin, A. E. (1985) An inventory to assess psychopathology of mentally retarded adults. *Am. J. Ment. Defic.*, **89**, 459–66.

Series, H. G. (1992) Drug treatment of depression in medically ill patients. *J. Psychosom. Res.*, **36**, 1–16.

Sethnna, E. R. (1974) A study of refractory cases in depressive illness and their response to combined antidepressant treatment. *Br. J. Psychiat.*, **124**, 265–72.

Sevin, J. A., Matson, J. L., Coe, D. A. *et al.* (1991) A comparison and evaluation of three commonly used autism scales. *J. Aut. Devel. Disord.*, **21**, 417–32.

Shafer, S., Hauser, W. A., Annegers, J. F., Klass, D. W. (1988) EEG and other early predictors of later epilepsy remission: a community study. *Epilepsia.*, **29**, 590–600.

Shaffer, D. (1973) The association between enuresis and emotional disorders: a review of the literature. In *Bladder Control & Enuresis* (ed. I. Kolvin, R. McKeith & S. R. Meadow). Clinics in Developmental Medicine, **48**(9) SIMP/Heinemann, London.

Shaffer, D. (1994a) Attention deficit hyperactivity disorder in adults. *Am. J. Psychiat.*, **151**, 633–8.

Shaffer, D. (1994b) Enuresis. In *Child and Adolescent Psychiatry: Modern Approaches*, 3rd edn. (ed. M. Rutter, E. Taylor & L. Hersov). Blackwell Scientific, Oxford, pp. 505–19.

Shaffer, D. & Piacentini, J. (1994) Suicide and attempted suicide. In *Child and Adolescent Psychiatry: Modern Approaches*, 3rd edn. (ed. M. Rutter, E. Taylor & L. Hersov). Blackwell Scientific, Oxford, pp. 407–24.

Shafii, M., Carrigan, S., Whittinghilld, R. & Derrick, A. (1985) Psychobiological autopsy of completed suicides in children and adolescence. *Am. J. Psychiat.*, **142**, 1061–4.

Sham, P. C., O'Callaghan, E., Takei, N. (1992) Schizophrenia following prenatal exposure to influenza epidemics between 1939 and 1960. *Br. J. Psychiat.*, **160**, 461–6.

Shamash, K., O'Connell, K., Lewy, M. & Katona, Ch. F. (1992) Psychiatric morbidity and outcome in elderly patients undergoing emergency hip surgery. A one-year follow-up study. *Int. J. Geriat. Psychiat.*, **7**, 505–10.

Shanks, S. (1992) *Coding and Mental Health Information Systems*. Report produced by the Research Unit of the Royal College of Psychiatry for the Department of Health.

Shapiro, S., Skinner, E., Kramer, M. *et al.* (1985) Measuring need for mental health services in a general population. *Med. Care*, **23**, 1033–43.

Shapiro, E. S., Shapiro, A. K., Fulop, G. *et al.* (1989) Controlled study of haloperidol, primozide and placebo for the treatment of Gilles de la Tourette's syndrome. *Arch. Gen. Psychiat.*, **46**, 722–30.

Shapland, J., Willmore, J. & Duff, P. (1985) *Victims in the Criminal Justice System.* Gower, Aldershot.

Sharma, U. (1990) Using Alternative Therapies. In *New Directions in the Sociology of Health* (ed. P. Abbot & G. Payne). Falmer Press, Lander.

Sharp, D. (1992) *A prospective longitudinal study of childbirth related emotional disorders in primary care.* PhD thesis, London University.

Sharp, D. & Morrell D. (1989) The psychiatry of general practice. In *Scientific Approaches on Epidemiological and Social Psychiatry. Essays in Honour of Michael Shepherd* (ed. P. Williams, G. Wilkinson & K. Rawnsley). Routledge, London.

Sharpe, M. & Bass, C. (1992) Pathophysiological mechanisms in somatisation. *Int. Rev. Psychiat.*, **81**, 81–97.

Sharpe, C. W. & Freeman, C. P. L. (1993) The medical complications of anorexia nervosa. *Brit. J. Psychiat.*, **162**, 452–62.

Sharpe, M., Hawton, K., Seagroatt, V. & Pasvol, G. (1992*a*) Follow-up of patients presenting with fatigue to an infectious diseases clinic. *Br. J. Med.*, **305**, 147–52.

Sharpe, M., Hawton, K., Simkin, S. *et al.* (1996) Cognitive behaviour therapy for chronic fatigue syndrome: a randomised controlled trial. *Brit. J. Med.*, **312**, 22–6.

Sharpe, M., Mayou, R. & Bass, C. (1995) Concepts, theories and terminology. In *Treatment of Functional Somatic Symptoms* (ed. R. Mayou, C. Bass & M. Sharpe). Oxford University Press, Oxford, pp. 3–16.

Sharpe, M., Peveler, R. & Mayou, R. (1992*b*) The psychological treatment of patients with functional somatic symptoms: a practical guide. *J. Psychosom. Res.*, **36**, 515–29.

Shaw, J., McKenna, J., Snowden, P. *et al.* (1994) The North-West region I: Clinical features and placement needs of patients detained in special hospitals. II: Patient characteristics in the research panels' recommended placement groups. *J. Forens. Psychiat.*, **5**, 93–122.

Shaw, J., McKenna, J., Snowden, P. R. *et al.* (1996) Clinical features and treatment needs of Northwest Region's patients currently in special hospitals. *J. Forens. Psychiat.*, in press.

Shaywitz, S. E., Escobar, M. D., Shaywitz, B. A. *et al.* (1992) Evidence that dyslexia may represent the lower tail of a normal distribution of reading ability. *N. Engl. J. Med.*, **326**, 145–50.

Sheehan, D. V., Ballenger, J. & Jacobsen, G. (1980) Treatment of endogenous anxiety with phobic, hysterical and hypochondriacal features. *Arch. Gen. Psychiat.*, **37**, 51–9.

Sheehan, D. V. & Sheehan, K. H. (1882) The classification of anxiety and hysterical states. Part I. Historical review and empirical delineation. *J. Clin. Psychopharmacol.*, **2**, 235–44.

Shenton, M. E., Kirkinis, R., Jolesz, F. A. (1992) Abnormalities of the left temporal lobe and thought disorder in schizophrenia. A quantitative magnetic resonance imaging study. *N. Engl. J. Med.*, **327**, 604–12.

Shepherd, G. (1988) The contributions of psychological interventions to the treatment and management of schizophrenia. In *Schizophrenia: The Major Issues* (ed. P. Bebbington & P. McGuffin). Heinemann, London.

Shepherd, M. (1957) A study of the major psychoses in an English County. *Maudsley Monograph.* Oxford University Press, Oxford.

Shepherd, M. (1961) Some clinical and social aspects of a psychiatric symptom. *J. Ment. Sci.*, **107**, 687–753.

Shepherd, M. (1961) Morbid jealousy: some clinical and social aspects of a psychiatric symptom. *J. Ment. Sci.*, **107**, 687–753.

Shepherd, M. (1994) ICD, mental disorder and British nosologists. *Br. J. Psychiat.*, **165**, 1–3.

Shepherd, M., Brooke, E. M., Cooper, J. E. & Lin, T. (1968) An experimental approach to psychiatric diagnosis. *Acta Psychiat. Scand.*, Suppl. 201.

Shepherd, M., Cooper, B., Brown, A. *et al.* (1966) *Psychiatric Illness in General Practice.* Oxford University Press, London.

Sherrington, R., Brynjolfsson, J., Petursson, H. *et al.* (1988) Localisation of a susceptibility locus for schizophrenia on chromosome 5. *Nature*, **336**, 164–7.

Shibuya, A., Yoshida, A. (1988) Genotypes of alcohol-metabolising enzymes in Japanese with alcohol liver diseases: a strong association of the usual Caucasian-type aldehyde dehydrogenase gene (ALDH2₁). *Am. J. Hum. Genet.*, **43**, 744–8.

Shichor, D. (1984) The extent and nature of lawbreaking by the elderly: a review of arrest statistics. In *Elderly Criminals* (ed. E. S. Newman, D. J. Newman, M. L. Gewirtz & Associates). Oelgeschlager, Gunn and Hain, Cambridge, Mass. pp. 17–32.

Shorter, E. (1992) *From Paralysis to Fatigue: A History of Psychosomatic Illness in the Modern Era.* MacMillan, New York.

Shrand, H. (1982) Agoraphobia and imipramine withdrawal? *Pediatrics*, **70**, 825.

Shulman, K. & Arie, T. (1991) UK survey of psychiatric services for the elderly: Directions for developing services. *Can. J. Psychiat.*, **36**, 169–75.

Shulman, K. & Post, F. (1980) Bipolar disorder in old age. *Br. J. Psychiat.*, **136**, 26–32.

Shulman, K. I., Silver, I. L., Hershberg, R. & Fisher, R. H. (1986) Geriatric psychiatry in the general hospital: the integration of services and training. *Gen. Hosp. Psychiat.*, **8**, 223–8.

Siatowsky, R. M., Zimmer, B. & Rosenberg, P. R. (1990) The Charles Bonnet syndrome. Visual perceptive dysfunction in sensory deprivation. *J. Clin. Neuro-Opthalmol.*, **103**, 215–18.

Sibbald, B., Addington-Hall, J., Brenneman, D. & Freeling, P (1993) Counsellors in English and Welsh general practices: their nature and distribution. *Br. Med. J.*, **306**, 29–33.

Siegler, M. & Osmond, H. (1974) *Models of Madness, Models of Medicine.* Collier Macmillan, London.

Siever, L. J. & Davis, K. L. (1985) Overview: toward a dysregulation hypothesis of depression. *Am. J. Psychiat.*, **142**, 1017–31.

Sifneos, P. E. (1972) *Short-term Psychotherapy and Emotional Crisis.* Harvard University Press, Cambridge, MA.

Sifneos, P. E. (1979) *Short-term Dynamic Psychotherapy: Evaluation and Technique.* Plenum, New York.

Sigerist, H. (1932) *Man and Medicine.* Norton & Co, New York.

Silfverskiold, P. & Risberg, J. (1989) Regional cerebral blood flow in depression and mania. *Arch. Gen. Psychiat.*, **46**, 253–9.

Silverstein, B., Peterson, B. & Perdue, L. (1986) Some correlates of the thin standard of bodily attractiveness for women. *Int. J. Eat. Disorders*, **5**, 907–16.

Silverstein, M. H., Fogg, L. & Harrow, M. (1991) Prognostic significance of cerebral status dimensions of clinical outcome. *J. Nerv. Ment. Dis.*, **179**, 534–9.

Silverstone, T. & Turner, P. (1982) *Drug Treatment in Psychiatry*, 3rd edn. Routledge & Kegan Paul, London.

Simeon, J. G., Dinicola, V. F., Ferguson, H. B. & Copping, S. (1990) Adolescent depression: a placebo-controlled fluoxetine treatment study and follow-up. *Prog. Neuro-Psychopharmacol. Biol. Psychiat.*, **14**, 791–5.

Simhandl, C. & Meszaro, K. (1992) The use of carbamazepine in the treatment of schizophrenic and schizoaffective psychoses: a review. *J. Psychiat. Neurosci.*, **17**, 1–14.

Simon, G. & VonKorff, M. (1991) Somatisation and psychiatric disorder in the NIMH Epidemiologic Catchment Area Study. *Am. J. Psychiat.*, **148**, 1494–500.

Simonoff, E., McGuffin, P. & Gottesman, I. I. (1994) Genetic influences on normal and abnormal development. In *Child and Adolescent Psychiatry: Modern Approaches*, 3rd edn. (ed. M. Rutter, E. Taylor & L. Hersov). Blackwell Scientific, Oxford, pp. 129–51.

Sims, A. (1987) Why the excess mortality from psychiatric illness? *Br. Med. J.*, **294**, 986–7.

Sims, A. (1988) *Symptoms in the Mind.* Baillière Tindall, London.

Sims. A. & O'Brien, K. (1979) Autokabalesis: an account of mentally ill people who jump from buildings. *Med. Sci. Law*, **19**, 195–8.

Sims, A. & Prior, P. (1978) The pattern of mortality in severe neuroses. *Br. J. Psychiat.*, **133**, 299–305.

Sipova, I. & Starka, L. (1977) Plasma testosterone levels in transexual women. *Arch. Sex. Behav.*, **6**, 477–81.

Siris, S. G., Bermanzohn, M. D., Gonzalez, A. *et al.* (1991) The use of antidepressants for negative symptoms in a subset of schizophrenic patients. *Psychopharmacol. Bull.*, **27**, 331–5.

Skinner, H. A., Holt, S., Sheu, W. J. & Israel, Y. (1986) Clinical versus laboratory detection of alcohol abuse: the alcohol clinical index. *Br. Med. J.*, **292**, 1703–8.

Skoog, I., Nilsson, L., Palmertz, B. *et al.* (1993) A population based study of dementia in 85 year olds. *N. Engl. J. Med.*, **328**, 153–8.

Skuse, D. (1988) Extreme deprivation in early childhood. In *Language Development in Exceptional Circumstances* (ed. K. Mogford & D. Bishop). Churchill Livingstone, Edinburgh, pp. 29–46.

Skuse, D. & Bentovim, A. (1994) Physical and emotional maltreatment. In *Child and Adolescent Psychiatry: Modern Approaches*, 3rd edn. (ed. M. Rutter, E. Taylor & L Hersov). Blackwell Scientific, Oxford, p. 209.

Skuse, D., Wolke, D. & Reilly, S. (1992) Failure to thrive. Clinical and developmental aspects. In *Child and Youth Psychiatry. European Perspectives. II. Developmental Perspectives* (ed. H. Remschmidt & M. Schmidt). Hans Huber, Stuttgart, pp. 46–71.

Slade, P. D. (1982) towards a functional analysis of anorexia nervosa and bulimia nervosa. *J. Clin. Psychol.*, **21**, 167–9.

Slade, P. D. & Bentall, R. P. (1988) *Sensory Deception*. Croom Helm, London.

Slater, E. (1965) Diagnosis of 'hysteria'. *Br. Med. J.*, **i**, 1395–99.

Slater, E. (1969) The schizophrenic like illnesses of epilepsy. In *Current Problems in Neuropsychiatry, Schizophrenia, Epilepsy and the Temporal Lobe* (ed. R. N. Herrington). British Journal of Psychiatry: Special Publication No. 4, Headley Bros., Ashford, pp. 77–81.

Slater, E., Beard, A. W. & Glithero, E. (1963) The schizophrenia-like psychoses of epilepsy. *Br. J. Psychiat.*, **109**, 95–150.

Slater, E. & Roth, M. (1969) *Clinical Psychiatry.*, Baillière, Tindall and Cassell, London.

Slavney, P. R. & McHugh, P. R. (1974) The hysterical personality: a controlled study. *Arch. Gen. Psychiat.*, **30**, 325–9.

Slone, D., Siskind, V., Heinonen, O. P. *et al* (1977) Antenatal exposure to the phenothiazines in relation to congenital malformations, perinatal mortality rate, birth weight, and intelligence quotient score. *Am. J. Obset. Gynaecol.*, **128**, 486–8.

Small, J. G., Klapper, M. H., Kellams, J. J. *et al.* (1988) Electroconvulsive treatment compared with lithium in the management of manic states. *Arch. Gen. Psychiat.*, **134**, 997–1001.

Small, J. G. & Small, I. F. (1967) A controlled study of mental disorders associated with epilepsy. *Rec. Adv. Biol. Psychiat.*, **9**, 171–81.

Smart, R. G. (1980) An availability-proneness theory of illicit drug use. In *Theories of Drug Abuse: Selected Contemporary Perspectives* (ed. D. J. Lettieri, M. Aayers & H. W. Pearson). National Institute of Drug Abuse Monograph, Rockville.

Smart, R. G. & Mann, R. E. (1993) Recent liver cirrhosis declines: estimates of the impact of alcohol abuse treatment and Alcoholics Anonymous. *Addiction*, **88**, 193–9.

Smith, A. L. & Weissman, M. M. (1991) Epidemiology. In *Handbook of Affective Disorders* (ed. E. S. Paykel). Churchill Livingstone, Edinburgh, pp. 111–30.

Smith, J. C. & Hogan, B. (1988) *Criminal Law*, 6th edn. Butterworths, London.

Smith, J. E. & Rachman, S. J. (1984) Non-accidental injury to children. II. A controlled evaluation of a behavioural management programme. *Behav. Res. Ther.*, **22**, 349–66.

Smith, K., Shah, A. J., Wright, K. & Lewis, G. (1995) The prevalence and costs of psychiatric disorders and learning disabilities. *Br. J. Psychiat.*, **166**, 9–18.

Smith, M. & Bentovim, A. (1994) Sexual abuse. In *Child and Adolescent Psychiatry: Modern Approaches* 3rd edn (ed. M. Rutter, E. Taylor & L. Hersov). Blackwell Scientific, Oxford, pp. 230–51.

Smith, M., Wolf, A. P., Brodie, J. D. *et al.* (1988) Serial [^{18}F]N-methylspiroperidol PET studies to measure changes in antipsychotic drug D-2 receptor occupancy in schizophrenic patients. *Biol. Psychiat.*, **23**, 653–63.

Smith, R. (1984) *Prison Health Care.* British Medical Association, London.

Smith, R. C., Baumgartner, R., Misra, C. H. *et al.* (1984) Haloperidol: Plasma levels and prolactin response as predictors of clinical improvement in schizophrenia: Chemical v radioreceptor plasma level assays. *Arch. Gen. Psychiat.*, **41**, 1945–49.

Smith, S. L. (1970) School refusal with anxiety: a review of sixty-three cases. *J. Can. Psychiat. Assoc.*, **15**, 257–64.

Snaith, P. (1987) The concepts of mild depression. *Br. J. Psychiat.*, **150**, 387–93.

Snaith, P. (1991) *Clinical Neurosis* (2nd edn). Oxford University Press, Oxford.

Snaith, P. (1993) What do depression rating scales measure? *Br. J. Psychiat.*, **163**, 293–8.

Snaith, R. P., Baugh, S. J. & Clayden, A. D. (1982) The Clinical Anxiety Scale: an instrument derived from the Hamilton Anxiety Scale. *Br. J. Psychiat.*, **141**, 518–23.

Snaith, R. P. & Owens, D. W. (1990) HAD and ROC. *Br. J. Psychiat.*, **156**, 744–5.

Sneddon, I. & Sneddon, J. (1975) Self-inflicted injury: A follow-up study of 43 patients. *Br. Med. J.*, **iii**, 527–30.

Snowden, P. R. (1985) A survey of the regional secure unit programme. *Br. J. Psychiat.*, **147**, 499–507.

Sokoloff, P., Giros, B. & Martres, M. P. (1990) Molecular cloning and characterisation of a novel dopamine receptor (D3) as a target for neuroleptics. *Nature*, **347**, 146–51.

Soloff, P. H., George, A., Nathan, R. S. *et al* (1986) Progress in pharmacotherapy of borderline disorders: a double-blind study of amitriptylline, haloperidol and placebo. *Arch. Gen. Psychiat.*, **43**, 691–97.

Solomon, P. (1956) Insomnia. *N. Eng. J. Med.*, **255**, 755–60.

Solomon, S., Gerrity, E. & Muff, A. (1992) Efficacy of treatments for post-traumatic stress disorder: an empirical review. *J. Am. Med. Assoc.*, **268**, 633–38.

Solomons, R. C. (1980) Emotion and choice. In *Explaining Emotions* (ed. A. O. Porty). University of California Press, pp. 251–81.

Solrush, L. (1988) Combat addiction: post-traumatic stress disorder re-explored. *Psychiat. J. Univ. Ottawa*, **133**, 177–20.

Solursh, L. (1989) Combat addiction: overview of implications in symptom maintenance and treatment planning. *J. Traum. Stress.*, **2**, 451–62.

Somander, L. & Rammer, L. (1991) Intra- and extra-familial child homicide in Sweden 1971–80. *Child Abuse and Neglect*, **15**, 45–55.

Song, F., Freemantle, N., Sheldon, T. A. (1993) Selective serotonin reuptake inhibitors: Meta-analysis of efficacy and acceptability. *Br. Med. J.*, **306**, 683–7.

Sonuga-Bark, E. J. S., Taylor, E., Sembi, S. & Smith, J. (1992) Hyperactivity and delay aversion I. The effect of delay on choice. *J. Child Psychol. Psychiat.*, **33**, 387–98.

Soni Raleigh, V. & Balarajan R. (1992) Suicide levels and trends among immigrants in England and Wales. *Health Trends.*, **24**, 91–4.

Soni Raleigh, V., Bulusu, L. & Balarajan, R. (1990) Suicides among immigrants from the Indian sub-continent. *Br. J. Psychiat.*, **156**, 46–50.

Sorensen, A. S., Hansen, H., Andersen, R. *et al.* (1989) Personality characteristics and epilepsy. *Acta Psychiat. Scand.*, **80**, 620–31.

Southall, D. P., Stebbens, V. A., Rees, S. V. *et al.* (1987) Apnoeic episodes induced by smothering: two cases identified by covert video surveillance. *Br. Med. J.*, **294**, 1637–41.

Sovner, R., Fox, C. J., Lowry, M. J. & Lowry, M. A. (1993) Fluoxetine treatment of depression and associated injury in two adults with mental retardation. *J. Intell. Disab. Res.*, **37**, 301–11.

Sovner, R. & Hurley, A. D. (1983) Do the mentally retarded suffer from affective illness? *Arch. Gen. Psychiat.*, **40**, 61–7.

Sowers, W. E. & Daley, D. C. (1933) Compulsory treatment of substance use disorders. *Crim. Behav. Ment. Health.*, **3**, 403–15.

Spector, S., Hirsch, C. W. & Brodie, B. B. (1963) Association of behavioural effects of clorgyline – a non hydrazine MAO inhibitor with increase in brain norepinephrine. *Int. J. Neuropharmacol.*, **2**, 81–93.

Spence, D. P. (1982) *Historical Truth and Narrative Truth*. Norton, New York.

Spence, D. P. (1986) When interpretation masquerades as explanation. *J. Am. Psychoanal. Assoc.*, **34**, 3–22.

Spielberger, C. D. (1983) *Manual for the State–Trait Anxiety Inventory (STAI)*. Consulting Psychologists Press, Palo Alto.

Spiegal, D. A., Bruce, T. J., Gregg, S. F. & Nuzzarello, A. (1994) Does cognitive behaviour therapy assist slow-taper alprazolam discontinuation in panic disorder? *Am. J. Psychiat.*, **151**, 876–81.

Spiegel, D., Bloom. J. R., Kraemer, H. C. & Gottheil, E. (1989) Effect of psychosocial treatment in survival of patients with metastatic breast cancer. *Lancet*, **ii**, 888–91.

Spitz, R. A. (1957) *No and Yes: On the Genesis of Human Communication*. International Universities Press, New York.

Spitz, R. A. (1965) *The First Year of Life: A Psychanalytic Study of Normal and Deviant Development of Object Relations*. International Universities Press, New York.

Spitzer, R. L. & Endicott, J. (1978) *Schedule of Affective Disorders and Schizophrenia* (3rd edn). Biometrics Research, New York.

Spitzer, R. L., Endicot, J. & Robins E. (1975) Clinical criteria for psychiatric diagnosis and DSM-III. *Am. J. Psychiat.*, **132**, 1187–92.

Spitzer, R. L., Endicott, J. & Robins, E. (1978a) Research diagnostic criteria: rationale and reliability. *Arch. Gen. Psychiat.*, **35**, 773–82.

Spitzer, R. L. Endicott, J. & Robins E. (1978b) *Research Diagnostic Criteria: Biometrics Research*. New York State Psychiatric Institute, New York.

Spitzer, R. L., William, J. B. W., Gibbon, M. *et al.* (1992) The structured clinical interview for DSM-IIIR (SCID). I: History, rationale and description. *Arch. Gen. Psychiat.*, **49**, 624–9.

Spitzer, R. L., Yanovski, S., Wadde, T. *et al.* (1993) Binge eating disorder: its further validation in a multisite study. *Int. J. Eat. Dis.*, **13**, 137–53.

Squire, L. R. (1986) Memory functions as affected by electroconvulsive therapy. *Ann. N. Y. Acad. Sci.*, **462**, 407–14.

Sroka, H., Elizan, T. S., Yahr, M. D. *et al.* (1981) Organic mental syndrome and confusional states in Parkinson's disease. *Arch. Neurol.* **38**, 339–42.

Srole, L., Langner, T., Michael, S. T. *et al.* (1962) *Mental Health in the Metropolis*. McGraw-Hill, New York.

St George Hislop, P., Tanzi, R., Polinsky, R. *et al.* (1987) The genetic defect causing familial Alzheimer's disease maps on chromosome 21. *Science*, **235**, 885–90.

Stallard, J. (1870) Pauper lunatics and their treatment. *Transactions on the National Association for the Promotion of Social Science*, p. 465.

Stampfl, T. J. & Levis, D. G. (1967) Essentials of implosive therapy: a learning theory based psychodynamic behaviour therapy. *J. Abnorm. Psychol.*, **72**, 496–503.

Stangl, D., Pfohl, B., Zimmerman, M. *et al.* (1985) A structured interview for the DSM-III personality disorders. *Arch. Gen. Psychiat.*, **42**, 591–6.

Stanovich, K. E. (1994) Does dyslexia exist? *J. Child Psychol. Psychiat.*, **35**, 579–95.

Stansfield, S., Davey Smith, G. & Marmot, M. (1993) Association between physical and psychological morbidity in the Whitehall II Study. *J. Psychosom. Res.*, **37**, 227–38.

Stansfield, S. & Marmot, M. (1992) Deriving a survey measure of social support: the reliability and validity of the Close Persons Questionnaire. *Soc. Sci. Med.*, **35**, 1027–35.

Stanton, D. & Todd, T. C. (1982) *The Family Therapy of Drug Abuse and Addiction*. Guilford, New York.

Starkstein, S. E. & Robinson, R. G. (1989) Effective disorders and cerebral vascular disease. *Br. J. Psychiat.*, **154**, 170–82.

Stattin, H., Magnusson, D. & Reichel, H. (1989) Criminal activity at different ages: a study based on a Swedish longitudinal research population. *Br. J. Criminol.*, **29**, 368–85.

Stavrakaki, C. & Vargo, B. (1986) The relationship between anxiety and depression: a review of the literature. *Br. J. Psychiat.*, **149**, 7–16.

Steadman, H., McCarty, D. W. & Morrissey, J. P. (1989) *The Mentally Ill in Jail*. Guilford Press, New York.

Steadman, H. J., Monahan, J., Appelbaum, P. J. *et al.* (1994) Designing a new generation of risk assessment research. In *Violence and Mental Disorder. Developments in Risk Assessment* (ed. J. Monahan & H. J. Steadman). University of Chicago Press, Chicago, pp. 297–318.

Steel, T. D., McCann, U. & Ricaurte, G. (1994) 3,4-Methylenedioxymethamphetamine (MDMA, 'Ecstasy'): pharmacology and toxicology in animals and humans. *Addiction*, **89**, 539–51.

Steffenburg, S. & Gillberg, C. (1986) Autism and autistic-like conditions in Swedish rural and urban areas: a population study. *Br. J. Psychiat.*, **149**, 81–7.

Stein, A. S., Woolley, H., Cooper, S. D. & Fairburn, C. G. (1994) An observational study of mothers with eating disorders and their infants. *J. Child Psychol. Psychiat.*, **35**, 733–48.

Stein, D. J., Hollander, E., Simeon, D. *et al.* (1993) Pregnancy and obsessive-compulsive disorder. *Am. J. Psychiat.*, **150**, 1131–2.

Steinhausen, H. C., Rauss-Mason, C. & Seidel, R. (1991) Follow-up studies of anorexia nervosa: a review of four decades of outcome research. *Psychol. Med.*, **21**, 447–54.

Stengal, E. (1959) Classification of mental disorders. *Bulletin of the WHO*, **21**, 601–63.

Stern, R. (1985) *The Interpersonal World of the Infant: A View from Psychoanalysis and Developmental Psychology*. Basic Books, New York.

Stern, R. & Marks, I. M. (1973) Brief and prolonged flooding: a comparison in agoraphobic patients. *Arch. Gen. Psychiat.*, **28**, 270–6.

Stevens, A. & Gabbay, J. (1991) Needs assessment, needs assessment. *Health Trends.*, **23**, 20–3.

Stevens, J. R. & Hermann, B. P. (1981) Temporal lobe epilepsy, psychopathology and violence: the state of the evidence. *Neurology.*, **31**, 1127–32.

Stevenson, J. (1988) Which aspects of reading ability show a 'hump' in their distribution: *Appl. Cogn. Psychol.*, **2**, 77–85.

Stevenson, J., Batten, N. & Cherner, M. (1992) Fears and fearfulness in children and adolescents: a genetic analysis of twin data. *J. Child Psychol. Psychiat.*, **33**, 977–85.

Stevenson, J., Richman, N. & Graham, P. (1985) Behaviour problems and language abilities at three years and behavioural deviance at eight years. *J. Child Psychol. Psychiat.*, **26**, 215–30.

Stewart, D. (1990) The changing face of somatisation. *Psychosomatics.*, **31**, 153–8.

Steward, D. E., Klompenhouwer, J. L., Kendell, R. E. & Van Hulst, A. M. (1991) Prophylactic lithium in puerperal psychosis. The experience of three centres. *Br. J. Psychiat.*, **158**, 393–7.

Stewart, D., Raskin, J., Garfinkel, P. E. *et al.* (1987) Anorexia nervosa, bulimia, and pregnancy. *Am. J. Obstet. Gynecol.*, **257**, 1194–8.

Stierlin, H. (1975) *Psychoanalysis and Family Therapy: Selected Papers*. Jason Aronson, New York.

Stimson, G. V. (1995) AIDS and injecting drug use in the United Kingdom. 1987–1993 the policy response and the prevention of the epidemic. *Soc. Sci. Med.*, **41**, 699–716.

Stimson, G. V. & Oppenheimer, E. (1982) *Heroin Addiction Treatment and Control*. Tavistock Publications, London.

Stirrat, G. M. (1990) Recurrent miscarriage. II: Clinical associations, causes, and management. *Lancet* **336**, 728–33.

Stirtzinger, R. & Robinson, G. E. (1989) The psychologic effects of spontaneous abortion. *Can. Med. Assoc. J.*, **140**, 799–801.

Stocking, B. (1985) *Initiative and Inertia*. Nuffield Hospital Trust, London.

Stockwell, T. & Bolderston, H. (1987) Alcohol and phobias. *Br. J. Addict.*, **82**, 971–9.

Stockwell, T., Hodgson, R., Edwards, G. *et al.* (1979) The development of a questionnaire to measure severity of alcohol dependence. *Br. J. Addict.*, **74**, 79–87.

Stone, C. (1988) *Bail Information for the Crown Prosecution Service*. Association of Chief Officers of Probation, Wakefield, W. Yorks (England) & The Vera Institute, New York.

Stone, C. (1989) *Public Interest Case Assessments*. Vera Institute, New York.

Stone, K. (1989) Mania in the elderly. *Br. J. Psychiat.*, **155**, 220–4.

Stores, G. (1981) Problems of learning and behaviour in children with epilepsy. In *Epilepsy and Psychiatry* (ed. E. H. Reynolds & M. R. Trimble). Churchill Livingstone, Edinburgh, pp. 33–48.

Stores, G. & Piran, N. (1978) Dependency of different types of school children with epilepsy. *Psychol. Med.*, **8**, 441–5.

Storr, A. (1979) *The Art of Psychotherapy*. Secker & Warburg, London.

Strachey, J. (1934) The nature and the therapeutic action of psycho-analysis. *Int. J. Psycho-Analysis*, **15**, 127–59; Reprinted in 1969, **50**, 275–92.

Strain, E. C., Stitzer, M. L. & Bigelow, G. E. (1991) Early treatment time course of depressive symptoms in opiate addicts. *J. Nerv. Ment. Dis.*, **179**, 215–21.

Strain, J. J. (1981) Diagnostic considerations in the medical setting. *Psychiat. Clin. N. Am.*, **4**, 287–300.

Strakowski, S. M. (1994) Diagnostic validity of schizophreniform disorder. *Am. J. Psychiat.*, **151**, 815–24.

Strang, J. (1992) Drug use and harm reduction. Responding to the challenge. In *Psychoactive Drugs and Harm Reduction – From Faith to Science* (ed. P. O'Hare, N. Heather & A Wodak). Whurr, London, pp. 3–20.

Strang, J., Bradley, B. & Stockwell, T. (1989) Assessment of drug and alcohol use. In *The Instruments of Psychiatric Research* (ed. C. Thompson). John Wiley and Sons Ltd, Chichester.

Strang, J. & Farrell, M. (1990) *Hepatitis*. ISDD, London.

Strang, J., Farrel, M. & Unithan, S. (1993*a*) Treatment of cocaine abuse: exploring the condition and selecting the response. In *Cocaine and Crack – Supply and Use* (ed. P. Bean). St Marks Press, London, pp. 146–67.

Strang, J. & Gossop, M. (1994) *The British System: A History of Drug Policy in the United Kingdom*. Oxford University Press, Oxford.

Strang, J., Gossop, M. & Stimson, G. (1990) Courses of drug use: the concepts of career versus natural history. In *Substance Misuse and Dependence: An Introduction for the Caring Profession* (ed. H. Ghodse & D. Maxwell). Macmillan Press, London.

Strang, J., Griffiths, P., Abbey, J. & Gossop, M. (1994) Survey of use of injected benzodiazepines by drug users in Britain – 1992. *Br. Med. J.*, **308**, 1082.

Strang, J., Johns, A. & Caan, W. (1993*b*) Cocaine in the UK – 1991. *Br. J. Psychiat.*, **162**, 1–13.

Strang, J., Ruben, S., Farrell, M. & Gossop, M. (1994) Prescribing heroin and other injectable drugs. In *Heroin Addiction and Drug Policy: The British System* (ed. J. Strang & M. Gossop). Oxford University Press, Oxford, pp. 192–203.

Strang, J., Sievewright, N. & Farrell, M. (1993*c*) Benzodiazepine dependence. In *Oral and Intravenous Abuse of Benzodiazepines* (ed. C. Hallstrom). Oxford Medical Publications, Oxford, pp. 128–42.

Strathdee, G. (1990) The delivery of psychiatric care. *J. Roy. Soc. Med.*, **83**, 222–5.

Strathdee, G. (1991) The interface between psychiatry and primary care in the management of schizophrenic patients in the community. In *The Primary Care of Schizophrenia* (ed. R. Jenkins, V. Field & R. Young). HMSO, London.

Strathdee, G. & Phelan, M. (1993) Editors of the Maudsley Practical Clinical Handbook Series for General Practitioners, published by Boots Pharmaceuticals, including (i) *Crisis Intervention* (in press); (ii) *Making Use of the Consultation* (In preparation); (iii) *Suicide (Health of the Nation)*; (iv) *Depression*; (v) *Anxiety*; (vi) *Organic Disorder*; (vii) *Drugs and Alcohol*; (viii) *Eating Disorders*.

Strathdee, G. & Thornicroft, G. (1992) Community sectors for needs-led mental health services. In *Measuring Mental Health Needs* (ed. G. Thornicroft, C. Brewin & J. K. Wing). Royal College of Psychiatrists, Gaskell Press, Chapter 8.

Strathdee, G. & Williams, G. (1984) A survey of psychiatrists in primary care: the silent growth of a new service. *J. Roy. Coll. Gen. Prac.*, **34**, 615–18.

Straus, E. W. (1948) On Obsession. *Nervous and Mental Disease Monographs*, No. 73.

Streissguth, A. P. (1990) Pre-natal alcohol induced brain damage and long-term post natal consequences – Editorial. *Alcoholism*, **14**, 648–9.

Striegel-Moore, R. H. (1993) Etiology of binge eating: a developmental perspective. In *Binge Eating, Nature, Assessment and Treatment* (ed. C. G. Fairburn & G. T. Wilson). Guilford Press, London, pp. 144–72.

Strober, M., Lampert, C., Morrell, W. *et al.* (1990) A controlled family study of anorexia nervosa: evidence of familial aggregation and lack of shared transmission with affective disorders. *Int. J. Eat. Disorders.*, **9**, 239–54.

Strober, M., Lampert, C., Schmidt, S. & Morrell, W. (1993) The course of major depressive disorder in adolescents. I. Recovery and risk of manic switching in a follow-up of psychotic and non-psychotic subtypes. *J. Am. Acad. Child & Adol. Psych.*, **32**, 34–42.

Strober, M., Morrell, W., Lampert, C. & Burroughs, J. (1990) Relapse following discontinuation of lithium maintenance therapy in adolescents with bipolar I illness: a naturalistic study. *Am. J. Psychiat.*, **147**, 457–61.

Strong, I., MacMillan, R. & Jennett, B. (1978) Head injuries in accident and emergency departments at Scottish hospitals, *Injury*, **10**, 154–9.

Strub, R. L. (1982) Acute confusional state. In *Psychiatric Aspects of Neurological Disease* (ed. D. F. Benson & D. Blumer). Grune and Stratton, New York, pp. 1–21.

Strupp, H. H. & Binder, J. L. (1984) *Psychotherapy is a New Key: A guide to time-limited dynamic psychotherapy*. Basic Books, New York.

Stuart, R. B. (1980) *Helping Couples Change*. Guilford Press, New York.

Studd, J. W. W. & Smith, R. N. (1994) Oestrogen and depression. *Menopause*, **1**, 33–7.

Sturmey, P., Carlson, A., Crisp, A. & Newton, J. I. (1988) The functional analysis of aberrant responses. A refinement and extension of Iwata *et al*'s (1982) methodology. *J. Ment. Defic. Res.*, **32**, 31–46.

Suddath, R. L., Christison, G. W., Torrey, E. F. *et al.* (1990) Anatomical abnormalities in the brains of monzygotic twins discordant for schizophrenia. *New Eng. J. Med.*, **322**, 789–94.

Sugrue, M. (1983) Can a unitary hypothesis for depression be valid? *Behav. Brain Sci.*, **4**, 559–60.

Summers, J., Alison, D., Lynch, P. & Sandler, L. (1995) Behaviour problems in Angelman Syndrome. *J. Intell. Disab. Res.*, **39**, 97–106.

Sunday, S. R., Levey, C. M. & Halmik, A. (1993) Effects of depression and borderline personality traits on psychological state and eating disorder symptomatology. *Compreh. Psychiat.*, **34**, 70–4.

Sunderland, T., Mueller, E., Cohen, R. M. *et al.* (1985) Tyramine suppressed sensitivity changes during deprenyl treatment. *Psychopharmacol.*, **86**, 432–7.

Suomi, S. J., Seaman, S. F., Lewis, J. K. *et al.* (1978) Effects of imipramine treatment on separation induced social disorders in rhesus monkeys. *Arch. Gen. Psych.*, **35**, 321–5.

Sullivan, H. S. (1953) *Conceptions of Modern Psychiatry*. W. W. Norton, New York.

Sulloway, F. J. (1979) *Freud, Biologist of the Mind: Beyond the Psychoanalytic Legend*. Basic Books, New York.

Surtees, P. G., Dean, C. Ingham, J. G. *et al.* (1983) Psychiatric disorder in women from an Edinburgh community: associations with demographic factors. *Br. J. Psychiat.*, **142**, 238–46.

Surtees, P. G. & Barcley, C. (1994) Future imperfect: the long-term outcome of depression. *Br. J. Psychiat.*, **164**, 327–41.

Surtees, P. G., Miller, P. Ingham, J. G. *et al.* (1986) Life events and onset of affective disorder: a longitudinal general population study. *J. Affec. Dis.*, **10**, 37–50.

Susser, E., Lin, S. P., Brown, A. S. (1994) No relation between risk of schizophrenia and prenatal exposure to influenza in Holland. *Am. J. Psych.*, **151**, 922–4.

Susser, E. & Wanderling, J. (1994) Epidemiology of nonaffective acute remitting psychosis vs schizophrenia. Sex and sociocultural setting. *Arch. Gen. Psych.*, **51**, 294–301.

Sutherby, K., Srinath, S. & Strathdee, G. (1991) The Domiciliary Consultation Service: outdated anachronism or essential part of community psychiatric outreach? Unpublished research report.

Sutherland, G., Edwards, G., Taylor, C. *et al.* (1987) the measurement of opiate dependence. *Br. J. Addic.*, **81**, 485–94.

Swanson, J. W., Holzer, C. E., Ganju, V. K. & Jono, R. T. (1990). Violence and psychiatric disorder in the community: evidence from the epidemiologic catchment area surveys. *Hosp. Comm. Psychiat.*, **41**, 761–70.

Swedo, S. E. Rapoport, J. L., Leonard, H. *et al.* (1989) Obsessive' compulsive disorder in children and adolescents: clinical phenomenology of 70 consecutive cases. *Arch. Gen. Psych.*, **46**, 335–41.

Swadi, H. (1988) Drug and substance use among 3333 London adolescents. *Br. J. Addic.*, **83**, 935–42.

Swadi, H. & Zeitlin, H. (1988) Peer influence and adolescent substance abuse: a promising side. *Br. J. Addic.*, **83**, 153–7.

Sytema, S., Balestrieri, M., Giel, R. *et al.* (1989) Use of mental health services in south-Verona and Groningen. *Acta Psych. Scand.*, **79**, 153–62.

Szasz, T. S. (1960) The myth of mental illness. *Am. Psychol.*, **15**, 113–18.

Szasz, T. (1961) *The Myth of Mental Illness*. Hoeber–Harper.

Szasz, T. S. (1972) Bad habits are not diseases. *Lancet*, **ii**, 83–4.

Szasz, T. S. (1974) *The Second Sin*. Routledge and Kegan Paul, London.

Szatmari, P., Bartolucci, G. & Bremner, R. (1989*a*) Asperger's syndrome and autism: Comparison of early history and outcome. *Develop. Med. Child Neurol.*, **31**, 709–20.

Szatmari, P., Offord, D. R. & Boyle, M. H. (1989*b*) Ontario Child Health Study: prevalence of attention deficit disorder with hyperactivity. *J. Child Psychol. Psychiat.*, **30**, 219–30.

Szmukler, G. (1985) The epidemiology of anorexia nervosa and bulimia. *J. Psychiat. Res.*, **19**, 143–53.

Szmukler, G. (1989) Anorexia nervosa and eating disorders. In *The Instruments of Psychiatric Research* (ed. C. Thompson). John Wiley and Sons, Chichester, pp. 177–94.

Szmukler, G., Bird, A. S. & Button, E. J. (1981) Compulsory admissions in a London Borough: 1. Social and clinical features and a follow-up. *Psychol. Med.*, **11**, 617–36.

Szmukler, G. & Dare, C. (1991) The Maudsley study of family therapy in Anorexia nervosa. In *Family Approaches to Eating Disorders* (ed. D. B. Woodside & L. Shekter-Wolfson). American Psychiatric Press, Inc., Washington DC.

Szmukler, G. I., Eisler, I., Russell, G. F. M & Dare, C. (1985) Anorexia nervosa, prenatal expressed emotion and dropping out of treatment. *Br. J. Psychiat.*, **147**, 265–71.

Szmukler, G. I., McCance, C. & McCrone, L. (1986) Anorexia nervosa: a psychiatric case register study from Aberdeen. *Psychol. Med.*, **16**, 49–58.

Szmukler, G. I. & Patton, G. (1995) Sociocultural models of anorexia nervosa. In *Handbook of Eating Disorders. Theory Treatment & Research* (ed. G. Szmukler, C. Dare & J. L. Treasure). Wiley, Chichester.

Szmukler, G. I. & Tantam, D. (1984) Anorexia nervosa: starvation dependence. *Br. J. Med. Psychol.*, **57**, 303–10.

Szmukler, G. I., Young, G. P., Lichtenstein, M. & Andrews, J. T. (1990) A serial study of gastric emptying in anorexia nervosa and bulimia nervosa. *Aus. NZ J. Med.*, **20**, 220–4.

Szymanski, L. S. & Biederman, J. (1984) Depression and anorexia nervosa of persons with Down syndrome. *Am. J. Ment. Def.*, **89**, 246–51.

Tabakoff, B., Hoffman, P. L., Lee, M. *et al.* (1988) Differences in platelet enzyme activity between alcoholics and non-alcoholics. *New Engl. J. Med.*, **318**, 134–9.

Takei, N., Sham, P., O'Callaghan, E. *et al.* (1995) Increased risk associated with winter and city birth. A case-control study in 12 regions within England and Wales. *J. Epidemiol. Comm. Health.*, **49**, 106–9.

Tambs, K. & Moum, T. (1993) Low genetic effect and age-specific family effect for symptoms of anxiety and depression in nuclear families, halfsibs and twins. *J. Affec. Dis.*, **27**, 183–95.

Tansella, M. (1986) Community psychiatry without mental hospitals – the Italian experience: a review. *J. Roy. Soc. Med.*, **79**, 664–9.

Tansella, M. (1989) Evaluating community psychiatric services. In *Scientific Approaches in Epi-*

demiological & Social Psychiatry. Essays in Honour of Michael Shepherd (ed. P. Williams, G. Wilkinson & K. Rawnsley). Routledge, London, pp. 386–403.

Tansella M., de Salvia D. & Williams, P. (1987) The Italian psychiatric reform: some quantitative evidence. *Soc. Psychiat.*, **22**, 37–48.

Tansella, M. & Williams, P. (1989) The spectrum of psychiatric morbidity in a defined geographical area. *Psychol. Med.*, **19**, 765–70.

Tantam, D. (1985) Alternatives to psychiatric hospitalisation. *Br. J. Psychiat.*, **146**, 1–4.

Tantum, D. (1991) Asperger syndrome in childhood. In *Autism and Asperger Syndrome* (ed. U. Frith). Cambridge University Press, Cambridge, pp. 147–83.

Tantum, D. & Burns, B. J. (1979) An international comparison of two systems of community mental health care. *Psychol. Med.*, **9**, 541–50.

Tarnopolsky, A. & Berelowitz, M. (1987) Borderline personality: a review of recent research. *Br. J. Psychiat.*, **151**, 724–34.

Tarnopolsky, A., Watkins, G. & Hand, D. J. (1980) Aircraft noise and mental health. I: Prevalence of individual symptoms. *Psychol. Med.*, **10**, 683–98.

Tarrier, N., Harwood, S., Yusopoff, L. *et al.* (1990) Coping strategy enhancement: a method of treating residual schizophrenic symptoms. *Behav. Psychother.*, **18**, 283–93.

Tarsh, M. J. & Royston, C. (1985) A follow-up study of accident neurosis. *Br. J. Psychiat.*, **146**, 18–25.

Tarter, R. E., Jacob, T. & Brewer, D. A. (1989) Cognitive status of sons of alcoholic men. *Alcohol. Clin. Exp. Res.*, **13**, 232–5.

Taylor, A. R. & Bell, T. K. (1966) Slowing of cerebral circulation after concussional head injury. *Lancet*, **ii**, 178–80.

Taylor, C. (1994) What happens over the long term. *Br. Med. Bull.*, **50**, 50–67.

Taylor, C., Brown, D. Duckitt, A. *et al.* (1985) Patterns of outcome: drinking histories over 10 years among a group of alcoholics. *Br. J. Addic.*, **80**, 40–5.

Taylor, D. C. (1979) The components of sickness: diseases, illnesses and predicaments. *Lancet*, **ii**, 1008–10.

Taylor, D. & Lewis, S. (1993) Delirium. *J. Neurol. Neurosurg, Psychiat.*, **56**, 742–51.

Taylor, E. (1994) Syndromes of attention deficit and overactivity. In *Child and Adolescent Psychiatry: Modern Approaches* 3rd edn (ed. M. Rutter, E. Taylor & L. Hersov). Blackwell Scientific, Oxford, pp. 285–307.

Taylor, E., Sandberg, S., Thorley, G. & Giles, S. (1991) *The Epidemiology of Childhood Hyperactivity.* Maudsley monographs No. 33. Oxford University Press, Oxford.

Taylor, F. (1972) Part 2. A logical analysis of the medico-psychological concept of disease. *Psychol. Med.*, **2**,1, 7–16.

Taylor, F. K. (1982) Depersonalisation in the light of Brentano's phenomenology. *Br. J. Med. Psychol.*, **55**, 297–306.

Taylor, M. A. (1992a) Are schizophrenia and affective disorder related? A selective literature review. *Am. J. Psychiat.*, **149**, 22–32.

Taylor, M. F. (ed). (1992b) *British Household Panel Survey User Manual.* University of Essex, Colchester.

Taylor, P. J. (1983) Consent, competency and ECT: a psychiatrist's view. *J. Med. Ethics.*, **9**, 146–51.

Taylor, P. J. (1985) Motives for offending among violent and psychotic men, *Br. J. Psych.*, **147**, 491–8.

Taylor, P. J. (1990) Schizophrenia and ECT: a case for a change in prescription? In *Dilemmas and Difficulties in the Management of Psychiatric Patients* (ed. K. Hawton & P. Cowen). Oxford University Press, Oxford, pp. 143–55.

Taylor, P. J. (1993) Schizophrenia and crime: distinctive patterns in association. In *Crime and Mental Disorder*, (ed. S. Hodgins). Sage, Beverley Hills, CA. pp. 63–85.

Taylor, P. J., Barry, M., Gudjonsson, G. *et al.* (1993a) The mentally disordered offender in non-medical settings. In *Forensic Psychiatry, Clinical, Legal and Ethical Issues* (ed. J. Gunn & P. J. Taylor). Butterworth–Heinemann, Oxford. pp. 732–93.

Taylor, P. J., Butwell, M., Dacey, R. & Kaye, C. (1991) *Within Maximum security Hospitals. A Survey of Need.* Special Hospital Services Authority, London.

Taylor, P. J., d'Orbán, P., Gunn, J. *et al.* (1993b) Organic disorders, mental handicap and offending. In *Forensic Psychiatry: Clinical, Legal and Ethical Issues* (ed. J. Gunn & P. J. Taylor). Butterworth–Heinemann, Oxford,pp. 286–325.

Taylor, P. J. & Fleminger, J. J. (1980) ECT for schizophrenics. *Lancet*, i, 1380–2.

Taylor, P. J., Garety, P., Buchanan, A. *et al.* (1994) Delusions and violence. In *Violence and Mental Disorders. Developments in Risk Assessment* (ed. J. Monahan & H. J. Steadman), Chicago University Press, Chicago, pp. 161–82.

Taylor, P. J. & Gunn, J. (1984) Violence and Psychosis. *Br. Med. J.*, **288**, 1945–9; **289**, 9–12.

Taylor, P. G., Gunn, J., Browne, F. W. A. *et al.* (1993c) Principles for treatment for the mentally disordered offender. In *Forensic Psychiatry: Clinical, Legal and Ethical Issues* (ed. J. Gunn & P. J. Taylor). Butterworth–Heinemann, Oxford, pp. 646–90.

Taylor, P. J., Hamilton, J., Kopelman, M. D. *et al.* (1993d) Addictions and Dependencies: their association with offending. In *Forensic Psychiatry: Clinical, Legal and Ethical Issues* (ed. J. Gunn & P. J. Taylor). Butterworth–Heinemann, Oxford, pp. 435–89

Taylor, P. J. & Hodgins, S. (1994) Violence and Psychosis: Critical Timings. *Crim. Behav. Ment. Health.*, **4**, 266–89.

Taylor, P. J., Mullen, P. E. & Wessely, S. (1993a) Psychosis, violence and crime. In *Forensic Psychiatry: Clinical, Legal and Ethical Issues* (ed. J. Gunn & P. J. Taylor). Butterworth–Heinemann, Oxford, pp. 329–71.

Taylor, P. J. & Parrott, J. M. (1988) Elderly offenders: a study of age-related factors among custodially remanded prisoners. *Br. J. Psychiat.*, **152**, 340–6.

Teasdale, G. & Jennet, B. T. (1974) Assessment of coma and impaired consciousness. *Lancet*, ii, 81–4.

Teasdale, J. D. (1993) Emotion and two kinds of meaning: Cognitive therapy and applied cognitive science. *Behav. Res. Ther.*, **31**, 339–54.

Teasdale, J. D., Fennell, M. J. V., Hibbert, G. A. & Amies, P. L. (1984) Cognitive therapy for major depressive disorder in primary care. *Br. J. Psych.*, **144**, 400–6.

Temoche, A., Pugh, T. F. & McMahon, B. (1964) Suicide rates among current and former mental institution patients. *J. Nerv. Ment. Dis.*, **138**, 124–31.

Tennant, C., Smith, A., Bebbington, P. *et al.* (1979) The contextual threat of life events: the concept and its reliability. *Psychol. Med.*, **9**, 525–8.

Tennant, C., Smith, A., Bebbington, P. & Hurry, J. (1981a) Parental loss in childhood: relationship to adult psychiatric impairment and contact with psychiatric services. *Arch. Gen. Psych.*, **38**, 309–14.

Tennant, C., Bebbington, P. & Hurry, J. (1981b) The short-term outcome of neurotic disorders in the community. The relationship of remission to clinical factors and to 'neutralising' life events. *Br. J. Psych.*, **139**, 213–20.

Teplin, L. A. (1985) The criminality of the mentally ill: a dangerous conception. *Am. J. Psych.*, **142**, 593–9.

Termelin, M. K. (1968) Suggestion effects in psychiatric diagnosis. *J. Nerv. Ment. Dis.*, **147**, 349–53.

Tessler, R. & Goldman, H. (1982). *The Chronic Mentally Ill, Assessing the Community Support Programme.* Ballinger, Cambridge.

Test, M. A. & Stein, L. J. (1980) Alternative to mental hospital treatment. 3, Social Cost. *Arch. Gen. Psychiat.*, **37**, 409–12.

Thapar, A., Gottesman, I. I., Owen, M. J. *et al.* (1994) The genetics of mental retardation. *Br. J. Psychiat.*, **164**, 747–59.

Thapar, A. & McGuffin, P. (1996) Genetic influences on life events in childhood. *Psychol. Med..*, **26**, 813–20.

Thapar, A. K. & Thapar, A. (1992) Psychological sequelae of miscarriage: a controlled study using the general health questionnaire and the hospital anxiety and depression scale. *Br. J. Gen. Pract.*, **42**, 94–6.

The Brewers' Society (1992) *Brewers' Society Statistical Handbook*. Brewing Publications Ltd, London.

Theander, S. (1985) Outcome and prognosis in anorexia and bulimia: some results of previous investigations, compared with those of a Swedish long-term study. *J. Psychiatr. Res.*, **19**, 493–508.

Theander, S. (1970) Anorexia nervosa: a psychiatric evaluation of 94 female patients. *Acta Psych. Scand.* Supp 214. Munksgard, Copenhagen.

Theander, S. (1994) The essence of anorexia nervosa: comment on Gerald Russell's 'Anorexia Nervosa Through Time' pp. 27–32. In *Handbook of Eating Disorders Theory Treatment and Research* (ed. G. Szmukler, C. Dare & J. L. Treasure). Wiley, Chichester, pp. 27–32.

Theilgaard, A. (1984) A psychological study of the personalities of XYY and XXY men. *Acta Psych. Scand. Suppl.* 315, Vol. 69.

Thom, B. (1986) Sex differences in help-seeking for alcohol problems. 1 The barriers to help seeking. *Br. J. Addic.*, **81**, 777–88.

Thom, B. (1987) Sex differences in help-seeking for alcohol problems. 2 Entry into treatment. *Br. J. Addic.*, **82**, 989–97.

Thomas, A. & Chess, S. (1984) Genesis and evolution of behavioural disorders: from infancy to early adult life. *Am. J. Psych.*, **141**, 1–9.

Thomas, D. A. (1979) *Principles of Sentencing*, 2dn edn. Heinemann, London.

Thomas, H. (1993) Psychiatric symptoms in cannabis users. *Br. J. Psychiat.*, **163**, 141–9.

Thomas, R. K., Cameron, D. J. & Fahs, M. (1988) A prospective study of delirium and prolonged hospital stay. *Arch. Gen. Psych.*, **45**, 937–40.

Thompson, C. (ed) (1989) *The Instruments of Psychiatric Research*. John Wiley & Sons, Chichester.

Thompson, C. (1994) The use of high-dose antipsychotic medication. *Br. J. Psychiat.*, **164**, 448–58.

Thompson, C. & Issacs, G. (1988) Seasonal affective disorder – a British sample. *J. Affec. Dis.*, **14**, 1–11.

Thompson, D. J. & Goldberg, D. (1987) Hysterical personality disorder: the process of diagnosis in clinical and experimental settings. *Br. J. Psych.*, **150**, 241–5.

Thompson, L. W., Gallagher, D. & Breckenridge, J. S. (1987) Comparative effectiveness of psychotherapies for depressed elders. *J. Consult. Clin. Psychol.*, **55**, 385–90.

Thompson, W. D. & Weissman, M. M. (1981) Quantifying lifetime risk of psychiatric disorder. *J. Psych. Res.*, **2**, 113–26.

Thomsen, I. (1974) The patient with severe head injury and his family. *Scand. J. Rehab. Med.*, **6**, 180–3.

Thomsen, P. H. (1990) The prognosis in early adulthood of child psychiatric patients: a case register study in Denmark. *Acta Psychiat. Scand.*, **81**, 89–93.

Thomsen, P. H. (1991) Obsessive-compulsive symptoms in children and adolescents. A phenomenological analysis of 61 Danish cases. *Psychopathol*, **24**, 12–18.

Thomsen, P. H. (1993) Obsessive-compulsive disorder in children and adolescents. Self-reported obsessive symptoms and traits in Danish pupils. *Acta. Psych. Scand.*, **88**, 212–17.

Thomsen, P. H. (1994a) Obsessive-compulsive disorder in children and adolescents. A review of the literature. *Eur. Child Adol. Psych.*, **3**, 138–58.

Thomsen, P. H. (1994b) Obsessive-compulsive disorder in children and adolescents. An analysis of sociodemographic characteristics. A case-control study. *Psychopathol.*, **27**, 303–11.

Thomsen, P. H. & Mikkelsen, H. U. (1993) Development of personality disorders in children and adolescents with obsessive-compulsive disorder. A 6 to 22 year follow-up study. *Acta Psych. Scand.*, **87**, 456–62.

Thorndike, E. L. (1898) *Animal Intelligence*. New York.

Thornicroft, G. (1988) Progress towards D.H.S.S. targets for community care. *Br. J. Psych.*, **153**, 257–8.

Thornicroft, G. (1991) Social deprivation and rates of treated mental disorder: developing statistical models to predict psychiatric service utilisation. *Br. J. Psych.*, **158**, 475–84.

Thornicroft, G. & Bebbington, P. (1989) Deinstitutionalisation: from hospital closure to service development. *Br. J. Psych.*, **155**, 739–53.

Thornicroft, G. & Strathdee, G. (1991) The health of the nation: mental health. *Br. Med. J.*, **303**, 1511.

Thornton, D. & Hogue, T. (1993) The large scale provision of programmes for imprisoned sex offenders: issues, dilemmas and progress. *Crim. Behav. Ment. Health.*, **3**, 371–80.

Thorpy, M. J. (1988) Diagnosis, evaluation and classification of sleep disorders, In *Sleep Disorders: Diagnosis and Treatment* (ed. R. Williams, I. Karacan & C. A. Moore). Wiley, New York, pp. 9–25.

Tienari, P. (1991) Interaction between genetic vulnerability and family environment: the Finnish adoptive family study of schizophrenia. *Acta Psychiat. Scand.*, **84**, 460–5.

Tiller, J., Schmidt, U. & Treasure, J. (1993) Compulsory treatment for anorexia nervosa: compassion or coercion? *Brit. J. Psychiat.*, **162**, 679–80.

Tizard, B. (1962) The personality of epileptics: a discussion of the evidence. *Psychol. Bull.*, **59**, 196–210.

Tober, G. & Raistrick, D. (1990) Development of a district training strategy. *Br. J. Addiction*, **85**, 1563–70.

Tobin, D. L. (1994) Psychodynamic psychotherapy and binge eating. In *Binge Eating, Nature Assessment and Treatment* (ed. C. G. Fairburn & G. T. Wilson). Guilford Press, New York, pp. 287–313.

Tohen, M., Tsuang, M. T. & Goodwin, D. C. (1992) Prediction of outcome in mania by mood-congruent or mood-incongruent psychotic features. *Am. J. Psych.*, **149**, 1580–4.

Tomlinson, B. (1992) *Report of the Inquiry into London's Health Service, Medical Education and Research.* HMSO, London.

Tomlinson, B., Blessed, G. & Roth, M. (1970) Observations on the brains of demented old people. *J. Neurol. Sci.*, **11**, 205–42.

Toone, B. K. (1981) Psychosis of epilepsy. In *Epilepsy and Psychiatry* (ed. E. H. Reynolds & M. R. Trimble). Churchill Livingstone, Edinburgh, pp. 113–37.

Torgerson, S. (1979) The nature and origin of common phobic fears. *Br. J. Psych.*, **134**, 343–51.

Torgersen, S. (1985) Hereditary differentiation of anxiety and affective neuroses. *Brit. J. Psych.*, **146**, 530–4.

Torgersen, A. (1986) Genetic factors in moderately severe and mild affective disorders. *Arch. Gen. Psych.*, **43**, 222–6.

Toro, G. & Roman, G. (1978) Cerebral malaria. *Arch. Neurol.*, **35**, 271–5.

Torre, E. & Marinoni, A. (1985) Register studies: data from four areas in Northern Italy. *Acta Psychiat. Scand.*, (Suppl. 136). 87–94.

Torrey, E. F. (1988) *Surviving Schizophrenia: A Family Manual.* Harper & Row, London.

Torrey, E. F., Stieber, J., Ezekiel, J. *et al.* (1992) *Criminalization of The Seriously Mentally Ill. The Abuse of Jails as Mental Hospitals.* Public Citizens Health Research Group, Washington DC.

Torrey, F. (1986) Continuous treatment teams in the care of the chronic mentally ill. *Hosp. Comm. Psych.*, **37**, 1243–7.

Traskman, L., Asberg, M., Birtleson, L. & Sjostrand, L. (1981) Monomine metabolites in CSF and suicidal behaviour. *Arch. Gen. Psych.*, **38**, 631–6.

Treasure, J. L. & Campbell, I. (1994) The case for biology in the aetiology of anorexia nervosa. *Psychol. Med.*, **24**, 3–8.

Treasure, J. L. & Holland, A. J. (1988) Genetic vulnerability to eating disorders: evidence from twin and family studies. In *Anorexia nervosa* (ed. H. Remschmidt & M. H. Schmidt). Hofrefe & Huber, Toronto, pp. 59–68.

Treasure, J. & Holland, A. J. (1993) What can discordant twins tell us about the aetiology of anorexia nervosa? In *Advances in the Neurosciences Vol. 90. Primary Approach* (ed. F. Ferrari & S. B. Solerte). Pergamon Press, Oxford, pp. 113–22.

Treasure, J. & Holland, A. J. (1995) Genetic factors in eating disorders. In *Handbook of Eating Disorders* (ed. G. Szmukler, C. Dare & J. L. Treasure). Wiley, London, pp. 65–82.

Treasure, J., Schmidt, U., Troop, N. *et al.* (1994) The first step in the management of bulimia nervosa. A controlled trial of a therapeutic manual. *Br. Med. J.*, **308**, 686–9.

Treasure, J., Schmidt, U., Troop, N. *et al.* (1996) Sequential treatment for bulimia nervosa incorporating a self-care manual. *Br. J. Psychiat.*, **168**, 94–8.

Treasure, J. L. & Szmukler, G. (1995) Medical complications of chronic anorexia nervosa. In *Handbook of Eating Disorders* (ed. G. Szmukler, C. Dare & J. Treasure). Wiley, Chichester, pp. 197–220.

Treasure, J., Todd, G., Brolly, M. *et al.* (1995) A pilot study of a randomised trial of cognitive analytical therapy vs educational behaviour therapy for adult anorexia nervosa. *Behav. Res. Ther.*, **33**, 363–7.

Tremblay, R. E., McCord, J., Boileau, H. *et al.* (1991) Can disruptive boys be helped to become competent? *Psychiatry*, **54**, 148–61.

Trevor, A. J. & Way, W. L. (1988) Drugs used for anxiety states and sleep problems. In *Review of General Psychiatry* 2nd edn. (ed. H. H. Goldman). Prentice Hall International Inc, London, pp. 600–13.

Trimble, M. (1981) *Post-Traumatic Neurosis*. John Wiley, New York.

Trotter, T. (1804) *An Essay, Medical, Philosophical and Chemical, on Drunkenness and its Effects on the Human Body*. T. N. Longman & O. Rees, London.

Trower, P., Bryant, B. & Argyle, M. (1978) *Social Skills and Mental Heath*. Methuen, London.

Truax, C. B., Wargo, D. G., Frank, J. D. *et al.* (1966) Therapist's empathy, genuineness, and warmth and patient therapeutic outcome. *J. Consult. Clin. Psychol.*, **27**, 395–401.

Truckle, S. (1992) *Psychoanalytic Politics: Jacques Lacan and Freud's French Revolution*. Guilford Press, New York.

True, W., Rice, J. Eisen, S. *et al.* (1993) A twin study of genetic and environmental contributions to liability for posttraumatic stress symptoms. *Arch. Gen. Psychiat.*, **50**, 257–64.

Trzepacz, P. T., Baker, W. & Greenhouse, J. (1988) A symptom rating scale for delirium. *Psych. Res.*, **23**, 89–97.

Tsuang, D. & Coryell, W. (1993) An 8-year follow-up of patients with DSM-IIIR psychotic depression, schizoaffective disorder, and schizophrenia. *Am. J. Psychiat.*, **150**, 1182–8.

Tsuang, M. T. (1978) Suicide in schizophrenics, manics, depressives and surgical controls. *Arch. Gen. Psych.*, **35**, 153–5.

Tsuang, M. T. (1983) Risk of suicide in the relatives of schizophrenics, manics, depressives, and controls. *J. Clin. Psych.*, **44**, 396–400.

Tsuang, M. T. (1991) Morbidity risks of schizophrenia and affective disorders among first-degree relatives of patients with schizoaffective disorders. *Br. J. Psych.*, **158**, 165–70.

Tsuang, M. T., Simpson, J. C. & Fleming, J. A. (1992) Epidemiology of suicide. *Int. Rev. Psych.*, **4**, 117–29.

Tsuang, M. T., Simpson, J. C. & Kronfol, Z. (1982) Subtypes of drug abuse with psychosis. *Arch of Gen. Psych.*, **39**, 141–47.

Tsuang, M. T. & Winokur, G. (1974) Criteria for subtyping schizophrenia. *Arch. Gen. Psych.*, **31**, 43–7.

Tsuang, M. T., Woolson, R. F. & Fleming, J. A. (1979) Long-term outcome of major psychoses. *Arch. Gen. Psych.*, **36**, 1295–301.

Tsuang, M. T., Woolson, R. F. & Fleming, J. A. (1980) Cause of death in schizophrenia and manic depression. *Br. J. Psychiat.*, **136**, 239–42.

Tuinier, S. & Verhoeven, W. M. A. (1993) Psychiatry in mental retardation: towards a behavioural pharmacological concept. *J. Intell. Dis. Res.*, Supplement 37, 16–25.

Tunnadine, P., Morrow, C. S. & Hutchinson, F. D. (1981) Sex problems in practice: training and referral. Institute of Psychosexual Medicine, Margaret Pyke Centre and Brook Advisory Centres. *Br. Med. J.*, **282**, 1669–72.

Turk, J. (1992*a*) The fragile X syndrome: recent developments. *Curr. Opin. Psych.*, **5**, 677–82.

Turk, J. (1992*b*) The fragile X syndrome: On the way to a behavioural phenotype. *Br. J. Psych.*, **160**, 24–35.

Turner, M. J., Flannelly, G. M., Wingfield, M. *et al.* (1991) The miscarriage clinic: an audit of the first year. *Br. Obstet. Gynaecol.*, **98**, 306–8.

Turner, R. J. & Wagenfeld, M. O. (1967) Occupational mobility and schizophrenia: an assessment of the social causation and social selection hypotheses. *Am. Sociol. Rev.*, **32**, 104–13.

Turner, T. H. (1989) Schizophrenia and mental handicap: an historical review, with implications for further research. *Psychol. Med.*, **19**, 301–14.

Turner, W. M. & Tsuang, M. T. (1990) Impact of substance abuse on the course and outcome of schizophrenia. *Schiz. Bul.*, **16**, 87–95.

Turrina, C., Siciliani, O., Dewy, M. E. *et al.* (1992) Psychiatric disorders among elderly patients attending a geriatric medical day hospital: Prevalence according to clinical diagnosis (DSM-IIIR) and Agecat. *Int. J. Geriat. Psych.*, **7**, 499–504.

Tweed, L., Schoenbach, V., George, L. & Blazer, D. (1989) The effects of childhood parental death and divorce on six-month history of anxiety disorders. *Br. J. Psych.*, **154**, 823–8.

Tym, E. (1991) A rural service in East Anglia. In *Psychiatry in the Elderly* (ed. R. Levy & C. Oppenheimer) Oxford University Press, Oxford, pp. 313–22.

Tyrer, P. J. (1973) Are monoamine oxidase inhibitors antidepressants? *Proc. Roy. Soc. Med.*, **66**, 950–1.

Tyrer, P. (1978) Drug treatment of psychiatric patients in general practice. *Br. Med. J.*, **2**, 1008–10.

Tyrer, P. (1984) Psychiatric clinics in general practice: an extension of community care. *Br. J. Psych.*, **145**, 9–14.

Tyrer, P. (1985a) The 'hive' system: a model for a psychiatric service. *Br. J. Psych.*, **146**, 571–5.

Tyrer, P. (1985b) Neurosis divisible. *Lancet*, **i**, 685–8.

Tyrer, P. (1989) *Classification of Neurosis.* John Wiley, Chichester.

Tyrer, P. (1992) Flamboyant, erratic, dramatic, borderline, antisocial, sadistic, narcissistic, histrionic and impulsive personality disorders: who cares which? *Crim. Behav. Ment. Helath*, **2**, 95–104.

Tyrer, P. & Alexander, J. (1979) Classification of personality disorder. *Br. J. Psych.*, **135**, 163–7.

Tyrer, P., Alexander, M. S., Cicchetti, D. *et al.* (1979) Reliability of a schedule for rating personality disorders. *Br. J. Psych.*, **135**, 168–74.

Tyrer, P. & Ashton, H. (1989) Controversies in therapeutics: risks of dependence on benzodiazepine drugs. *Br. Med. J.*, **298**, 102–5.

Tyrer, P., Casey, P. & Ferguson, B. (1991) Personality disorder in perspective. *Br. J. Psych.*, **159**, 463–71.

Tyrer, P., Casey, P. & Gah, J. (1983) Relationship between neuroses and personality disorder. *Br. J. Psych.*, **142**, 404–8.

Tyrer, P., Ferguson, B. & Alexander, J. (1988) Personality Assessment Schedule (4th edition). In *Personality Disorder: Diagnosis, Management and Course.* John Wright, Bristol.

Tyrer, R. & Hallstrom, C. (1993) Antidepressants in the treatment of anxiety disorder. *Psych. Bul.*, **17**, 75–6.

Tyrer, P., Marsden, C. A., Casey, P. *et al.* (1987) Clinical efficacy of paroxetine in resistant depression. *J. Psychopharmacol.*, **1**, 251–7.

Tyrer, P., Rutherford, D. & Huggett, T. (1981) Benzodiazepine withdrawal symptoms and propranodol. *Lancet*, **i**, 520–2.

Tyrer, P., Sievewright, N., Murphy S. *et al* (1988) The Nottingham Study of neurotic disorder: comparison of drug and psychological treatments. *Lancet*, **ii**, 235–40.

Tyrer, P., Sievewright, N. & Wollerton, S. (1984) General practice psychiatric clinics. Impact on psychiatric services. *Br. J. Psych.*, **145**, 15–9.

Tyrer, P., Turner, R. & Johnson, A. (1989) Integrated hospital and community psychiatric services and use of inpatient beds. *Br. Med. J.*, **299**, 198–300.

Tyrer, S. & Shakour, Y. (1990) The effect of lithium in the periodicity of aggressive episodes. In *Key Issues in Mental Retardation Research* (ed. W. Fraser). Routledge, London, pp. 121–9.

Tyrer, S., Walsh, A., Edwards, D. E. *et al.* (1984) Factors associated with a good response to lithium in aggressive mentally handicapped subjects. *Prog. Neuropsychopharmacol.*, **8**, 751–9.

Udry, J. R., Talbert, L. M. & Morris, N. M. (1986) Biosocial foundations for adolescent female sexuality. *Demography*, **23**, 217–27.

Uhl, G., Blum, K., Noble, E. & Smith, S. (1993) Substance abuse vulnerability and D2 receptor genes. *Trends in Neurosci.*, **16**, 83–8.

Ullman, L. P. & Krasner, L. (1975) *A Psychological Approach to Abnormal Behaviour*, 2nd edn. Prentice-Hall, Englewood Cliffs.

United States Department of Health & Human Services (1988) *Study Findings: Study of the National Incidence and Prevalence of Child Abuse and Neglect*. US Department of Health & Human Services, Washington DC.

United States Department of Health and Human Services (1991) *Healthy People 2000: National Health. Promotion and Disease Prevention Objectives*. Government Printing Office, Washington DC.

Urwin, P. & Gibbons, J. L. (1979) Psychiatric diagnosis in self-poisoning patients. *Psychol. Med.*, **9**, 501–7.

Usdin, C. (1978) Metabolic pathways of antipsychotic drugs. In *Psychopharmacology: A Generation of Progress* (ed. M. A. Lipton, A. DiMascio & K. F. Killam). Raven Press, New York, pp. 895–905.

Vaillant, G. E. (1973) A 20-year follow-up of New York narcotic addicts. *Arch. Gen. Psych.*, **29**, 237–41.

Vaillant, G. E. (1979) Natural history of male psychologic health: Effects of mental health on physical health. *N. Engl. J. Med.*, **301**, 1249–54.

Vaillant, G. E. (1983) *The Natural History of Alcoholism. Causes, Patterns and Paths to Recovery*. Harvard University Press, Cambridge.

Vaillant, G. (1986) Cultural factors in the etiology of alcoholism: a prospective study. *Ann. N. Y. Acad. Sci.*, **472**, 142–8.

Vallada, H., Gill, M., Sham, P. *et al.* (1995) Linkage analysis of schizophrenia on chromosome 22 in familial schizophrenia. *Am. J. Med. Genet (Neuropsych. Genet.)*, **60**, 139–46.

Van Den Berg, J. H. (1982) On hallucinations: critical-historical overview. In *Phenomenology and Psychiatry* (ed. A. J. DeKoning & F. A. Jenner). Academic Press, London, pp. 92–110.

Van den Hout, M., Arntz, A. & Hoekstra, R. (1994) Exposure reduced agoraphobia but not panic, and cognitive therapy reduced panic but not agoraphobia. *Behav. Res. Ther.*, **32**, 447–51.

Van Duijn, C., Stijinen T. & Hofman, A. (1991) Risk factors for Alzheimer's disease: Overview of the EURODEM collaborative re-analysis of case control studies. *Int. J. Epidemiol.*, **20** (supplement 2) S4–S12.

Van Eerdewegh, M. M., Bieri, M. D., Parrilla, R. H. & Clayton, P. J. (1982) The bereaved child. *Br. J. Psych.*, **140**, 23–9.

Van Furth, E. F. (1991) Parental expressed emotion and eating disorders. PhD thesis. University of Utrecht.

Van Hemert, A., Hengeveld, M., Bolk J. *et al.* (1993) Psychiatric disorders in relation to medical illness among patients of a general medical out-patient clinic. *Psychol. Med.*, **23**, 167–173.

Van Oppen, P., de Haan, E., Balkom, A. J. L. M. *et al.* (1995) Cognitive therapy and exposure *in vivo* in the treatment of obsessive-compulsive disorder. *Behav. Res. Ther.*, **33**, 379–90.

Van Os, G., Fahy, T., Bebbington, P. *et al.* (1994) Influence of life events on subsequent course of psychotic illness. *Psychol. Med.*, **24**, 503–13.

Van Os, J., Fahy, T., Jones, I. *et al.* (1996*a*) Tardive dyskinesia: effect of medication or illness deterioration: *Schiz. Bul.*, (in press).

Van Os, J., Fahy, T., Jones, P. *et al.* (1996*b*) Psychopathological syndromes in the functional psychoses: associations with course and outcome. *Psychol. Med.*, **26**, 203–8.

Van Putten, T., Marder, S. & Mintz, J. (1990) A controlled dose comparison of haloperidol in newly admitted schizophrenic patients. *Arch. Gen. Psychiat.*, **47**, 754–8.

Van Putten, T. V. & May, P. R. A. (1976) Milieu therapy of the schizophrenias. In *Treatment of Schizophrenia: Progress and Prospects* (ed. L. J. West & D. E. Flinn). Grune & Stratton, New York, pp. 217–43.

Van Tol, H. H. M., Bunzow, J. R., Guan, H. C. *et al.* (1991) Cloning of the gene for a human dopamine D4 receptor with high affinity for the antipsychotic clozapine. *Nature*, **350**, 610–14.

Van Valkenburg, C. & Clayton, P. J. (1985) Electroconvulsive therapy in schizophrenia. *Biol. Psych.*, **20**, 699–700.

Varan, L. R., Gillieson, M. S., Skene, D. S. & Sarwer-Foner, G. J. (1985) ECT in an acutely psychotic pregnant woman with actively aggressive (homicidal) impulses. *Can. J. Psychiatry-Revue Canadienne de Psychiatrie*, **30**, 363–7.

Vassilas, C. A. & Morgan, H. G. (1993) General practitioners' contact with victims of suicide. *Br. Med. J.*, **307**, 300–1.

Vaughn, C. & Leff, J. P. (1976) The influence of family and social factors on the course of psychiatric illness. *Br. J. Psychiat.*, **129**, 125–37.

Vazquez-Barquero, J. F., Diez-Manrique, J. F., Pena, C. *et al* (1986) Two stage design in a community survey. *Br. J. Psych.*, **149**, 88–97.

Veiel, H. O. F. (1985) Dimensions of social support: a conceptual framework for research. *Soc. Psychiat.*, **20**, 156–62.

Velleman, R. & Orford, J. (1993) The importance of family discord in explaining childhood problems in the children of problem drinkers. *Addic. Res.*, **1**, 39–57.

Victor, M., Adams, R. & Collins, G. (1981) *Wernicke–Korsakoff Syndrome*. F. A. Davis, Philadelphia.

Vigersky, R. A. & Loriaux D. L. (1977) The effect of cyproheptidine in anorexia nervosa: A double blind trial, In *Anorexia Nervosa* (ed. R. Vigersky). Raven Press, New York, pp. 349–56.

Villeponteaux, V. A., Lydiard, R. B., Laraia, M. T. *et al.* (1992) The effects of pregnancy on preexisting panic disorder. *J. Clin. Psych.*, **53**, 201–3.

Virag, R. (1982) Intracavernous injection of papaverine for erectile failure. *Lancet*, **ii**, 938.

Virchow, R. (1847) Standpoints in scientific medicine. In *Diseases, Life and Man* selected essays by Rudolf Virchow, translated by L. J. Rather 1958. Stanford University Press, Palo Alto.

Virkkunen, M. (1976) Attitude to psychiatric treatment before suicide in schizophrenia and paranoid psychoses. *Br. J. Psych.*, **128**, 47–9.

Vitiello, B., Spreat, S. & Behar, D. (1989) Obsessive-compulsive disorder in mentally retarded patients. *J. Nerv. Ment. Dis.*, **17**, 232–6.

Vizard, E. (1991) Interviewing children suspected of being sexually abused: a review of theory and practice. In *Clinical approaches to Sex Offenders and their Victims* (ed. C. R. Hollin & K. Howells). John Wiley, Chichester, pp. 117–48.

Volavka, J., Cooper, T., Czobor, P. *et al.* (1992). Haloperidol blood levels and clinical effects. *Arch. Gen. Psych.*, **49**, 354–61.

Von Knorring, A.-L., Andersson, O. & Magnusson, D. (1987) Psychiatric care and course of psychiatric disorders from childhood to early adulthood in a representative sample. *J. Child Psychol. Psychiat.*, **28**, 329–41.

Von Knorring, A.-L., Cloninger, C. R., Bohman, M. & Sigvardsson, S. (1983) An adoption study of depressive disorder and substance abuse. *Arch. Gen. Psych.*, **40**, 943–50.

Vygotsky, L. S. (1978) *Mind in Society. The Development of Higher Psychological Processes*. Harvard University Press, Cambridge, Mass.

Wadsworth, M. (1979) *Roots of Delinquency*. Martin Robertson, London.

Wagner, G. & Brindley, G. S. (1980) The effect of atropine and alpha-blockers on human penile erection. In *Vasculogenic Impotence* (ed. A. W. Zorgniotti & G. Rossi). C. C. Thomas, Springfield.

Wahler, R. G. & Dumas, J. E. (1985) Maintenance factors in coercive mother–child interactions: the compliance and predictability hypothesis. *J. Appl. Behav. Anal.*, **19**, 13–22.

Wald, A., Chandra, R., Chiponis, D. & Gabel, S. (1986) Anorectal function and continence mechanisms in childhood encopresis. *J. Ped. Gastroenterol. Nutr.*, **5**, 346–51.

Walk, D. (1967) Suicide and community care. *Br. J. Psychiat.*, **113**, 1381–91.

Walker, E. & Lewine, E. J. (1990) Prediction of adult-onset schizophrenia from childhood movies of the patients. *Am. J. Psychiat.*, **147**, 1052–6.

Walker, M. & Armfield, A. (1981) What is Makaton vocabulary? Special Education. *Forward Trends*, Vol. 8, No. 3.

Wallace, S. A., Crown, J. M., Cox, A. D., & Berger, M. (1996) *Epidemiologically-based Needs Assessment: Child and Adolescent Mental Health*. Radcliffe Medical Press, Oxford.

Wallace, P., Cutler, S. & Haines, A. (1988) Randomised controlled trial of general practitioner intervention in patients with excessive alcohol consumption. *Br. Med. J.*, **277**, 663–8.

Wallack, J. J., Snyder, S., Bialer, P. A. *et al.* (1991) An Aids bibliography for the general psychiatrist. *Psychosomatics*, **32**, 243–54.

Wallerstein, R. S. (1986) *Forty-two lives in Treatment: a Study of Psychoanalysis and Treatment.* Guilford Press, New York.

Wallis, N. C. J. *et al.* (1993) Magnetic resonance for detection of abnormalities in partial epilepsy. *Lancet*, **342**, 1252.

Walsh, D. (1987) Mental health service models in Europe. In *Mental Health Services in Pilot Study Areas: Report on a European Study.* WHO, Copenhagen.

Walsh, T. B., Hadigan, C. M., Devlin, M. J. *et al.* (1991) Long-term outcome of antidepressant treatment for bulimia nervosa. *Am. J. Psychiat.*, **148**, 1206–12.

Walton, H. J. & Presly, A. S. (1973) Use of a category system in the diagnosis of abnormal personality. *Br. J. Psych*, **122**, 259–68.

Wanigaratne, S., Wallace, W., Pullin, J. *et al.* (1990). *Relapse Prevention for Addictive Disorders.* Blackwell Scientific Publications, Oxford.

Ward, C. H., Beck, A. T., Mendelson, M. *et al.* (1962) The psychiatric nomenclature. *Arch. Gen. Psychiat.*, **7**, 198–205.

Waring, E. M. (1985) Measurement of intimacy: conceptual and methodological issues of studying close relationships. *Psychol. Med.*, **15**, 9–14.

Warner, P. & Bancroft, J. (1988) Mood, sexuality, oral contraceptives and the menstrual cycle. *J. Psychosom. Res.*, **32**, 417–27.

Warner, V., Weissman, M. M., Fendrich, M. *et al.* (1992) The course of major depression in the offspring of depressed parents: incidence, recurrence and recovery. *Arch. Gen. Psych.*, **49**, 795–801.

Warr, P. B. (1987) *Work, Unemployment and Mental Health.* OUP, Oxford.

Warrington, E. K. & Weiskrantz, L. (1982) Amensia: a disconnection syndrome. *Neuropsychologia*, **20**, 233–48.

Warwick, H. M. C. & Marks, I. M. (1988) Behavioural treatment of illness phobia. *Br. J. Psych.*, **152**, 239–41.

Warwick, H. & Salkovskis, P. (1990) Hypochondriasis. *Behav. Res. Ther.*, **28**, 105–17.

Wasserman, I. M. (1984) Imitation and suicide: a re-examination of the Werther effect. *Am. Soc. Rev.*, **49**, 427–36.

Watanabe, H. & Azuma, Y. (1989) A proposal for a classification of enuresis based on overnight simultaneous monitoring of electroencephalography and cystometry. *Sleep*, **12**, 257–64.

Watkins, S. E., Callender, K. Thomas, D. R. *et al.* (1987) The effect of carbamazepine and lithium on remission from affective illness. *Br. J. Psych.*, **150**, 180–2.

Watson, J. P. & Marks, I. M. (1971) Relevant and irrelevant fear in flooding – a crossover study in phobic patients. *Behav. Ther.*, **2**, 275–93.

Watson, J. & Rayner, R. (1920) Conditioned emotional responses. *J. Exp. Psychol.*, **3**, 1–14.

Watts, F. N. (1982) Attributional aspects of medicine. In *Attributions and Psychological Change* (ed. C. Antaki & C. Brewin). Academic Press, London, pp. 135–55.

Waxman, S. G. & Geschwind, N. (1975) The interictal behaviour syndrome of temporal lobe epilepsy. *Arch. Gen. Psychiat.*, **32**, 1580–6.

Weatherall, D. (1983) *The New Genetics and Clinical Practice.* Nuffield Provincial Hospital Trust, Oxford.

Webb, T., Crawley, P. & Bundey, S. (1990) Folate treatment of a boy with Fragile-X syndrome. *J. Ment. Defic. Res.*, **34**, 67–73.

Weaver, S. M., Armstrong, N. E., Broome, A. K. & Stewart, L. (1978a) Behavioural principles applied to a security ward. *Nursing Times*, **5**, 22–4.

Weaver, S. M., Broome, A. K. & Kat, B. J. B. (1978b) Some patterns of disturbed behaviour in a closed ward environment. *J. Adv. Nursing*, **3**, 251–63.

Webb, T. & Bundey, S. (1991) Prevalence of Fragile-X syndrome. *J. Med. Genet.*, **28**, 358–61.

Webb, T., Bundey, S., Thake, A. & Todd, J. (1986) The frequency of FRAX among schoolchildren. *J. Med. Genet.*, **23**, 396–9.

REFERENCES

Weber, M. (1930) *The Protestant Ethic and the Spirit of Capitalism.* Allen & Unwin, London.

Webster, L., Dean, C. & Kessel, N. (1987) Effect of the 1983 Mental Health Act on the management of psychiatric patients. *Br. Med. J.*, **295**, 1529–32.

Webster-Stratton, C. (1990) Stress: a potent disrupter of parent perceptions on family interactions. *J. Clin. Child Psychol.*, **19**, 302–12.

Webster-Stratton, C. (1991) *The Dinosaur Videotape Curriculum for Young Children.* Seth Enterprises, Seattle.

Webster-Stratton, C. & Herbert, M. (1993) *Troubled Families – Problem Children.* Wiley, Chichester.

Wechsler, A. F., Verity, A., Rosenschein, S. *et al.* (1982) Pick's disease. *Arch. Neurol.*, **39**, 287–90.

Wechsler, D. (1958) *The Measurement and Appraisal of Adult Intelligence* 4th edn. Williams and Wilkins, Baltimore.

Wehrspann, W. H., Steinhauer, P. D. & Klajner-Diamond, H. (1987) Criteria and methodology for assessing credibility of sexual abuse allegations. *Can. J. Psych.*, **32**, 615–23.

Weil, R. J. & Tupper, C. (1960) Personality, life situation and communication: a study of habitual abortion. *Psychosom. Med.*, **22**, 448–55.

Weinberger, D. R. (1987) Implications of normal brain development for the pathogenesis of schizophrenia. *Arch. Gen. Psychiat.*, **44**, 660–9.

Weinberger, D. R. Delisi, L. Perman, G. P. *et al.* (1982) Computered tomography in schizophreniform disorder and other acute psychiatric disorders. *Arch. Gen. Psych.*, **39**, 778–83.

Weindling, P. (1992) From infectious to chronic diseases: changing patterns of sickness in the nineteenth and twentieth centuries. In *Medicine in Society* (ed. A. Wear). Cambridge University Press, Cambridge, pp. 303–16.

Weiner, B. A. (1980) Cognitive (attribution) – emotion-action model of motivated behaviour: an analysis of judgements of help giving. *J. Personality & Soc. Psychol.*, **39**, 186–200.

Weinstein, M. (1977) Recent advances in clinical pharmacology. I. Lithium carbonate. *Hosp. Form*, **12**, 759–62.

Weinstein, M. (1980) Lithium treatment of women during pregnancy and in the post-delivery period. In *Handbook of Lithium Therapy* (ed. F. N. Johnson). University Park Press, Baltimore, pp. 421–9.

Weiss, G. & Hechtman, L. T. (1986) *Hyperactive Children Grown Up.* Guilford Press, New York.

Weiss, R. (1974) The provisions of social relationships. In *Doing Unto Others* (ed. Z. Rubin). Prentice-Hall, Englewood Cliffs, NJ, pp. 17–26.

Weiss, R., J. & Bergen, B. J. (1968) Social supports and the reduction of psychiatric disability. *Psychiatry*, **31**, 107–15.

Weissman, M. M. Leaf, D. J., Tischler, G. L. *et al.* (1988) Affective disorders in five United states communities. *Psychol. Med.*, **18**, 141–53.

Weissman, M. M. & Myers, J. (1978) Rates and risks of depressive symptoms in a United States urban community. *Acta Psych. Scand.*, **57**, 219–31.

Weissman, M. M. & Paykel, E. S. (1974) *The Depressed Woman: a Study of Social Relations.* University of Chicago Press, Chicago.

Wells, B. (1987) Narcotics Anonymous (NA) the phenomenal growth of an important resource. *Br. J. Addiction*, **82**, 581–2.

Wells, J. E., Coope, P. A., Gabb, D. C. *et al.* (1985) The factor structure of the eating attitudes test with adolescent schoolgirls. *Psychol. Med.*, **15**, 141–6.

Wells, K., Stewart, A., Hays, R. *et al.* (1989) The functioning and well-being of the depressed: results from the medical out-patients study. *J. Am. Med. Assoc.*, **262**, 914–19.

Wender, P., Kety, S., Rosenthal, D. *et al.* (1986) Psychiatric disorders in the biological and adoptive families of adopted individuals with affective disorders. *Arch. Gen. Psych.*, **43**, 923–9.

Werner, E. E. (1987) Vulnerability and resiliency in children at risk for delinquency: a longitudinal study from birth to young adulthood. In *Prevention of Delinquent Behaviour* (ed. J. D. Burchard & S. N. Burchard). Sage, Beverly Hills, CA.

Werner, P. D., Rose, T. L., Yesavage, J. A. & Seeman, K. (1984) Psychiatrists' judgements of dangerousness in patients on an acute care unit. *Am. J. Psych.*, **141**, 263–2.

Werry, J. (1968) Developmental hyperactivity. *Ped. Clin. N. Am.*, **15**. 581–99.

Wessely, S. (1990) Old wine in new bottles: neurasthenia and ME. *Psychol. Med.*, **20**, 35–53.

Wessely, S. (1994) Neurasthenia and chronic fatigue syndrome: theory and practice. *Transcult. Psych. Rev.*, **31**, 73–209.

Wessely, S. (1995) The epidemiology of chronic fatigue syndrome. *Epidemiol. Rev.*, **17**, 139–51.

Wessely, S., Buchanan, A., Reed A. *et al.* (1993) Acting on delusions 1: Prevalence. *Br. J. Psychiat.*, **163**, 69–76.

Wessely, S., Butler, T., Chalder, T. & David, A. (1991) The cognitive behavioural management of the Post-Viral Fatigue Syndrome. In. *Post-Viral Fatigue Syndrome* (ed. R. Jenkins & J. Mowbray). John Wiley & Sons, Chichester.

Wessely, S., Chalder, T., Hirsch, S. *et al.* (1996) Psychological symptoms, somatic symptoms and psychiatric disorder in chronic fatigue and chronic fatigue syndrome: a prospective study in primary care. *Am. J. Psych.* (in press)

Wessely, S., Castle, D., Der, G. & Murray, R. M. (1991) Schizophrenia and Afro-Caribbeans: a case control study. *Br. J. Psych.*, **159**, 795–801.

Wessely, S. C., Castle, D., Douglas, A. J. & Taylor, P. J. (1994) the criminal careers of incident cases of schizophrenia. *Psychol. Med.*, **24**, 483–502.

Wessely, S. & Lewis, G. (1989) The classification of psychiatric morbidity in attenders at the dermatology clinic. *Br. J. Psych.*, **155**, 686–91.

Wessely, S. & Taylor, P. J. (1991) Madness and crime: criminology versus psychiatry. *Crim. Behav. Ment. Health.*, **1**, 193–228.

West, D. J. (1982) *Delinquency: Its Roots, Careers and Prospects.* Heinemann, London.

West, D. J. & Farrington, D. P. (1977) *The Delinquent Way of Life.* Heinemann, London.

West, D. J., Grubin, D., Gudjonsson, G. & Gunn, J. (1993) Disordered and offensive sexual behaviour. In *Forensic Psychiatry: Clinical, Legal and Ethical Issues* (ed. J. Gunn & P. J. Taylor). Butterworth–Heinemann, Oxford, pp. 522–66.

West, D. J. & Walk, A. (eds) (1977) *Daniel McNaughton. His Trial and the Aftermath.* Gaskell Books, Headley Brothers, Ashford, Kent.

West, E. D. & Dally, P. J. (1959) Effects of iproniazid in depression syndromes. *Br. Med. J.*, i, 1491–4.

Whipple, S. C. & Noble, P. (1991) Personality characteristics of alcoholic fathers and their sons. J. Stud. Alcohol., **52**, 331–7.

Whitehouse, A. M., Cooper, P. J., Vize, C. V. *et al.* (1992) Prevalence of eating disorders in three Cambridge general practices: Hidden and conspicuous morbidity. *Br. J. Gen. Prac.*, **42**, 57–60.

Whitehouse, P., Price, D., Struble, R. *et al.* (1982) Alzheimer's disease in senile dementia: loss of neurons in the basal forebrain. *Science*, **215**, 1237–9.

Whitlock, F. A. & Edwards, J. E. (1968) Pregnancy and attempted suicide. *Compr. Psych.*, **9**, 1–12.

Whittaker, J. J. (1989) Postoperative confusion in the elderly. *Int. J. Ger. Psych.*, **4**, 321–6.

Wickramaratne, P. J., Weissman, M. M., Leaf, P. J. & Holford, T. R. (1989) Age, period and cohort effects on the risk of major depression: results from five United States communities. *J. Clin. Epidemiol.*, **42**, 333–43.

Widom, C. S. (1989) The cycle of violence. *Science*, **244**, 160–6.

Widom, C. S. (1991) Avoidance of criminality in abused and neglected children. *Psychiatry*, **54**, 162–74.

Wieck, A., Kumar, R., Hirst, A. D. *et al.* (1991) Increased sensitivity of dopamine receptors and recurrence of affective psychosis after childbirth. *Br. Med. J.*, **303**, 613–16.

Wiersma, D., Giel, R., de Jong, A. & Slooff, C. (1983) Social class and schizophrenia in a Dutch cohort. *Psychol. Med.*, **13**, 141–50.

Wieselberg, M. (1993) Classification and epidemiology. In *Seminars in Child and Adolescent Psychiatry* (ed. D. Black & D. Cottrell). Gaskell, London, pp. 54–74.

Wikler, A. (1965) Conditioning factors in opiate addiction and relapse. In *Narcotics* (ed. D. I. Willner & G. G. Kassenbaum). McGraw Hill, New York, pp. 85–100.

Wikstrom, P. O. (1987) *Patterns of Crime in a Birth Cohort*. University of Stockholm Department of sociology, Stockholm.

Wilcox, D. E. (1985) The relationship of mental illness to homicide. *Am. J. Foren. Psych.*, **6**, 3–15.

Wilde, E. J., Kienhorst, I. C. W. M., Diekstra, R. F. W. & Wolters, W. H. G. (1992) The relationship between adolescent suicidal behaviour and life events in childhood and adolescence. *Am. J. Psych.*, **149**, 45–51.

Wilhelm, K. & Parker, G. (1989) Is sex necessarily a risk factor for depression? *Psychol. Med.*, **19**, 401–13.

Wilkinson, G. (1985) *Mental Health Practices in Primary Care Settings*. Tavistock Publications, London.

Wilkinson, G. (1989) Referrals from general practitioners to psychiatrists and paramedical mental health professionals. *Br. J. Psych.*, **154**, 72–6.

Wilkinson, G., Allen, P., Marshall, E. *et al.* (1993) The role of the practice nurse in the management of depression in general practice: treatment adherence to antidepressant medication. *Psychol. Med.*, **23**, 229–37.

Wilkinson, G. & Bacon, N. A. (1984) A clinical and epidemiological survey of parasuicide and suicide in Edinburgh schizophrenics. *Psychol. Med.*, **14**, 899–912.

Wilkinson, G., Balestrieri, M., Ruggeri, M. & Bellantuomo, C. (1991) Meta-analysis of double blind placebo controlled trials of anti-depressants and benzodiazepines for patients with panic disorders. *Psychol. Med.*, **21**, 991–8.

Wilkinson, G. & Williams, P. (1985) Priorities for research on mental health in primary care settings. *Psychol. Med.*, **15**, 509–14.

Wilkinson, M. J. B. & Barczak, P. (1988) Psychiatric screening in general practice: comparison of the General Health Questionnaire and the Hospital Anxiety Depression Scale. *J. Roy. Coll. Gen. Pract.*, **38**, 311–13.

Willi, J., Giacometti, G. & Limacher, B. (1990) Update of the epidemiology of anorexia nervosa in a defined region of Switzerland. *Am. J. Psychiat.*, **140**, 564–7.

Williams, H. V., Lipman, R. S., Rickels, K. *et al.* (1968) Replication of symptom distress factors in anxious neurotic out-patients. *Multiv. Behav. Res.*, **3**, 199–211.

Williams, J. B. W., Gibbon, M., First, M. B. *et al.* (1992) The Structured Clinical Interview for DSM-III-R (SCID). II: Multi-site test-retest reliability. *Arch. Gen. Psych.*, **49**, 630–6.

Williams, J. M. G. & Moorely, S. (1989) The wider application of cognitive therapy: the end of the beginning. In *Cognitive Therapy in Clinical Practice: An Illustrative Casebook* (ed. J. Scott, J. M. G. Williams & A. T. Beck). Routledge, London, pp. 227–50.

Williams, M. (1991) Antianxiety agents: A historical perspective. In *Current and Future Trends in Anticonvulsant, Anxiety and Stroke Therapy* (ed. B. S. Meldrum, & M. Williams). Wiley-Liss (Pubs), New York, pp. 131–45.

Williams, P. & Clare, A. J. (1979) *Psychosocial Disorders in General Practice*. Academic Press, London.

Williams, P., De Salvia, D. & Tansella, M. (1986) Suicide, psychiatric reform, and the provision of psychiatric services in Italy. *Soc. Psych.*, **21**, 89–95.

Williams, P., Hand, D. & Tarnopolsky, A. (1982) The problem of screening for uncommon disorders – a comment on the Eating Attitudes Test. *Psychol. Med.*, **12**, 431–4.

Williams, P. & King, M. (1987) The epidemic of anorexia nervosa: another medical myth? *Lancet*, **i**, 205–7.

Williams, P., Tarnopolsky, A. & Hand, D. (1980) Case definition and case identification in psychiatric epidemiology: review and assessment. *Psychol. Med.*, **10**, 101–14.

Williams, P., Tarnopolsky, A., Hand, D. *et al.* (1988) Minor psychiatric morbidity and general practice consultations: the West London survey. *Psychol. Med.*, Monograph Supplement 9.

Williams, R. & Richardson, G. (eds) (1995) *Child and Adolescent Mental Health Services: Together We Stand*. HMSO, London.

Williams, S., Anderson, J., McGee, R. & Silva, P. A. (1990) risk factors for behavioural and emotional disorder in preadolescent children. *J. Am. Acad. Child Adol. Psych.*, **29**, 413–19.

Williamson, T. M. (1993) From interrogation to investigative interviewing: strategic trends in police questioning. *J. Comm. App. Soc. Psychol.*, **3**, 89–99.

Willett, W. C., Stampfer, M. J., Colditz, G. A. *et al* (1987) Moderate alcohol consumption and the risk of breast cancer. *New Engl. Med.*, **316**, 1174–80.

Willner, P. (1990*a*) Animal models of depression: an overview. *Pharmacol, Therap.*, **45**, 425–55.

Willner, P. (1990*b*) The role of slow changes in catecholamine receptor function in the action of antidepressant drugs. *Int. Rev. Psych.*, **2**, 141–56.

Willner, P., Sampson, D., Papp, M., Phillips, G. & Muscat, R. (1991) Animal models of anhedonia. In *Anxiety, Depression and Mania*, vol. 3 (ed. P. Soubrie). Karger, Basel, pp. 71–00.

Wilsher, C. R. & Taylor, E. A. (1994) Piracetam in developmental reading disorders: a review. *Eur. Child Adol Psych.*, **3**, 59–71.

Wilson, I. C., Vernon, T. J. & Guin, T. (1963) A controlled study of treatments of depression. *J. Neuropsych.*, **4**, 331–7.

Wilson, J. P. & Zigelbaum, S. D. (1983) The Vietnam veteran on trial: the relation of post-traumatic stress disorder to criminal behaviour. *Behav. Sci. Law*, **1**, 69–83.

Wilson, L. G. (1976) Viral encephalopathy mimicking functional psychosis. *Am. J. Psychiat.*, **133**, 165–70.

Wilson, M. S. & Meyer, E. (1962) Diagnostic consistency in a psychiatric liaison service. *Am. J. Psychiat.*, **119**, 207–9.

Wilson, R. S. Kaszniak, A. W., Klawans, H. L. & Garron, D. C. (1980) High speed memory scanning in Parkinsonism. *Cortex*, **16**, 67–72.

Wing, J. (1971) How many psychiatric beds? *Psychol. Med.*, **1**, 189–190.

Wing, J. K. (1978*a*) *Reasoning about Madness*. Oxford University Press, Oxford.

Wing, J. K. (1978b) *Schizophrenia: Towards a New Synthesis*. Academic Press, London and Orlando.

Wing, J. K. (1982) Course and prognosis of schizophrenia. In *Handbook of Psychiatry*, vol. 3 (ed. J. K. Wing & L. Wing). Cambridge University Press, Cambridge, pp. 33–41.

Wing, J. K. (1983) Use and misuse of the PSE. *Br. J. Psychiat.*, **143**, 111–17.

Wing, J. (1989) Editor. *Health Services Planning and Research. Contributions from Psychiatric Case Registers*. Gaskell, London.

Wing, J. (1993) Institutionalism revisited. *Crim. Behav. Ment. Health.*, **3**, 441–51.

Wing, J. K., Babor, T., Brugha, T. *et al.* (1990) SCAN: Schedules for clinical assessment in neuropsychiatry. *Arch. Gen. Psychiat.*, **47**, 589–93.

Wing, J. K., Bebbington, P. & Robins L. N. (eds) (1981) *What is a Case?* Grant McIntyre, London.

Wing, J. K., Birley, J. L. T., Cooper, J. E *et al.* (1967) Reliability of a procedure for measuring and classifying 'present psychiatric state'. *Br. J. Psychiat.*, **113**, 499–515.

Wing, J. K. & Brown, G. W. (1970) *Institutionalism and Schizophrenia*. Cambridge University Press, Cambridge.

Wing, J. K., Cooper, J. E. & Sartorius N. (1974) *The Measurement and Classification of Psychiatric Symptoms*. Cambridge University Press, Cambridge.

Wing, J. K. & Furlong, R. (1986) A haven for the severely disabled. Context of a comprehensive psychiatric community service. *Br. J. Psychiat.*, **149**, 449–58.

Wing, J. K., Mann, S. A., Leff, J. P. *et al.* (1978) The concept of a 'case' in psychiatric population surveys. *Psychol. Med.*, **8**, 203–17.

Wing, J. K. & Sturt, E. (1978) *The PSD-ID-CATEGO System Supplementary Manual* (mimeo). Medical Research Council, London.

Wing, J. K. & Wing, L. (1976) In *Early Childhood Autism* (ed. L. Wing). Pergamon Press, Oxford, p. 313.

Wing, L. (1991) The relationship between Asperger's syndrome and Kanner's Autism. In *Autism and Asperger's Syndrome* (ed. U. Frith). Cambridge University Press, Cambridge, pp. 93–121.

Wing, L. & Gould J. (1979) Severe impairments of social interactions and associated abnormalities in children: epidemiology and classification. *J. Autism Devel. Dis.*, **9**, 11–29.

Winick, C. (1962) Maturing out of narcotic addiction. *Bull Narcotics*, **142**, 1–7

Winnicot, D. W. (1958) *Collected Papers*. Basic Books, New York.

Winokur, G. (1975) The Iowa 500: heterogeneity and course in manic-depressive illness – bipolar. *Compr. Psychiat.*, **16**, 125–131.

Winokur, G. (1977) Delusional disorder (paranoia). *Comp. Psychiat.*, **18**, 511–21.

Winokur G. & Coryell, W. (1991) Femilial alcoholism in primary unipolar major depressive disorder. *Am. J. Psychiat.*, **148**, 184–8.

Winokur, G., Clayton, P. J. & Reich, T. (1969) *Manic Depressive Illness*. C. V. Mosby, St Louis.

Winston, A. (1985) (ed.) *Clinical and Research Issues in Short-term Dynamic Psychotherapy*. American Psychiatric Press, Washington DC.

Winston, A., Pollack, J., McCullough, L. *et al.* (1991) Brief psychotherapy of personality disorders. *J. Nerv. Ment. Dis.*, **179**, 188–93.

Winters, K. C. & Neale, J. M. (1993). Delusions and delusional thinking in psychotics: a review. *Clin. Psychol. Rev.*, **3**, 227–53.

Wisdom, J. O. (1967) Testing an interpretation within a session. *Int. J. Psycho-Analysis*, **48**, 44–52.

Wise, R. A. (1987) the role of reward pathways in the development of drug dependence. *Pharmacol. Therap.*, **35**, 227–63.

Wiseman, M. R., Vizard, E., Bentovim, A. & Leventhal, J. (1992) Reliability of videotaped interviews with children suspected of being sexually abused. *Br. Med. J.*, **304**, 1089–91.

Wisner, K. L. & Perel, J. M. (1988) Psychopharmacologic agents and electroconvulsive therapy during pregnancy and the puerperium. In *Psychiatric Consultation in Childbirth Settings* (ed. R. L. Cohen). Plenum, New York.

Wisner, K. L., Perel, J. M. & Wheeler, S. B. (1993) Tricyclic dose requirements across pregnancy. *Am. J. Psychiat.*, **150**, 1541–42.

Wittchen, H. -U., Robins, L. N., Cottler, L. B. *et al.* (1991) Cross-cultural feasibility, reliability and sources of variance of the Composite International Diagnostic Interview (CIDI). *Br. J. Psychiat.*, **159**, 645–53.

Wittchen, H. -U., Zhao, S., Kessler, R. C. & Eaton, W. W. (1994) DSM-IIIR Generalised anxiety disorder in the National Comorbidity Survey. *Arch. Gen. Psychiat.*, **51**, 355–64.

Wittenborn, J. R., McDonald, D. C. & Maurer, H. S. (1977). Persisting symptoms in schizophrenia predicted by background factors. *Arch. Gen. Psychiat.*, **34**, 1057–61.

Wittgenstein, L. (1966) *Wittgenstein: Lectures and Conversations* (ed. C. Barrett). Blackwell, Oxford.

Woff, K., Goldberg, D, & Fryer, T. (1988) The practice of community psychiatric nursing and mental health social work in Salford. *Br. J. Psychiat.*, **152**, 783–92.

Wolff, P. H., Gardner, J., Paccia, J. & Lappen, J. (1989) The greeting behaviour of Fragile-X. *Am. J. Ment. Retard.*, **95**, 406–11.

Wolfgang, M. E., Thornberry, T. P. & Figlio, R. M. (1987) *From Boy to Man, from Delinquency to Crime*. University of Chicago Press, Chicago.

Wolkin, A., Barouche, F., Wolf, A. P. *et al.* (1989) Dopamine blockade and clinical response: evidence for two biological subgroups of schizophrenia. *Am. J. Psych.*, **146**, 905–8.

Wolpe, J. (1958) *Psychotherapy by Reciprocal Inhibition*. Standard University Press, Palo Alto.

Wolraich, M., Drummond, T., Salomon, M. *et al.* (1978) Effects of methylphenidate alone and in combination with behaviour modification procedures on the behaviour and academic performance of hyperactive children. *J. Abnorm. Child Psych.*, **6**, 149–61.

Wonderlich, S. A., Swift, W. J., Slotnick, H. B. *et al.* (1990) DSM-IIIR personality disorder in eating disorder subtypes. *Int. J. Eat. Disorders.*, **9**, 607–16.

Wong, D. F., Wagner, H. N. & Tune, L. E. (1986) Positron emission tomography reveals elevated D2 dopamine receptors in drug-naive schizophrenics. *Science*, **234**, 1558–63.

Wood, R. L. & Eames, P. (1989) *Models of Brain Injury Rehabilitation*. Chapman & Hall, London.

Woody, G. E., Luborsky, L., McLellan, A. T. *et al.* (1983) Psychotherapy for opiate addicts: Does it help? *Arch. Gen. Psychiat.*, **40**, 639–45.

Wootton, B. (1959) *Social Science and Social Pathology*. George Allen, London.

Workman-Daniels, K. L. & Hesselbrock, V. M. (1987) Childhood problem behaviour and neuro-psychological functioning in persons at risk for alcoholism. *J. Stud. Alcohol.*, **48**, 187–93.

World Health Organization (annual publication) *World Health Statistics Annual*. WHO, Geneva.

World Health Organization (1973*a*) *International Pilot Study of Schizophrenia*, WHO, Geneva.

World Health Organization (1973*b*) *Report of the Eighth Seminar on Standardisation of Psychiatric Diagnosis, Classification and Statistics*. WHO, Geneva.

World Health Organization (1973*c*) *Report on Working Group, Psychiatry and Primary Care*. WHO, Copenhagen.

World Health Organization (1974) *Glossary of mental disorders and guide to their classification for use in conjunction with the International Classification of Diseases, 8th Revision*. WHO, Geneva.

World Health Organization (1978) *Mental Disorders Glossary and Guide to their Classification in Accordance with the Ninth Revision of the International Classification of Diseases*. WHO, Geneva.

World Health Organization (1980) *International Classification of Impairments, Disabilities and Handicaps*. WHO, Geneva.

World Health Organization (1983) *First Contact Mental Health Care*. WHO Regional Office for Europe, Copenhagen.

World Health Organization (1987) *Tenth Revision of the International Classification of Diseases*. WHO, Geneva.

World Health Organization (1992*a*) *The ICD-10 Classification of Mental and Behavioural Disorders. Clinical descriptions and diagnostic guidelines*. WHO, Geneva.

World Health Organization (1992*b*) *Mental Disorders: Glossary and Guide to their Classification in Accordance with the Tenth Revision of the International Classification of Diseases (ICD-10)*. WHO, Geneva.

World Health Organization (1992*c*) *Targets for Health for all. The Health Policy for Europe*. World Heath Organization Regional Office for Europe, Copenhagen.

World Health Organization (1993) *The ICD-10 Classification of Mental and Behavioural Disorders. Diagnostic Criteria for Research*. WHO, Geneva.

World Psychiatric Association (1990) WPA statement and viewpoints on the rights and legal safeguards of the mentally ill. *WPS Bull.*, **1**, 32–3.

Wragg, R. & Jeste, E. (1989) Overview of depression and psychosis in Alzheimer's disease. *Am. J. Psychiat.*, **146**, 577–87.

Wright, A. F., Crichton, D. N., Loudon, J. B. *et al.* (1984) B-adrenoceptor binding defects in cell lines from families with manic-depressive disorder. *Ann. Hum. Genet.*, **48**, 201–14.

Wright, P., Donaldson, P., Underhill, J. *et al.* (1995) Schizophrenia, an HLA Class I and II association study. *Psych. Genet.*, **5**(1), 35.

Wright, S. P. (1978) Hazards with monoamine oxidase inhibitors: a persistent problem. *Lancet*, **i**, 284–5.

Wrightsman, L. S. & Kassin, S. M. (1993) *Confessions in the Courtroom*. Sage, Newbury Park, CA.

Wulff, M. (1932) Lieber einen interessen oralen syptomenkomplex und seine Beziehung zur Sucht. *Internat. Psychoanal.*, **18**, 13–16.

Wundt, W. (1903) *Grundriss der Psychologie*. Engelmann, Struttgart.

Wyatt, G. E. & Peters, S. D. (1986) Issues in the definition of child sexual abuse in prevalence research. *Child Abuse and Neglect*, **10**, 231–40.

Wykes, T. (1992) The assessment of severely disabled psychiatric patients for rehabilitation. In *Schizophrenia: an Overview and Practical Handbook* (ed. D. Kavanagh). Chapman & Hall, London.

Wykes, T. & Hurry, J. (1991) Social behaviour and psychiatric disorders. In *Social Psychiatry: Theory, Methodology and Practice* (ed. P. E. Bebbington). Transaction, New Brunswick, NH.

Wykes, T. & Sturt, E. (1986) The measurement of social behaviour in psychiatric patients: an assessment of the reliability and validity of the SBS schedule. *Br. J. Psychiat.*, **148**, 1–11.

Xenophon (1923) *Memorabilia* (with an English translation by E. G. Marchant). Leob Classical Library, London.

Yager, J., Landsverk, J. & Edelstein, C. K. (1987) A 20-month follow-up study of 628 women with eating disorders. 1: Course and severity. *Am. J. Psychiat.*, **144**, 1172–7.

Yamaguchi, S., Kobayashi, S., Koide, H. & Tsunematsu, T. (1992) Longitudinal study of regional blood flow change in depression after stroke. *Stroke*, **23**, 1716–22.

Yap, P. M. (1967) Classification of the culture-bond syndromes. *Aus. N.Z. J. Psychiat.*, **1**, 172–9.

Yassa, R., Noir, V., Nastase, C. *et al.* (1988) Prevalence of bipolar disorder in a psychogeriatric population. *J. Affect. Disorders*, **14**, 197–201.

Yates, W. R., Sieleni, B., Reich, J. & Brass, C. (1989) Co-morbidity of bulimia nervosa and personality disorder. *J. Clin. Psychiat.*, **50**, 57–9.

Yehuda, R., Giller, E., Southwick, S. *et al.* (1991) Hypothalamic–pituitary–adrenal dysfunction in post-traumatic stress disorder. *Biol. Psychiat.*, **30**, 1031–48.

Yesavage, J., Brooks, J., Taylor, J. & Tinklanberg, J. (1993) Development of aphasia apraxia and agnosia and decline in Alzheimer's disease. *Amer. J. Psychiat.*, **150**, 742–7.

Yellowlees, P. M. & Page, T. (1990) Safe use of electroconvulsive therapy in pregnancy. *Med. J. Aust.*, **153**, 679–680.

Yevich, J. (1991) Drug development from discovery to marketing. In *A Textbook of Drug Design and Development* (ed. P. Krogsgaard-Larsen & H. Bundgard). Harwood Academic Publishers, UK.

Yokel, R. A. (1987) Intravenous self-administration: response rates, the effects of pharmacological challenges and drug preference. In *Methods of Assessing the Reinforcing Properties of Abused Drugs* (ed. M. A. Bozarth). Springer-Verlag, New York, pp. 1–35.

Yoshida, A., Huang, I. Y. & Ikawa, M. (1984) Molecular abnormality of an inactive aldehyde dehydrogenase variant commonly found in Orientals. *Proc. Nat. Acad. Sci.*, **81**, 258–61.

Yoss, R. E. & Daly, D. D. (1960) Narcolepsy. *Arch. Intern. Med.*, **106**, 168–71.

Yost, E. B., Bleuler, L. E. Carbishley, M. A. & Allender, J. R. (1986) *Group Cognitive Therapy: A Treatment Approach for Depressed Older Adults*. Pergamon Press, New York.

Young, G. C. & Morgan, R. T. T. (1972) Overlearning in the conditioning treatment of enuresis. *Behav. Res. Ther.*, **10**, 147–51.

Young, J. P. R., Lader, M. H. & Hughes, W. C. (1979) Controlled trial of imipramine, monoamine oxidase inhibitors and combined treatment in depressed subjects. *Brit. Med. J.*, **2**, 1315–17.

Young, R. C., Biggs, J. T., Ziegler, V. E. *et al.* (1978) A rating scale for mania. *Br. J. Psychiat.*, **133**, 429–35.

Yule, W. (1994) Post traumatic stress disorders. In *Child and Adolescent Psychiatry: Modern Approaches*, 3rd edn (ed. M. Rutter, M. Taylor & L. Hersov). Blackwell Scientific, Oxford, pp. 392–406.

Yule, W. & Carr, J. (1980) (eds) *Behaviour Modification for the Mentally Handicapped*. Croom Helm, London.

Yule, W. & Udwin, O. (1991) Screening child survivors for post-traumatic stress disorders: experiences from the 'Jupiter' sinking. *Br. J. Clin. Psych.*, **30**, 131–8.

Zarkowska, E. & Clements, J. (1988) *Problem Behaviour in People with Severe Learning Difficulties: A Practice Guide to a Constructional Approach*. Croom Helm, London.

Zeitlin, H. (1986) *The Natural History of Psychiatric Disorder in Children*. Maudsley Monograph, No 29. Oxford University Press, Oxford.

Zeitlin, H. (1994) Children with alcohol misusing parents. *Br. Med. Bull.*, **50**, 139–51.

Zielinsky, J. J. (1982) Epidemiology of epilepsy. In *Textbook of Epilepsy* (ed. J. Laidlaw & A. Richens). Churchill Livingstone, Edinburgh, pp. 16–33.

Zigmond, A. S. & Snaith, R. P. (1982) The hospital anxiety and depression scale. *Acta Psych. Scand.*, **67**, 361–70.

Zimmerman, M., Pfohl, B., Stangl, D. *et al.* (1986) Assessment of DSM-III personality disorders: the importance of interviewing the informant. *J. Clin. Psychiat.*, **47**, 261–3.

Zitrin, C., Kelin, D. & Woerner, M. (1980) Treatment of agoraphobia with group exposure *in vivo* and imipramine. *Arch. Gen. Psych.*, **37**, 63–72.

Zitrin, C., Klein, D., Woerner, M. & Ross, D. (1983) Treatment of phobias. Comparison of imipramine hydrochloride and placebo. *Arch Gen Psychiat.*, **40**, 125–38.

Zoccolillo, M., Pickles, A., Quinton, D. & Rutter, M. (1992) The outcome of childhood conduct disorder: implications for defining adult personality disorder and conduct disorder. *Psychol. Med.*, **22**, 971–86.

Zohar, A. H., Ratzoni, G., Pauls, D. L. *et al.* (1992) An epidemiological study of obsessive-compulsive disorder and related disorders in Israeli adolescents. *J. Am. Acad. Child Adol. Psychiat.*, **31**, 1057–61.

Zolese, G. & Blacker, C. V. R. (1992) The psychological complications of therapeutic abortion. *Br. J. Psychiat.*, **160**, 742–49.

Index